OXFORD MEDICAL PUBLICATIONS

Imaging in liver disease

From diagnosis to treatment

Imaging in Liver Disease

From Diagnosis to Treatment

KENICHI TAKAYASU

Department of Diagnostic Radiology, National Cancer Center Hospital, Tokyo, Japan

and

KUNIO OKUDA

Emeritus Professor of Medicine, Chiba University School of Medicine, Chiba, Japan

Oxford New York Tokyo
OXFORD UNIVERSITY PRESS
1997

Oxford University Press, Great Clarendon Street, Oxford OX2 6DP
Oxford New York
Athens Auckland Bangkok Bogota Bombay Buenos Aires
Calcutta Cape Town Dar es Salaam Delhi Florence Hong Kong
Istanbul Karachi Kuala Lumpur Madras Madrid Melbourne
Mexico City Nairobi Paris Singapore Taipei Tokyo Toronto
and associated companies in
Berlin Ibadan

Oxford is a trade mark of Oxford University Press

Published in the United States
by Oxford University Press Inc., New York

This publication was supported by generous donations from the Daido Life Foundation, the Naito Foundation, and the Foundation for Promotion of Cancer Research, Japan. Originally published as Imaging in Liver Disease (in Japanese) by Bunkodo Co. Ltd, Japan

A catalogue record for this book is available from the British Library

Library of Congress Cataloging in Publication Data
Takayasu, Kenichi, Dr.
Imaging in liver disease: from diagnosis to treatment/Kenichi Takayasu and Kunio Okuda
(Oxford medical publications)
Updated English version of the first author's work in Japanese published in 1991
Includes bibliogaphical references and index.
1. Liver—Imaging. I. Okuda, Kunio. II. Series
[DNLM: 1. Liver Diseases—diagnosis. 2. Diagnostic Imaging.
3. Liver Diseases—therapy. WI 700 T1362i 1997]
RC847.5.I42T35 1997 616.3'620754—dc20 96–8949
ISBN 0–19–262634–5 (hbk)

Typeset by Footnote Graphics, Warminster, Wilts
Printed in Hong Kong

Preface

Hepatology, the study of liver diseases, is a relatively new discipline. The American Association for the Study of Liver Diseases (AASLD) was created in 1950, the first organization in the world for the advancement of this new field of learning. Earlier, the liver was regarded and investigated as a functional organ by Anglo-American and Germanic countries. Improved communication after the end of World War II resulted in an upsurge of interest in various aspects of the liver. Eight years after the establishment of the AASLD, the International Association for the Study of the Liver (IASL) was organized under the leadership of the late Hans Popper and Dame Sheila Sherlock. In this Society, the study of basic aspects of the liver was emphasized and the word 'diseases' was not used in its name. Radiological study of the patient was not part of liver diagnosis until radionuclide scintigraphy came to be used clinically.

In 1976, one of the authors (KO) published a monograph entitled *Radiological aspects of the liver and biliary tract. X-ray and radioisotope diagnosis* (Igaku-Shoin, Tokyo and Year-Book Chicago). This was the first textbook to deal with radiological diagnosis of the liver. In the Foreword to this book, Hans Popper stated: 'I have claimed for many years that the progress in physical methods, particularly radiologic technique, will eventually attain superiority in many aspects of the differential diagnosis of liver disease where they will partly replace the presently used biochemical and immunological methods in liver function test or the histological diagnosis of liver biopsy.' He not only praised the diagnostic power of the 'skinny needle' developed at Chiba University where the current authors both worked, but also emphasized better correlation of clinical manifestations with gross abnormalities than with microscopic and fine structural analysis. The authors of the current book strongly agree. The previous book emphasized gross abnormalities of the liver and biliary tract, because in the early 1970s only a limited number of radiological techniques were available. Percutaneous transhepatic portography was in a fledging state, and only one portogram was shown in the book. Radiological methodology has since made remarkable progress with the development of such new techniques as endoscopic cholangiography, real-time ultrasonography, computed tomography, digital subtraction angiography, and magnetic resonance imaging. Instrumentation has also been vastly improved. The role of imaging in diagnosis has expanded, and the need for needle biopsy has been considerably, if not totally, reduced.

The current book is an updated English version of *Imaging in liver disease* which was published with the subtitle 'From detection of small liver cancer to its treatment', by one of the authors (KT) by Bunkodo, Tokyo, in 1991. This new English version has a separate new chapter on MR imaging, and more emphasis is placed on the diagnosis of localized hepatic lesions, particularly liver cancer and its differential diagnosis, bearing in mind the prevalence of primary liver cancer, which kills more than one million people every year worldwide. The recent progress, made particularly in the Far East, in the imaging diagnosis of asymptomatic hepatocellular carcinoma now permits its treatment. In order to help inexperienced radiologists and hepatologists learn about the early diagnosis and treatment of hepatocellular carcinoma we introduce in this book not only the use of various new imaging techniques, such as portal-CT and Lipiodol-CT, but also interventional therapy such as transcatheter arterial embolization (TAE), Lipiodol-TAE, percutaneous ethanol injection, and a discussion of systematic subsegmentectomy, heavy particle irradiation, etc. as carried out in Japan. Our understanding of molecular events leading to hepatocarcinogenesis will soon enable us to distinguish preneoplastic and early neoplastic lesions with confidence; so that chemoprevention and gene therapy of hepatocellular carcinoma may no longer be only a dream.

The authors felt that to present actual cases with the imaging findings and the outcome was the most effective method of presentation. Most of the patients described in the book, therefore, were fully discussed preoperatively by a team consisting of internists, radiologists, and surgeons at the regular conference of the National Cancer Center Hospital (NCCH), Tokyo, and the resected specimens were compared and assessed with the preoperative imaging diagnosis at the pathological conference. The interpretation of imaging findings always improved if resected and autopsied specimens were compared with the imaging features. Recurrence of cancer in the liver after treatment is one of the major problems closely related to pretreatment diagnosis, and some pages are devoted to this problem, along with the discussion on multidisciplinary therapy; most long-term survivors in our experience had received such treatment. We sincerely hope that our experience will assist readers elsewhere to practise liver diagnosis.

The authors wish to express their gratitude to Mr Toyoshi Onji, Oxford University Press, and Mrs Kyoko Kasami, Bunkodo, for the publication, to Mrs Yoshie Kataoka, and Miss Fumiko Shiga for their able secretarial assistance, to NCC President Emeritus Takashi Sugimura and Keiichi Suemasu, and NCCH Director Tadao Kakizoe for their continuous support and encouragement.

Tokyo K. T.
Chiba K. O.
December 1996

Acknowledgements

The authors are deeply indebted to the following collaborators without whose assistance the preparation of this book would not have been possible.

Masatoshi Makuuchi, M.D., University of Tokyo, Tokyo
Hiroshi Hasegawa, M.D. and Nobuo Okazaki, M.D., Ibaragi Central Hospital, Tomobe
Masatoshi Okazaki, M.D., Fukuoka University Hospital, Fukuoka
Kiyozo Kishi, M.D., Saitama Cancer Center, Ina
Chizuko Kobayashi, M.D., Takanobu Yoshida, M.D., and Hirotaka Musha, M.D., National Chiba Hospital, Chiba
Yasuyuki Akine, M.D., Tsukuba University Hospital, Tsukuba
Kiyoaki Iwashita, M.T., National Sakura Hospital, Sakura
Hidemitsu Ohkado, M.D., Saiseikai Kumamoto Hospital, Kumamoto
David J. Brandt, M.D., Department of Radiology, Mayo Clinic, Rochester, MN, USA
Noriyuki Moriyama, M.D., Shigeru Nawano, M.D., Ryuzou Sekiguchi, M.D., Yasuo Shima, M.D., Masahiro Yoshino, M.D., and Hisao Tajiri, M.D., National Cancer Center Hospital East, Kashiwa

The following are at the National Cancer Center Hospital:
Susumu Yamasaki, M.D., Tomoo Kosuge, M.D., Tadatoshi Takayama, M.D., Junji Yamamoto, M.D., Kazuo Shimada, M.D., and Yoshihiro Moriya, M.D., Surgery
Michiie Sakamoto, M.D., Setsuo Hirohashi, M.D., Pathology
Shuichi Okada, M.D., Haruhiko Nose, M.D., Hiroshi Ishii, M.D., and Hisanao Ohkura, M.D., Medicine
Yukio Shimosato, M.D., Clinical Pathology
Jun Takayama, M.D., Pediatrics
Kyosuke Ushio, M.D., Hiroto Matsue, M.D., Shoji Terui, M.D., Yukio Muramatsu, M.D., Tsutomu Ishikawa, M.D., Yasunori Mizuguchi, M.D., Hiroyoshi Furukawa, M.D., Fumihiko Wakao, M.D., and Yoshiko Iwata, M.D., Diagnostic Radiology

Contents

Notice to readers

Usage of anatomical, radiological, and other terms and abbreviations used in this book are as follows:

1. Anatomical terms—P, portal vein; A, artery; B, bile duct; S, subsegment corresponding to the sector proposed by Couinaud. The Roman numeral as its superscript corresponds to the number of the subsegment, and subscripts a, b, c, d are the distribution of branching. L (l), left; R (r), right; t, trunk; M (med), medial; sup, superior; dor, dorsal; inf, inferior (cf. pp.34, 35).

The designation of the first-, second-, and third-order branches of the portal vein system is the one proposed by Takayasu (*Radiology* 1985, **154**, 31) which is somewhat different from the previous ones (cf. p.36).

2. CT angiography—although new abbreviations such as CTAP and CTA are becoming popular, the original procedure was carried out by one of the authors with the term 'angio-CT'. Therefore, the terms 'portal-CT' and 'arterial-CT' will also be used alternatively in this book.

3. Histopathology of hepatocellular carcinoma—Edmondson (and Steiner) grading is used. Edmondson's II>III means that a greater part of the tumor was grade II, and a lesser portion grade III.

4. Frequently used names for diseases or lesions—HCC, hepatocellular carcinoma; AH, adenomatous hyperplasia; AAH, atypical adenomatous hyperplasia, (these may be re-termed 'dysplastic nodules' internationally in future); FNH, focal nodular hyperplasia.

5. Other abbreviations:

AFP	alpha-fetoprotein
A-V	arterio-venous
CEA	carcinoembryonic antigen
CT	computed tomography
DIC	drip infusion cholecystocholangiography
DSA	digital subtraction angiography
ERC	endoscopic retrograde cholangiography
ERCP	endoscopic retrograde cholangiopancreatography
Gd-DTPA	gadolinium diethylene-triaminepentaacetate
HBsAg	hepatitis B surface antigen
HCV	hepatitis C virus
IVC	inferior vena cava
LIP-CT	Lipiodol-CT
MR	magnetic resonance
PEI	percutaneous ethanol injection
PTC	percutaneous transhepatic cholangiography
PTCD	percutaneous transhepatic cholangiodrainage
PTP	percutaneous transhepatic portography
SE	spin echo
TAE	transcatheter arterial embolization
TVDT	tumor volume doubling time
US	ultrasound

Dose schedules are being continually revised and new side effects recognized. Oxford University Press makes no representation, express or implied, that the drug dosages in this book are correct. For these reasons the reader is strongly urged to consult the pharmaceutical company's printed instructions before administering any of the drugs recommended in this book.

1

Anatomy of the liver

1.1 Gross anatomy

Anatomy and physiology of the liver

The liver is the largest parenchymal organ in the abdomen, located under the right diaphragm. It weighs 1200–1500 g, about 2 per cent of the whole body weight of an adult, with three dimensions of an average of 15 cm in length (vertical), 20 cm in width (transverse) and 15 cm in thickness (sagittal). It receives a dual blood supply, via the hepatic artery and the portal vein. Blood that has perfused the hepatic lobules enters the inferior vena cava through the hepatic veins. The blood flow volume is about 30 per cent of cardiac output, an average of 1500 ml/min, 25 per cent coming from the hepatic artery and 75 per cent from the portal vein, whereas oxygen supply is about 50 per cent from each. Beside the vascular system, the liver contains the biliary tract, the excretory route for bile, and the lymphatics. These vessels are situated in the fibrous portal tract (Glisson's sheath) which is also called the portal triad because it encompasses three vessels, the artery, portal vein, and bile duct.

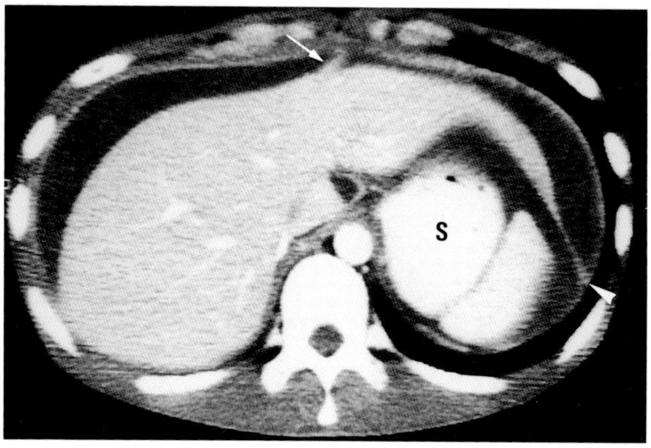

Fig. 1.1 Fixation of the liver. Anatomical assessment of the liver attachment is possible with a CT image in a patient with ascites. The falciform ligament (→) and left triangular ligament (▶) are identifiable in the frontal and lateral aspects of the liver. The spaces surrounding the liver are filled by fluid except for the posterior aspect of the right lobe which corresponds to the bare area.

Fixation of the liver

The liver is covered by the peritoneum except for the following three parts: (1) the bare area that connects the diaphragm and the dorsal surface of the liver; (2) the inferior vena cava that runs within the bare area; and (3) the gallbladder bed. The supporting tissue for the liver consists of the falciform ligament, and the right and left triangular ligaments (Fig. 1.1). The ligamentum teres, the obliterated remnant of the left umbilical vein, extends from the porta hepatis where it attaches to the left portal vein, out through the fissure of the ligamentum teres and the falciform ligament, up to the umbilicus. The remnant of the ductus venosus (duct of Arantius), which once connected the left umbilical vein and the inferior vena cava during fetal development, runs as the ligamentum venosus toward the left triangular ligament.

1.2 The vascular system

Hepatic artery

The origin and course of the hepatic artery may vary from person to person with many variations. According to Michels (1955), aberrant arteries are seen in 45 per cent of individuals (Fig. 1.2) with a normal anatomy in only 55 per cent (Fig. 1.3). It has been suggested that such variations are due to the irregularity in the process of the disappearance of communicating branches between the ventral and dorsal aortas when the former disintegrates during fetal life. When opacification of the hepatic artery is inadequate during celiac arteriography, one has to look for a replacment artery with an aberrant origin and branching. Occasionally, there is an accessory artery providing a dual blood supply to an area normally supplied by one artery; it has to be taken into consideration when the arteriogram is interpreted. It occurs more often in areas smaller than subsegments.

A variation of the left hepatic artery in which all or part of its branches arise from the left gastric artery occurs in about 25 per cent of people. By contrast, in 45 per cent the middle hepatic artery orginates from the left hepatic, in about 45 per cent from the right hepatic, and from another artery such as the proper hepatic, gastroduodenal, or right gastric in 10 per cent (Reuter and Redman 1977). One has to be cautious not to mistake the accessory left gastric artery (Nakamura *et al.* 1980) arising from the root of the left hepatic and supplying the gastric fundus for the left lateral inferior branch of the left hepatic (A^{III}) (Fig. 1.4). Variation in the anterior and posterior branches of the right hepatic artery is relatively uncommon. However, we have seen variations in which all (Fig. 1.5) or some (Fig. 1.6) of the right posterior branches arise from the superior mesenteric artery.

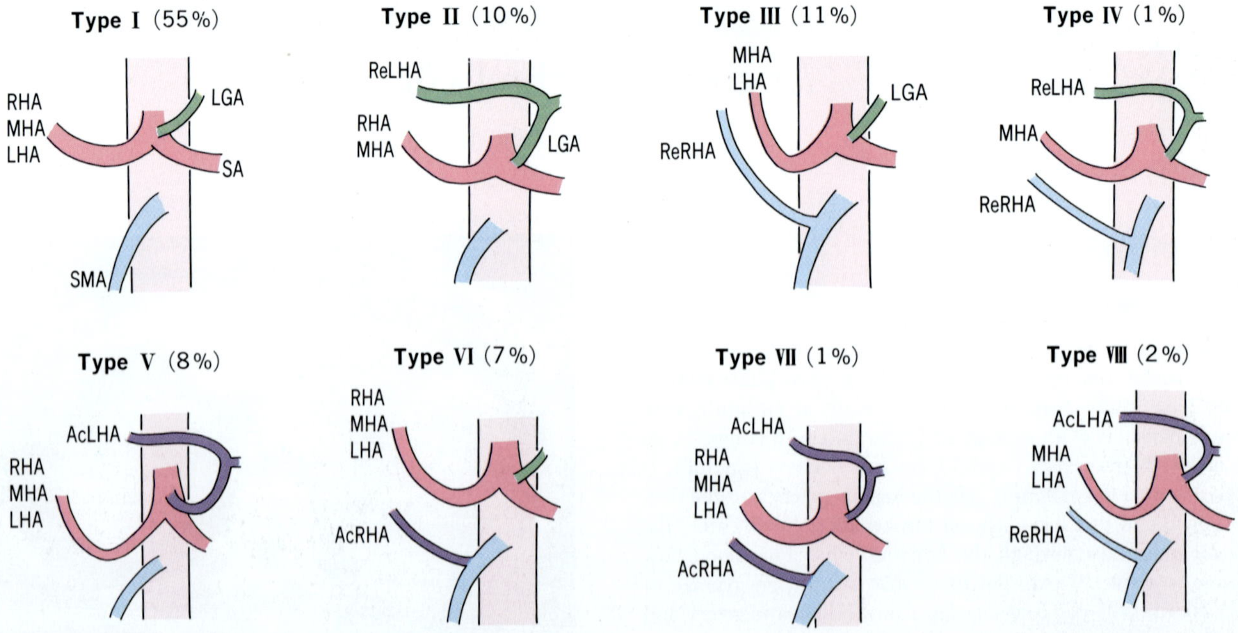

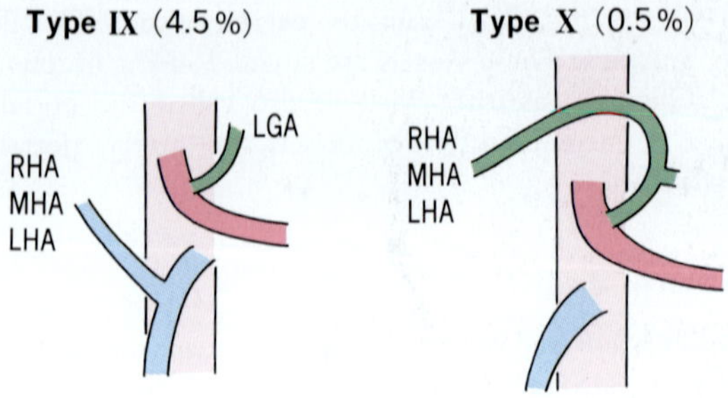

Type I: The typical or most common pattern in which the right hepatic artery (RHA), middle hepatic artery (MHA), and left hepatic artery (LHA) are distributed through the common hepatic and the proper hepatic artery. LGA, left gastric artery; SA, splenic artery; SMA, superior mesenteric artery.
Type II: The left hepatic artery is replaced by the left gastric artery.
Type III: The right hepatic artery is replaced by the superior mesenteric artery.
Type IV: The left hepatic artery is replaced by the left gastric, and right hepatic by the superior mesenteric or the common hepatic artery.
Type V: Only the accessory artery of the left hepatic artery arises from the left gastric. In practice, this occurs in much fewer than 8 per cent, the figure given by Michels.
Type VI: Only the accessory artery of the right hepatic arises from the superior mesenteric artery. In our experience, the frequency of this type is slightly less than 7 per cent, the figure given by Michels.
Type VII: The accessory arteries of the right and left hepatic arteries arise from the superior mesenteric and the left gastric, respectively.
Type VIII: Type a—superior mesenteric artery replacing the right hepatic and left accessory arising from the left gastric. Tybe b—the right accessory artery arising from the superior mesenteric and the left hepatic being replaced by the left gastric. The frequency of these two types is 2 per cent.
Type IX: All hepatic arteries derive from the superior mesenteric artery.
Type X: All hepatic arteries come from the left gastric artery.

Numbers in parentheses denote the frequencies of these types. The scheme given by Michels (1955) has been modified.

Fig. 1.2 Variation in the derivation of hepatic arteries from the aorta.

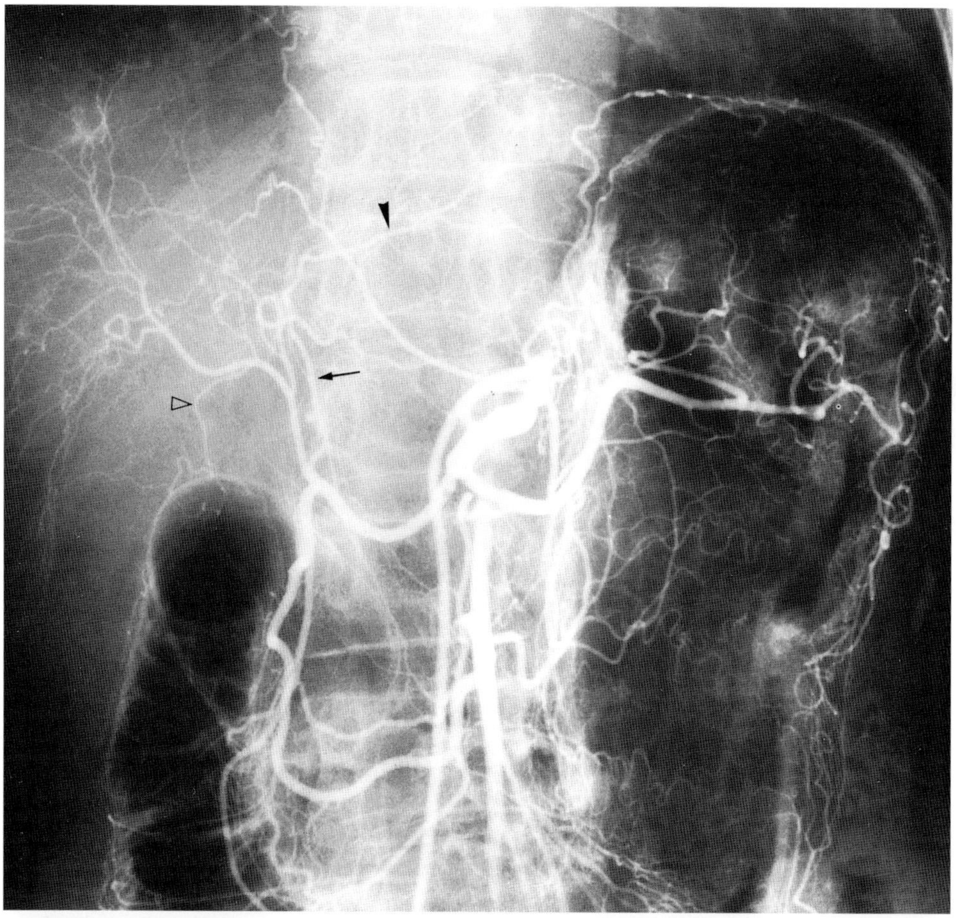

Fig. 1.3 Branching and course of the hepatic artery. Celiac arteriogram: the superior mesenteric artery is also opacified. From the beginning of the celiac artery first come off the inferior phrenic arteries, followed by the left gastric and the common hepatic/splenic artery in most cases. The common hepatic artery sends off the gastroduodenal and the proper hepatic, then the right and left hepatic arteries. The distribution of the extrahepatic arteries varies considerably from person to person. This particular patient has aberrant branching in which the left lateral superior branch A^{II} (▶) arises from the common trunk of one of the left hepatic arteries (→) and the right gastric artery. The cystic artery (▷) is normal coming from the right hepatic.

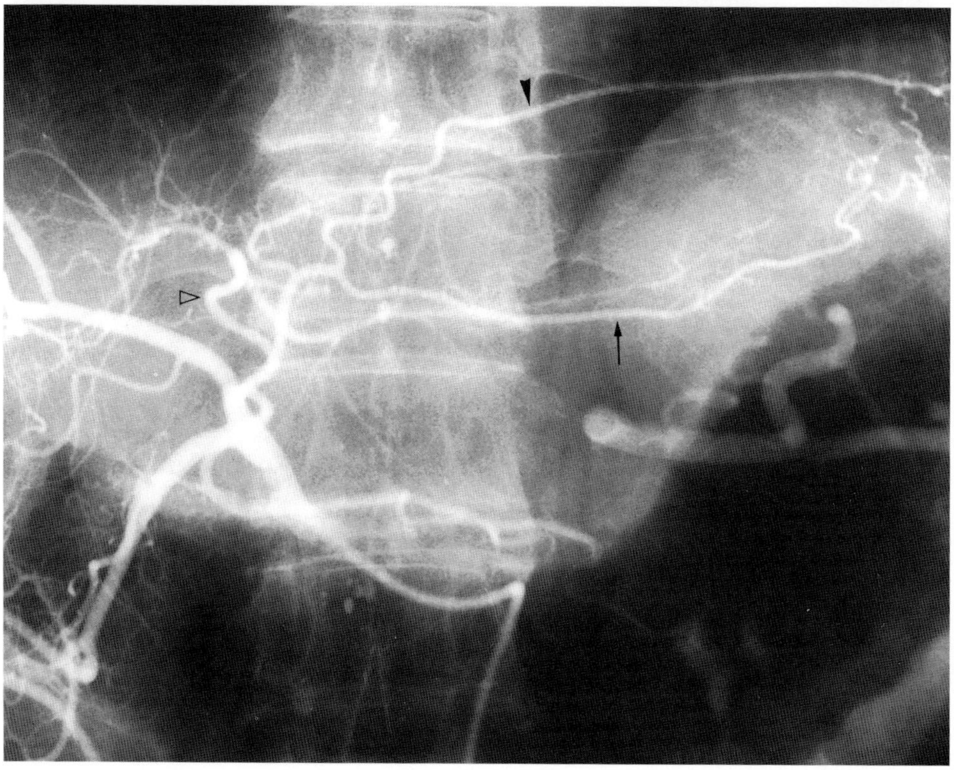

Fig. 1.4 Accessory left gastric artery. The left hepatic artery and the right gastric artery form a common channel. An accessory left gastric (→) and left inferior phrenic (▶) artery come from the right gastric, whereas the left hepatic (▷) ramifies branches that reach A^{III} and A^{IV}. The accessory left gastric artery is often superimposed on A^{III}, but may be identified by following its course with reference to the portal branch that accompanies it.

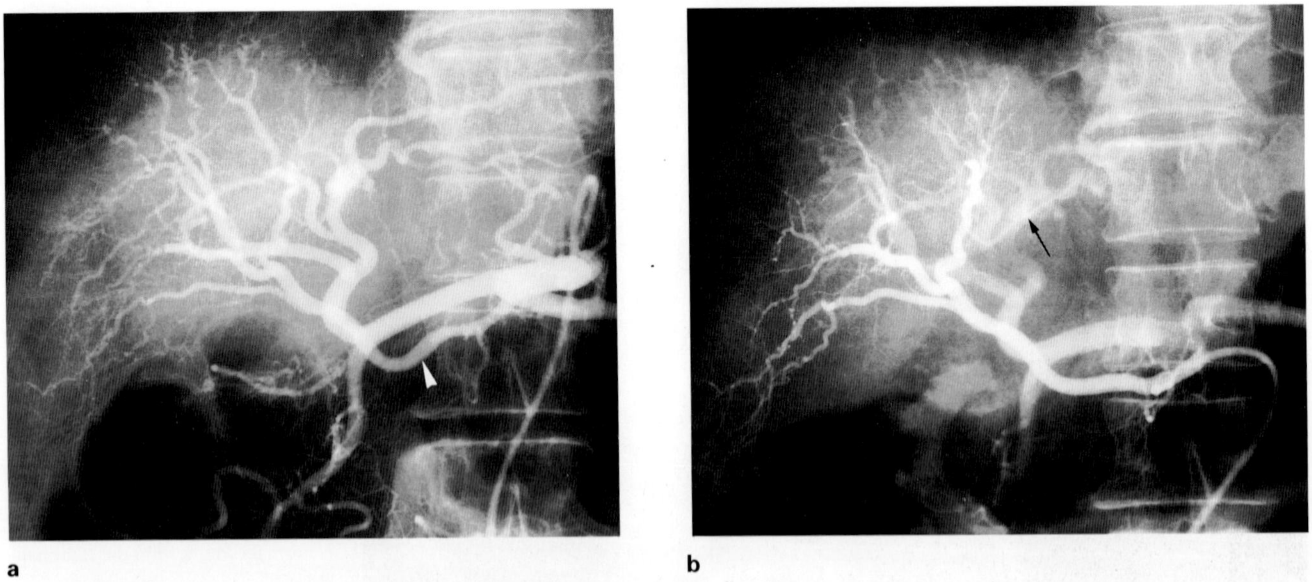

Fig. 1.5 Aberrant posterior branches of the right hepatic artery.
(a) Celiac arteriogram: the right posterior segment artery (▶) arises early from the dorsal pancreatic artery.
(b) Selective dorsal pancreatic arteriography: the area supplied by this artery is the posterior region as seen in this angiogram. This artery (→) was identified as the left caudate lobe branch from arterial-CT shown in (c).
(c) Arterial-CT: arterial-CT was made at the catheter position of (b). Only the posterior region was opacified from cranial to caudal in sequence (1–8 sections). ▶: the right hepatic vein. The left caudate lobe is also opacified to the left of the inferior vena cava. Comparing this with the arteriogram of the posterior segment artery (b), → branch is determined to be the left caudate artery.

The caudate lobe is divided into three parts in the USA where Healey's segmentation scheme is adopted (1953). These parts are the caudate process, right part, and left part, and are contiguous from the right lobe through the caudate process. According to Michels (1955), the three parts are supplied by three caudate arteries in 30 per cent, and by two arteries in 45 per cent. In the latter case, the caudate process and the right part of the caudate lobe are supplied by one caudate artery, and the left part by another caudate artery. In 23 per cent, the entire caudate lobe is supplied by one caudate artery, and 2 per cent have four arteries. In 35 per cent all caudate arteries derive from the right hepatic artery (Fig. 1.7) and all from the left hepatic artery in 12 per cent. Among the Japanese, one caudate artery is from the left hepatic artery and the other from the right posterior segment artery in 32 per cent, one each from the middle and the right posterior segment artery in 26 per cent, one each from the left hepatic, right posterior segment and middle hepatic arteries in 21 per cent (Suzuki 1982). In the angiogram in Fig. 1.8, one can identify the caudate artery originating from the left hepatic artery and supplying a hemangioma that has developed in the left caudate lobe. In an ordinary angiogram, the caudate arteries are difficult to recognize. In rare instances, a caudate artery arises independently of other hepatic arteries (Fig. 1.9).

Sometimes, one may opacify the hepatic falciform artery (Fig. 1.10) (Williams *et al.* 1985) during arteriography. The periphery of this artery reaches the subcutaneous tissue near the umbilicus through the falciform ligament. If an anticancer agent is injected into the hepatic artery through a catheter or a pump, it may cause reddening or pain in the skin above the umbilicus. The incidence of this artery is about 2 per cent (Williams *et al.* 1985). The inferior phrenic arteries usually arise as the first branch of the celiac artery. Occasionally, however, the right inferior phrenic artery may come from the right adrenal artery (Fig. 1.11) or the dorsal pancreatic (Fig. 1.12), and the left inferior phrenic artery from the left hepatic or directly from the aorta. In the diagnosis of hepatocellular carcinoma (HCC) which is supplied by the inferior phrenic artery, and when embolization of this artery is required for treatment, these aberrant origins of the inferior phrenic artery are to be considered. It is to be noted also that the right inferior phrenic artery runs dorsal to the inferior vena cava near the porta hepatis (Fig. 1.13).

The cystic artery is a single artery in 75 per cent of individuals, and double arteries in 25 per cent (Michels 1951), the superficial artery supplying the serosa and the deep one the bladder bed. It arises from the right hepatic artery in 90 per cent, and from either the middle hepatic, left hepatic, gastroduodenal, or less commonly from the aorta in the remaining 10 per cent. The cystic vein (Fig. 1.14) runs either from the liver bed into an intrahepatic portal vein branch, from the Calot triangle along the hepatic artery into an intrahepatic portal branch, or both. According to Sato (1989), the cystic vein enters the right lobe in 40 per cent of people, the left lobe in 17 per cent, and into both lobes in the remainder. The portal branches that receives the cystic vein are commonly P^{V} and P^{VI} in the right lobe, and P^{IV} in the left.

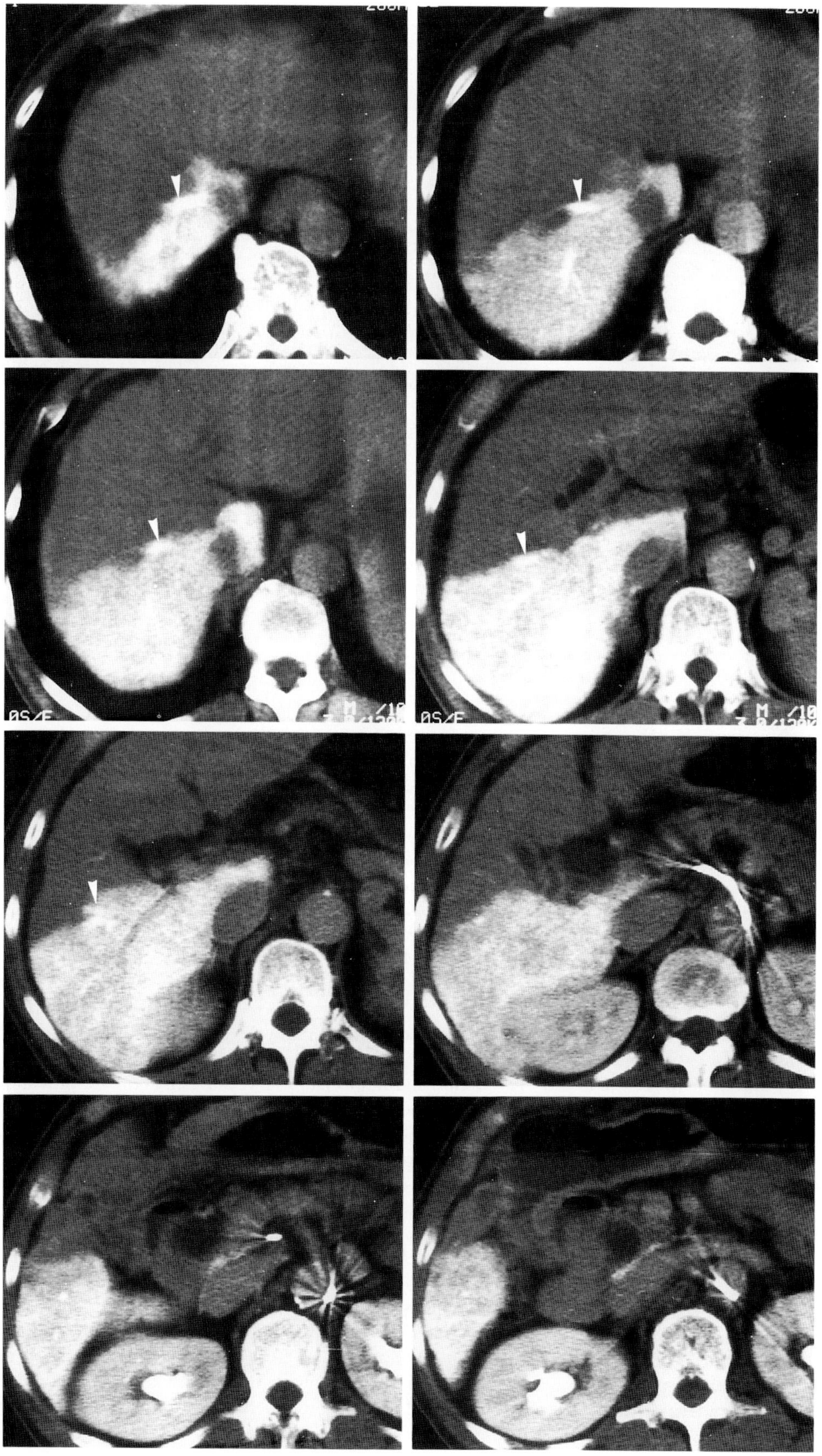

c

1	2
3	4
5	6
7	8

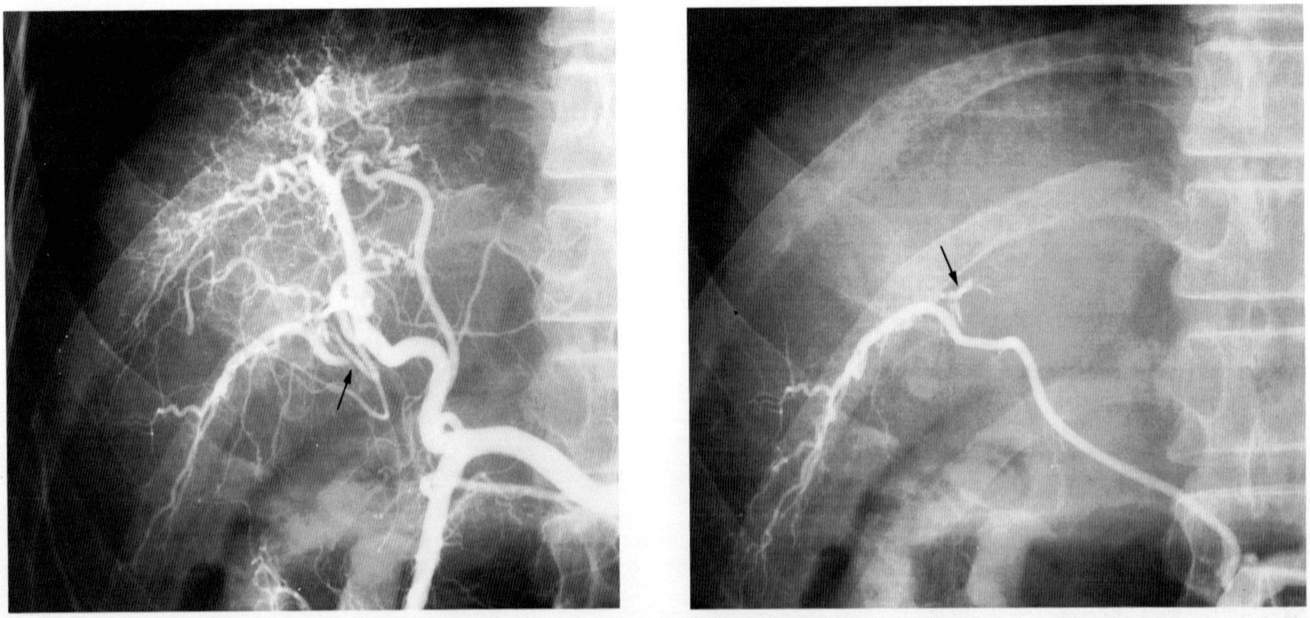

a b

Fig. 1.6 Aberrant posterior segment artery. A^{VI} alone originates from the superior mesenteric artery.
(a) Common hepatic arteriogram: as the proximal part of A^{VI} is not fully opacified (→), the possibility is suggested that this branch is replaced by another artery.
(b) Selective angiography for A^{VI} arising from the superior mesenteric artery: it is supplying only area S^{VI}, but is communicating with other intrahepatic arteries through a small anastomosis (→).

Portal vein

The portal vein trunk typically divides into the right and left first-order portal vein in 84–92 per cent (Fig. 1.15). The anterior and posterior segment branches of the right portal vein and left portal vein arise independently from the portal trunk without forming a common segment (triple branch type) in 4–12 per cent, and the posterior portal vein alone begins early in the portal trunk (independent branch type) (Fig. 1.16) in 3–6 per cent. A surgeon resecting the right lobe may inadvertently ligate the posterior portal vein mistaking it for the right portal vein if preoperative evaluation of the independent type of the posterior portal vein was inadequate. The variation in branching of the intrahepatic portal vein system is thought to be minimal. Yet, with increasing numbers of patients studied, we have seen cases in which the right anterior inferior portal vein (subsegment branch, P^{V}) arises early (Fig. 1.17), the anterior portal vein arises from the left portal vein (Fig. 1.18), and the right gastric vein directly enters the left lateral and medial portal vein (Fig. 1.19) (Takayasu *et al.* 1990*a*).

After division from the portal trunk, the right portal vein further divides into the anterior and posterior subsegmental portal veins (Fig. 1.20). In the lateral view, the anterior and the posterior portal veins are not on top of each other; rather the anterior portal vein is located more cranially as shown in Fig. 1.21. The anterior portal vein branches are arranged cranially in an arc shape, convex laterally (Fig. 1.20), with the periphery frequently ending in the anterior (P^{VIII}_{a}) and posterior (P^{VIII}_{c}) branches, or branching further into the lateral (P^{VIII}_{b}) and medial (P^{VIII}_{d}) branches. The anterior (P^{VIII}_{a}) and posterior (P^{VIII}_{c}) branches are often seen as a single branch as they overlie one another in the frontal view, but in the lateral view they are quite separate. The medial branch (P^{VIII}_{d}) originates near the area where the right and middle hepatic veins divide, and an HCC that has arisen in this region is difficult to resect despite its small size. Occasionally the medial branch (P^{VIII}_{d}) arises more centrally making it difficult to distinguish it from the superior branch of the right caudate lobe ($P^{I}_{r\text{-}sup}$). There is no hepatic vein that will assist in distinguishing these two branches.

The anterior inferior portal vein (P^{V}) is usually distributed as the first anterior branch in the lateral caudal area anteriorly. The calibre and number of branches of this vein are generally small compared with the anterior superior portal vein.

The posterior portal vein (Fig. 1.22), after separating from the anterior portal vein, runs vertical to the dorsum and sends off the caudal (P^{VI}), lateral (P^{VI}_{*}) and cranial (P^{VII}) branches in that order. The pattern of division in the lateral projection may resemble an opened fan with the P-point as the pivot (Takayasu *et al.* 1985*d*). As the posterior portal vein courses vertically to the frontal plane, it is seen as a high-density round point (P-point) on the portogram.

The left portal vein (Fig. 1.23) first forms the transverse portion, then the umbilical portion that ends as a cul-de-sac. It is the remains of the fetal umbilical vein which was in continuity with this blind end. The transverse portion after dividing from the right portal vein runs somewhat anteromedially. The umbil-

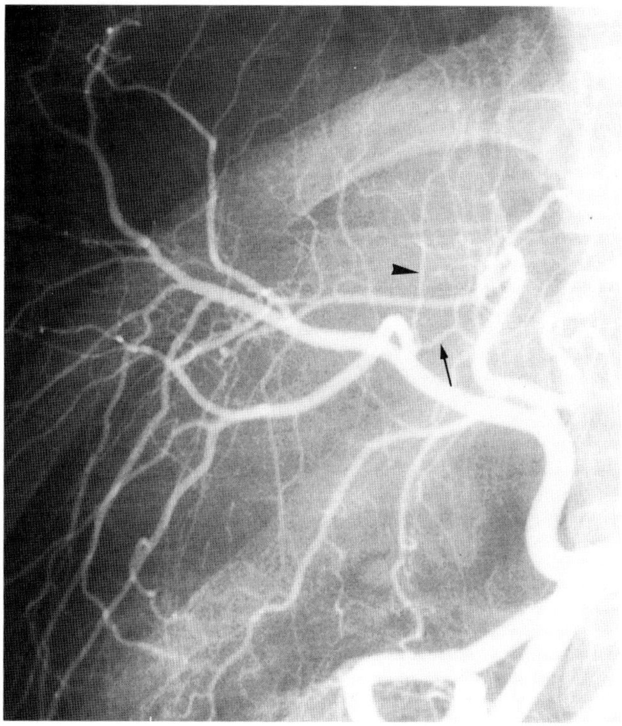

a

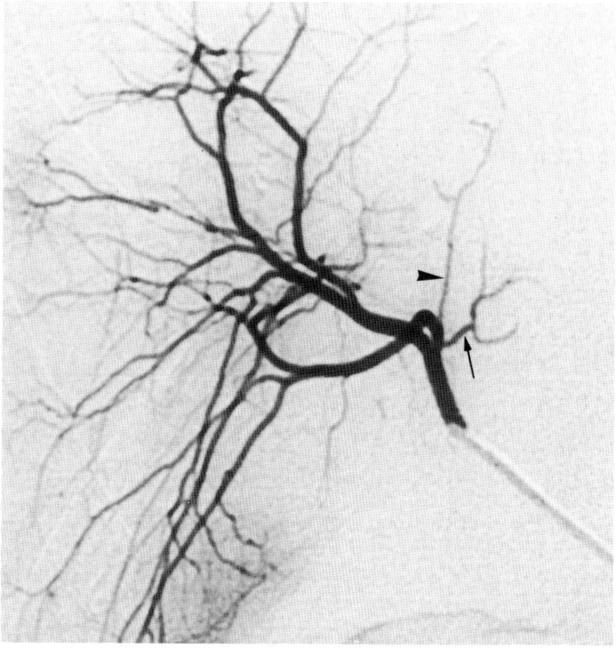

b

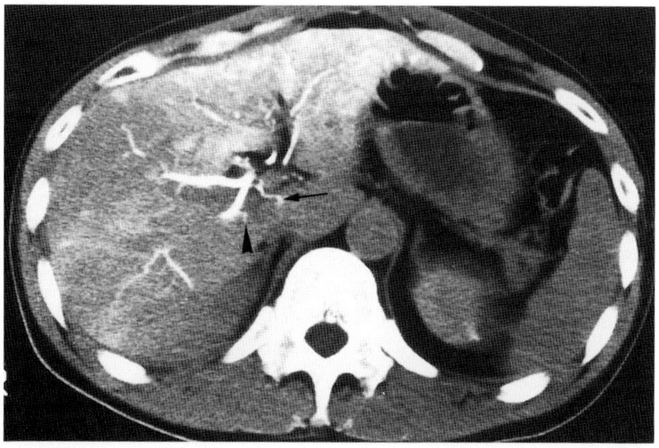

c

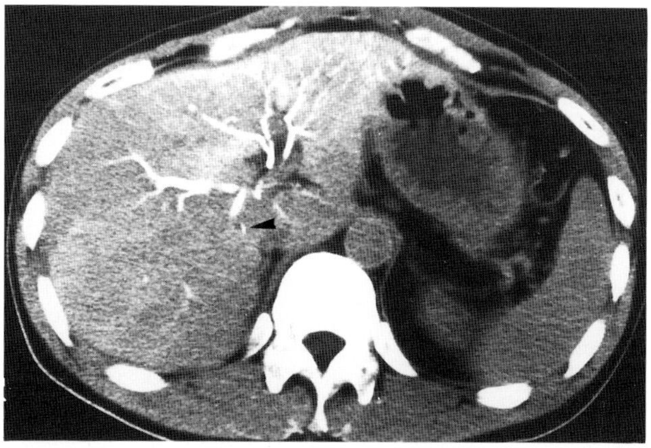

d

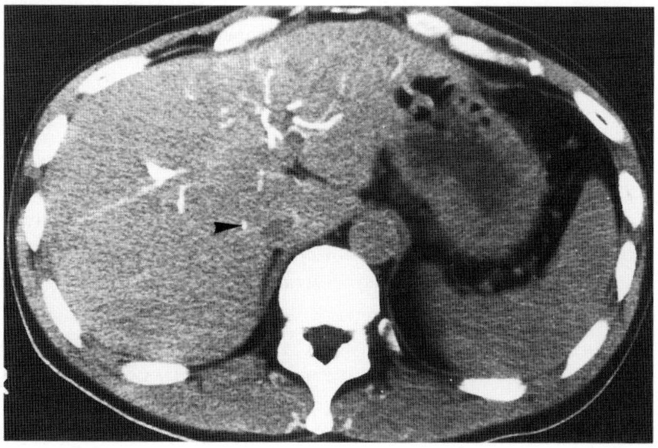

e

Fig. 1.7 Identification of caudate lobe arteries.

(a) Common hepatic arteriogram: the caudate arteries (▶; →) are not well identified as the left and right hepatic arteries are seen in close proximity in the area of the caudate lobe.

(b) DSA: with the catheter past the origin of the cystic artery, the left hepatic artery is avoided, and the right hepatic artery is clearly opacified by DSA. By stereo-vision, two arteries are seen coming off the posterior segment artery, one (▶) the cephalad branch of the caudate lobe artery posterior to the other (→) left medial branch.

(c), (d), (e) Arterial-CT: with the catheter in the proper hepatic artery, the liver was sliced from the level of the hilum moving cranially for 5 mm sections (c)–(e). One caudate lobe artery (→) that supplies both sides of the caudate lobe, and another artery (▶) that arises from the posterior segment artery, coursing to the right of the inferior vena cava and supplying the right part of the caudate lobe, are identified.

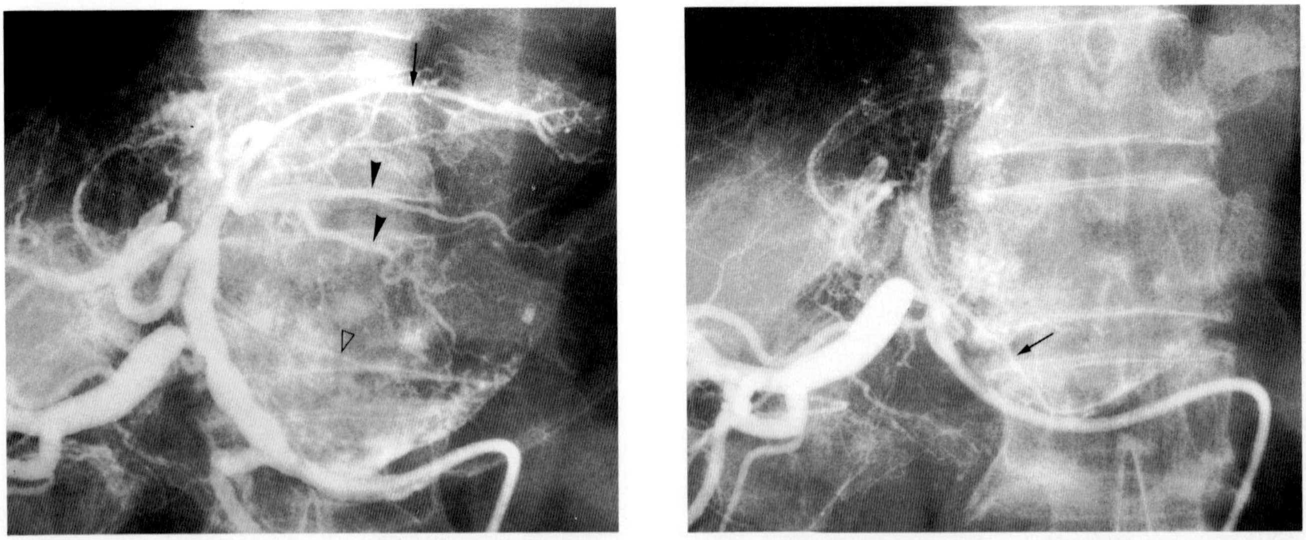

a b

Fig 1.8 A large left caudate artery (A^{I}_{l}) supplying a hemangioma that has arisen in the caudate lobe (cf. hepatic hemangioma, Case 14).
(a) Proper hepatic arteriogram: the left lateral superior branch A^{II} (→) displaced cranially and the inferior branch A^{III} (▶) are seen. A dilated left caudate branch A^{I}_{l} (▷) coming off the central part of the left hepatic artery is recognized caudal to A^{II} and A^{III}.
(b) Right hepatic arteriogram: the left hepatic is not opacified due to angiospasm and only the right hepatic is seen. In this film, a left caudate lobe branch (→) arising from the right hepatic is seen beside the left caudate lobe branch seen in (a).

ical portion usually runs vertically to the frontal plane and is seen as a dense round point (U-point) in the front view. The lateral superior portal vein (P^{II}) arises from the origin of the umbilical portion, from the end of which arise the lateral inferior portal vein (P^{III}) and the medial portal vein (P^{IV}). There are a number of small branches running cephalad from the umbilical portion which are called the dorsal branches (P^{IV}_{dor}) and are included in the medial branch for practical purposes. However, there is no anatomical means by which to distinguish them from the lateral branches. The authors prefer including them in the left medial portal vein (P^{IV}) since they are frequently distributed to the right of the sagittal plane at the U-point. With regard to the left lateral branches, an extra branch is occasionally seen between the superior (P^{II}) and inferior (P^{III}) branches; it is mostly part of the inferior branch.

The caudate branches (Fig. 1.24) generally arise from the right and left first-order portal vein, and occasionally from the portal trunk (P^{I}_{t}). The right caudate portal vein consists of the superior ($P^{I}_{r\text{-sup}}$) and the inferior ($P^{I}_{r\text{-inf}}$) branches, and the left caudate the superior ($P^{I}_{l\text{-sup}}$) and the medial ($P^{I}_{l\text{-med}}$) branches (Fig. 1.25). In a few cases the inferior branches of the right caudate portal vein overlie the inferior vena cava and are distributed in the region of the medial branches of the left caudate portal vein.

Hepatic vein

The major vessels that drain the liver, the right, middle, and left hepatic veins, open into the inferior vena cava immediately below the diaphragmatic level, and the inferior right (accessory right) hepatic vein enters the inferior vena cava 5–6 cm caudal to them (Figs. 1.26, 27). Whereas the right hepatic vein joins the inferior vena cava from the right, the middle hepatic vein joins the left hepatic vein near its opening into the inferior vena cava in 85 per cent of cases, forming a short common segment (Nakamura and Tuzuki 1981) that joins the vena cava slightly to the left of front (Fig. 1.28).

In the venogram seen from the front, the right hepatic vein runs nearly superimposed on the middle hepatic, and sends out many peripheral branches (Fig. 1.29). The left hepatic vein (Fig. 1.30) runs between P^{II} and P^{III} and divides into the ventral and dorsal branches. The left superficial hepatic vein runs in the superior posterior region (Fig. 1.28b). The angles that the right hepatic, middle hepatic, and left hepatic make with the inferior vena cava, when viewed from the right side, are increasingly wider (Fig. 1.31). The right superficial hepatic vein joins the right hepatic from behind in 96 per cent, and joins the vena cava directly in only 4 per cent (Nakamura and Tuzuki 1981).

The inferior right hepatic vein drains the posterior segment of the right lobe (Fig. 1.32) and several thin short hepatic veins (caudate lobe vein) drain the caudate lobe. These veins are seldom seen by imaging except when using dynamic CT, which occasionally opacifies them (Fig. 1.33). In Budd–Chiari syndrome, however, they are commonly identified as the caudate lobe is greatly hypertrophied. According to Healey and Schroy (1953), the inferior right hepatic vein can be demonstrated in only 17 per cent of individuals. It is enlarged when the hepatic portion of the inferior vena cava is blocked by tumor or a membrane (a type of Budd–Chiari syndrome), and becomes a collateral route (Makuuchi *et al.* 1984; Takayasu *et al.* 1994*b*), an important diagnostic clue. In extended medial bisegmentectomy

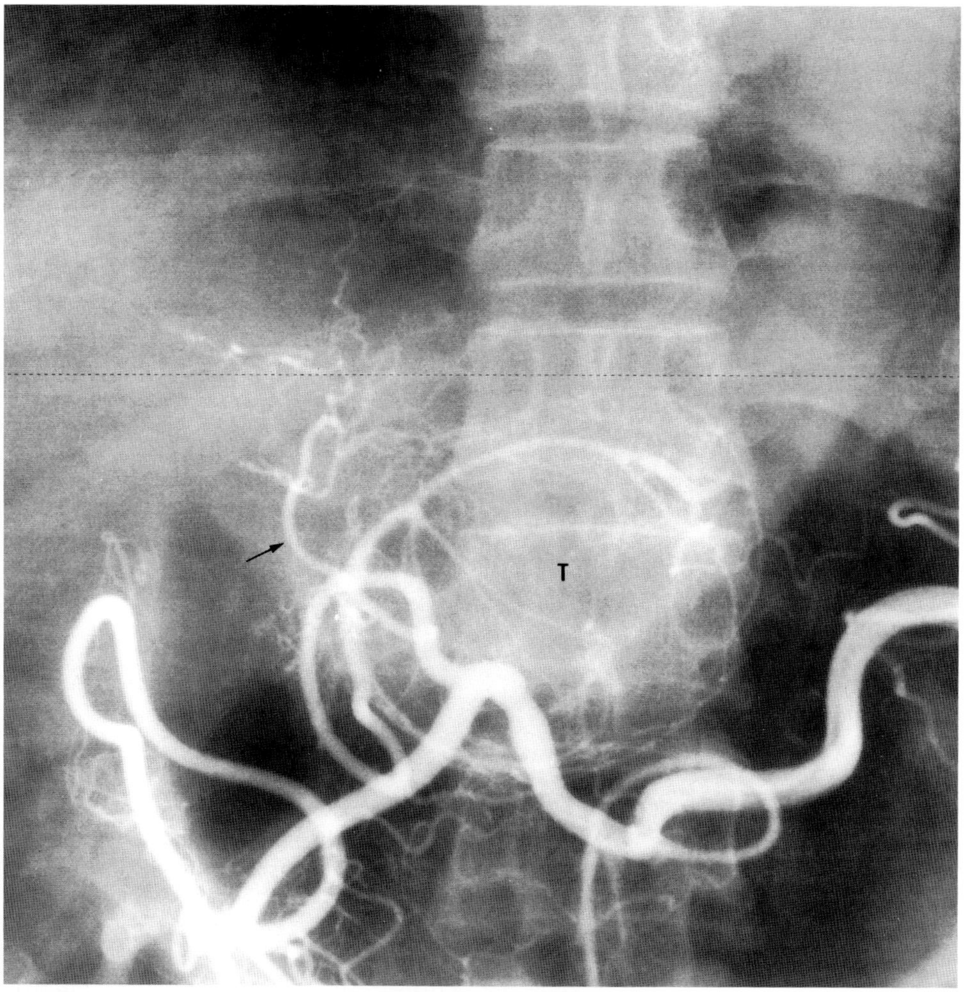

a

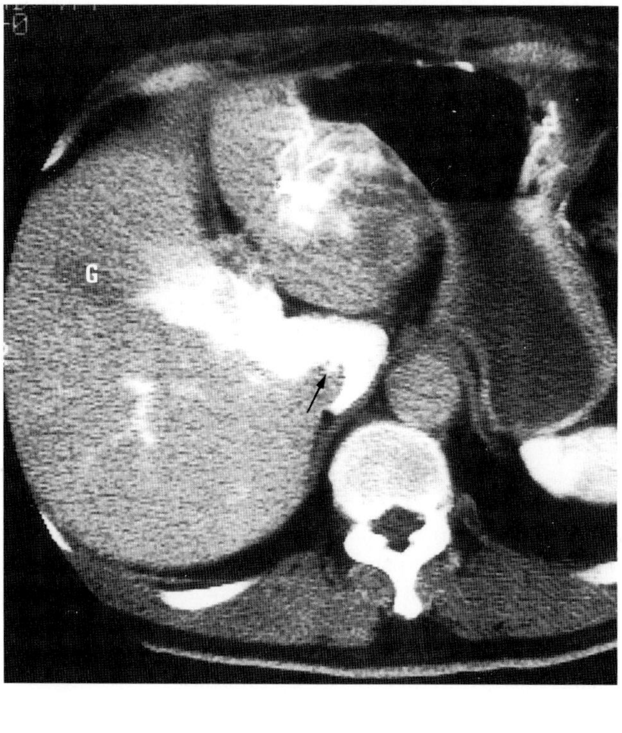

b

Fig. 1.9 Independent caudate lobe artery.

(a) Arteriogram: in this arteriogram done for a gastric leiomyosarcoma (T), an artery is seen (→) arising from the right gastric and running toward the hepatic hilum. In this patient, the right hepatic and left hepatic derive from the superior mesenteric and the left gastric artery respectively.

(b) Arterial-CT: arterial-CT was done with the catheter in the common hepatic artery for the estimation of tumor involvement. The CT scan clearly demonstrates the left and right parts of the caudate lobe. The level of this CT scan is shown by the interrupted line in (a). It cuts two thin arteries which are the left and right caudate lobe arteries. The right part of the caudate lobe is less clearly demarcated than the left, suggesting an additional arterial supply from the adjacent region. In the inferior vena cava, the short hepatic vein is seen as a dot of contrast (→). The stain in the left lateral region of the left lobe is part of the leiomyosarcoma. G, gallbladder.

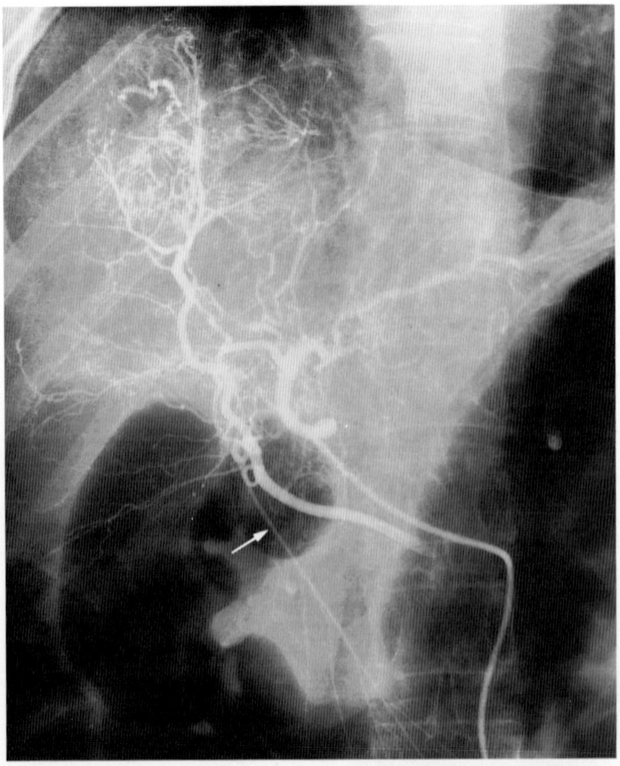

Fig. 1.10 Hepatic falciform artery. Selective left hepatic arteriogram: the hepatic falciform artery (→) is seen running from a branch of A^{IV} toward the umbilicus.

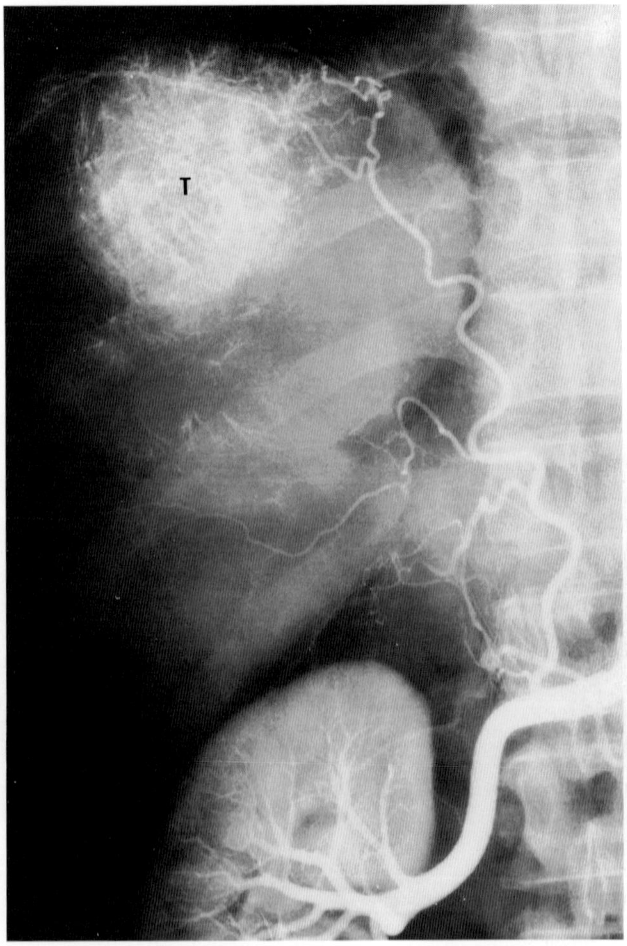

Fig. 1.11 The right inferior phrenic artery arising from the right renal artery. Right renal arteriogram: Lipiodol-TAE (transcatheter arterial embolization) was carried out for the treatment of HCC (T). As the treatment of the diaphragmatic side of the mass was inadequate, an attempt was made to embolize the tumor from the left inferior phrenic artery. It was not identified in the celiac arteriogram, but was seen by right renal arteriography permitting embolization of the right inferior phrenic artery.

conserving the posterior segment and the inferior right hepatic vein, this vein becomes an important draining vessel (Makuuchi *et al.* 1987*b*). Small peripheral communications between hepatic veins are common in healthy people (Fig. 1.34), but they are very much exaggerated in those with idiopathic portal hypertension (Okuda *et al.* 1981*a*).

Intrahepatic bile duct

The intrahepatic biliary tree may be divided into several types depending on the pattern of branching of the right posterior (segmental) branch at the hilum (Ohto *et al.* 1978). The most common type is one in which the posterior and anterior branches form a common channel which then joins the left hepatic (Fig. 1.35). In 11.5 per cent of individuals, three major branches join the principal junction simultaneously, the posterior branch joins it independently in 8.7 per cent, and the posterior branch joins the left hepatic duct in 8.7 per cent (Kida *et al.* 1987). In a patient with the last type, the posterior branch is not dilated on CT when the right hepatic duct is occluded, and only the ducts draining the anterior segment are dilated; a situation in which this kind of variation is a possibility. According to Michels (1955), the caudate lobe has three bile ducts in 44 per cent of people (each of the three parts of this lobe is drained separately by them) and two bile ducts in 26 per cent (the caudate process and right part are drained by one duct, and the left part by another). Most of these ducts draining the caudate lobe join both the left and right hepatic ducts in 78 per cent of people, the left hepatic duct in 15 per cent, and the right hepatic duct only in the remaining 7 per cent.

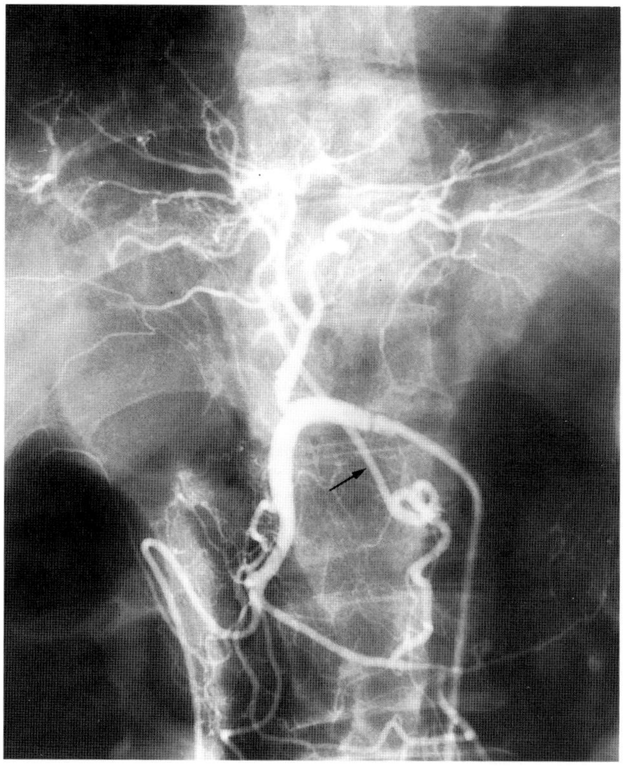

Fig. 1.12 The right inferior phrenic artery arising from the dorsal pancreatic artery. Common hepatic arteriogram: the dorsal pancreatic was opacified through the transverse pancreatic, and then the ascending right inferior phrenic artery (→). The right hepatic artery was not visualized because it was replaced by the superior mesenteric artery.

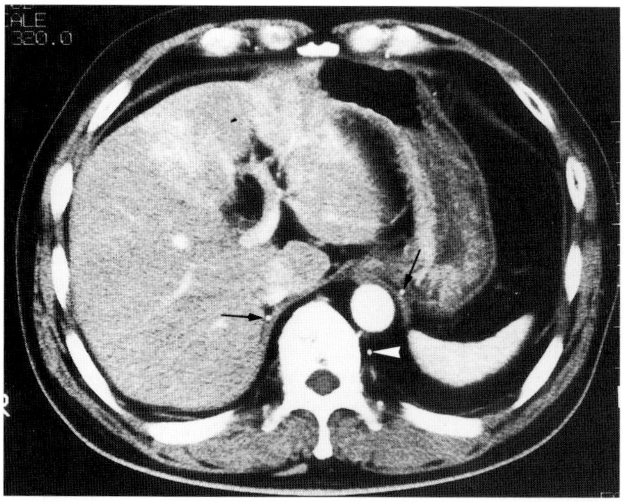

Fig. 1.13 Course of the inferior phrenic arteries. Dynamic CT: the inferior phrenic arteries (→) on both sides run anterior to the diaphragmatic crus. The right inferior phrenic artery is located posterior to the inferior vena cava and required differentiation from the vein (▶) that belongs to the azygos vein system lying posterior to the diaphragmatic crus.

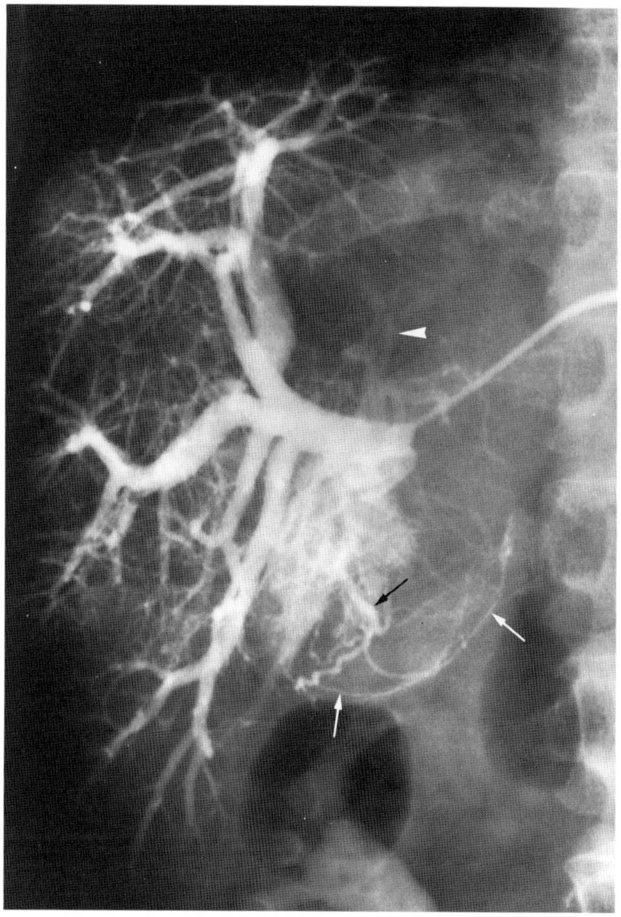

Fig. 1.14 The cystic vein communicating with the right anterior portal vein. Selective opacification of the right anterior portal vein by PTP: a dilated cystic vein (→) arising from the proximal P^{V} and its tributaries along the gallbladder wall are seen.

▶, the posterior portal vein is faintly opacified by the regurgitation of contrast medium.

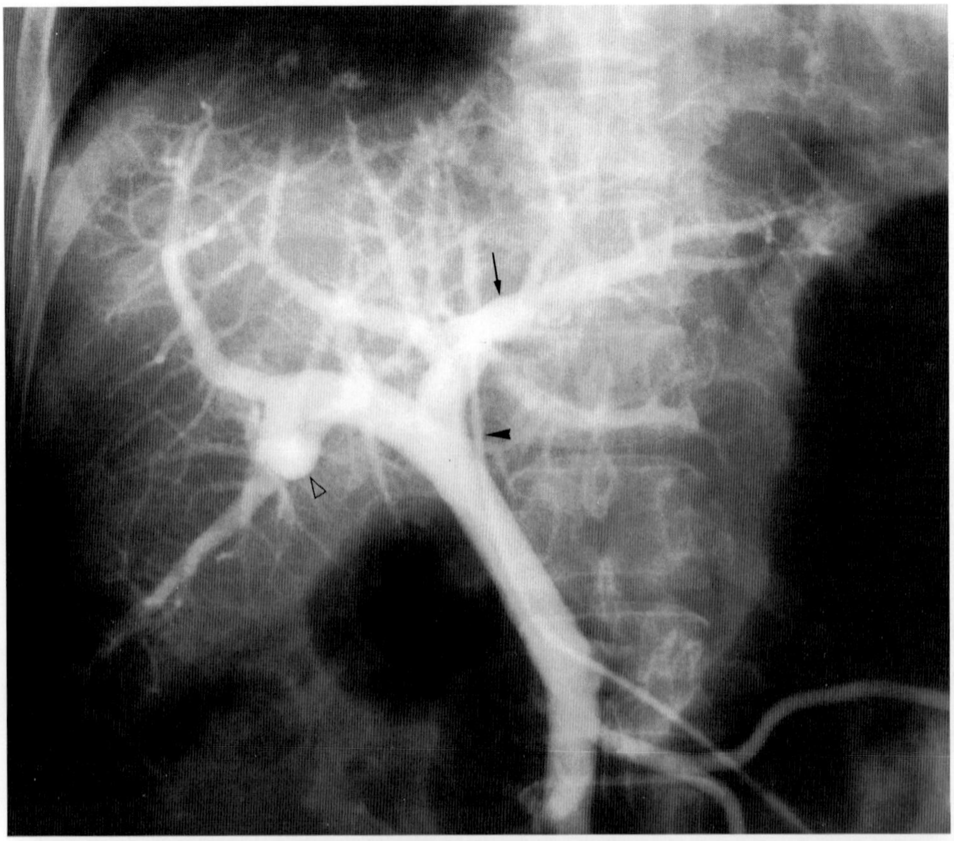

a

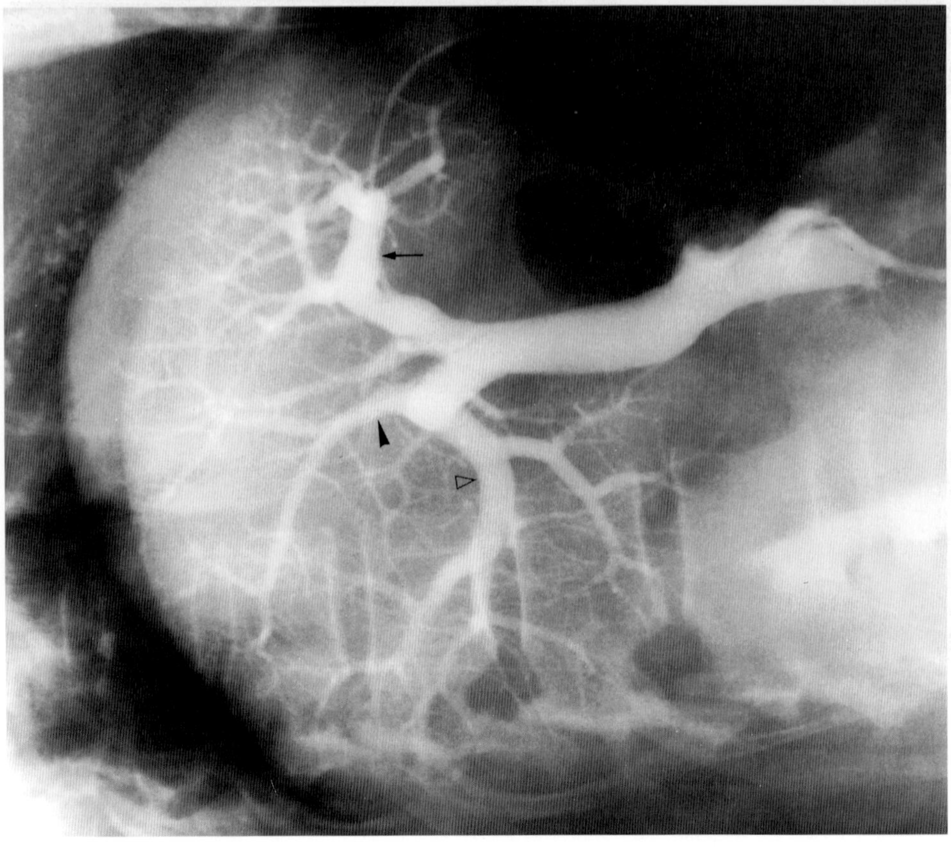

b

Fig. 1.15 Normal intraheptic portal vein branches.

(a) Antero-posterior view of the normal intrahepatic portal branches opacified by PTP: the umbilical portion along the left portal vein and the right posterior portal vein both run vertical to the frontal plane and are seen as a dense point: U-point (→) and P-point (▷). Both are useful markers in topographic diagnosis. ▶, the catheter.

(b) Lateral view of (a): the vertical course of the left umbilical portion (→) and the right posterior portal vein (▷) can be seen on this film. The areas supplied by the anterior (▶) and posterior portal veins are not separable by a horizontal plane; the separating plane is shifting cranially at an angle of about 45° against the dorsal plane.

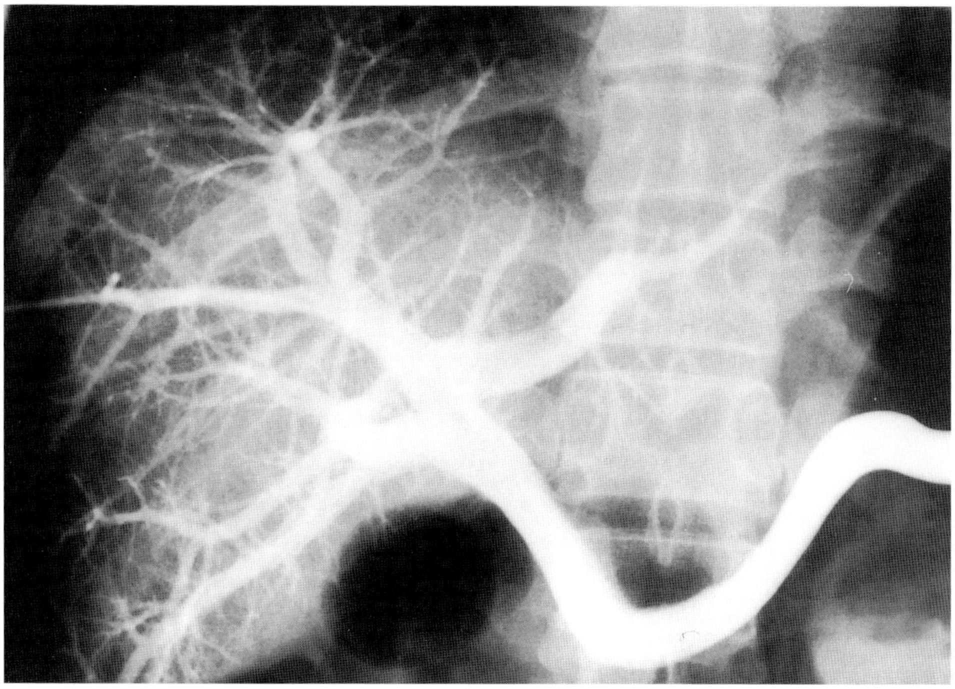

Fig. 1.16 A posterior portal vein of the independent type. The posterior portal vein branches off the portal trunk early, from the area where normally the right and left first veins divide.

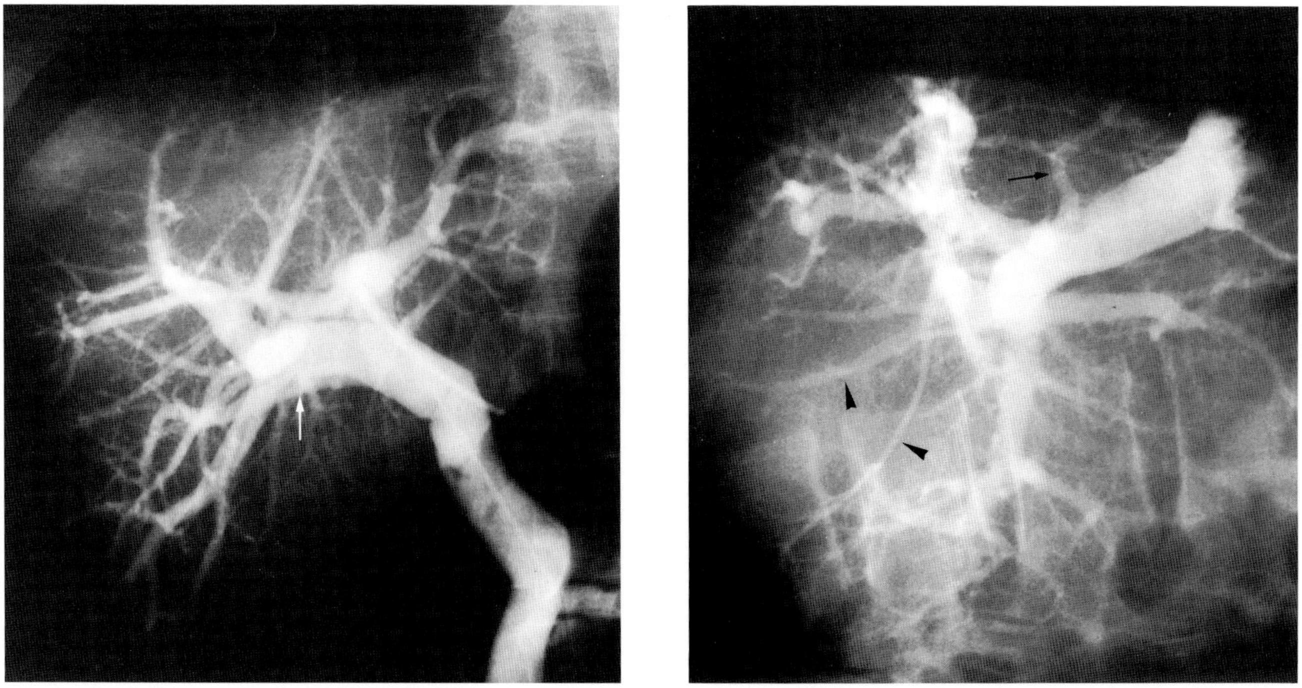

a b

Fig. 1.17 Aberrant right anterior inferior subsegment portal branch (P^{V}).
(a) Frontal view of PTP: a portal branch (P^{V}, →) is seen arising from the area where normally the right and left first-order portal veins divide.
(b) Right lateral view of PTP: the same portal branch (→) is situated anterior to the portal trunk, and also anterior to the right hepatic vein (not visualized) which was opacified later, supporting the diagnosis of this being P^{V}. The branches of P^{VIII} (▶) are displaced by an HCC occupying this region.

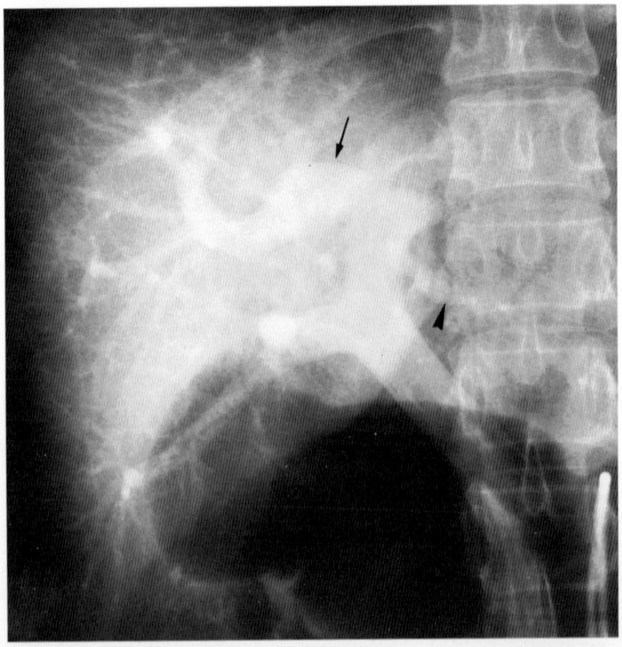

a

Fig. 1.18 Aberrant right portal vein arising from the left portal vein.

(a) Superior mesenteric arterial portogram: this major vein looks like an independent posterior portal vein, but actually it arises from an aneurysmal left portal vein (→). (▶) is a branch of P^{III} and the normally dense left umbilical portion is obscure (P^{II} is not opacified because of cholangiocarcinoma occupying the lateral portion of the left lobe).

(b)–(g) Dynamic CT: the study of the relationship between the portal and hepatic veins demonstrates that the left umbilical portion is obscure, and the right anterior portal (A) which is situated anterior to the middle hepatic vein (→), is distributed in the right anterior area through a markedly dilated portal vein (e), (f). The gallbladder has been removed and is not recognized. ▶ hepatic round ligament; ▷ right hepatic vein.

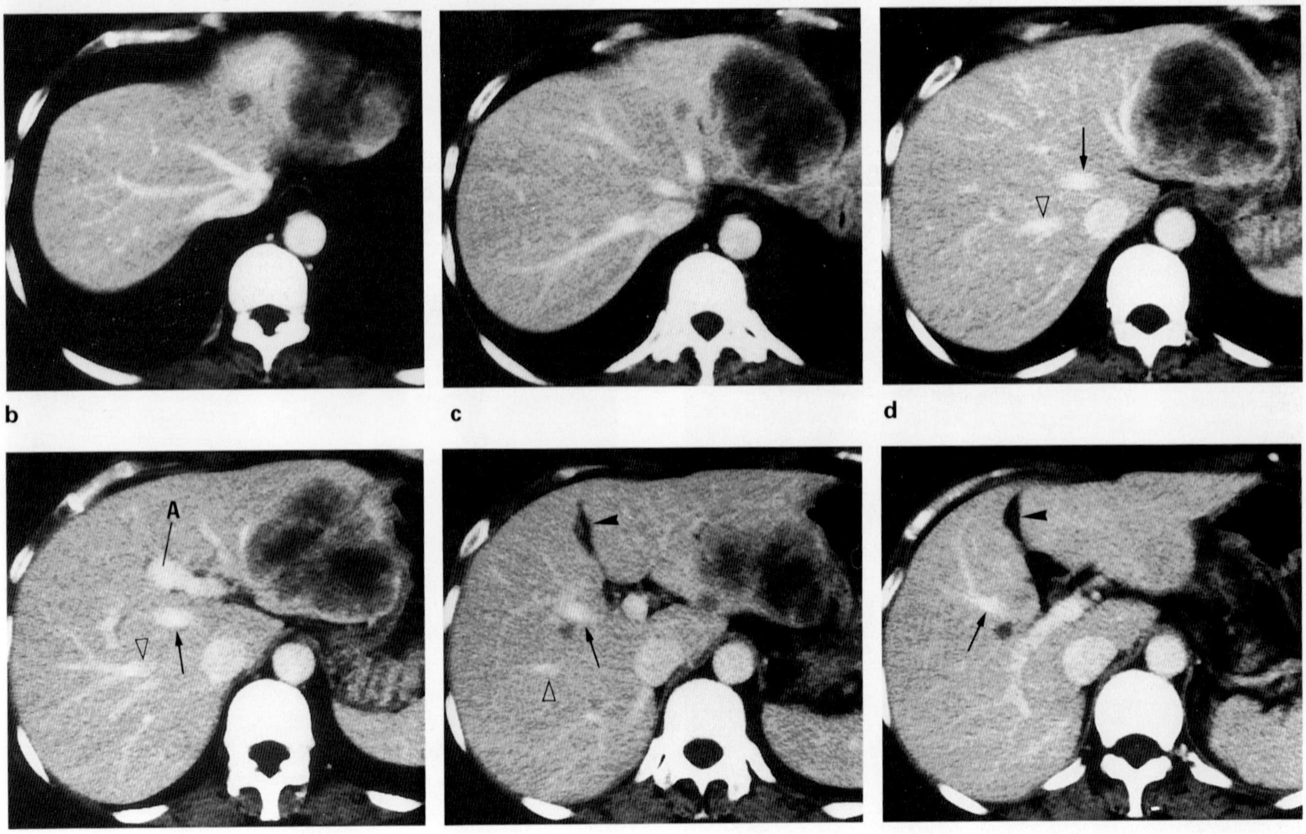

b c d e f g

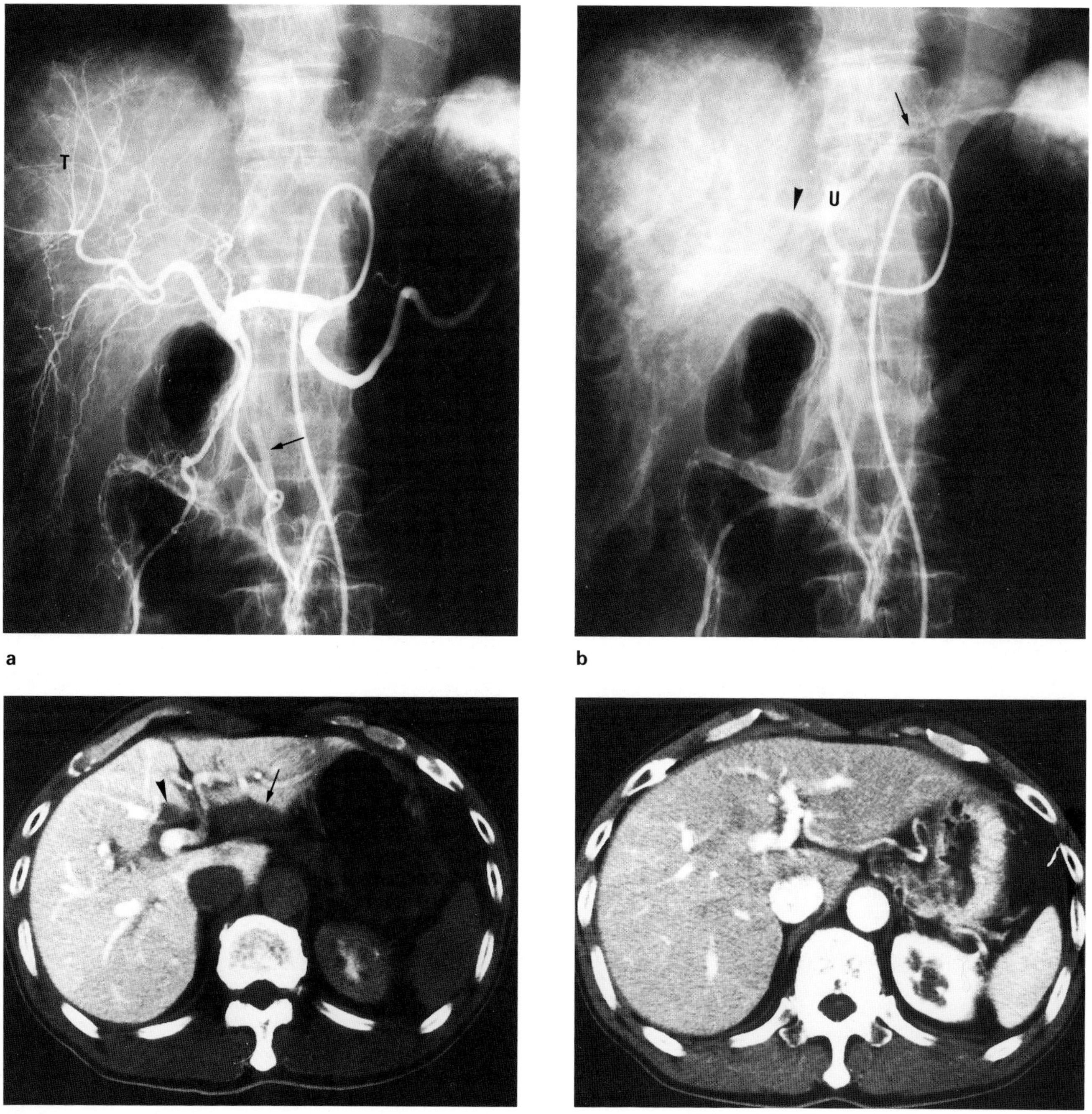

Fig. 1.19 Variation in which the right gastric vein directly enters the left portal vein (accessory portal vein).
(a) Common hepatic arteriogram (early phase): the right gastric vein (→) is opacified early. T, liver tumor.
(b) Common hepatic arteriogram (late phase): beside the portal vein opacified through the splenic artery, the left umbilical portion (U), the left lateral superior branch P^{II} (→) as its continuation, and part of the medial branch P^{IV} (▶) are clearly opacified.
(c) Portal-CT: there are areas in S^{II} of the left lobe (→) and in the posterior region of S^{IV} (▶) that were not opacified.
(d) Dynamic CT: contrast CT in the same slice as (b) shows normal S^{II} and S^{IV}. The non-opacified areas of S^{II} and S^{IV} in (c) are thought to be supplied by the right gastric vein that enters the intraphepatic portal vein directly.

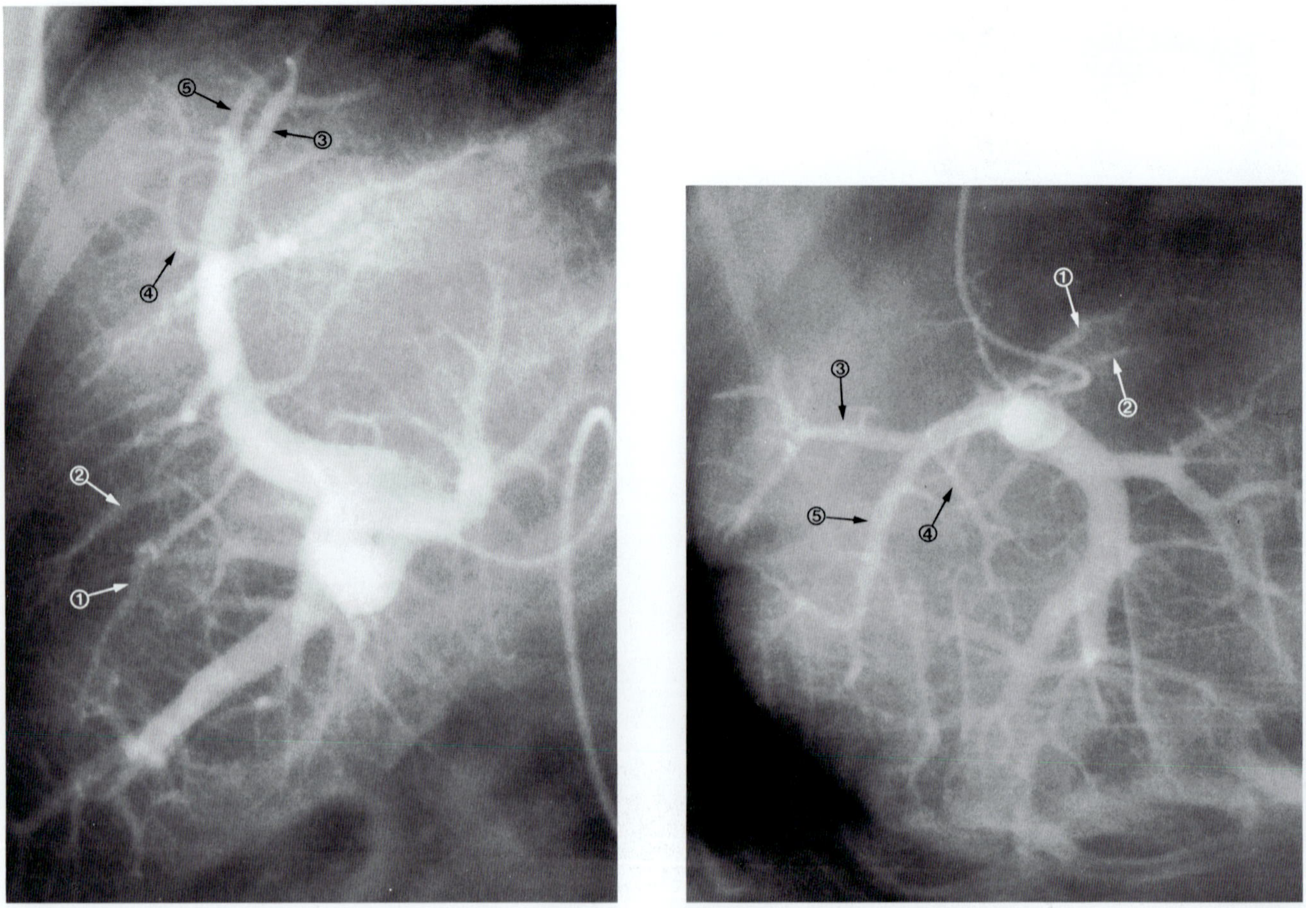

a b

Fig. 1.20 Selective right portal venography.

(a) Anterior view: the right anterior and posterior segments supplied by the portal vein are shifted cranial and caudal to each other, in the frontal plane. (1), P^{V}_{a}; (2), P^{V}_{b}; (3), P^{VIII}_{a}; (4), P^{VIII}_{b}; (5), P^{VIII}_{c}.

(b) Right lateral view: as illustrated in Fig 1.21, the anterior and posterior segments are shifted cephalad and caudad respectively, and their boundary is oblique; almost all of the right lobe immediately below the diaphragm is the anterior segment. For that reason, in the diagnosis of a tumor located in the anterior segment there may be a discrepancy in segment diagnosis between CT scan that emphasizes hepatic veins and angiography that delineates the portal tract containing the arteries and portal veins (cf. Fig. 1.58).

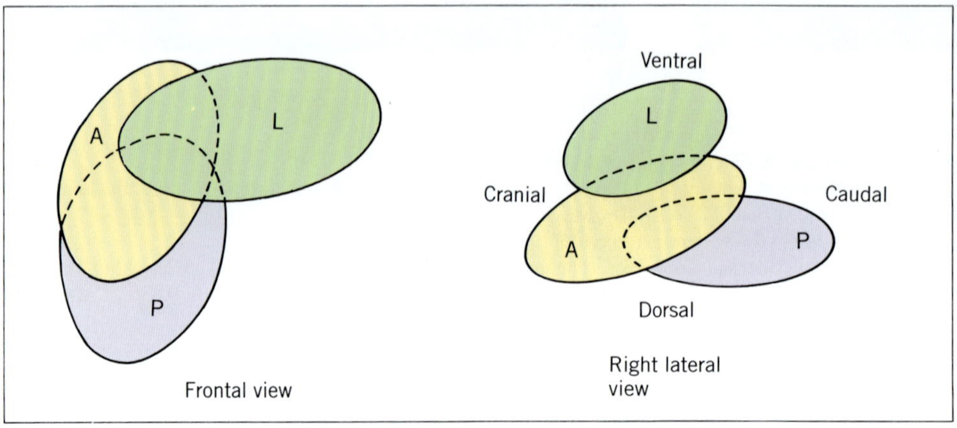

Fig. 1.21 Spatial relation between the anterior, posterior, and lateral areas supplied by portal veins. The anterior (A) and the posterior (P) segment of the right lobe are shifted cephalad and caudad, respectively, and the medial segment of the left lobe (L) is located ventral to the anterior segment.

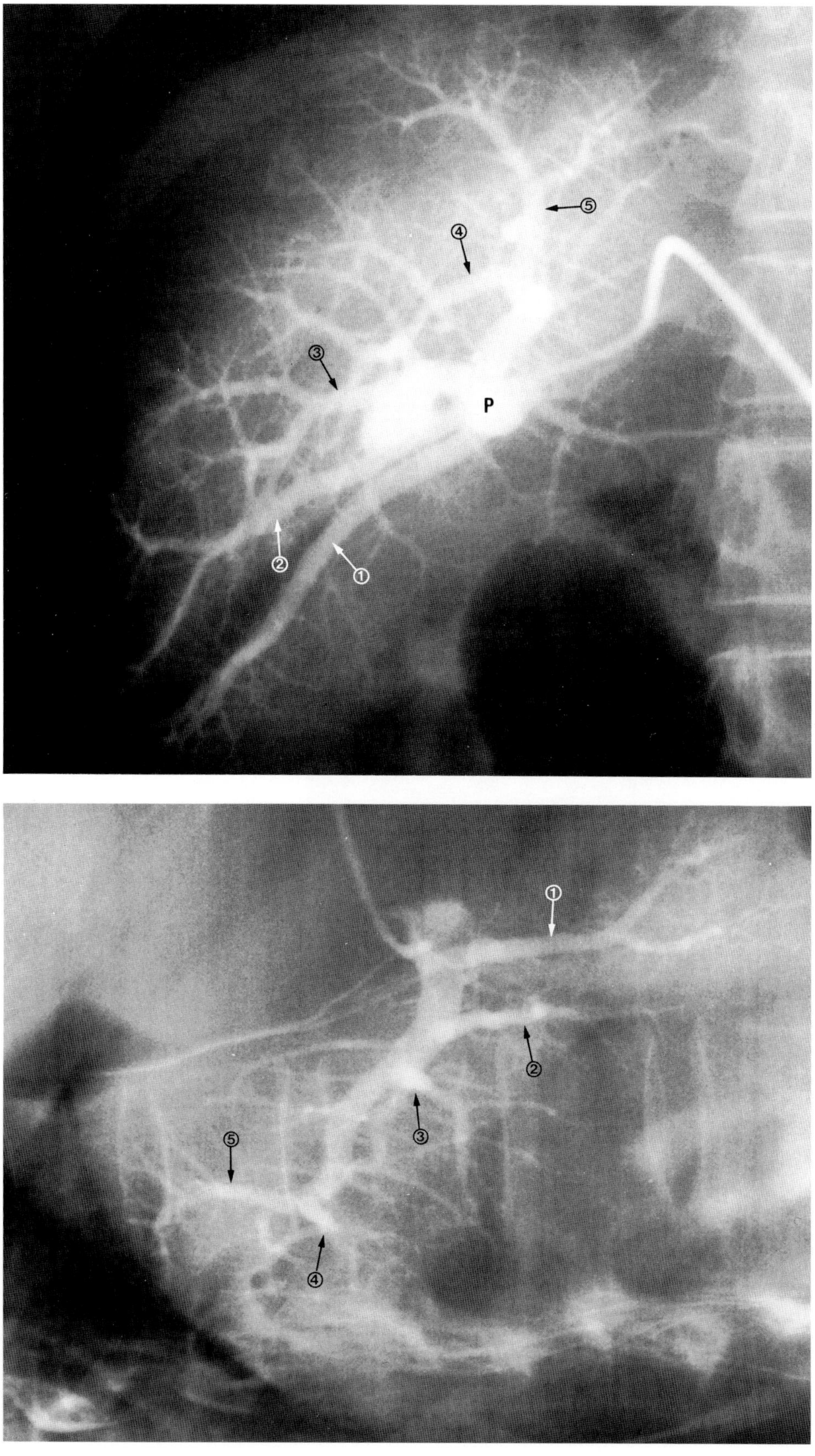

a

b

Fig. 1.22 Selective opacification of the right posterior portal vein.
(a) Frontal view: clockwise arrangement of branches of the posterior portal vein with the P-point (P) as their pivot, first P^{VI}_{a} (1), then P^{VI}_{b} (2) P^{VI}_{*} (3) running laterally, and a common channel that sends out P^{VII}_{a} (4) and P^{VII}_{b} (5). The pool of contrast lateral to the P-point is an artefact due to catheterization.
(b) Right lateral view: one can identify the five branches seen in the frontal view (a).

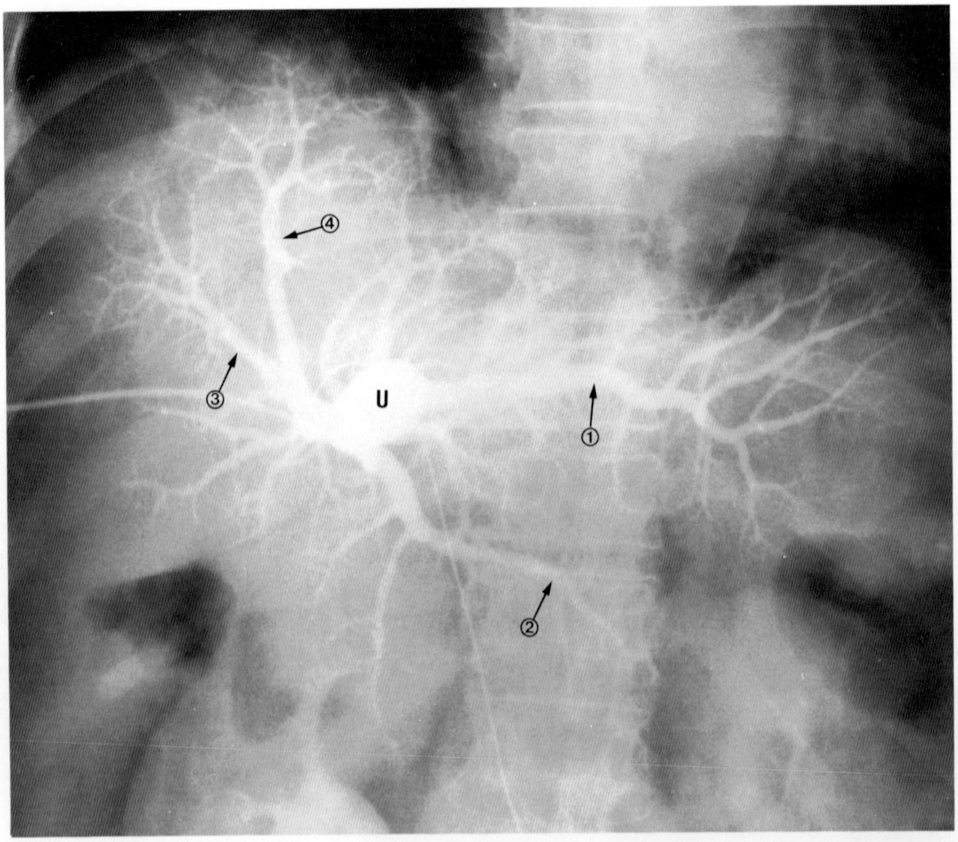

a

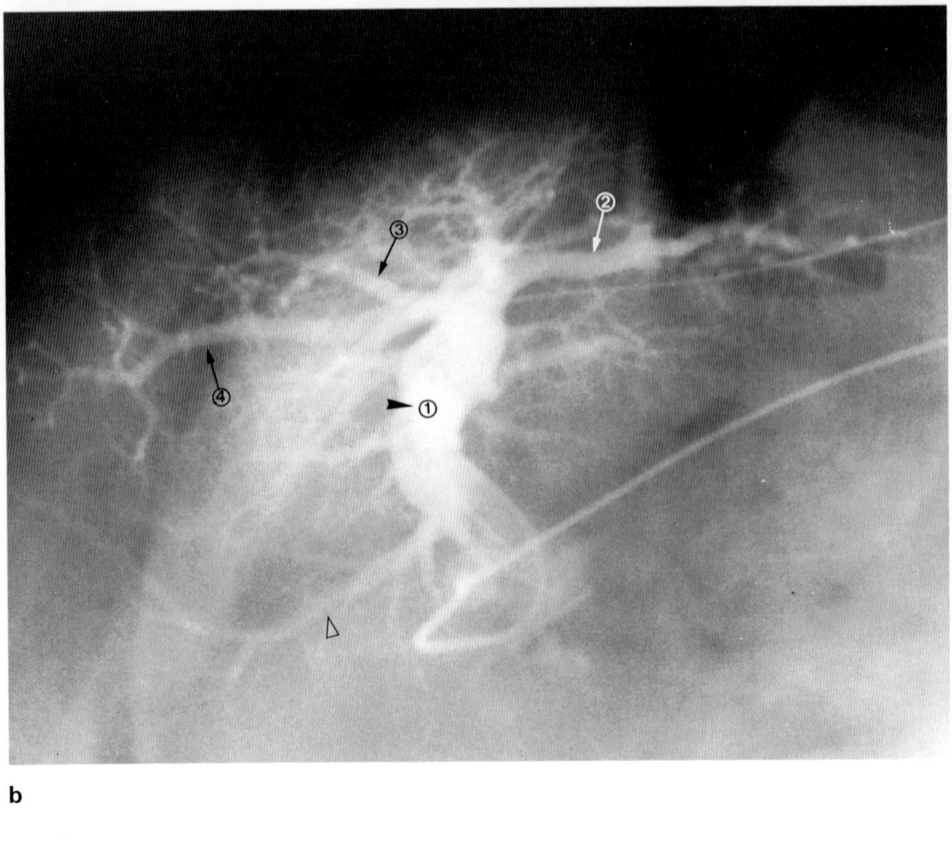

b

Fig. 1.23 Selective opacification of the left portal vein.

(a) Frontal view: one can identify the portal branches in the left lobe fanning out laterally and medially from the U-point (U). The transverse portion is not seen in this view. (1), P^{II}; (2), P^{III}; (3), $P^{IV}{}_{a}$; (4), $P^{IV}{}_{b}$.

(b) Right lateral view: from the faintly opacified transverse portion comes off the superior branch for the left part of the caudate lobe $P^{I}{}_{I\text{-sup}}$ (▷), followed by the lateral superior P^{II} (1) which is seen as a round dense object (▶) superimposed on the umbilical portion. The umbilical portion sends out at its blind end the medial portal vein $P^{IV}{}_{a}$ (3) and $P^{IV}{}_{b}$ (4) cranially, and the lateral inferior P^{III} (2) caudally. Posterior to the medial portal vein several small tributaries arise from the umbilical portion running cephalad, which we call the dorsal group of branches ($P^{IV}{}_{dor}$). As P^{II} supplies the dorsal area of the left lobe, and P^{III} and P^{IV} the ventral area, Couinaud (1981) proposed the possibility of combining S^{III} and S^{IV} to be separated from S^{II}.

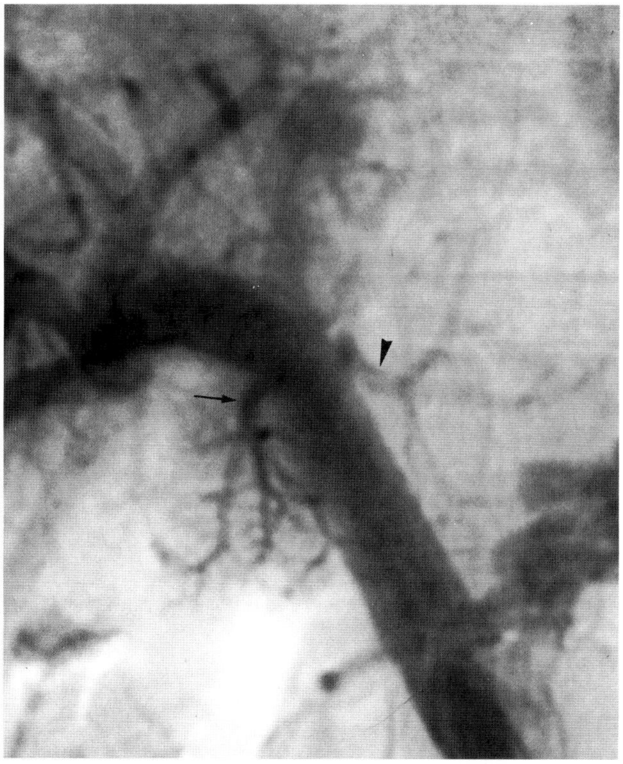

Fig. 1.24 The portal vein (caudate portal veins). Portogram: hypertrophied caudate lobe in a patient with cirrhosis. An enlarged inferior branch $P^{I}_{r\text{-}inf}$ (→) of the right caudate portal vein and the medial branch $P^{I}_{l\text{-}med}$ (▶) of the left caudate portal vein are recognized.

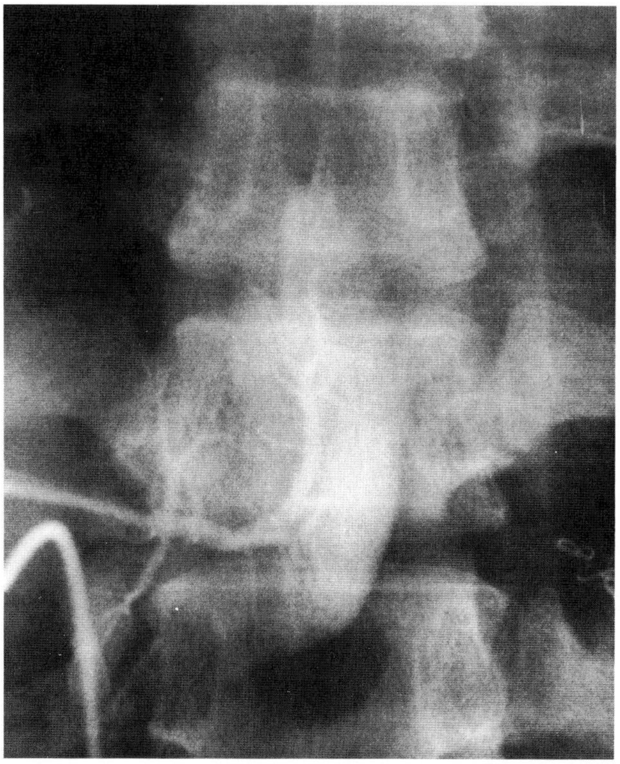

Fig. 1.25 The medial branch of the left caudate portal vein. Selective opacification of the medial branch ($P^{I}_{l\text{-}med}$) of the left caudate portal vein by PTP: the edge of the left caudate lobe is usually seen rounded as in this radiograph.

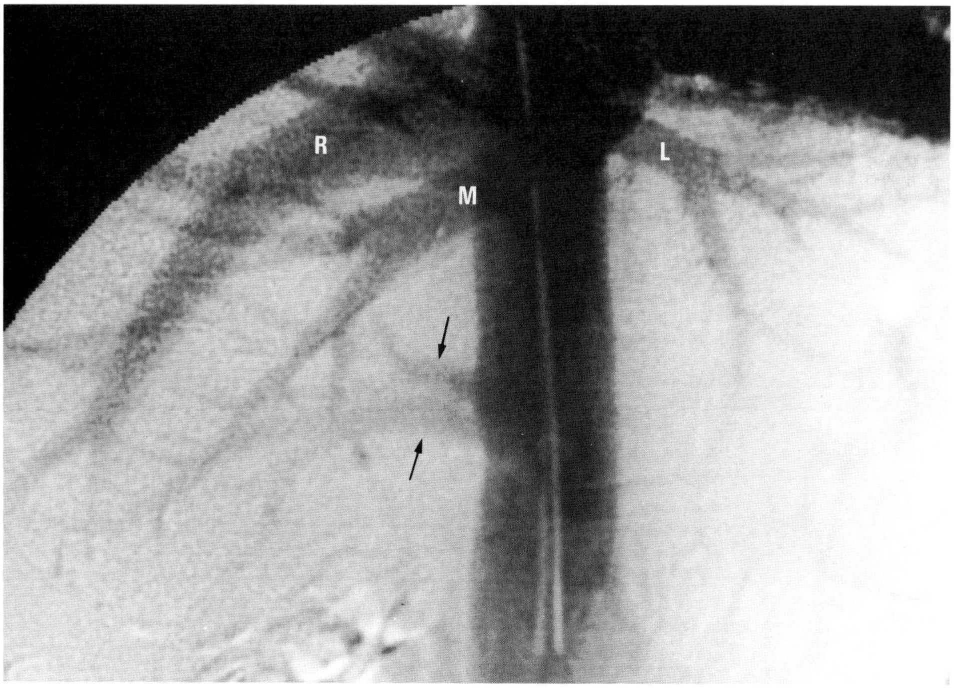

Fig. 1.26 Pan-hepatic venogram and inferior cavogram. Besides the three major veins, the right (R), middle (M), and left (L) hepatic veins, two inferior right hepatic veins (→) are recognized. In this patient, the middle hepatic runs slightly caudad to the right hepatic vein with no superposition, both being seen separately. This rare radiograph was obtained when all hepatic veins happened to be opacified during in-ferior cavography due to arrythmia. R, right hepatic vein; M, middle hepatic vein; L, left hepatic vein.

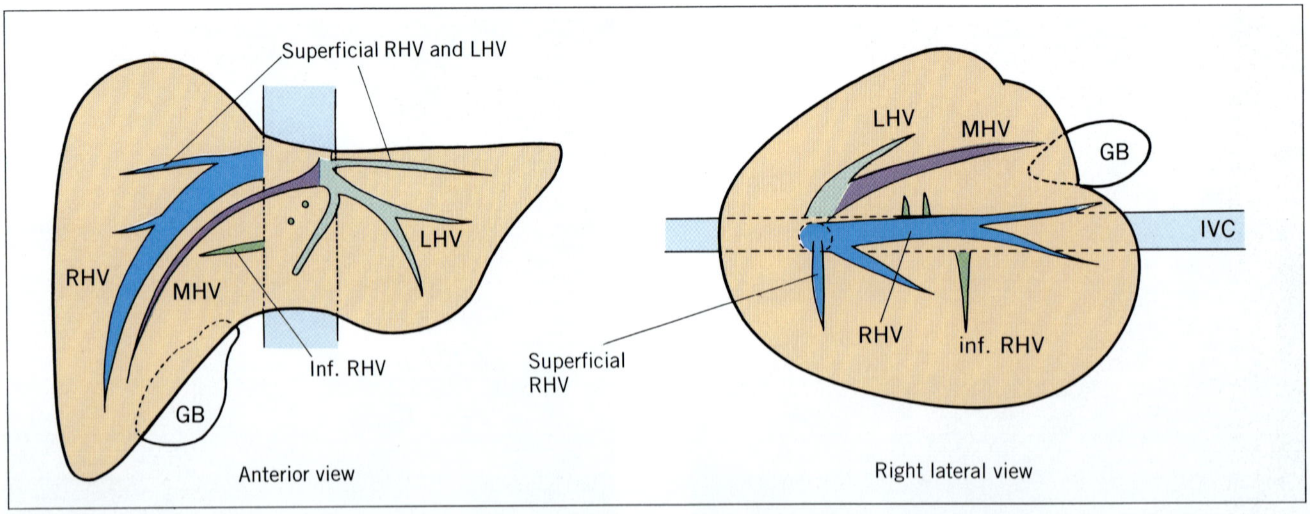

Fig. 1.27 Spatial relationships between the hepatic veins. On the venogram, the right and middle hepatic veins are often superimposed on the frontal view, but the middle hepatic can be distinguished from the right hepatic because it joins the left hepatic, forming a short common channel which enters the vena cava anteriorly and somewhat to the left in the majority of cases (85 per cent). In the lateral view, the right hepatic is at about the same level as the vena cava to which enter the right hepatic, middle hepatic, and left hepatic from the back towards the front in this order.

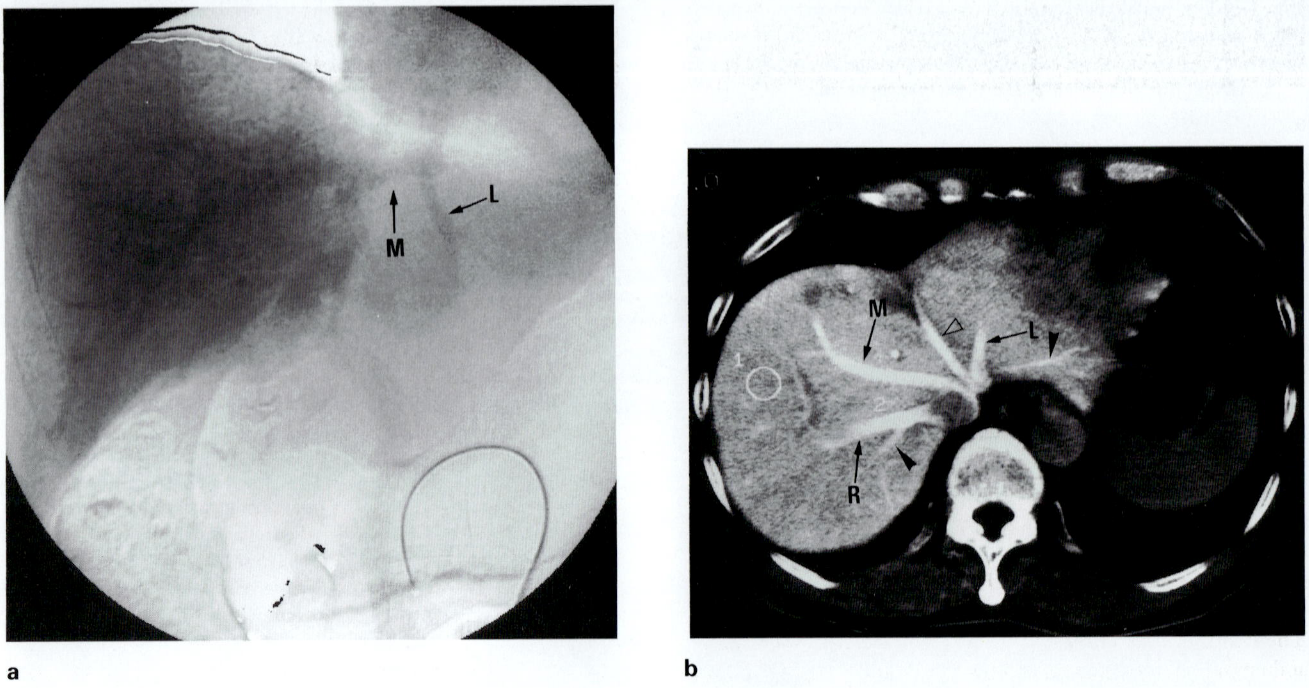

Fig. 1.28 Site of junction of the hepatic veins and inferior vena cava.
(a) Late phase of a superior mesenteric arterial portogram made by DSA: the hepatic veins are recognized if studied carefully. The right hepatic and middle hepatic are usually superimposed and seen as one vessel. However, the middle (M) and left (L) hepatic join to form a short channel that enters the vena cava from the left anteriorly. Thus, it can be distinguished from the right hepatic. The portal vein is faintly discerned.
(b) Hepatic veins at the level of their entry into the vena cava (portal-CT): the veins seen in the angiogram (a) can be identified in the CT scan. The middle hepatic (M) joins the left hepatic (L) and enters the vena cava from left opposite to the right hepatic. The right branch of the left hepatic (▷) seen on the angiogram (a) comes from the area of the left umbilical portion; in addition, the left and superficial right hepatic veins (▶) are seen in this CT scan.

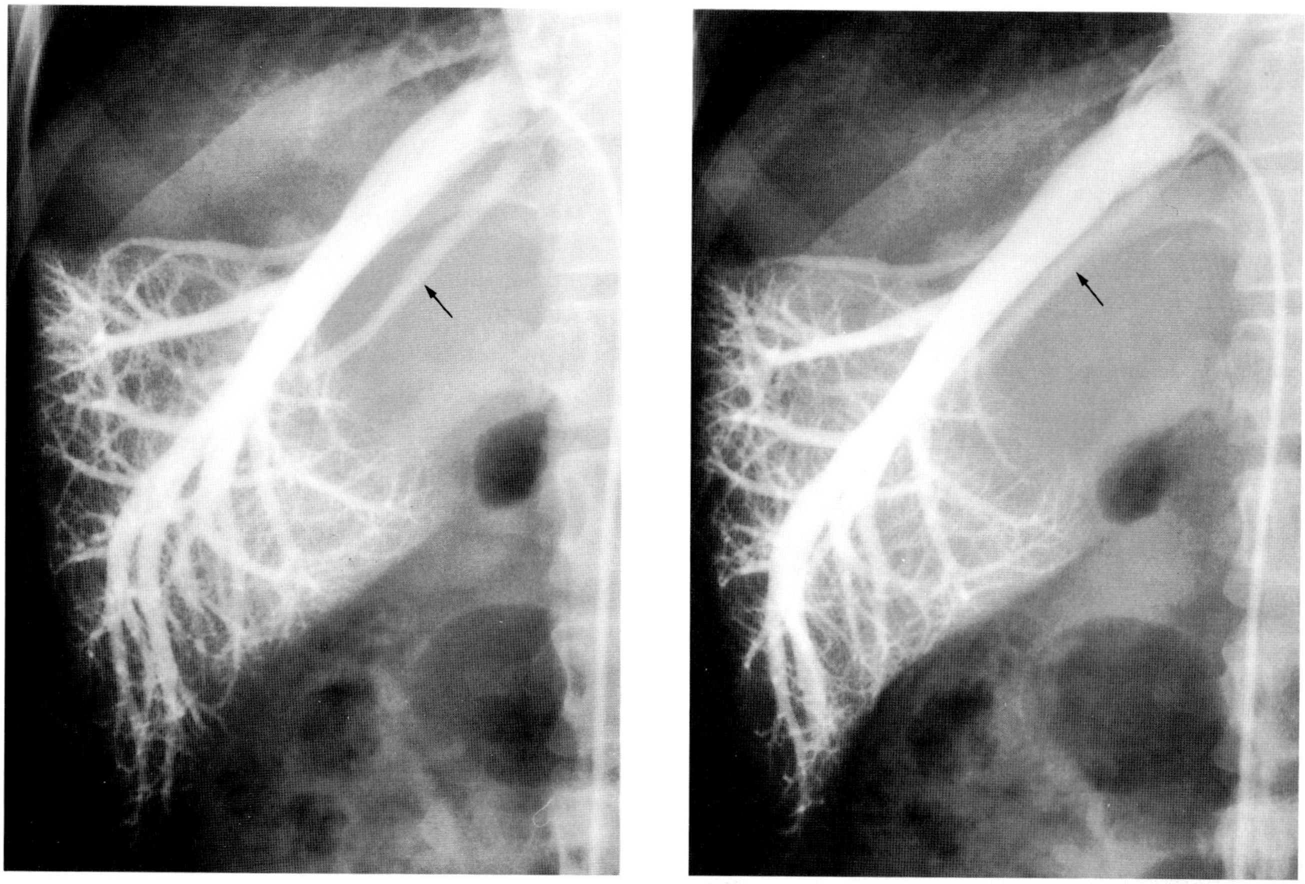

a b

Fig. 1.29 Selective right hepatic venography.
(a) Right anterior oblique view: the right hepatic vein of large caliber and a thin middle hepatic vein (→) are seen. The right hepatic sends out many tributaries in its periphery. The catheter is placed in the right hepatic vein.
(b) Frontal view: this and (a) make up a stereoscopic display.

Lymphatics

The hepatic lymphatics are not visualized by conventional imaging. However, during the procedure for percutaneous transhepatic cholangiography (PTC) (Okuda *et al.* 1974) and percutaneous transhepatic portography (PTP) (Lunderquist, and Vang 1974; Okuda *et al.* 1982*b*), the hepatic lymphatics may be incidentally opacified (Okuda *et al.* 1976*c*). There are three lymphatic routes that drain the liver: (1) parallel to the portal tracts; (2) beneath the liver capsule toward the hilum; and (3) along the hepatic veins toward their openings into the inferior vena cava. The lymphatics of (1) and (2) join the lymph nodes within the abdominal cavity. Understanding the course of hepatic lymphatics is important in the study of lymphatic spread of liver cancer. In patients with cirrhosis, lymph flow is much augmented with visibly dilated lymph vessels in the mesentery.

Fine structure of intraheptic vessel systems

One has to be well versed in the microscopic vascular structure, particularly the relationship between different vascular systems, in order to understand physiologic and pathologic changes affecting the vascular/ductal systems, such as arterioportal communications incidentally found by hepatic arteriography and complications that follow transcatheter arterial embolization (TAE). Figure 1.36 schematically depicts the microscopic biliary system in its relation to vascular supplies. Cho and Lunderquist (1983) described the arteries around the bile duct as the peribiliary arterial plexus, but this seems to encompass the epicholedochal plexus as well as the intramural plexus (Parke *et al.* 1963). Cho and Lunderquist (1983) suggested three possible ways for the formation of arterioportal communications in a diseased liver: (1) transsinusoidal, (2) transvasal, and (3) transplexal. The transsinusoidal route forms to allow arterioportal communication when the hepatic vein is closed or stenosed (cirrhosis, Budd-Chiari) with increased resistance to outflow within the vein, when the portal vein pressure decreases and retrograde portal flow occurs as a result of a large spontaneous portal-systemic shunt, or following porta-caval shunt surgery. Another opinion is that of Bookstein *et al.* (1982) who think that the transvasal route is the most likely explanation for arterioportal shunt that occurs in HCC and hemangioma. The

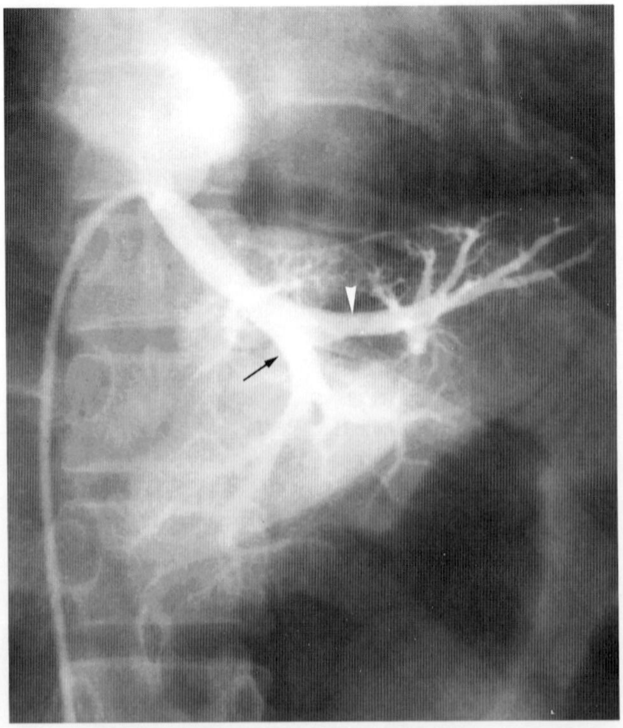

Fig. 1.30 Selective left hepatic venography. The ventral (→) and dorsal branches (▶) are opacified.

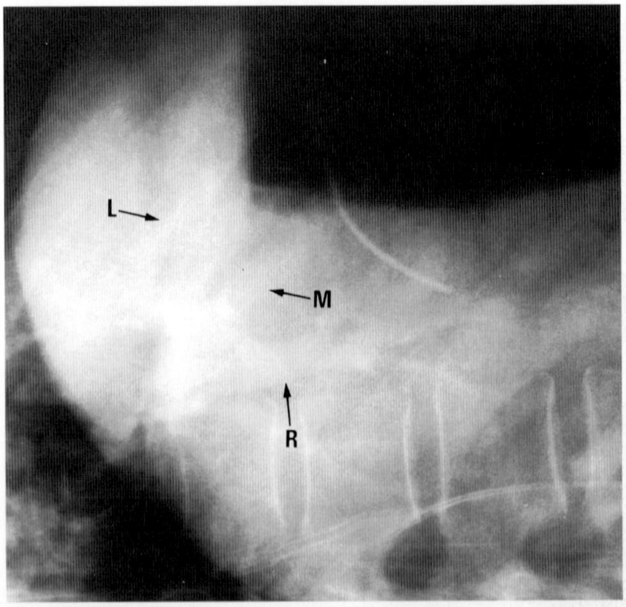

Fig. 1.31 Major hepatic veins in the right lateral view (late phase of PTP). The right hepatic vein (R) runs nearly parallel to the body axis and is the largest. The middle hepatic (M) is located anterior to it and its peripheral branches are in the area of the gallbladder. The left hepatic (L) is further anterior to the other two.

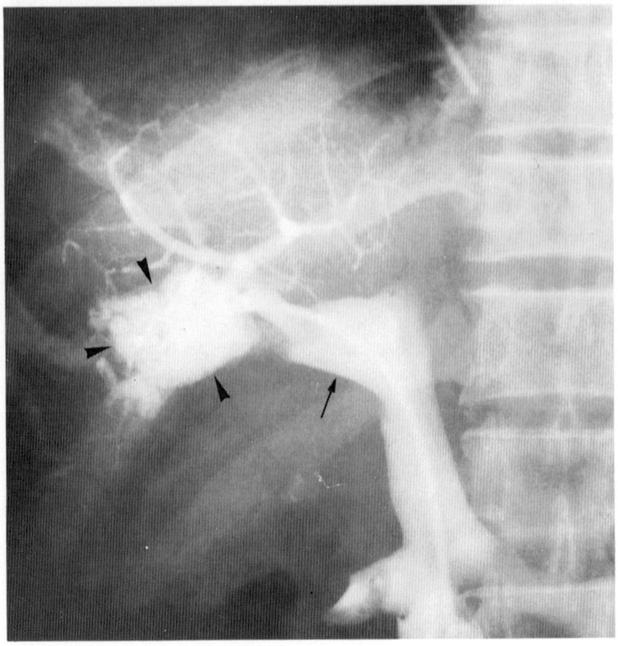

a

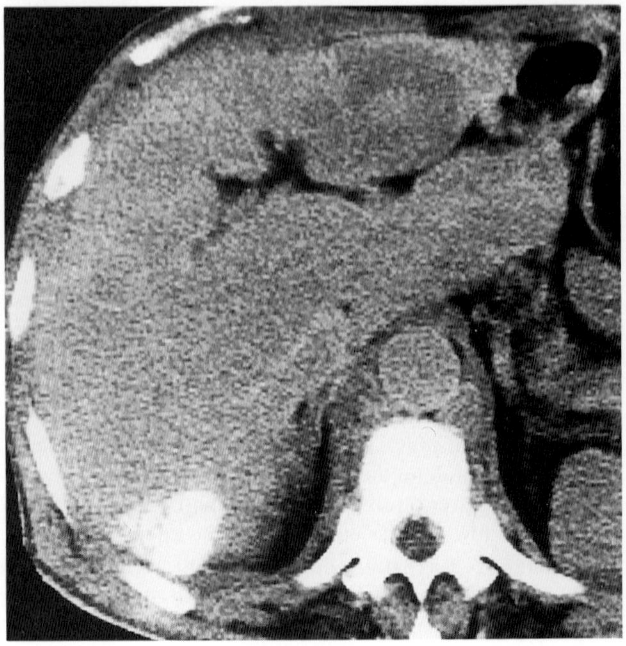

b

Fig. 1.32 The area drained by the inferior right hepatic vein.
(a) Retrograde portal venography: retrograde portal venography was carried out in this patient with Budd–Chiari syndrome (Case 3, p. 395) through an enlarged inferior right hepatic vein (→). The pool of contrast medium (▶) in the parenchyma and the posterior portal vein, particularly the branches of P^{VII}, are delineated clearly.
(b) CT scan: plain CT carried out immediately following retrograde portography. The contrast pooling is in the posterior segment near the liver surface.

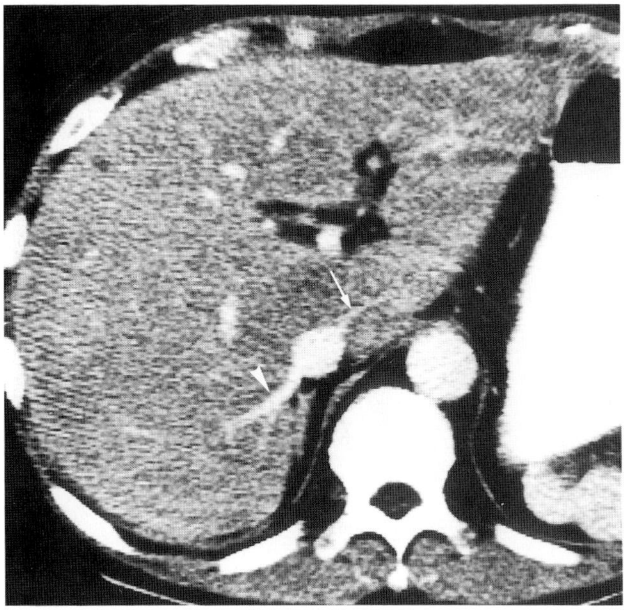

Fig. 1.33 The inferior right hepatic vein and short hepatic veins (caudate lobe veins) seen on CT. In this dynamic CT scan, the short hepatic (→) and the inferior right hepatic veins (▶) are seen flowing into the inferior vena cava.

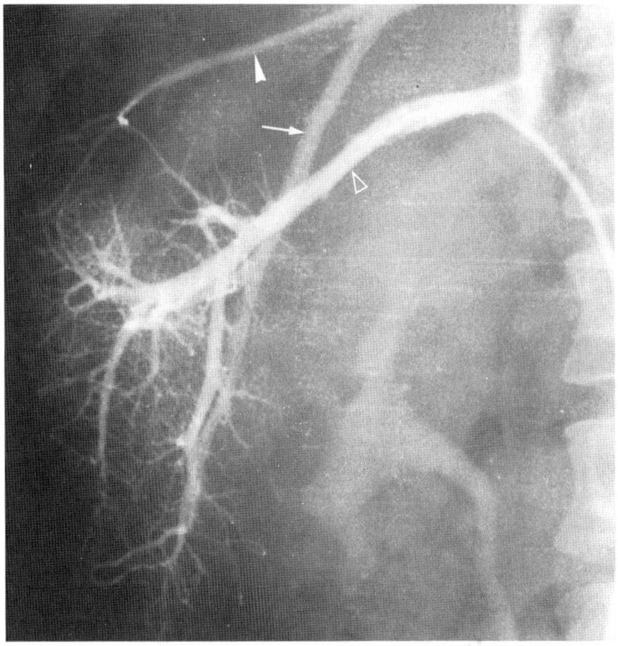

Fig. 1.34 Peripheral anastomoses between hepatic veins. Selective inferior right hepatic venography (▷): the right hepatic vein (→) and its superficial branches (▶) are faintly opacified.

transplexal route was suggested by Cho and Lunderquist (1983) based on their rabbit study. Whereas this route is frequently observed in rabbits, it is not clear whether it applies to human cases. Injection of Lipiodol into the hepatic artery is a recent practice in the management of HCC, and this oil contrast medium is frequently retained in the portal vein system following intraarterial injection, but the exact route through which the contrast oil passes into the portal vein is yet to be determined. It is possible that as small arteries are occluded by Lipiodol, a route other than the transsinusoidal comes to operate.

In HCC, the tumor tissue growing within the portal vein (Okuda *et al.* 1977*a*) and bile duct (Kojiro *et al.* 1982) come to be supplied by the vasa vasorum and peribiliary arterial plexus (Nakashima 1976). Arteriography carried out after TAE frequently delineates thin winding arteries that run along the occluded arteries; they are peribiliary arterial plexuses supplying the biliary tract (Fig. 1.37) as clearly identified in the microangiogram made in a resected specimen (Fig. 1.38). Use of Gelfoam powder and ethanol in TAE frequently causes bile duct necrosis (Makuuchi *et al.* 1985*b*). Intraarterial injection of 5FU and FUDR through a catheter placed in the hepatic artery for a long period causes intrahepatic sclerosing cholangitis (Pien *et al.* 1985; Botet *et al.* 1985). Infarction of the biliary tract as a result of occlusion of the peribiliary arterial plexus is thought to be responsible. Sclerosing cholangitis as a complication of arterial infusion of anticancer agents gives rise to portal vein thrombosis (Takayasu *et al.* 1990*d*), and it is a likely consequence of pylephlebitis due to cytotoxic agents that flow into the portal vein system through the peribiliary arterial plexus and vasa vasorum. When the extrahepatic hepatic artery is occluded, arterial collaterals form through the epicholedochal arterial plexus (Fig. 1.39) similar to the cavernous transformation that develops following occlusion of the extrahepatic portal vein (Parker and Seal 1955). Following embolization of intrahepatic portal veins and subsequent recanalization of these veins, one or two thin portal branches develop along the once occluded portal veins (Fig. 1.40). It is likely that these collateral routes have developed through the peribiliary venous plexus, turning into neovasculature. The same finding is frequently seen in idiopathic portal hypertension (Futagawa *et al.* 1980). A similar phenomenon in which cavernous transformation develops following thrombosis and tumor invasion (Ohnishi *et al.* 1984*b*) in the extrahepatic portal vein is also thought to be through the peribiliary venous plexus. It explains why cavernous transformation occurs in closer association with the biliary tract than with the portal vein.

Spatial relationship between the intrahepatic portal veins, bile ducts, and arteries

The spatial relationship between the three vessel systems may be described as 'thin arteries and bile ducts creeping on a thick portal vein as ivy does on trees'. The common bile duct, right hepatic artery, and portal trunk are situated from anterior toward posterior at the porta hepatis (Fig. 1.41), with the proper hepatic artery running slightly dorsal and medial to the bile duct (Fig. 1.42). However, the lower common bile duct runs dorsal to the portal trunk (Fig. 1.43). In the right lobe, the

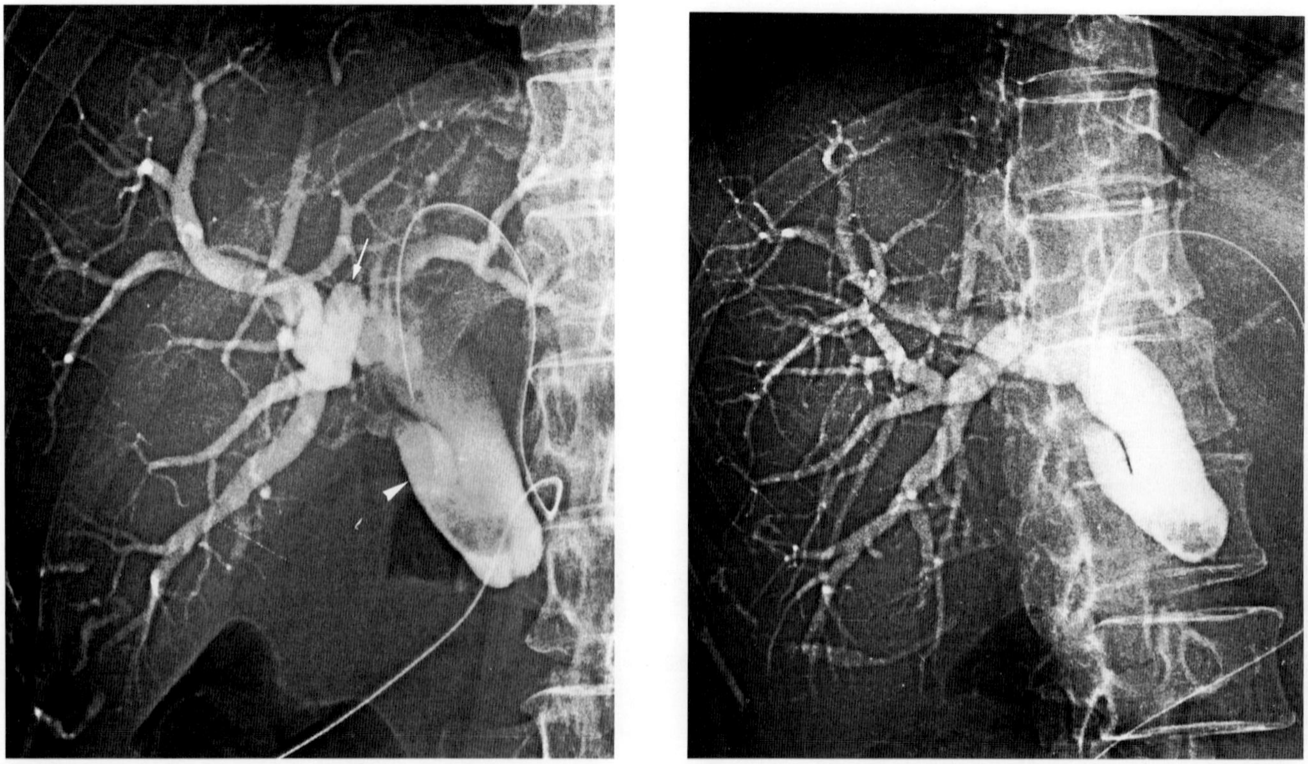

a b

Fig. 1.35

(a) Frontal view of the biliary tree opacified through the catheter in a patient with common bile duct occlusion: the bile duct draining the right posterior area runs in the anterior posterior direction over the right anterior portal vein and is seen protruding cephalad (→). The P-point seen on the portogram does not usually exist in the cholangiogram. (▶), cystic duct.

(b) Right anterior oblique projection of (a): the distribution of intrahepatic bile ducts is very similar to that of portal vein branches except for the pattern of division at the beginning of the bile ducts draining the posterior area.

posterior segment bile duct runs cephalad to the portal vein and turns downward to course laterally to the posterior portal vein (Figs. 1.44, 45). In the anterior segment, the bile duct runs medial to the portal vein (Fig. 1.44) in most cases, which is why one can easily puncture the portal vein during the PTP procedure. The right hepatic artery runs between the common hepatic duct and the bifurcation of the portal vein (Fig. 1.42) ; this explains why hilar bile duct carcinoma invades the artery first and then the portal vein, seen as an encasement on angiography.

In the left lobe, the left hepatic duct runs slightly cephalad to the transverse portion of the portal vein, sends off its left medial branch, and passes cephalad to the umbilical portion, then between the lateral portal veins P^{II} and P^{III} along them (Fig. 1.45).

If the left lobe is supplied solely by the left hepatic artery, this artery runs to the left of the umbilical portion of the portal vein, and if the middle hepatic artery is present in this lobe, the umbilical portion is sandwiched between the two arteries (Fig. 1.46). In the right lobe, if there is only the posterior segment artery, it usually turns around to the right, lateral to the portal vein at a point proximal to the P-point as does the bile duct. If the posterior segment artery is divided into the posterior superior subsegment branch (A^{VII}) and posterior inferior subsegment branch (A^{VI}), A^{VII} may leave proximal to the point where the anterior and posterior segment arteries divide; it may be mistaken for the caudate branch.

The intrahepatic artery system and biliary tree do not have a portion that runs vertical to the frontal plane like the P- and U-points in the portal vein system, and identification of branches is more difficult than in the portal system, but it can be improved if the portal vein system is used as a reference. For identification of the caudate lobe arteries, one should compare the portogram and arterial-CT as well as superselective caudate arteriography. Normally, the portal tract has one each of the - portal vein, artery, and bile duct, but occasionally it may contain two arteries (Fig. 1.47).

Differences in the spatial relation of intrahepatic vasculature between cast study and imaging

Prior to modern imaging, knowledge of the hepatic vasculature was derived from case studies of cadaveric liver. An injection corrosion cast of an excised liver on a flat surface does not give a true representation of the hepatic vasculature in a living body. One typical example is the portal vein in the right lobe. The right anterior portal vein may be mistaken for the posterior portal vein and the posterior portal vein for the anterior (Fig. 1.48).

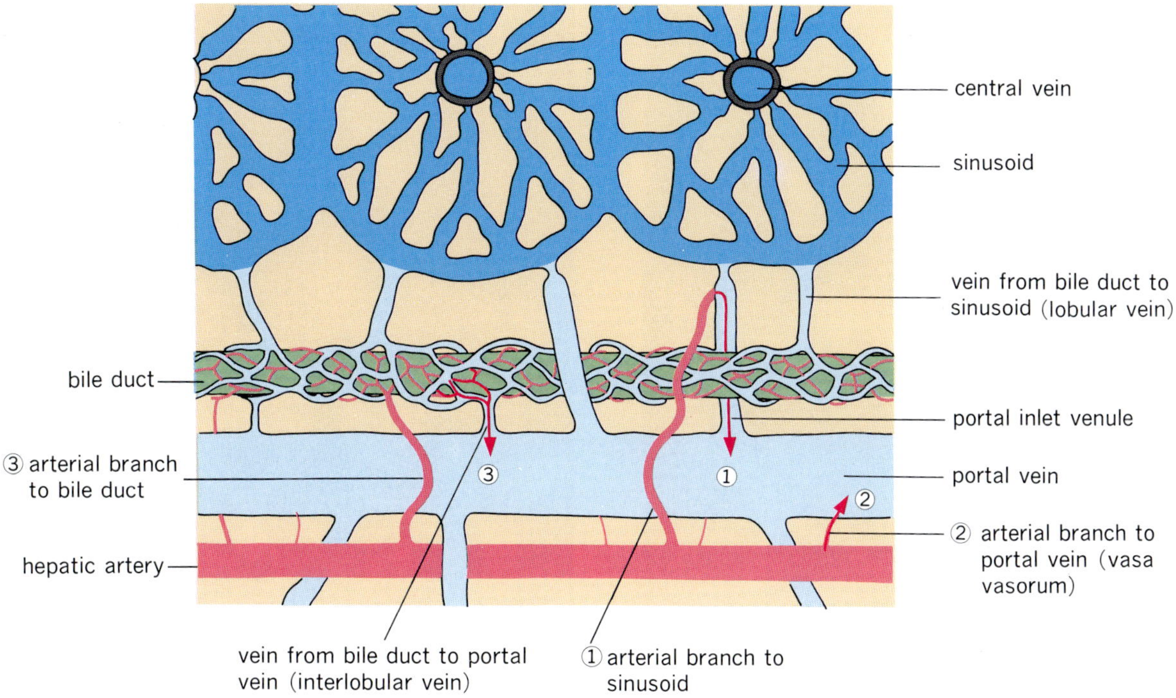

Fig. 1.36 Arterial and venous plexuses associated with the bile duct and the three routes that will contribute to the development of arterio-portal communications. Intrahepatic arteries are distributed to the (a) sinusoid, (b) portal vein, and (c) bile duct, and bile duct veins drain into the portal vein via the interlobular vein and into the sinusoid via the lobular vein. Arterial blood enters the portal vein (1) through the sinusoid (transsinusoidal), (2) through the vasa vasorum that nourishes the portal vein (transvasal), and (3) through the peribiliary venous plexus and interlobular vein (transplexal): these three routes are thought to contribute to the formation of arterio-portal shunts.
[From Cho and Lunderquist (1983), with modification.]

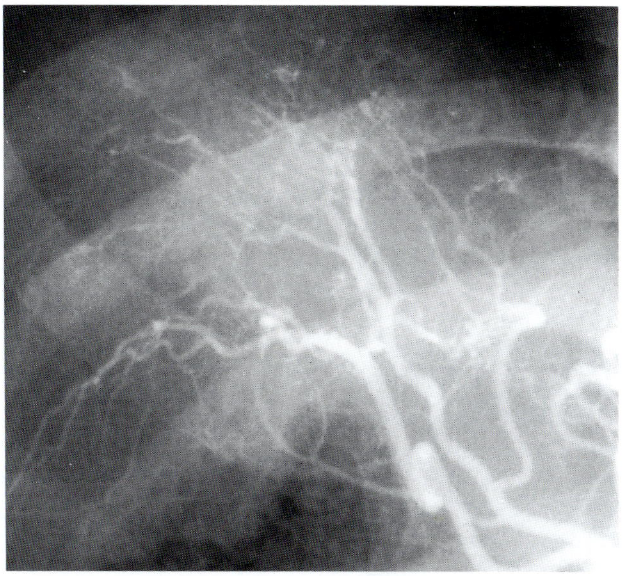

Fig 1.37 Reopening of the hepatic artery following transcatheter arterial embolization (TAE). The arteries supplying the right lobe, particularly A^{VIII}, show interruptions and irregularities due to TAE carried out earlier. Reopening perhaps occurred through the peribiliary arterial plexus (Case 5, p. 490).

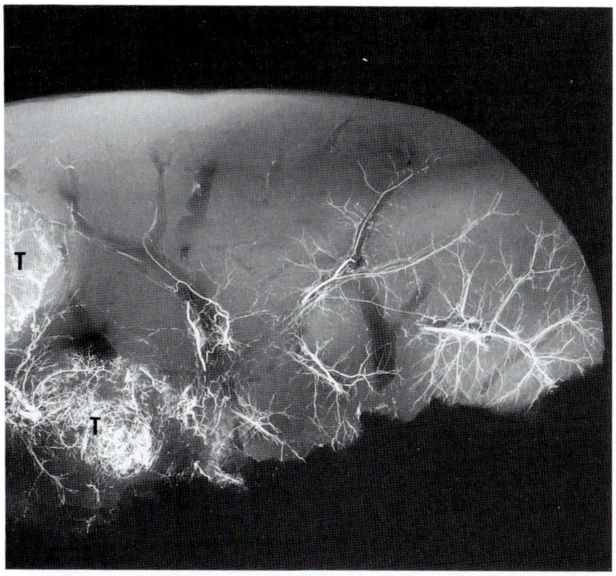

Fig. 1.38 The peribiliary arterial plexuses seen in the microangiogram of a resected liver specimen. In this microangiogram of liver parenchyma (non-tumor liver), one or two thin peribiliary arterial plexuses are seen running along the normal arteries. T, tumor.

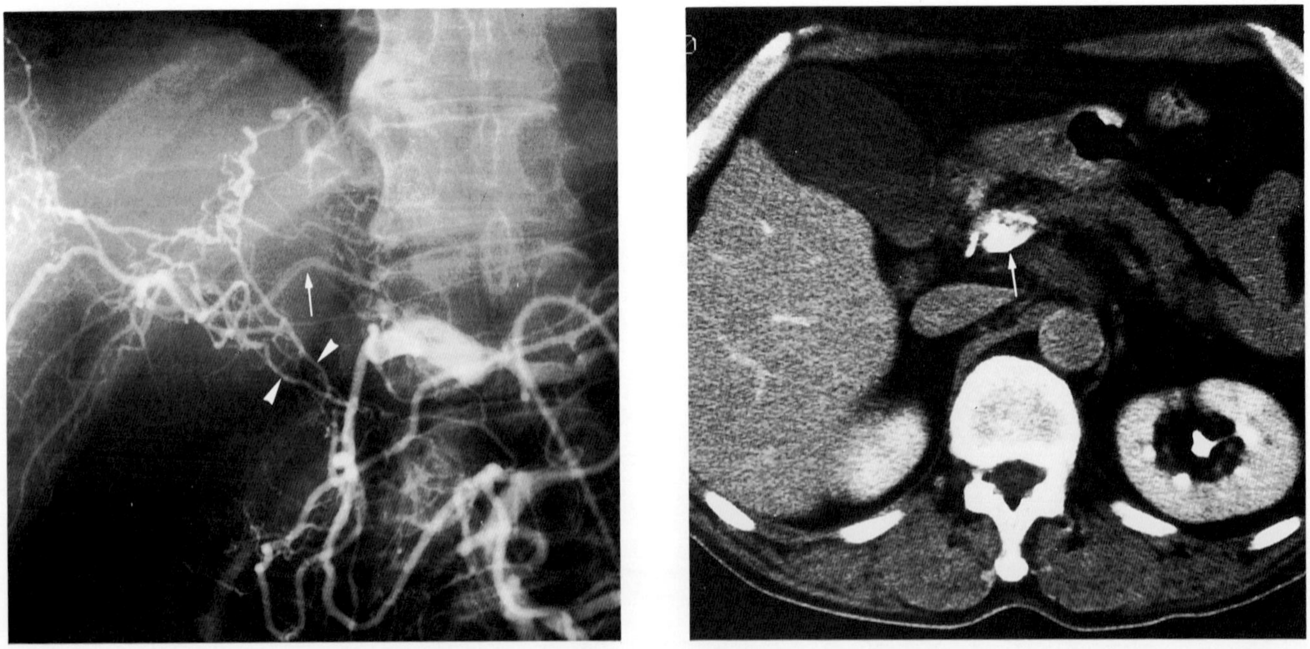

a b

Fig. 1.39 Subintimal injury of the common hepatic artery and enlargement of the epicholedochal or peribiliary arterial plexus.
(a) Superior mesenteric arteriography: the common hepatic artery was occluded as a technical complication of catheterization, and the epicholedochal arterial plexus (▶) has been enlarged providing communications between the gastroduodenal artery and intrahepatic arteries. →, partially opacified proper hepatic artery.
(b) Arterial-CT: with the catheter at the same position as in (a) an arterial-CT scan was made. Superior mesenteric arteriographic portogram in the area of the head of the pancreas, and a number of small arteries (epicholedochal arterial plexuses) are seen anterior and lateral to the portal vein (→).

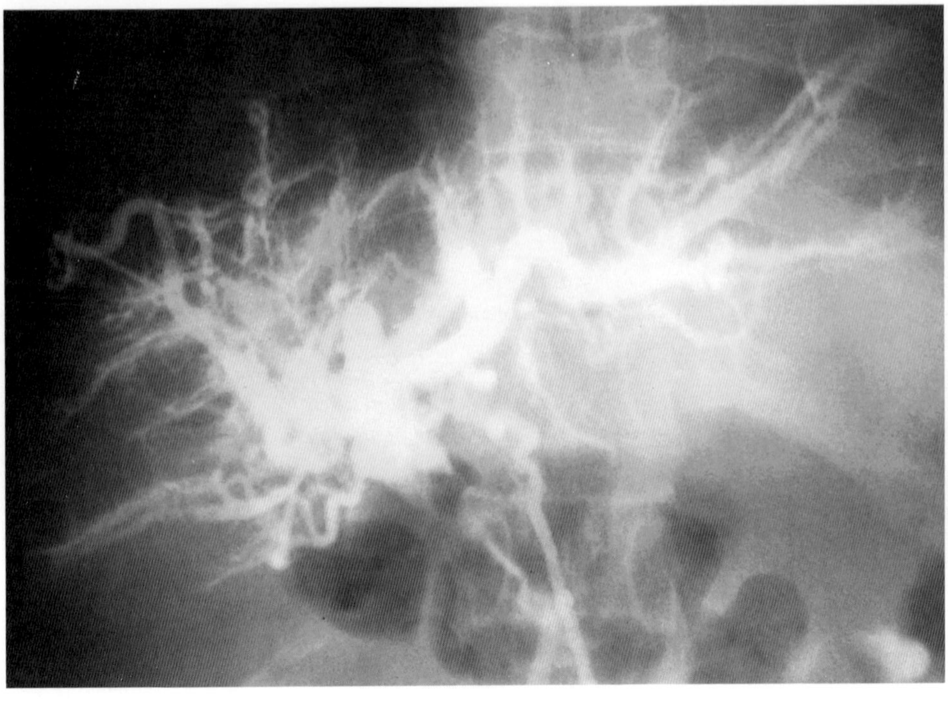

Fig. 1.40 Reopening of an intrahepatic portal vein thrombosis through the peribiliary venous plexuses. PTP: PTP was carried out on a patient who had had hematemesis after splenectomy. The left umbilical portion, P^{II}, and P^{III} are barely identifiable. Thin vessels accompanying the intrahepatic portal veins seem to have developed from the peribiliary venous plexuses; it is suggested that they were thrombosed and reopened through the peribiliary venous plexuses.

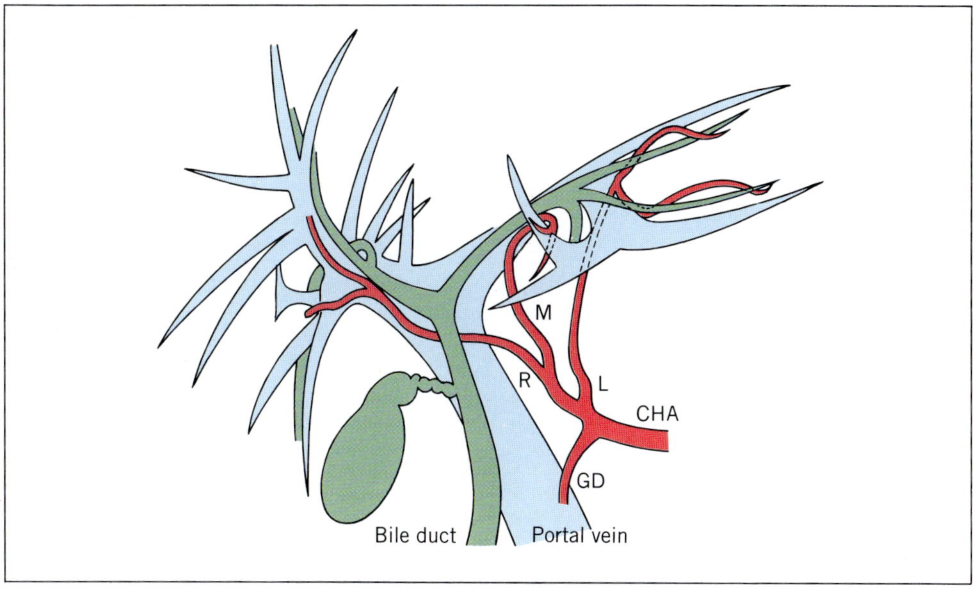

Fig. 1.41 Spatial relationship between intrahepatic portal veins, bile ducts, and arteries. The umbilical portion of the left portal vein is depicted in a slanted position for ease of understanding. R, M, L, right, middle, left hepatic arteries; GD, gastroduodenal artery; CHA, common hepatic artery.

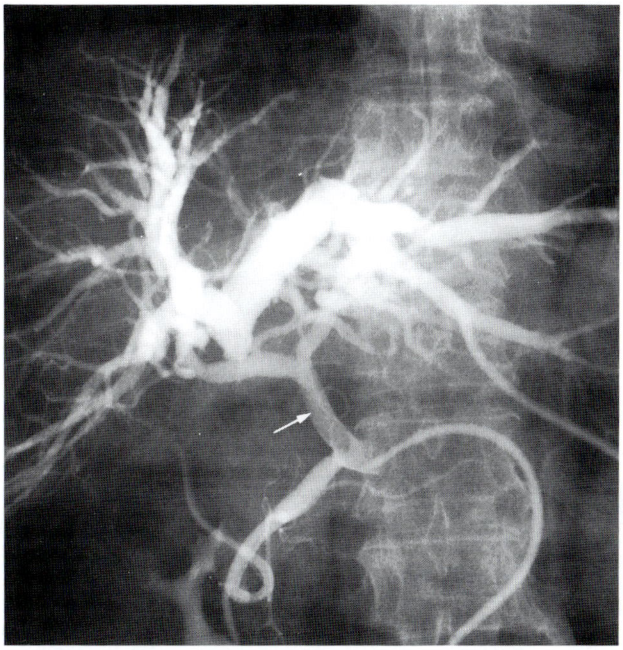

Fig. 1.42 Spatial relationship between the biliary tract and hepatic arteries. Cholangiogram made through percutaneous transhepatic cholangio drainage (PTCD): cholangiography was done through the catheter prior to hepatic arteriography. The proper hepatic artery (→) runs left to the common bile duct (not opacified), and the right hepatic artery posterior to the occluded common bile duct crossing it.

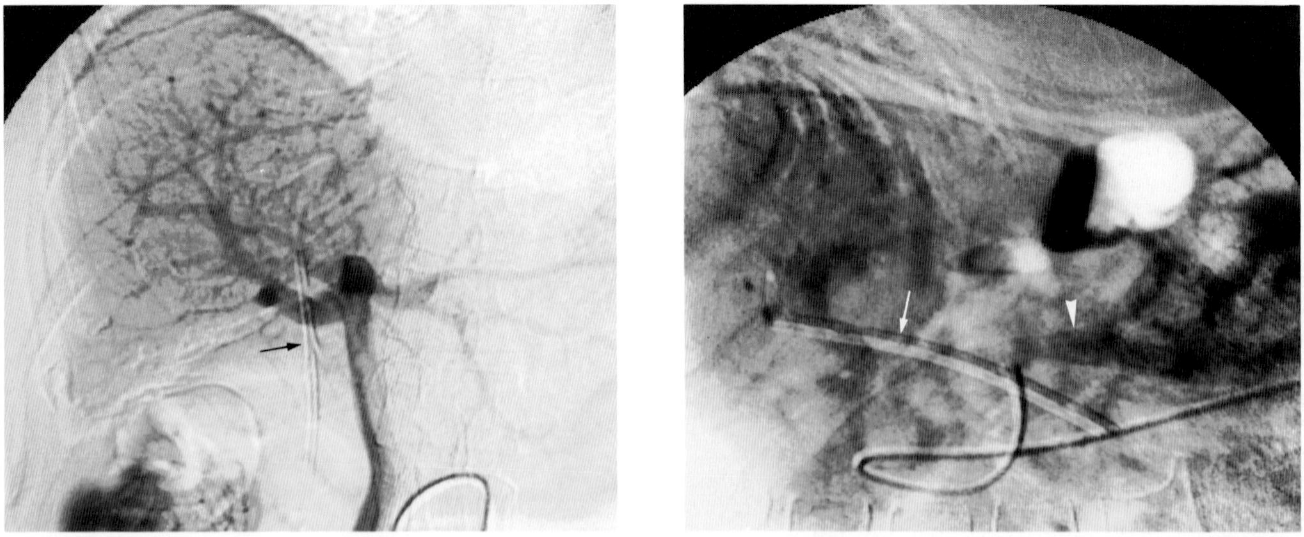

a b

Fig. 1.43 Spatial relationship between the extrahepatic bile duct and portal vein (superior mesenteric arterial portogram and stent).
(a) Frontal view: the common bile duct (stent, →) runs to the right of the portal vein trunk.
(b) Right lateral view: the common bile duct (stent, →) slowly deviates posterior to the portal trunk (▶) in order to open into the duodenum.

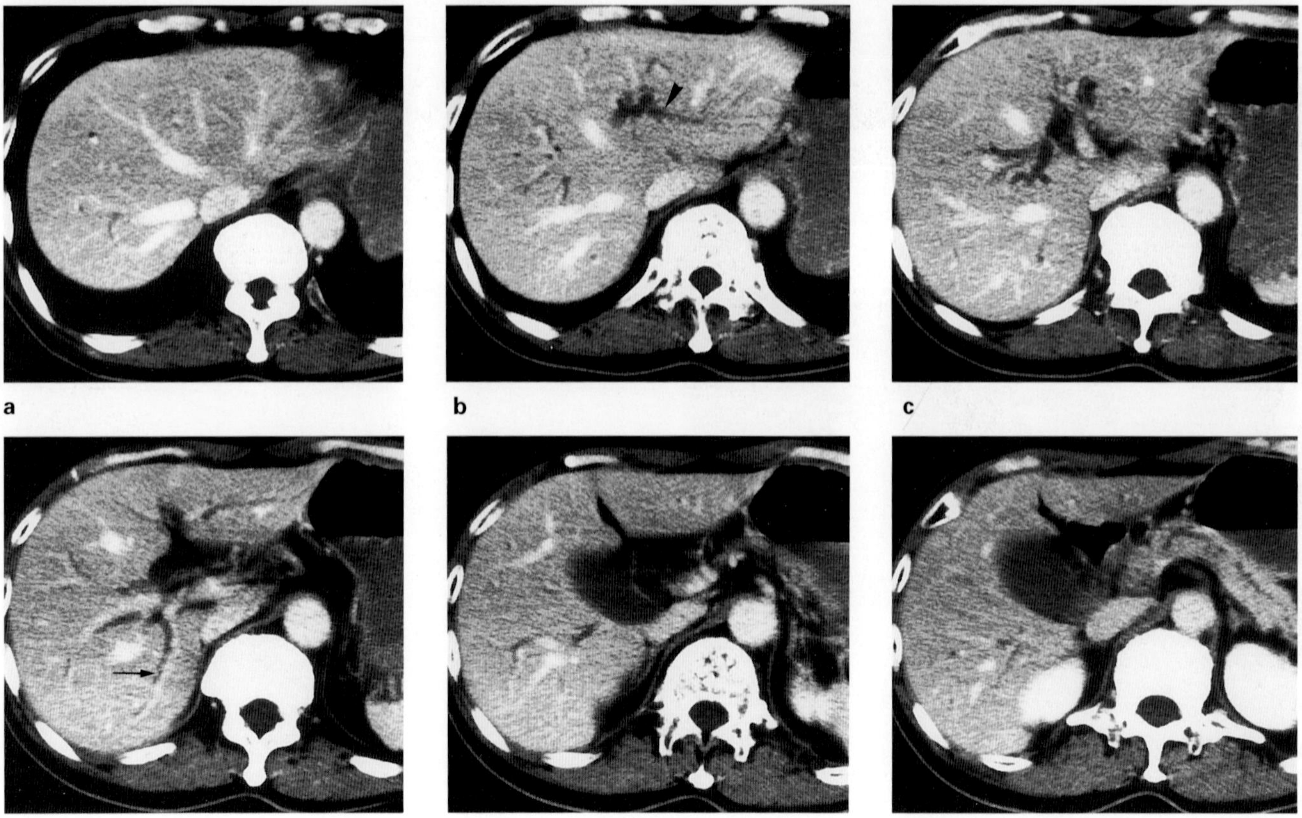

a b c d e f

Fig. 1.44 Spatial relationship between the biliary tract and portal vein (dynamic CT). Dynamic CT with shifting the level of section in a patient with intrahepatic bile duct dilatation: the bile duct (→) runs lateral to the portal vein in the posterior area (d) of the right lobe, and in the anterior area (b) it courses medial to the portal vein. Since the lateral branch of the left hepatic duct (▶) is seen in the section (b) 1 cm cranial to the umbilical portion of the portal vein (c), it can be assumed that this bile duct turns around cranial to the umbilical portion and runs between P^{II} and P^{III}.

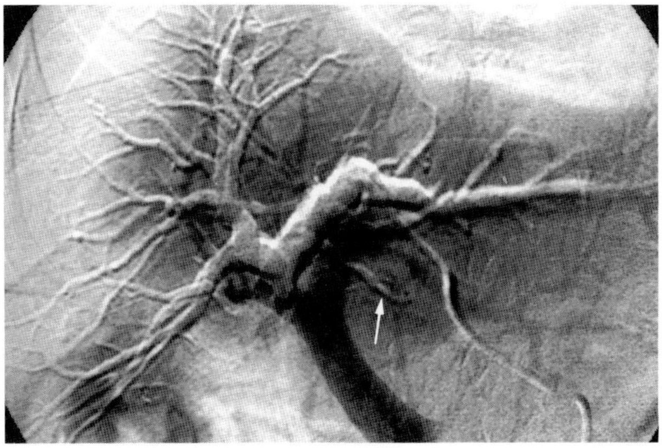

Fig. 1.45 Spatial relationship between the biliary tract and portal vein. Cholangiogram (white tree) made through the PTCD catheter and simultaneous arterial portogram (black tree): a spatial relationship similar to that shown in Fig. 1.44 is recognized in the antero-posterior view. Bile duct B^{III} which should accompany P^{III} is not visualized due to insufficient contrast medium. $B^{I}_{l\text{-med}}$ (→), the bile duct draining the left part of the caudate lobe and $P^{I}_{l\text{-med}}$ supplying the same area can be seen. $B^{I}_{l\text{-med}}$ reaches the left caudate lobe along the posterior aspect of the transverse portion of the left portal vein.

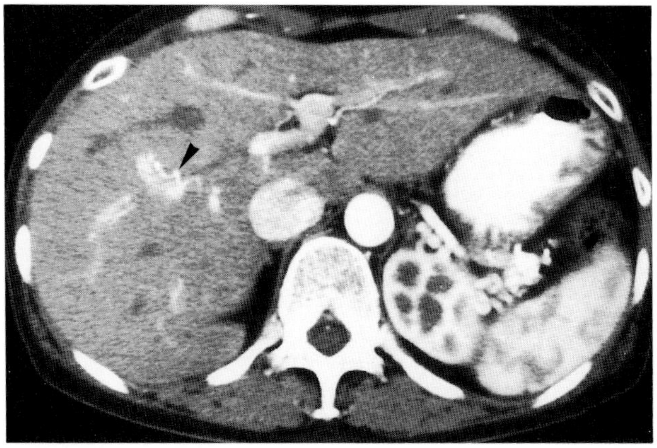

Fig. 1.46 The portal vein and hepatic artery. Early phase dynamic CT: thin caliber arteries of high density and the portal vein system of a lower density are seen. The left and middle hepatic arteries run on both sides of the umbilical portion of the left portal vein. An artery closely and medially accompanying the right anterior vein is seen (▶).

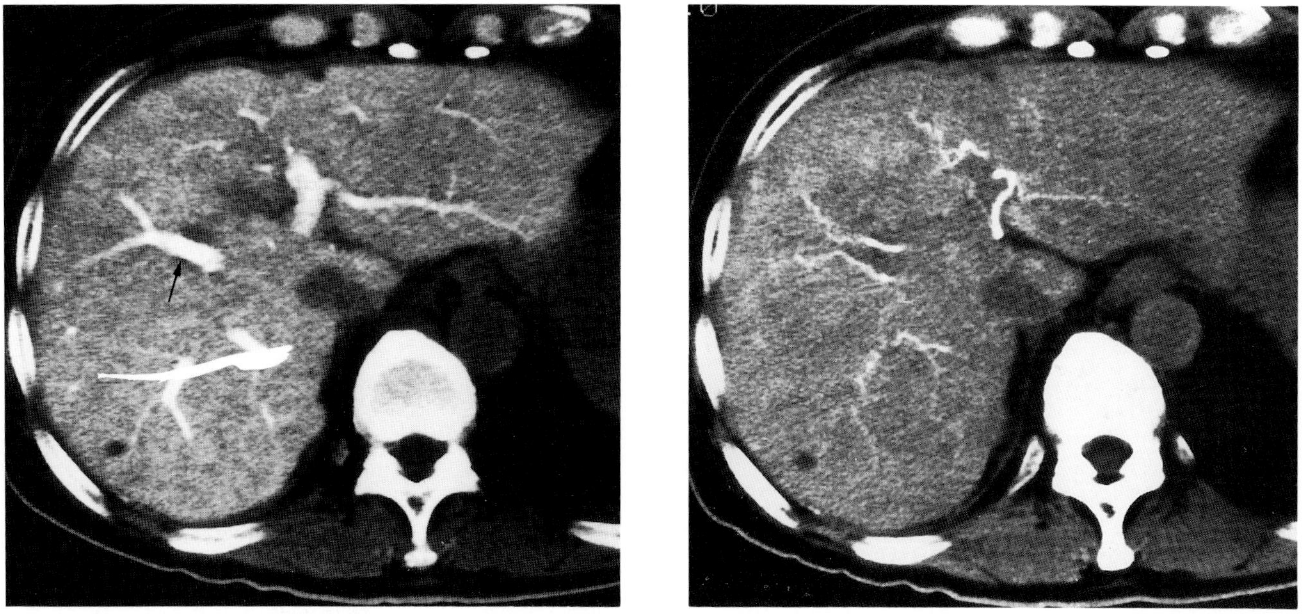

a b

Fig. 1.47 The portal vein and hepatic artery.
(a) Portal-CT (CTAP): the arrow (→) points at the portal vein supplying the right anterior segment.
(b) Arterial-CT (CTA): the arteries that correspond to the portal vein in (a) shown by → run anterior and posterior to it, sandwiching it.

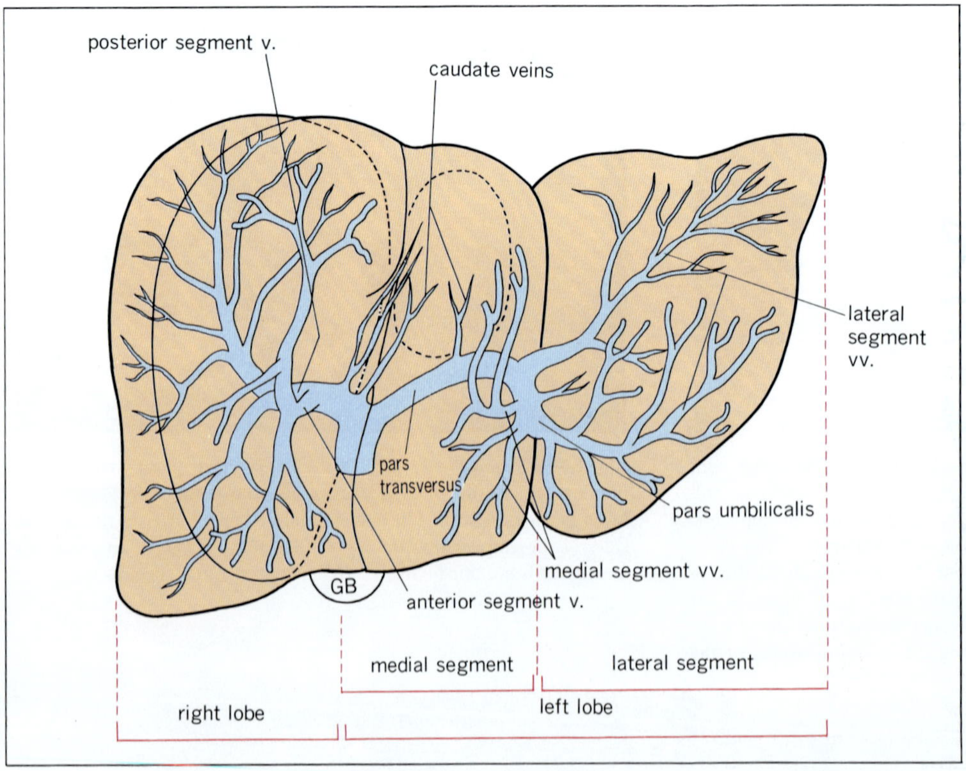

Fig. 1.48 The courses of intrahepatic portal veins based on an injection corrosion cast. This schema itself is not erroneous, but if a portogram made in a living person is interpreted from this schema, the relationship between the anterior segment portal vein and posterior segment portal vein in the right lobe is reversed. In this schema depicted by Healey (1954) and modified by the authors, the umbilical portion of the left portal vein is slanted anteriorly, which seldom occurs in a living person.

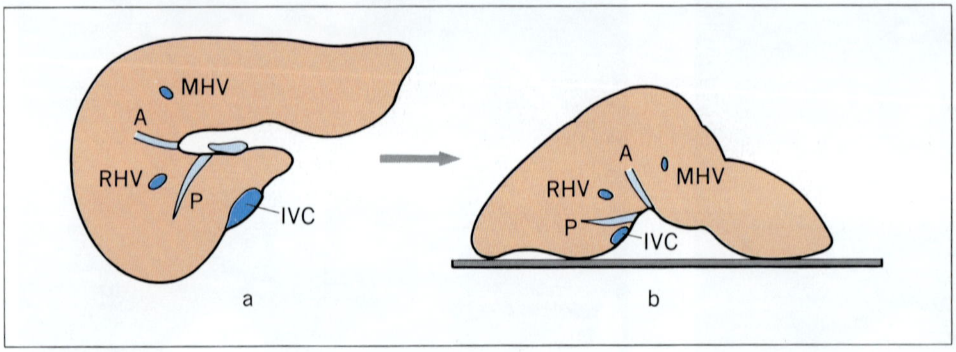

Fig. 1.49 Differences between the liver in a living person and a corrosion cast in the course of intrahepatic vessels. In a liver removed (b) from the body and placed on a plane, the posterior segment extends laterally to the right and comes to be located lateral to the anterior segment compared with the liver in a living body (a). The inferior portion of the left lobe falls down (slanting caudally) with a removed liver.

The liver in a living body is covered by a cylinder-shaped torso and hence is hemispherical (Fig. 1.49a). Out of the body and during preparation of an injection corrosion cast, the liver is expanded sideways and the hemisphere becomes flatter, displacing the posterior portal vein laterally to the right of the anterior portal vein (Fig. 1.49b). The specimen is placed on a flat surface causing the liver to be slanted anteriorly, as if bowing. The vertically positioned umbilical portion of the left portal vein comes to be slanted anteriorly, and the anterior portal vein, which is normally higher along the vertical axis than the posterior portal vein (Fig. 1.20), becomes about the same in level (Fig. 1.48).

Similar differences are noted in the depiction of the hepatic vein system between the cast and the liver in the body (Fig. 1.50). In the frontal view, the right and middle hepatic veins are nearly superimposed (Fig. 1.28, 29) whereas a schema depicted from a cast shows these two vessels wide apart with the middle hepatic displaced further to the left, caused by the lateral displacement of the right posterior segment in the excised liver during cast preparation. More recently, efforts have been made to minimize such a drawback in the cast study by maintaining the natural position of the liver during the preparation. Such efforts will certainly improve our understanding of the spatial relationship between the three intrahepatic vessel systems. As there is a certain restriction in the use of whole liver at the sacrifice of tissue, we are using steel wire to reproduce the three-dimensional positions of these vessel as an aid to imaging diagnosis (Fig. 1.51).

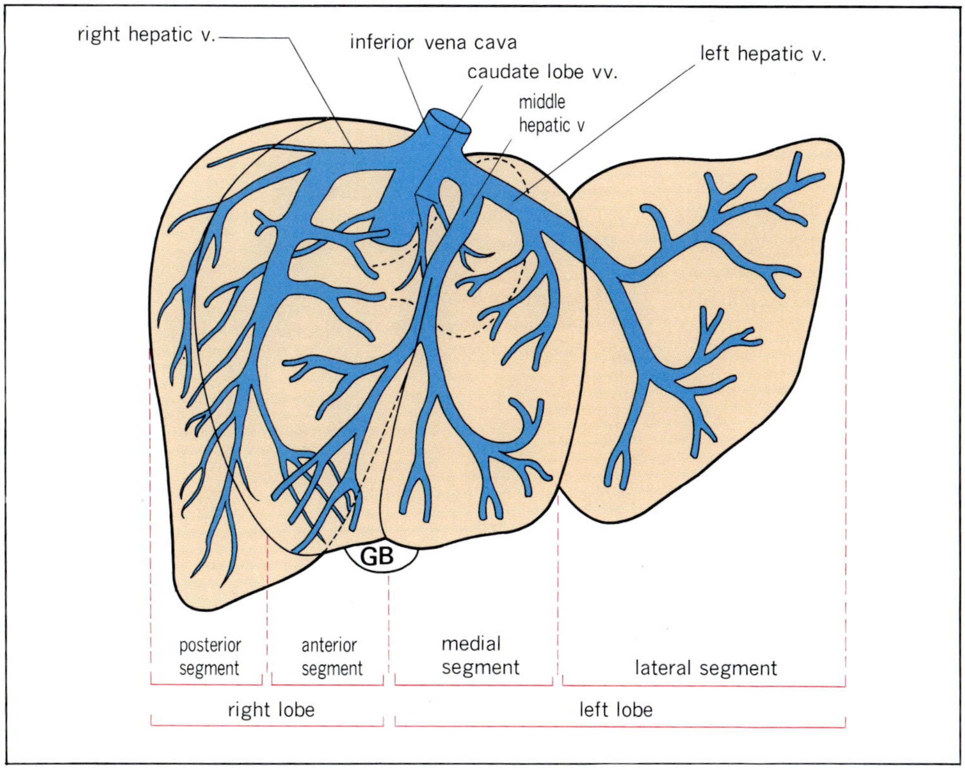

Fig. 1.50 The courses of hepatic veins based on a cast. As the posterior segment of the right lobe is rotated laterally, the frontal view is that of a right anterior oblique projection of the liver in a living body. (Scheme of Healey (1954), modified by the authors.)

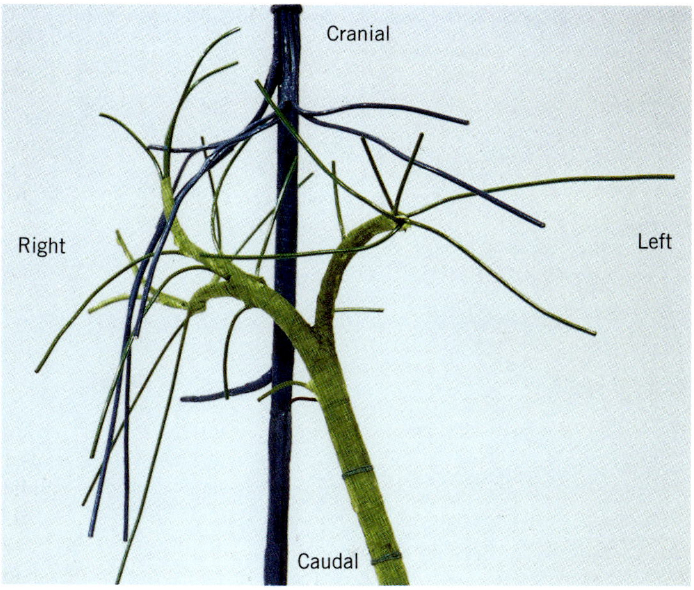

a (a) Anterior view

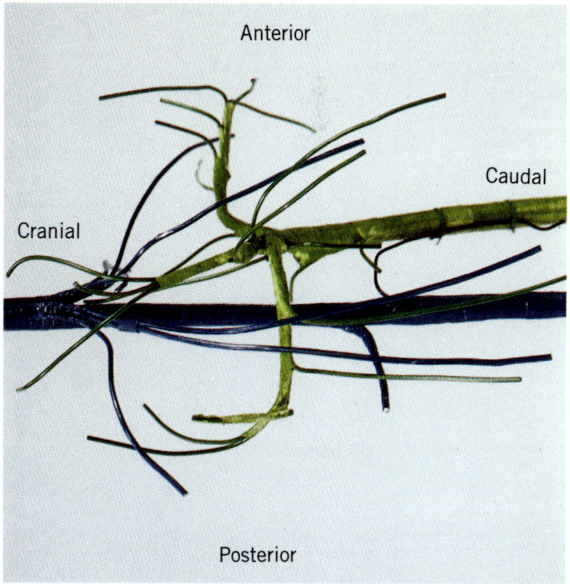

b (b) Right lateral view

Fig. 1.51 A model of hepatic vasculature made of wire:
(a) Frontal view, (b) right lateral view. This is very useful in the understanding of the spatial relationship between the portal vein and hepatic vein systems, and between the hepatic veins and the inferior vena cava. Portal vein, light green; hepatic vein, blue; inferior vena cava, the thick blue vessel.

1.3 Liver segments

Chronologic changes in the concept of liver segments

Segmental division of the liver is a three-dimensional concept of the parenchymal parts of the liver based on vasculature. In the past, spatial understanding of hepatic vasculature was not possible without the aid of a cast model made from the liver removed at autopsy. With the progress made in imaging techniques, it has become possible to grasp the three-dimensional structure of the liver non-invasively. To understand the hepatic segments one needs to grasp the course of hepatic vasculature, particularly the portal and hepatic veins, in individual cases. The merits of understanding the hepatic segments are itemized in Table 1.1. It is important for the diagnostician and the surgeon to be able to determine the location of an intrahepatic lesion.

Historically, an early attempt at segmentation was made by Cantlie in 1898 who functionally divided the liver into the left and right lobes along the line that connects the gallbladder fossa and the inferior vena cava at its emergence from the liver surface (Cantlie line). Prior to this, the liver was anatomically divided into the left and right lobes using an obvious marker, the falciform ligament, as the dividing line. Cantlie's segments were based on vasculature, and his concept left a strong impact on subsequent studies for hepatic surgery.

In the late 1940s, injection corrosion cast study using a cadaveric liver became popular, and the first segmentation scheme based on the portal veins was proposed by Hjortsjö in Sweden in 1951 (Fig. 1.52). It was followed in 1953 by another proposal from the USA by Healey and Schroy (1953) (Fig. 1.53), and by Couinaud in France (Couinaud 1954) (Fig. 1.54). Healey and Schroy divided the left and right lobes into two areas each, which they further divided into two parts, cranial and caudal. They divided the caudate lobe into a left part, right part, and caudate process. Thus, there were 11 areas in their segmentation scheme. If the two areas divided in the left medial

Table 1.1 Concept of liver segments and its significance

1. For diagnosis

(a) Systematic diagnosis based on vasculature, particularly the portal vein system, reduces the chance of overlooking pathologic lesions.

(b) If multiple lesions found by several different imaging modalities were compared, determined for the exact location, and numbered, the diagnosis would become more definitive.

(c) In the follow-up of detected lesions, if they were numbered, they would be more accurately evaluated.

2. For surgery

(a) Understanding of the spatial relation of a lesion to the vascular system enables the surgeon to decide on the most appropriate operation method.

(b) Recognition of the lesion and its relation to the vascular system by intraoperative US improves the results of resection.

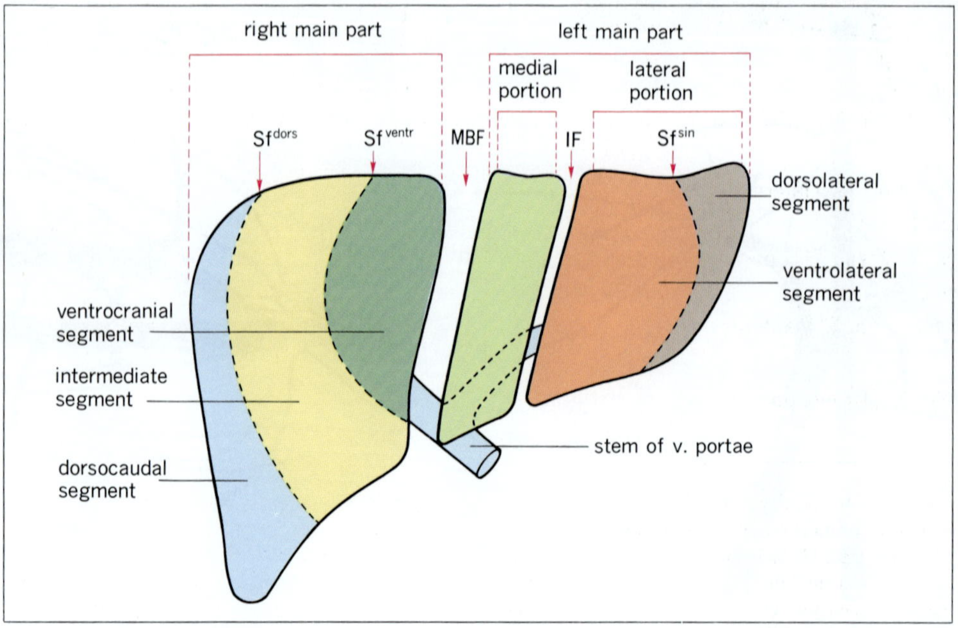

Fig. 1.52 Segments proposed by Hjortsjö (1951). Six segments are separated based on stereoscopic cholangiograms ($n = 12$). He called the Cantlie line the 'main boundary fissure' (MBF) and the boundary between the lateral and medial portions 'incidental fissure' (IF). This separation scheme is the same as the current one. The lateral portion of the left lobe is divided vertically into the left and right subportions by a line which he termed 'segment fissure sinistra (Sf^{sin}); it is divided horizontally in the current scheme. The right lobe is divided into three segments by two segment fissures (Sf^{dors}, Sf^{ventr}). His ventrocranial segment roughly corresponds to Couinaud's S^{V}, the ventrocranial and intermediate segments combined correspond to the current anterior segment, and the dorsocaudal segment to the current posterior segment. Thus, Hjortsjö's segmentation is similar to the current scheme. The caudate lobe is not shown in this schema.

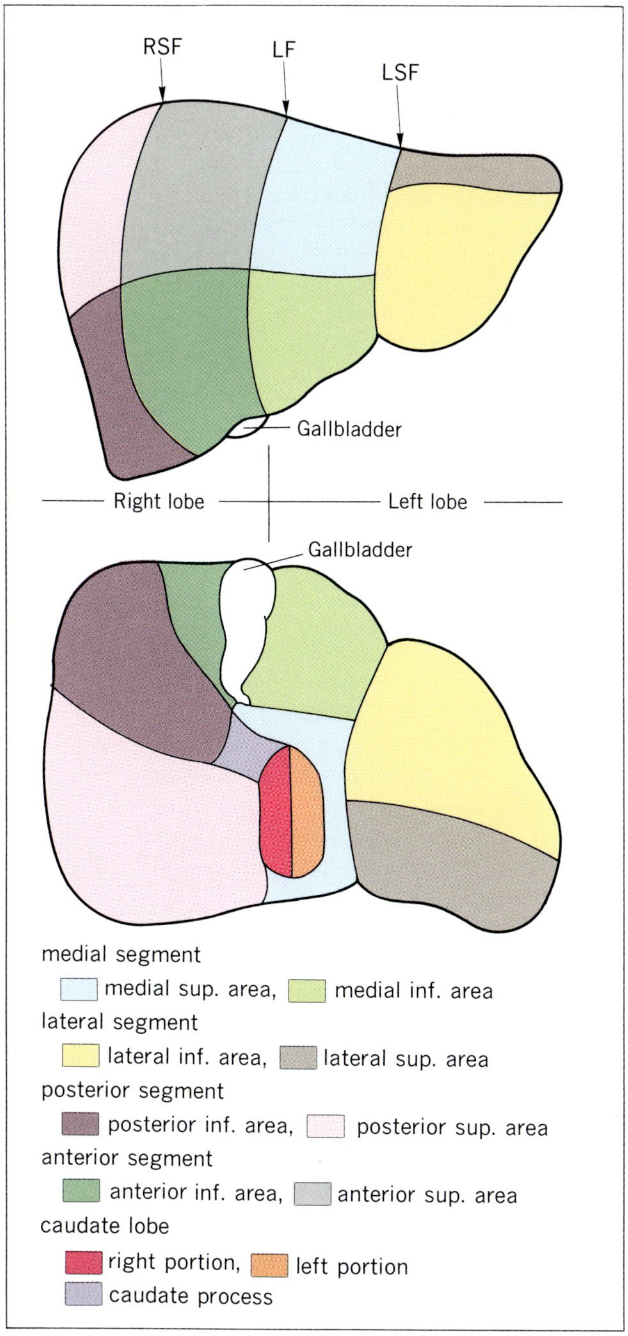

Fig. 1.53 Segments proposed by Healey (1953). Healey divided the liver into 11 segments based on injection corrosion models made with the hepatic artery and biliary tree. His scheme was commonly used in the USA until recently. The Cantlie line corresponds to the lobar fissure (LF), the boundary between the left medial and left lateral segments is the left segmental fissure (LSF), and the boundary between the right anterior and right posterior segments is the right segmental fissure (RSF). The caudate lobe is divided into three portions. It is continuous with the right lobe through the caudate process, but no mention is made of the vessel that assists in the segmentation of this lobe.

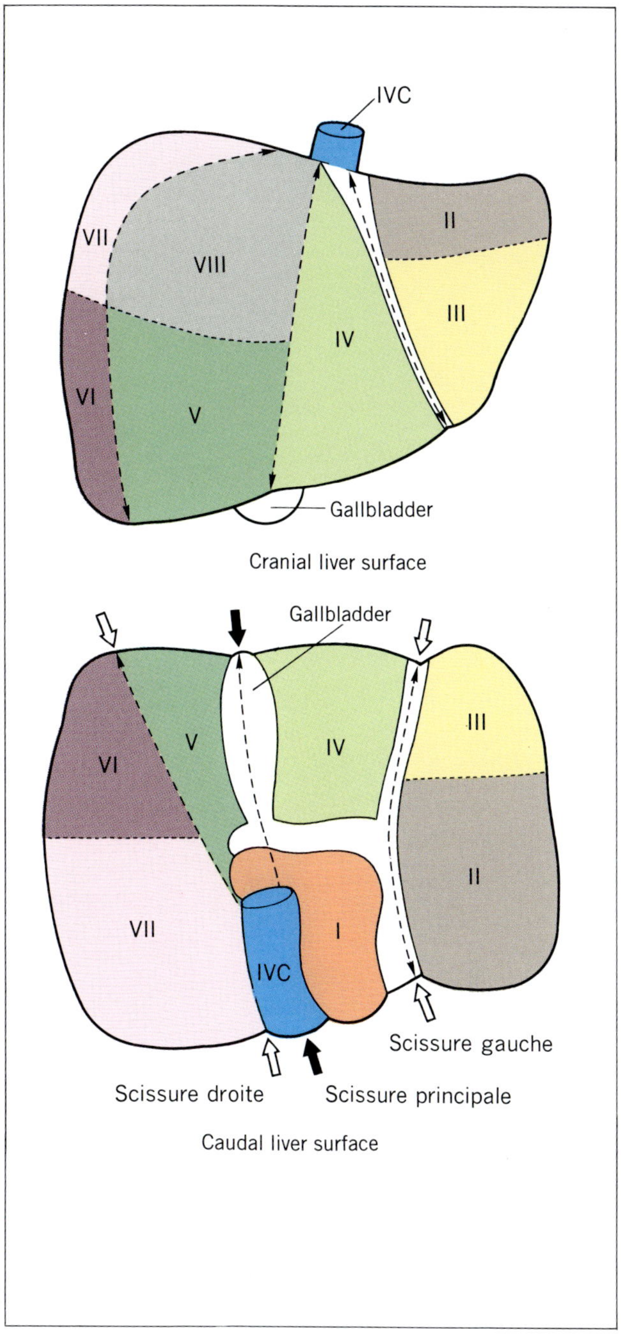

Fig. 1.54 Segments proposed by Couinaud (1954). Couinaud divided the liver into eight segments based on the injection corrosion model made from the portal vein system. In Healey's scheme, if the two areas of the left lobe were combined, and three areas of the caudate lobe made into one, this scheme would become essentially the same as Couinaud's. Even in Couinaud's scheme, the right boundary of the caudate lobe is obscure. Numbering of the segments begins from the caudate lobe (I) and goes anticlockwise on the liver placed with the anterior surface down. Segment VIII is not seen from the caudal surface.

Table 1.2 Division of intrahepatic portal vein branches, areas they supply, and their relation to the hepatic vein system

order of portal vein	1st order branch (main portal vein)	2nd order branch (segment portal vein)	3rd order branch (subsegment portal vein)		hepatic vein	Couinaud's segment No.
territory	lobe	segment	subsegment			
portal vein trunk	right main portal vein	posterior portal vein (P-point)	superior portal vein	P^{VII}_{a}, P^{VII}_{b}		VII
			inferior portal vein	P^{VI}_{a}, P^{VI}_{b}, $P^{VI}_{※}$		VI
			- - - - - - - - - -		right hepatic vein	
		anterior portal vein	superior portal vein	P^{VIII}_{a}, P^{VIII}_{b}, P^{VIII}_{c}, P^{VIII}_{d}		VIII
			inferior portal vein	P^{V}_{a}, P^{V}_{b}		V
	caudate portal vein (P^{I}_{t})	right caudate portal vein (P^{I}_{r})				
			- - - - - - - - - -		middle hepatic vein	
	transverse portion (left main portal vein)	left caudate portal vein (P^{I}_{l})				
		umbilical portion (U-point)	medial portal vein	P^{IV}_{a}, P^{IV}_{b}, P^{IV}_{dor}		IV
			—·—·—·—		falciform ligament	
			lateral portal vein	P^{III}	left hepatic vein	III
				P^{II}		II

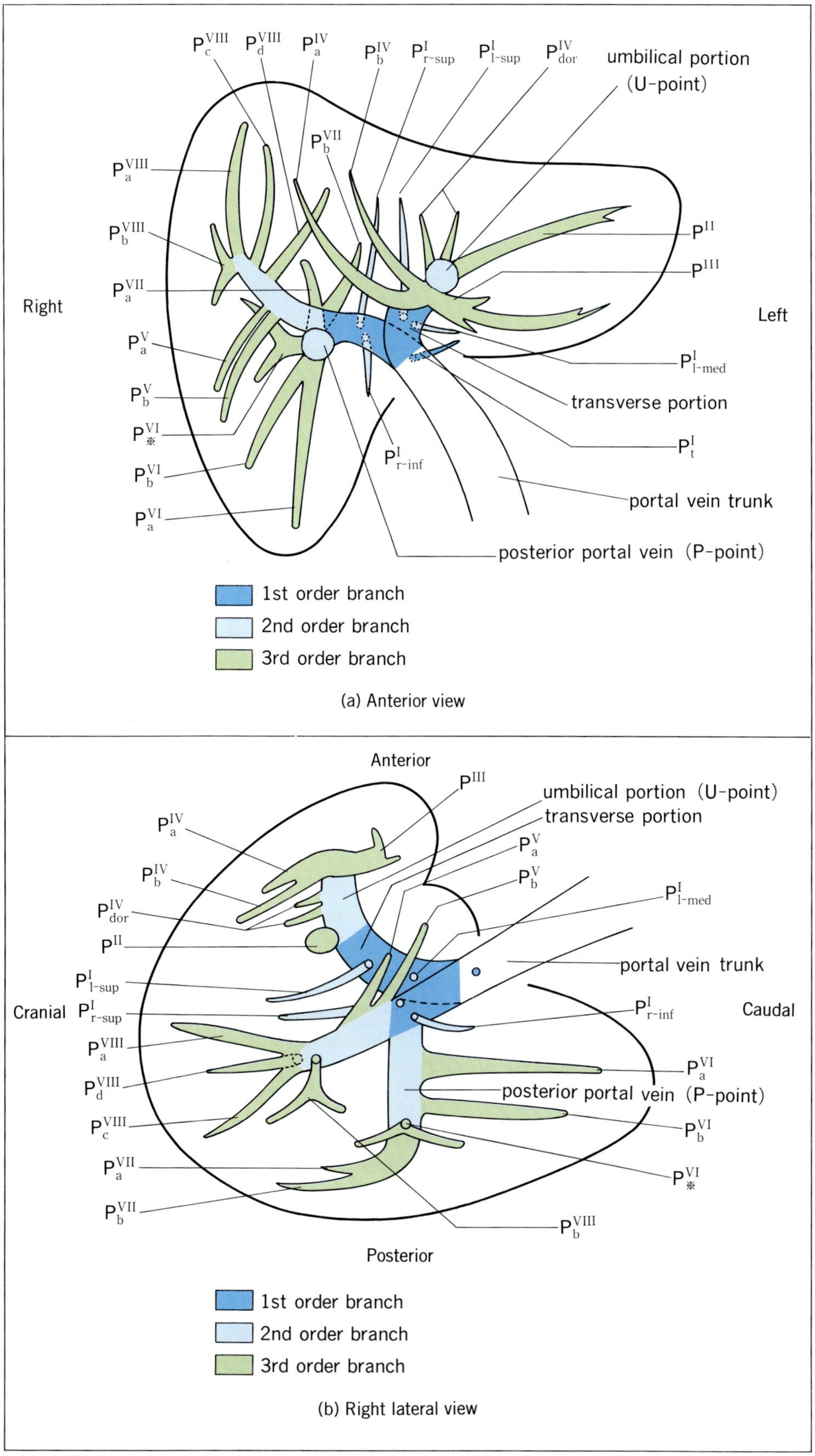

a

b

Fig. 1.55 The numbering scheme for the order of division and naming of subsegments based on intrahepatic portal vein branches proposed by Takayasu *et al.* (1985):
(a) Anterior view, (b) Right lateral view.

area were combined as one segment, and three parts of the caudate lobe made into one segment, then their scheme is very similar to that of Couinaud. In Japan, Couinaud's eight segments are commonly adopted because of the simplicity of his scheme.

However, in the 1980s, along with the remarkable progress in imaging diagnosis, small liver cancers have come to be detected and resected in Japan, requiring a more detailed and accurate three-dimensional anatomy and segmentation scheme. In 1985, we proposed a new system of segmentation based on intrahepatic portal branches and the order of their branching (Takayasu *et al.* 1985*d*). In this scheme, the subsegments frequently identified by PTP are named alphabetically from **a** to **c**, or to **d**, starting from the ventral to dorsal areas. This permits naming of small areas that correspond to the supplying portal branches. This scheme may be likened to a street address with house numbers. Table 1.2 puts forward the individual portal veins, branching orders, and areas they supply in relation to the hepatic veins (Fig. 1.55). There is no anatomical marker for dividing the anterior and posterior segments into the superior and inferior subsegments; the scheme of Healey and Schroy, and of Couinaud, necessarily depended on the anterior view of these segments. In our scheme, however, the level at which the first branch of the anterior portal vein divides is used for the separation of the superior and inferior subsegments. In the posterior segment, the P-point is used for practical purposes to separate the superior and inferior subsegments. In the posterior segment, the branch situated between the superior and inferior subsegments is named $P^{VI}{}_{*}$.

Problems with the currently used segmentation schemes and possible improvement

If our scheme given in Table 1.2 is correlated with Couinaud's segment numbers, segments II (S^{II}) to VIII (S^{VIII}) are supplied by the third-order branches, but S^{I} is supplied mainly by second-order branches ($P^{I}{}_{r}$ and $P^{I}{}_{l}$), or occasionally by the first-order portal vein ($P^{I}{}_{t}$). S^{II} and S^{III} are supplied by further peripheral branches coming off the third-order branches. Thus, Couinaud's segments do not fit the order of portal vein branching (Takayasu *et al.* 1985*d*). With respect to the hepatic vein system, the right hepatic and middle hepatic veins are good markers for dividing the anterior and posterior segments, and the anterior segment and left medial subsegment respectively. However, the left hepatic vein divides only a small left subsegment; it does not assume the same status as does the right or the middle hepatic vein.

Another problem is that the four segments in the Healey-Schroy scheme, namely the right anterior, right posterior, left medial, and left lateral, are not quite equal in weight and volume. The left lateral and medial segments, if combined (excluding the caudate), may become similar to the anterior and the posterior segment of the right lobe (Stone *et al.* 1969; Torres *et al.* 1986). In surgical practice, resection of the left lateral segment (left lateral segmentectomy) is easy, and the amount of tissue removed is much less than in right anterior or right posterior segmentectomy. The term 'segmentectomy' in this case may not be equivalent to other segmentectomies. To summarize the above discussion, the liver may be divided into three large areas, the right anterior segment, right posterior segment, and left lobe, with the addition of the caudate lobe (Takayasu *et al.* 1985*d*). As long as the caudate lobe has its own independent afferent (artery and portal vein) and efferent vessels (short hepatic vein), it may be regarded, despite its small size, as an independent region with its own vasculature, like other lobes. A new concept of segmentation that considers the vasculature, order of branching, and volume should be developed in the future with proper treatment of the left hepatic vein.

Segment diagnosis based on imaging using Couinaud's segmentation scheme

Figure 1.56 represents the eight subsegments of Couinaud in spatial relation to the portal and hepatic veins.

Segment diagnosis based on CT images

Dynamic CT is very useful in making segment diagnosis because the portal vein, hepatic vein, and inferior vena cava are opacified simultaneously (Pagani 1983) (Fig. 1.57).

In the slices cranial to the hilum the lines connecting the major hepatic veins and the inferior vena cava are the markers for individual segments, except for the left lobe in which the medial and lateral subsegments may be divided by the U-point or the falciform ligament. In the slices caudal to the hilum, segment diagnosis is made with reference to the portal veins that supply the liver and to the hepatic veins that drain it. The inferior vena cava is the vein that drains the organs caudal to the liver, not the liver itself, and should not be used as a reference for segment identification. It is used in the cranial slices simply because the portal vein is not clearly identified cranial to the porta hepatis. The gallbladder bed and the middle hepatic vein are in a fixed position in most cases and the Cantlie line connecting them is fairly constant. However, a large branch of the middle hepatic often lies lateral and posterior to the gallbladder bed (in the right anterior segment). Discrepancy occurs rather seldom between the segment diagnosis made based on the vasculature within the portal tract (hepatic artery and portal vein) and one based on the hepatic vein. However, it occasionally occurs in S^{VIII} as shown in Fig. 1.58 because the anterior segment lies cranial to the posterior segment in the right lobe near the diaphragm. The inferior right hepatic vein is recognized on ultrasound (US) in about 10 per cent of patients (Makuuchi *et al.* 1983), but it is more often delineated on portal-CT scan than plain CT or US.

Segment division of the caudate lobe is often problematic. For practical purposes the left part of the caudate lobe is considered to be situated to the left of the middle of the inferior vena cava with a discrete left end (Fig. 1.59). However, the right side is poorly demarcated because it is in continuity with the right lobe and left side of the caudate lobe, and it has no discrete draining hepatic vein. During arterial-CT the right side of the caudate lobe may be enhanced by chance (Fig. 1.9); this enabled us to identify the right side of the caudate lobe in a patient with marked atrophy of the right lobe (see p.311). In either case, the right border of the caudate lobe is irregular, perhaps due to the complicated blood supply coming from the adjacent area.

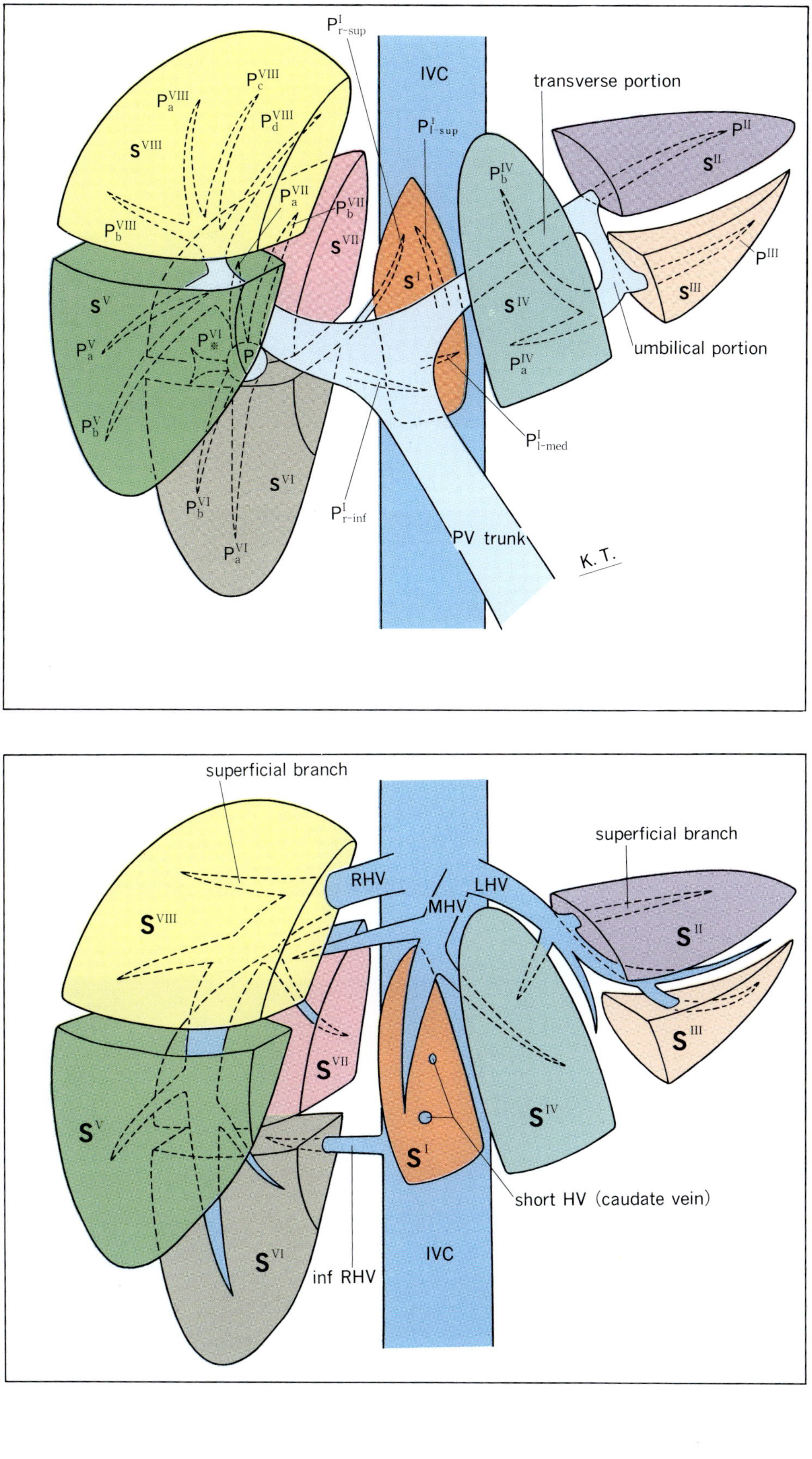

Fig. 1.56 (a) The subsegments proposed by Couinaud and their relation to the portal vein system. (b) The eight subsegments proposed by Couinaud and their relation to the hepatic vein system.

Fig. 1.57 (a)–(l) Identification of subsegments on CT.

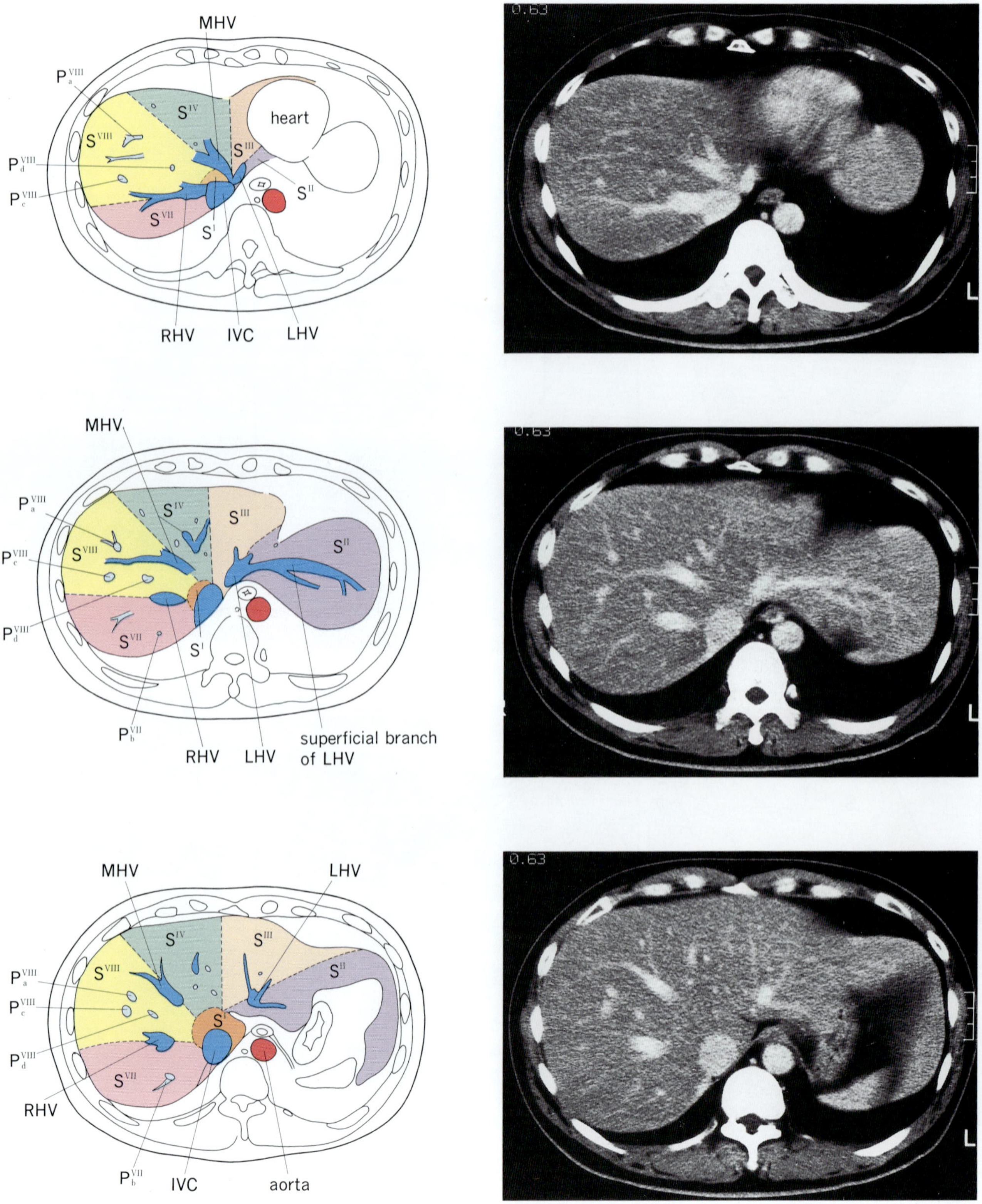

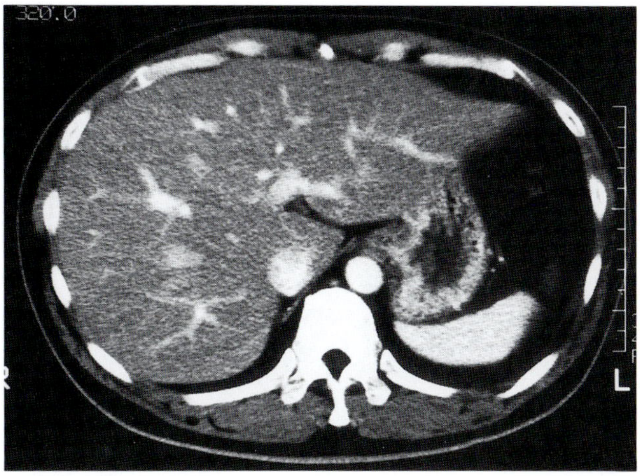
320.0
L

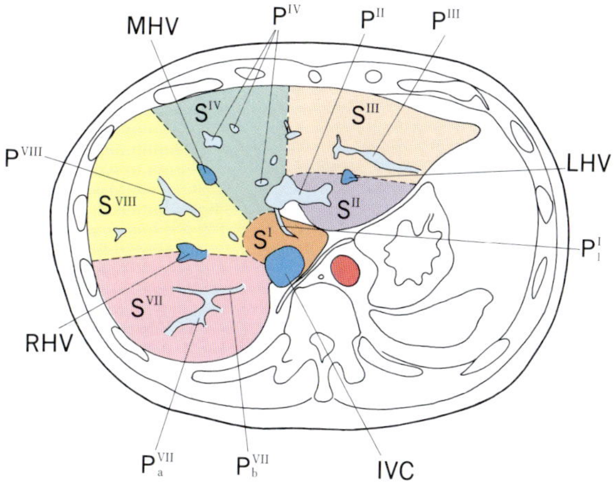
MHV
P^{IV}
P^{II}
P^{III}
S^{IV}
S^{III}
P^{VIII}
LHV
S^{VIII}
S^{II}
S^{I}
P^{I}_{l}
S^{VII}
RHV
P^{VII}_{a}
P^{VII}_{b}
IVC

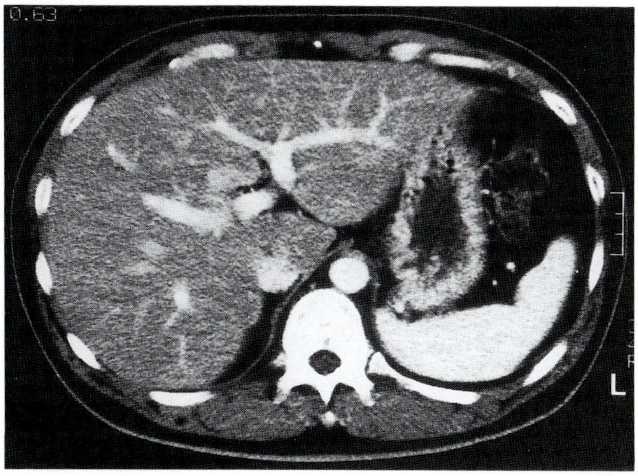
0.63
L

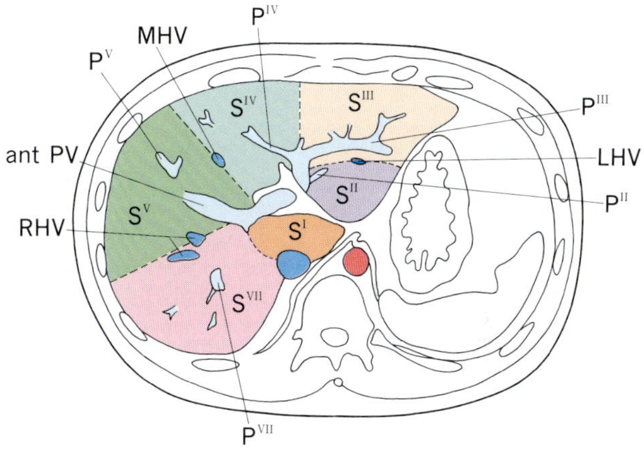
P^{IV}
MHV
P^{V}
S^{IV}
S^{III}
P^{III}
ant PV
LHV
S^{II}
P^{II}
S^{V}
RHV
S^{I}
S^{VII}
P^{VII}

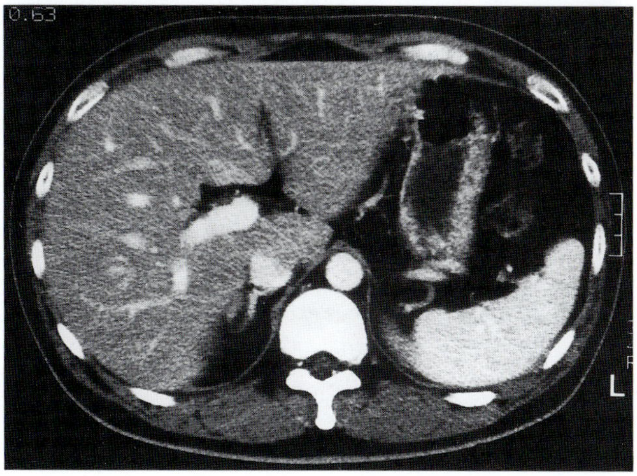
0.63
L

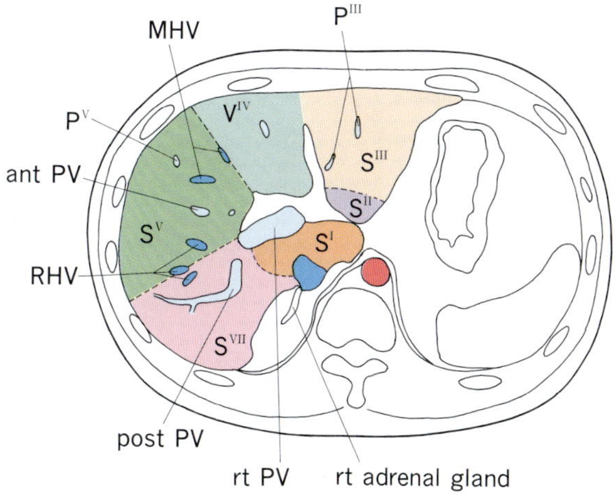
MHV
P^{III}
P^{V}
V^{IV}
ant PV
S^{III}
S^{II}
S^{V}
S^{I}
RHV
S^{VII}
post PV
rt PV
rt adrenal gland

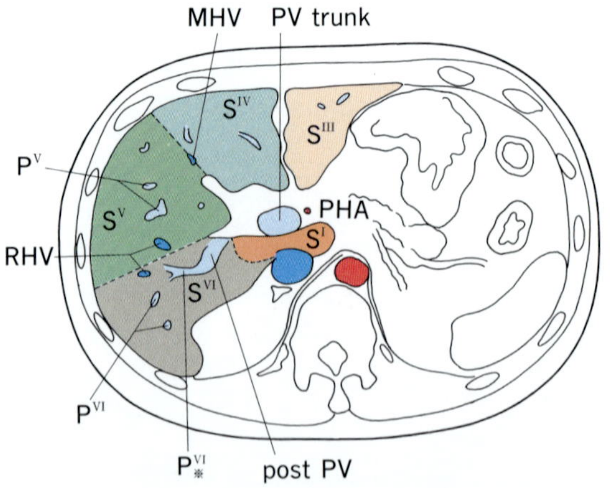
MHV
PV trunk
SIV
SIII
PV
PHA
SV
RHV
SI
SVI
PVI
P*VI
post PV

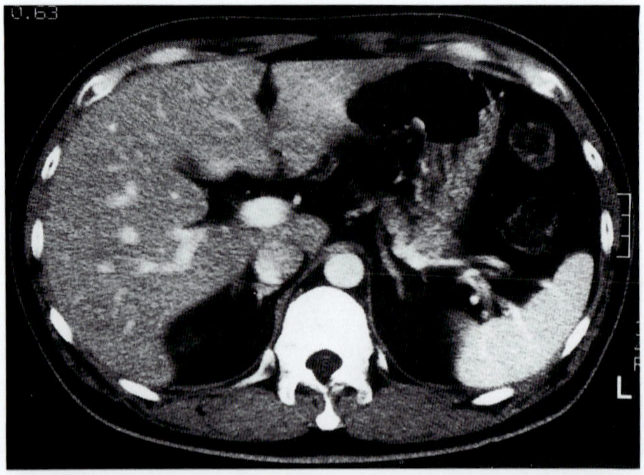
0.63
L

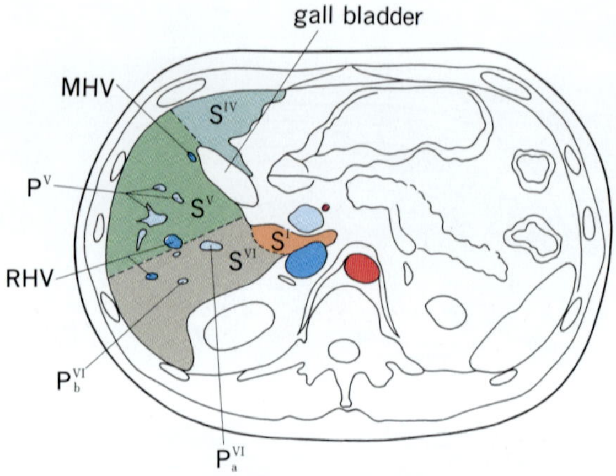
gall bladder
MHV
SIV
PV
SV
SI
RHV
SVI
PVIb
PVIa

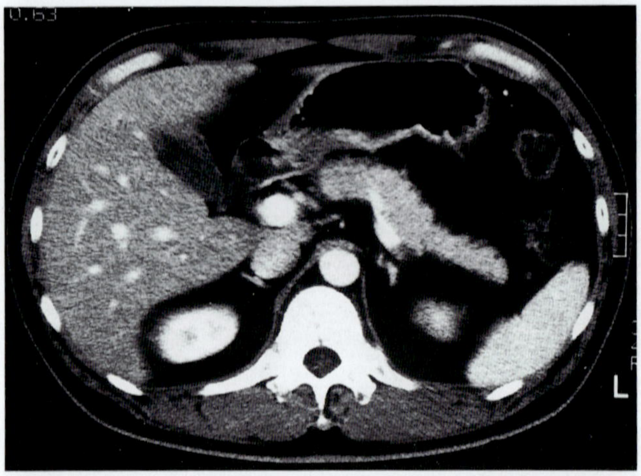
0.63
L

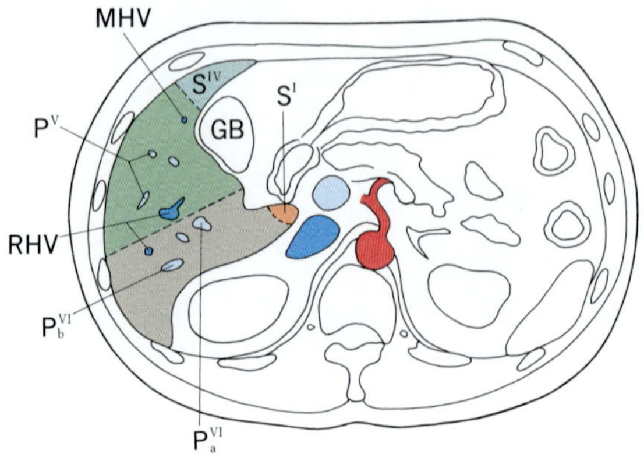
MHV
SIV
SI
GB
PV
RHV
PVIb
PVIa

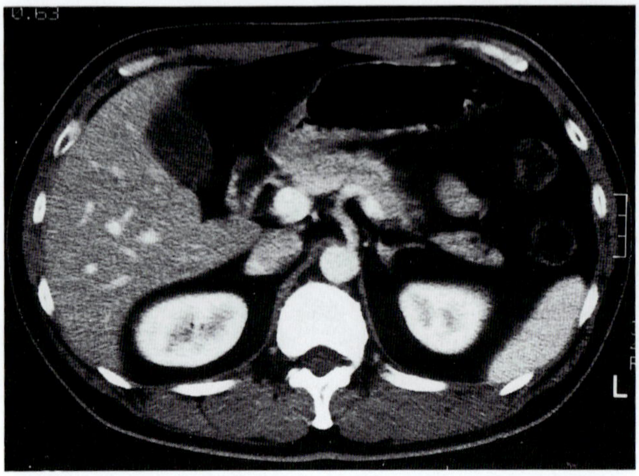
0.63
L

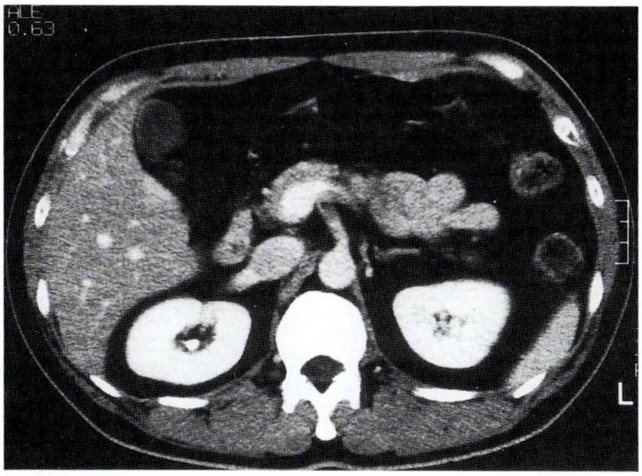

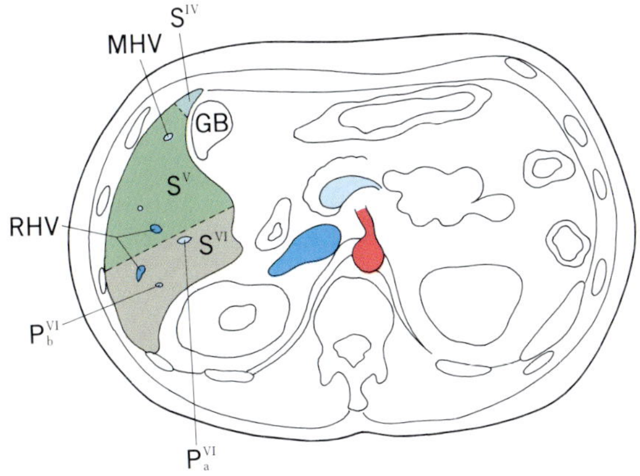
S^IV
MHV
GB
S^V
RHV
S^VI
P_b^VI
P_a^VI

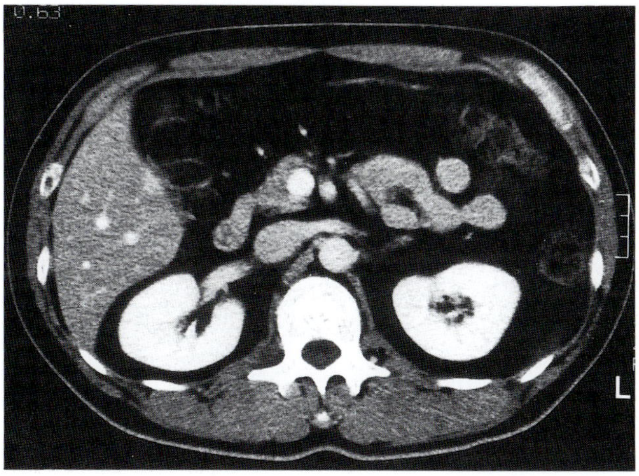

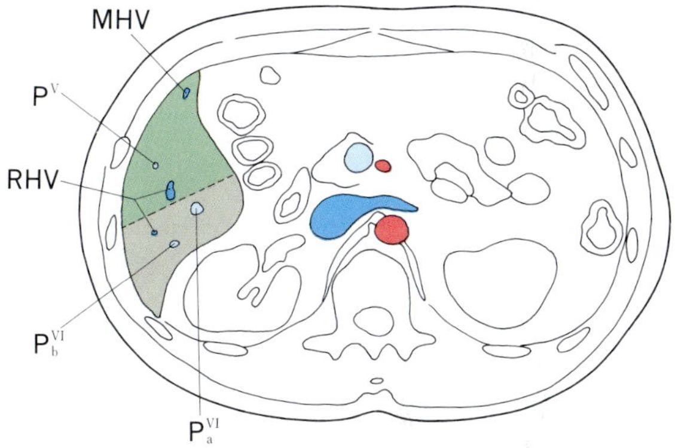
MHV
P^V
RHV
P_b^VI
P_a^VI

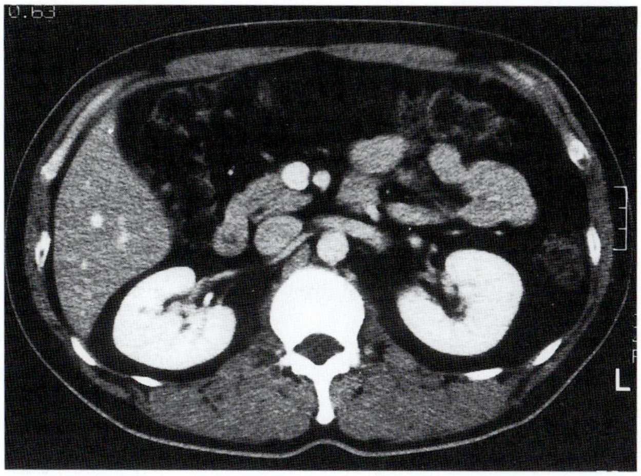

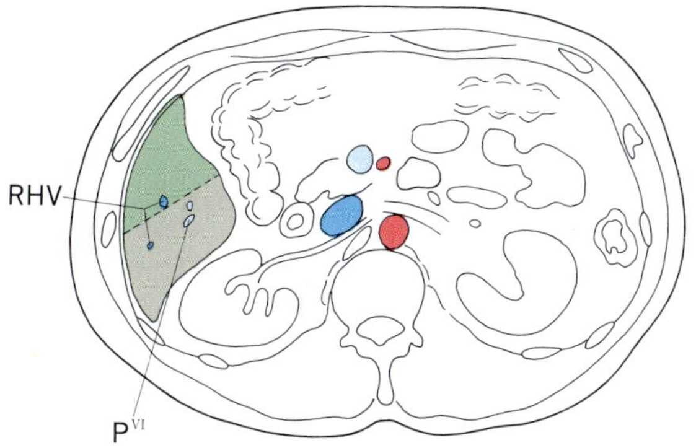
RHV
P^VI

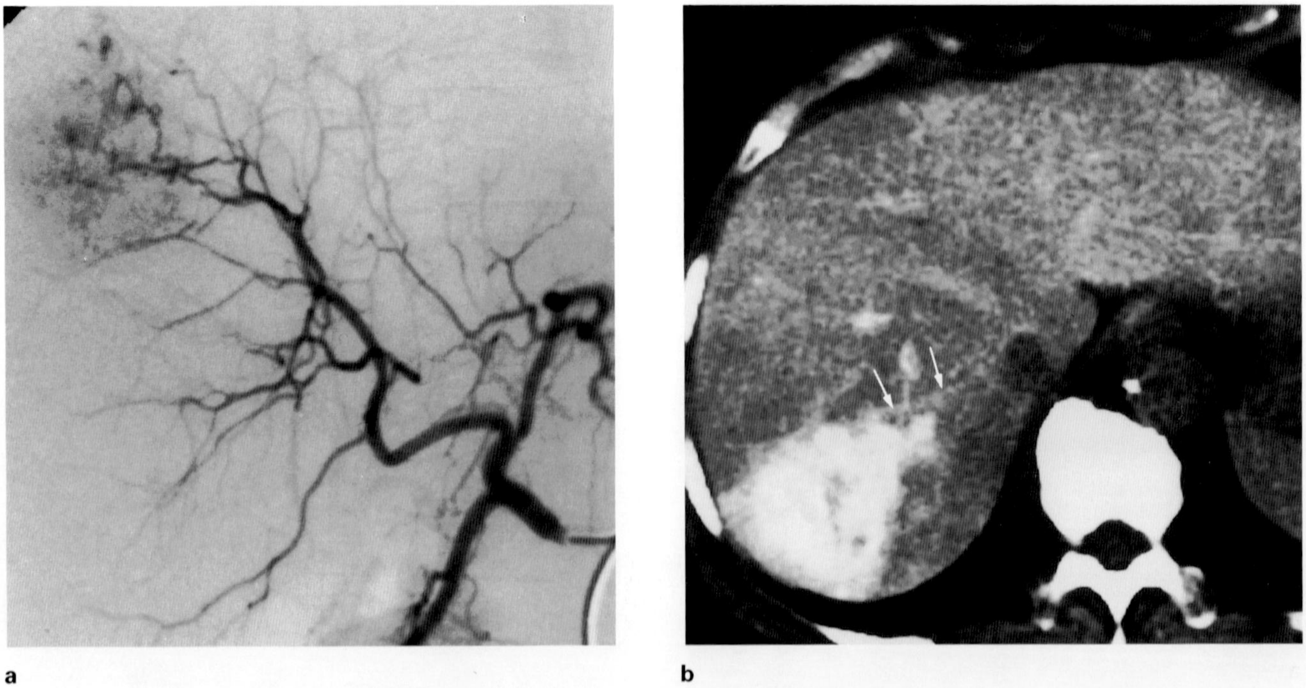

Fig. 1.58 Discrepancy between the angiogram and CT in segment diagnosis.
(a) Hepatic arteriogram: a 4 cm HCC is found in subsegment S^{VIII}. Segment diagnosis was the same when made with the portogram.
(b) Arterial-CT: on this arterial-CT, the opacified tumor is behind the right hepatic vein (→), and therefore CT segment diagnosis should be S^{VII}.

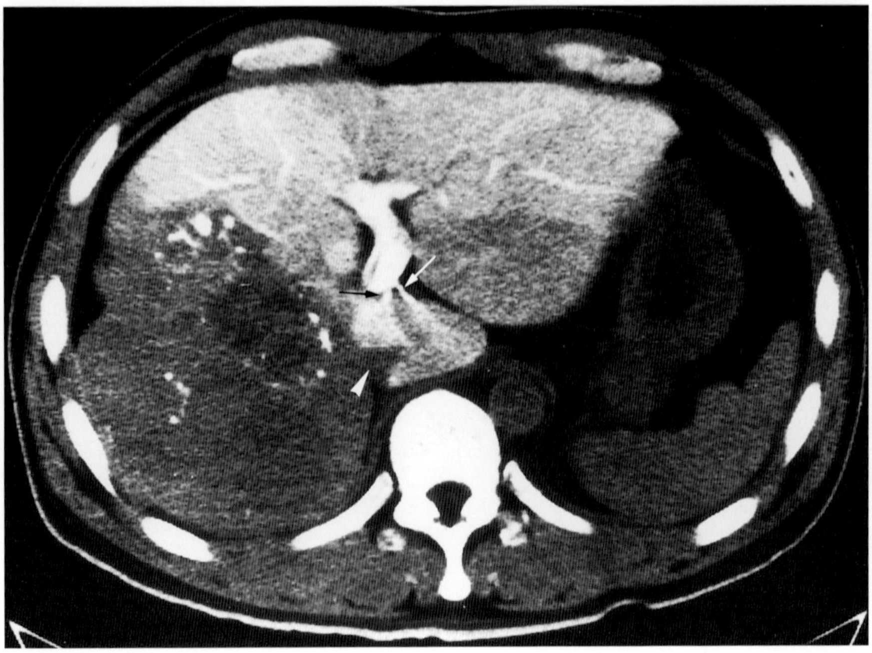

Fig. 1.59 The areas of the left caudate lobe. Portal-CT: portal-CT was made in this patient with HCC which was completely occluding the right main portal vein. The left lobe and left side of the caudate lobe was opacified. The left side of the caudate lobe was supplied by two caudate lobe portal branches (→), and the right border of the opacified area lies in the right lobe beyond the inferior vena cava (▶). From this CT, it is not clear whether the opacified area corresponds to the entire caudate lobe, or whether it represents a phenomenon in which blood supply coming from the left has increased, compensating for the decreased blood in the right side. More study is necessary for the determination of the boundary between the right and left sides of the caudate lobe.

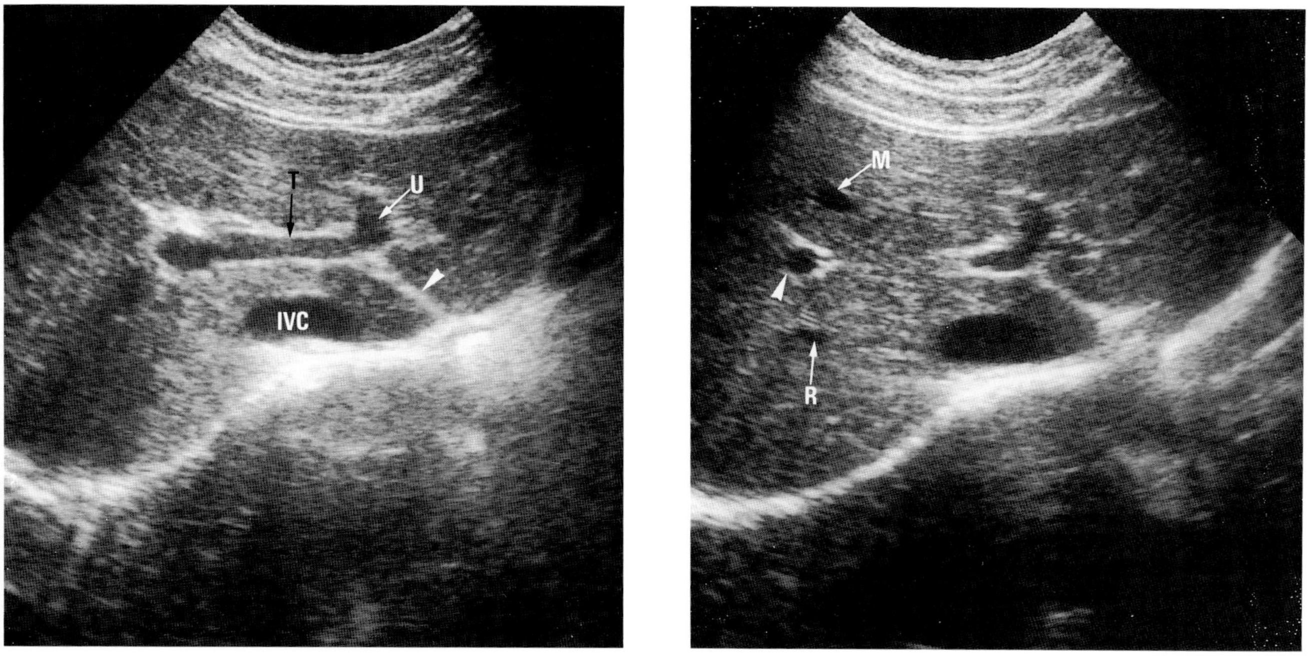

a b

Fig. 1.60 Segment diagnosis by US.
(a) In this section, the transverse (T) and umbilical (U) portions and the first order branch of the right portal vein are seen. This is somewhat similar to a CT section as shown in Fig. 1.57(e). The caudate lobe is seen anterior to the inferior vena cava (IVC). ▶, remnant ductus venosus.
(b) Slanting the transducer cranially, one can identify the right hepatic vein (R) and middle hepatic vein (M). The slicing plane is close to that shown in Fig. 1.57(d). (▶), anterior segment branch of the portal vein.

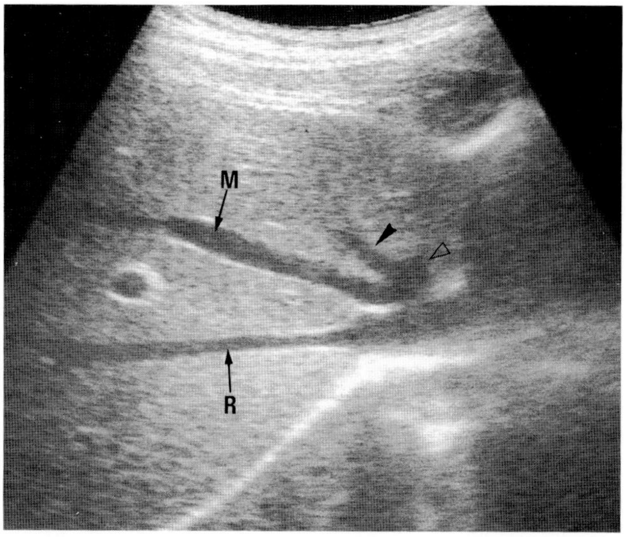

Fig. 1.61 Segment diagnosis by US (visualization of the hepatic veins by subcostal scan). In this US scan, the right hepatic vein (R), middle hepatic vein (M) and its branch (▶), and the opening of the left hepatic vein to its left (▷) are recognized. This scan corresponds to a CT section shown in Figs. 1.57 (a) and (b). In this scan, the probe is somewhat sagittal, enabling recognition of the periphery of the right and middle hepatic veins.

Segment diagnosis by ultrasound imaging

Ultrasonic waves do not penetrate bone or air, and so scanning must be done with the probe placed in the intercostal and subcostal spaces when the entire liver is to be evaluated. One can scan in any plane, and so ultrasound scanning can give variable results. Expertise varies a great deal with the examiner, and US records tend to be biased with emphasis on the diseased areas of the liver. As a result, retrospective evaluation of US images which have poor reproducibility may not be as useful as with CT and angiography. Assessment of the course of the portal vein and its ramification often varies between sonographers.

If one attempts to make a US section of the liver similar to CT, the costal margin gets in the way, and one is forced to place the probe (transducer) subcostally along the costal margin in a slanted plane in which the transverse portion, umbilical portion, and the first-order portal branch are seen in continuity (Fig. 1.60a). By cranially slanting the probe placed in the same position, one can obtain a section in which the right hepatic vein and middle hepatic vein are seen, somewhat similar to a CT section (Fig. 1.60b).

In the right subcostal scan, the liver is seen in a plane that is partially sagittal and partially coronal, and the right hepatic and middle hepatic veins are seen separately in the same plane (Fig. 1.61); they are usually superimposed on a late phase angiogram.

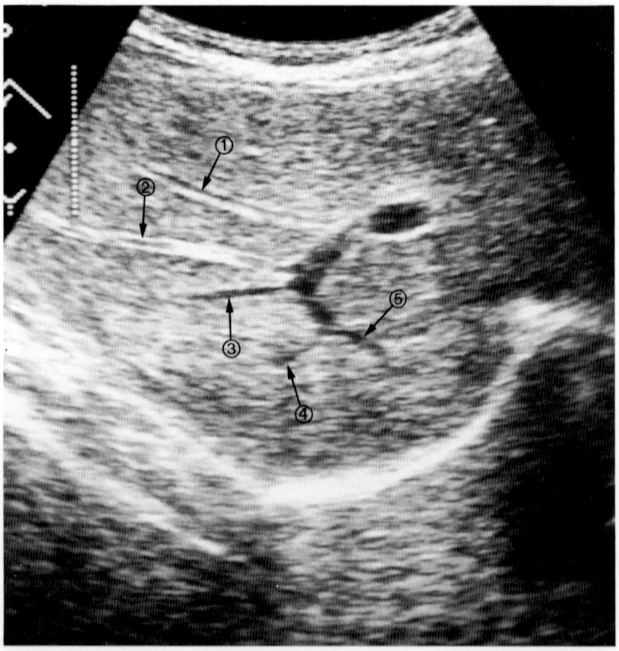

Fig. 1.62 Segment diagnosis by US (visualization of the right posterior portal vein by right subcostal scan). The branches are seen coming off the right portal vein in an arc shape: P^{VI}_{a} (1), P^{VI}_{b} (2), P^{VI}_{*} (3), P^{VII}_{a} (4) P^{VII}_{b} (5).

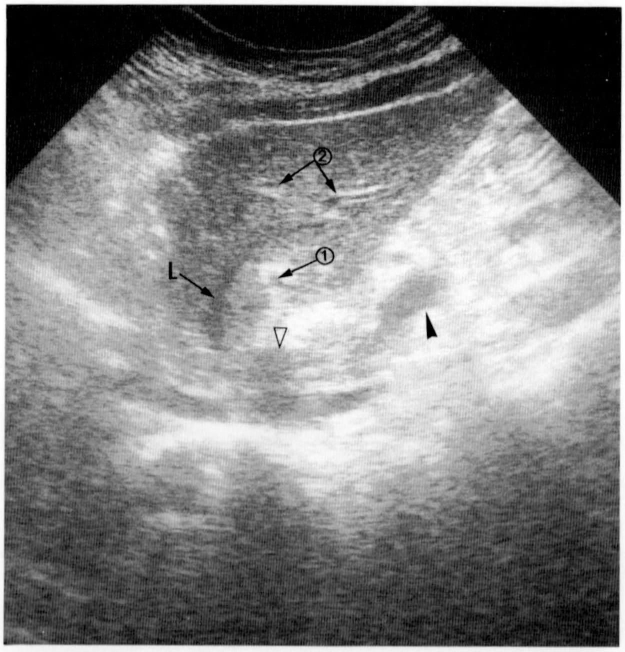

Fig. 1.63 Segment diagnosis by US (epigastric sagittal scan). In this scan, the left hepatic vein (L) is seen between the left superior branch (P^{II}) (1) and inferior branch P^{III} (2). ▷, inferior vena cava; ▶, portal trunk.

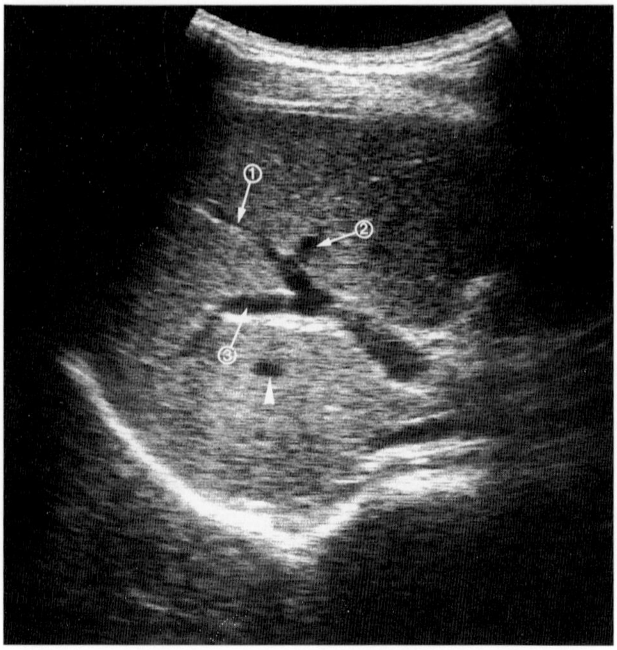

Fig. 1.64 Segment diagnosis by US (visualization of the anterior portal vein by right intercostal scan). Branches supplying the anterior segment are clearly identified in this scan. P^{VIII}_{a} (1) and P^{VIII}_{c} (3) are seen in the anterior and posterior areas respectively. The branch (2) coming of P^{VIII}_{a} may be P^{VIII}_{b}, but may also be P^{V}, but no clear distinction is possible because there is no hepatic vein that will help distinguish them. ▶, right hepatic vein.

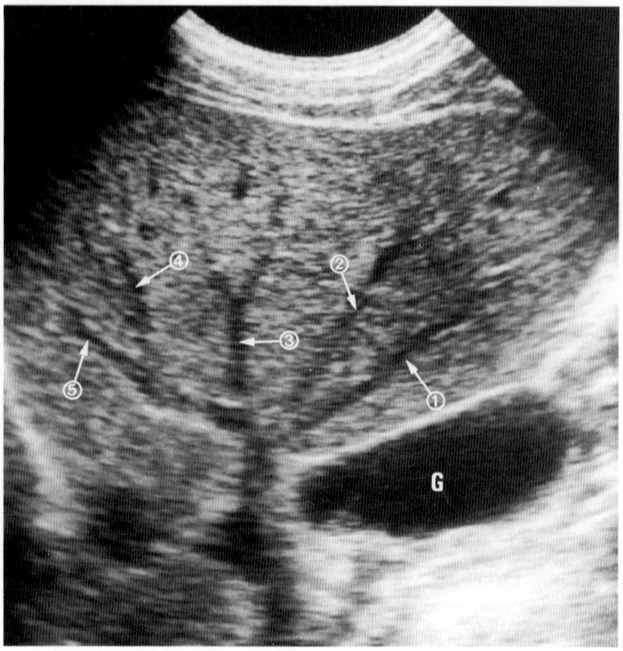

Fig. 1.65 Segment diagnosis by US (visualization of the posterior portal vein by right intercostal scan). A scan was made in the right dorsal area and the gallbladder (G) is seen in the lower area of the image. The right posterior portal vein is seen sending off P^{VI}_{a} (1), P^{VI}_{b} (2), P^{VI}_{*} (3), P^{VII}_{a} (4), and P^{VII}_{b} (5).

In the same scan made in the left decubitus position and on deep inspiration, the right posterior segment may be observed as shown in Fig. 1.62. Under these conditions, the scanning plane is close to sagittal. In the epigastric sagittal scan, the US image is very similar to that from sagittal MR imaging (Fig. 1.63). In the intercostal scan, the ribs are at an angle of 20–45 degrees to the table surface, and the images thus obtained are somewhat similar to the coronal section made at that angle on MR imaging, good for visualization of the right anterior segment portal branches (Fig. 1.64). Furthermore, the right hepatic vein that divides the anterior and posterior segments is readily recognized. Angling the probe slightly posteriorly, the posterior segment can be seen. Whereas the Cantlie line is clearly identified by CT, and the main lobar fissure and the intersegmental plane can be drawn on the image with reference to it, it is difficult to have the same orientation by US. The examiner has to visualize these anatomical markers and locations from many US images.

For the surgeon, intraoperative US is a most important and indispensable procedure, and expertise is required for preoperative US identification of segments and vasculature.

I. Diagnosis

2

Diagnosis of hepatic tumors and histological classification

2.1 Diagnosis of liver tumors

Accurate diagnosis is essential for the selection of the best treatment and for the prediction of prognosis. Diagnosis of liver disease, particularly of tumors, consists of the following: (1) diagnosis of disease existence, (2) quality diagnosis, (3) estimation of degree of spread, and (4) prediction of prognosis.

Diagnosis of disease existence

It is essential first to determine whether there is disease in the liver. If there is one, the size and number of lesions have to be determined. One should not be satisfied by just detecting disease. Effort has to be made to explore the entire liver; it is also important to keep a detailed record of the findings and to report them. For the description of the lesion, one has to consider the vascular systems as already discussed in Chapter 1 for more accurate diagnosis. For the determination of the size of a mass, US and CT give relatively accurate measures, if section is made in the center. On angiograms, there is certain artificial enlargement depending on the distance between the lesion and the film, and an average factor of 1.2 is usually used for correction.

Quality diagnosis

This includes not only differentiation between benign and malignant disease but also determination of the nature of the lesion, etc. The interior of a section of the lesion presents various characteristics on US, CT, and MR imaging, and if contrast enhancement is made in addition, more information is provided such as blood flow and hemodynamics. The examiner is required to be familiar with the gross features of various tumors in cut sections. If the tumor size is less than 2 cm or so, the internal structure is not well delineated, and quality diagnosis becomes difficult because information may be limited only to differences in temporal changes in staining on contrast enhancement, and echogenicity.

The individual imaging modalities vary considerably in their value in quality diagnosis. Angiography provides more information for quality diagnosis than does US, whereas the latter is better for diagnosis of existence but not of quality. Portal-CT has a high sensitivity in existence diagnosis, but is poor in quality diagnosis with low specificity. One has to be well versed in the individual modalities to appreciate their merits and demerits.

Determination of extent of involvement

Accurate existence and quality diagnoses permit accurate assessment of the extent of involvement within the liver, and if combined with a diagnosis of extrahepatic involvement, they will provide the basis on which the most appropriate treatment can be selected.

Prediction of prognosis

When the extent of involvement is determined, the responsible team of physicians should study reports on the efficacy of individual treatments and must be well informed about the biological characteristics and behavior of each type of tumor. It has to be expected that some patients succumb earlier or live longer postoperatively then generally expected due to early recurrence, rapid growth, slow growth, changes in degree of malignancy, etc.

With progress in understanding of tumor biology, selection of a therapeutic modality and prognostic prediction will improve. Molecular biological techniques will greatly facilitate investigations in tumor biology and hasten progress in the future.

2.2 Histological classification of liver tumors

The histological classification of liver tumors recommended by WHO (Gibson and Sobin 1978) is widely used throughout the world. In Japan, the classification adopted by the Liver Cancer Study Group of Japan (1989) in the General Rules for the Clinical and Pathological Study of Primary Liver Cancer is also based on it. In the oncological practice for the liver, one has to be familiar with the tumors listed in the WHO classification (Table 2.1). One should also know the frequency with which they occur. For instance, hemangioma and cysts are commonly encountered in imaging of the liver, whereas adenoma and angiosarcoma are very rare, particularly in the Orient. HCC is endemic in the Far East, including China, Japan and South-east Asia; in the western countries, by contrast, secondary cancers far exceed HCC in frequency. Since 1978, when the WHO classification was published, several new types of liver neoplasms have been identified. For instance, fibrolamellar carcinoma of the liver which occurs in young individuals with a relatively good prognosis (Craig *et al.* 1980) and a sclerosing type of liver carcinoma characterized by hypercalcemia (Omata *et al.* 1981) may or may not need a new place in this classification scheme.

Table 2.1 Histological classification of tumors of the liver (1978)

I. Epithelial tumors
A. Benign
  1. Liver cell adenoma (hepatocellular adenoma)
  2. Intrahepatic bile duct adenoma
  3. Intrahepatic bile duct cystadenoma
B. Malignant
  1. Hepatocellular carcinoma (liver cell carcinoma)
  2. Cholangiocarcinoma (intrahepatic bile duct carcinoma)
  3. Bile duct cystadenocarcinoma
  4. Combined hepatocellular and cholangiocarcinoma
  5. Hepatoblastoma
  6. Undifferentiated carcinoma

II. Non-epithelial tumors
A. Hemangioma
B. Infantile haemangioendothelioma
C. Hemangiosarcoma
D. Embryonal sarcoma
E. Others

III. Miscellaneous tumors
A. Teratoma
B. Carcinosarcoma
C. Others

IV. Unclassified tumors
V. Hemopoietic and lymphoid tumors

VI. Metastatic tumors
VII. Epithelial abnormalities
A. Liver cell dysplasia
B. Bile duct abnormalities

VIII. Tumor-like lesions
A. Hamartoma
  1. Mesenchymal hamartoma
  2. Biliary hamartoma (microhamartoma, von Meyenburg complex)
B. Congenital biliary cysts
C. Focal nodular hyperplasia
D. Compensatory lobar hyperplasia
E. Peliosis hepatis
F. Heterotopia
G. Others

The revised version of the WHO classification now includes them (Ishak *et al.* 1994). It leaves some questions unanswered, such as the difference between sclerosing carcinoma and scirrhous type HCC, which some pathologists consider to be the same. Epithelioid hemangioendothelioma (Ishak *et al.* 1984) which was known to be associated with the lung is now recognized in the liver. It is usually classified with hemangiosarcoma, but is of low-grade malignancy. Should this be treated as an independent tumor or included in hemangioma? Lipoma and angiomyolipom are being found in the liver in increasing numbers, and in the WHO classification, they are summarily placed in the category of 'others' in *II. Non-epithelial tumors*. They may need independent places. Undifferentiated sarcoma that occurs in children is now thought to be the same as *II.D. Embryonal sarcoma*. We have seen carcinoid tumor and lymphoma,although the incidence is low; the former is included in *III. Miscellaneous tumors*, and the latter in *V. Hemopoietic tumors and lymphoid tumors*. Ciliated hepatic foregut cyst which derives from the embryonal foregut is placed in *VIII. Tumor-like lesions, B. Congenital biliary cyst*. There are several such problems.

3

Benign liver tumors

3.1 Hemangioma of the liver

Of the primary liver tumors, hemangioma (Fig. 3.1) is the most frequent with an incidence of about 4 per cent in autopsied livers (Edmondson 1958). Unless otherwise specified, it means cavernous hemangioma. With the recent progress in imaging diagnosis, it is incidentally found quite frequently in asymptomatic individuals (Case 1). More reports suggest that hemangioma is more common in females than in males. A large hemangioma that requires resection is absolutely more common in females, and a hormonal relationship is suspected in its etiology. In autopsy material, this tumor is more frequently solitary, multiple hemangiomas occurring in only about 10 per cent. However, in the clinical setting, more than one lesion is seen in about 60 per cent of the cases in our experience.

Clinical symptoms

Hemangiomas smaller than 5 cm are usually free of symptoms, but those greater than 10 cm may cause abdominal complaints, such as pain and a sensation of fullness (60 per cent) (Table 3.1). Hemangiomas larger than 15 cm are frequently associated with consumption coagulopathy, typified by Kasbach-Merritt syndrome (Kasbach and Merritt 1940) of various degrees, requiring treatment. Rupture of a hemangioma into the abdominal cavity has been described (Yamamoto *et al.* 1991), but is very rare.

Table 3.1 Size of hemangioma in relation to clinical symptoms and frequency of consumption coagulopathy ($n = 40$)

Tumor diameter (cm)	Number of cases	Symptom [No. of cases]	Consumption coagulopathy (No. of cases)
<5	18	Right upper quadrant pain [1]	0
5–10	9		0
10–15	3	Right upper quadrant pain [1]	0
15–20	5	Upper abdominal full sensation [2] protrusion [3]	3 (2)*
20–25	3		2 (2)*
25≤	2	Abdominal mass [2]	2 (1)*
Total	40	[9]	7 (5)*

* Numbers in parentheses denote those who presented features of diffuse intravascular coagulation with marked thrombocytopenia and increased fibrin degradation products, although not typical of consumption coagulopathy.

The natural history of hemangioma of the liver is not well known. While the tumor size remains unchanged for 10 years in some patients (Gibney *et al.* 1987), the mass could be enormous at the time the patient comes to hospital. We have seen several cases in which the tumor size increased during a relatively short follow-up period (Takayasu *et al.* 1990*e*; Yoshida *et al.* 1991). The natural history and histological growth mechanism are of great interest. It is expected that study of the natural history of hepatic hemangioma using various imaging techniques will increase in the near future. Although our experience is limited, we have seen an hemangioma which ordinarily has an abundant blood supply or almost completely replaced by fibrous tissue (Case 4) and one in which the entire tumor was calcified (Case 5). These changes clearly suggest that hemangioma ages in various fashions. Hemangioma does not turn into its malignant counterpart, angiosarcoma. Angiosarcoma is known to be associated with vinyl chloride monomer and Thorotrast (Case 1, p.246).

Imaging diagnosis

Hemangiomas of the liver may be grossly divided into (1) nodular (Case 6), (2) massive (Case 2) and (3) diffuse (Case 7) as are HCCs. It is easy to diagnose a typical hemangioma by imaging, but there is considerable variation in individual cases, such as differences in tissue ageing, hence differences in histology, size of vascular lumina, thrombus formation, degree of fibrosis, and calcification; all are variable and imaging findings depend on them. Thus, there are atypical cases that pose problems in diagnosis (Takayasu *et al.* 1986*d*; Itai *et al.* 1987*b*).

Ultrasound

Ultrasound beams are reflected more irregularly as the blood spaces and intervening stromata are mixed in a complex fashion, interfering with each other in beam reflections and producing high echoes as a net effect. A hemangioma that has wider blood spaces and little stroma is less echogenic (Case 8). Such masses are also seen to be hypervascular upon angiography (Toboury *et al.* 1983). Some hemangiomas show high echoes only in the periphery of the mass resulting in the appearance of a hyperechoic rim (Case 9), while in others the entire mass may be hyperechoic. Usually, as the mass increases in size, the echo pattern becomes more complex making quality diagnosis difficult (Case 2). Another situation where quality diagnosis is difficult is the background of fatty liver; hemangiomas are seen as relatively hypoechoic (Case 10).

CT

The characteristic features of hemangioma on contrast enhancement CT are: (1) early enhancement of the tumor periphery and (2) progressive enhancement toward the center (the fill-in phenomenon) resulting in iso- or slightly high density of the mass compared with the surrounding parenchyma in the delayed phase after 10 min or so (Freeny *et al.* 1979; Itai *et al.* 1980*b*). In occasional cases, the whole mass is enhanced from its center (Case 11). Some large hemangiomas have hyalinizing degeneration in the interior which may not be stained even after 15 min (Case 2) (Scatarige *et al.* 1987).

The fill-in phenomenon is also seen in the delayed phase in metastatic tumors from the breast (Case 12) and the lung. However, it may be distinguished from the fill-in phenomenon seen in hemangioma by the following features: (1) there is no early cotton wool enhancement in the periphery, (2) the periphery is ripple shaped, and (3) peripheral low density (Muramatsu *et al.* 1986) is rather common.

Angiography

Angiography was the most reliable diagnostic technique before the advent of US and CT. It was generally believed that if the cotton wool appearance thought to be characteristic was demonstrated, the diagnosis was nearly established (McLoughlin 1971; Freeny *et al.* 1979). However, when the diagnostic accuracy was compared between US, CT, and angiography, it became clear that there are cases that are not delineated by angiography (Case 4) (Takayasu *et al.* 1986*d*). The reason is that the length of time during which films are made following contrast injection in angiography is usually only about 20 s, which is a little too short for demonstrating high enhancement. We have seen a patient in whom the lesion became enhanced on CT after 30 min from contrast injection (Case 13). Conversely, there are cases in which CT/US fails to delineate the lesion which is detectable by angiography. Therefore, it is important to use various imaging modalities with full understanding of the merits and drawbacks of the individual modalities, and make a collective diagnosis.

Some angiographers maintain that intra-arterial Lipiodol injection may facilitate differential diagnosis between a small hemangioma and HCC if the shape and duration of Lipiodol retention are considered. However, this is not always the case; we feel that this should not be done, because retention of Lipiodol within the tumor makes subsequent examination difficult (Case 14). We have experienced a case in which Lipiodol did not disappear from the hemangioma for at least a year and a half (Case 15).

MR imaging

A hemangioma is demonstrated as a hypointense mass on T1-weighted spin echo (SE) images and a hyperintense lesion on T2-weighted images (Itai *et al.* 1985; Stark *et al.* 1985). If the size of lesion is small, about 3 cm in diameter, the lesion intensity is homogeneous. With an increasing size, hyalinized degeneration and fibrous changes occur, and the intensity becomes inhomogeneous (Choi *et al.* 1989; Semelka *et al.* 1994). Using gadolinium-DTPA (Gd-DTPA), the lesion is well enhanced from the periphery to the central area (fill-in appearance) and the whole of the lesion is enhanced within 15 min or so. Hyalinized degeneration and hemorrhage are not enhanced by Gd-DTPA.

Other features include arterio-portal fistula formation (Case 16), which though uncommon mimics an HCC on dynamic CT and angiography. One has to be careful not to mistake it for HCC. Rare but problematic cases may present a 'halo' on US (Case 6), and fluid in the interior (Case 17) (Takayasu *et al.* 1986*d*). When a hemangioma expands to occupy the whole of one lobe, it may compress and even occlude the major portal vein supplying that lobe. If a major portal vein is occluded by PTP for therapeutic purposes in HCC, the non-tumorous lobe supplied by that portal vein undergoes marked atrophy with a compensatory increase of arterial supply (Makuuchi *et al.* 1990). Judging from such observations, a similar phenomenon is expected to occur following portal vein occlusion by hemangiomas; it might affect the growth of the mass itself. In our analysis, the first-order portal vein was occluded in 60 per cent of the patients with a hemangioma greater than 10 cm in diameter.

Treatment

The important question is whether or not to treat a hemangioma incidentally found in an adult, and if so, how. Operation is indicated for spontaneous rupture, but in reality it is extremely uncommon. Therefore, it seems that only large hemangiomas that exert symptomatic compression or present consumption coagulopathy should be treated.

For treatment, surgery, irradiation (Case 18), hepatic arterial embolization (Sato *et al.* 1987) (Case 19), and corticosteroids may be considered. As long as this neoplasm is benign, there is no need for radical resection. If multiple, only reduction surgery is indicated in most instances. For an extremely large hemangioma that defies resection, irradiation was the choice in the past. However, some hemangiomas are not sensitive to radiation and there is no consensus today on the most appropriate therapeutic approach. Transcatheter arterial embolization has recently become a common practice in the management of liver tumors, and it is expected that this modality may prove useful in the treatment of certain cases of huge hemangiomas.

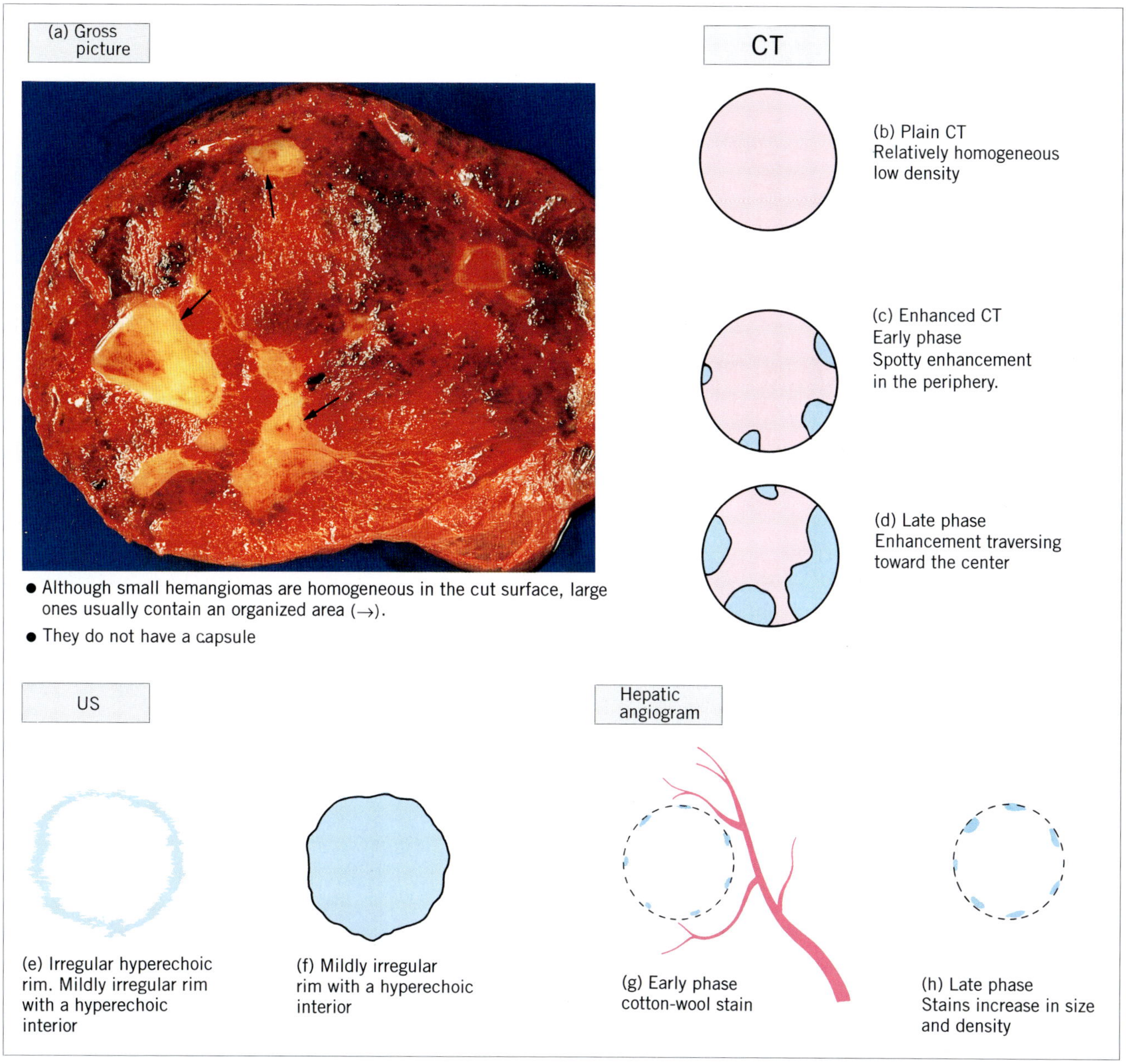

Fig. 3.1 Imaging characteristics of hepatic hemangioma.

Hepatic hemangioma—Case 1: Hepatic hemangioma incidentally found at a so-called human dock (medical examination taken by adults for early detection of adult disease).

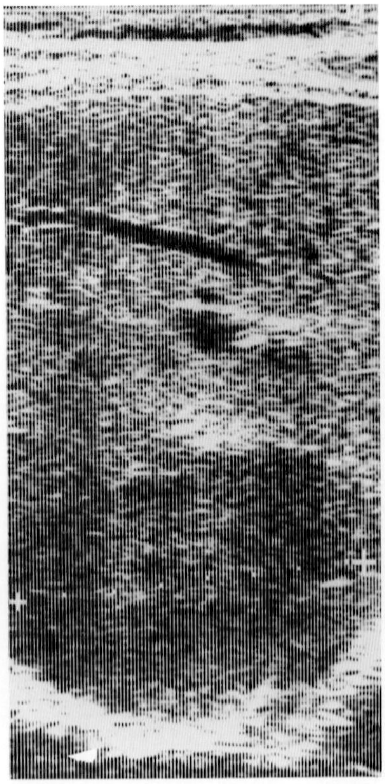

a

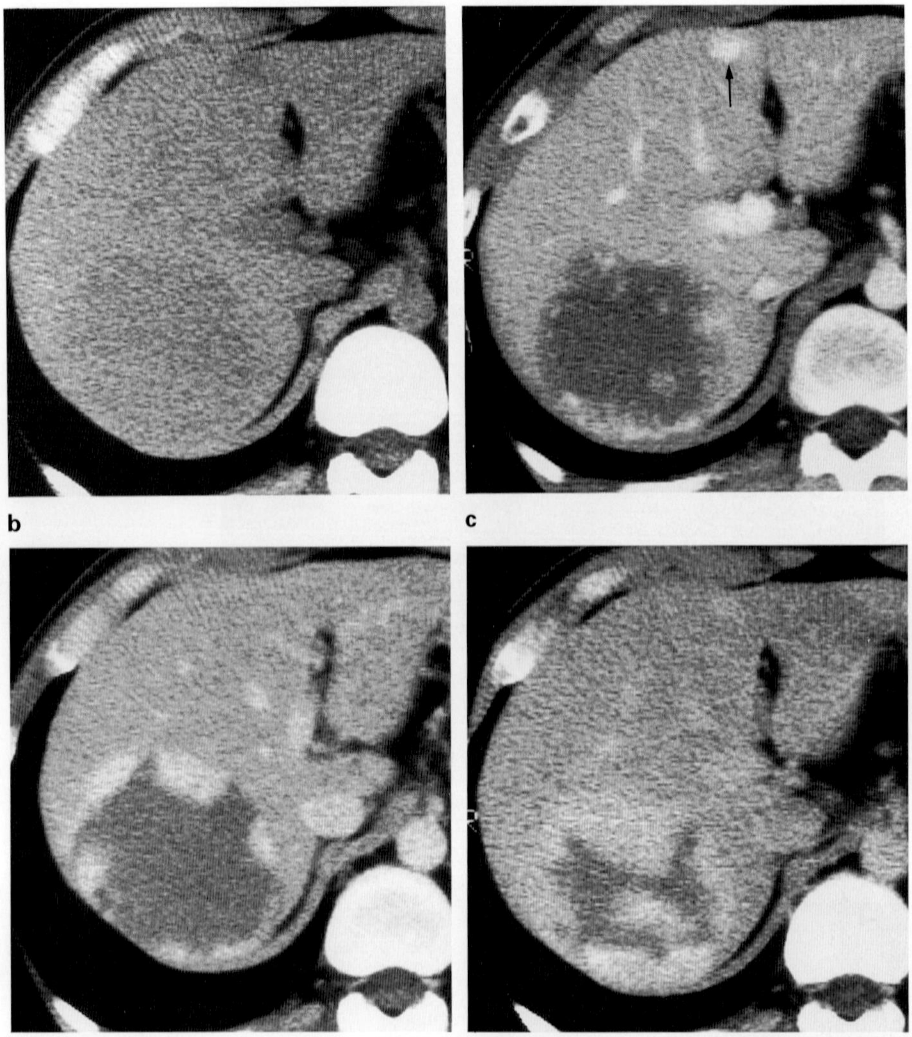

b c d e

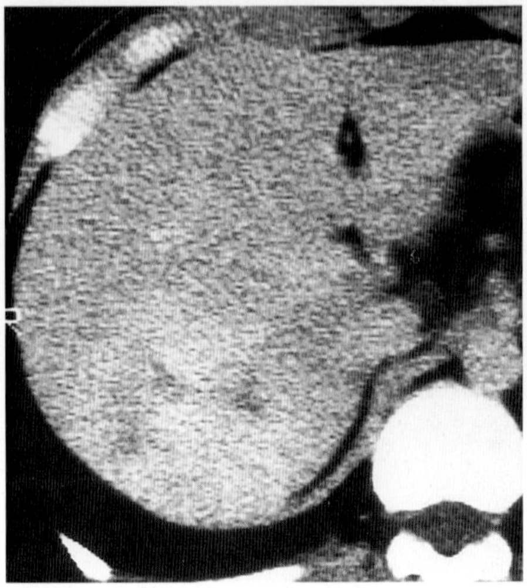

f

(a) US, right subcostal scan: a 8.5 × 7 cm hypoechoic mass was found in S^{VII}. It has areas of high echoes. In general, hemangiomas greater than 5 cm show an inhomogeneous interior with infrequent peripheral high echoes which are common in small hemangiomas.

(b–f) CT images: in a plain CT (b) a homogeneous low-density lesion was seen in S^{VII}. At the same level, on dynamic CT (c)–(e), spotty stains appeared early in the periphery. They expanded toward the center slowly, and in the late phase (f) (15 min after i.v. injection), nearly the entire mass became enhanced, denser than the surrounding parenchyma. A 1.5 hemangioma (→) found in S^{IV} was diffusely enhanced in the early phase (c) turning isodense in the late phase (f).

Case 1 (contd.)

(g–h) On hepatic angiography, small spotty dense stains (so-called cotton-wool appearance) were seen in the early phase, and in the late phase (20s) (h) the individual stains were expanded and seen more clearly. →, hemangioma in S^{IV}.

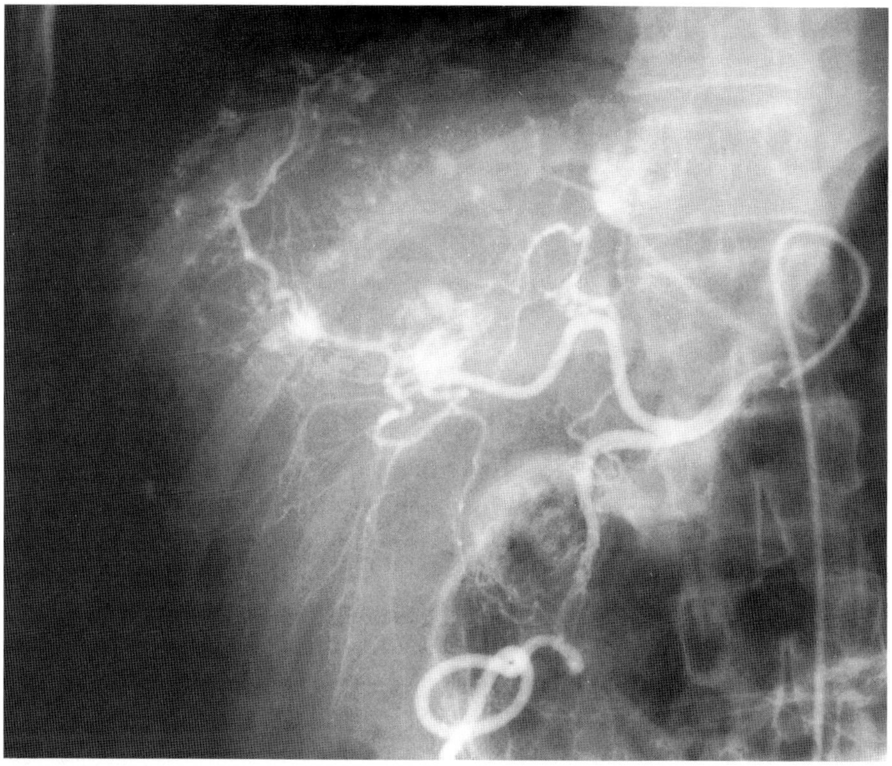

g

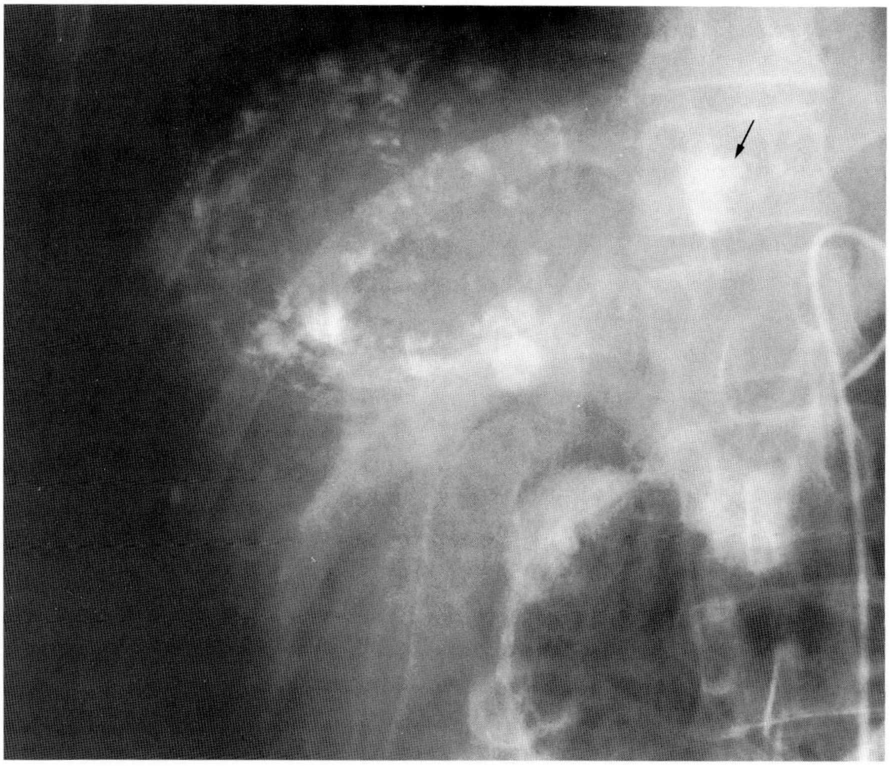

h

Hepatic hemangioma—Case 2: Massive hemangioma of the liver occupying the right lobe.

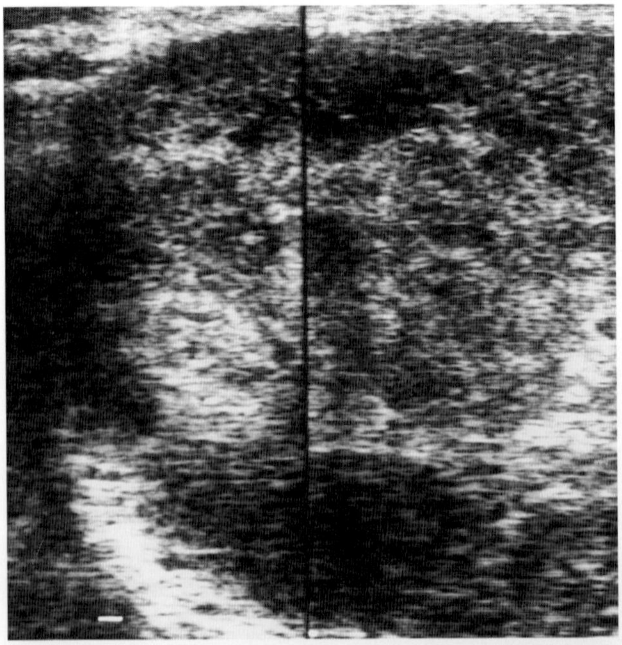

(a) US: the mass presents mixed high and low echoes. If the mass becomes so large as to occupy one whole lobe, the characteristic US features of hemangioma are not seen, and differential diagnosis from HCC is difficult.

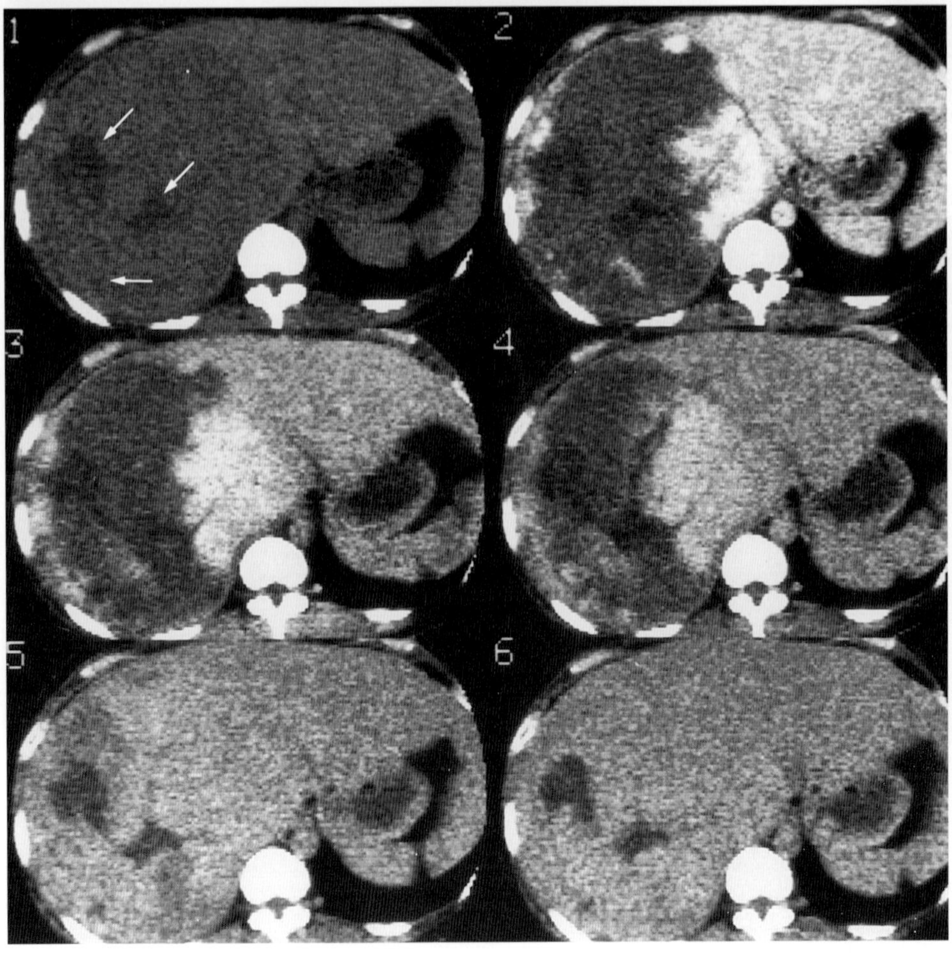

(b) Dynamic CT: on plain CT (1), a large lesion is seen occupying the entire right lobe. It has three low-density areas (→). Dynamic CT (2–6) in the same level demonstrates dense stains starting from the periphery and slowing progressing toward the center.

Case 2 (contd.)

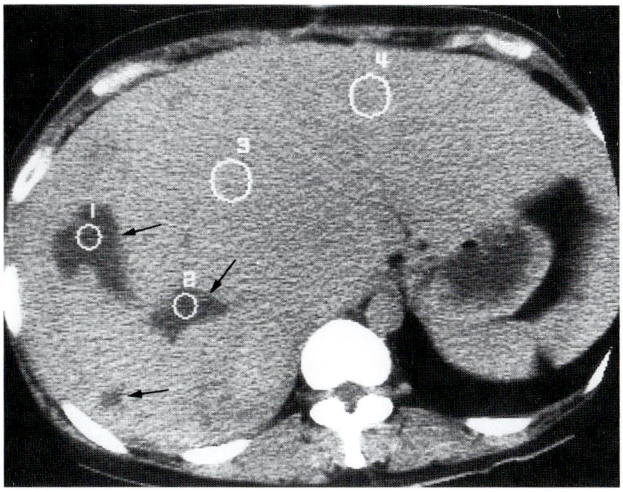

(c) CT at 15 min: the mass is now isodense showing three non-enhanced areas (→). CT values (HU) are: 1 = 36, 2 = 33, 3 (enhanced area)= 91, 4 (non-tumor area) = 84.

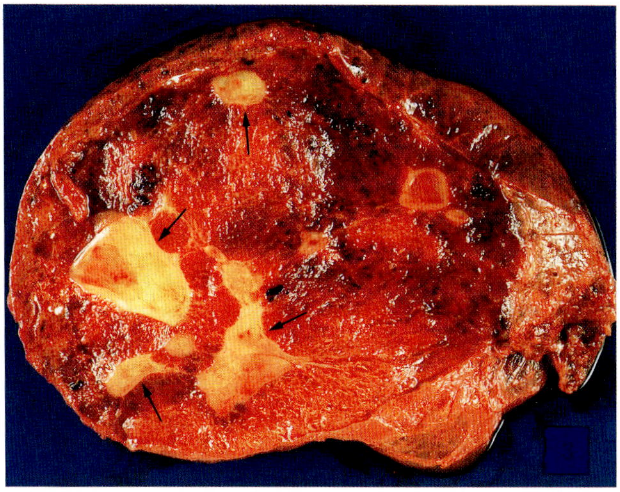

(d) Hepatic arteriogram: this shows typical cotton-wool stains. As seen on CT (b), the mass is more densely opacified in the hilar areas where blood supply is more abundant.

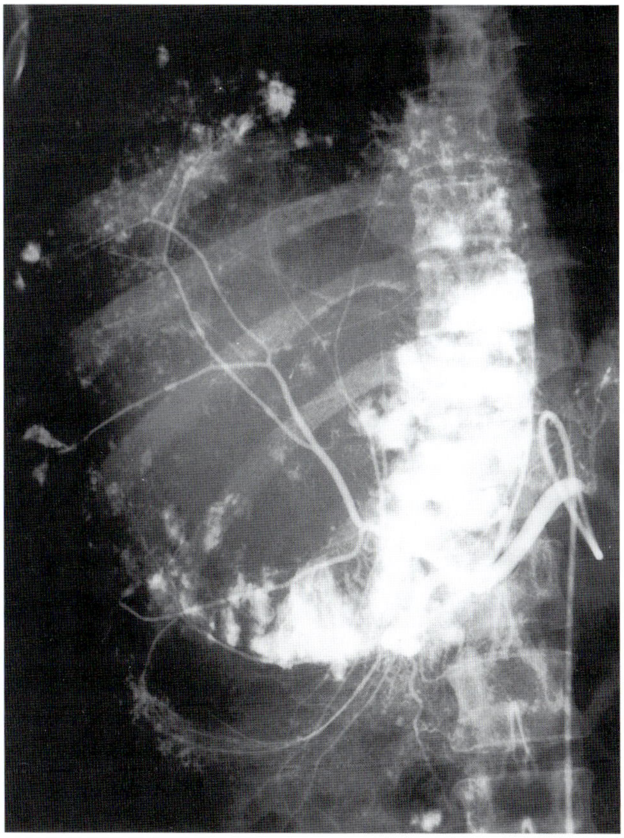

(e) Cut surface of resected specimen: extended right lobectomy was carried out (2300 g). Almost the entire right lobe was replaced by a reddish brown cavernous hemangioma which contained areas of yellowish firm organized tissue. They corresponded to the unenhanced areas on dynamic CT. Such findings are common in large hemangiomas.

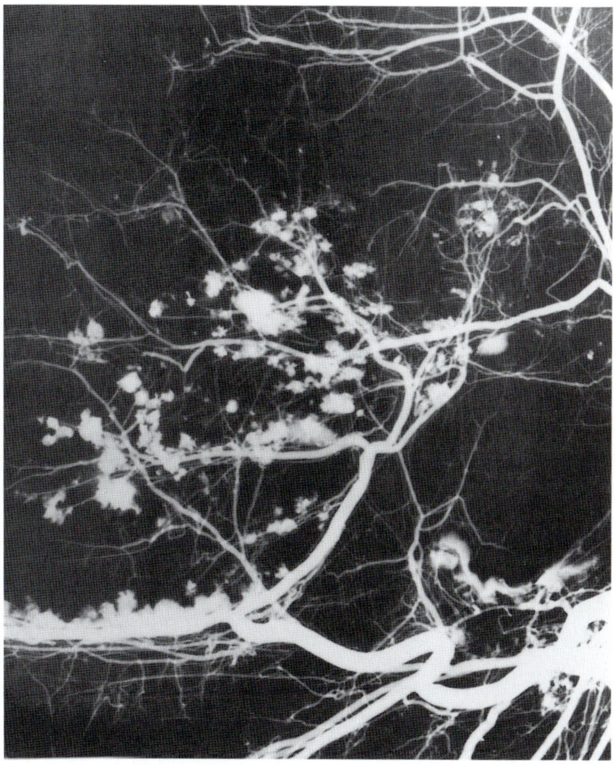

(f) Microangiogram made with the resected specimen: arterially injected barium leaking into the tumor from the peripheral arteries produced the cotton-wool appearance or multiple spots looking like babies' breath. As more barium was injected, the cotton wool expanded, confirming the angiographic interpretation.

Hepatic hemangioma—Case 4: Hemangioma which angiography failed to delineate and dynamic CT did not enhance. A 5 cm hypervascular renal cell carcinoma was found in the upper pole of the right kidney (not shown). There was an hepatic mass continuous with it.

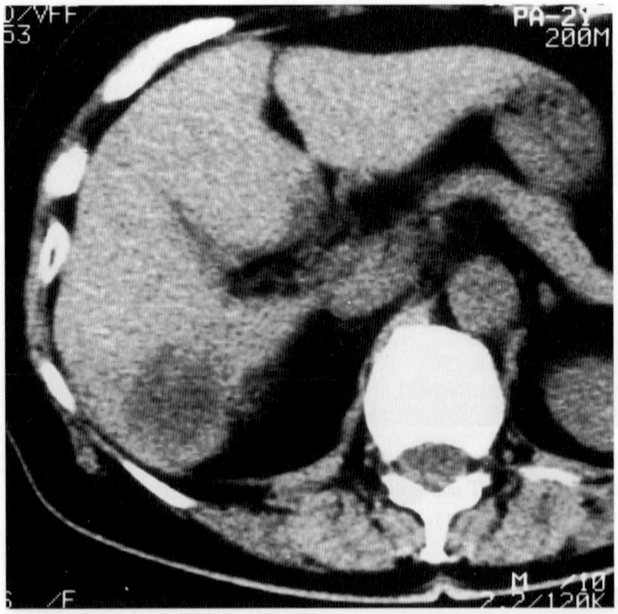

(a) Plain CT: a 4 cm low-density mass was found in S^{VI}.

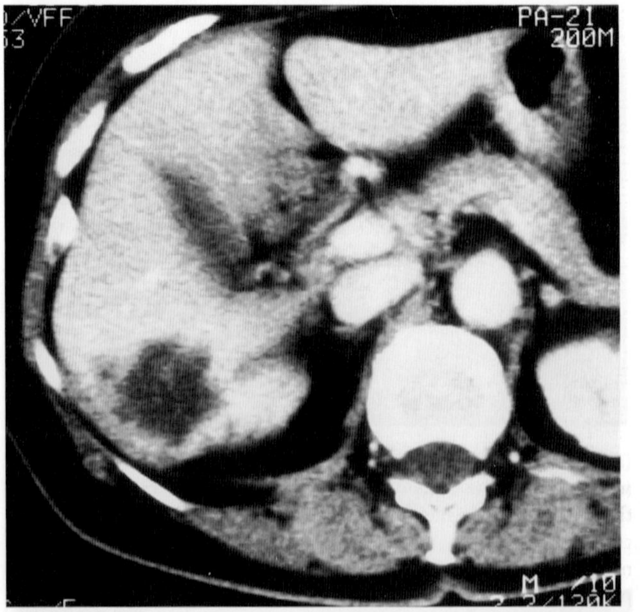

b

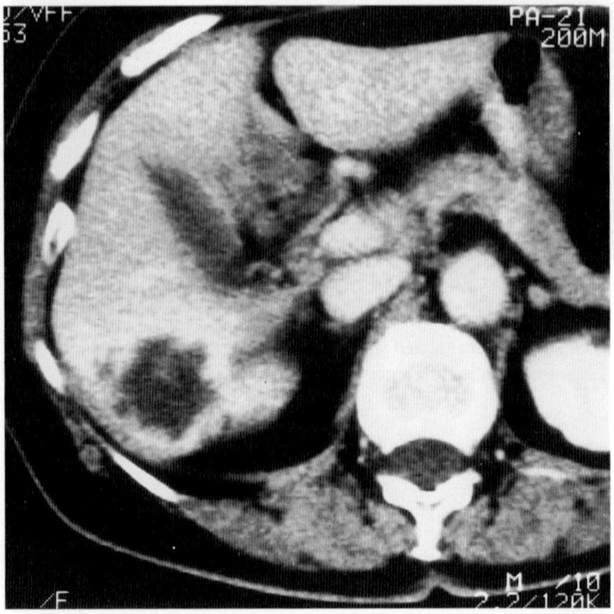

c

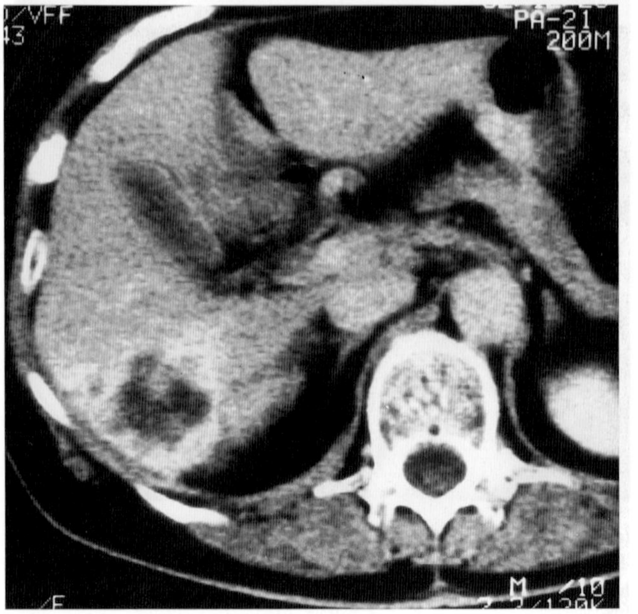

d

(b–d) Dynamic CT: dynamic CT made in the same slice barely stained the mass. CT at 8 min from contrast injection only minimally stained the lateral periphery and interior.

Case 4 (contd.)

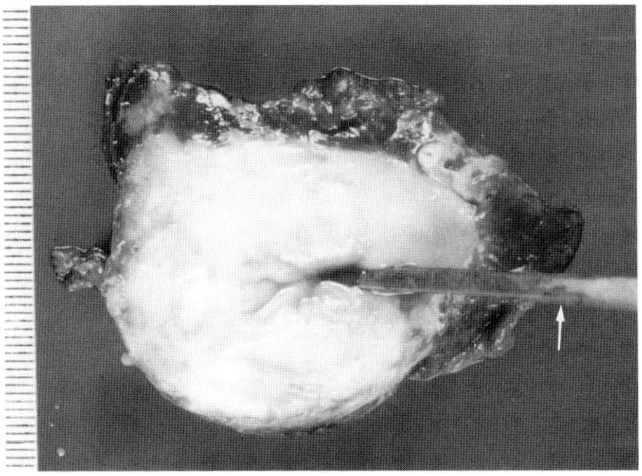

(e) Cut surface of resected tumor: following right nephrectomy, resection of S^{VI} was carried out. The cut surface was white, soft, and so elastic that a metal bar could be pushed in without penetration. There was no continuity with the renal cancer, and grossly a hamartoma was suspected.

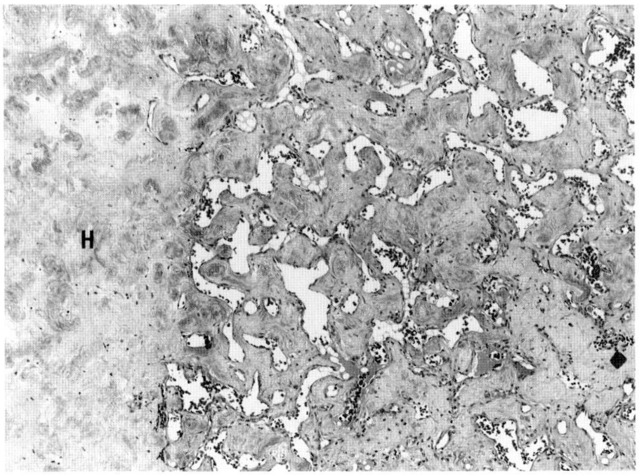

(f) Histology: a large part of the mass was hyalinized tissue (H). A small area showed a wide stroma and narrow blood spaces. The diagnosis was hemangioma.

Hepatic hemangioma—Case 5: Large hemangioma seen as multiple calcification in the right lobe.

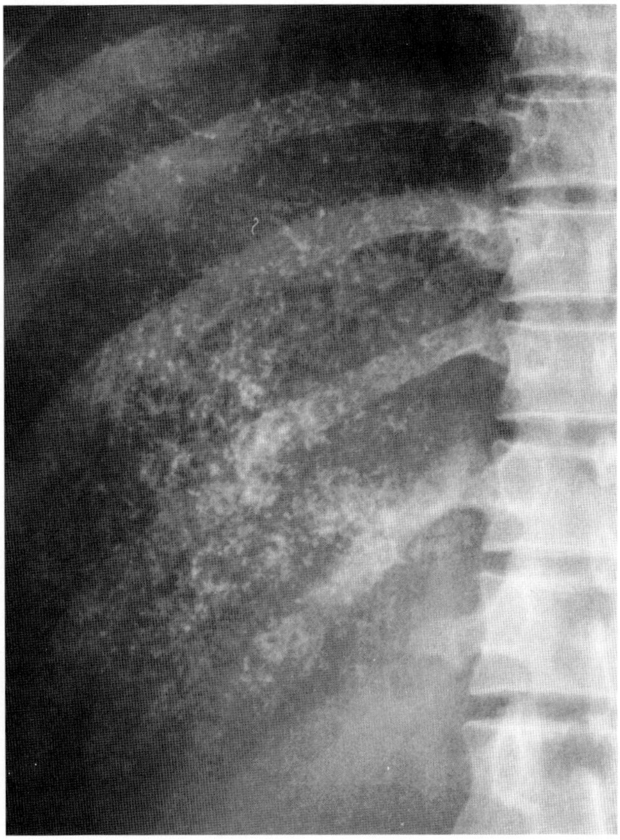

Plain roentgenogram: small dots of calcification are seen throughout the right lobe. Angiography did not produce tumor stains. Extended right lobectomy was carried out, demonstrating a huge hemangioma with fine calcific lesions within it.

Hepatic hemangioma—Case 6: Small nodular hemangioma seen by US as a mass with a halo.

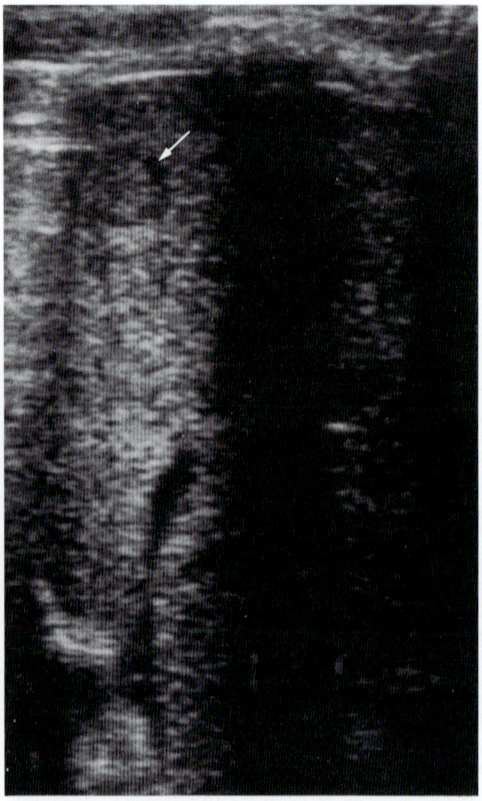

(a) US: a 1.5 cm isoechoic mass (→) that has a halo was found in S^{VIII}. The interior was mosaic, and an HCC was strongly suspected.

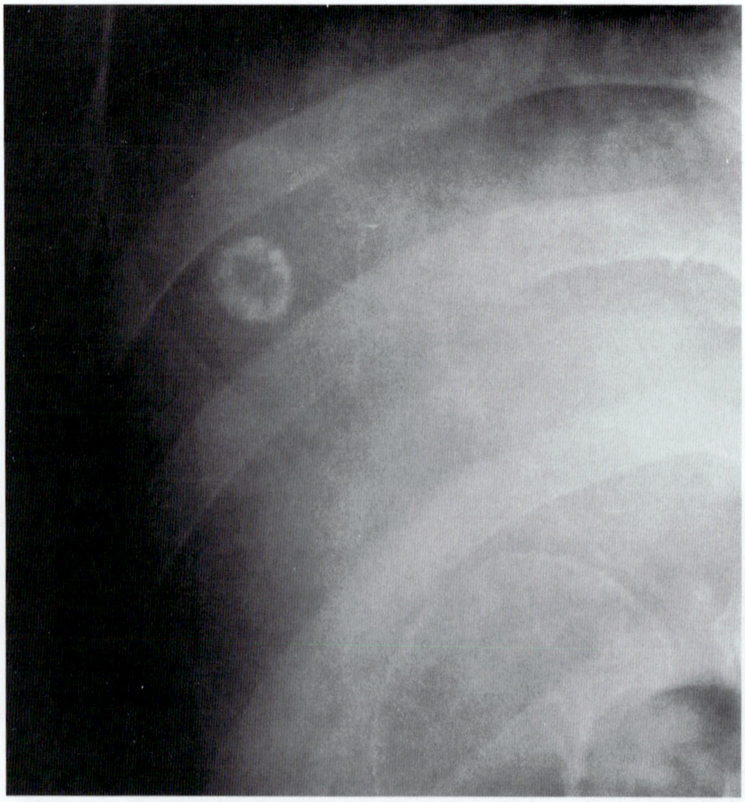

(b) Angiogram (late phase): the S^{VIII} tumor showed a ring stain typical of hemangioma, making the diagnosis likely. However, dynamic CT failed to confirm the diagnosis, and it was resected.

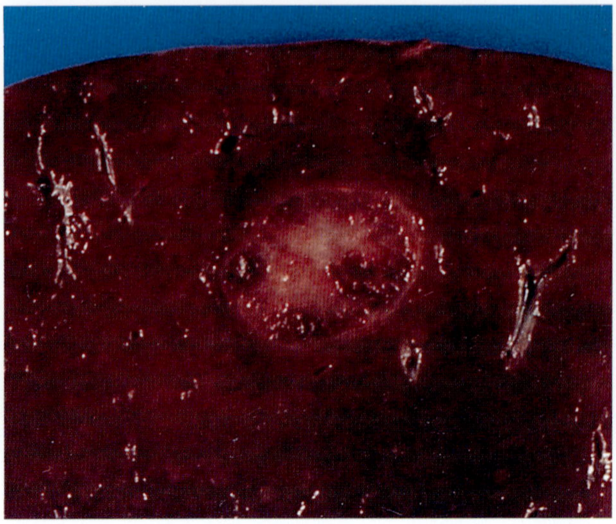

(c) Cut surface of resected specimen: the interior had dark red hemangioma tissue and the periphery was a capsule-like structure.

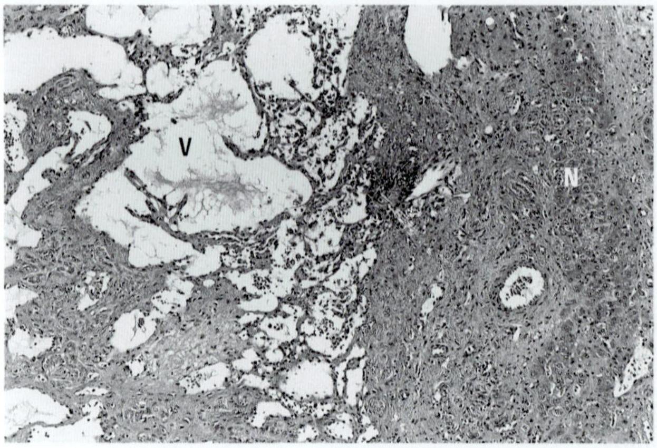

(d) Histology: hemangioma in a liver with micronodular cirrhosis. Many dilated vascular spaces and cirrhotic tissue were seen with intervening fibrous tissue. The latter was perhaps seen as a halo on US.

Hepatic hemangioma—Case 7: Diffuse type hemangioma occupying the entire liver and obstructing the portal vein.

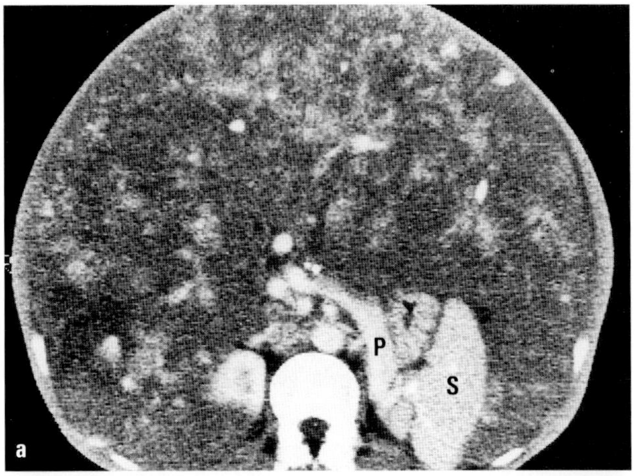

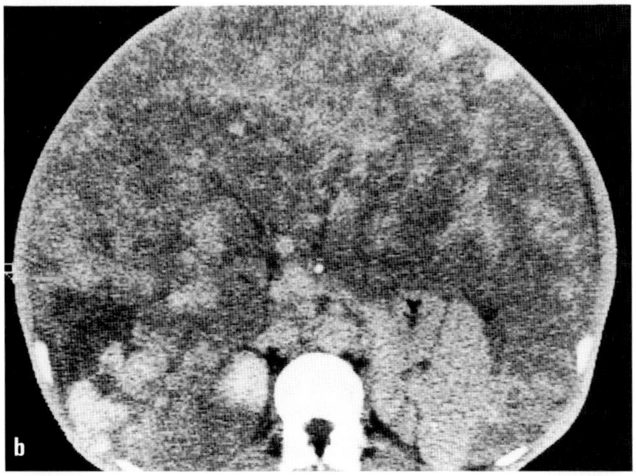

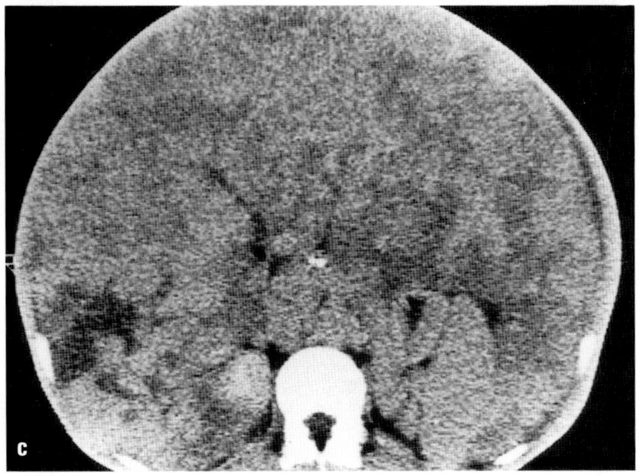

(a)–(c) Dynamic CT: a huge liver mass is occupying the entire abdomen. Early phase CT (a) shows multiple snow-flake stains, and in the late phase (b,c), these stains are slowly expanding. The pancreas (P) and spleen (S) are displaced dorsally.

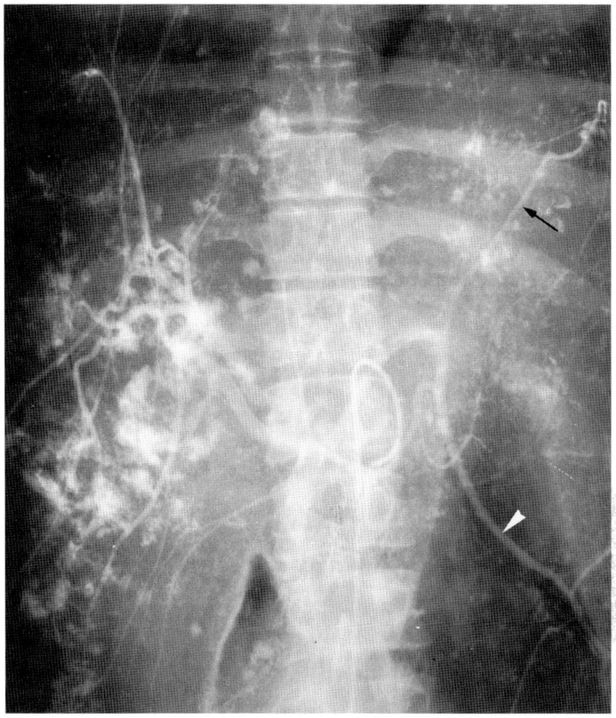

(d) Arteriogram (early phase): most lesions are in the right lobe, but there are small lesions in the other parts of the liver. The left hepatic arteries (→ A^{II}, ▶A^{III}) are wide apart in the frontal plane, suggesting compensatory hypertrophy of the left lobe.

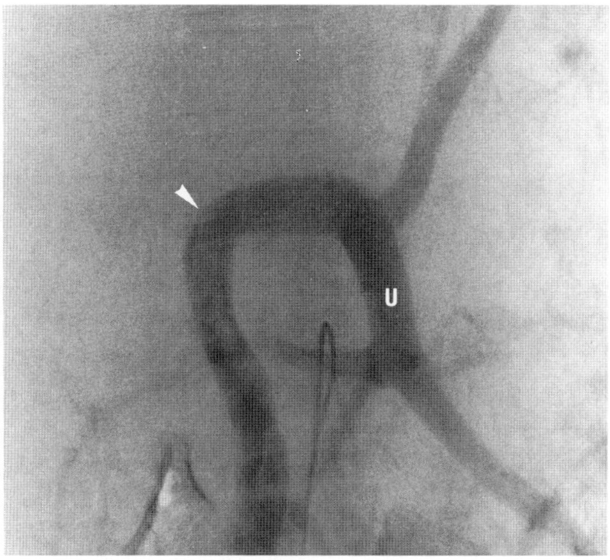

(e) Superior mesenteric arterial portogram: the right portal vein is completely occluded at its beginning (▶), and compensatory hypertrophy of the left lobe is evident. The umbilical portion (U) of the left portal vein normally seen as U-point is slanted forward due to hypertrophy.

Hepatic hemangioma—Case 8: Hemangioma seen as a hyperechoic and angiographically nodular mass that required differentiation from HCC. A 69-year-old woman. An hepatic mass was incidentally found by US.

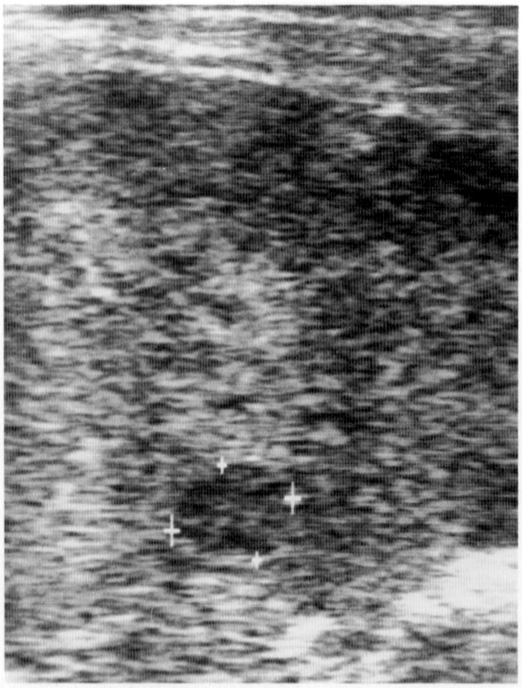

(a) US: a 2.3 cm hypoechoic mass was seen in S^{VIII} (within marks).

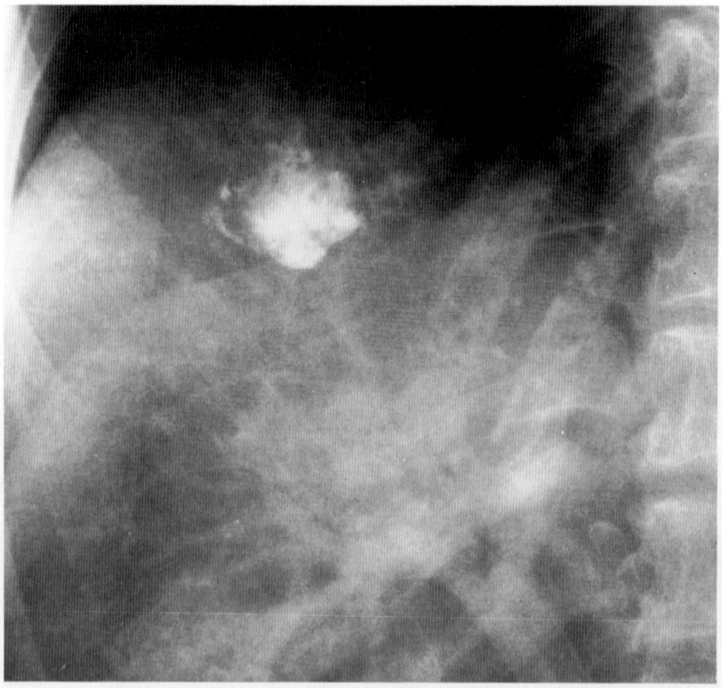

(b) Celiac arteriogram (late phase): the mass was seen as a dense nodular stain. HCC generally does not show such a strong stain, and is rather seen as a light stain in the late phase. A hemangioma with large vascular spaces was the diagnosis. The tumor size did not change during follow-up.

Hepatic hemangioma—Case 9: Hemangioma with a high echo ring in its periphery. A 55-year-old man. A mass was discovered at the annual medical examination.

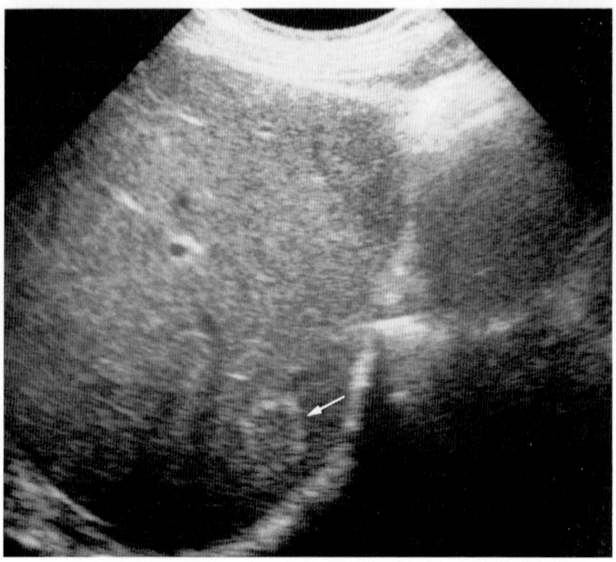

US (right subcostal scan): a typical 2.8 cm hemangioma with a hyperechoic irregular border (→) was found in S^{VII}. Dynamic CT demonstrated typical features of hemangioma.

Hepatic hemangioma—Case 10: Hemangioma for which quality diagnosis by US was difficult due to fatty liver. A 51-year-old woman with a history of operation for rectum carcinoma. US examination demonstrated a mass in the liver. Metastasis was suspected.

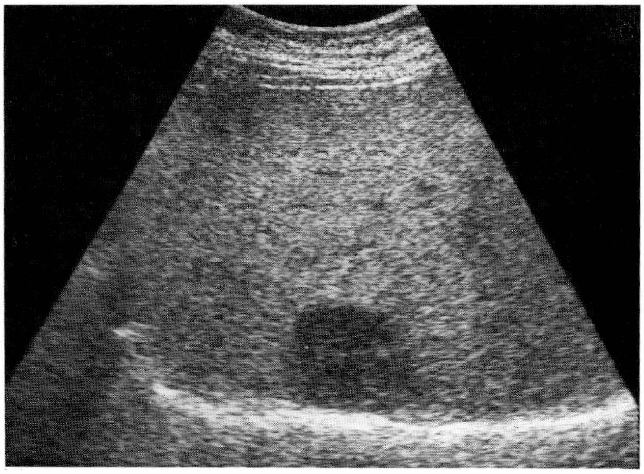

(a) US (right subcostal scan): a hypoechoic mass was found immediately below the diaphragm. Liver parenchyma is echogenic and white due to fat.

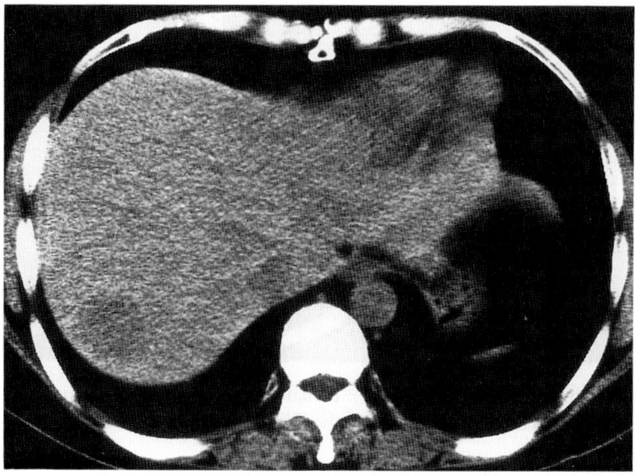

(b) Plain CT: a mass of homogeneously low density was seen in $S^{VII-VIII}$. Mild steatosis was an additional finding.

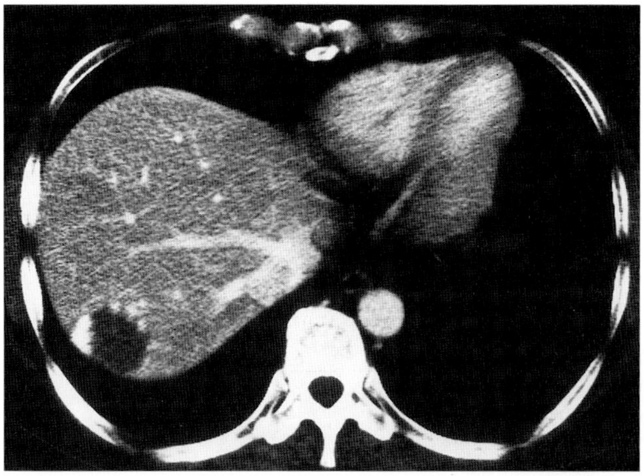

(c) Dynamic CT (early phase): this mass was densely stained from the periphery.

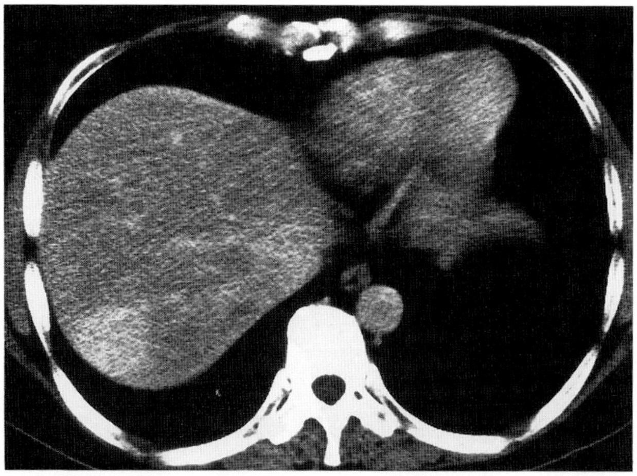

(d) Dynamic CT (late phase, 6 min): the entire mass was seen enhanced, presenting a typical feature of hemangioma. The difference in density was exaggerated in this case because of the parenchymal fat.

Case 13 (contd.)

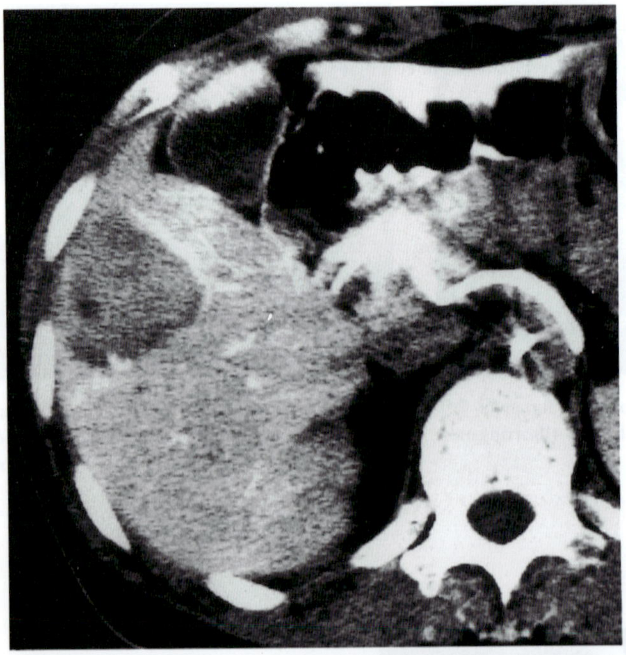

(c) Hepatic arterial-CT: hepatic arteriography failed to clearly demonstrate the mass, necessitating arterial-CT. It only stained an artery in the periphery and liver parenchyma, but the tumor interior was not stained at all.

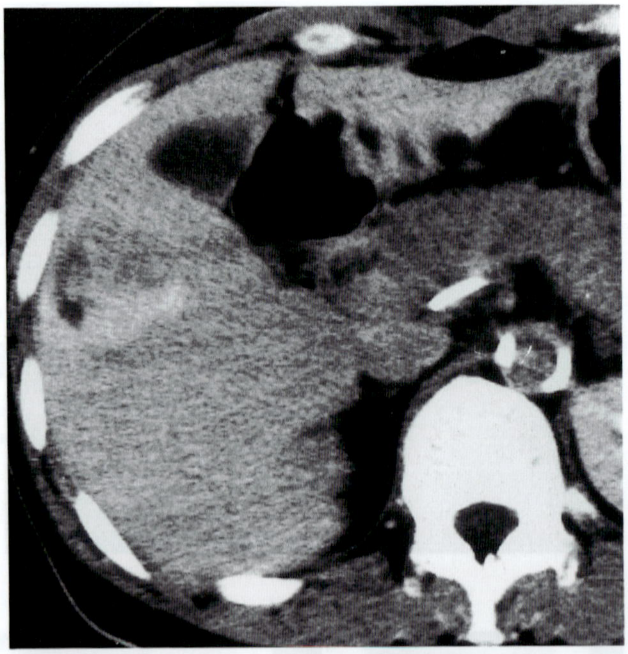

(d) Arterial-CT (30 min later): after 30 min from (c), the lower half of the mass was enhanced. In retrospect, this finding was strongly suggestive of hemangioma. Some of the other CT images showed peripheral low densities, suggesting primary or secondary adenocarcinoma.

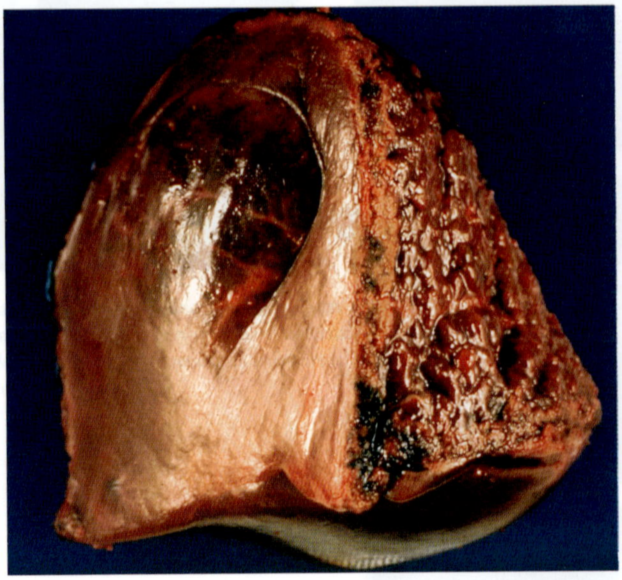

(e) Surface of resected specimen: opening the abdomen, a spherical protruding dark reddish mass was recognized in region S^V. Partial resection of S^V was carried out. The tumor surface was soft and bulging.

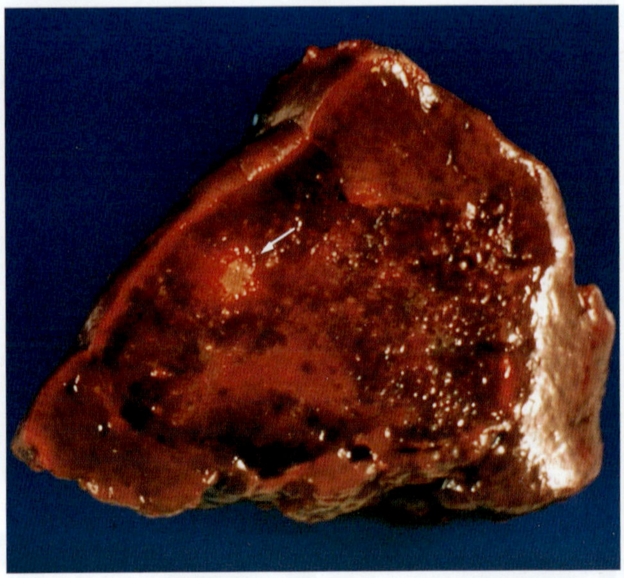

(f) Cut surface of specimen: the cut surface was grossly typical of hemangioma, and histologically as well. The well-demarcated area in the center (→) seen as a spot on imaging was hyalinized.

Hepatic hemangioma—Case 14: Hemangioma in the caudate lobe for which quality diagnosis was hampered by earlier Lipiodol injection. This patient was given Lipiodol intra-arterially at another hospital. The right and left sides of the caudate lobe was occupied by a 6 × 5 cm mass with retained Lipiodol (▶).

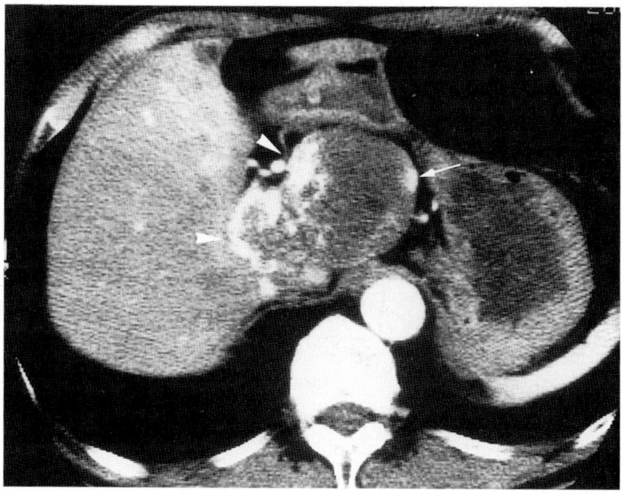

(a) Dynamic CT (early phase): there is a dense spot of contrast retention in the left margin of the mass (→).

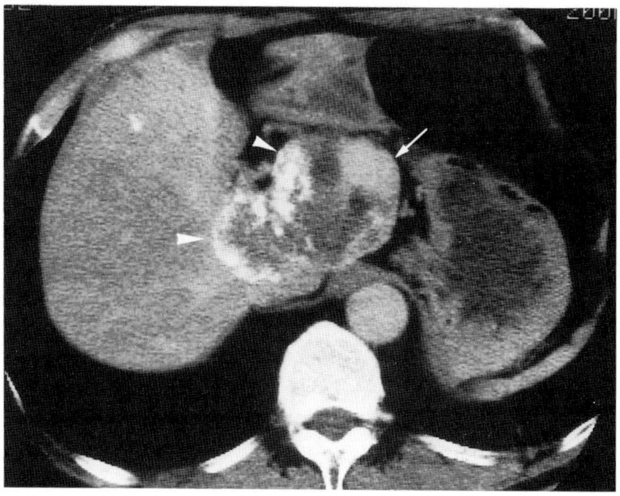

(b) Dynamic CT (late phase): from this spot, staining slowly proceeded toward the interior making a diagnosis of hemangioma possible.

Hepatic hemangioma—Case 15: Hemangioma retaining arterially administered Lipiodol for more than a year.

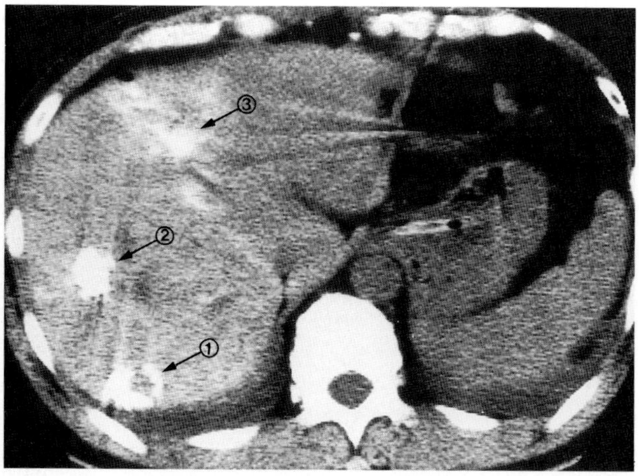

(a) Plain CT: CT image 7 days after arterial injection of Lipiodol. Lipiodol retention is seen in 3 areas: 1, S^{VII}; 2, S^{VIII}; 3, S^{IV}.

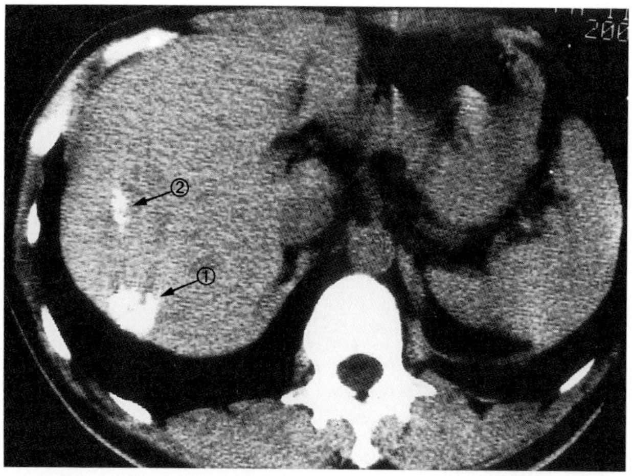

(b)Plain CT (1.5 years later): Some Lipiodol is still present in area 1, but has disappeared in area 3. Area 2 has lost most of its Lipiodol.

Hepatic hemangioma—Case 16: Hemangioma with an arterio-portal fistula.

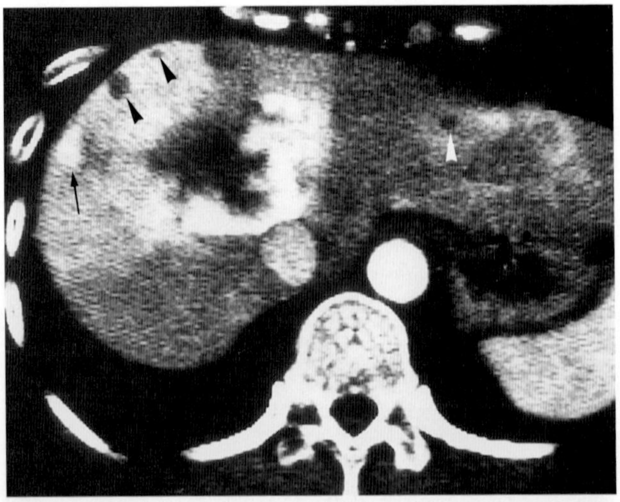

(a) Dynamic CT (early phase): this large mass occupying S^{VIII}–S^{IV} was enhanced in its periphery and some inner parts; a less dense stain was seen in the periphery in a fan-like shape. The interior of the mass was not yet stained. Another hemangioma (→) and several cysts (▶) are additional findings.

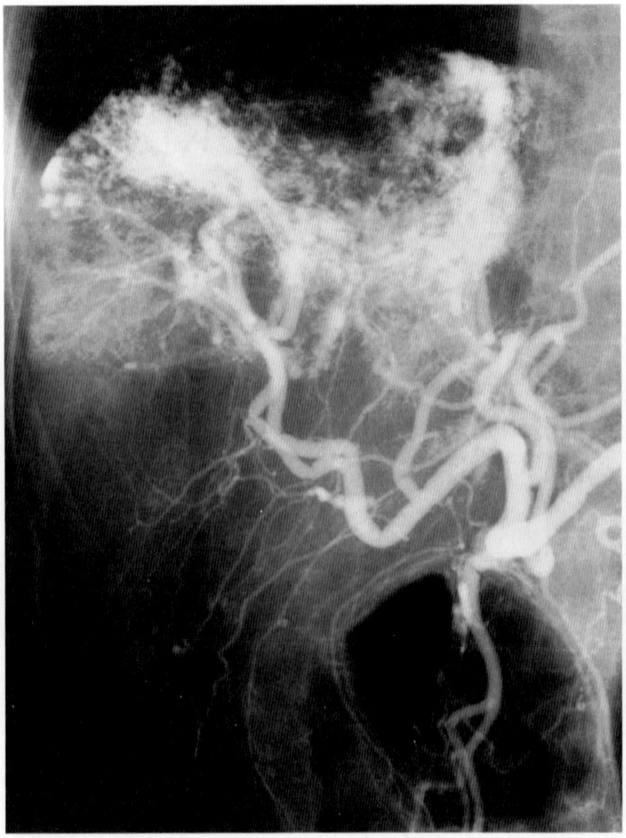

(b) Angiogram (early phase): cotton-wool appearance and opacification of the portal vein accompanying an artery are evident (arterio-portal shunt).

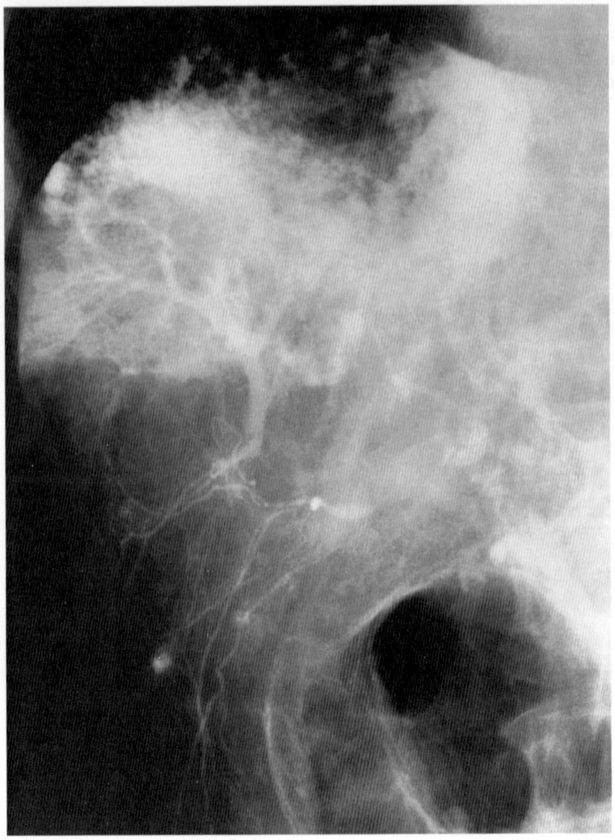

(c) Angiogram (late phase): the portal vein is opacified further proximally toward the hilum, and the liver parenchyma supplied by that portal branch has received the contrast material.

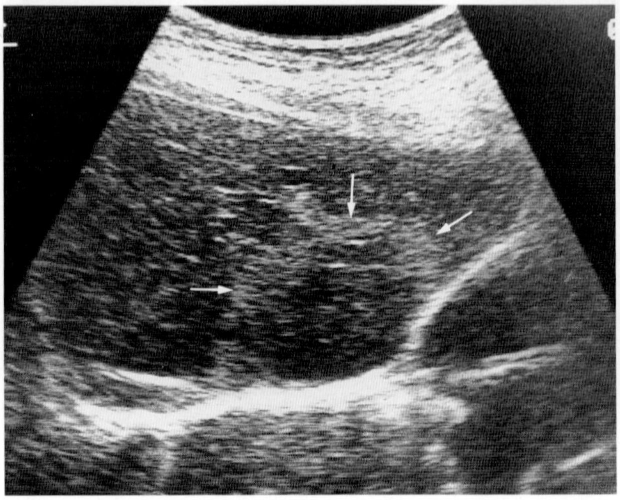

(d) US: it is not easy to measure the size of a mass in the presence of arterio-portal communication on CT, but US permits accurate measurement (→) (6 × 5 cm) because the arterio-portal shunt is not

Hepatic hemangioma—Case 17: Hemangioma containing a fluid necessitating differentiation from sarcoma.

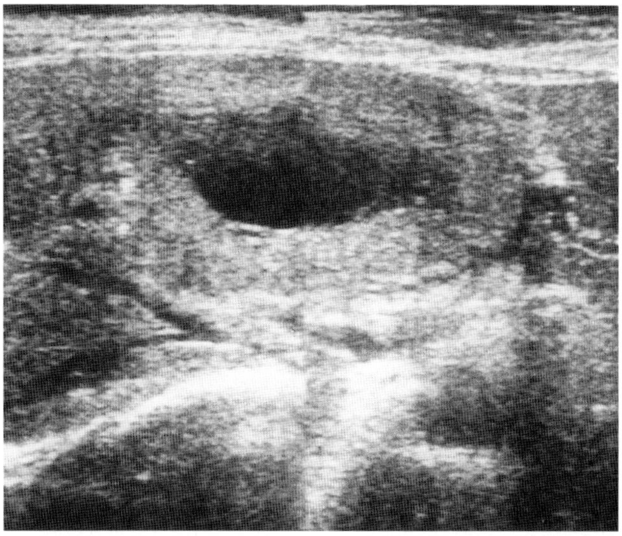

(a) US (transverse scan): a spheroidal isoechoic mass is seen in S^{IV}. The interior is free of echo with posterior echo enhancement, suggesting a mass containing a fluid.

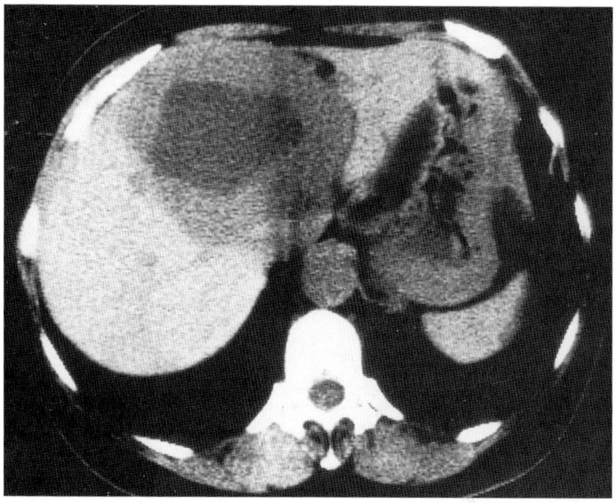

(b) Plain CT: a low-density mass with an interior having the density of water is recognized.

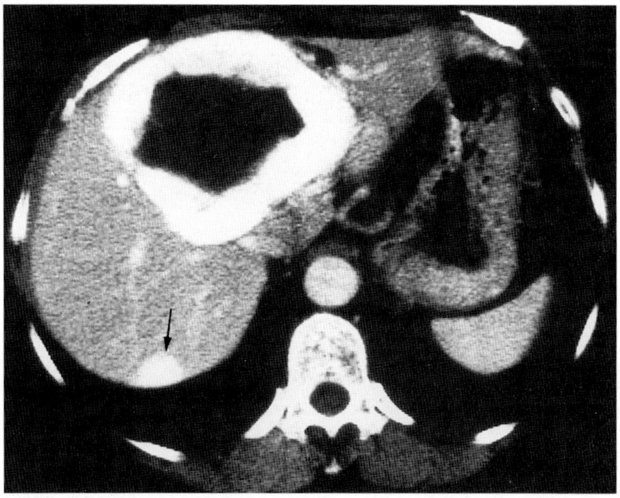

(c) Dynamic CT (early phase): the whole mass except the interior was enhanced quickly. Another small enhanced lesion is recognized (→) in S^{VII}.

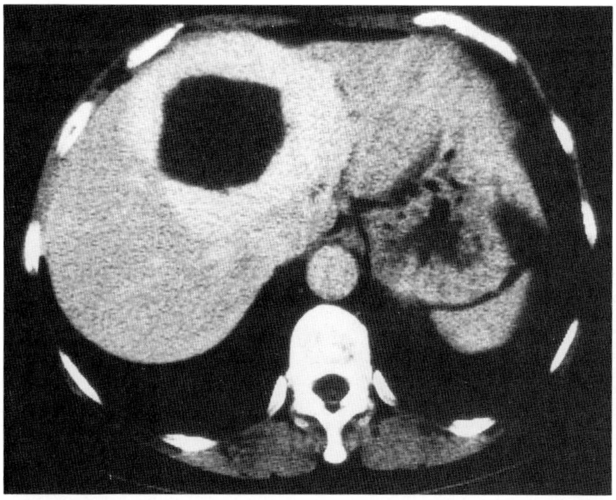

(d) Dynamic CT (late phase, 5 min): the mass still retains some contrast. The lesion in S^{VII} has become isodense, a finding compatible with the CT of hemangioma.

Case 17 (contd.)

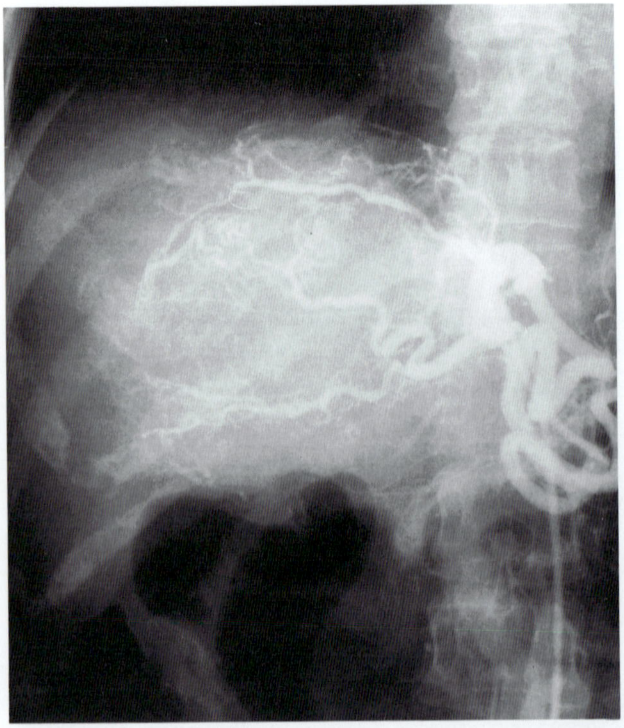

(e) Left hepatic arteriogram (early phase): dilated arteries and some neovascularization are seen.

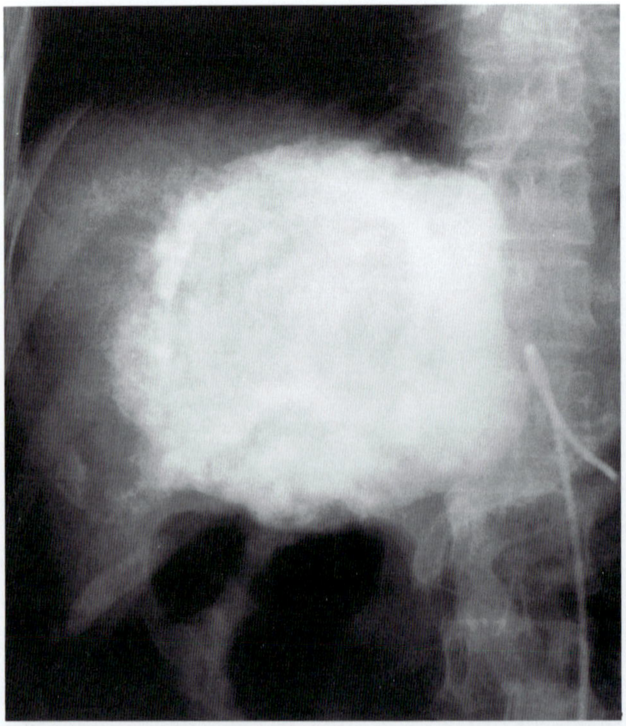

(f) Left hepatic arteriogram (late phase): homogeneous tumor stain with a less intensely stained center. The right half of the mass is supplied by the right hepatic artery replaced from the superior mesenteric artery. Angiography made from this artery yielded the same finding.

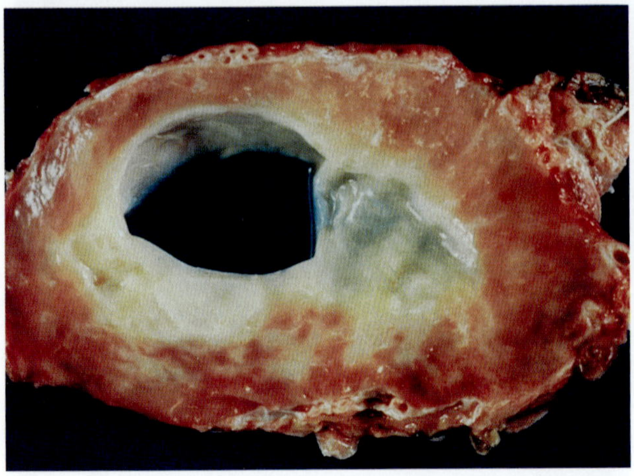

(g) Section of resected specimen: on cutting the mass, a light yellow fluid came out. The mass had a central cavity and the surrounding portion of the tumor was soft.

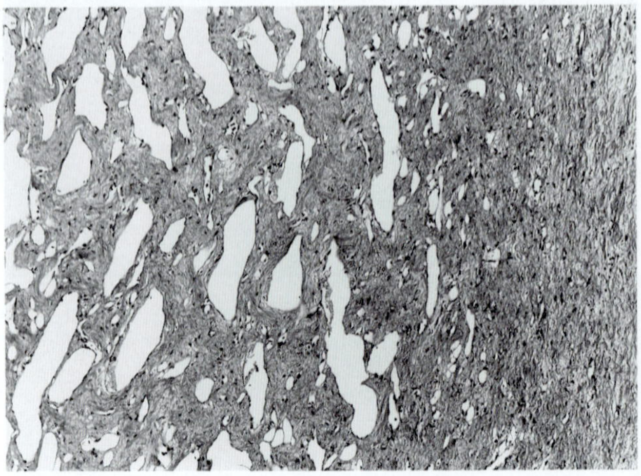

(h) Histology: typical cavernous hemangioma (left side). Vascular spaces as they moved toward the center (right) became smaller, and then turned to fibrous tissue to surround the cavity that contained fluid.

Hepatic hemangioma—Case 18: Shrinking of a hemangioma by irradiation that also induced atrophy of liver parenchyma. A 49-year-old man. A total dose of 3450 rad was given to a diffuse hemangioma that occupied the entire liver.

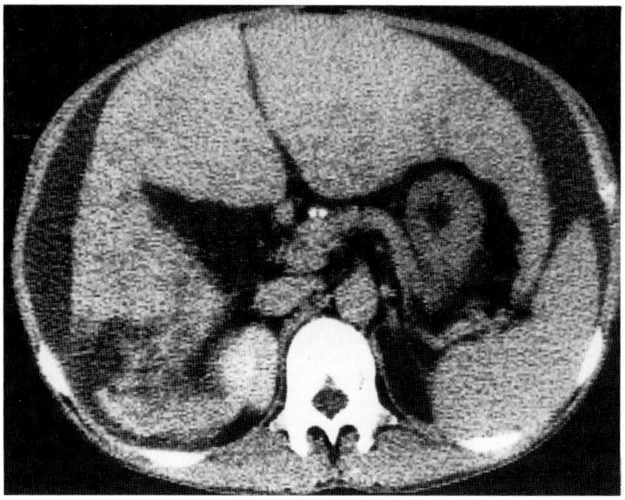

Enhanced CT: CT made 1 year and 7 months after the irradiation. The mass that occupied the entire abdomen has shrunk remarkably, and there is no more compression on the surrounding organs. However, the patient developed ascites and splenomegaly, and bled from esophageal varices. It is likely that marked atrophy of the liver with normal histology (fibrosis?) and tumor reduction have caused portal hypertension (same as Case 7, p.63).

Hepatic hemangioma—Case 19: Hepatic hemangioma that has been markedly reduced in size following transcatheter arterial embolization (TAE). A 48-year-old woman. An upper abdominal mass was found by a physician whom she visited because of abdominal discomfort.

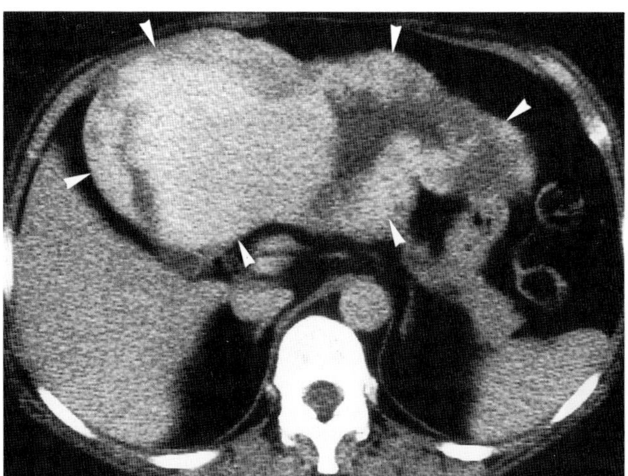

(a) CT before arterial embolization (TAE): an 18 cm hemangioma (longest axis) is seen occupying the entire left lobe (▶). Transcatheter arterial embolization was carried out from the left hepatic artery using Gelfoam sponge particles.

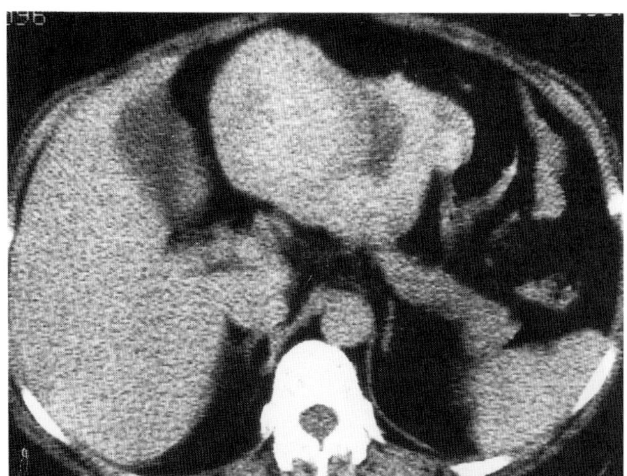

(b) CT 3 months after TAE: the hemangioma in the left lobe has been reduced in size (10 cm) with improvement of complaints.

3.3 Hepatocellular adenoma

Hepatocellular adenoma (HCA) (Fig. 3.2) is a benign tumor derived from the hepatocyte, most common in middle aged women. Unlike focal nodular hyperplasia (FNH), it is closely associated with the use of oral contraceptives (Edmondson *et al.* 1976; Rooks *et al.* 1979). Some patients are rushed to hospital because of shock caused by spontaneous bleeding into the free abdominal cavity or into the tumor. With progress in imaging diagnosis, patients with incidentally discovered HCA are now seen in increasing numbers. Surgery is positively recommended in many institutions because differentiation from HCC by imaging is not always certain; even with histological examination the differential diagnosis is difficult, it readily bleeds, and it may also have a malignant potential (Kerlin *et al.* 1983).

Whereas HCA is frequently associated with contraceptives in the western countries, pill-associated HCA is very uncommon in Japan where women have no legal access to oral contraceptives (spontaneous HCA).

Gross appearance

As evident from the cut surface (Case 1), the interior is homogeneous unlike HCC which is often mosaic. One-third of the cases may show a rim by MR imgaing, but it is not a true capsule (fibrous capsule composed of poorly cellular collagenous connective tissue) according to Arrivé *et al.* (1994). However, none of the three HCAs we studied had a true capsule.

Imaging features

Imaging features reflect the gross picture. The lesion has homogeneous internal echoes on US and homogeneous dense staining on angiography; irregularly winding dilated vessels commonly seen in HCC are not present. On dynamic CT, the time-related stain pattern of HCA is somewhat similar to that of HCC, but it lacks the nodule-in-nodule structure.

Some HCAs have a high fat content, creating a problem in differential diagnosis from hemangioma and lipoma, or even from HCC with a high fat content. US does not contribute much to making such a distinction.

There are conflicting reports on the uptake of radiocolloid by adenoma. Most studies showed photon deficiency on ^{99m} Tc colloid, but in one study (Lubbers *et al.* 1987) 3 of 13 cases took up the colloid. Kupffer cells were present in all these cases as studied histochemically. Adenoma takes up ^{99m}Tc-*n*-pyridoxyl-5-methyltryptophan (PMT) suggesting that it is a tumor derived from hepatocytes. However, some HCCs and focal nodular hyperplasias (FNH) behave similarly, and radionuclide imaging alone is not sufficient for differential diagnosis. Hemorrhage at different stages and fatty changes result in a varying intensity of MR images. In a large series of patients with hepatic adenoma, the lesion was mainly demonstrated as a hyperintense mass (59–77 per cent) on T1-weighted images and a hyperintense one (67–74 per cent) on T2-weighted images (Arrivé *et al.* 1994; Paulson *et al.* 1994). Fatty changes of the lesion have been suggested as the reason for hyperintensity of hepatic adenoma on T1-weighted images (Paulson *et al.* 1994). The capsule is demonstrated as a hypointense ring on T1-weighted images. The frequency of the lesion being shown as hypointensity on T2-weighted images is very low (Gabata *et al.* 1990; Arrivé *et al.* 1994). Hepatic adenoma is well enhanced by Gd-DTPA.

Differential diagnosis of HCA from HCC is difficult using MR imaging alone, because both tumors have hemorrhage, fatty changes, and a capsule around the lesion. HCC is much more frequently associated with cirrhosis and seropositivity for HBsAg or anti-HCV antibodies than is adenoma.

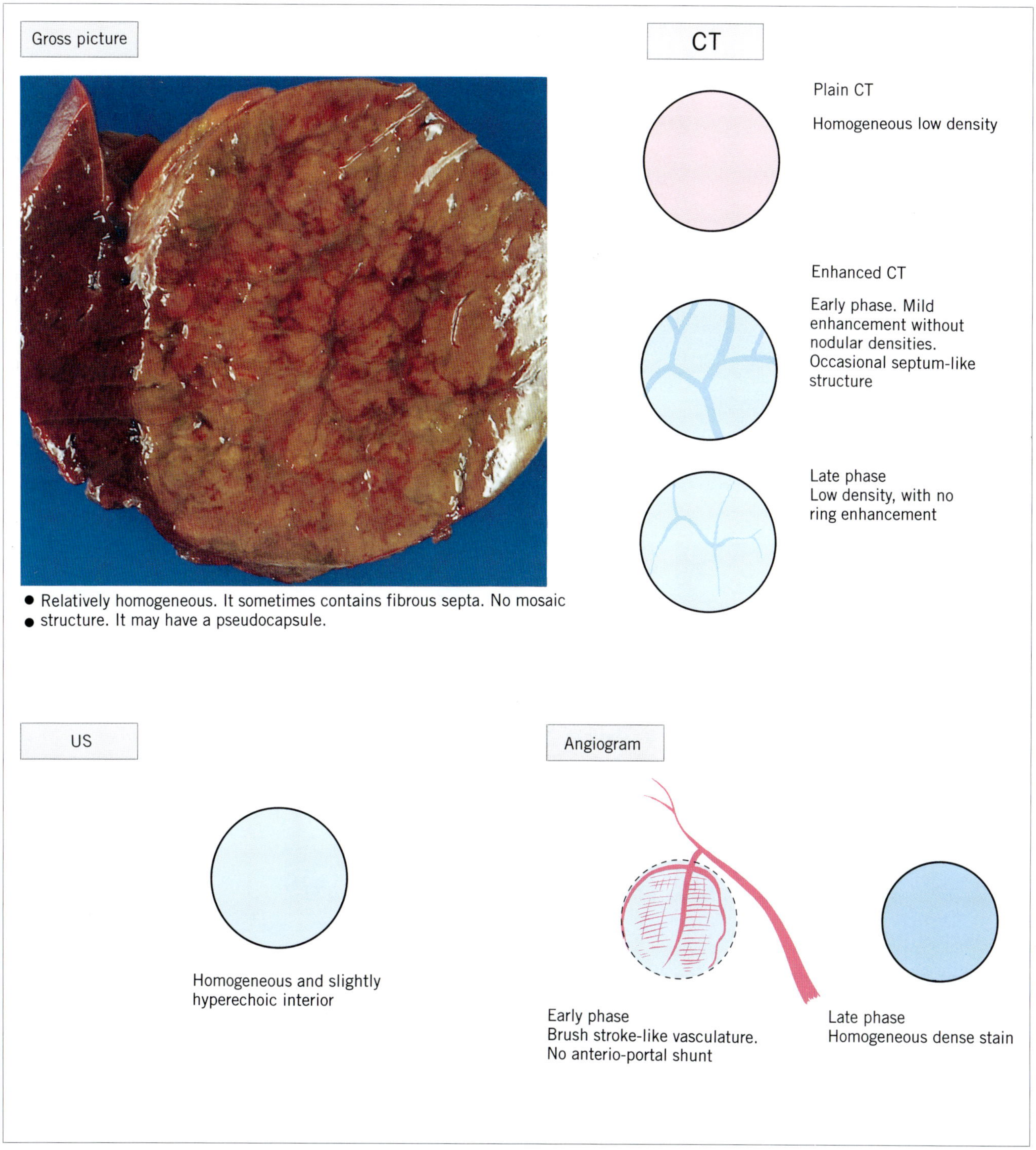

Fig. 3.2 Imaging features of hepatocellular adenoma.

Hepatocellular adenoma—Case 1: Radionuclide scanning was useful in differential diagnosis. A 41-year-old woman. AFP (−), HBsAg (−), normal liver tests, no oral contraceptive use.

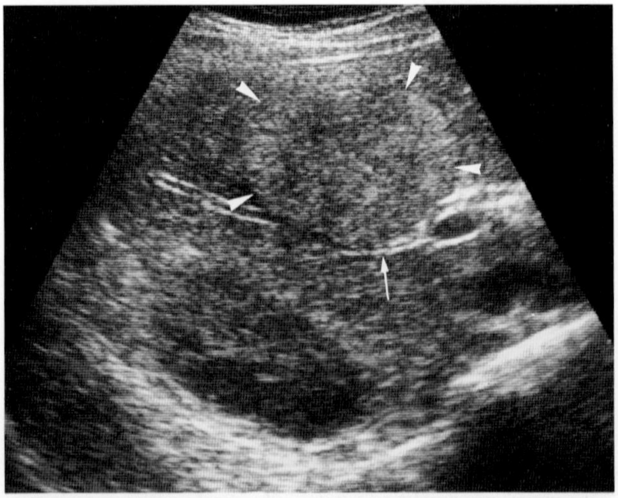

(a) US (right subcostal scan): an 8 cm mass is seen in S^{V} that has slightly increased echoes in the periphery and an isoechoic interior (▶). There is no halo or a mosaic interior pattern. The portal tract (→) in S^{VI} is shifted dorsally due to compression by the mass.

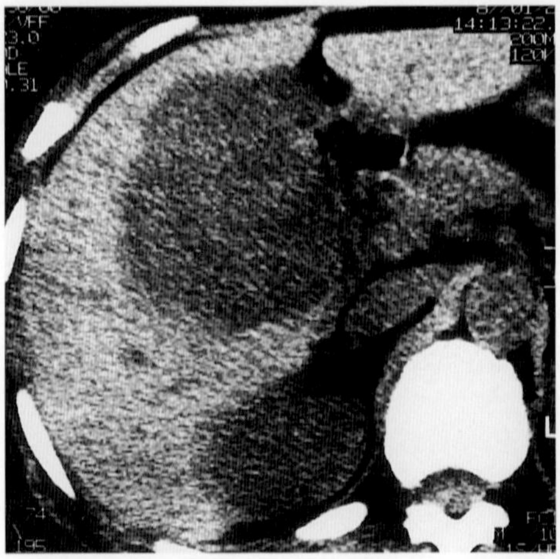

b

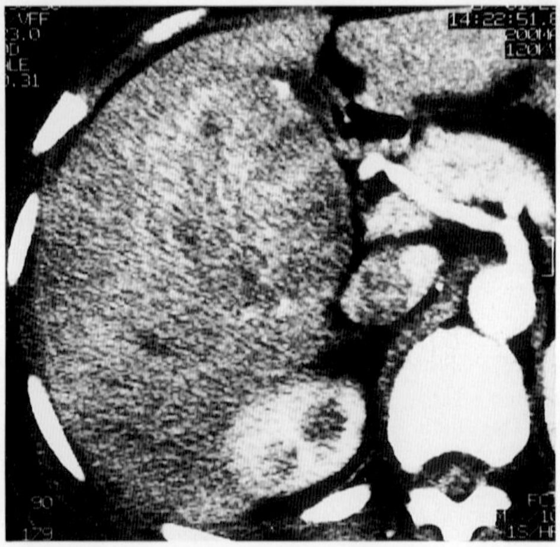

c

(b) Plain CT: the mass is seen as a lesion of homogeneous low density.

(c) Dynamic CT (early phase): the mass is isodense except for several areas of increased density.

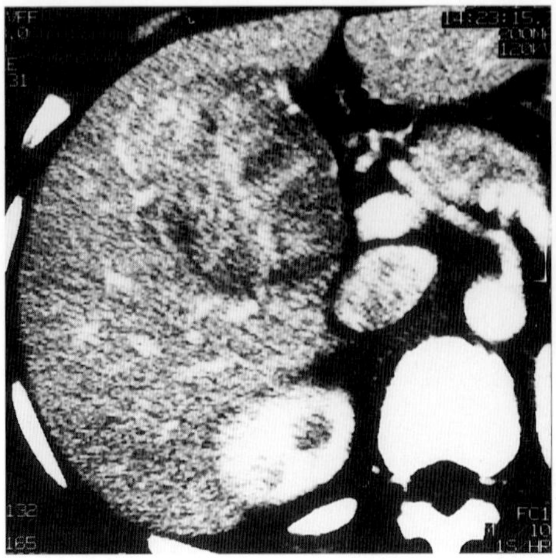

d

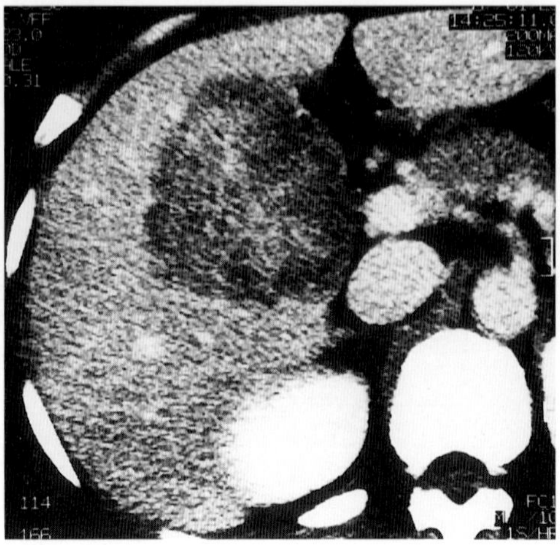

e

(d) Dynamic CT (slightly delayed phase): stellate high densities in the interior.

(e) Dynamic CT (late phase): the whole mass has turned hypodense, but no ring enhancement is seen.

Case 1 (contd.)

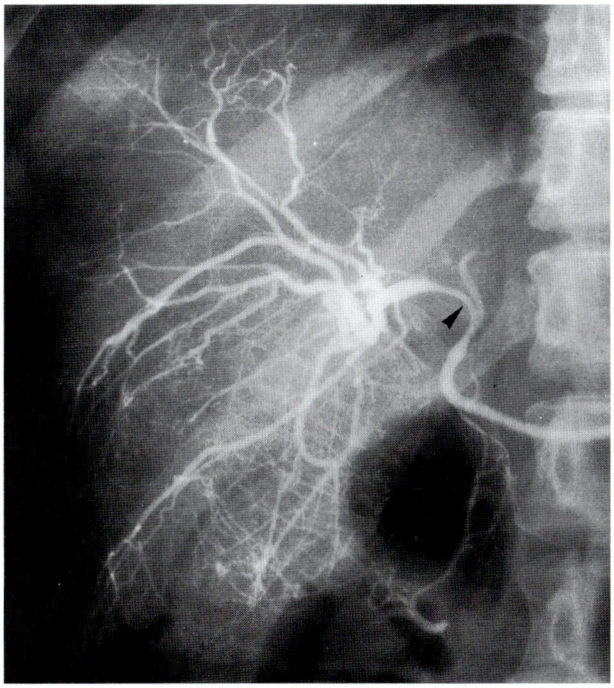

(f) Hepatic angiogram (early phase): many fine tumor vessels looking like a brush-stroke are seen in the area supplied by S^V arteries. (▶), angiospasm due to catheterization.

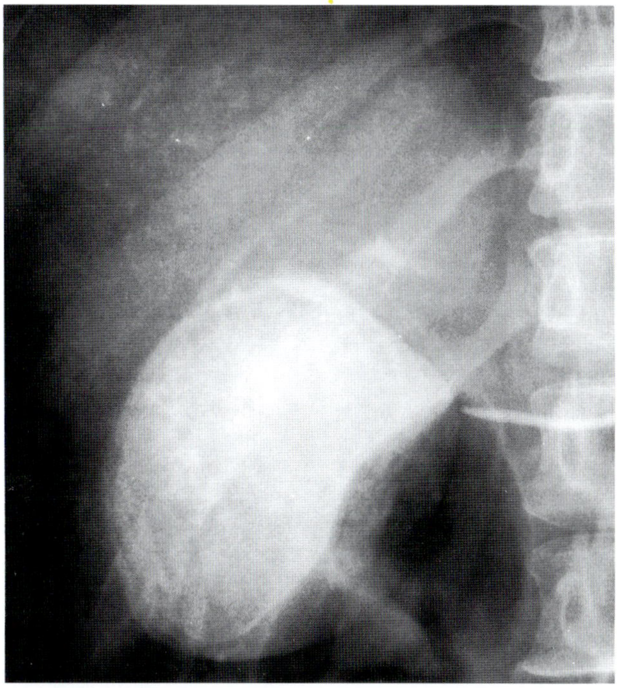

(g) Hepatic angiogram (late phase): the whole mass is homogeneously stained. There is no arterio-portal shunt or tumor thrombus.

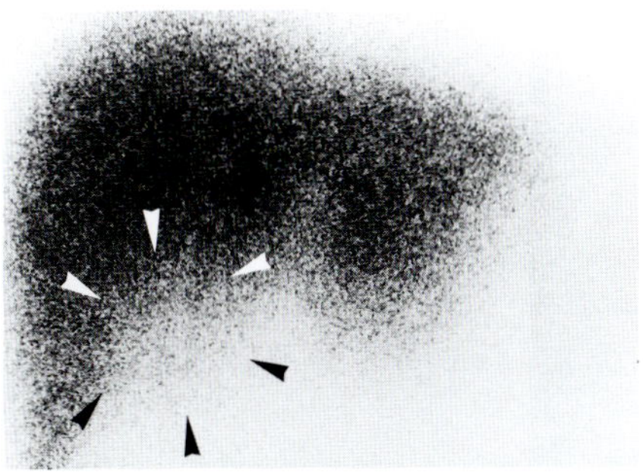

(h) ^{99m}Tc-phytate scintiscan: the mass in S^V is seen as a cold area (▶).

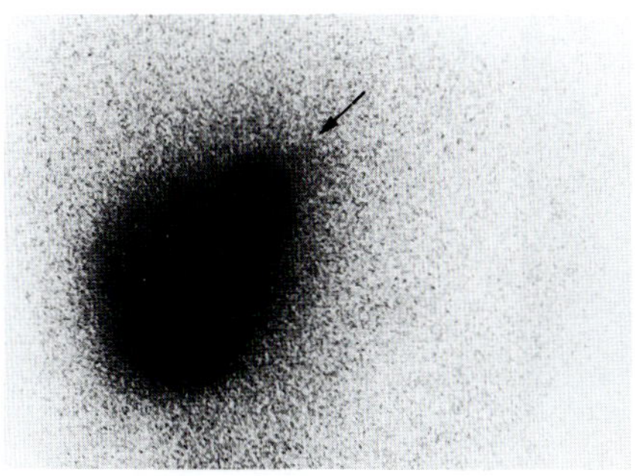

(i) ^{99m}Tc-PMT scintiscan (late phase): the mass is seen as a hot area. Due to the nuclide excreted into the gallbladder, the shape of the tumor is distorted (→).

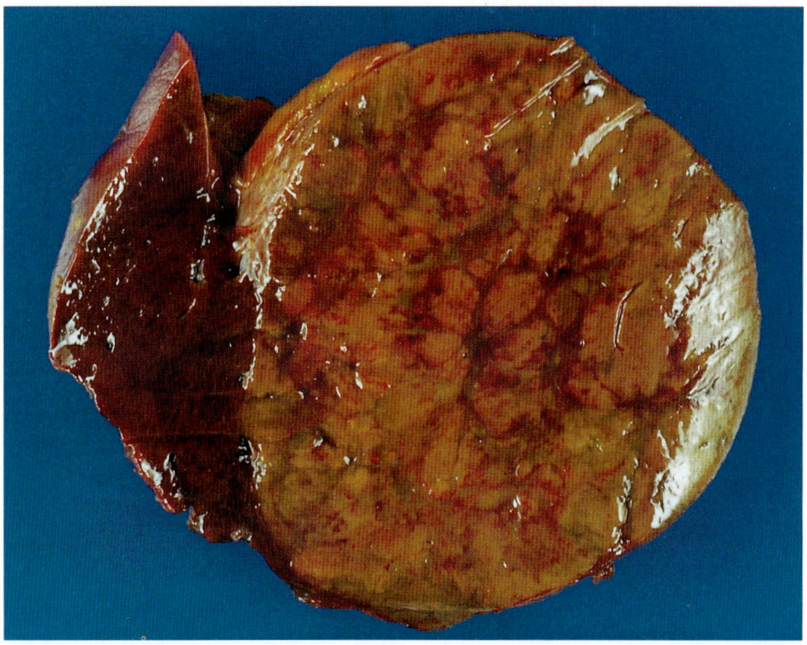

(j) Cut surface of the mass: opening the abdomen, a hemispherical mass was seen protruding from the inferior surface of the right liver, and a partial resection including S^V and S^{VI} was carried out. The cut surface was reddish brown showing a relatively homogeneous interior. In the center, thin fibrous tissues were separating nodular parenchymal tissues, and there were bleeding areas. Histologically, there were no portal tracts in the tumor nor a covering capsule. It lacked a malignant feature, and the diagnosis was 'hepatocellular adenoma with normal parenchyma'.

Hepatocellular adenoma—Case 2: Adenoma containing fat, first diagnosed as a hemangioma by US, but was resected as it grew in size. A 26-year-old man. US found an incidental hepatic mass (8 mm). It was followed as a hepatic hemangioma. The tumor grew to 32 mm in 19 months. AFP (−), HBsAg (−), normal liver tests.

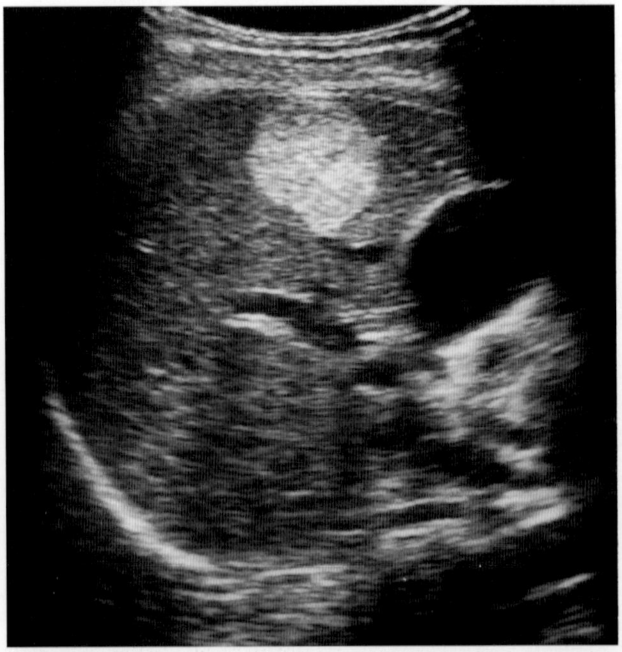

(a) US (right intercostal scan): a well demarcated hyperechoic mass is seen in S^{V}.

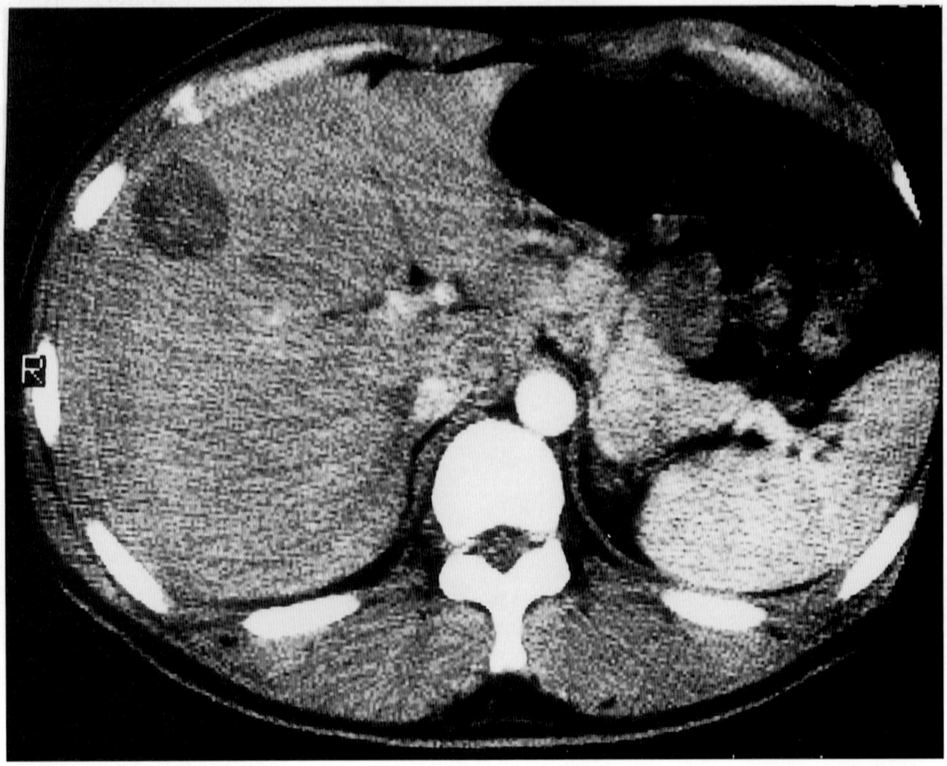

(b) Dynamic CT: the mass is not enhanced and seen as a low-density lesion.

Case 2 (contd.)

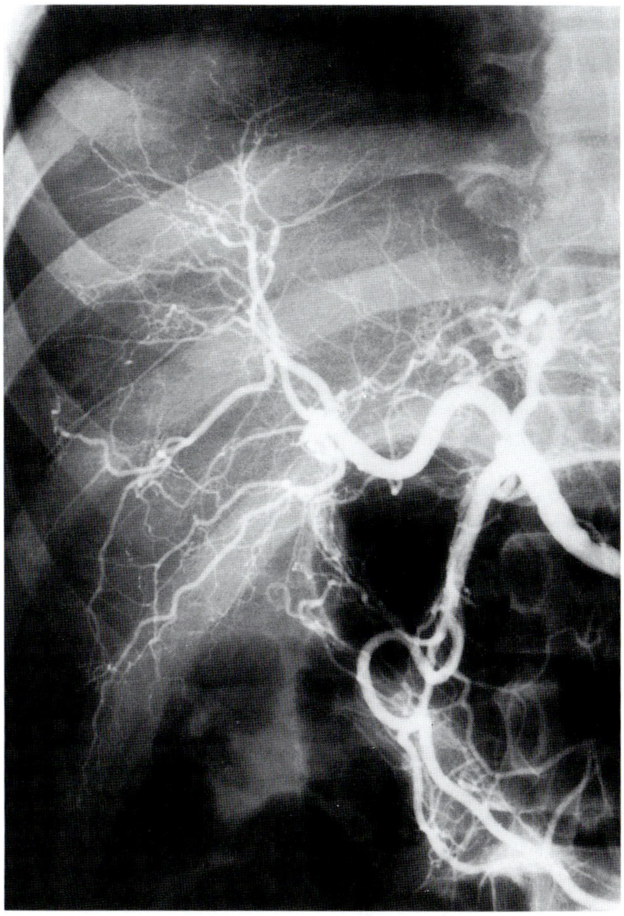

(c) Angiogram (early phase): the mass cannot be recognized.

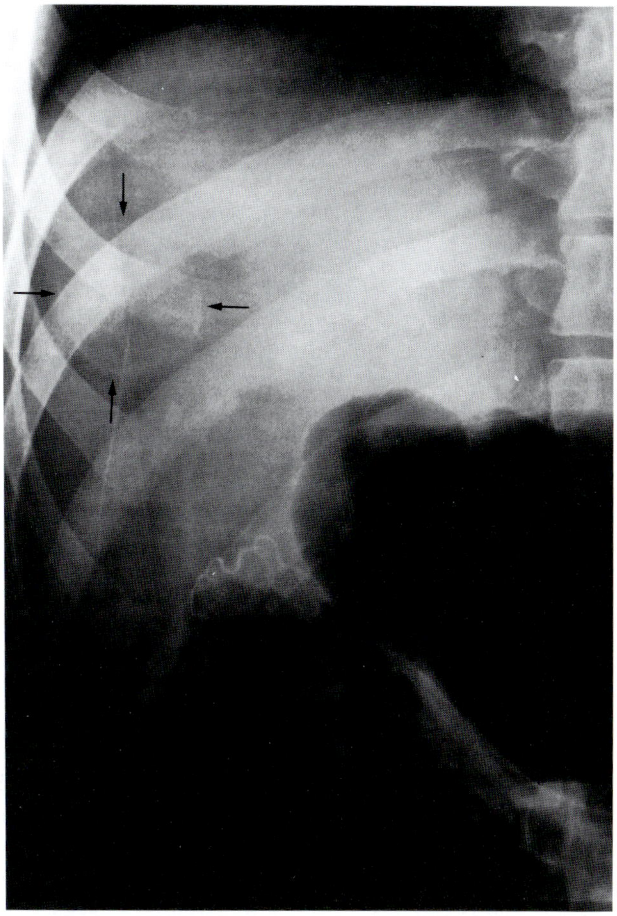

(d) Angiogram (late phase): the periphery of the mass (→) is stained slightly, and the interior shows homogeneous faint staining.

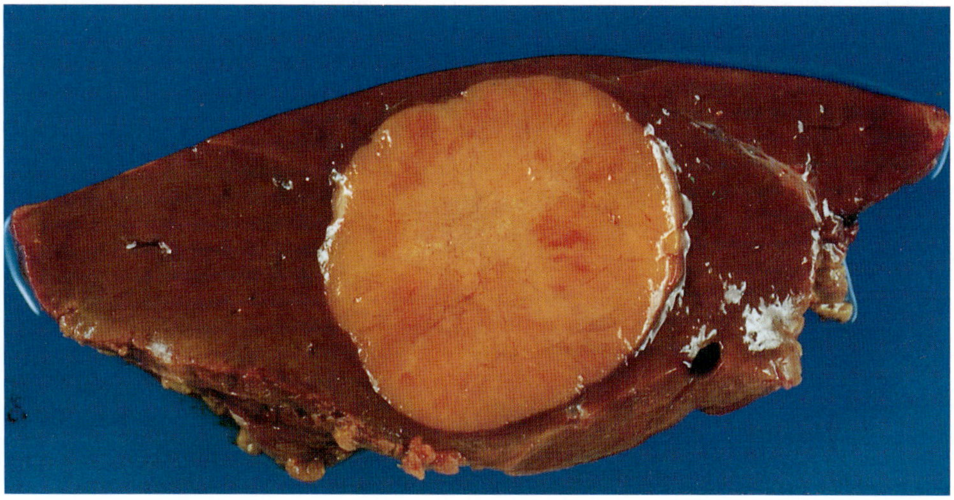

(e) Cut surface of resected specimen: the tumor has no capsule but is discretely bounded from the parenchyma. The border is mildly irregular in places. The central area is whitish in an irregular shape, but there is no central scar. Tumor cells were large hepatocytes containing fat, and bile production was recognized making the diagnosis of hepatocellular adenoma possible. The non-tumor parenchyma was normal.

3.4 Focal nodular hyperplasia (FNH)

This benign tumor (Fig. 3.3) is grossly characterized by a stellate scar in the center. Some pathologists consider focal nodular hyperplasia (FNH) to be a hamartoma or a lesion that develops as a reaction associated with vascular malformation (Whelan *et al.* 1973). Unlike the case of hepatocellular adenoma, contraceptive steroids do not cause this lesion although they may act as a trophic factor (Ross *et al.* 1976). In the western countries, FNH occurs in both sexes, somewhat more frequently in females. The age of onset varies from infancy to very advanced ages above 90, but more often between 20 and 50 years (Ishak and Rabin 1975; Knowles and Wolff 1976). At the National Cancer Center Hospital, Tokyo, resection was carried out in 9 patients, 6 males and 3 females with an average age of 43.3 years. The event or process that led to the diagnosis was mild abdominal pain in 2 and incidental detection by US in 7. None of them had a history of sex hormone intake. Tumor markers such as AFP and CEA were negative and liver function tests were normal in all.

Imaging diagnosis

The important features include a spoke-wheel appearance (Fechner and Roehm 1977) (Case 1) on angiography (spoke-wheel shaped stains radiating from the tumor center toward the periphery) and uptake of ^{99m}Tc-phytate (Case 2) suggesting the presence of Kupffer cells. When these two are demonstrated, this disease is suspected. However, the spoke-wheel appearance is not always present and arterial-CT should be done when this disease is possible, in order to study the direction of blood flow (centrifugal) within the neovasculature. Arterial-CT may demonstrate a lobulated structure of the mass (Case 1), a septum-like structure (Case 3), and lack of stain of the center of the mass in an early phase (Takayasu *et al.* 1992*b*). ^{99m}Tc-PMT uptake simply suggests that the tumor has hepatocytes or hepatocyte derived cells, but the same uptake is seen in HCC and adenoma, and it does not assist much in differential diagnosis.

More recently, Kudo *et al.* (1992*a*) emphasized the usefulness in differential diagnosis of FNH of sonographic angiography in which CO_2 microbubbles are injected into the hepatic artery. On MR imaging, the central stellate scar is depicted as an isointensity mass, occasionally hypointense relative to the surrounding hepatic parenchyma on T1-weighted images. On T2-weighted images, the mass is seen as an isointense one, occasionally of hyperintensity. The central stellate scar is hypointense on T1-weighted and hyperintense on T2-weighted images (Rummeny *et al.* 1989). The lesion is markedly enhanced by the intravenous administration of Gd-DTPA. Superparamagnetic iron oxide (SPIO) is taken up in this mass which contains Kupffer cells, and the contrast of the lesion against liver parenchyma becomes low.

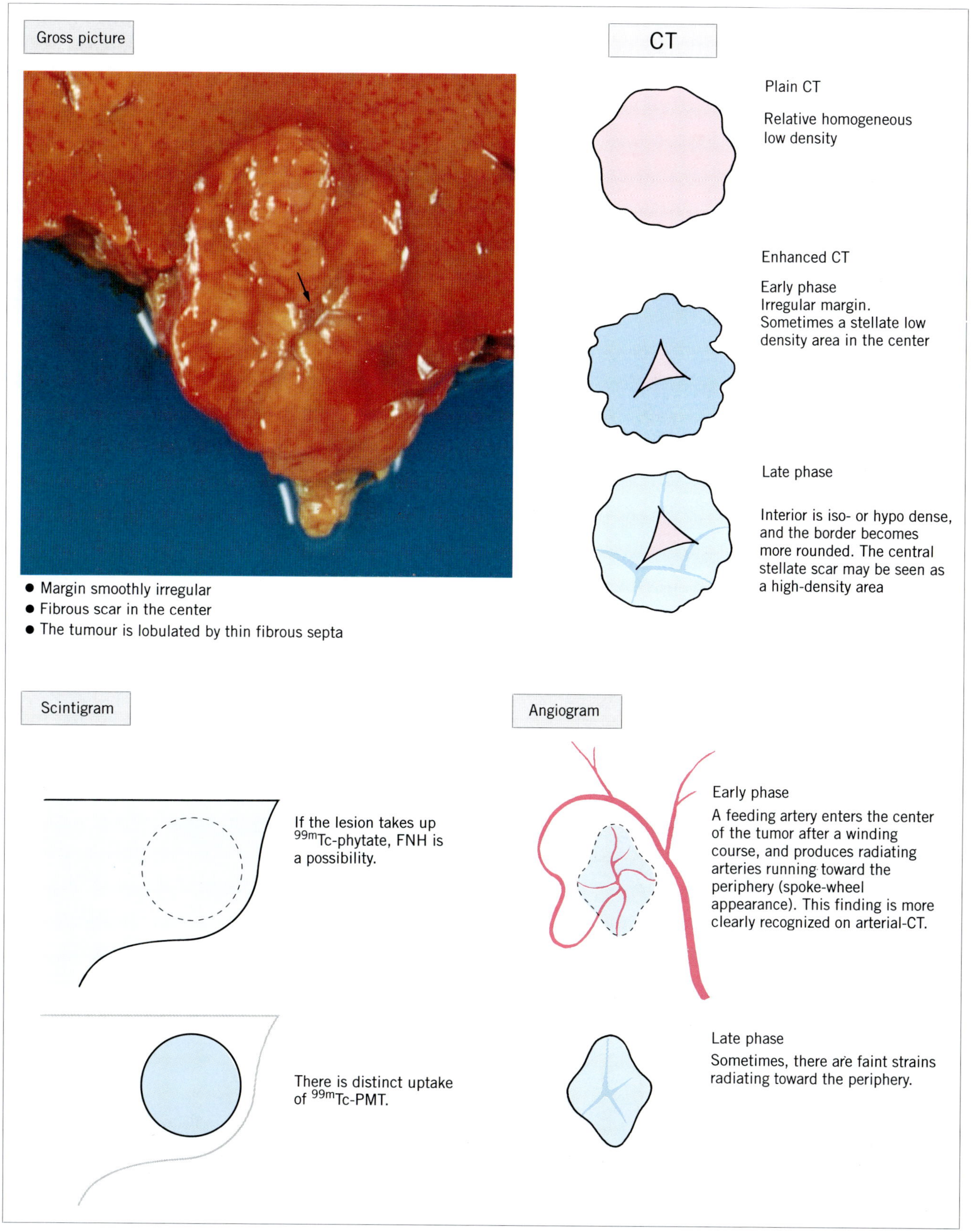

Fig. 3.3 Imaging characteristics of FNH.

FNH—Case 1: FNH for which arterial-CT was diagnostically useful. An 18-year-old man. An hepatic tumor was incidentally found by US. All tumor markers and HBV serology were negative.

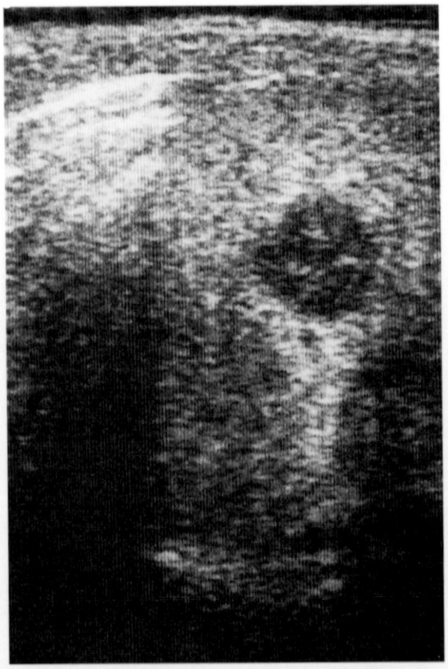

(a) US: the mass is seen as a homogeneous hypoechoic lesion within a hyperechoic fatty liver. Several high-echo dot structures are seen in the center of the lesion. The tumor border is irregular.

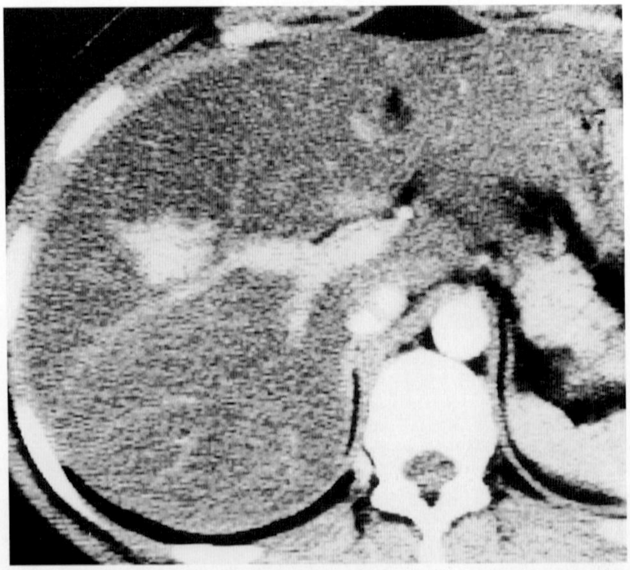

(b) Dynamic CT (early phase): the tumor in S^{V} is seen as a high-density lesion with an irregular margin against fatty liver parenchyma.

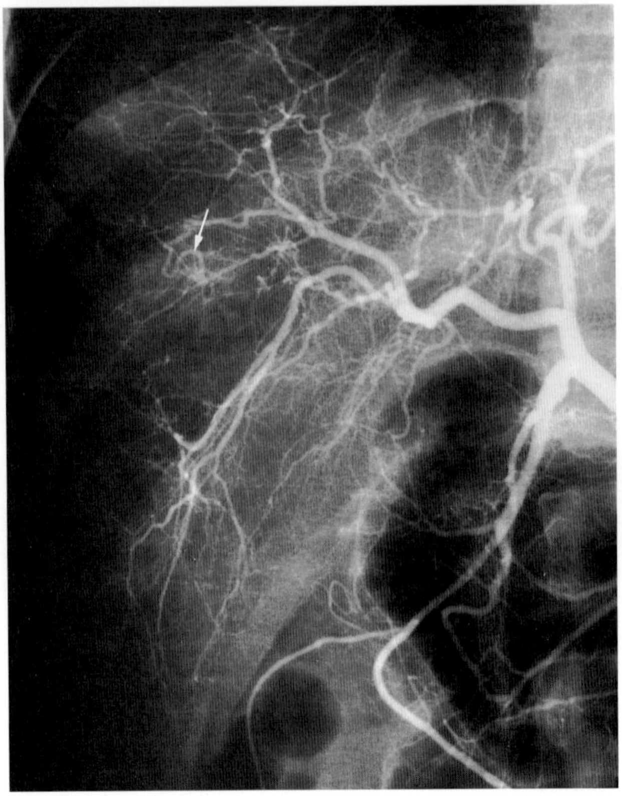

(c) Angiogram (early phase): a thick artery, winding and coursing

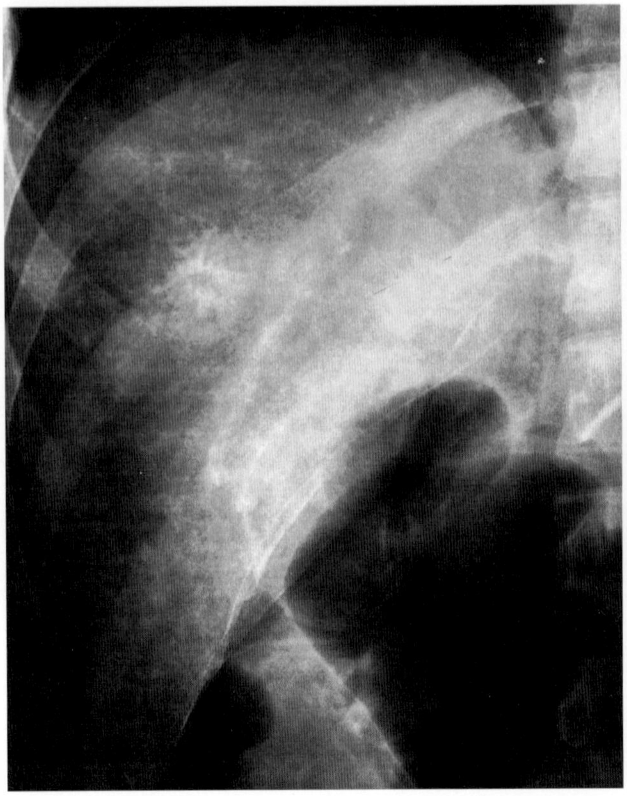

(d) Angiogram (late phase): tumor vessels running centrifugally (from

Case 1 (contd.)

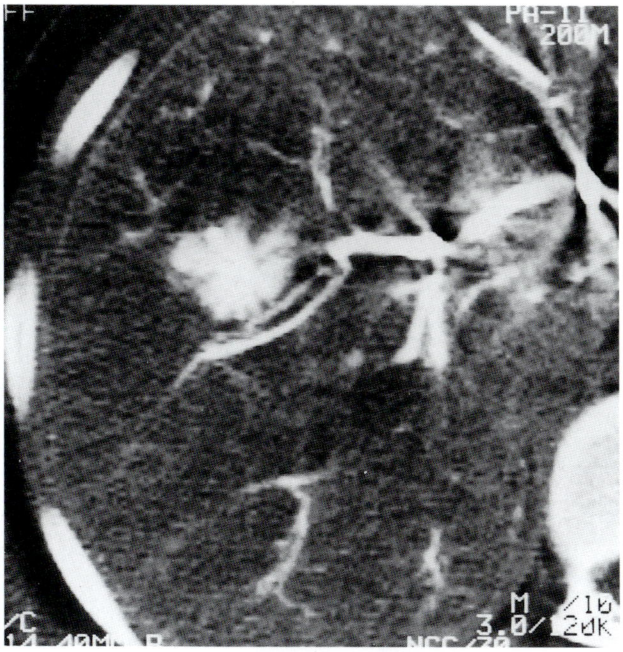

(e) Arterial-CT (early phase): the mass is clearly opacified delineating lobular structures in the periphery of the mass.

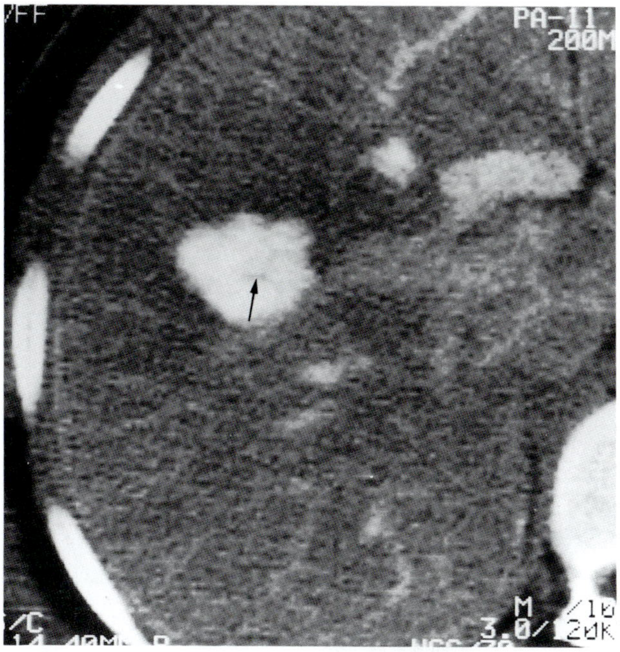

(f) Arterial-CT (late phase): the tumor border is somewhat rounded and there is a low-density spot (→) in the center.

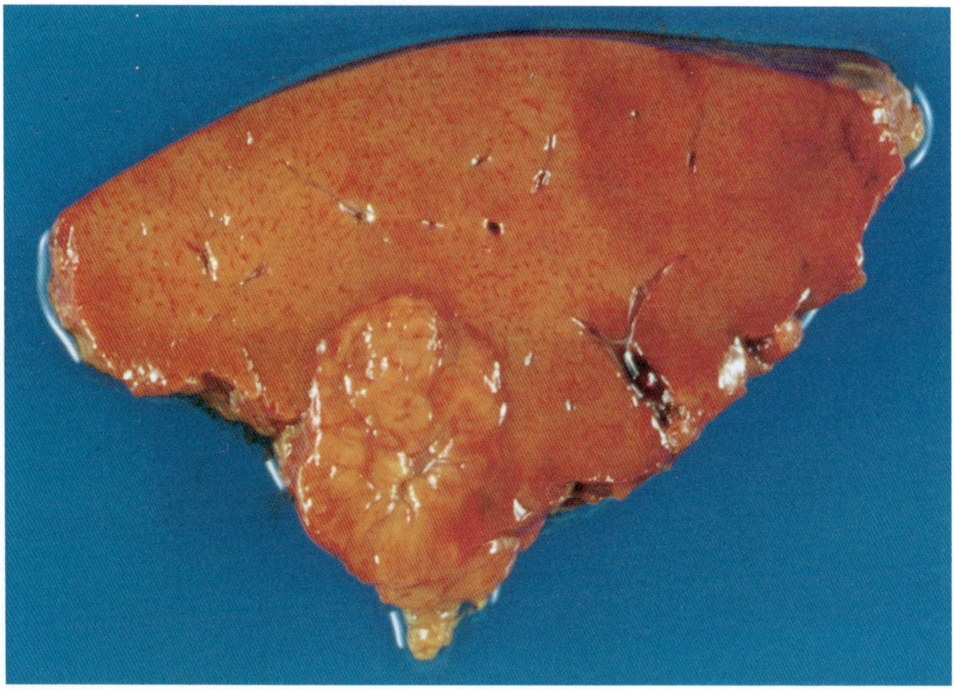

(g) Cut surface of resected specimen: the periphery of this 2.3 × 2.0 cm tumor is smoothly irregular with no apparent fibrous capsule. Lobular structures are seen being separated by thin fibrous septa, and there is a scar in the center. The non-tumor parenchyma shows steatosis.

FNH—Case 2: Three FNH lesions for which ^{99m}Tc-phytate proved useful for differential diagnosis. A 64-year-old man. He had been followed because of elevated gamma-GTP, and then a liver mass was discovered. AFP (−), HBsAg (−), and anti-HBs (+), and anti-HBc (+).

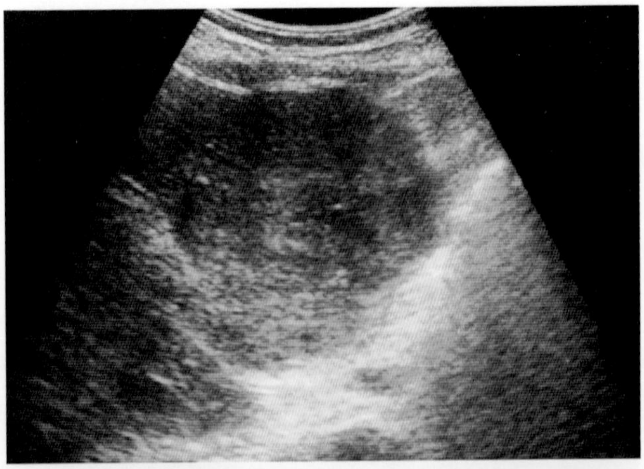

a

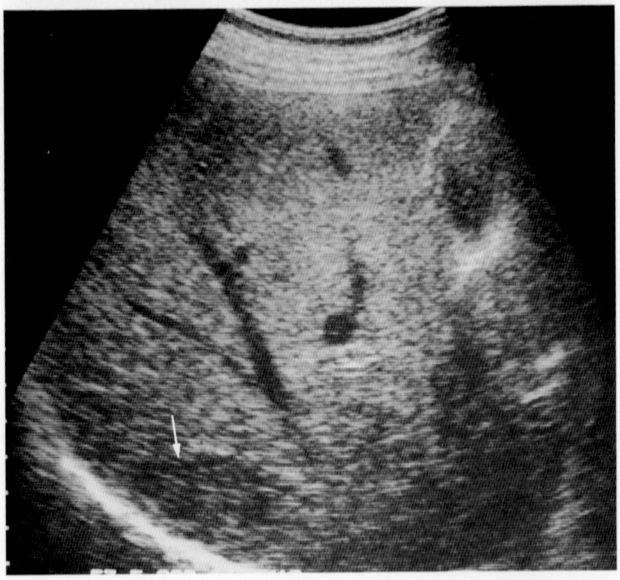

b

(a),(b) US: a 9 cm lesion, mostly hypoechoic with an irregular boundary, is seen in the left lobe laterally (a). In addition, two 3 cm lesions in S^{VII} (b) (→) and a 0.5 cm hyperechoic lesion in S^{IV} are recognized.

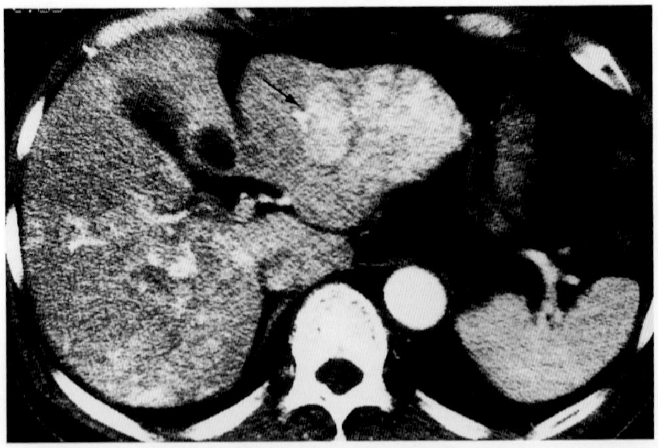

(c) Dynamic CT (early phase): the tumor is homogeneously enhanced. A nodular stain to the right of the main mass (→) may be interpreted as a nodule within the mass or a daughter nodule.

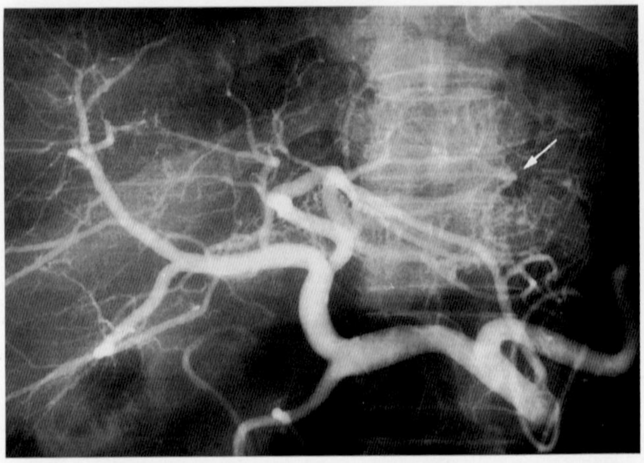

(d) Celiac arteriogram (early phase): a mass mainly supplied from A^{II} is seen in the left lobe laterally. Tumor vessels radiating from the center (→) toward the periphery are recognized (spoke-wheel appearance).

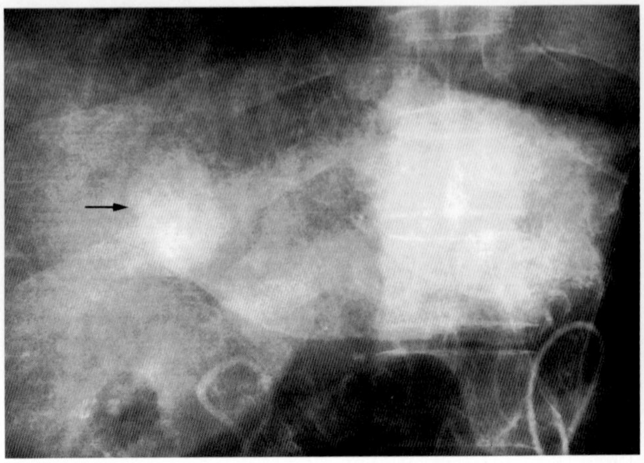

(e) Celiac arteriogram (late phase): a round tumor stain (→) is seen in S^{VII} beside the one in the lateral region of the left lobe.

Case 2 (contd.)

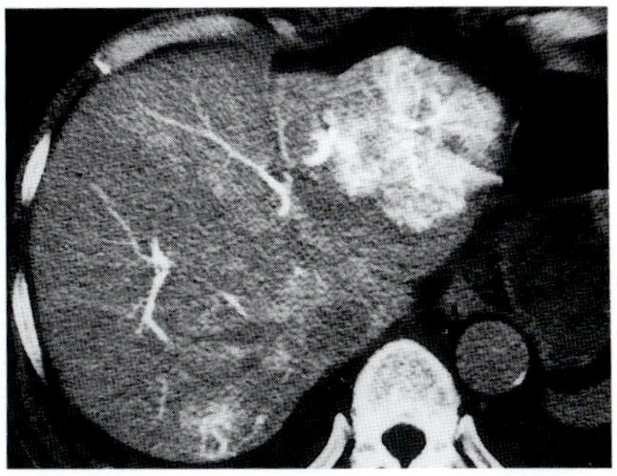

f

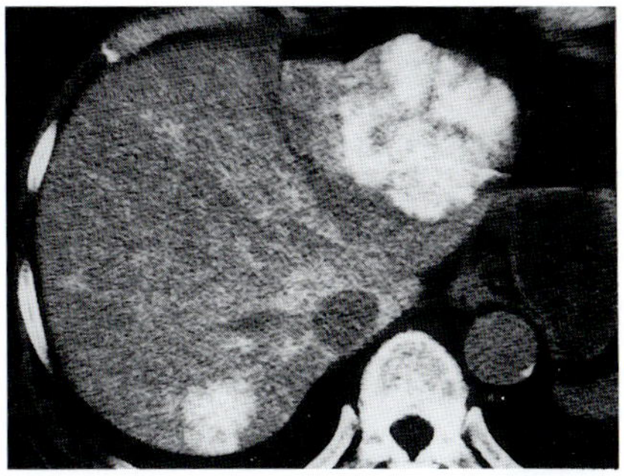

g

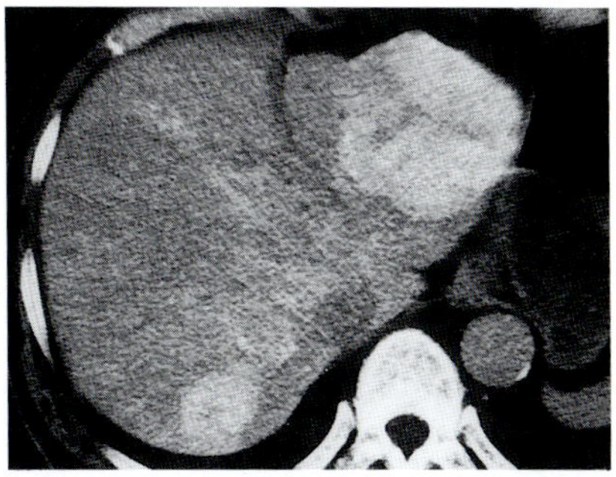

h

(f)–(h) Arterial-CT: the tumor shows a lobular structure and the border is irregular. In the early phase (f) neovasculature is seen in the center of the mass. In the late phase (h), linear low-density areas are seen in the center. As the mass in S^{VII} demonstrated the same imaging features (centrifugal staining) and hemodynamics as the main one, FNH was the most likely diagnosis.

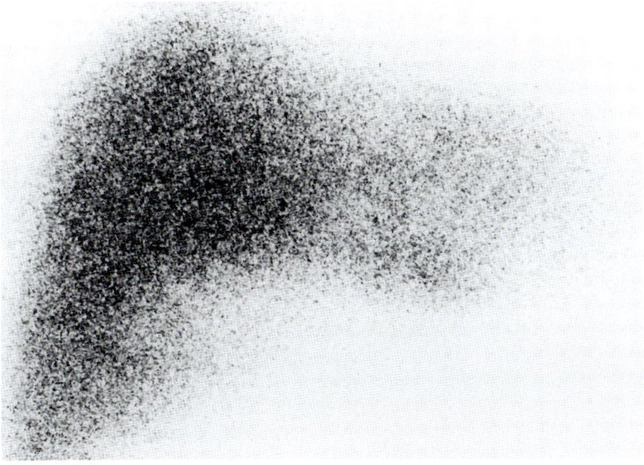

(i) ^{99m}Tc-phytate scintiscan: although the uptake of this nuclide is somewhat low in the left lobe laterally, considering the presence of an unquestionable large mass in the same location, it is assumed that the mass takes up ^{99m}Tc-phytate slightly.

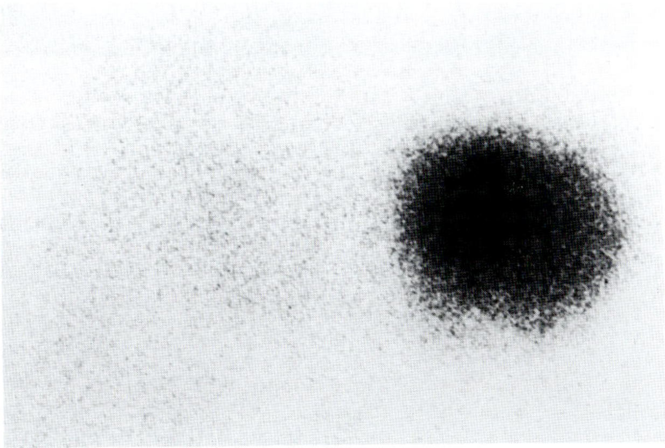

(j) ^{99m}Tc-PMT scan (anterior view): a marked uptake was seen in the main mass in the left lobe. In the posterior view (not shown), the other two mass lesions also showed a similar uptake.

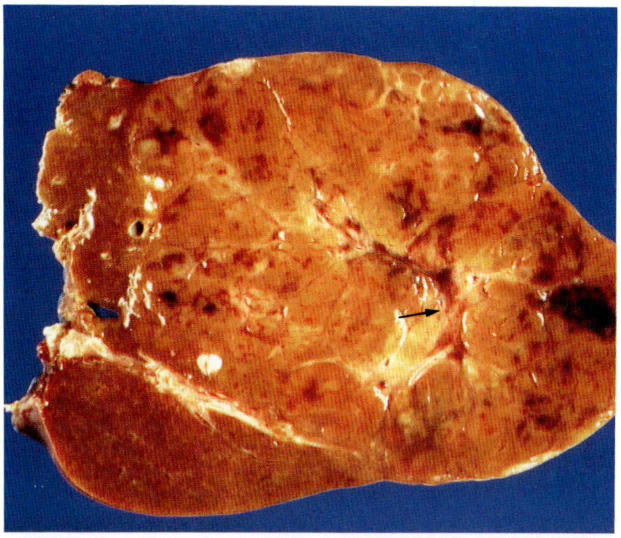

k

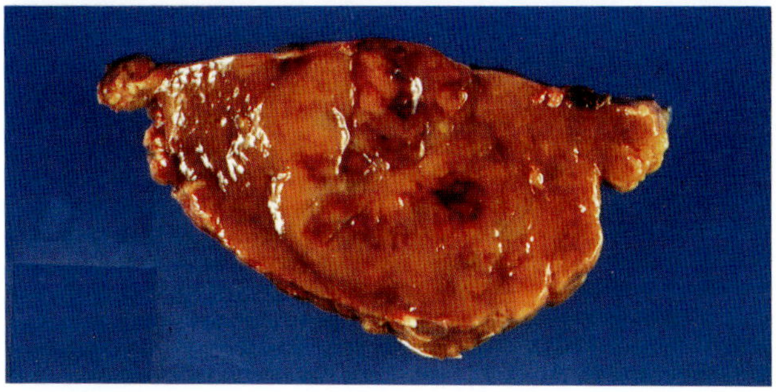

l

(k),(l) Cut surface of resected specimen: beside left lateral resection, partial resections for S^{VII} and S^{IV} were carried out. The tumor in the left lateral area was relatively well demarcated from liver parenchyma, but there was no capsule formation. The tumor was divided into several nodules containing typical central scar (→). The other two masses were grossly similar. The non-tumor liver parenchyma was normal.

FNH—Case 3: A dumb-bell shaped FNH occupying through S^{I} and S^{VIII}. A 22-year-old woman. A liver mass was found incidentally by US. AFP (−), CEA (−), HBsAg (−), no history of oral contraceptive intake, normal liver function tests.

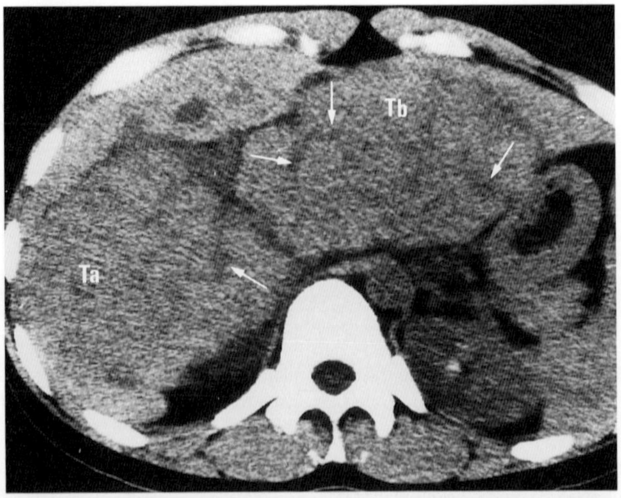

(a) Plain CT: there are two masses (Ta, Tb). They are low in density with several septum-like structures (→).

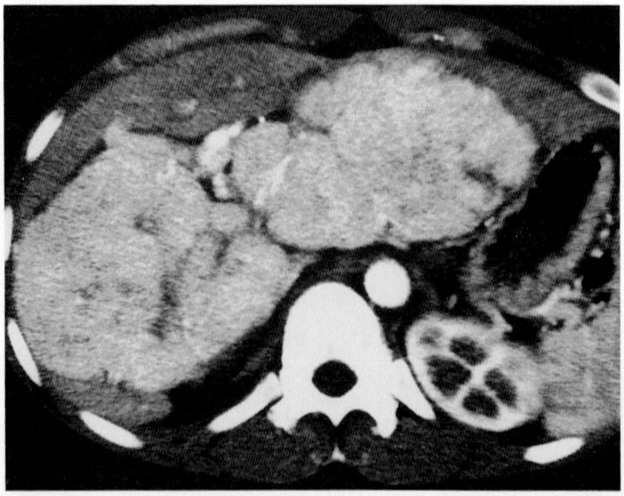

(b) Dynamic CT (early phase): both tumors are stained well. Tb is more irregularly bounded than Ta.

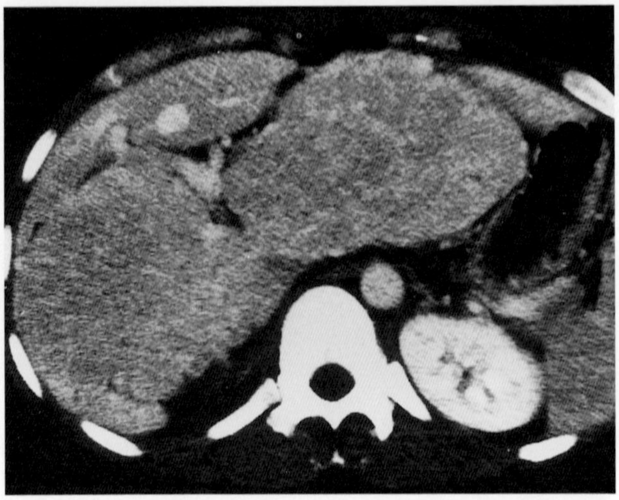

(c) Dynamic CT (1 min): the masses are homogeneously isodense.

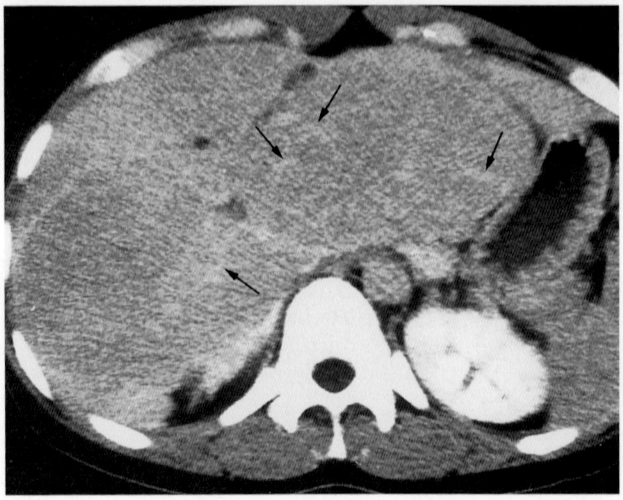

(d) Late enhanced CT (10 min): the tumors are more isodense. The low-density structures within the mass have turned hyperdense (→), suggesting that these structures contain fibrous elements.

Case 3 (contd.)

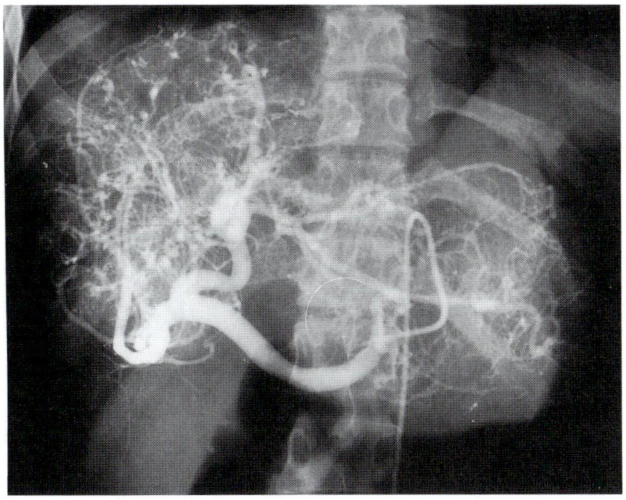

(e) Celiac arteriogram (early phase): all hepatic arteries are markedly dilated, and hypervascular tumors are seen in the right anterior area and the caudate lobe. However, the spoke-wheel appearance was not present. As most arterial flow enters the masses, the non-tumor area is receiving little blood [cf. portogram (g)].

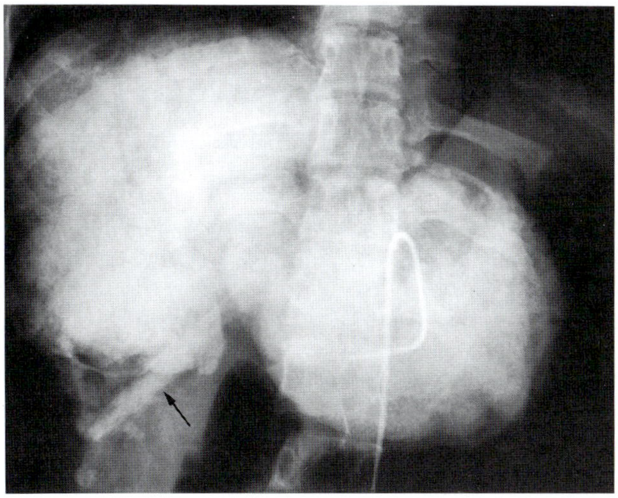

(f) Celiac arteriogram (late phase): the tumors are stained homogeneously and heavily, with opacification of an hepatic vein (→).

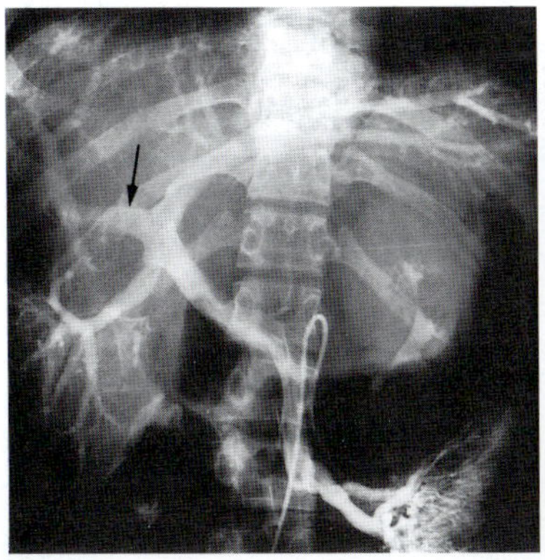

g

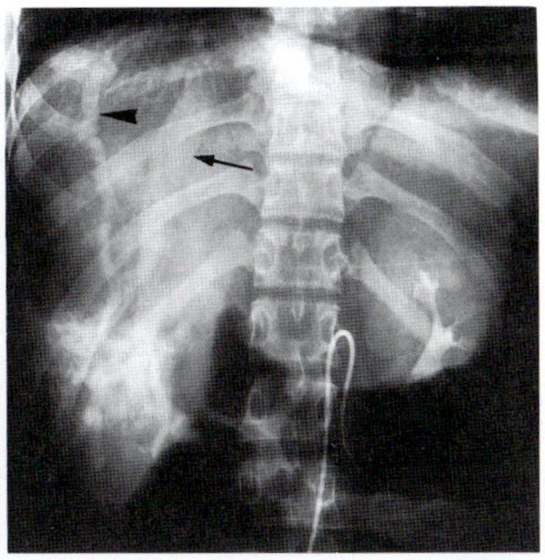

h

(g) Portogram (early phase): a malignant tumor was suspected from the arteriogram. This superior mesenteric arterial portogram demonstrates compression of the right anterior segment branch (→) by the mass.

(h) Portogram (late phase): as the hepatic veins as well as the portal veins were opacified a low-grade malignancy was suspected. →, middle hepatic vein; ▶, right hepatic vein.

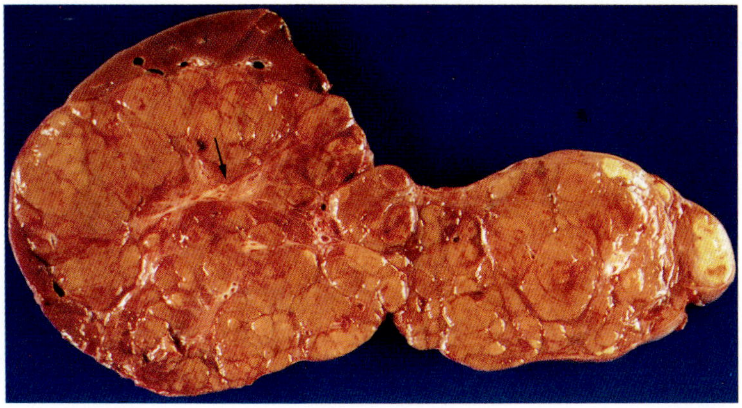

(i) Cut surface of resected specimen: extended right hepatectomy including the caudate lobe was carried out (1130 g). The longest axis of the tumor was 21 cm. The mass was pushing the right anterior and posterior segments, and was continuous with the left part of the caudate lobe. Therefore, it was suspected that each developed from the caudate lobe (the right and left parts). A scar is seen in the center of the right tumor (→), and the mass consisted of many lobular structures making somewhat irregular. The diagnosis was FNH, and the non-tumor part of the liver was normal.

3.5 Nodular regenerative hyperplasia (NRH)

This is a benign condition in which multiple hepatocellular nodules form with intervening areas of hepatic atrophy. It occurs at any age (8 months–82 years) (Goodman 1987) with no sex difference. It is frequently associated with various non-hepatic chronic diseases. These include myeloproliferative disorders (chronic myelogenous leukemia, polycythemia vera, myeloid metaplasia), lymphoproliferative disorders (Hodgkin's and non-Hodgkin's lymphomas, chronic lymphocytic leukemia, plasma cell dyscrasia), and collagen-vascular diseases (rheumatoid arthritis, polyarteritis nodosa, Felty's syndrome, CREST syndrome, lupus erythematosus), etc. Nodules are usually small, but they may coalesce and form large masses, and could rupture into the peritoneal cavity (Stromeyer *et al.* 1981).

The etiology is unknown. One theory suggests that this is a neoplastic process, because the nodules are similar to those produced in animals treated with various carcinogens, which are called 'hyperplastic nodules', 'hepatocellular foci', or 'neoplastic nodules'. Many patients with these diseases are on various drugs, and steroids. The evidence that NRH is preneoplastic is weak, but HCC that develops following NRH has been described (Stromeyer and Ishak 1981). The other more recent theory is a vascular one proposed by Wanless (1990). He suggests that reduction of blood flow for various reasons induces parenchymal atrophy which in turn results in compensatory hyperplasia in the areas where blood supply is adequate. Obliterative portal venopathy has been suggested as a cause of reduced blood flow. Idiopathic portal hypertension in Japan (Okuda *et al.* 1984*a*) is occasionally accompanied by NRH as well as larger nodule formation. Partial nodular transformation described by Sherlock *et al.* (1966) falls into the same category. According to Stromeyer and Ishak (1981), portal hypertension is associated in more than 60 per cent of the cases. In our Case 1, NRH was incidentally discovered following irradiation and chemotherapy with cytotoxic agents (Feng *et al.* 1991). There was no portal hypertension.

NRH—Case 1: NRH that developed after chemotherapy for a non-Hodgkin lymphoma and proved difficult to differentiate from its metastasis. A 61-year-old man. Non-Hodgkin lymphoma that originated from the tonsil was treated (chemotherapy and steroids following irradiation), and US done 6 months later demonstrated multiple tumors in the liver.

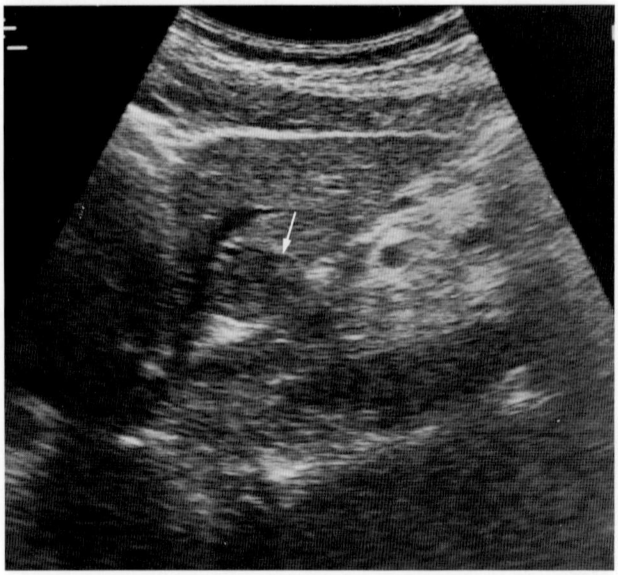

(a) US (epigastric sagittal scan): A 2 cm hypoechoic lesion (→) is seen dorsal to the left hepatic vein. There is no posterior echo enhancement or a halo.

Case 1 (contd.)

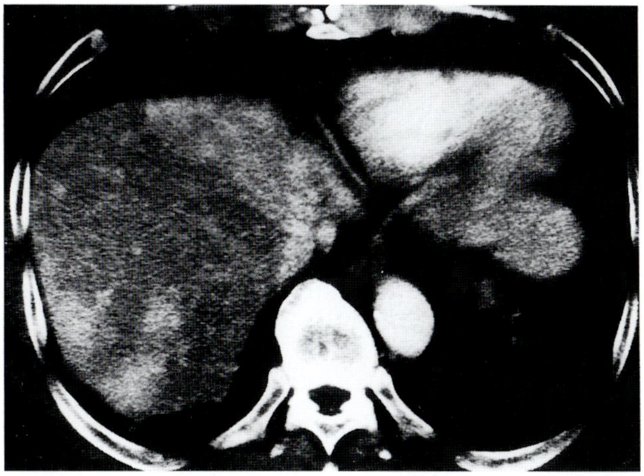

(b) Dynamic CT (early phase): there are multiple enhanced lesions in the right lobe and increased enhancement in the left lobe with the Cantlie line as its border. In the late phase, both lobes were isodense. On angiography, many tumor stains were seen in both lobes with an arterio-portal anastomosis in the left lobe.

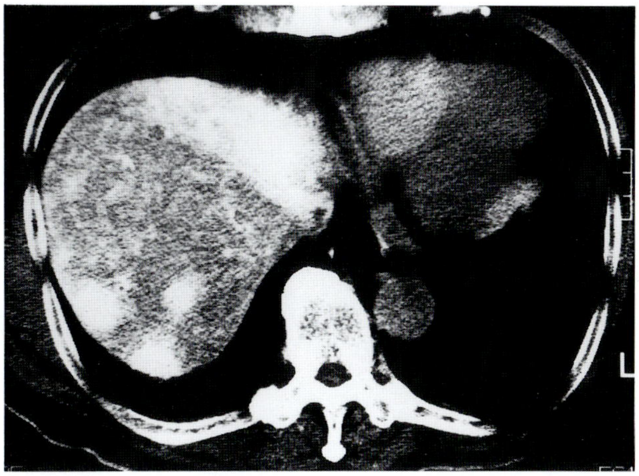

(c) Arterial-CT: this demonstrated mutiple densely stained lesions of about 2 cm in the right lobe. It was found that the increased stain of the left lobe with the Cantlie line as its border was due to an arterio-portal communication.

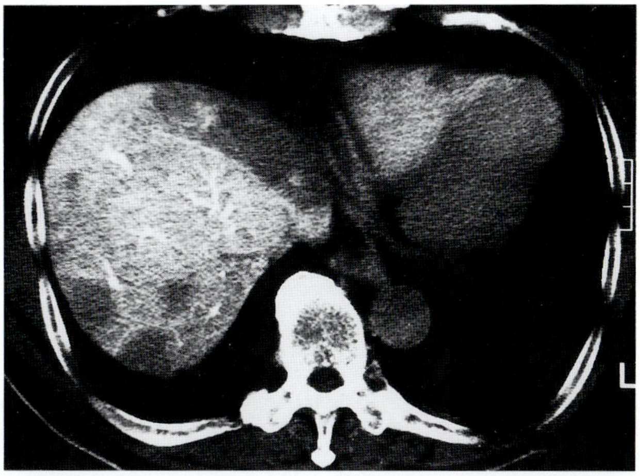

(d) Portal-CT: the lesions in the right lobe were identified as low-density masses. Since there was no portal vein flow, the left lobe was hypodense.

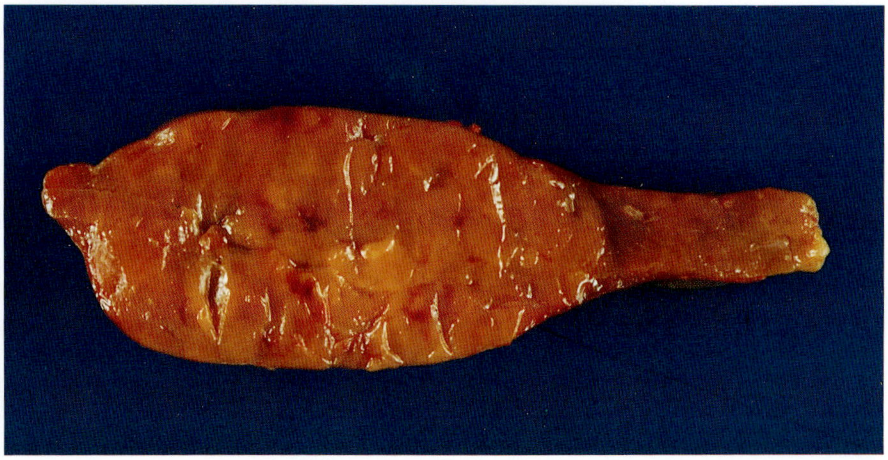

(e) Cut surface of resected specimen: with a diagnosis of multiple metastases from non-Hodgkin lymphoma, exploratory left lateral subsegmentectomy was carried out. On the cut surface, the nodule was oval in shape showing an expanding growth. There was no scar or fibrous capsule. Histologically, portal tracts were seen within the nodule with proliferating small hepatocytes; no lymphoid cell infiltration was present. There was no malignant feature, and the diagnosis was NRH occurring in a normal liver.

3.6 Hepatic cyst

Hepatic cyst (Fig. 3.4) is a congenital malformation derived from bile duct epithelia which should disappear during the development of the biliary tract during fetal growth. Hepatic cyst is either single or multiple. It occurs four to five times more frequently in females than in males. Diagnosis is easy with CT and US if it is large. Angiography provides only indirect findings such as a deviated course of vessels as a result of compression, and is not very diagnostic. Small cysts, less than 1 cm in size, may mimic a hypovascular HCC or metastasis requiring careful differentiation. Thin CT sectioning and follow-up may be necessary in such cases (Fig. 13.7, p.408).

Solitary cyst (Case 1)

A solitary cyst generally lacks septa within the cyst and is rarely associated with renal cyst. The cyst is lined with a single layer of cuboidal or cylindrical epithelium that somewhat resembles bile duct epithelium. As the size of the cyst increases, the patient commonly complains of a feeling of abdominal compression. A pedunculated cyst sometimes causes torsion of the pedicle requiring emergency laparotomy. The lining epithelium may turn malignant, but the incidence of this is very low.

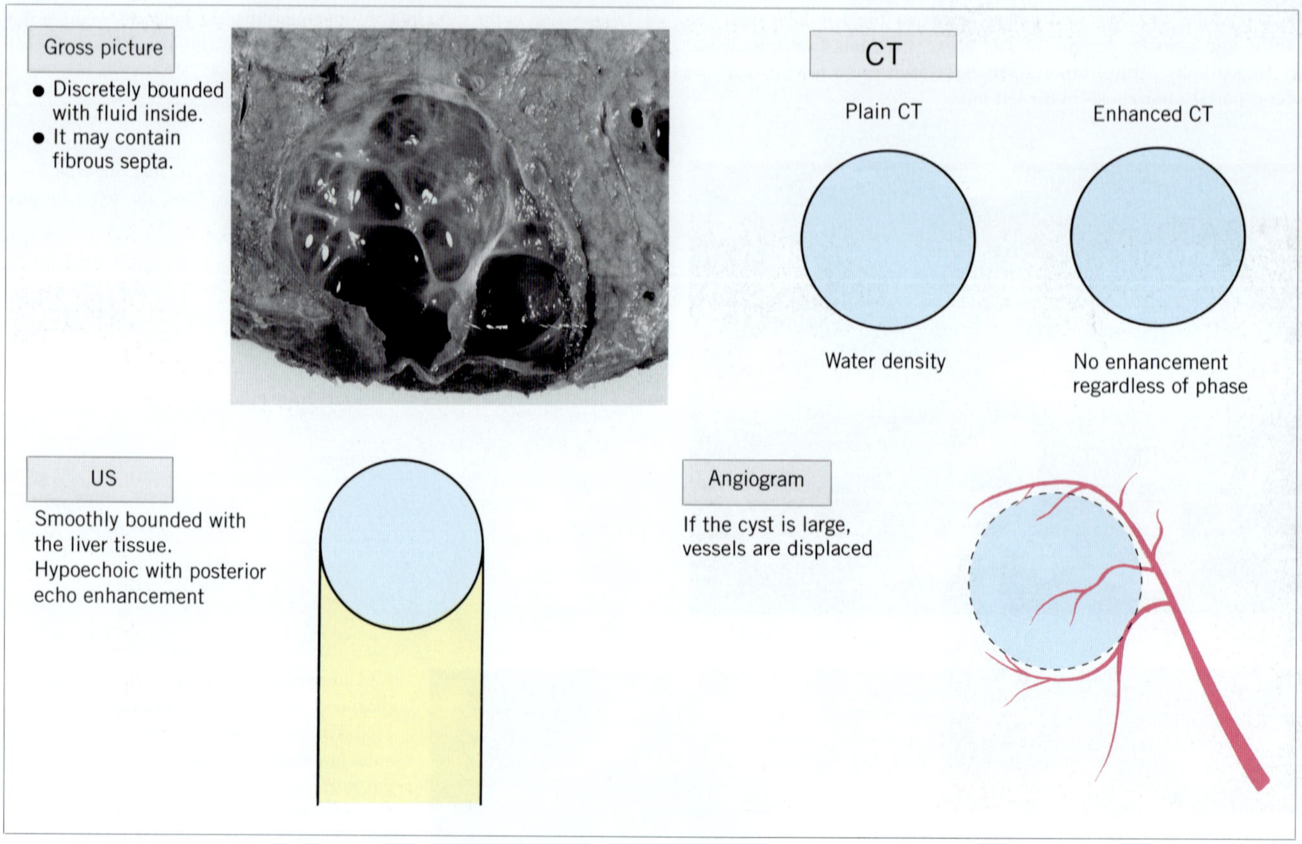

Fig. 3.4 Imaging features of hepatic cyst.

Hepatic cyst—Case 1: Huge solitary cyst occupying the left lobe.

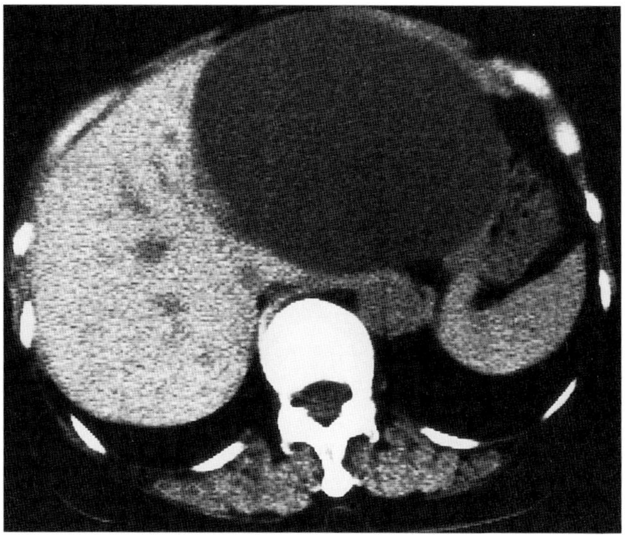

(a) Plain CT: a 12 cm cyst in the left lobe.

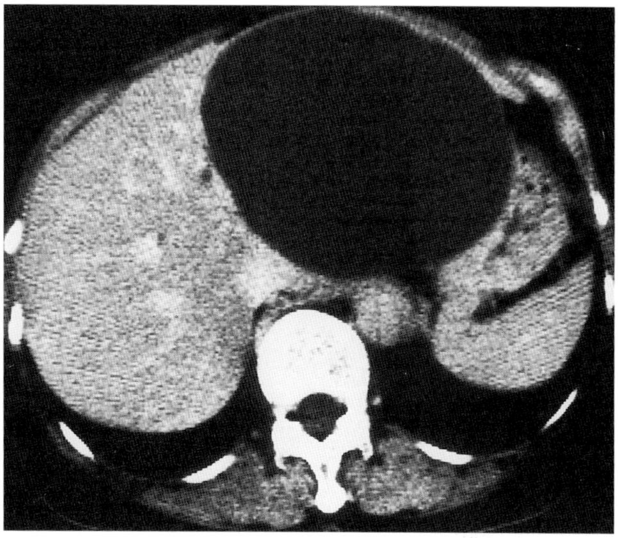

(b) Enhanced CT: the boundary and interior of the cyst are not enhanced at all. Enhanced CT is important for the differentiation from a malignant transformed cyst (mural nodules) and metastasis of a cystic malignancy.

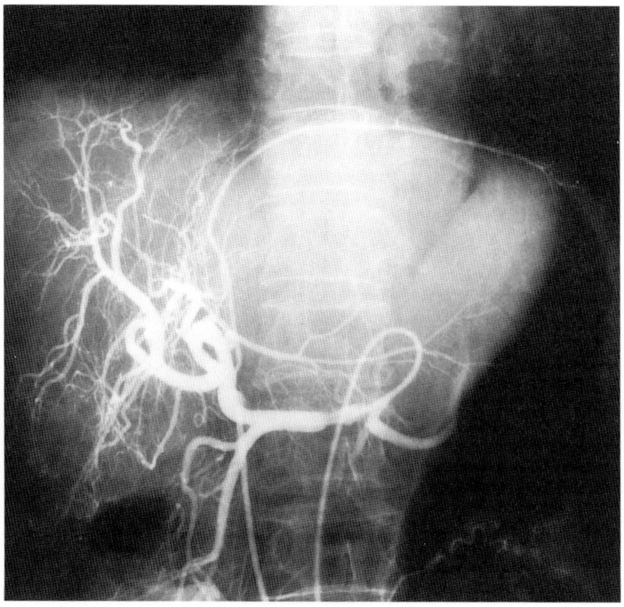

(c) Hepatic arteriogram: displaced arteries are seen in the left lobe laterally, but there is no encasement or neovasculature.

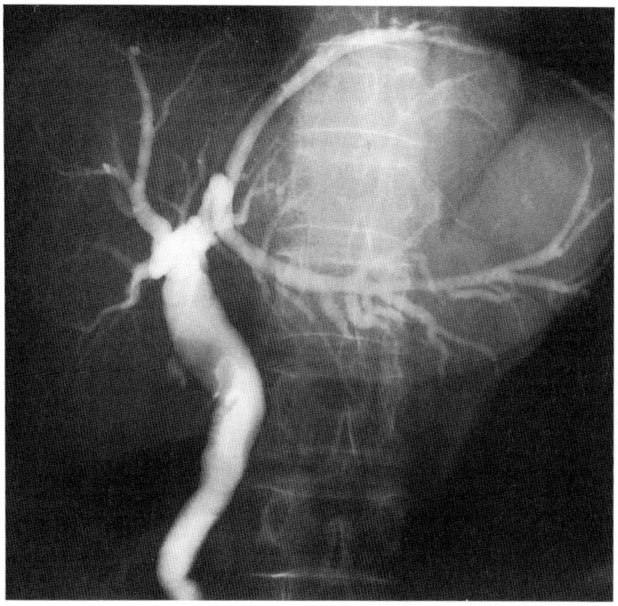

(d) ERC: bile ducts in the left lobe are displaced as are the arteries. There is no communication between the cyst and biliary tract.

Hepatic cyst—Case 2: Congenital multiple cysts with bleeding. A 45-year-old woman. She came to the hospital complaining of abdominal distension. During the follow-up, the number and sizes of cysts did not change. One day, she suddenly developed right upper quadrant pain, and a diagnosis of bleeding into the cyst was made by MR imaging. No associated renal or pancreas cyst.

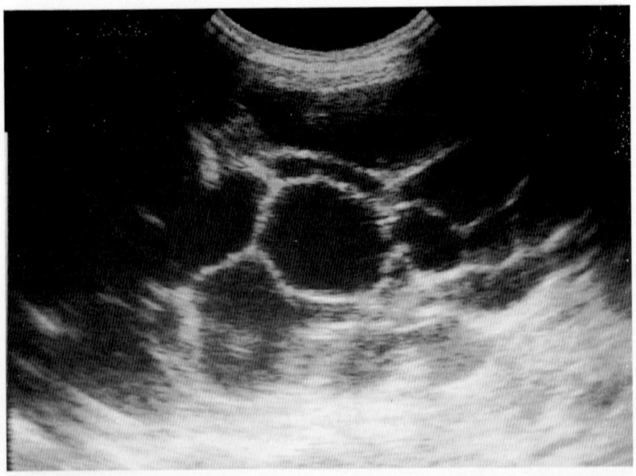

(a) US (transverse scan): honeycomb-like multiple cystic lesions are recognized.

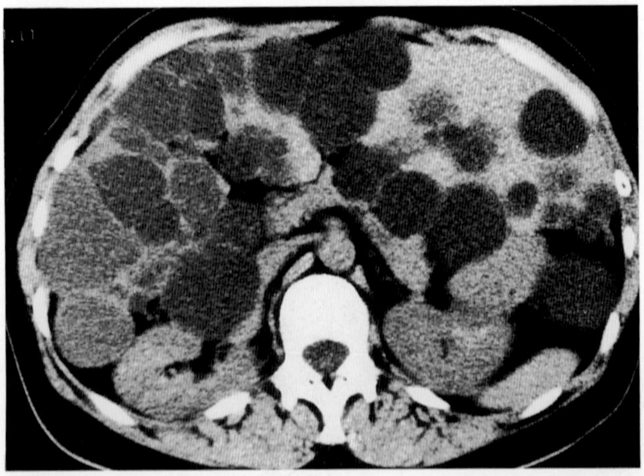

(b) Plain CT: multiple, variously sized cystic lesions are seen throughout the liver. The CT values of the cyst contents varied from 9 HU to 36 HU, suggesting varying densities of the contents. It seems that some of the septa were formed as the cysts expanded and the sandwiched parenchyma disappeared.

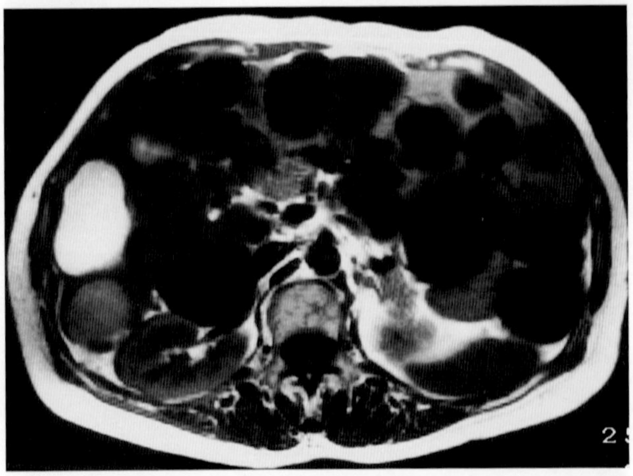

(c) MR imaging (T1-weighted image): emergent T1-weighted MR imaging (TR 600/TE 20) done for acute abdominal pain showed the majority of cysts to be of low intensity, except for two cysts.

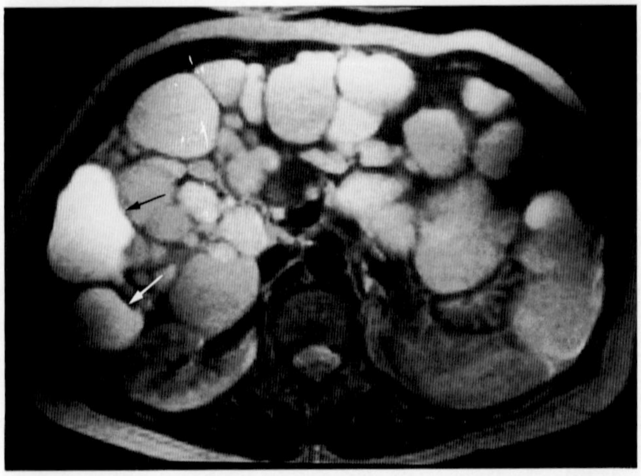

(d) MR imaging (T2-weighted image): T2-weighted image (2400/60) demonstrates that all lesions are of high intensity. However, two lesions indicated by arrows are of high intensity both in T1- and T2-weighted images. The diagnosis was bleeding in the cyst.

Case 2 (contd.)

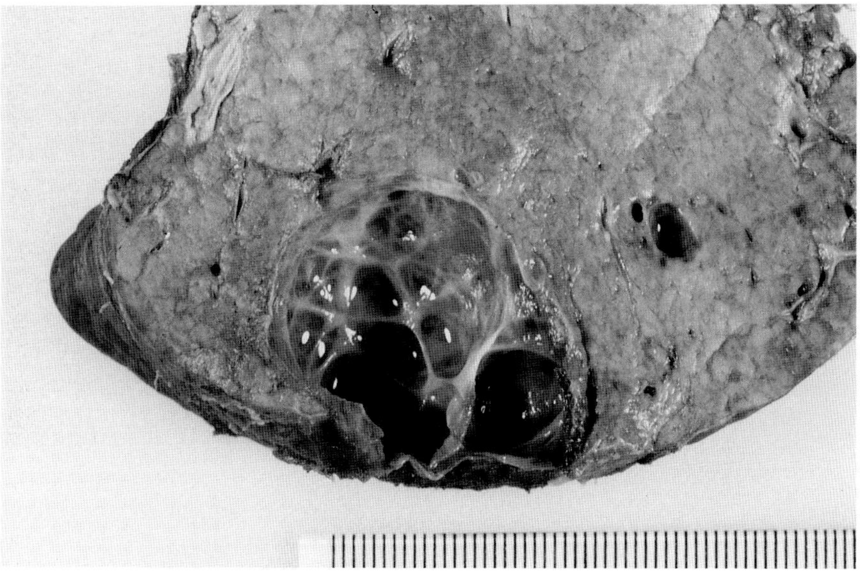

(e) Cut surface of a resected cyst (another case): this is one of the multiple cysts incidentally found in a liver resected for HCC. The interior is separated into a number of lumina by fibrous septa. Histologically, the cyst was surrounded by fibrous tissue, and the cyst was lined by a layer of columnar or low cylindrical epithelium.

Multiple cysts (Case 2)

Multiple cysts occur in both infants and adults. Infantile multiple cystic disease is transmitted by an autosomal recessive trait and has a rather poor prognosis, whereas adult disease is transmitted by an autosomal dominant trait. The frequency of adult multiple cysts is less than 0.6 per cent in autopsy cases (Melnick 1955), and about half of them have associated cystic kidney disease (Walt 1977). Sometimes bleeding occurs within a cyst causing abdominal pain. Diagnosis with CT and MR imaging (Case 2) becomes important. Malignant transformation rarely occurs, but the patient may succumb to hematemesis due to portal hypertension and chronic renal failure.

Differential diagnosis and treatment

Cystic metastatic cancer resulting from internal bleeding (ovarian carcinoma, esophageal cancer, carcinoid tumor, leiomyosarcoma, etc.) requires differential diagnosis. Such cancers are not enhanced on contrast CT and the CT value is low, making distinction rather difficult. Other diseases that required differential diagnosis include cystadenoma, cystadenocarcinoma, hydatid cyst, etc., and delineation of the detailed internal structure becomes necessary.

Hepatic cysts are thought to grow very slowly, and sometimes they spontaneously regress (Case 3). For symptomatic cysts, US guided catheterization may be done for removal of fluid followed by injection of absolute ethanol to damage the lining epithelium; fluid production will cease.

Ciliated hepatic foregut cyst

With advanced imaging practice, increasing numbers of rare cystic diseases are now being found. Ciliated hepatic foregut cyst is a solitary cyst without a septum, derived from the foregut, and lined by a single layer of ciliated epithelium (Case 4).

Similar disorders have been reported in the esophagus and bronchus, but modern imaging techniques have shown that it also occurs in the liver (Kadoya *et al.* 1990; Kimura *et al.* 1990). The imaging features of this cyst include a high density of the content which is mucin on plain CT, and multiple floating hyperechoic spots on US. This cyst may be mistaken for a hypovascular solid tumor. It is surrounded by fibrous tissue, and usually located immediately beneath the hepatic capsule and segment 4. Resection is easy because of its surface location.

Hepatic peribiliary cysts

This is a recently recognized cystic disease in which multiple small cysts are distributed along the intrahepatic biliary tract (Baron *et al.* 1994; Itai *et al.* 1994). It is derived from the periductal gland (Nakanuma *et al.* 1984).

Hepatic cyst—Case 3: Spontaneously regressed cyst.

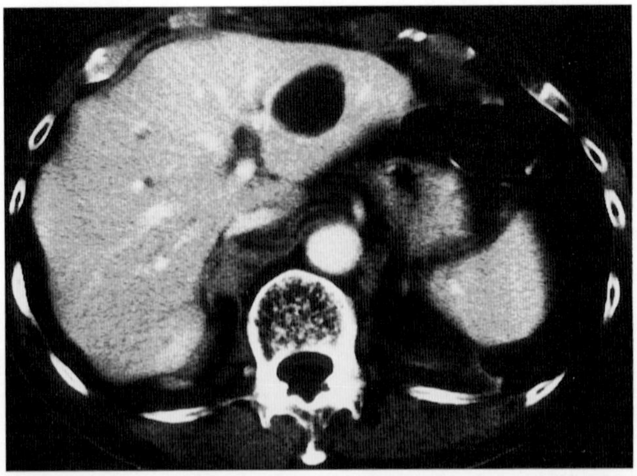

(a) Enhanced CT: a 3 cm cyst is seen in the left lobe laterally.

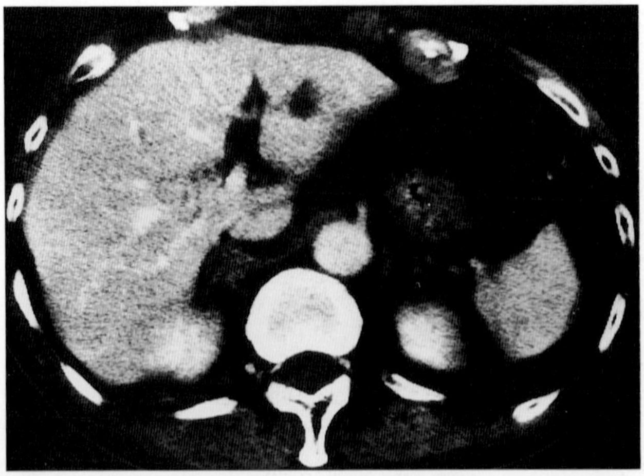

(b) Enhanced CT (1.5 years later): the cyst has been reduced in size to 1.3 cm without treatment.

Hepatic cyst—Case 4: Ciliated hepatic foregut cyst requiring differentiation from a solid tumor. A 67-year-old man. An hepatic mass was found at the annual health check. AFP (−), CEA (−), HBV seromarkers all negative.

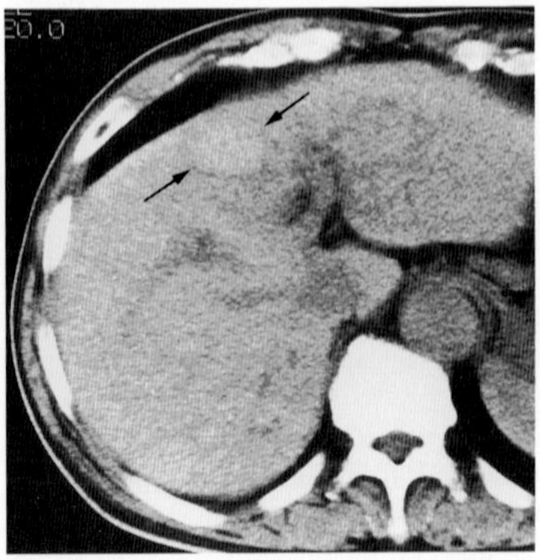

(a) Plain CT: a 2.5 cm round tumor of a slightly high density (→) is seen in S^{IV} (CT value = 74 HU). The non-tumor parenchyma has a CT value of 66 HU.

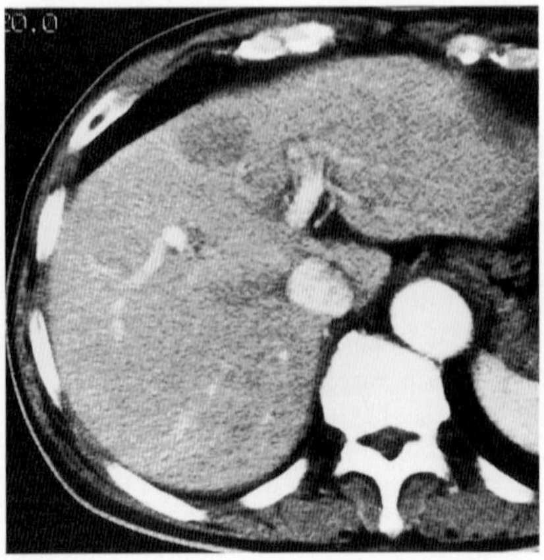

(b) Enhanced CT (early phase): the mass is not enhanced.

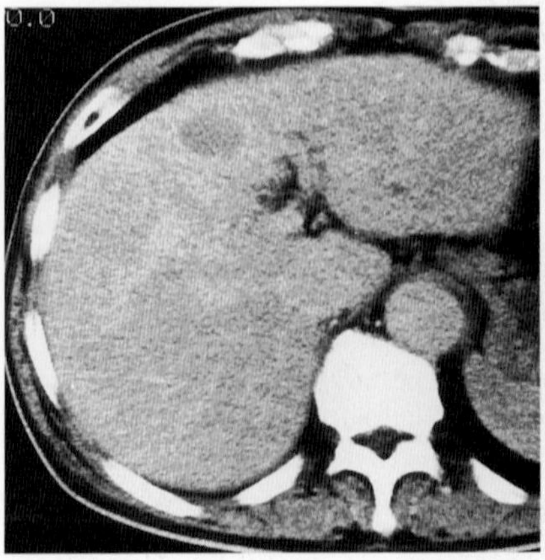

(c) Enhanced CT (late phase, 10 min): the tumor is not enhanced, although the periphery seems to be minimally enhanced.

Case 4 (contd.)

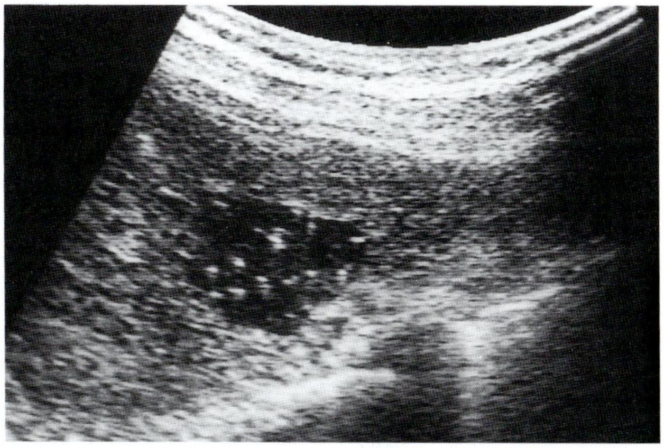

(d) US: the lesion seems to be cystic, and contains many hyperechoic spots with a comet-like tail.

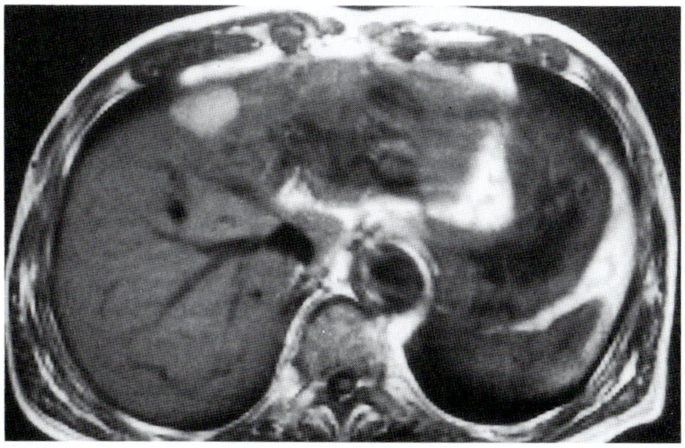

e

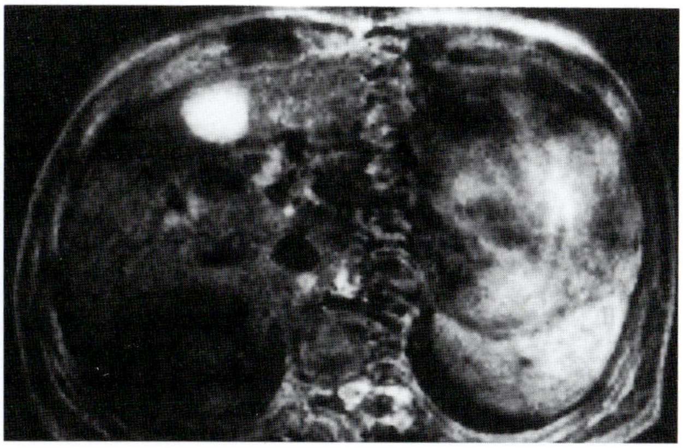

f

(e),(f) MR imaging: on both T1- (e) and T2-weighted (f) images, the tumor is of high signal intensity, suggesting a lesion with a high fat content or hemorrhage. However, because of discrepancies among various imaging findings, an operation was carried out. Opening the abdomen, the mass was protruding from the liver surface, and it was easily enucleated.

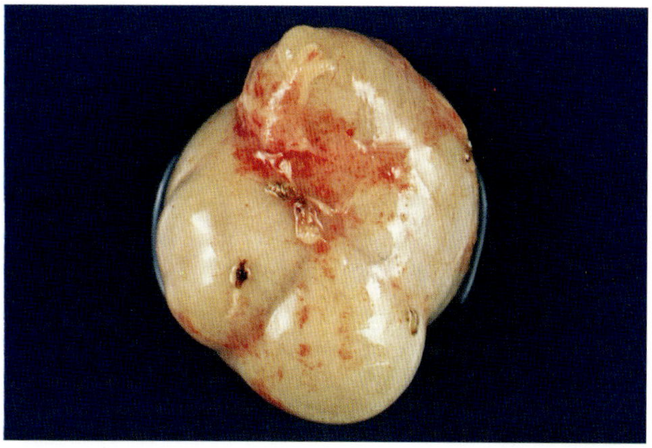

(g) Surface of the removed tumor: gross appearance of the removed tumor as seen from the liver surface.

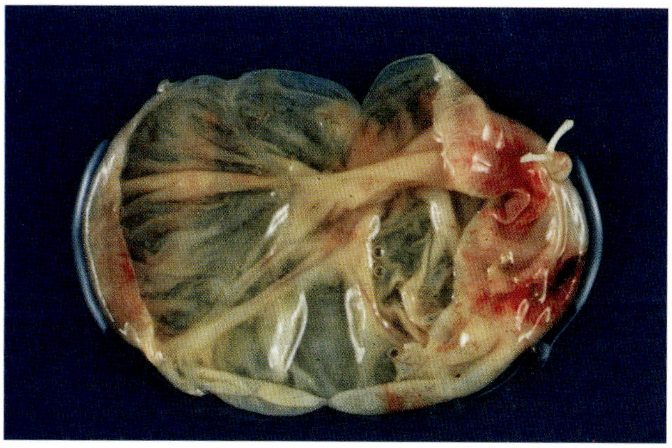

(h) Cut specimen: when the tumor was cut, brownish yellow mucin came out. There was no solid mass in the interior.

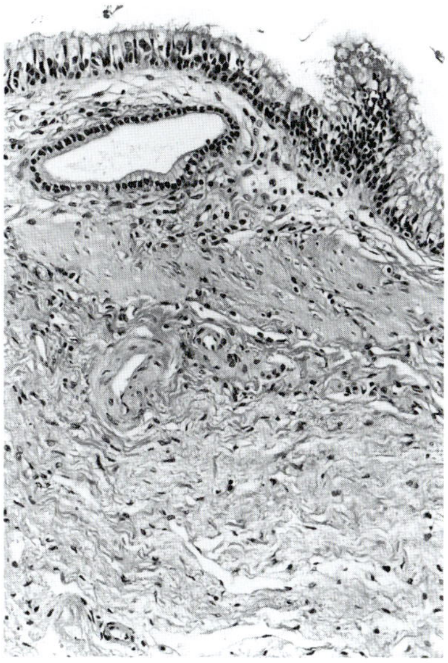

(i) Histopathology: the cyst is lined by ciliated high columnar epithelium, below which there is a layer of smooth muscle, and fibrous tissue further below it.

3.7 Adipose tumors

Fat cell or adipose tumors (Fig. 3.5) primary to the liver are very rare and used to be found incidentally at autopsy. In recent years, they have come to be detected more frequently due to improved imaging techniques; diagnosis of the fat element of the tumor is now possible with CT which thus contributes to differential diagnosis (Kawarada and Mizumoto 1983; Roberts *et al.* 1986; Takayasu *et al.* 1987*b*). The typical fat tumors are lipoma (Case 1) and angiomyolipoma (Case 2), but other types such as angiomyelolipoma (Peters WM *et al.* 1983) and adeno-lipoma (Kurdziel *et al.* 1984) have also been described. Those with a high fat content are readily diagnosed by imaging, but those with little fat are difficult to be differentiate from other solid tumors. Occasional cases of HCC and hepatocellular adenoma that contain fat may require differential diagnosis from localized fatty liver.

Lipoma

Lipoma composed of mature lipocytes alone is very rare, and as of 1985 the survey of the world literature showed no more than 10 cases reported.

Case 1. US and CT demonstrated a tumor which consisted of fat, but the angiogram showed many fine tumor vessels making differentiation from liposarcoma difficult. However, in view of the extreme rarity of primary hepatic liposarcoma, and the possibility that feeding vessels were exaggerated on angiography in the background of fat, the likely diagnosis was lipoma. The resected pure lipoma was perhaps the largest ever reported.

Angiomyolipoma

The tumor consists of three tissue elements, fat, blood vessels, and smooth muscle. It may be differentiated from lipoma by imaging with a demonstration of non-fat elements within the mass. If the fat content is low, identification of the fat element by imaging is not possible, making differential diagnosis from other solid neoplasms difficult. Renal angiomyolipoma is a relatively common benign tumor, and frequently (40–50 per cent) associated with tuberous sclerosis, but hepatic angiomyolipoma is not known to have a similar association.

Case 2. A physician who carried out barium examination on himself for upper abdominal pain, found a hepatic mass. It was subsequently found by US to be an adipose tumor in the left lobe. The CT value of the mass was low (-66 HU) and some areas within the mass were enhanced on contrast injection. Angiomyolipoma was the likely diagnosis, but the tumor was resected because there were many tumor vessels on the angiogram and some of them appeared interrupted; there was a possibility of this being malignant.

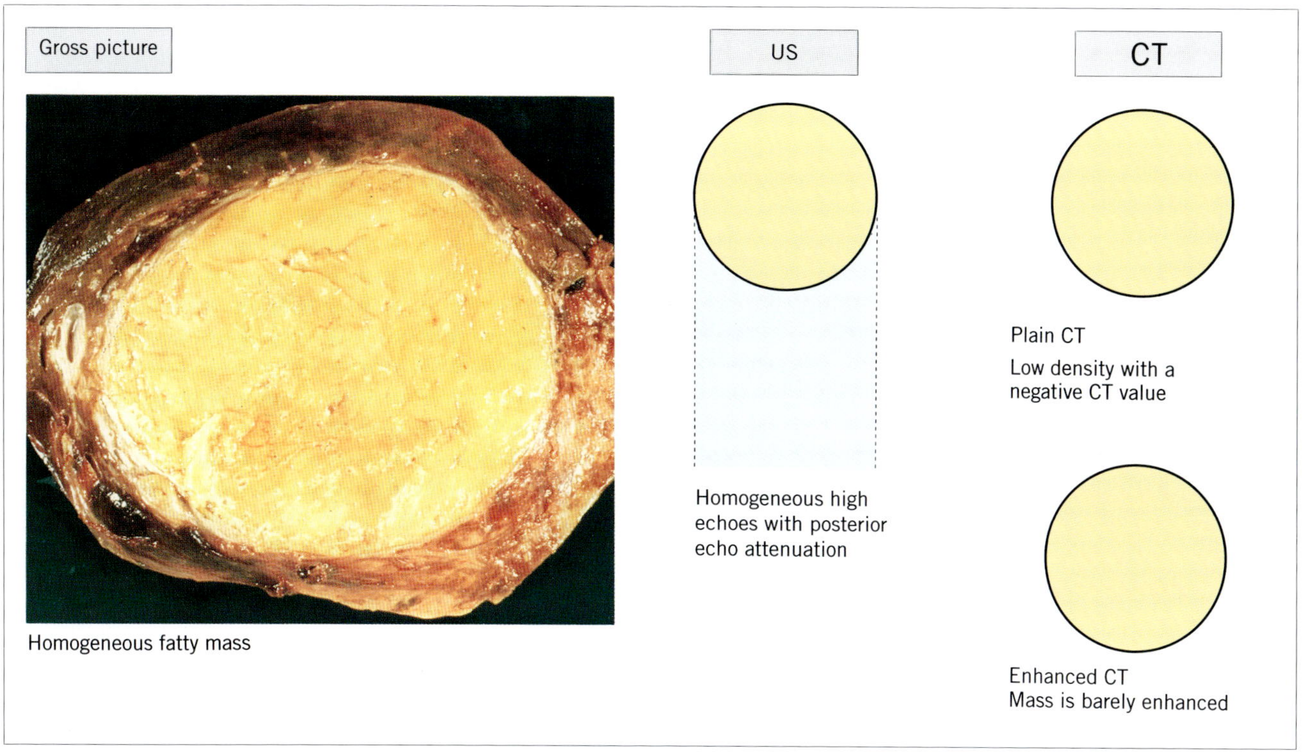

Fig. 3.5a Imaging features of lipoma.

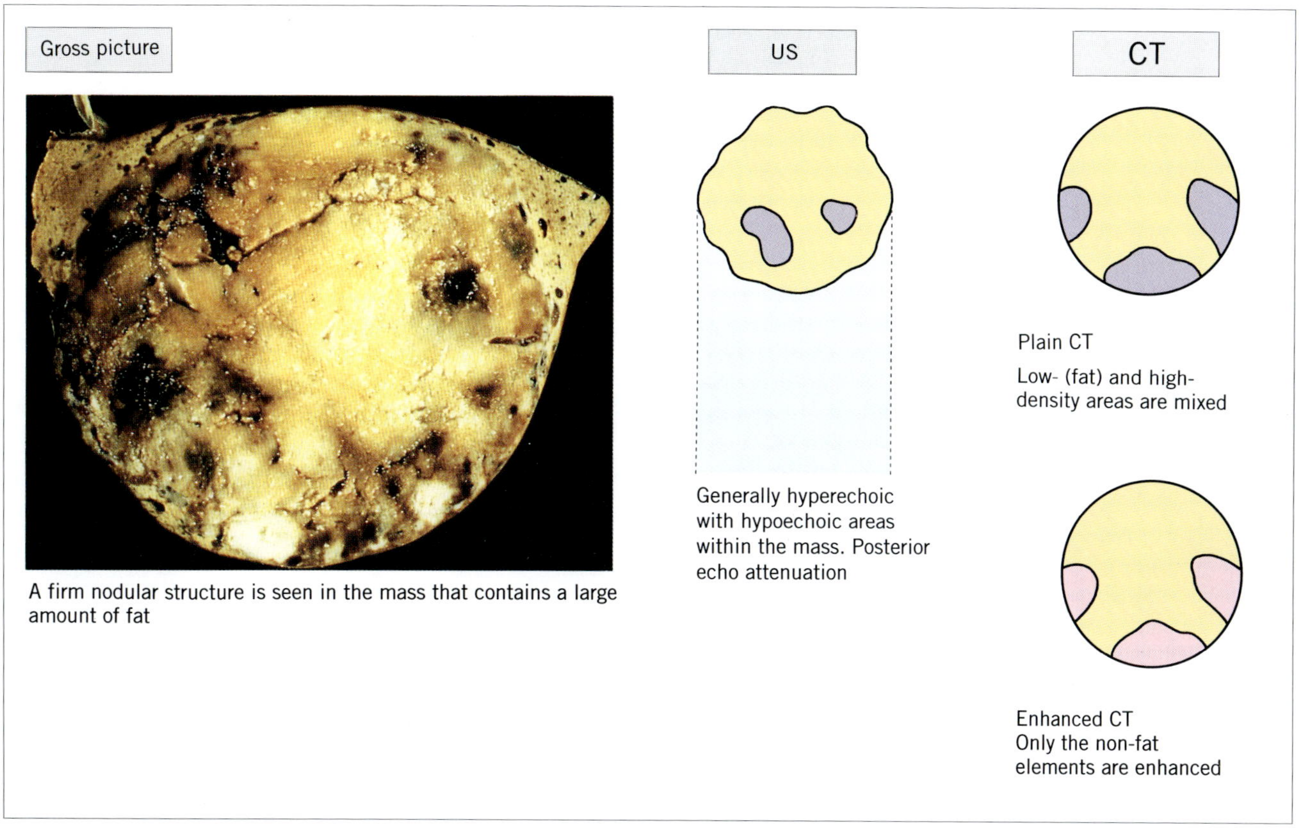

Fig. 3.5b Imaging features of angiomyolipoma.

Adipose tumor—Case 1: A large lipoma occupying the right lobe that required differential diagnosis from liposarcoma. A 63-year-old woman. An abdominal mass was found by a physician whom she visited for abdominal discomfort. During a six-year follow-up the tumor slowly expanded and she was referred to us.

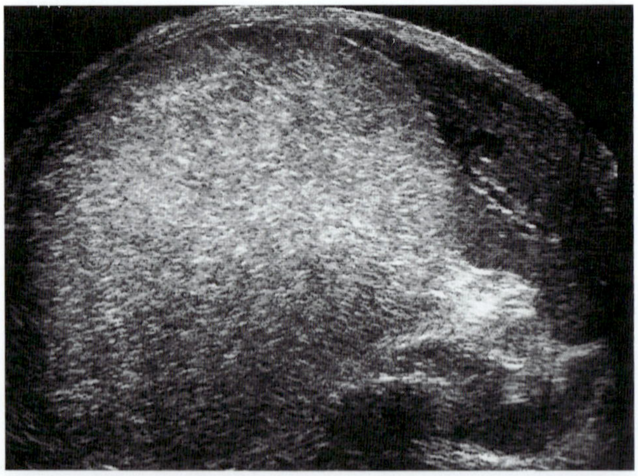

(a) US (transverse scan): a hyperechoic mass is seen in the right lobe. The posterior half of the mass is hypoechoic (reduced echogenicity) due to attenuation of the beam by fat.

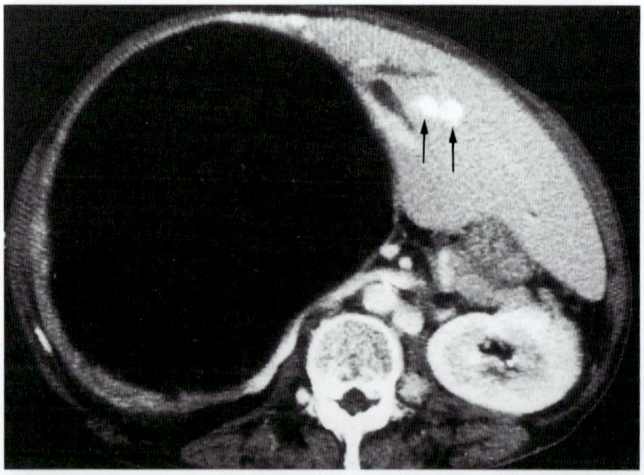

(b) Dynamic CT (early phase): the tumor is not enhanced. The CT value on plain (not shown) CT is −96 HU, suggesting fat as the main component. →; dilated left hepatic vein.

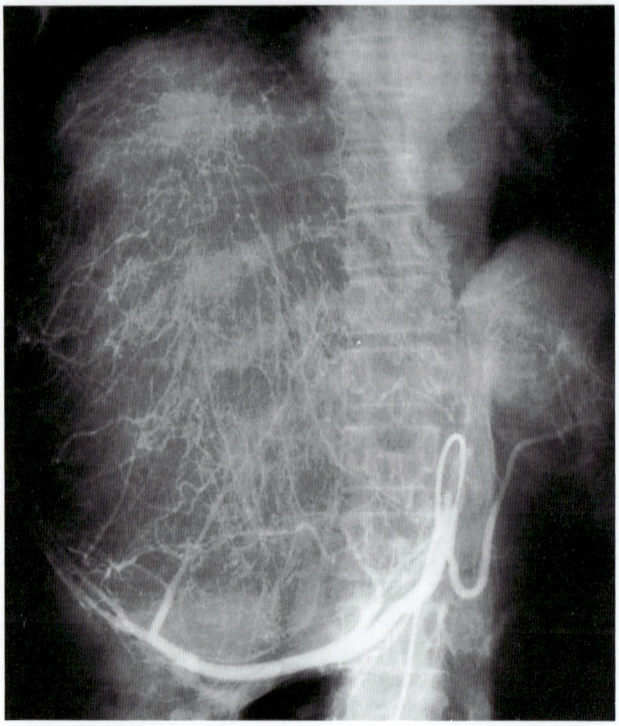

(c) Celiac arteriogram (early phase): the tumor is supplied by meshes of many distended thin tumor vessels.

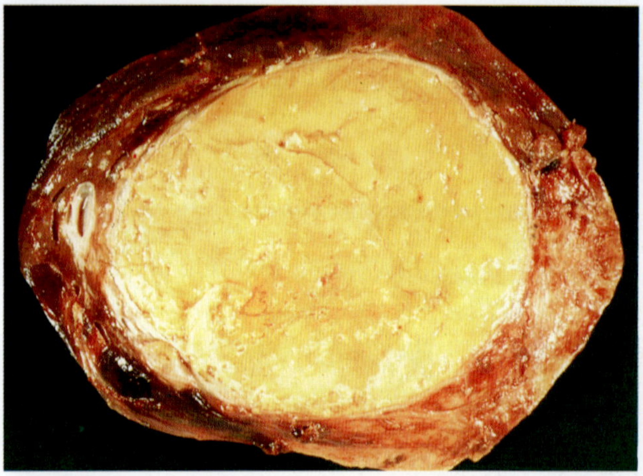

(d) Cut surface of the tumor: extended right lobectomy was carried out (3100 g). It was a lipoma that showed homogeneous yellow fatty tissue on the cut surface.

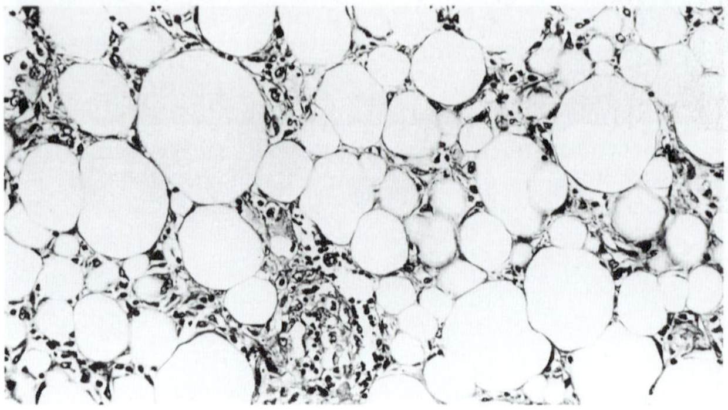

(e) Histology: it consisted of mature lipocytes, and the non-tumor area was normal. The mass was surrounded by a fibrous capsule.

Adipose tumor—Case 2: Hepatic angiomyolipoma requiring differentiation from liposarcoma. A 39-year-old man. Barium examination of the stomach showed a compression by an extra-gastric mass, and US demonstrated a tumor in the left lobe of the liver.

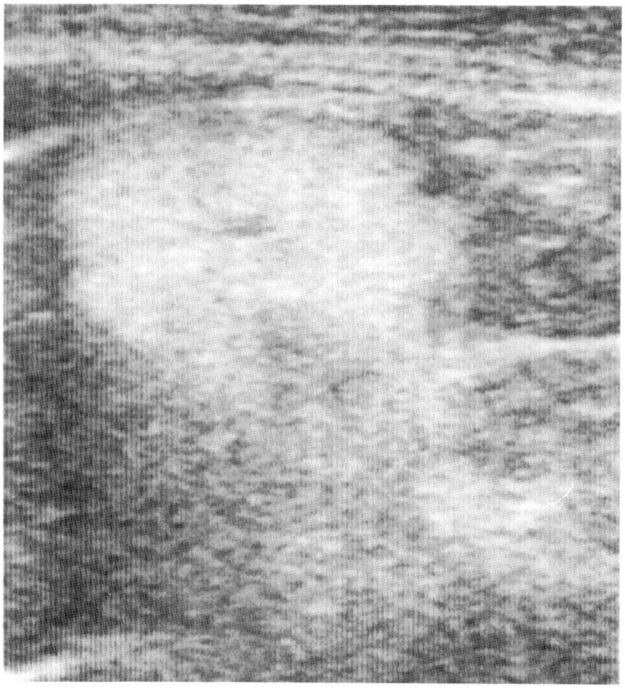

(a) US (transverse scan): a tumor with a high-echo interior and an irregular border was found in the left lobe. The center and a posterior area of the mass are hypoechoic.

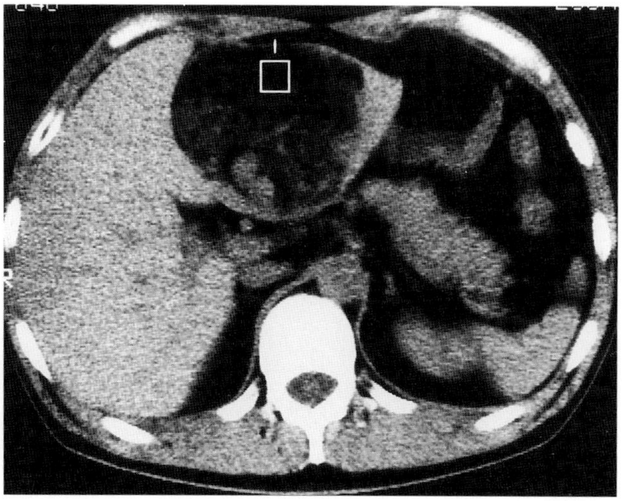

(b) Plain CT: the density of this 9 cm tumor was −66 HU with a nodular inward protrusion in the posterior aspect of the tumor.

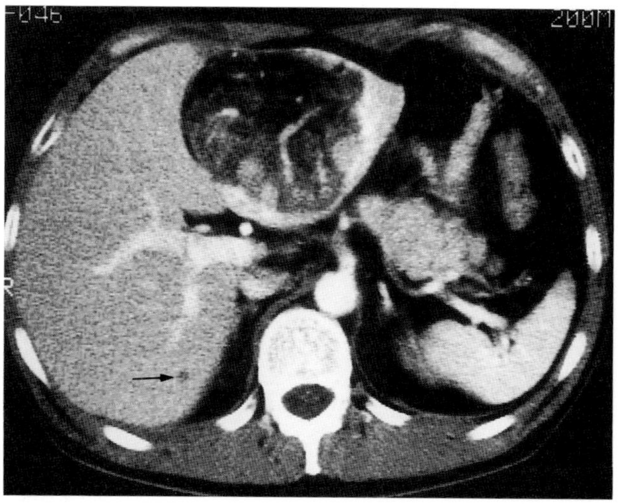

(c) Dynamic CT (early phase): the nodular and string-like structures within the mass were enhanced well. A small unenhanced lesion was found in the right posterior area (→).

Case 2 (contd.)

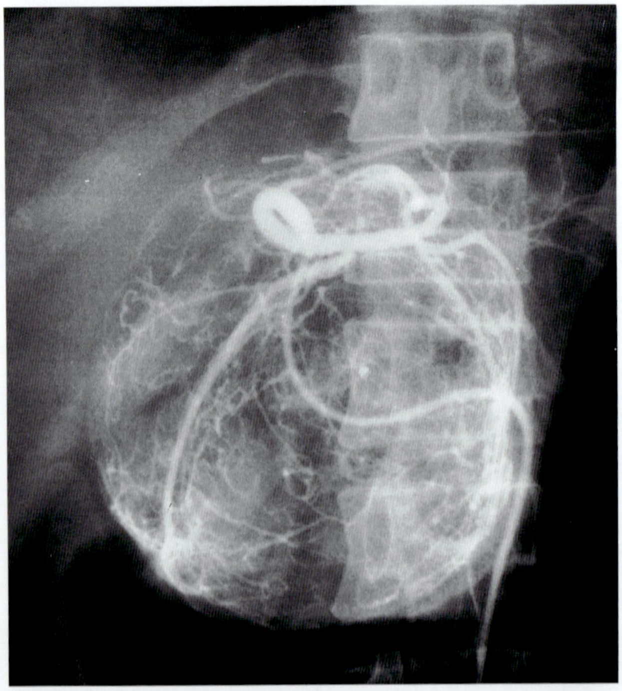

(d) Left hepatic arteriogram (early phase): a hypervascular tumor with many tumor vessels is apparent.

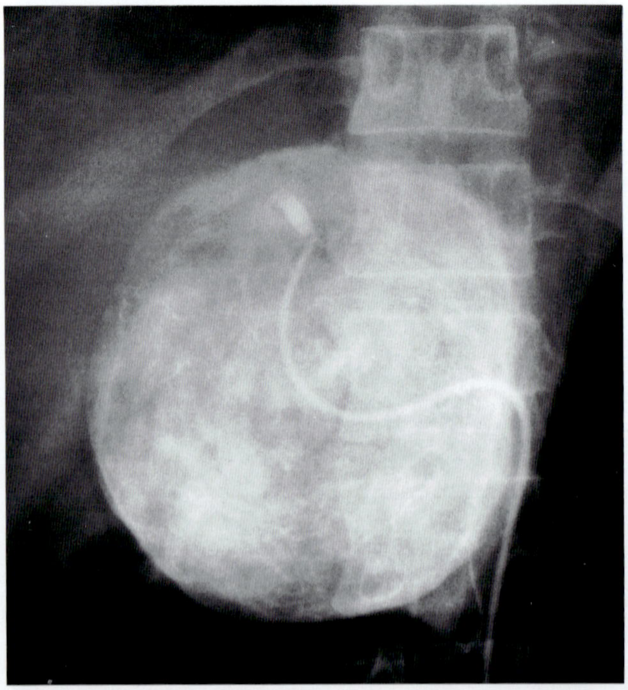

(e) Left hepatic arteriogram (late phase): several nodular stains are seen.

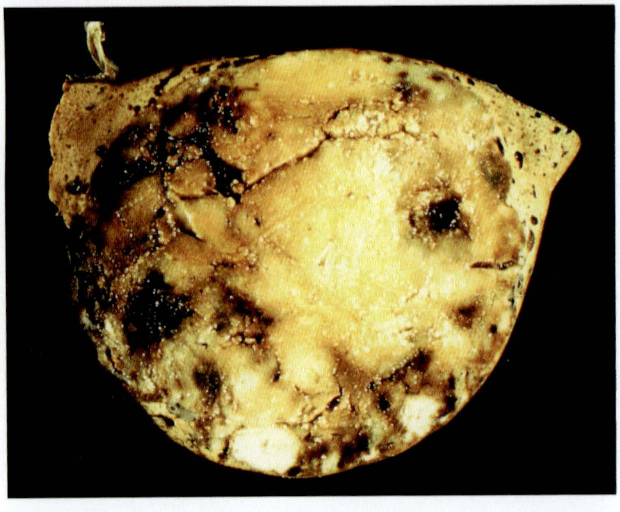

(f) Cut surface of resected specimen: extended left hepatectomy was carried out. This formalin-fixed specimen shows soft fat tissue in the center, black bleeding in the periphery, and several nodular lesions that consist of firm whitish non-fat tissues.

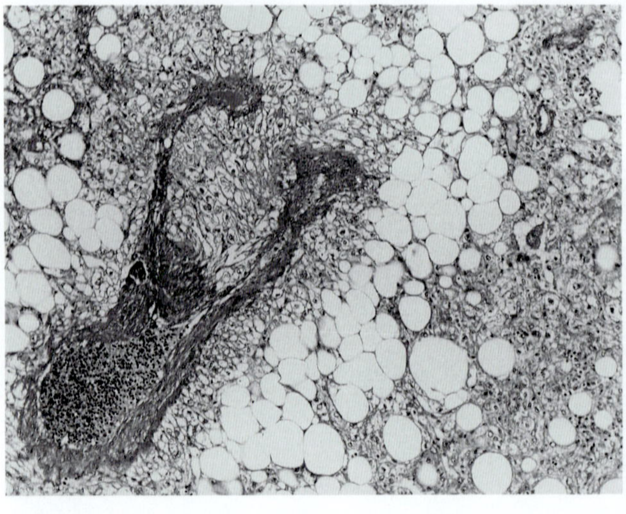

(g) Histology: it consisted of mature lipocytes, winding blood vessels, and smooth muscle surrounding them. Histological diagnosis was angiomyolipoma. There was no fibrous capsule, and the non-tumor parenchyma was normal.

3.8 Other benign hepatic tumors

The other benign hepatic neoplasms include biliary cystadenoma (Ishak *et al.* 1977; Korobkin *et al.* 1989), bile duct adenoma, mesenchymal hamartoma (Ros *et al.* 1986), leiomyoma (Herzberg *et al.* 1990), etc.

Biliary cystadenoma

A multilocular tumor lined by cylindrical epithelium that secretes mucin. It is similar to pancreatic mucinous cystadenoma, and the interior of the cyst can be discerned by US. If it contains protruding structures, carcinoma is likely, and a positive therapeutic approach is required.

Bile duct adenoma

This is mostly found at the time of hepatic surgery as a small whitish firm mass immediately beneath the liver capsule. It is often mistaken as a metastatic lesion. Histologically, the diagnosis is easy if one sees many small benign bile ducts proliferating within a fibrous tissue.

Mesenchymal hamartoma

Mostly occurs in infants younger than 2 years. It is seen as multiple cysts or a multilocular mass by US and CT. It is regarded as a benign counterpart of undifferentiated mesenchymal sarcoma of the liver (Case 1, p.244).

4

Malignant hepatic tumors

4.1 Introduction

Historical background of liver cancer classification

The first attempt to grossly classify liver cancer was made by Eggel in 1901 who proposed three gross types, 'nodular', 'massive' and 'diffuse.' This classification is still used throughout the world, including Japan. However, he had only two cases of his own, and his classification was based on the published reports which lacked morphologic details. A massive tumor almost always has other smaller nodular tumors within the same liver, and one or two of nodular tumors may be so large as to be classified as 'massive.' Nakashima, Okuda and their group felt that mode of growth seen at the tumor boundary should be just as important, and proposed in 1974 a more detailed classification in which eight types were separated (Nakashima *et al.* 1974; Peters 1976). They distinguished the expanding and infiltrating growth patterns and an encapsulated type. Acquisition of a fibrous capsule is a result of slow expanding growth (Okuda *et al.* 1977*c*) more commonly seen in Japan than anywhere else. Okuda, Peters, and Simson (Okuda *et al.* 1984*b*) subsequently proposed another classification in which expanding and infiltrating (spreading) growth patterns were distinguished, and global differences in their incidences were emphasized. These classifications were based on autopsied livers which frequently have advanced cirrhosis, and questions may be asked whether or not the frequency of each type is influenced by the underlying cirrhosis. The relative frequencies may vary between the clinical and autopsy settings, because autopsy cases more often died from hepatic failure as a result of advanced cirrhosis; advanced cirrhosis may have nodular cancer more often than otherwise. Classification based on autopsy does not provide information on the question of whether frequent massive and diffuse types in patients who died from cancer rather than from cirrhosis are simply due to more advanced cancer or to differing degrees of tumor malignancy.

With the progress in imaging techniques, increasing numbers of small HCCs, frequently less than 3 cm, have come to be diagnosed and resected. Classification based on autopsy livers may not be applicable to such tumors, and we now need a classification for small cancers that reflects their biological characteristics. The Japanese version of the *General Rules for the Clinical and Pathological Study of Primary Liver Cancer*, 2nd Edition (Liver Cancer Study Group of Japan 1987) uses Eggel's classification with a modification for the nodular type, considering small cancers. Namely, the nodular type was further divided into four subtypes in order to assist classification of small HCCs. However, these four subtypes are not necessarily independent because mutual transition may occur. In this classification, small HCCs less than 2 cm with an ill-defined tumor boundary are called 'massive' by definition. This deviates from the original definition of 'massive' proposed by Eggel that the mass occupies the whole or nearly the entire lobe. A slight modification was introduced in the 3rd Edition (Liver Cancer Study Group of Japan 1992) in which the 'multinodular' type within the subtypes of the nodular HCC has been deleted with the argument that the individual nodules can be grossly described (Fig. 4.1). It has added an 'infiltrative' type as a subtype within the nodular type for a minute cancer of less than one subsegment that has an irregular and indistinct boundary with the non-cancerous parenchyma. The note to this definition states that the word 'node' means a binding knot on a cord with no intention of describing its periphery whether it is smooth or irregular. The editors comment that that is the reason for making the 'infiltrative' type a subtype rather than an independent type. Some of cholangiocarcinomas [Case 2, (b) p.227], are included in the infiltrative type. However, some other cholangiocarcinomas [Case 1, (f) p.212], and sclerosing HCC [Case 12, (d) p.194], may have an irregular but discrete boundary, and do not fall into any of the given subtypes—a problem to be solved in the future. This classification is for advanced liver cancers, and does not apply to early HCC. In a late stage of diffuse type HCC, a similar infiltrating picture may be seen in autopsy livers. Eggel (1901) defined the diffuse type as 'numerous small tumors indistinguishable from cirrhosis nodules seen throughout the liver with no discernible main tumor,' but in reality such cases are seldom operated and grossly studied. One of the present authors (KO) has seen only one case of strictly diffuse HCC autopsied by the late Professor Peters in Los Angeles, and all other diffuse HCCs had one or two main HCCs with extensive portal infiltration giving rise to diffuse portal spread occurring within a rather short period of time. The clinical course after such intrahepatic spread is rapidly downhill (Okuda *et al.* 1981*b*).

Staging of liver cancer

Staging of liver cancer should vary with the histological type. Most HCC develops on the basis of cirrhosis, and more often the degree of cirrhosis determines the prognosis rather than the tumor itself, whereas the prognosis of cholangiocarcinoma largely depends on its site of origin, and presence or absence of major bile duct obstruction more directly affects the prognosis. The purpose of staging is two-fold. One is for comparison of the efficacy of different treatment modalities; one has to have patients of a comparable stage for comparison. The other is to study the effect of surgical treatment in relation to the stage.

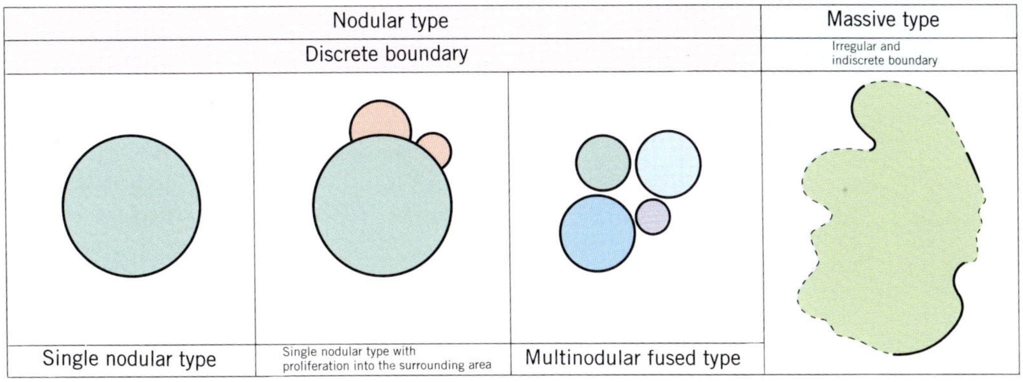

Fig. 4.1 Gross classification of advanced HCC (schema of the three subtypes of nodular form, and massive type). (Cited from the 3rd edition of *General Rules for the Clinical and Pathological Study of Primary Liver Cancer*, edited by the Liver Cancer Study Group of Japan (1992).)

Table 4.1 Staging scheme proposed by Okuda *et al.* (1985*c*)

Stage	Tumor size		Ascites		Albumin		Bilirubin	
	>50%	<50%			<3g/dl	>3g/dl	>3mg/dl	<3mg/dl
	(+)	(−)	(+)	(−)	(+)	(−)	(+)	(−)
I	(−)		(−)		(−)		(−)	
II	1 or 2(+)							
III	3 or 4(+)							

The TNM staging scheme was initially developed for the latter purpose.

The first staging attempt for HCC was proposed at the international meeting held in Kampala, Uganda, in 1971, based on 72 untreated patients seen in Uganda (Primack *et al.* 1975). The prognosis in these patients was very poor with a median survival of only one month, because the diagnosis was made at an advanced stage. In the proposed three stages, weight loss, ascites, signs of portal hypertension, and serum bilirubin were considered. This classical staging system no longer applies to the current practice in which the diagnosis is made much earlier with modern diagnostic procedures, such as AFP and imaging. In 1985, a new more practical staging scheme was proposed (Okuda *et al.* 1985*c*) based on 850 cases in which tumor size, ascites, albumin and bilirubin are considered (Table 4.1). More recently, an attempt was made by a group at the National Cancer Center Hospital (Yamasaki *et al.* 1990) to adopt the TNM system to liver cancer staging at the recommendation of UICC (International Union Against Cancer 1987), and the Japanese recommendation was formally adopted by UICC (Table 4.2). This staging is meant for HCC as are the classifications of gross pathology, since more than 90 per cent of primary liver cancers are HCC, but it can also be used for intrahepatic bile duct carcinoma.

The TNM classification emphasizes the T factor. It considers the size (larger or smaller than 2 cm), vascular invasion and its degree, and number of tumors (single or multiple) (Table 4.3). In many cases, T numbers correspond to stage numbers. In this scheme, major vessels for vascular invasions mean the central part of the right and left first order portal vein branch and major hepatic veins from immediately before entry into the inferior vena cava up to the right atrium. For the N factor, the presence of metastasis in the TNM lymph nodes (hilar and suprahepatic infradiaphragmatic) or lymph nodes beyond them classifies the tumor into Stage III or IV. For the M factor, extrahepatic metastasis is called M1, and the tumor is staged as IV-B. Current imaging techniques permit such classification.

Imaging diagnosis of degree of gross cancer progression

Diagnosis of tumor existence (segment diagnosis) and quality (differential) diagnosis constitutes imaging diagnosis of the T factor. Early diagnosis of HCC depends on collective diagnosis mobilizing various imaging modalities including MR imaging. For the assessment of vascular invasion, a similar approach in which diagnosis of the order of the branch involved and differentiation from thrombosis are required. Lobar attenuation differences between the right and left lobes in dynamic CT are an important diagnostic finding closely associated with occlusion of a large portal vein branch or an arterio-portal communication.

For the diagnosis of the N factor, CT is better than other modalities, but Gastrografin must be used for differentiating the lymph node from the bowel.

If the size of the lymph node is less than 1 cm, differential diagnosis between metastasis and relative enlargement of the lymph node is required. The possibility of metastasis increases

Table 4.2 Classification of degree of liver cancer progression

Stage	Factor		
	T	N	M
I	T1	N0	M0
II	T2	N0	M0
III	T3	N0	M0
	T1–3	N1	M0
IV-A	T4	N0-1	M0
IV-B	T1-4	N0-1	M1

Table 4.3 Breakdown of the T factor in the Japanese General Rules for Cancer Study

<table>
<tr><td colspan="2" rowspan="2">Item</td><td colspan="4">Largest diameter</td></tr>
<tr><td colspan="2">≤2 cm →</td><td colspan="2">2 cm<</td></tr>
<tr><td colspan="2">Vascular invasion</td><td>(−)</td><td>(+)→</td><td>(−)</td><td>(+)</td></tr>
<tr><td colspan="2">Solitary</td><td>T1</td><td colspan="2">T2</td><td></td></tr>
<tr><td rowspan="2">Multiple</td><td>One lobe</td><td>T2</td><td colspan="3">T3</td></tr>
<tr><td>Two lobes</td><td colspan="4" rowspan="2">T4</td></tr>
<tr><td colspan="2">Major vessel invasion</td></tr>
</table>

as the size exceeds 1.5 cm, and careful intraoperative identification of the node seen by imaging is necessary. In enhanced CT, lymph node metastasis of HCC is frequently enhanced to some extent.

Of the extrahepatic metastases (M factor), lung metastasis is the most common; this is usually associated with large (more than 10 cm) HCC in the liver and seen as bilateral multiple coin lesions. In the area which is superimposed on the mediastinal lymph node metastasis or the heart, CT is most diagnostic. Bone metastasis is more common in the spine and rib, seen as a osteolytic lesion. Occasionally, bone metastasis is the first symptom that leads to the discovery of the primary, fracture of the femur facilitates the diagnosis of bone metastasis, or spinal metastasis is incidentally found on a CT film made for other purposes. When bone metastasis is suspected, or for preoperative screening of the bone, scanning using ^{99m}Tc-hydroxymethylene diphosphonate is useful.

Adrenal metastasis is more frequently discovered at the time of liver imaging without previous knowledge; upon angiography, it appears similar to HCC. If the size is as small as 2 cm or so, it could also be an incidental adrenal adenoma, calling for differentiation.

4.2 Small hepatocellular carcinoma

Small liver cancer has recently come to be detected by modern imaging in increasing numbers of patients who have no tumor-associated symptoms. The name and definition of small liver cancer have undergone changes in the past. In 1977, Okuda *et al.* (1977*e*) used the term 'minute hepatocellular carcinoma' for HCC smaller than 4.5 cm if solitary, or less than 3.5 cm for HCCs less than four in number. Subsequently, Chen *et al.* (1982) proposed that HCC smaller than 3 cm in the largest diameter be called 'small HCC.' In the following year, the Liver Cancer Study Group of Japan defined small liver cancer as a solitary cancer with its largest diameter less than 2 cm. These decreasing sizes in definition reflect the limit of imaging capability at these times; improvement in imaging capability is apparent.

Currently, lesions as small as 1 cm are detectable, and in fact, are being detected. Histopathological diagnosis of such small lesions whether benign or malignant, is not always easy, and it is one of the major tasks that liver pathologists are facing at the moment.

In this book, a tumor smaller than 3 cm is called 'small' liver cancer or HCC for practical reasons, and imaging diagnosis of such lesions shall be discussed in more detail.

Detection method and the process leading to definitive diagnosis

In our experience at the National Cancer Center Hospital, 89 per cent (89 of 100 cases) of the cases of small HCC, less than 3 cm, were found during the follow-up of chronic liver disease (chronic hepatitis and cirrhosis) having no symptom (Takayasu *et al.* 1990*f*). The number of patients who had objective and subjective symptoms was very few. Classical HCC in which AFP elevation above 400 ng/ml during the follow-up led to diagnosis, constituted 21 per cent. Diagnosis was made in the remainder by US (56 per cent) or CT (20 per cent) (Table 4.4).

There were more males than females with an M:F ratio of approximately 5:1. Associated liver cirrhosis was demonstrable histopathologically in about 80 per cent. Clearly, the background of small HCC is chronic liver disease, the same as that of advanced HCC, and HCC develops among the high-risk group of patients (Kubo *et al.* 1978; Obata *et al.* 1980; Shinagawa *et al.* 1984; Kobayashi *et al.* 1985).

Alpha-fetoprotein (AFP) and other tumor markers

The AFP levels at the time of imaging diagnosis of small HCC were normal, less than 20 ng/ml, in 41 per cent (40/97 cases), and only 16 per cent of the cases showed levels above 400 ng/ml. When the relationship of AFP levels and tumor size was

Table 4.4 Methods by which small HCC (≤3 cm) was detected and the diagnostic process

Tumor size	No. of	Methods used for the first detection			
cm	cases	AFP	US	CT	Angiography
≤1	4	0	2	1	1
1–2	43	8	23	10	2
2–3	53	13	31	9	0
Total	100 (89)	21 (20)	56 (48)	20 (18)	3 (3)

( ): Number of cases found to have small HCC during follow-up for chronic liver disease.

Table 4.5 AFP levels in relation to tumor size in small HCC (≤3 cm)

Tumor size (cm)	No. of cases	AFP levels (ng/ml)			
		<20	20–400	400–1000	≥1000
≤1	4	4	0	0	0
1–2	45	23	16	4	2
2–3	48	13	25	2	8
Total	97	40	41	6	10

analyzed, the number of cases having normal valus increased as the tumor size decreased (Table 4.5), suggesting the limitations of AFP measurement in its diagnostic capability (Takayasu *et al.* 1990*f*). Thus, it is obvious that AFP measurement alone is not sufficient for early detection of HCC. HCC specific AFP subspecies can now be quantified (Taketa *et al.* 1993) and may assist in early detection of HCC in patients with mildly elevated AFP. Des-γ-carboxy prothrombin (PIVKA-II) is more specific than AFP (Okuda H *et al.* 1991), but is less sensitive, and has not contributed much to early diagnosis of HCC although this test is widely used.

Imaging diagnosis

Currently, US, CT, angiography and MR imaging are used for the diagnosis of liver cancer. However, if an operation is being considered in the patient, these routine examinations are inadequate, and more sophisticated and meticulous examination is desirable. Particularly, in the presence of certain discrepancies between various imaging findings, all the possible diagnostic approaches are to be mobilized, because the selection of the operative procedure may vary with the findings.

Existence diagnosis

Correct existence diagnosis for small HCC with each imaging technique At the Cancer Center Hospital, Tokyo, arterial-CT, portal-CT, and/or Lipiodol-CT (Lip-CT) are carried out in patients scheduled for surgery. The rates of correct diagnosis of disease existence with individual imaging modalities are given in Table 4.6. In a total of 135 cases of small HCC, the rate of correct diagnosis was 84 per cent both with US and CT which was slightly better than that with angiography (81 per cent) and arterial-CT (82 per cent); an even better rate was obtained with portal-CT (91 per cent) and Lip-CT (93 per cent), both above 90 per cent (Takayasu *et al.* 1990*f*).

As regards the diameter of the tumor and diagnosis rate, there was little difference between these modalities for tumors between 1 and 3 cm, but for a tumor smaller than 1 cm, they differed, correct diagnosis rates with US and CT being less than 50 per cent, whereas portal-CT (67 per cent) and Lip-CT (83 per cent) were much better, and more effective. The diagnosis rate with intraoperative US is given for comparison in table 4.6. It is more accurate than any other modality, but is not to be compared with imaging from outside the body; it is carried out with direct contact with the liver under laparotomy. In table 4.6, the denominator consists of the number of lesions found by intraoperative US plus those found in the resected specimens. Thus, there is certain bias in case selection. We have experienced several cases in which arterial-CT and MR imaging demonstrated a lesion but intraoperative US failed to do the same. However, the figures in table 4.6 are the best results that specialists in each imaging modality obtained with histological confirmation. A more recent problem is differential diagnosis of preneoplastic nodules and early HCC found by intraoperative US.

False negative and false positive results with each imaging modality There are two factors which reduce the detection rate for small HCC; one is the anatomical characteristics of the liver and the other the physical characteristics of the individual imaging instrument. Figure 4.2 depicts the anatomical region within the liver where each of US, CT, and angiography has difficulties in diagnosing small HCC.

For US, the area immediately below the diaphragm is frequently a dead angle, and lesions in S^{VII} and the lateral aspect of the left lobe are often overlooked. With the advent of the convex transducer, the dead angle below the diaphgram has been reduced. In cirrhosis, however, the liver configuration is much altered and the bowels are elevated as a result; the area visible with US thus becomes much smaller.

On CT images, the cranial and caudal rims of the liver may produce the partial volume phenomenon causing false negative and false positive imaging. In the area in the left lobe immediately below the diaphragm contiguous to the heart contrast medium in the ventricle of the heart in the early phase of enhancement may be mistaken for a tumor stain. The most common cause of false negative results in CT imaging may be incomplete slicing due to irregular breathing movements on the

Table 4.6 Detection rates for small HCC (≤3 cm) with individual imaging modalities

Tumor size (cm)	No. of lesions	Imaging modality						
		US	CT	Angiography	Arterial-CT	Portal-CT	Lipiodol-CT	Intraoperative US
≤1	22	7/19 (37)	8/19 (42)	12/22 (55)	0/1 (0)	2/3 (67)	10/12 (83)	19/22 (86)
1–3	113	101/110 (92)	100/110 (91)	97/112 (87)	14/16 (88)	19/20 (95)	45/47 (96)	110/113 (98)
Total	135	108/129 (84)	108/129 (84)	109/134 (81)	14/17 (82)	21/23 (91)	55/59 (93)	130/135 (96)

Figures in parentheses are percentage values.

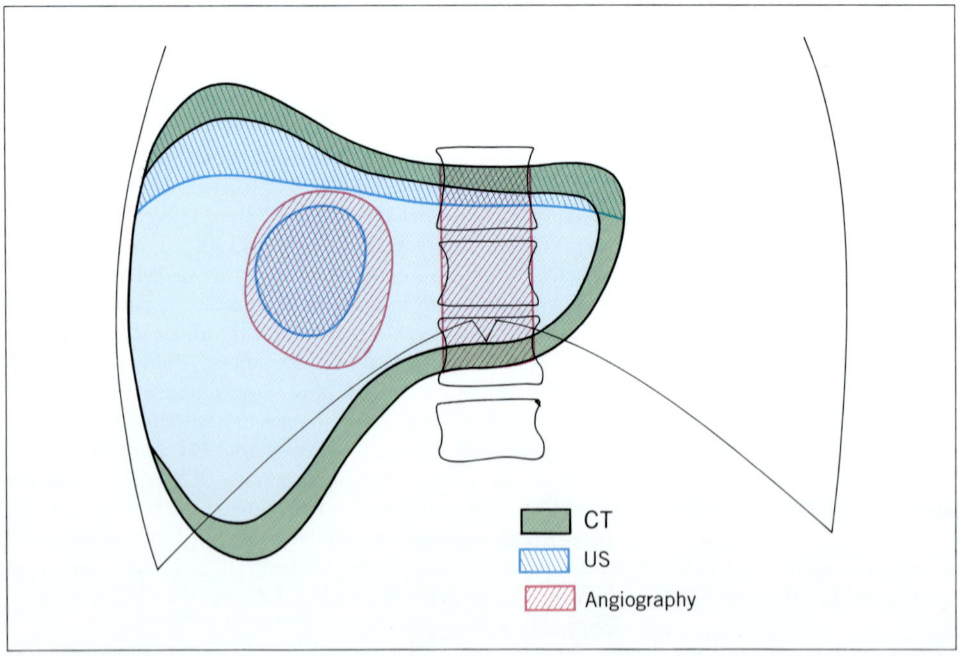

Fig. 4.2 The area where a small lesion is difficult to detect by various imaging modalities.

part of the patient. At the time of interpretation, some areas appear to be missing, to the dismay of the radiologist, although continuous sectioning was done. This kind of difficulty has been overcome with the advent of high-speed CT/ helical CT in which the CT table shifts while CT slices are being made. During one breath hold, eight to ten slices or all slices for the entire liver can be made, and slicing failure is very uncommon.

In angiography, difficulty was encountered in the past in identifying small lesions in the lateral area of the left lobe, because the vertebral column is superimposed. This problem has now largely been solved with the introduction of DSA. In angiography, most HCCs are seen as hypervascular lesions as they are supplied predominantly by arteries. Although they receive arteries, the amount of arterial blood inflow may not be much higher or may be even less than the surrounding parenchyma. In such a situation, the lesion is not recognizable, with a false negative result. This phenomenon is seen in extremely well differentiated HCC (Edmondson-Steiner's grade I) (Takayasu *et al.* 1986*e*; Takayasu, Okuda 1987*e*) (Case 1), HCC with fatty changes (Yoshikawa *et al.* 1988) (Case 2), and less frequently HCC with spontaneous necrosis (Case 3). When small lesions are located behind a large tumor, naturally they are not recognized (Case 4). We have experienced a 1.5 cm HCC which was masked because there was a large arterio-portal communication resulting in regurgitation of contrast medium into the portal trunk (cf. Case 22 in the section on tumor thrombus, p.177).

Although Lip-CT is generally very sensitive and capable of detecting small HCC, false results, though uncommon, are also experienced, for example no Lipiodol retention in a 3 cm HCC even immediately after Lipiodol injection (Merine *et al.* 1990) (Case 5), and false positive retention in a regenerative nodule (Case 6). The CT image made shortly after Lipiodol injection may show non-specific retention immediately beneath the liver surface, in the gallbladder bed, and along the Cantlie line (cf. Lipiodol-CT, Section 13.5, Figs 28, 29, and 30, p.424–5). Therefore, one has to be careful in interpreting Lipiodol retention in the caudal border of the S^{VI} segment and around the gallbladder; repeat CT after some interval may be required. Even intraoperative US may have difficulty in identifying small lesions occurring in a liver with macronodular cirrhosis (Case 7). For such a liver, it is desirable to study the resected specimen with soft X-rays to determine whether or not an HCC was present in the specimen.

How high-tesla MR imaging compares with CT in the diagnosis of small HCC is a recent question. Although some reports indicate an equally high detection rate with MR imaging, detection of a mass in the left lobe is hampered by the movement of the heart and aorta. With new contrast agents for MR imaging (compounds containing paramagnetic atoms such as Gd, Mn, and Fe), its diagnostic acuity is improving. There have been some early HCCs only MR imaging could detect, and MR imaging may be regarded as being complementary to CT.

Quality diagnosis (differential diagnosis)

A nodular HCC, 2–3 cm in size, with a surrounding fibrous capsule demonstrates typical imaging features of a nodule-in-nodule interior and the presence of a capsule on US (Tanaka *et al.* 1983), CT, and angiography. In such cases, quality diagnosis is not difficult at all. Namely, US frequently shows a mosaic internal structure and posterior acoustic accentuation, along with a lateral shadow or a halo derived from the capsule (Case 8).

On plain CT, HCC is seen as a low-density lesion unless bleeding or calcification is present, but the capsule is seldom discerned (Case 9). In the early phase of dynamic CT, the individual nodules within the mass are seen in differing densities,

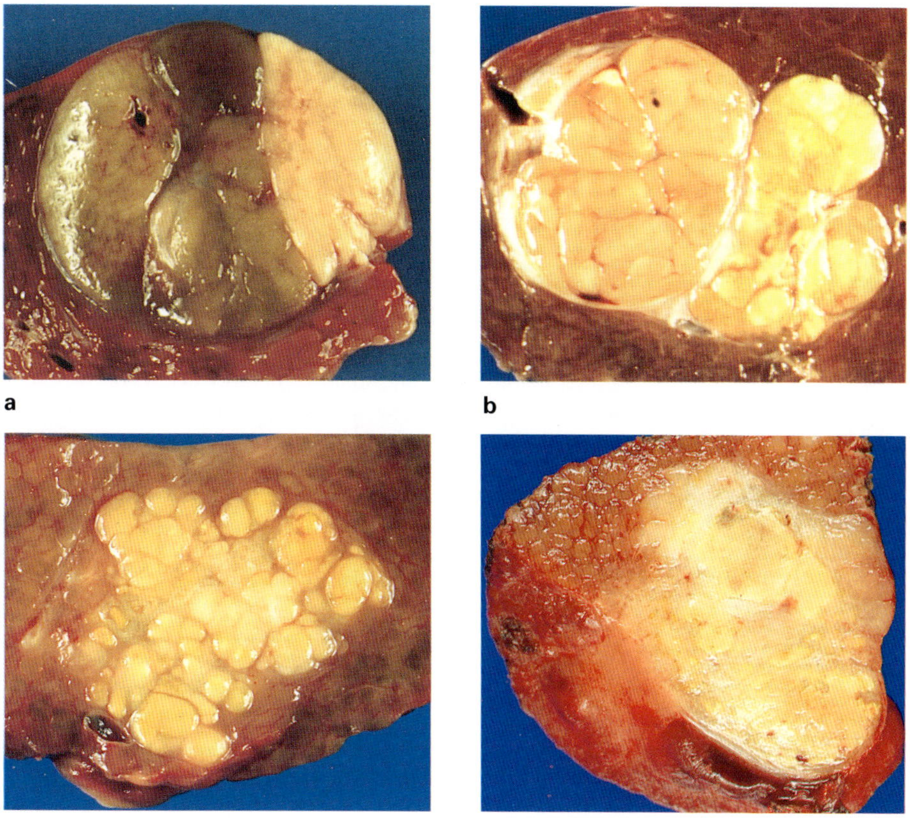

a b c d

Fig. 4.3 Gross appearance of nodular types of small HCC (the infiltrative type (d) is a mixed type): (a) single nodular type; (b) single nodular type with proliferation into the surrounding area; (c) multinodular fused type; (d) infiltrative type.

and the entire mass is de-enhanced, becoming low in density in the late phase after 3 min (Araki *et al.* 1980) (Case 10). The high-density rim around the mass strongly suggestive of a capsule, is not commonly seen. On angiography, extensive neovasculature with winding new vessels is seen in the arterial phase, and the pre-existing artery or arteries feeding the tumor are dilated. In the parenchymal phase, uneven nodular stains are seen within the mass (Takayasu *et al.* 1986*e*). The capsule may be suggested from a translucent rim (Okuda *et al.* 1977*c*) surrounding the tumor (Case 11).

One can clearly delineate tumor nodules within the mass and septa separating them using DSA (Case 12) which provides improved quality diagnosis of HCC. Some small HCCs may already have arterio-portal shunts, and small shunts in the real periphery or near the liver capsule, can only be demonstrated by angiography (Case 1).

In the diagnosis of HCC smaller than 1 cm, the diagnostic features are quite different. US and CT are not capable of delineating the internal structure of the tumor. On US, it is seen either as a homogeneously low-density lesion, or less commonly as a high-density lesion. Quality diagnosis is difficult. Even dynamic CT fails to discern the internal structure and a contrast agent may become necessary for temporal changes in staining for quality diagnosis (Case 13). We carry out arterial-CT for quality diagnosis when tumor stain is equivocal (Case 14). An HCC of about 1 cm in size gives only a mild stain without showing tumor vessels on angiography, and a translucent rim is rarely discerned.

On MR imaging small HCC gives varying intensities in T1-weighted spin echo images; low intensity is more common but high and isointensities are also seen in some cases. In T2–weighted images, the majority of small HCCs show high intensity (Itoh *et al.* 1987; Kadoya *et al.* 1992) (Case 15). The capsule is delineated much better than with CT.

The above discussion is mainly for nodular type small HCC. Imaging diagnosis of the single nodular type with proliferation into the surrounding area (type 2) and multinodular fused type (type 3) will be discussed in the next section on gross pathological features and imaging diagnosis of small HCC.

Gross pathology and imaging features of small HCC

Gross pathological classification of small HCC is basically the same as that for HCC in general (Fig. 4.1). However, to determine the basic types of small HCC, it is more desirable to study a small HCC of an early stage rather than a small metastatic HCC within the liver with advanced HCC and vascular invasion. Small HCC may be classified into four types as illustrated in Fig. 4.3. However, the infiltrative type is rather uncommon in Japan as a small HCC. The single nodular type with proliferation into the surrounding area (type 2) is perhaps a more advanced stage of the single nodular type (type 1), but whether the multiple nodular fused type is a totally different growth type or an outcome of expansion of the single nodular type is not clear. Some suggest that the prognosis and degree of malignancy may be predicted from the gross anatomical features and attempts have been made to determine the gross types by imaging (Okuda *et al.* 1977*f*; Kanai *et al.* 1987), although accurate assessment is not easy by any modality. Dynamic CT perhaps provides more information because it reflects the gross features better than the other modalities.

(i) Type 1 small HCC. If it is larger than 2 cm, dynamic CT may demonstrate nodular stains within the tumor in the early phase, and a high density ring in the late phase (Case 10).

(ii) Type 2 small HCC. Dynamic CT may show the main mass and nodular stains in the perphery as its continuation. However, a small tumor budding from the main mass may be difficult to discern by US and CT, depending on the direction of the beam or section.

(iii) Type 3 small HCC. Dynamic CT demonstrates an irregular contour (Case 17), and the tumor is seen as a fused multiple nodules by Lip-CT (Case 18) and angiography.

Small HCC followed for a long time

One can seldom follow a small lesion for which quality diagnosis could not be made until it becomes an overt classical HCC.

Case 19. The follow-up CT made 4 years postoperatively showed multiple small low-density tumors in the remnant liver. Tumor recurrence was strongly suspected, but angiography, arterial-CT, and Lip-CT all failed to demonstrate tumor stain or Lipiodol retention. Existence diagnosis was made only by portal-CT. Subsequent angiography made the diagnosis of HCC recurrence in the remnant liver. The small lesions first found postoperatively were deemed to represent either very early HCCs or adenomatous hyperplasias which turned into classical HCC in 1 year and 7 months. To our regret, these lesions did not respond to repeated Lip-TAE.

Case 20. In this patient, a lesion that was not detectable by enhanced CT, angiography or arterial-CT, grew to 2.5 × 2.0 cm in size in 8 months to be delineated by angiography and arterial-CT.

In addition, we have also seen a case in whom a lesion showing typical imaging features of HCC slowly diminished in size and eventually disappeared (Case 8 in Section 4.6, p.190).

Tumor volume doubling time (TVDT)

The time required for a mass to double its volume is called the tumor volume doubling time (TVDT). TVDT may be calculated from the following formula proposed by Schwartz and Gerstenbery, provided that the Collins' conditions (Collins 1956) are met:

$$\text{TVDT} = t/10\,(\log_{10}d_1 - \log_{10}d_0)$$

where t is the number of days during which the initial diameter (d_0) has grown to d_1.

If the largest diameter (a) on its section and the shorter diameter (b) at right angles to it are not equal, an averaged diameter $\sqrt{a \times b}$ is used. With the measurement of TVDT, it has become apparent that the growth speed of HCC varies considerably from case to case. According to Okazaki *et al.* (1989), the average TVDT is about 100 days. This and other studies based on US (Sheu *et al.* 1985; Ebara *et al.* 1986*a*), have laid the ground for the current screening program for early HCC detection (Okuda 1986) in which imaging is done every 3 months in order to detect a 2 cm HCC growing from 1 cm. It has also been found by repeated TVDT measurements that TVDT becomes shorter as the tumor size increases.

Small HCC—Case 1: Well differentiated HCC not enhanced even by arterial-CT. A 51-year-old man. During the follow-up of chronic liver disease, US detected a solitary mass, and dynamic CT found another lesion.

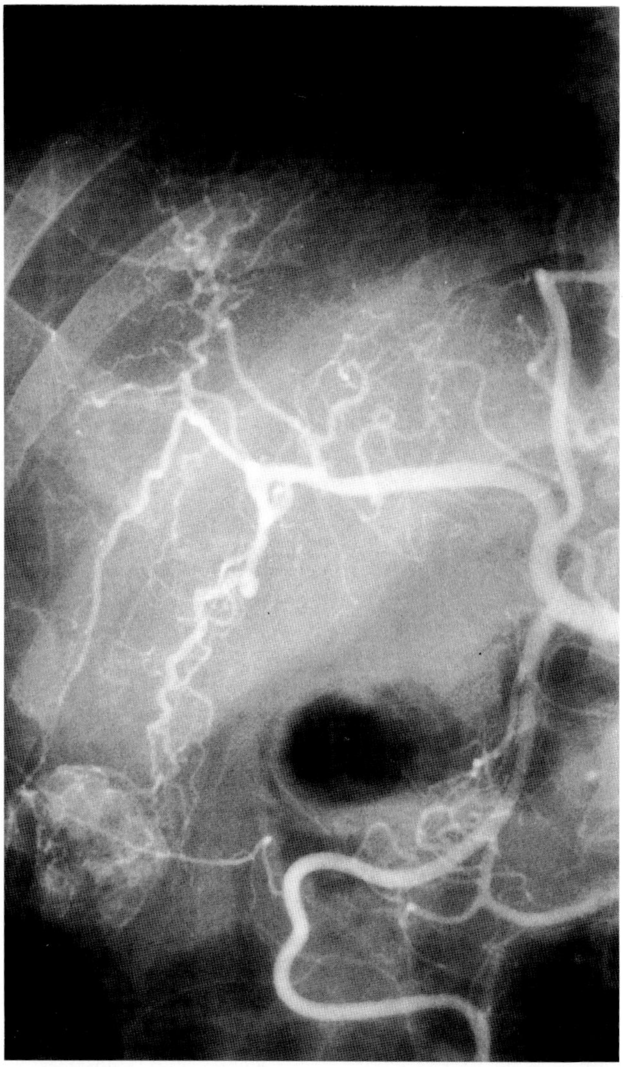

(a) Arteriography (early phase): a 3 cm hypervascular tumor with distinct neovasculature is seen in S^{VI}.

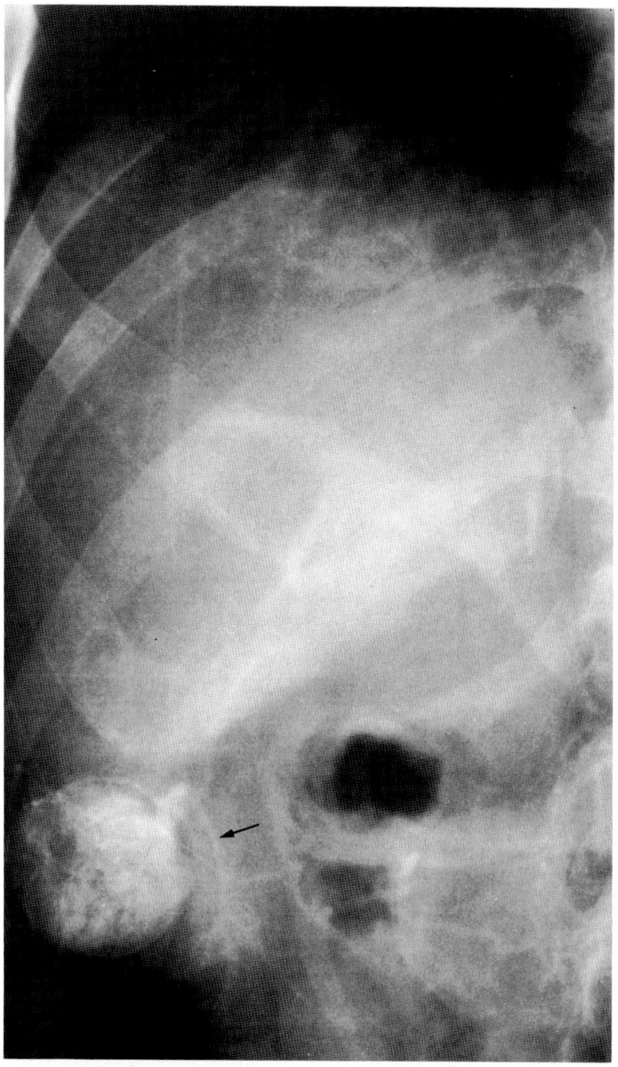

(b) Arteriography (late phase): a nodule-in-nodule stain within the tumor and a small arterio-portal shunt (→) are seen.

Case 1 (contd.)

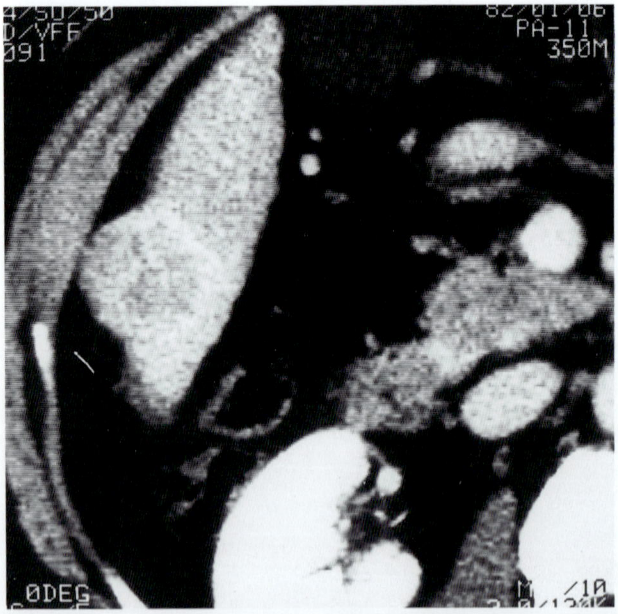

(c) Dynamic-CT (early phase): the same lesion in S^{VI} as seen by angiography is now diagnosed as HCC from the peripheral ring stain and a somewhat mosaic internal structure.

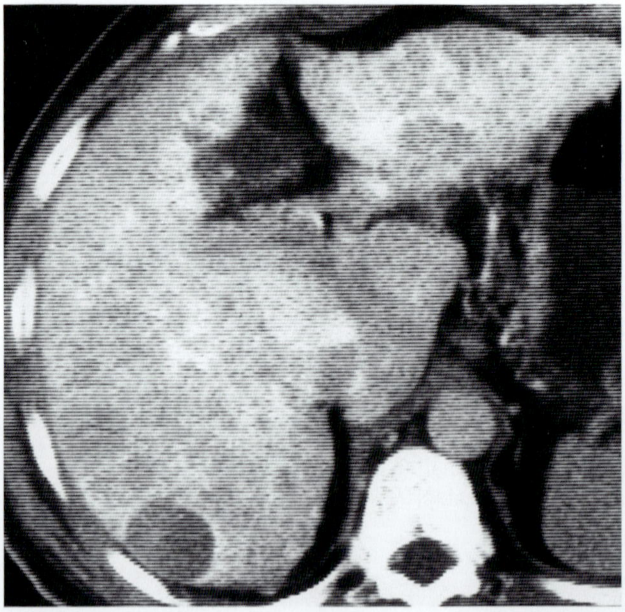

(d) Arterial-CT: in a slice further cranial, another 3 cm low-density lesion was found in S^{VII}. This lesion was not stained despite adequate contrast enhancement in the non-tumor parenchyma.

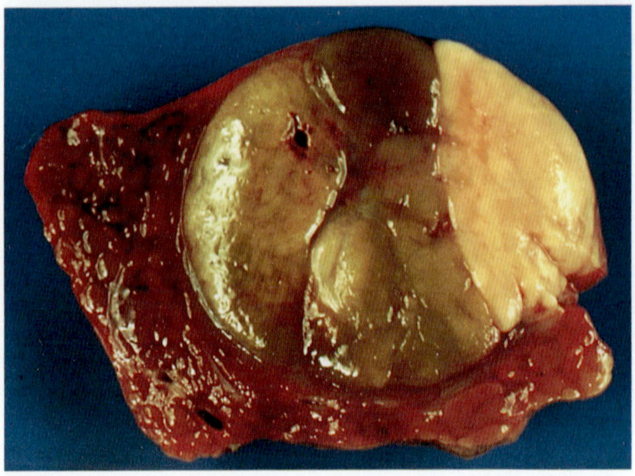

(e) Cut surface of resected specimen (S^{VI}).

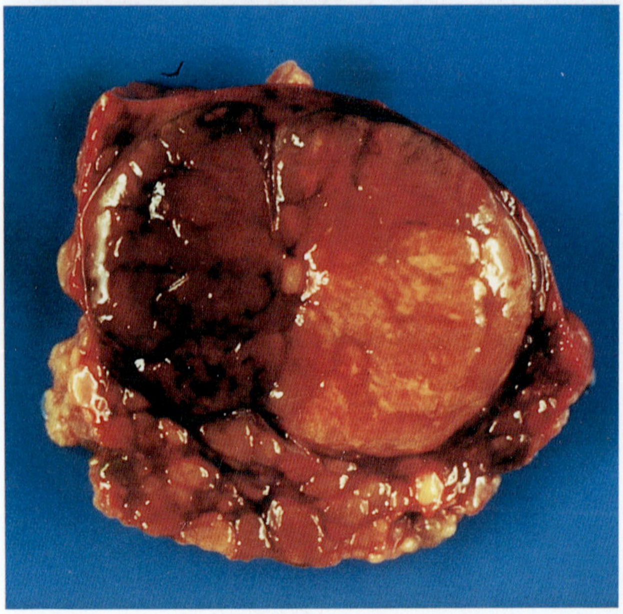

(f) Cut surface of resected specimen (S^{VII}). Partial resection was carried out for both tumors. The S^{VI} mass (e) was grade II > I on Edmondson's scale, and the S^{VII} mass (f) Edmondson's grade I, well differentiated HCC. Both were of the single nodular type having a capsule.

Small HCC—Case 2: Marked fatty changes within the tumor. A 49-year-old man.

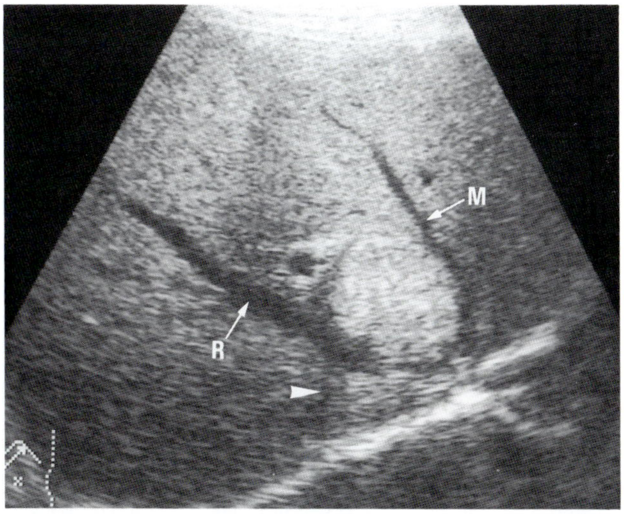

(a) US (right subcostal scan): a 4 cm hyperechoic mass is seen in S^{VIII}, but the interior structure is obscure. R, right hepatic vein; M, middle hepatic vein; ▶, lateral shadow.

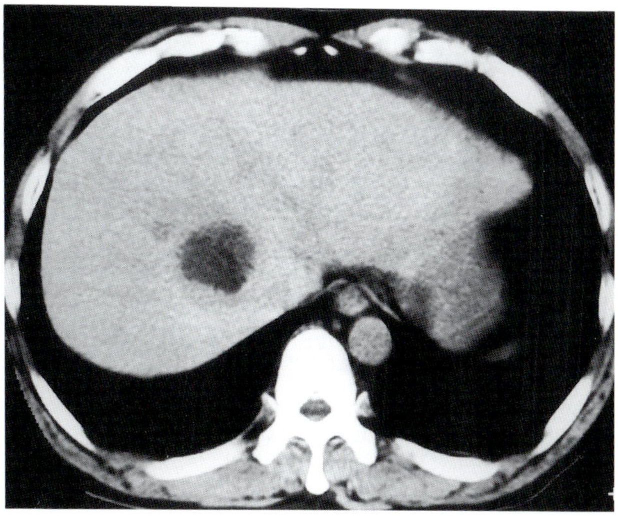

(b) Plain CT: the tumor is of low density containing within it a further low-density area (−23 HU), and the possibility of an HCC rich in fat is suggested.

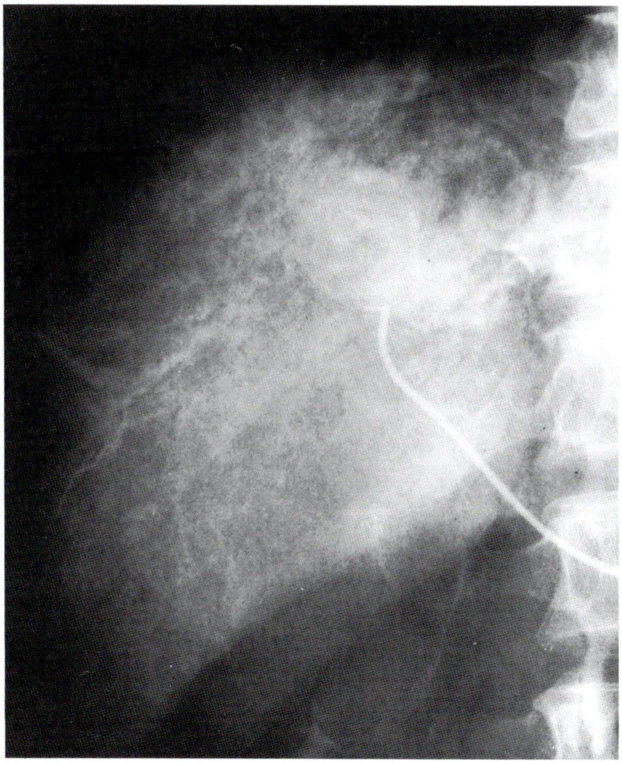

(c) Right hepatic arteriography: common hepatic arteriography did not produce staining, but selective right hepatic arteriography heavily stained the tumor.

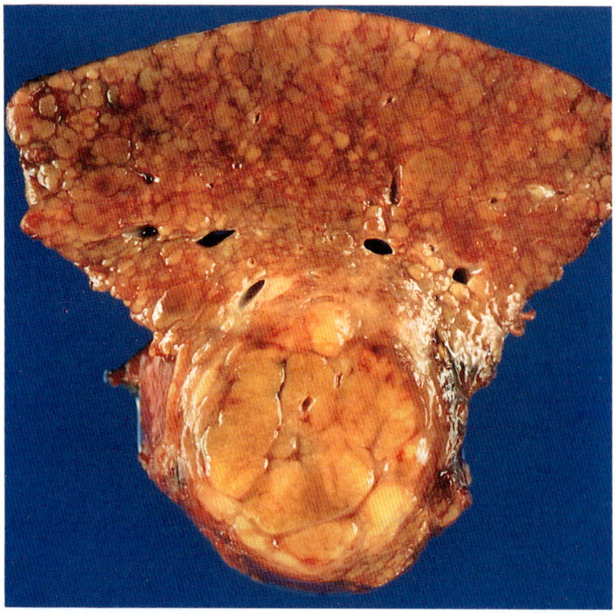

(d) Cut surface of resected specimen: subsegmentectomy for S^{VIII} was carried out. The tumor was a single nodular type (type 1) with a fibrous capsule around it. Histologically, it was HCC of Edmondson's grade II > I with marked fatty changes. The cirrhotic liver also had fatty changes.

?Small HCC—Case 6: A regenerative nodule that retained Lipiodol. A 77-year-old woman.

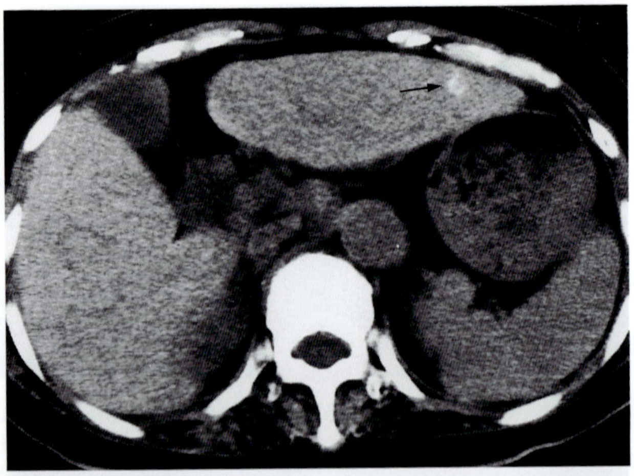

(a) Plain CT made 1 month after Lipiodol (8 ml) and adriamycin (30 mg) were injected into the proper hepatic artery: beside the main mass in the right lobe, a 1 cm lesion with Lipiodol retention was seen in S^{III}.

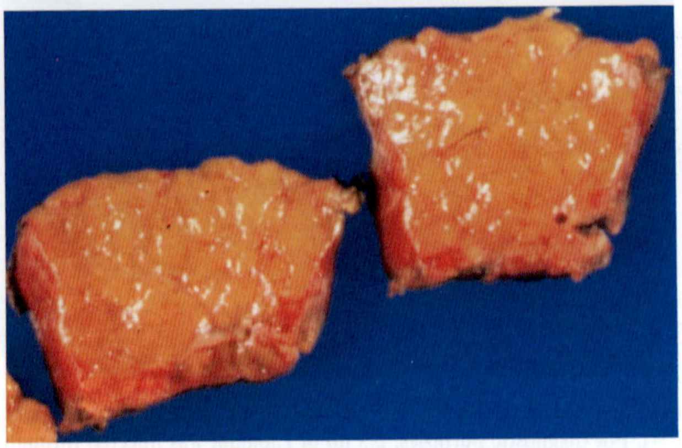

(b) Cut surface of resected specimen: the resected S^{III} lesion was cut into 5 mm slices, but no gross tumor was found.

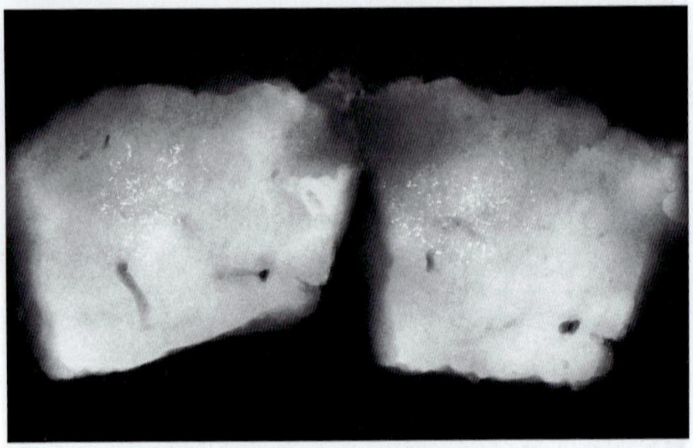

(c) Low-voltage radiograph: two slices of the resected specimen showed dots of retained Lipiodol, but histologically only regenerative nodules with fatty changes were recognized with no malignant feature.

Small HCC—Case 7: Small HCC developing in a liver with macronodular cirrhosis (soft X-ray of the resected specimen proved useful in confirming successful resection of small lesions).

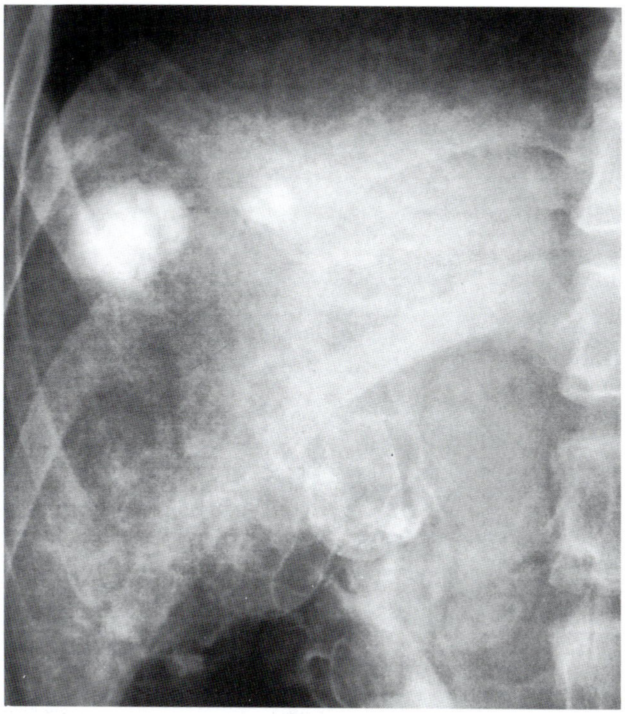

(a) Angiography (late phase): two lesions, large and small, were found in S^{VIII} and S^{VII}, and Lipiodol was injected for diagnostic purposes.

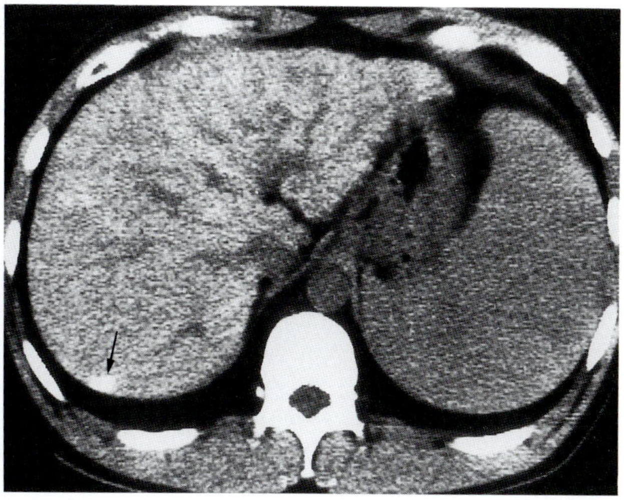

(b) Plain CT made 10 days after hepatic arterial injection of Lipiodol: a large and a small lesion (→) were found. The small S^{VII} lesion could not be identified by intraoperative US, while the large S^{VIII} lesion was readily recognized. Soft X-ray film (c) was made with the resected specimen during the operation, and it did contain the tumor in question; a further resection was called off.

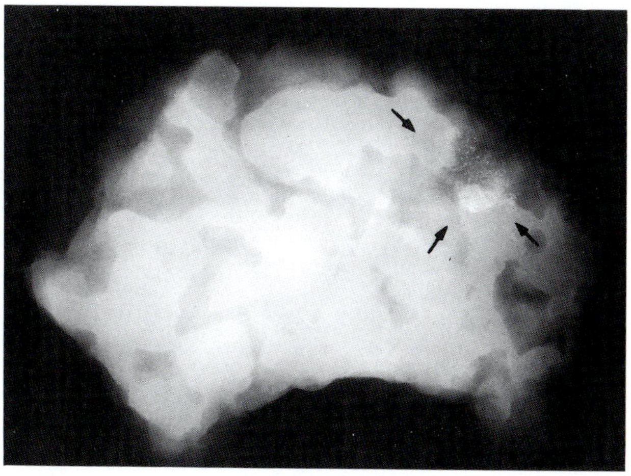

(c) Soft X-ray film of the resected specimen demonstrating the lesion (→).

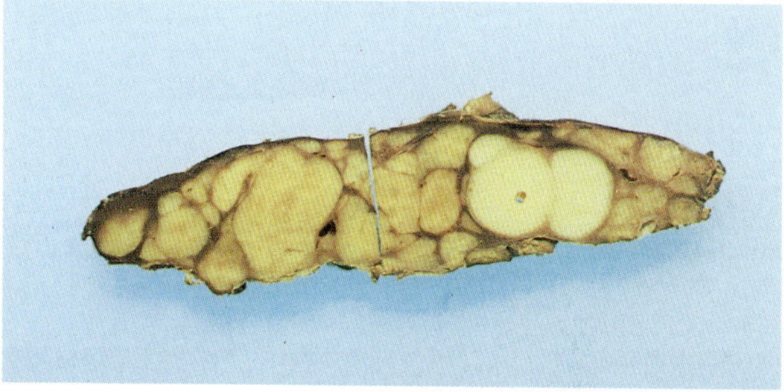

(d) Cut surface of resected specimen: the S^{VII} lesion consisted of two yellowish white lesions of about the same size as the surrounding regenerative nodules.

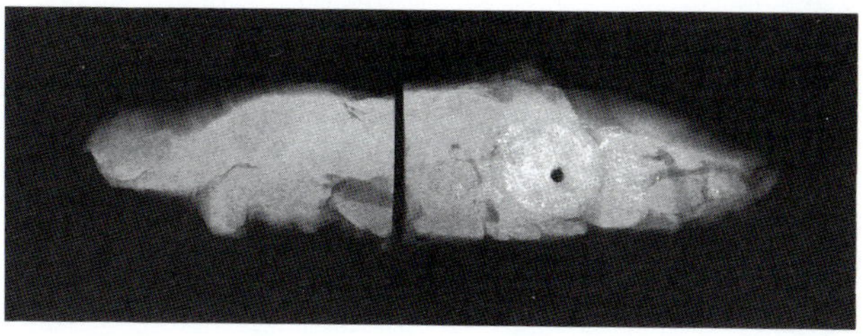

(e) Low-voltage radiograph film of (d): Lipiodol retention is seen in the tumor.

Small HCC—Case 8: Encapsulated nodular type HCC.

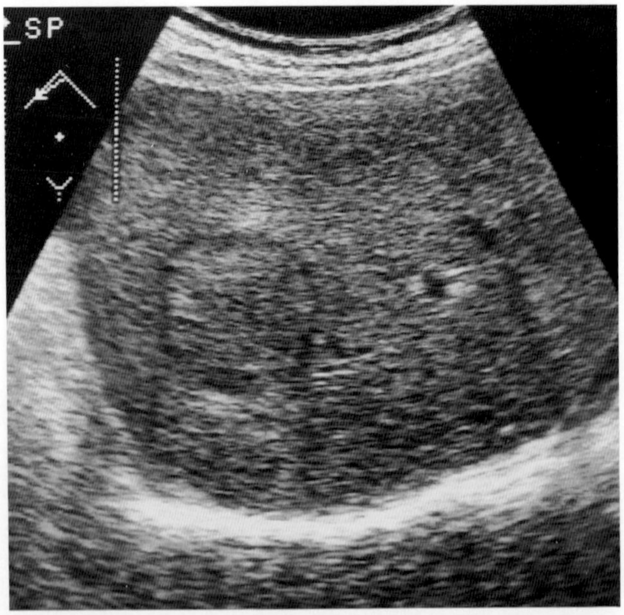

US (right subcostal scan): a 4 cm mass with a homogeneous internal echo is seen in S^{VI}. It is surrounded by a single layer of halo with two lateral shadows.

Small HCC—Case 9: HCC with a peripheral capsule seen in plain CT.

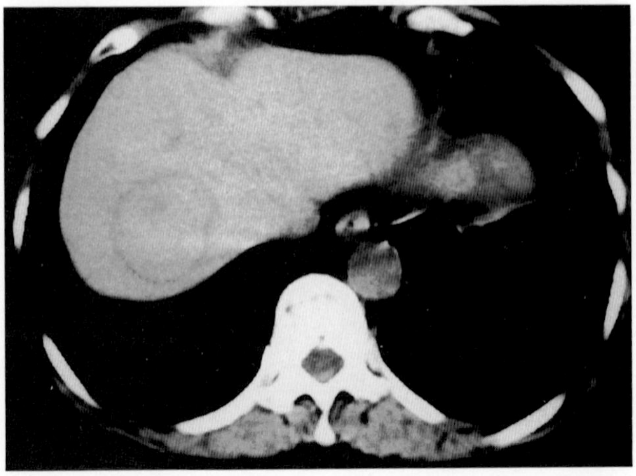

Plain CT: a 4 cm isodense tumor is seen in the border of S^{VIII} and S^{VII}. It is surrounded by a layer of low density. On resection, it was found to be an HCC of Edmondson's grade II covered by a thick fibrous capsule. The non-cancerous parenchyma showed chronic mild hepatitis. Isodense HCC on CT is rather uncommon.

Small HCC—Case 10: A pattern of enhancement in a small HCC on dynamic CT.

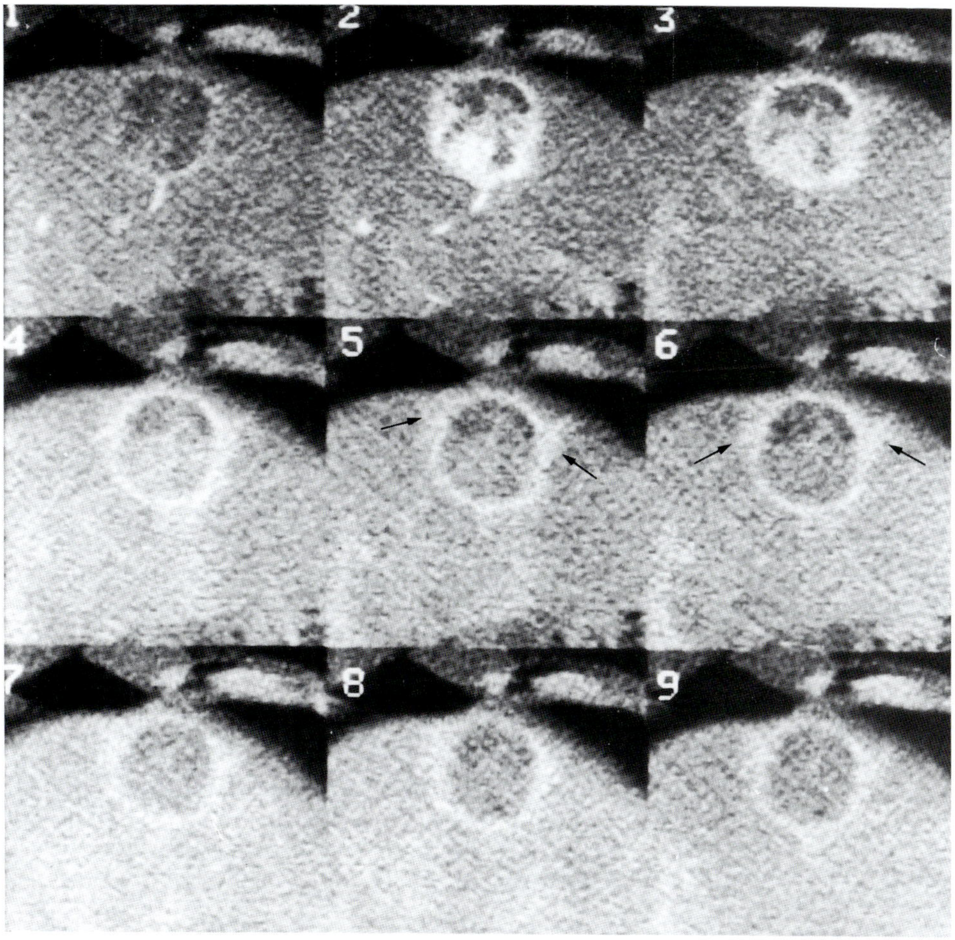

(a) Same level slices: the sequence of enhancement starting from the periphery is clearly recognized. The interior was enhanced nodule by nodule, and the area that was not enhanced early was eventually enhanced in the late phase. After 1 min the whole mass becomes homogeneously low in density with a contrasting high density ring. After slice #4 wedge-shaped high-density areas are seen outside the capsule in contact, and it was thought to represent the transport of contrast medium from the interior toward the periphery.

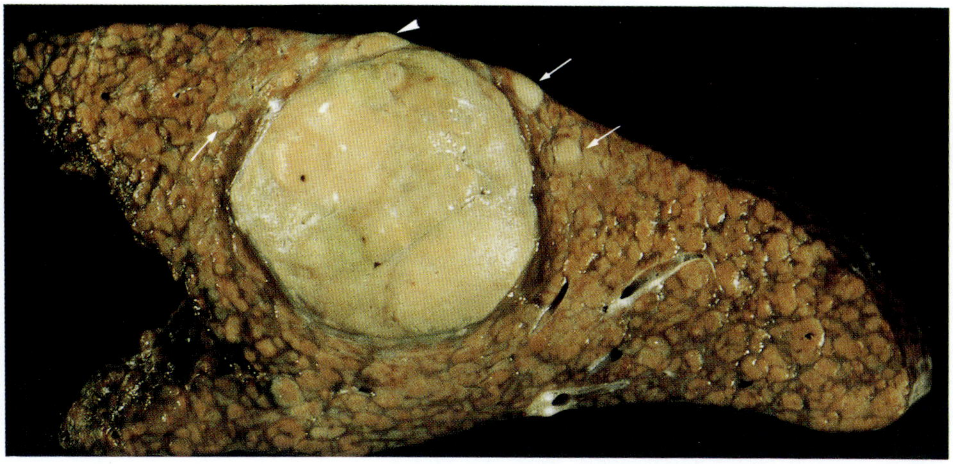

(b) Cut surface of resected specimen: a typical HCC with a fibrous capsule and a mosaic structure of the interior. There were small daughter nodules in the areas where late wedge-shaped stains were seen on dynamic CT (→). The gross type of this HCC was the single nodular one with proliferation into the surrounding areas, since there was a small nodule (▶) that seems to have grown in continuity with the main mass.

Small HCC—Case 11: Encapsulated HCC with a translucent rim on angiography.

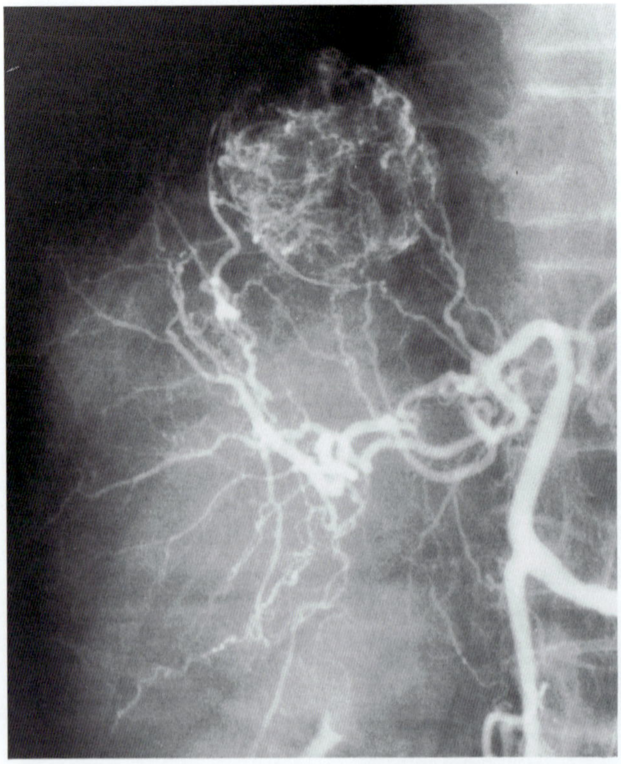

(a) Hepatic arteriography (early phase): a 3 cm hypervascular mass supplied from both the right and middle hepatic arteries is seen in $S^{IV-VIII}$ (on the Cantlie line). In the arterial phase, dilated feeding arteries are distributed around the mass, and numerous tumor vessels are supplying individual tumor nodules.

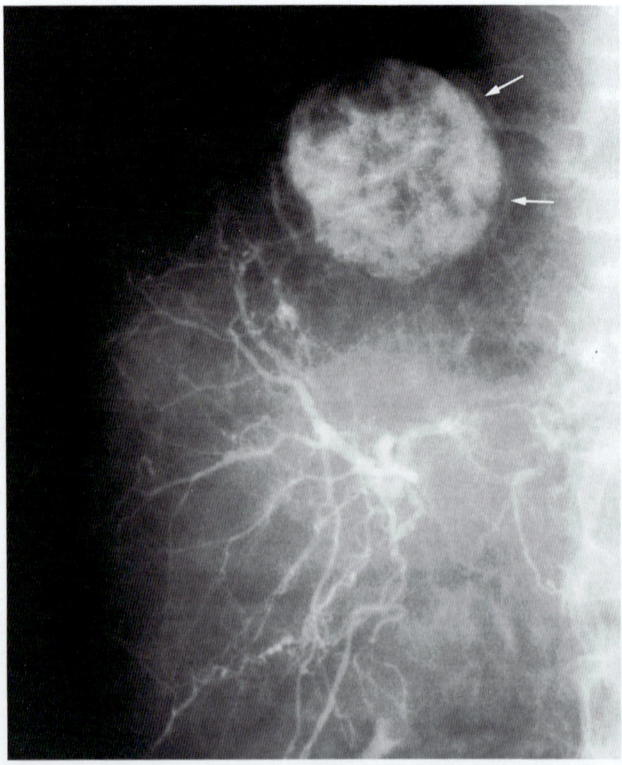

(b) Hepatic arteriography (late phase): the whole mass is seen as a nodule that is unevenly stained. This may correspond to slices #2 and #3 of Case 10. A thin translucent unstained rim and a ring stain (→) in its outside are recognized.

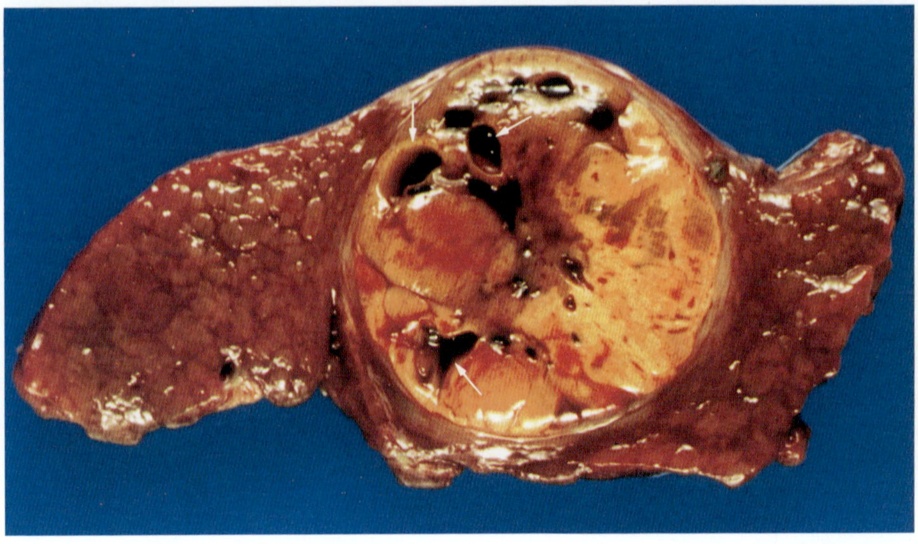

(c) Cut surface of resected specimen: the mass bulges slightly from the cut surface suggesting constraint against tumor expansion by the capsule. The interior is mosaic with many nodules and vascular lakes (→) that retain blood. A fibrous capsule around the mass is obvious. The mass usually bulges on cutting if the tumor cells are viable, but it does not when they are necrotic as after TAE. The pressure of a viable interior is greater than that of the surrounding parenchyma.

Small HCC—Case 12: Small HCC in which DSA demonstrated a translucent rim as well as intratumor septa.

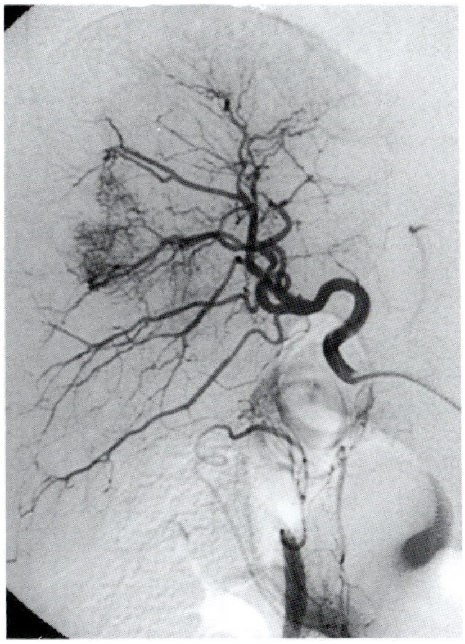

(a) Right hepatic arteriography by DSA (arterial phase, 5.3 s): a hypervascular mass is seen in S^{V-VIII}.

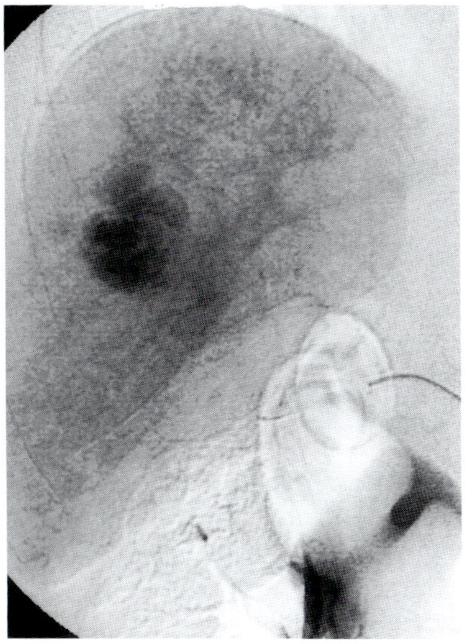

(b) Right hepatic arteriography by DSA (venous phase, 9.7 s): there are at least three nodules which are separated by a transculent structure which was thought to correspond to septa. The two cranially located nodules are supplied by A^{VIII} and the caudal one by A^{V}.

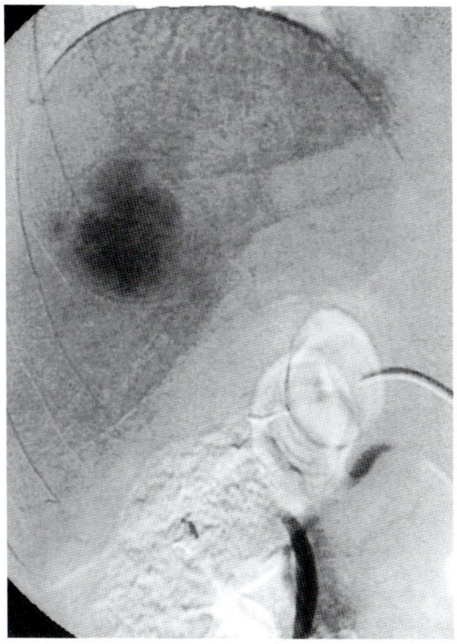

(c) Right hepatic arteriography by DSA (late phase, 15.6 s): in the further late phase, the intratumor lucent structure became obscure, and a thin layer of translucent rim surrounding the tumor came to be recognized surrounded by a ring stain.

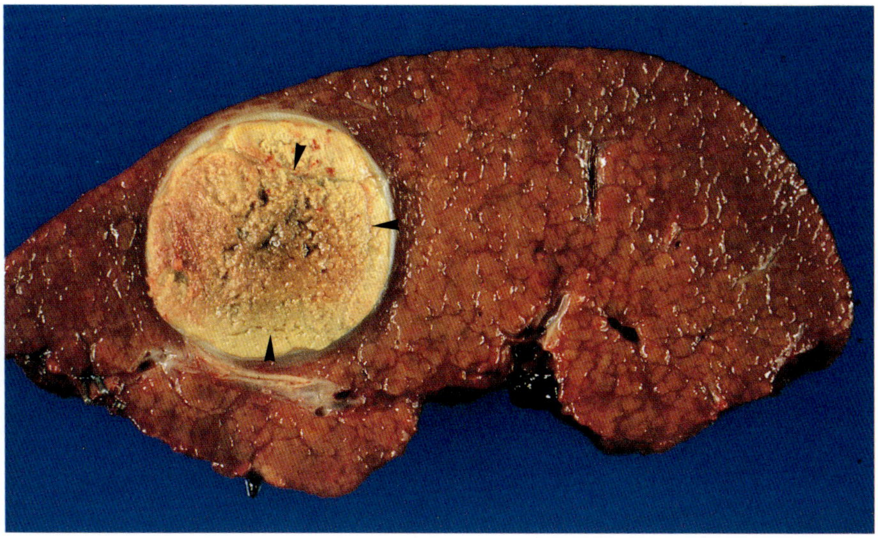

(d) Cut surface of resected specimen: the interior was totally necrotized by Lipiodol-TAE with remaining septa (▶). A thick fibrous capsule was also recognized.

Small HCC—Case 13: Differential diagnosis of small HCC based on enhanced pattern of dynamic CT stains.

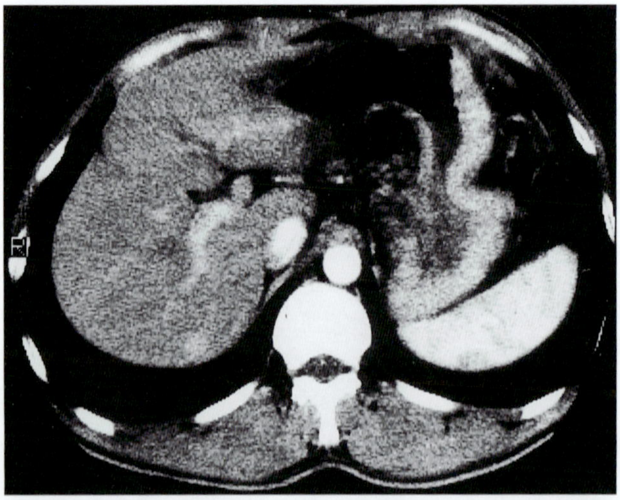

(a) Dynamic CT (early phase): a 1.5 cm highly stained lesion was found in S^{VI-VII} in the remnant liver after resection. Since the size is small, the internal structure is obscure.

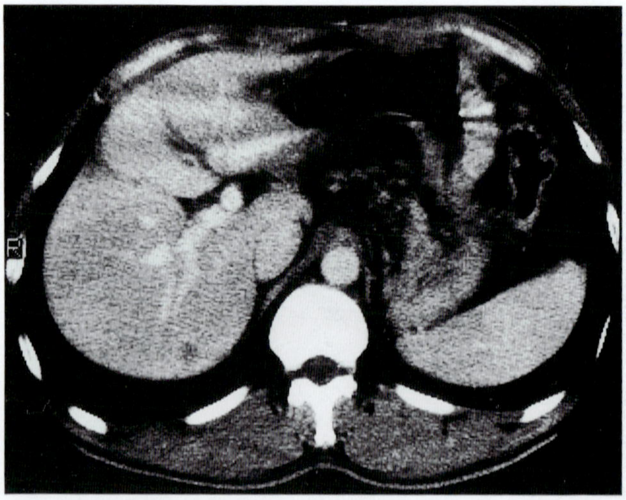

(b) Dynamic CT (late phase, 30 s): since the mass turned low density, the diagnosis is clearly HCC.

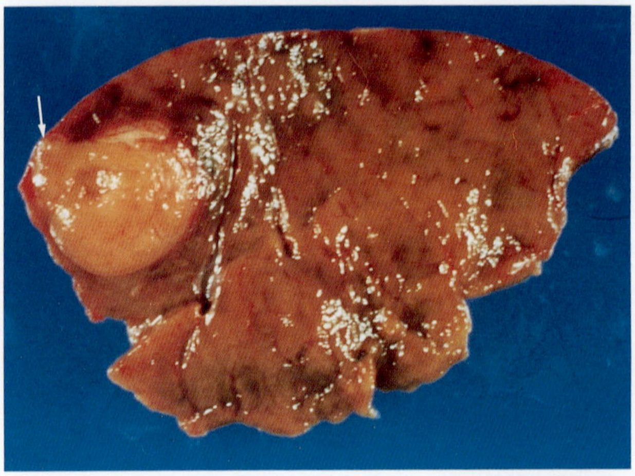

(c) Cut surface of resected specimen: the mass is surrounded by a fibrous capsule with a small extracapsular growth (→), and the type diagnosis is 'single nodular type with proliferation into the surrounding areas'. The histology was Edmondson's grade II, very similar to that of the specimen resected 11 months earlier; the diagnosis was recurrence of the primary HCC.

Small HCC—Case 14: Quality diagnosis made by arterial-CT.

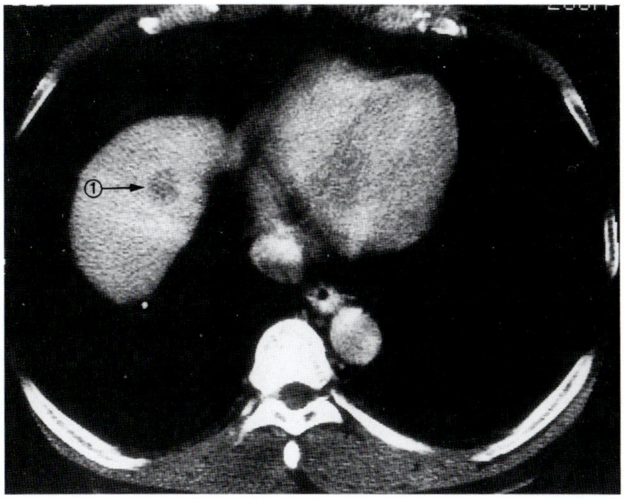

a

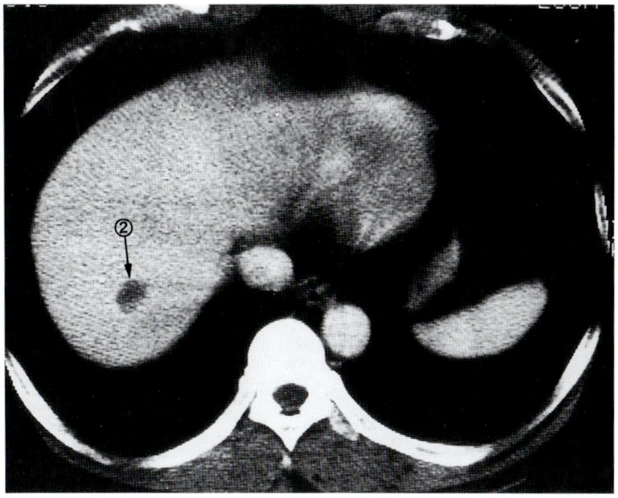

b

(a,b) Enhanced CT: in a slightly late arterial phase, a 1.5 cm low-density lesion was seen in S^{IV} (1) and S^{VIII} (2), but quality diagnosis was not feasible.

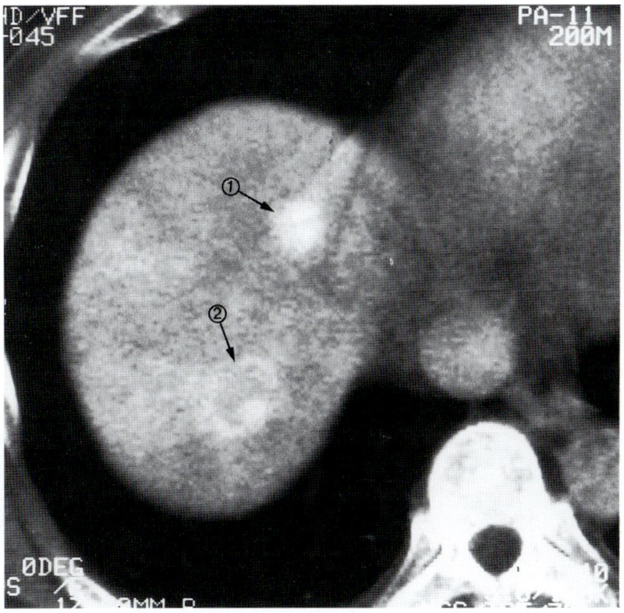

(c) Arterial-CT: since arteriography failed to stain these lesions, arterial-CT was carried out, which demonstrated a round stain (1) in S^{IV} and another lesion (2) in S^{VIII} which showed peripheral stains and a partial nodular stain of the interior.

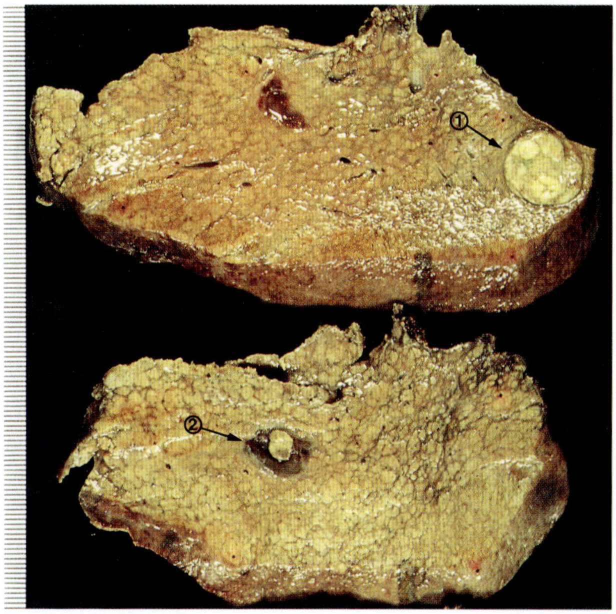

(d) Cut surface of resected specimens: both were histologically of Edmondson's grade II > I. The lesion in S^{IV} had a typical mosaic internal structure, but the S^{VIII} lesion was in large part degenerate with colloidal appearance. The latter contained a small tumor nodule closely reflecting the arterial-CT finding shown in (c).

Small HCC—Case 15: MR imaging (1.5 T) of small HCC.

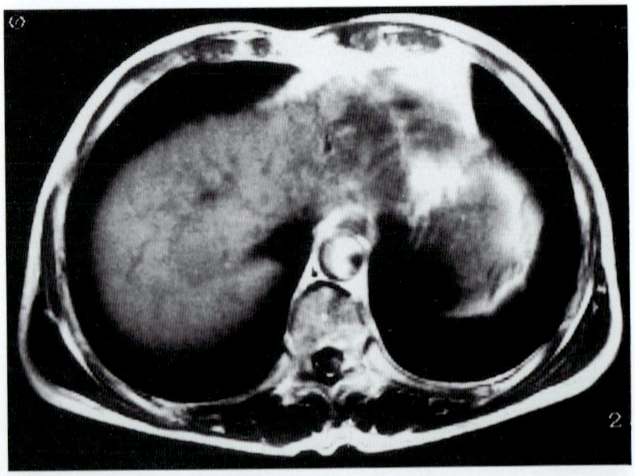

(a) MR imaging (T1-weighted, 600/15): T1-weighted spin echo image shows the lesion in S^{VIII} as a low intensity mass; it was seen on enhanced CT as a hypervascular HCC of 3 cm (not shown).

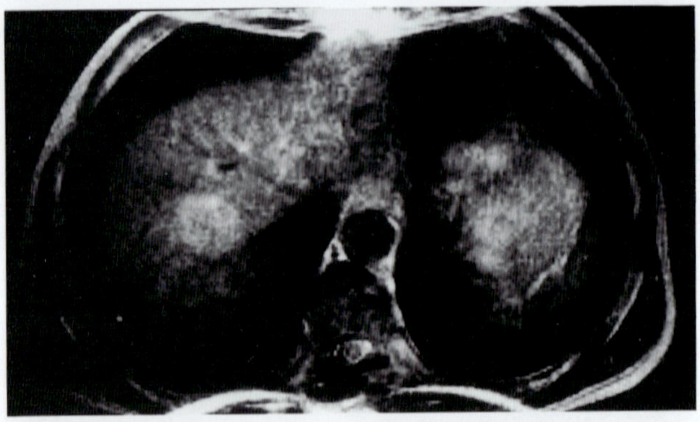

(b) MR imaging (T2-weighted, 2400/60): the same mass is seen as a high-intensity lesion.

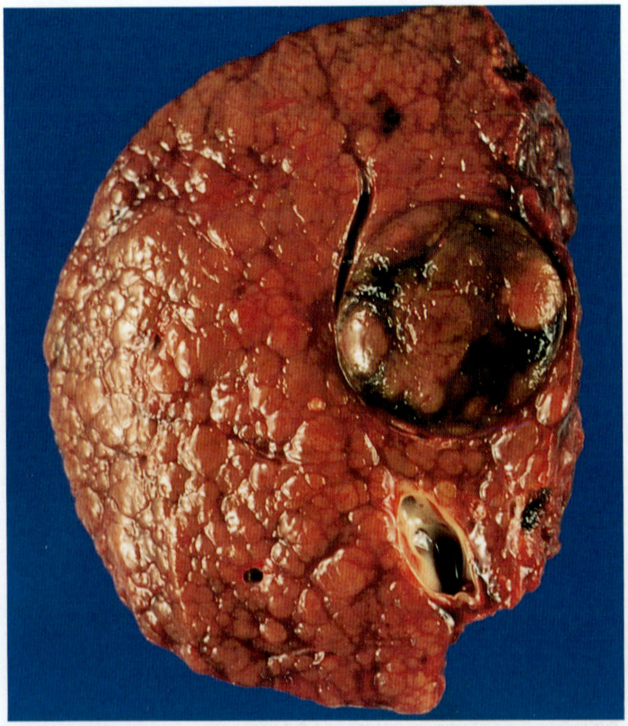

(c) Cut surface of resected specimen: a typical encapsulated single nodular type HCC, but MR imaging failed to demonstrate the capsule.

Small HCC—Case 16: Dynamic CT of an HCC of the single nodular type with proliferation into the surrounding areas (type 2).

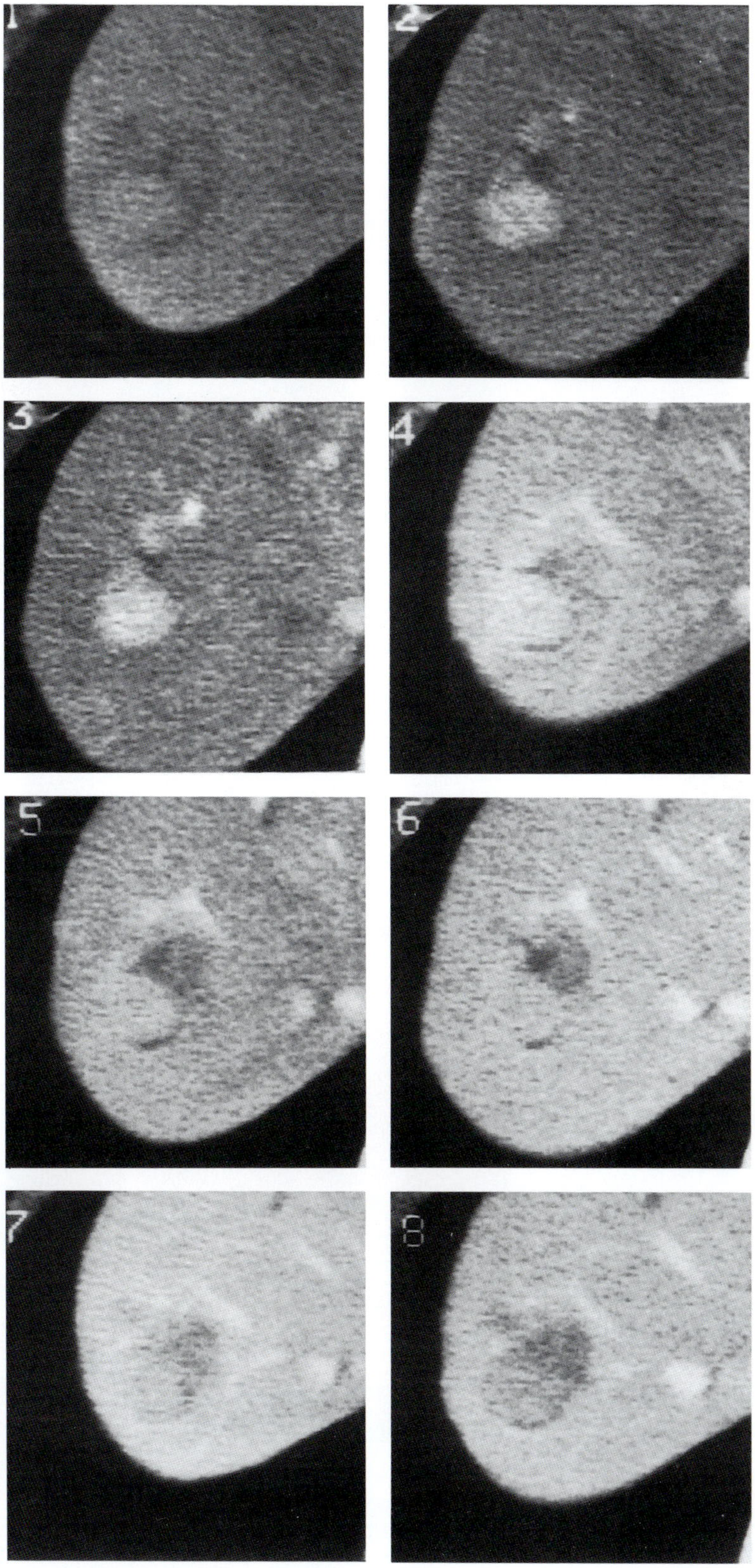

(a) Dynamic CT (single slice level): the individual tumor nodules are stained one after another and then turn low density. Late phase images (slice #8) most closely reflect the cut surface structure (b). Imaging diagnosis of type 2 HCC is not very easy. If the tumor growth continues from the periphery of the main mass is small, it is difficult to differentiate it from the single nodular type (type 1). In this case, dynamic CT was done in the same section level and comparison with the resected specimen was possible.

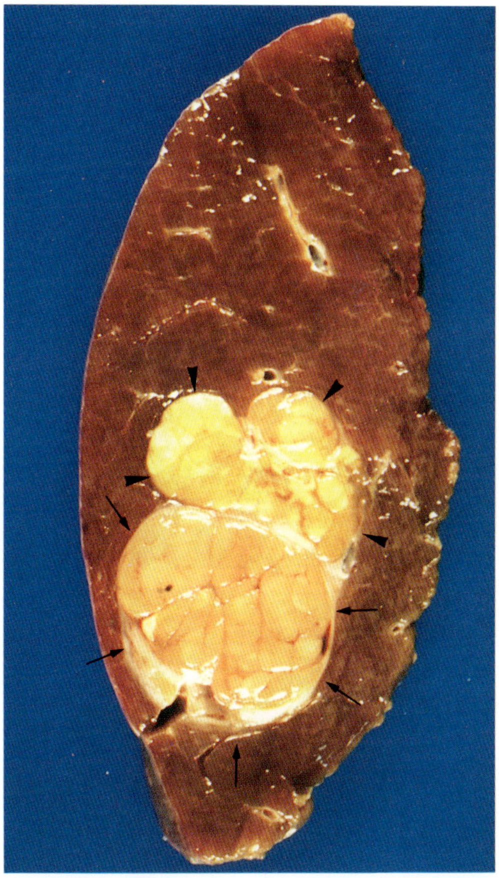

(b) Cut surface of resected specimen: →, main mass; ▶, growth outside the main mass. Both closely correspond with the CT images.

Small HCC—Case 17: Dynamic CT of HCC of the multinodular fused type (type 3).

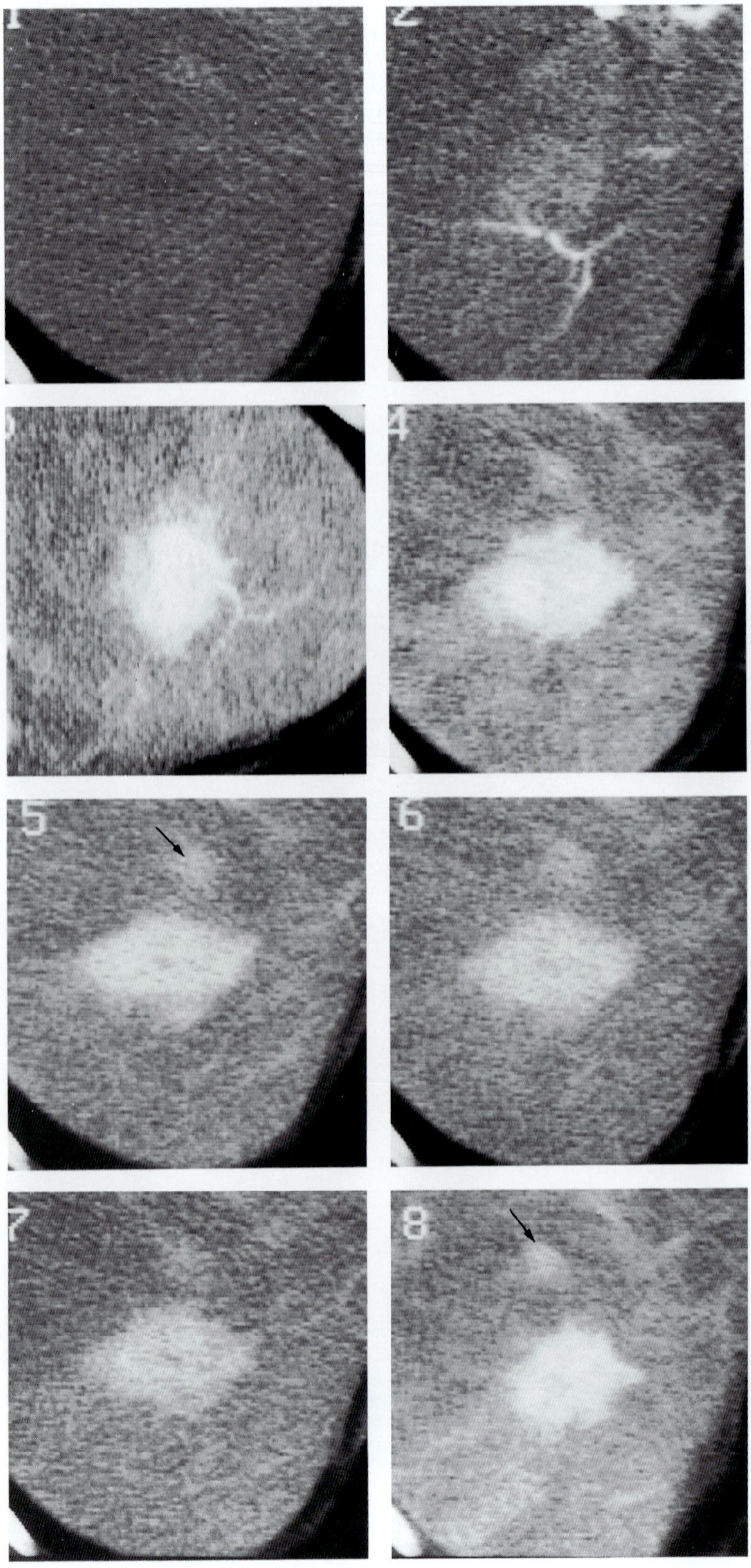

(a) Dynamic CT (single slice level): the mass in S^{VII} is slowly stained revealing a mass of rhomboid shape. Even the late phase image does not show a high-density ring. (→), right hepatic vein.

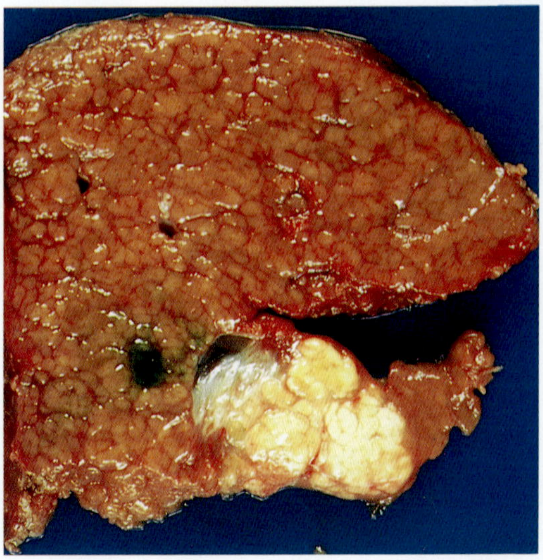

(b) Cut surface of resected specimen: subsegmentectomy of S^{VII} was carried out. The mass, as dynamic CT suggested, consisted of fused small multiple nodules which were of Edmondson's grade III histologically.

Small HCC—Case 18: Lipiodol-CT of HCC of the multinodular fused type (type 3).

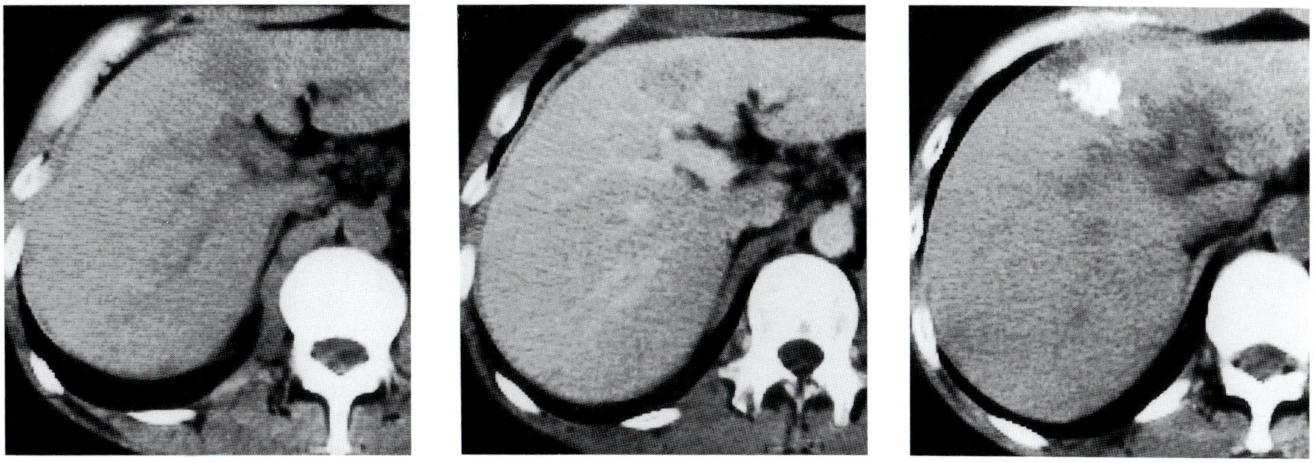

(a) Plain CT: the mass has an irregular boundary and the internal structure is obscure.

(b) Enhanced CT (late phase): the same as plain CT.

(c) Lipiodol CT: Lipiodol is retained in the mass as a collection of dots, suggesting confluent nodular tumors.

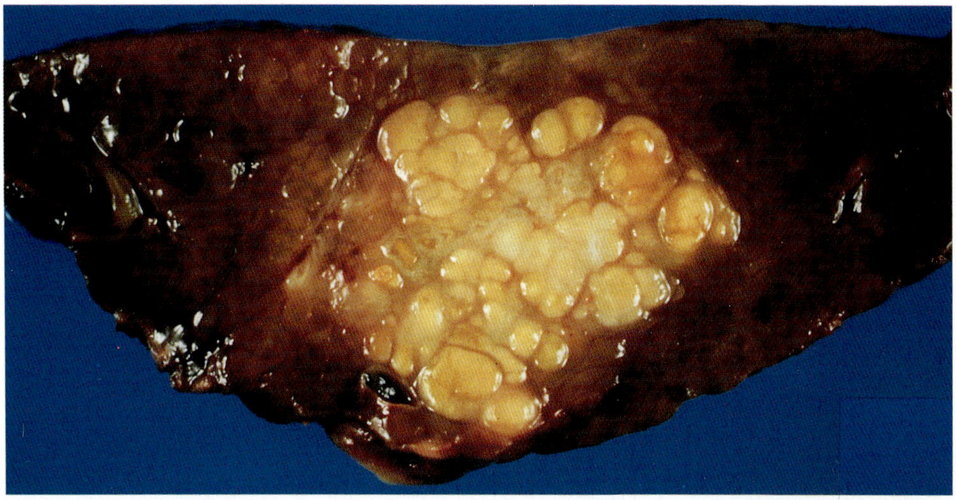

(d) Cut surface of resected specimen: many small tumor nodules coalesced without a capsule (type 3). This was an HCC of Edmondson's grade II > III. The preoperative Lipiodol-TAE killed only 10 per cent of the mass.

Small HCC—Case 19: Recurrent HCC in the remnant liver that was followed up.

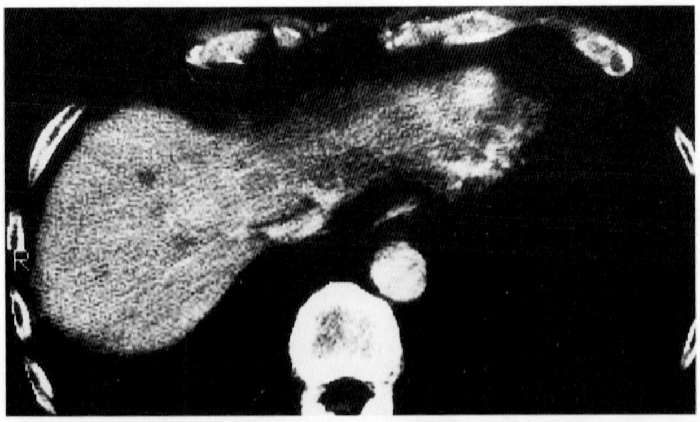

(a) Enhanced CT: resection was done for HCC in S^{VII} and S^{IV} 4 years earlier. Subsequent CT demonstrated multiple low-density lesions in the right lobe.

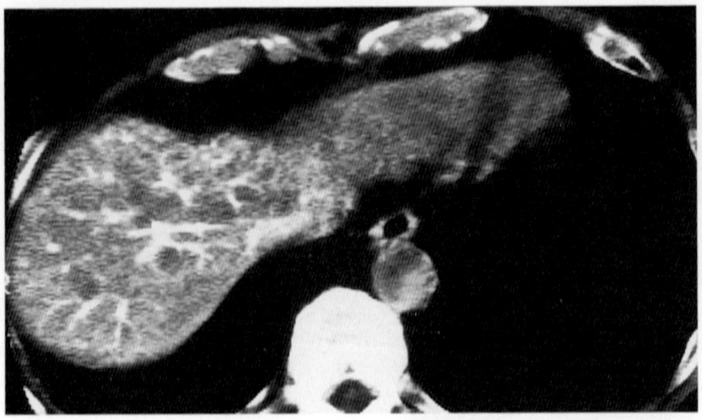

(b) Portal-CT: these lesions were not stained by angiography carried out 1 month later. Subsequent portal-CT reconfirmed the presence of multiple low-density lesions in the right lobe.

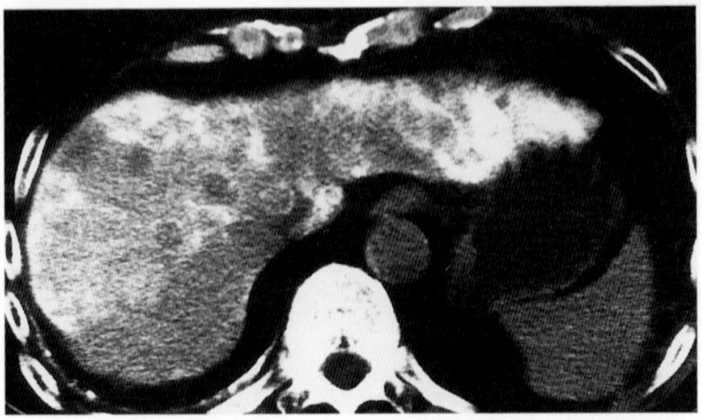

(c) Lipiodol-CT: angiography was repeated 8 months later, but no lesion was stained, and Lipiodol was injected into the hepatic artery. CT made immediately after Lipiodol injection failed to show uptake by the lesions despite retention by the non-cancerous parenchyma; they were seen as low-density areas relative to the parenchyma.

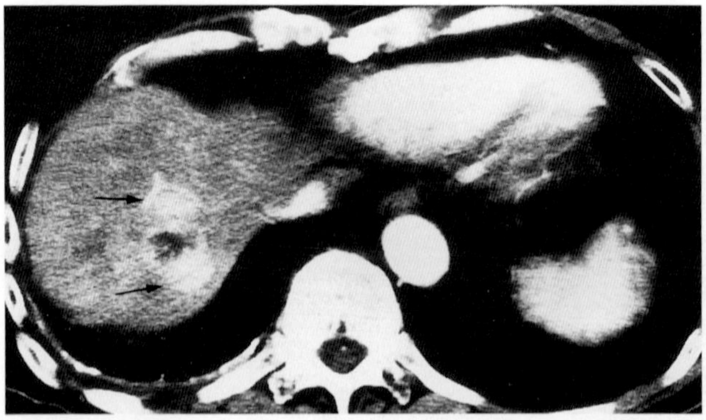

(d) Enhanced CT [10 months after (c)]: enhanced CT was repeated 10 months later. This time, new enhanced lesions (→) were found beside non-enhanced ones. It was thought that some of the non-enhanced lesions found by the previous enhanced CT examination (a) and portal-CT (b) came to be stained near the inferior vena cava.

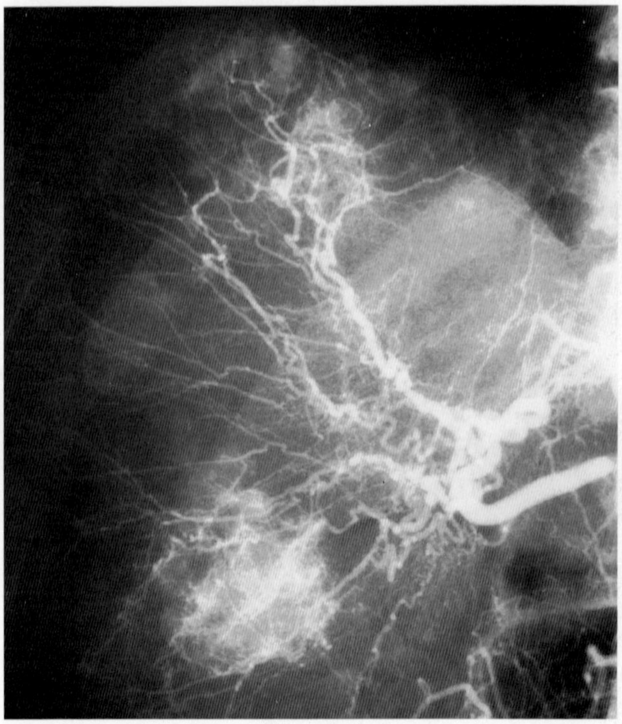

(e) Angiography: angiography carried out shortly thereafter demonstrated advanced HCC not only in S^{VIII} but also in S^{VI}. The interval between (a) and (e) was 1 year and 7 months. US provided the same information as CT, but no definitive diagnosis could be made. Serum AFP remained normal during this period.

Small HCC—Case 20: Small HCC that visibly grew in a short period. In this patient with chronic liver disease, serum AFP rose to 37 ng/ml during the follow-up. With a suspicion of HCC, enhanced CT, US, and angiography were done, but they did not demonstrate any lesion in the liver. Arterial-CT also failed to reveal a lesion.

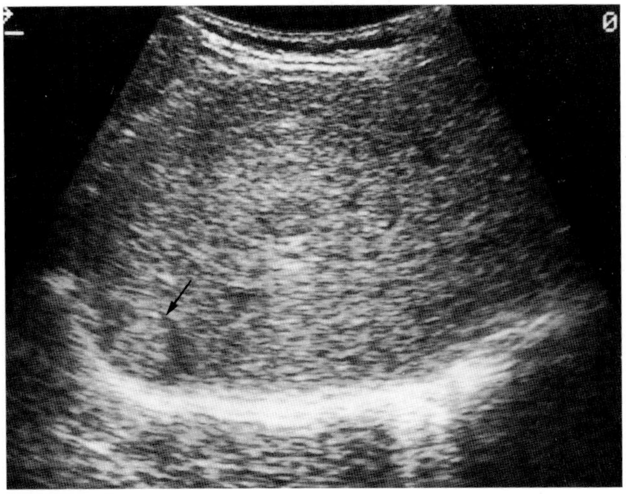

(a) US: a 2 cm lesion with a peripheral halo was found by US done 8 months later.

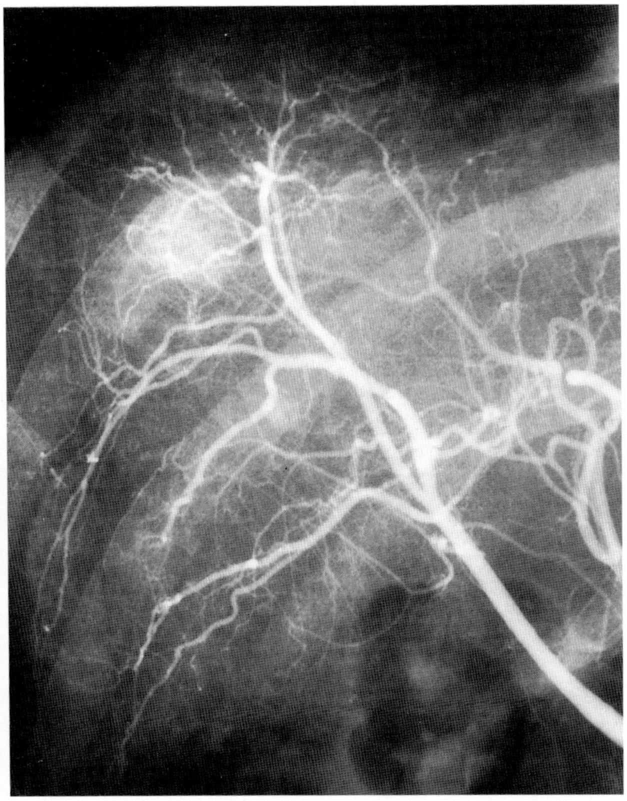

(b) Angiography: angiography demonstrated a tumor stain in S^{VIII}.

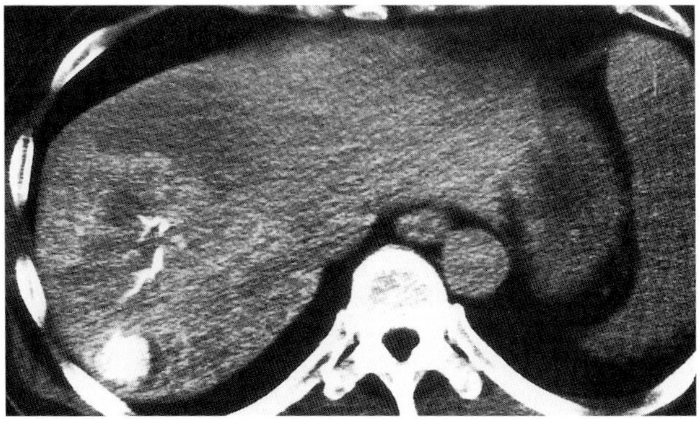

(c) Arterial-CT (early phase): for comparison with the previous arterial-CT (e), repeat arterial-CT was carried out. It clearly demonstrated a 2 cm lesion supplied by the $A^{VIII}{}_b$ artery.

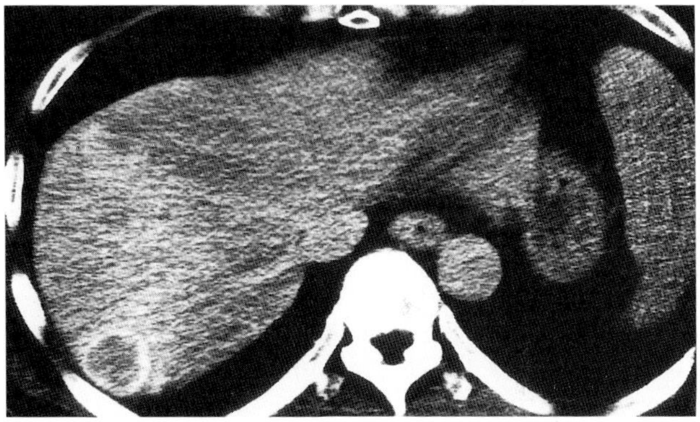

(d) Arterial-CT (late phase): with clearly stained ring density a diagnosis of HCC was made. The same examination done 8 months earlier (e) did not show this, and a rapidly growing HCC was the diagnosis.

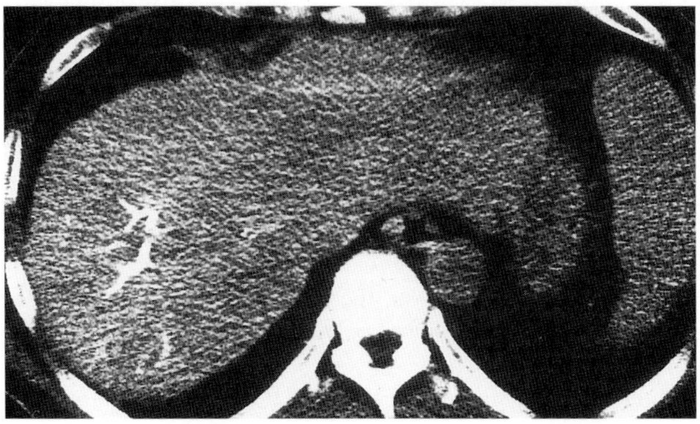

(e) Arterial-CT (8 months earlier): no lesion is seen.

4.3 Early hepatocellular carcinoma and adenomatous hyperplasia (dysplastic nodule)

As increasing numbers of small HCCs came to be resected and the sections of cirrhotic livers were studied, it slowly became clear that the histology of some of the nodules was suggestive of early HCC (Arakawa *et al.* 1986*a*). Grossly, such lesions are light yellow or the same in color as the surrounding parenchyma, retaining the lobular structure. Occasionally, they contain a discrete nodule (mostly well differentiated but overt HCC) or a small nodule only microscopically identifiable (Kanai *et al.* 1987) (Case 1). Such lesions have been termed 'early HCC' in Japan, meaning that they are in an early clinical stage. These early HCCs usually lack a fibrous capsule, have portal tracts within the tumor and adenomatous hyperplasia in the surrounding area (Sakamoto *et al.* 1991). Such early HCC is often found as an accessory lesion beside the main HCC by US or intraoperative US (Matsui *et al.* 1989, 1991; Takayasu *et al.* 1990*f*; Choi *et al.* 1993). These observations have recently been confirmed by American investigators in a transplant study in which small malignant lesions were found in an explant with large nodules (Ferrell *et al.* 1992; Theise *et al.* 1992).

Imaging diagnosis

Early HCC is usually seen as a low-density lesion rarely stained by dynamic CT, angiography, or arterial-CT (Takayasu *et al.* 1989*a*, 1990*f*, 1995*a*,*b*; Choi *et al.* 1993) (Case 2). Arterially injected Lipiodol is not retained after intraarterial injection, and therefore Lipiodol-CT is seldom diagnostic (Takayasu *et al.* 1993) (Case 3). Occasional cases may show partial staining which is overt HCC histologically (Takayasu *et al.* 1995*a*, *b*) (Case 4) or a grossly discrete nodule (nodule in nodule) which is less well differentiated (Mitchell *et al.* 1991; Nomura *et al.* 1993; Winter *et al.* 1994), or an advanced HCC (Case 5). The latter lesion is called 'early advanced HCC' and is distinguished from early HCC at the National Cancer Center Hospital, Tokyo, because the former is more advanced than the latter which does not have such a well differentiated lesion. It was subsequently found that small liver cancer, defined in the General Rules for the Clinical and Pathological Study (Liver Cancer Study Group of Japan 1989) as a lesion less than 2 cm in size, frequently belongs to advanced HCC while some HCCs as large as 3 cm may be early HCC (Case 6). It is to be remembered, however, that early HCC does not mean a good prognosis, unlike the case early stomach cancer which has an excellent prognosis if treated early. Even with resection carried out for an early HCC, postresection recurrence is not infrequent, and early death may occur—in the current usage of the word, 'recurrence' can be another primary rather than recurrence from remaining HCC cells.

Along with experience with early HCC, a lesion commonly called in Japan 'adenomatous hyperplasia'(AH) has come to be found in the same resected specimens. Malignant transformation from AH to overt HCC was clinically confirmed in 9 of 18 nodules during a follow-up of 6 months to 4 years (Takayama *et al.* 1990). The first study on the nodule-in-nodule evolution of HCC reported by Arakawa *et al.* (1986*a*) used the term 'adenomatous hyperplastic nodule' avoiding the term adenomatous hyperplasia, which was used by Edmondson in 1976 without clear definition. The international working party on the terminology of nodular hepatic lesions organized by the World Organization of Gastroenterology (OMGE) on the occasion of its 10th Congress (chairman I. Wanless) now recommends 'dysplastic nodule' (Wanless 1995) instead. In his recommendation, dysplastic lesions are defined histologically by the presence of cytoplasmic and/or nuclear variations and the topographic clustering of such variations to form recognizable subpopulations of cells without definite histologic criteria of malignancy. At the time of writing the term 'dysplastic nodule' has not yet been generally accepted, and therefore we will use the term AH. The frequency with which AH is found by various imaging methods is given in Table 4.7. Intraoperative US detected 36 per cent of AHs while none of the other modalities that use contrast medium could detect AH (Takayasu *et al.* 1989*a*). In other words, AH is not distinguishable from the non-cancerous parenchyma in vascular supply. Perhaps US is capable of demonstrating differences in acoustic impedance reflecting differences in cell density (Case 7). Histologically, AH is a nodular lesion that consists of small basophilic cells in high cellularity that lack cellular atypia or structural abnormality. Kondo *et al.* (1989) called a lesion containing increased cellularity, 'microacinus formation' and increased cytoplasmic basophilia 'borderline lesion.' Some are difficult to differentiate from HCC, and such atypical AH is generally larger than typical AH and may be seen on US (Case 8) and infrequently as a stain on enhanced CT or arterial-CT. It seems that the AHs that are not stained by contrast medium have not yet acquired neovasculature. From these discussions, the suggestion is that if a small lesion is clearly stained by contrast medium, it is more likely to have undergone transformation from a clinical point of view. In such situation, arterial-CT is recommended for determining whether the lesion is stainable or not (Takayasu *et al.* 1995*a*). Lipiodol-CT which has a high diagnostic capability and sensitivity for small HCC, detected none (0%) of AHs (Table 4.7); it is not useful for the diagnosis of AH.

These so-called borderline lesions (Kondo *et al.* 1989) need further study particularly of their pathophysiology and vascular structure using portal-CT and arterial-CT simultaneously. Progress is being made on this problem using new techniques in molecular biology and immunohistochemistry.

Problems in therapy

As early HCC lacks neovasculature, Lipiodol-TAE is usually of no avail for treatment (Takayasu *et al.* 1993) (Cases 3, 6). One could wait till it acquires neovasculature for Lipiodol-TAE or carry out percutaneous ethanol injection (PEI) (Ohto *et al.* 1987; Livraghi *et al.* 1989). Another problem is the obscurity of the boundary between the lesion and liver parenchyma when examined by intraoperative US, which sometimes makes inaccurate determination of the cutting edge, hence stump recurrence (Case 10). Meticulous and complete resection is required for the surgeon.

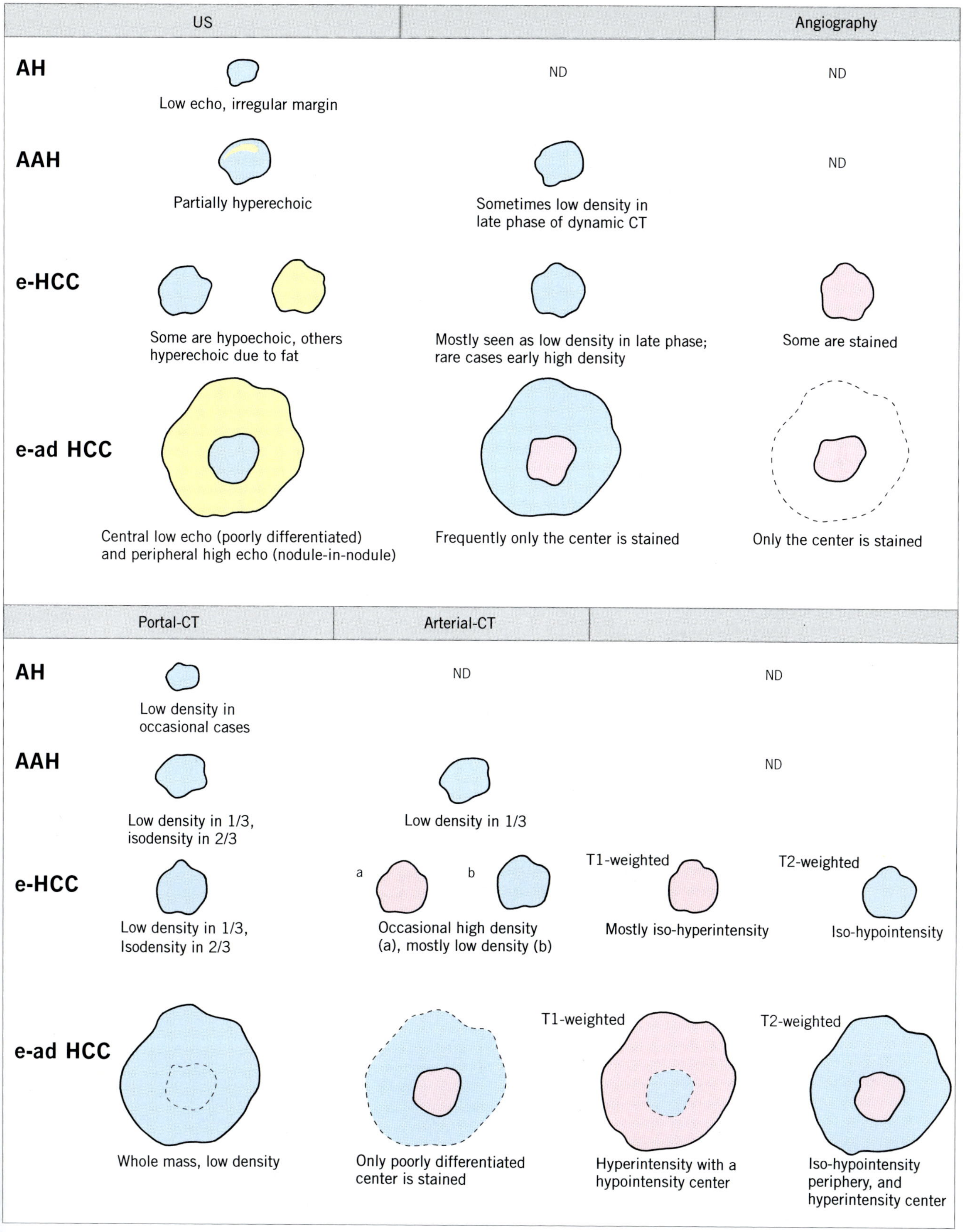

Fig. 4.4 Imaging features of borderline lesions including early HCC.

ND . not detected

Table 4.7 Detection rates (in per cent) in 54 reseced borderline lesions by various imaging techniques

Lesion	Number	Size (cm)	US	CT	Angiography	Arterial-CT	Portal-CT	Lipiodol-CT	Intraoperative US
AH[a]	14	0.8±0.3*	0 (0/14)	0 (0/12)	0 (0/10)	0 (0/1)	50 (1/2)	0 (0/10)	35.7 (5/14)
AAH[b]	12	1.2±0.3	50 (6/12)	9.1 (1/11)	0 (0/11)	33.3** (1/3)	33.3 (1/3)	0 (0/4)	75.0 (9/12)
Sub-total	26	1.0±0.4	23.1 (6/26)	4.3 (1/23)	0 (0/21)	25.0** (1/4)	40.0 (2/5)	0 (0/14)	53.8 (14/26)
e-HCC[c] (I)***	21	1.3±0.4	61.9 (13/21)	52.5 (10/19)	26.3 (5/19)	50.0** (2/4)	33.3 (1/3)	16.7 (1/6)	82.4 (14/17)
e-HCC (I>II)***	7	1.5±0.5	71.4 (5/7)	71.4 (5/7)	42.9 (3/7)	not done	100 (4/4)	50.0 (1/2)	100 (7/7)
Sub-total	28	1.4±0.5	64.3 (18/28)	57.7 (15/26)	30.8 (8/26)	50.0** (2/4)	71.4 (5/7)	25.0 (2/8)	87.5 (21/24)
Total	54	1.2±0.4	44.4 (24/54)	32.7 (16/49)	17.0 (8/47)	37.5** (3/8)	58.3 (7/12)	9.1 (2/22)	70.0 (35/50)

[a] Adenomatous hyperplasia (AH); [b] atypical AH; [c] early HCC; * AH versus other groups ($p<0.01$); **lesion was seen as a low-density mass; ***Edmondson's grade

MR imaging of early HCC and early advanced (overt) HCC

Recently, multistep progression of preneoplastic lesion to classical HCC has been demonstrated that begins with adenomatous hyperplasia progressing to early HCC, from early HCC to early advanced HCC and finally to advanced HCC (classical HCC) histopathologically (Sakamoto *et al.* 1991) as well as clinically (Takayama *et al.* 1990). Early HCC is an extremely well differentiated HCC that commonly develops within an adenomatous hyplastic lesions (Arakawa *et al.* 1986*a*); it frequently has fatty changes and is demonstrated on T1-weighted images as isointense (55 per cent) or hyperintense (45 per cent), and on T2-weighted images it is seen as an isointense (85 per cent), partially hyperintense (10 per cent), or hypointense (5 per cent) lesion (Case 9) (Muramatsu *et al.* 1991).

Early advanced HCC, which sounds paradoxical but is in use, is an intermediate between early HCC and advanced HCC with more differentiated HCC cells emerging in an early HCC lesion. It has a nodule-in-nodule appearance and shows central hypointensity and peripheral hyperintensity on T1-weighted images, and central hyperintensity and peripheral iso- or hypointensity on T2-weighted images are seen in one-third to one-half of the lesions of early advanced HCC (Winter *et al.* 1994). In other words, the signal behavior of early and advanced components of early advanced HCC was similar to that of isolated early HCC and isolated advanced HCC. Matsui *et al.* (1989) described the MR findings of two kinds of nodular lesions associated with cirrhosis: all adenomatous hyperplastic nodules without cellular atypia were hyperintense on T1-weighted images and hypointense on T2-weighted images, and adenomatous hyperplastic nodules with atypia or malignant foci were hyperintense on T1-weighted SE images and hypointense with central hyperintensity on T2-weighted images. The MR findings of the former and the latter nodular lesions are well consistent with early HCC and early advanced HCC, respectively, as proposed by us (Muramatsu *et al.* 1991). These discrepancies in MR imaging largely depend on the different scales for pathologic diagnosis at different institutions. An international consensus on the grading of nodular lesions seen in cirrhosis is badly required.

Early HCC—Case 1: Arterial-CT in early HCC.

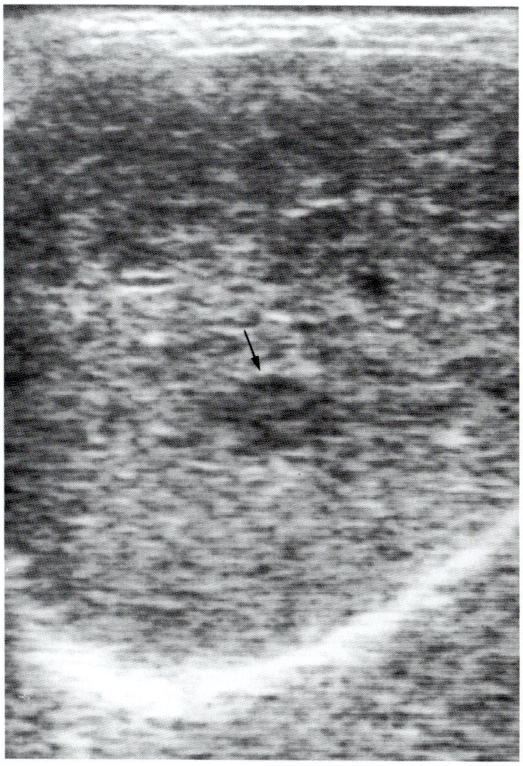

(a) US: an oval shaped low echo lesion (→) is seen in S^{VIII}, but no mosaic structure or halo is seen.

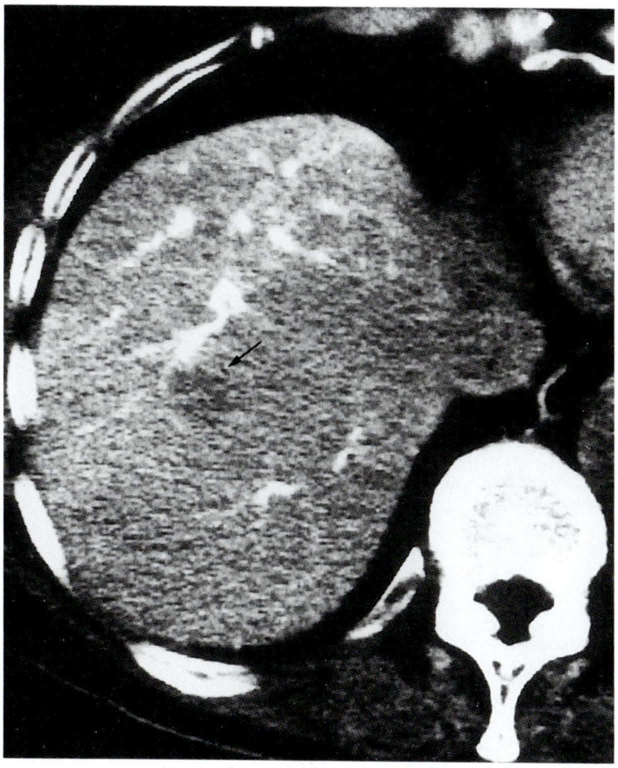

(b) Arterial-CT: since this lesion was not seen by arteriography, arterial-CT was done. The lesion is seen as a low-density area (→) although the intrahepatic arteries are clearly opacified.

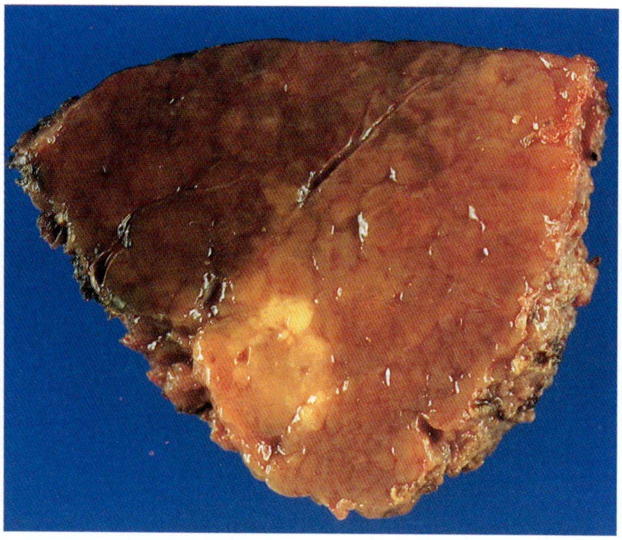

(c) Cut surface of resected specimen: a 1.2 cm light yellow lesion was seen in the resected specimen. The internal structure of the mass was very much the same as the other regenerative nodules, and contained portal tracts, a feature quite different from ordinary small HCC.

Early HCC—Case 2: Early HCC seen as a low or isodensity lesion on portal- and arterial-CT.

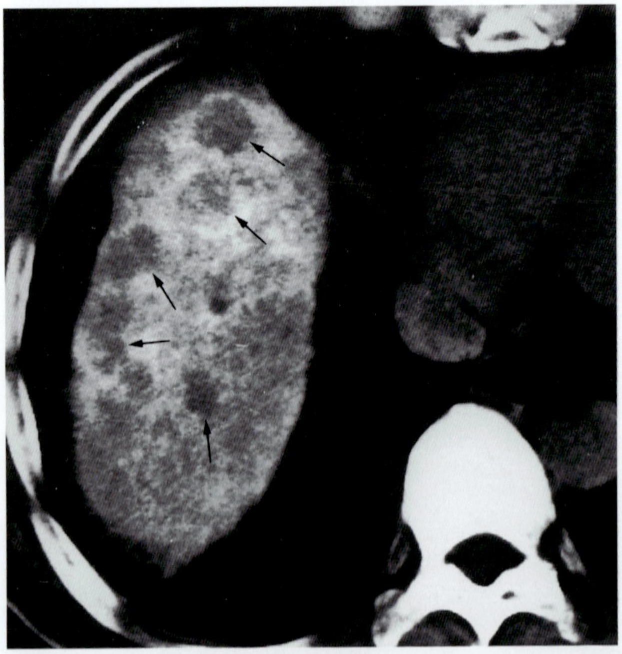

(a) Portal-CT: multiple small low-density lesions are seen in S^{VIII} (→).

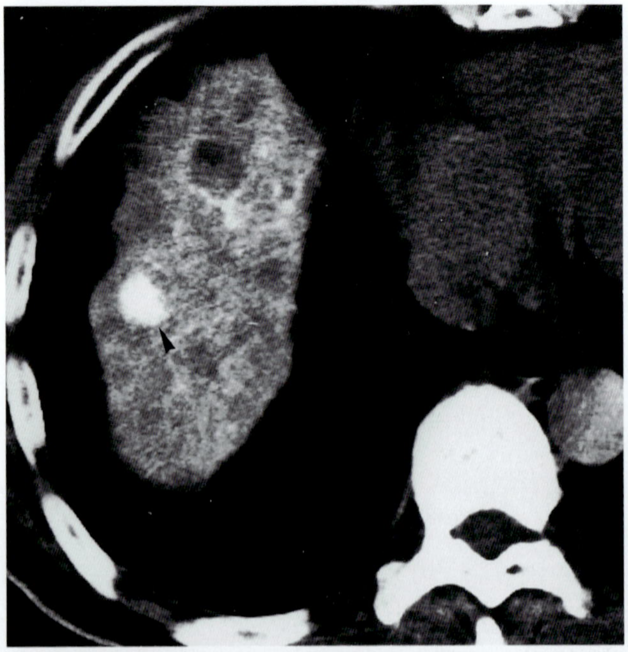

(b) Arterial-CT: except for one densely stained lesion (▶), all the other lesions are of low density or isodense.

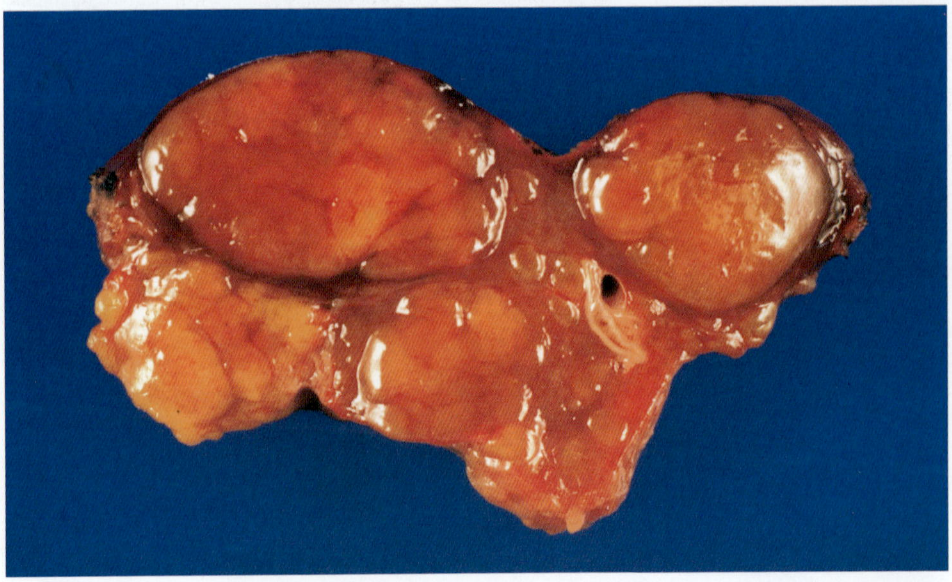

(c) Cut surface of resected specimen: multiple small nodular lesions were seen. Histologically, all of them including the stained one were early HCC.

Early HCC—Case 3: Lipiodol-CT in early HCC.

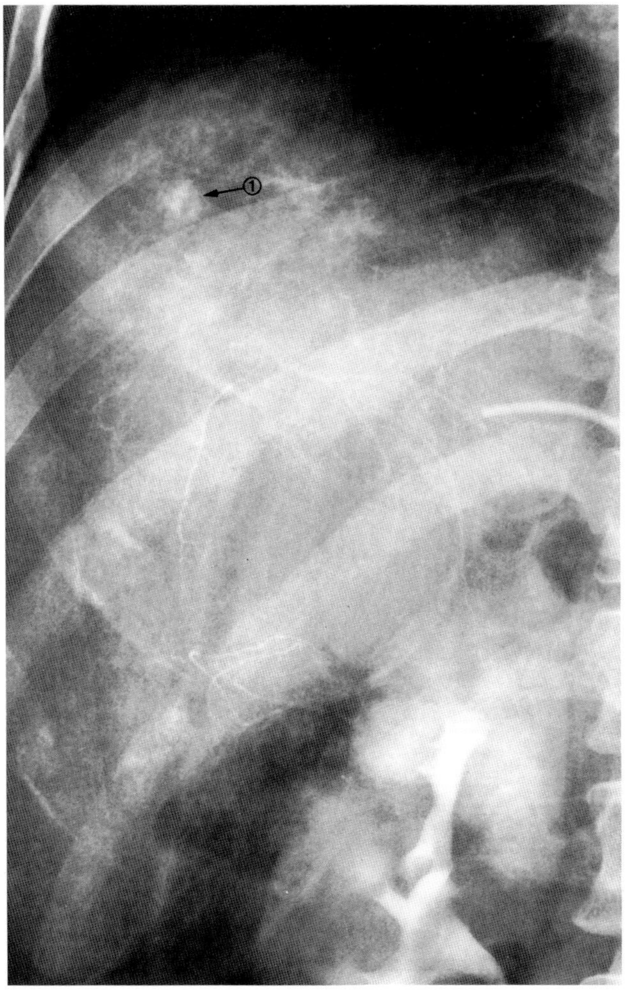

(a) Proper hepatic arteriogram: a 1.0 cm stain (1) was recognized in S^{VIII}.

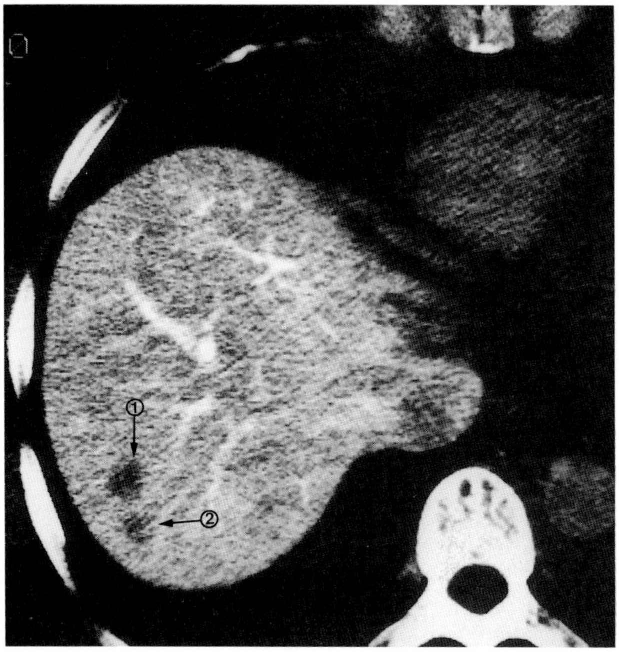

(b) Portal-CT: portal-CT delineated two low-density lesions (1) and (2).

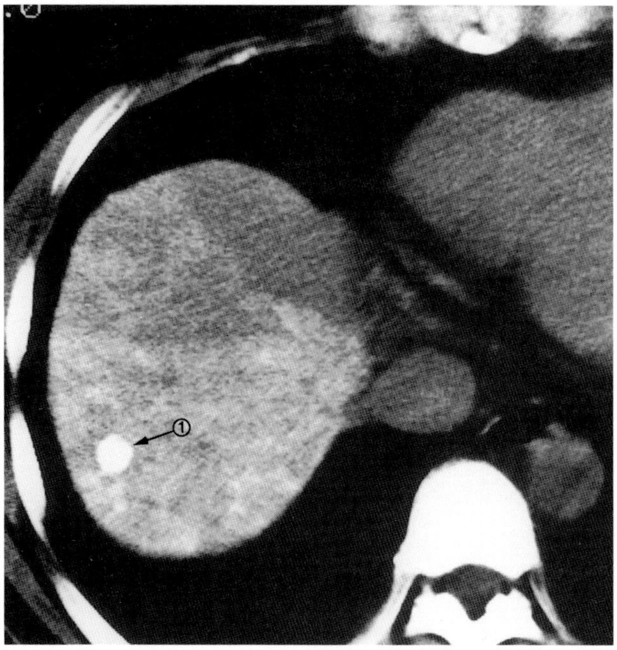

(c) Lipiodol-CT: the hepatic artery was recatheterized and Lipiodol was injected. CT made immediately thereafter demonstrated only (1).

Case 3 (contd.)

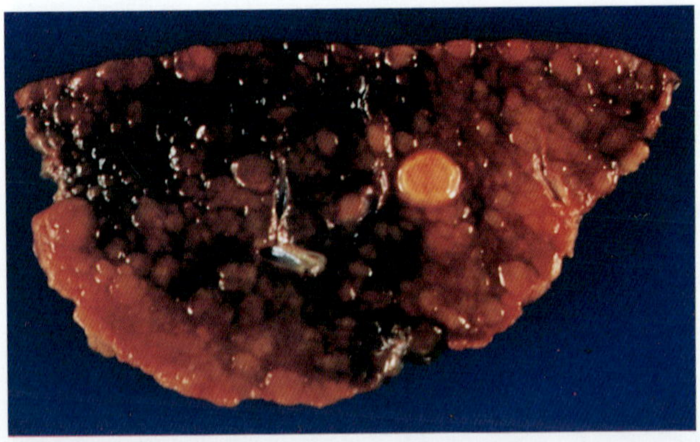

(d) Cut surface of resected specimen: S^{VIII} was partially resected. The cut section revealed two lesions (d, f). Lesion (1) was completely necrotized, and soft X-rays demonstrated retention of Lipiodol. Despite its small size, it had a capsule, and considering the ghost-cell feature, the diagnosis was 'highly differentiated HCC'.

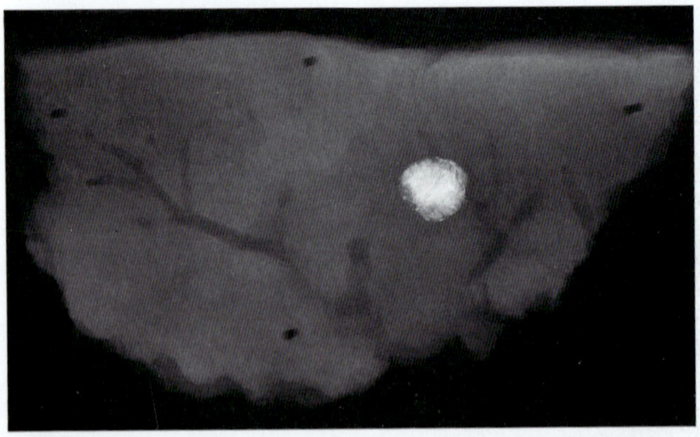

(e) Low-voltage radiograph of (d).

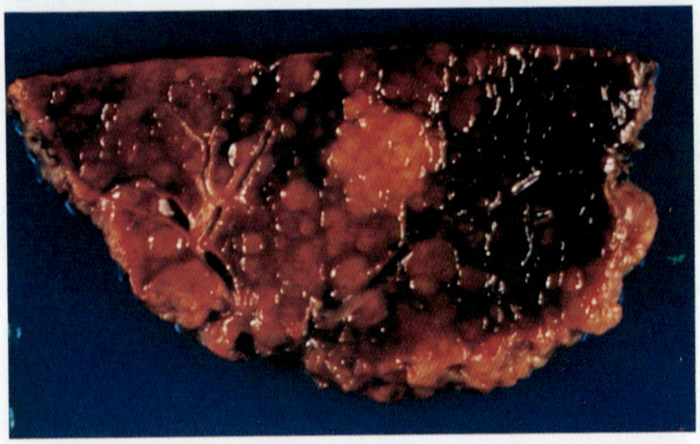

(f) Cut surface of resected specimen: lesion (2) measuring 0.9 cm was irregularly bounded, the internal structure resembled the surrounding liver parenchyma. Histologically it was HCC of Edmondson's grade I. The histologic diagnosis was adenomatous hyperplasia containing an HCC of Edmondson's grade I, consistent with early HCC. This lesion did not retain Lipiodol studied by soft X-ray.

Early HCC—Case 4: Early HCC which angiography stained partially.

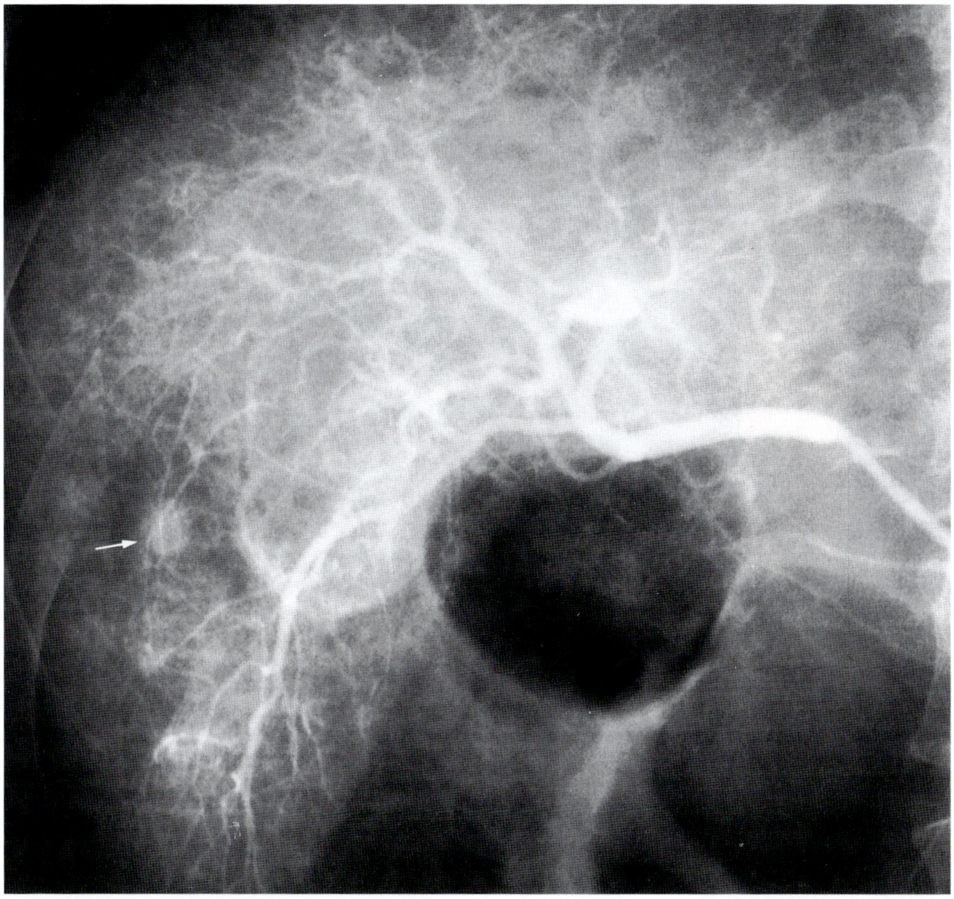

(a) Arteriography (late phase): a 0.8 cm tumor stain (→) was recognized.

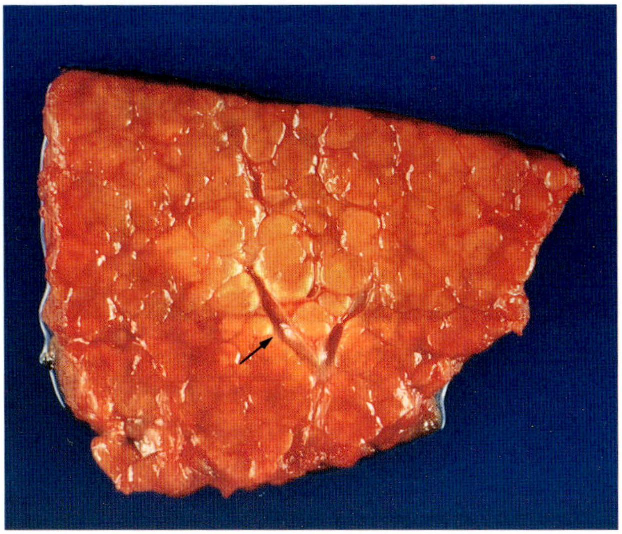

(b) Cut surface of resected specimen (one side): a 2 cm yellowish lesion with an internal structure resembling the surrounding parenchyma. An hepatic vein is seen running through it (→).

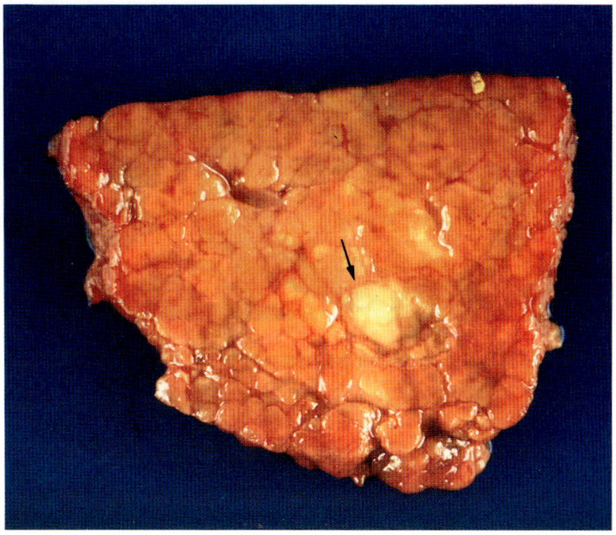

(c) Cut surface (the other side): a 0.7 cm whitish lesion is seen (→). This lesion was histologically HCC of Edmondson's grade I > II surrounded by small nodules of adenomatous hyperplasia.

Early HCC—Case 6: A 3 cm early HCC associated with an advanced HCC.

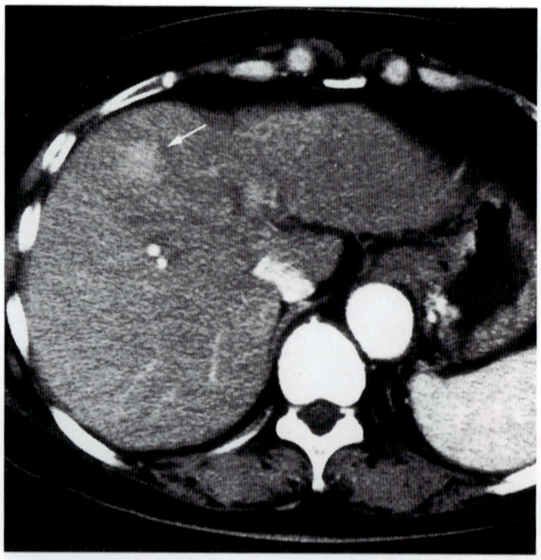

(a) Enhanced CT: on enhanced CT, beside a main mass another accessory lesion that was faintly stained was found (→). This lesion could not be recognized by angiography or US.

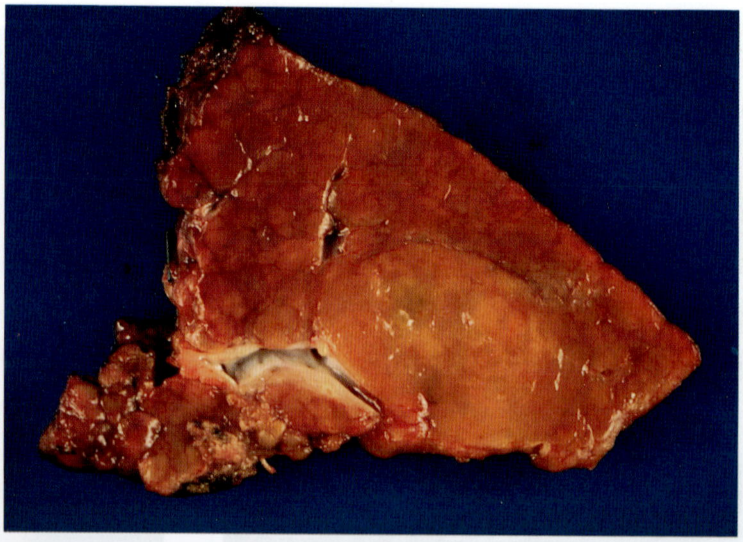

(b) Cut surface of resected specimen: a 3 cm early HCC with a homogeneous interior (Edmondson's grade I – II) was found. Since this lesion was not clearly recognized by intraoperative US, the surgical margin was found to have some tumor cells. As Lipiodol–adriamycin intra-arterial injection was carried out preoperatively, about 20 per cent of the main tumor was necrotized. Early HCC was not affected by this treatment at all.

Adenomatous hyperplasia—Case 7: Adenomatous hyperplasia associated with an advanced HCC.

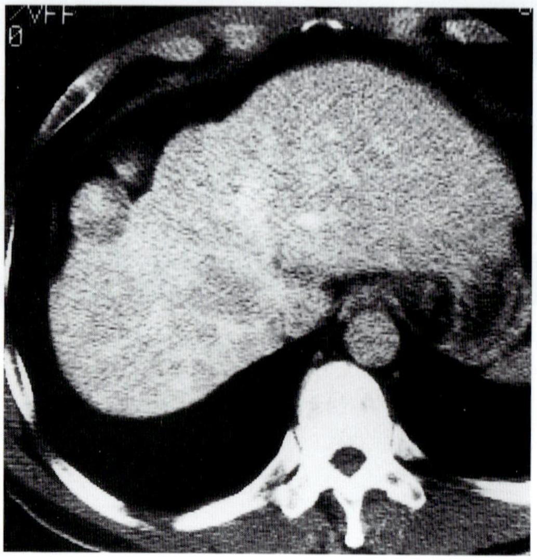

(a) Enhanced CT (late phase): a protruding advanced HCC is seen in S^{V}.

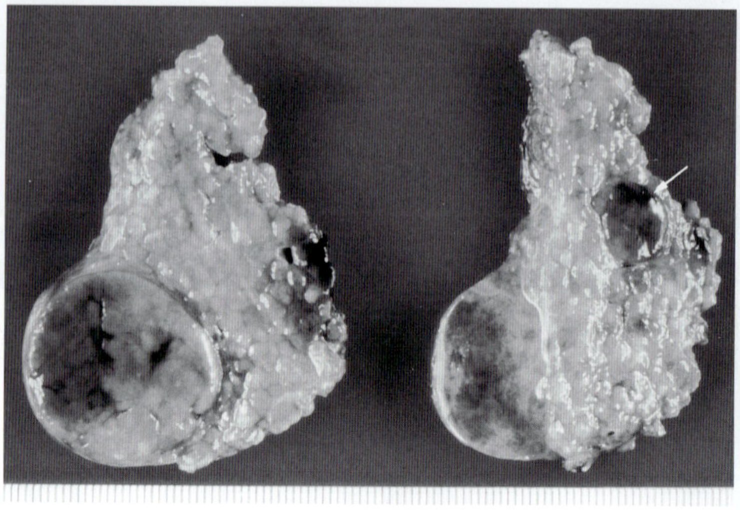

(b) Cut surface of resected specimen: when the resected specimen was cut, another small 1 cm lesion (→) in the vicinity of the main mass was formed. Histologically, it was adenomatous hyperplasia.

Atypical adenomatous hyperplasia—Case 8: Atypical adenomatous hyperplasia associated with cirrhosis.

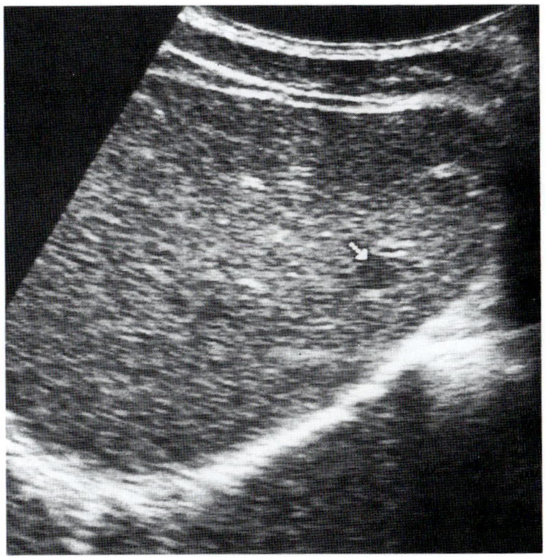

(a) US: during a follow-up of this patient at the out-patient clinic, a 1 cm low-echoic lesion was found (→) in S^{VIII}. In the ensuing 7 months, no change in size occurred.

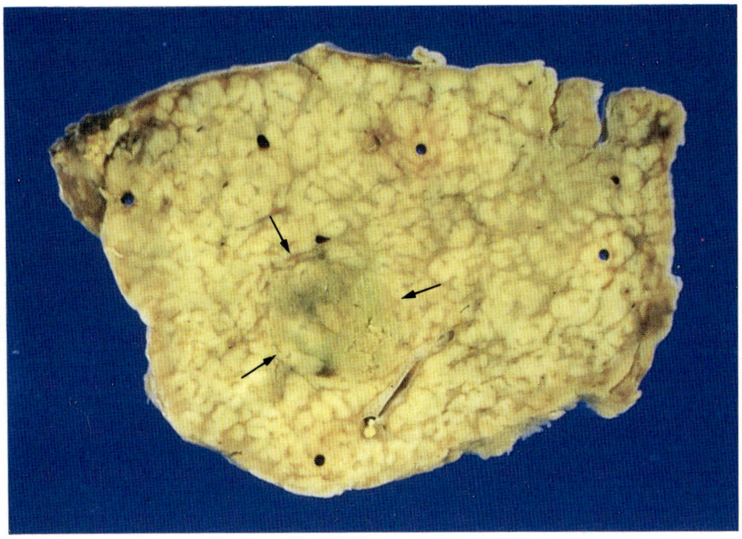

(b) Cut surface of resected specimen: another new small lesion (small HCC) was found during the follow-up in S^{IV} (not shown), and an operation was carried out. The original lesion that had been followed was also resected. It turned out to be atypical adenomatous hyperplasia (→) because the only abnormality of this lesion was increased cellularity; there was no evidence of malignancy.

Early HCC—Case 9: Early HCC that showed isointensity on T2-weighted MR imaging.

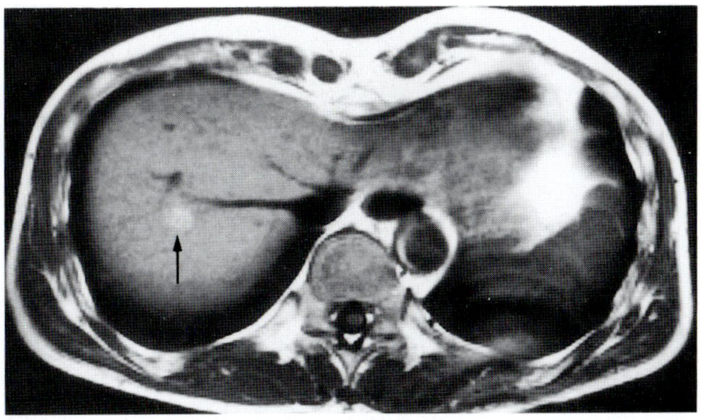

(a) MR imaging (T1-weighted, 600/15): a high-intensity mass (→) is seen in S^{VIII}.

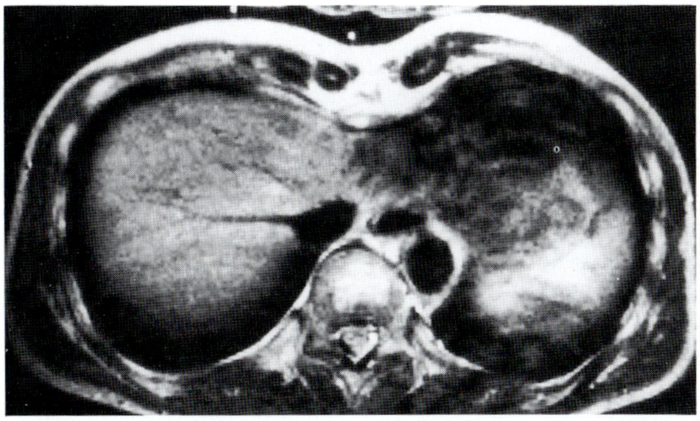

(b) MR imaging (T2-weighted, 2400/60): this tumor showed isointense signals.

Early HCC—Case 10: Stump recurrence after resection for an early HCC.

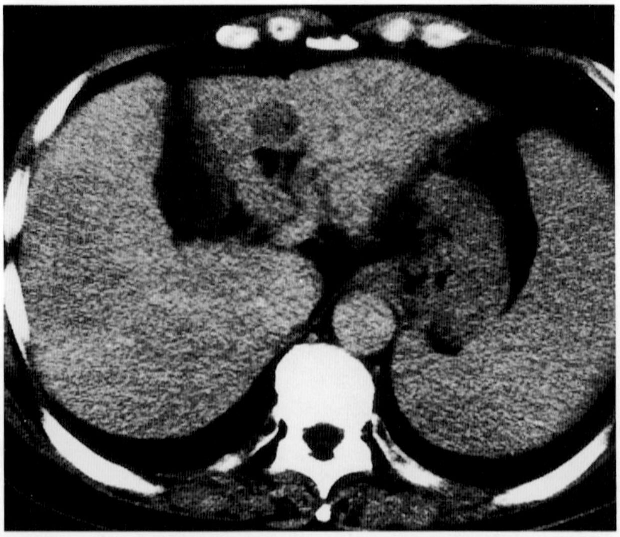

(a) Enhanced CT (late phase): a low-density lesion is seen in the left lobe. During the operation, intraoperative US failed to delineate the boundary between the mass and parenchyma, and the surgical margin was found to have tumor cells.

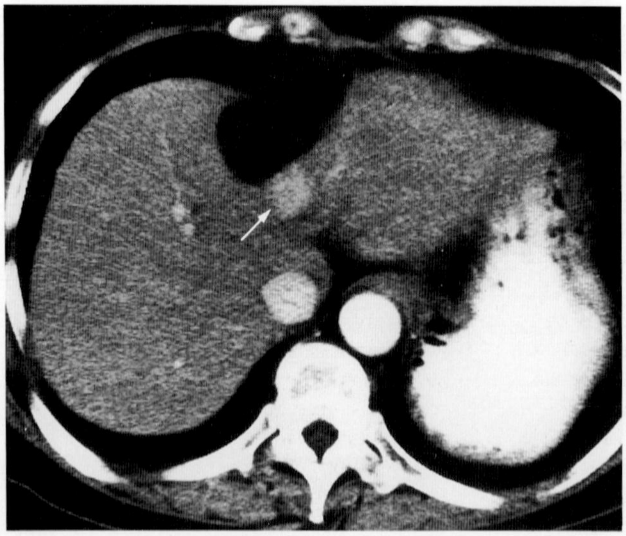

(b) Enhanced CT 6 months later: a recurrent lesion that was stained (→) was found at the surgical margin.

4.4 Medium- and large-sized hepatocellular carcinoma

In the section 4.2 we discussed HCC smaller than 3 cm. HCCs larger than 3 cm may be categorized into medium and large sizes with no clear-cut definition for separation. It is generally accepted that as a cancer grows larger, it will cause more infiltration into the surrounding parenchyma and more metastases with progressively poorer prognosis. In HCC, however, beside the size other factors influence prognosis. For instance, a liver with multiple small lesions and portal invasion and a liver in which single large encapsulated HCC occupies two segments without portal invasion may appear similar in the degree of cancer progression, yet the prognosis is much worse with the former; the treatment should not be the same. In other words, one should not be concerned about the tumor size only, but quality diagnosis and degree of advanced state have to be determined for the selection of appropriate treatment.

In the following discussion, HCCs larger than 10 cm in diameter will be called 'large' for the sake of convenience. The majority of large HCCs resected at the National Cancer Center Hospital were the nodular type (type 1), and a considerable proportion of them did not have portal invasion or intrahepatic spread, suggesting that some of the large HCCs are not biologically very malignant.

Our clinicopathological analysis of such large HCCs showed that some patients lack subjective complaints, less commonly have underlying cirrhosis (31 per cent) compared with small HCCs, and that the mass frequently has a capsule (95 per cent). It was suggested that these large HCCs had perhaps grown at a very slow rate. The prognosis of such large HCCs after resection was significantly better than comparably sized HCCs that defied resection. TAE and PEI are not very effective for large HCC, and resection should be considered positively. Recurrence in the remnant liver after resection for large HCC is almost as frequent as after resection for a small HCC, and therefore reduction surgery is of significance from the point of view of therapy. The important point in the diagnosis of large HCC is accurate quality diagnosis and diagnosis of small HCC in the lobe not to be resected.

Diagnosis of main mass

The internal structure of a 3–10 cm medium-sized HCC is essentially the same as that of a small HCC of the nodular type, except that in the former the nodule-in-nodule structure is more distinct and the presence of a fibrous capsule is more common. Such characteristics help CT and angiography delineate the typical HCC features (Case 1).

In general, as the tumor increases in size, central necrosis becomes more frequent, seen by CT as a stellate low-density area. This same area is seen as an avascular region by angiography (Case 2). A huge HCC, larger than 20 cm, can no longer be fully supplied by feeding arteries, and peripheral areas situated far from the feeding arteries undergo spontaneous necrosis. CT and angiography do not stain such areas (Case 3). However, some huge HCCs may receive arterial blood from the subphrenic and gastroduodenal arteries (development of parasitic arteries from the adjacent organs)(Case 4). Occasionally, a large HCC undergoes minimal central necrosis as a result of development of abundant feeding arteries (Case 5), requiring differential diagnosis from hepatocellular adenoma and focal nodular hyperplasia.

At MR imaging, advanced HCC is generally demonstrated either as an area of hypo- (41–51 per cent), iso- (17–24 per cent), or hyperintensity (31–34 per cent) on T1-weighted images, and most HCC is as a hyperintense mass (91–97 per cent) on T2-weighted images (Itoh *et al.* 1987; Kadoya *et al.* 1992). According to Ebara *et al.* (1991), hyperintensity on T1-weighted images of HCC less than 5 cm may be due to increased copper content. In encapsulated HCC, the fibrous capsule surrounding it is shown as hypointense on both T1- and T2-weighted images. According to Kadoya *et al.* (1992), the capsule is histologically composed of two layers, an inner layer rich in fibrous components and an outer layer containing varying numbers of compressed small vessels and newly formed bile ducts. A double-layered ring on T2-weighted imaged (hypointense inner layer and hyperintense outer layer) was observed in some large HCCs with a thick capsule (Itoh *et al.* 1987), but its incidence is not high. The sensitivity of MR imaging for the capsule was 66 per cent on T1-weighted image and 29 per cent on T2-weighted images in the study of Kadoya *et al.* (1992). The HCC structure consisting of internal nodules of different cell differentiation that contains necrosis, hemorrhage, and fatty changes assumes a mosaic appearance on MR imaging (Choi *et al.* 1990*b*). Fresh hemorrhage is generally thought to be hyperintense on both T1- and T2-weighted images, and necrosis hypointense on T1-weighted and hyperintense on T2-weighted images. Coagulative necrosis, however, is hypointense on T2-weighted images due to decrease of free water. A tumor thrombus which frequently develops in large vessels such as the portal vein and inferior vena cava, is seen as hypointense structures on T1-weighted images (Ohtomo *et al.* 1987).

Advanced HCC is usually well enhanced by Gd-DTPA. The lesion appears hyperintense in the early phase of enhancement, changing to a hypointense mass with an enhanced ring around it in the late phase on T1-weighted SE or gradient echo sequence images (Yoshida *et al.* 1989*b*). With SPIO as a contrast agent, an HCC is demonstrated as a hyperintense mass relative to the liver parenchyma because SPIO is not taken up by HCC which does not have Kupffer cells; parenchyma is enhanced producing a clear contrast.

Diagnosis of small HCC in the lobe not to be resected

A large nodular HCC usually receives a large feeding artery, hence an abundant arterial blood supply, and as a result the other lobe not containing the mass receives much less arterial blood. To make up for the reduction of arterial blood supply, the portal blood flow to that lobe increases (Case 6). Such hemodynamic changes make the diagnosis of small lesions in that lobe very difficult, because contrast medium preferentially goes to the lobe occupied by the HCC and the other lobe receives only a small amount of it on arterial-CT and Lipiodol-CT (Merine *et al.* 1990). We therefore believe that portal-CT is most suited for the diagnosis of small lesions in the contralateral lobe.

Vascular structure of HCC and delineation of the fibrous capsule

A typical HCC has many dilated and winding tumor vessels, but their stereoscopic distribution can not be grasped on the antiogram which is two dimensional. Arterial-CT provides a more objective view of vasculature in a living person (Case 7). The fibrous capsule, sometimes called a pseudocapsule (Edmondson and Steiner 1954), that surrounds a nodular HCC has certain biological significance and needs to be delineated by imaging. Dynamic CT is very useful in this respect because the capsule seen as a low-density ring in the early phase becomes a high-density ring with the passage of time, and the thickness of the ring somewhat increases (Case 8). The time when the translucent ring (Okuda *et al.* 1977*c*) is seen in the late phase of anteriography corresponds to the early phase of dynamic CT. Therefore, it seems that the low-density ring on dynamic CT corresponds to the angiographic translucent rim. Our interpretation is that in dynamic CT the parenchyma receives portal blood containing contrast medium and its density increases producing a low-density area sandwiched between the tumor and parenchyma (low-density ring) as a result of retention of contrast medium by the fibrous tissues; this results in the interior of a metastatic liver cancer becoming stained in a very late phase of CT. The slow and slight increase in the width of the high-density ring that follows may be due to increasing contrast retention by a coarse fibrous tissue in the non-cancerous parenchyma surrounding the capsule.

Mode of intrahepatic extension of HCC

Intrahepatic spread of a unicentric HCC may be either through the portal vein or via the artery that carries HCC cells coming from an extrahepatic metastasis. The latter is perhaps very uncommon. Transportal spread occurs when a cancer cell or a cluster of cancer cells enter the portal branch at the periphery of the tumor and are sent to the peripheral liver tissue where they settle. Transport of cancer cells to the other side of the liver readily occurs in the presence of an arterio-portal shunt, a frequent development in advanced HCC, through which contrast medium flows retrogradely (Okuda and Matsutani 1987). In liver cirrhosis with portal hypertension and extensive portal systemic collaterals, the flow in the portal trunk is frequently to-and-fro, sometimes retrograde (Okuda *et al.* 1973*b*; Takayasu *et al.* 1982*b*) (Case 12, p.370). If such a liver bears an HCC, spread of cancer to the other side of the liver can readily occur. Even a small HCC, less than 3 cm, may show portal invasion; there was gross portal invasion in 28 per cent of such HCCs in our experience (Kanai *et al.* 1987), and intrahepatic spread may be more frequent in the presence of arterio-portal shunts. When a large first- or second-order portal vein has a tumor thrombus, the ipsilateral lobe will have extensive tumor spread, and it is frequently difficult at the time of autopsy to identify the primary tumor and make measurements. Transarterial spread may produce multiple lesions of a similar size in both lobes, more heavily in the sucapsular area as in hepatic spread of lung and breast cancers, but in reality distinction between portal and arterial spreads is not easy. Should arterial spread occur, it would be preceded by portal spread in most instances, masking the feature of the former.

Medium- and large-sized HCC—Case 1: Typical nodular HCC seen by dynamic CT.

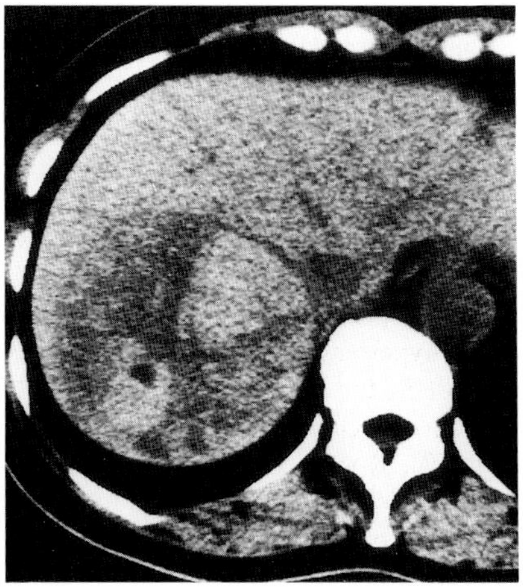

(a) Plain CT: a 7 cm mass with a discrete boundary is seen in S^{VII} and its vicinity. Part of the interior is of high density suggestive of bleeding.

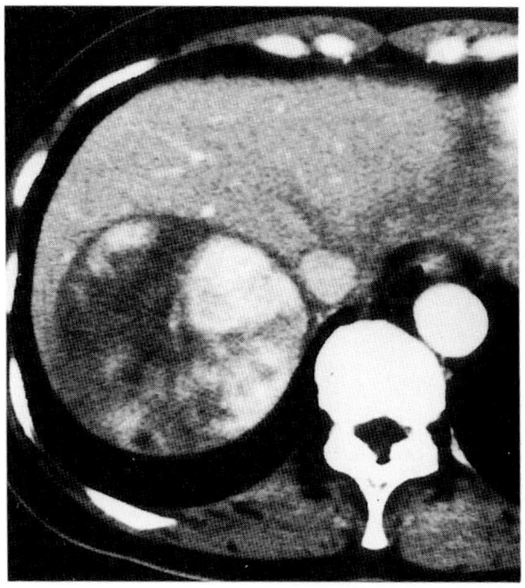

(b) Dynamic CT (early phase): however, on dynamic CT, the interior has several lobular stains, and the suspected bleeding necrosis now seems to represent a viable region.

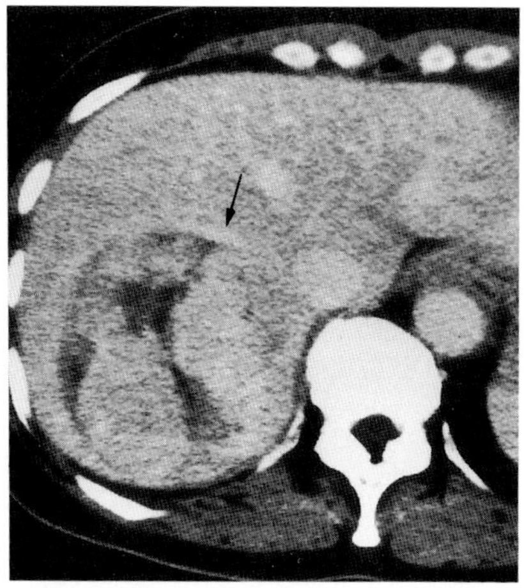

(c) Dynamic CT (late phase): the lobular stains have become more distinct, but several areas, two in the centre and one in the periphery to the right, are not stained. Beside, a ring stain in continuity with the right hepatic vein (→) is recognized, suggesting a capsule.

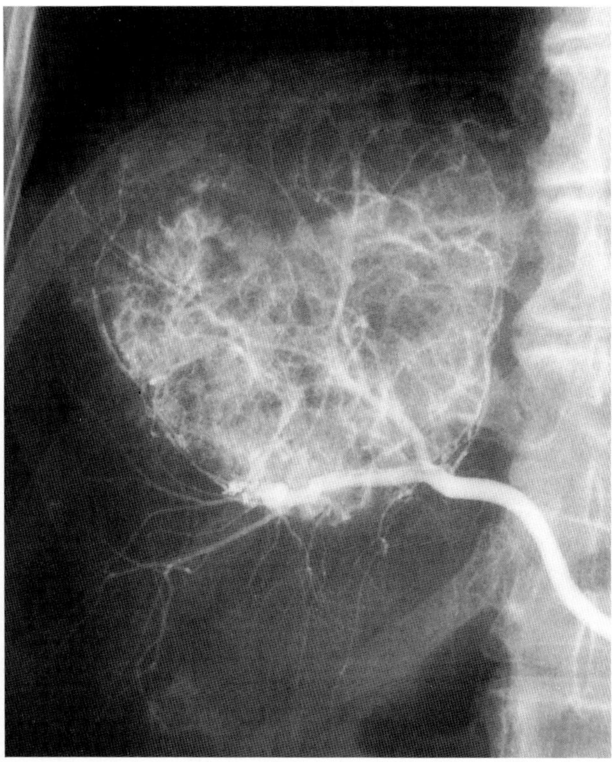

(d) Right hepatic arteriogram (early phase): the artery feeding the posterior segment and its numerous branches are forming tumor vessels.

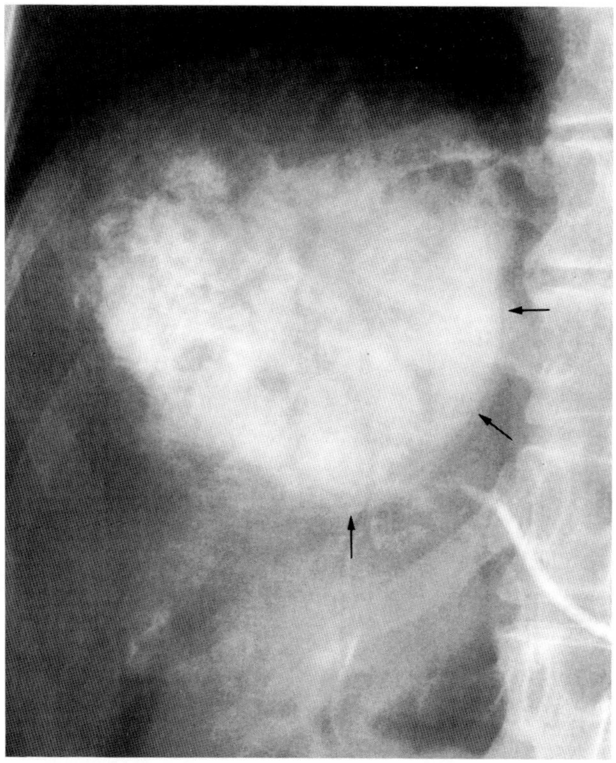

(e) Right hepatic arteriogram (late phase): the stain is inhomogeneous. The reduced stain in the area near the diaphragm suggested a supply coming from the inferior phrenic artery, but in a further late phase, this area was also stained. A thin lucent ring (→) is seen (translucent rim) between the tumor stain and a ring stain.

Case 1 (contd.)

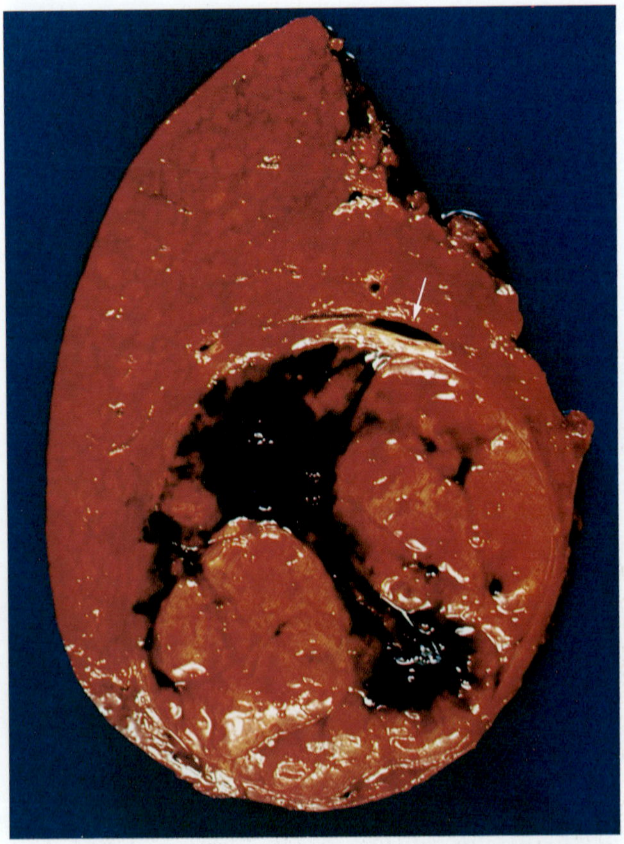

(f) Cut surface of resected specimen: right lobectomy was carried out. There was a bleeding area which corresponded to the unstained area on dynamic CT. The tumor had a nodule-in-nodule structure with a single layer of fibrous capsule. (→), right hepatic vein.

Medium- and large-sized HCC—Case 2: Large nodular HCC with a central coagulation necrosis.

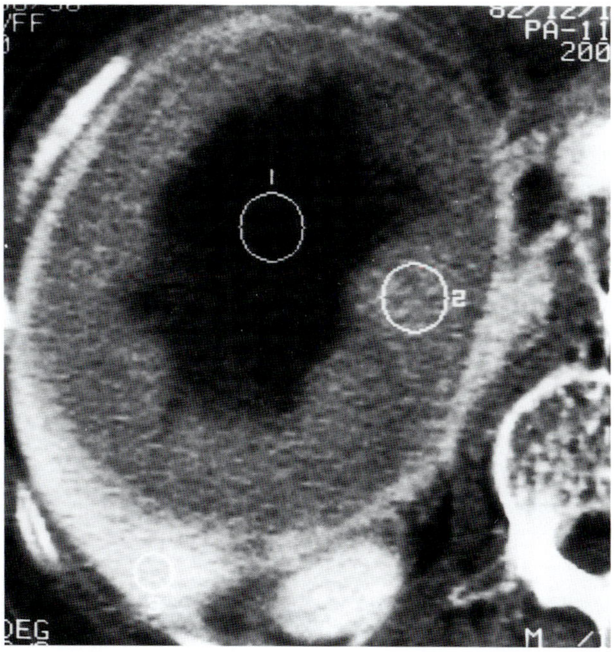

(a) Enhanced CT (late phase): the center of the mass is not stained, and the stellate shaped area (#1) has a density of 33 HU. The nodular area of the mass once enhanced is now of low density (#2).

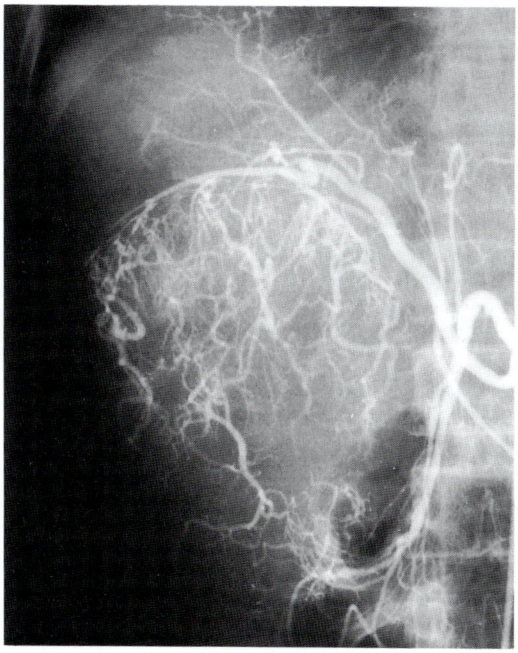

(b) Hepatic arteriogram (early phase): a hypervascular 11 cm mass with dilated and winding tumor vessels is recognized in S^{VI}. A parasitic pancreaticoduodenal artery is also recognized.

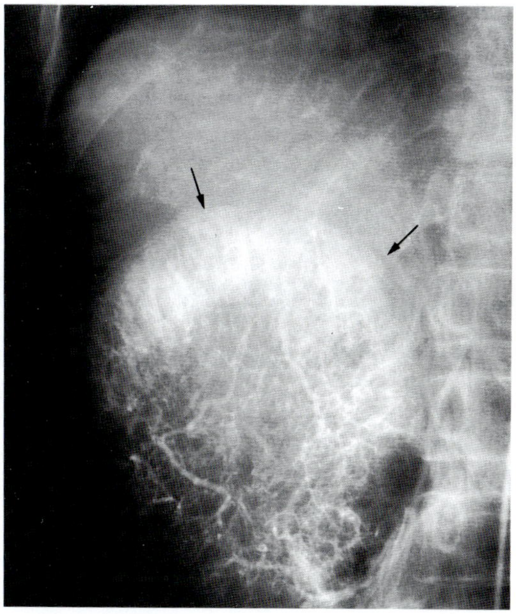

(c) Hepatic arteriogram (late phase): the nodules near the hilum are seen as stains resembling brush strokes. In addition, one thin layer of translucent rim is seen (→).

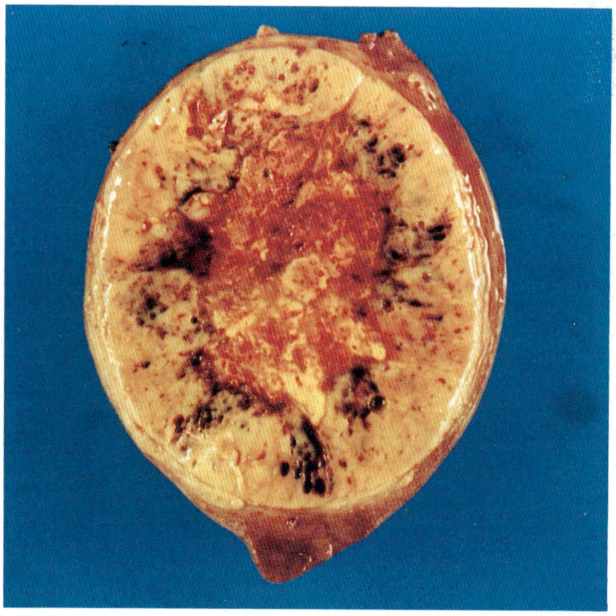

(d) Cut surface of resected specimen: a fibrous capsul^ and a stellate shaped necrotic area is seen in the center. This picture corresponds well to the CT finding. Many parasitic arteries derived from the pancreaticoduodenal artery were identified.

Medium- and large-sized HCC—Case 3: A massive HCC of a diameter of 20 cm.

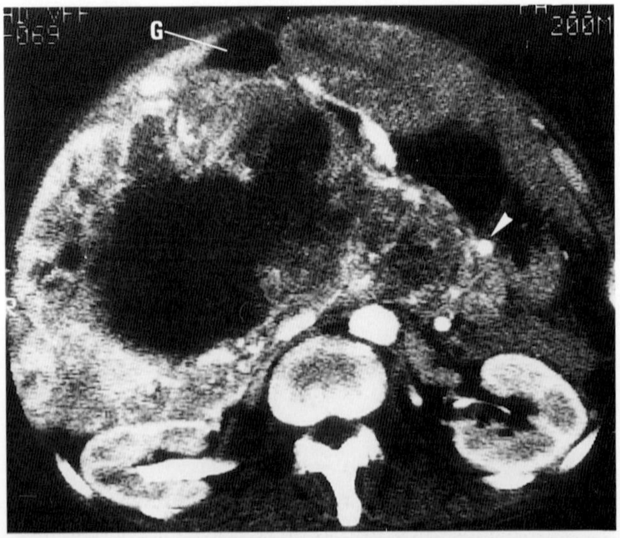

1

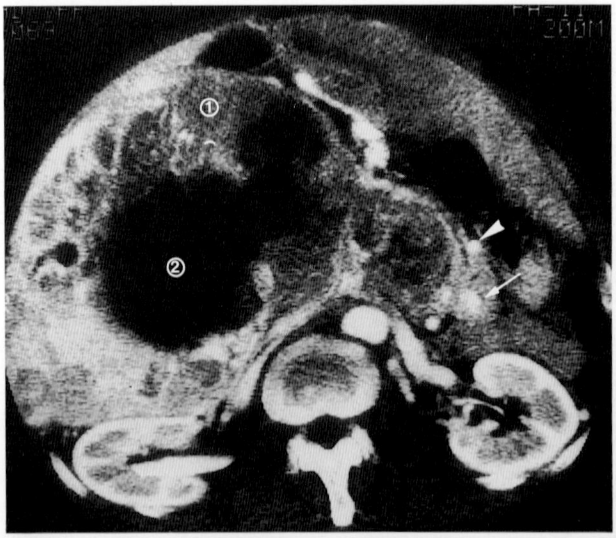

2

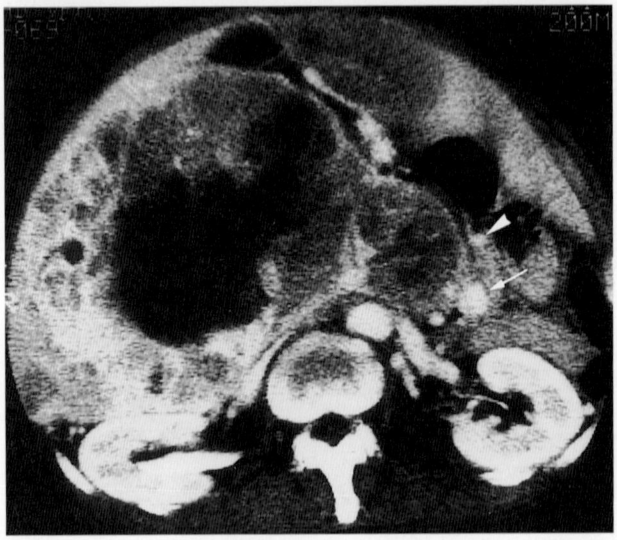

3

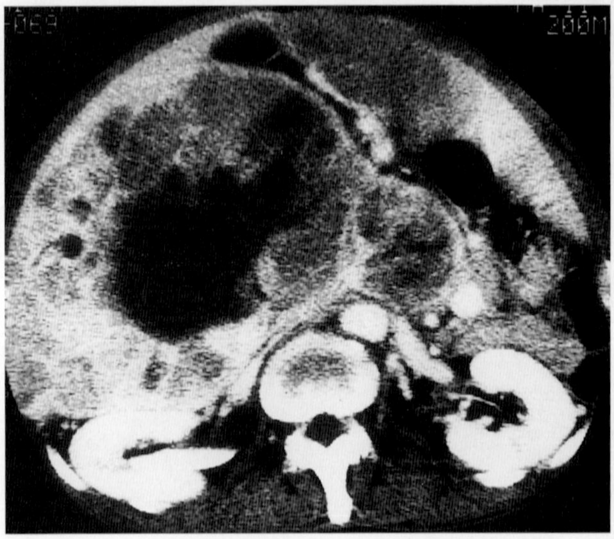

4

(a) Dynamic CT (same level slices): a large mass originating in the right lobe is seen. The superior mesenteric artery (▶) and vein (→) are displaced to the left, and the inferior vena cava is also flattened. The area in S^{IV} to the left of the gallbladder was of low density and diagnosed as tumor invasion. Upon opening the abdomen, there was in fact tumor invasion, but it was not in S^{IV} but in S^{V} which was hypertrophied as a compensation. The periphery of the mass was stained, but the interior was barely stained. The CT values of the stained area (1) was 63 HU and the unstained (2) 38 HU.

Case 3 (contd.)

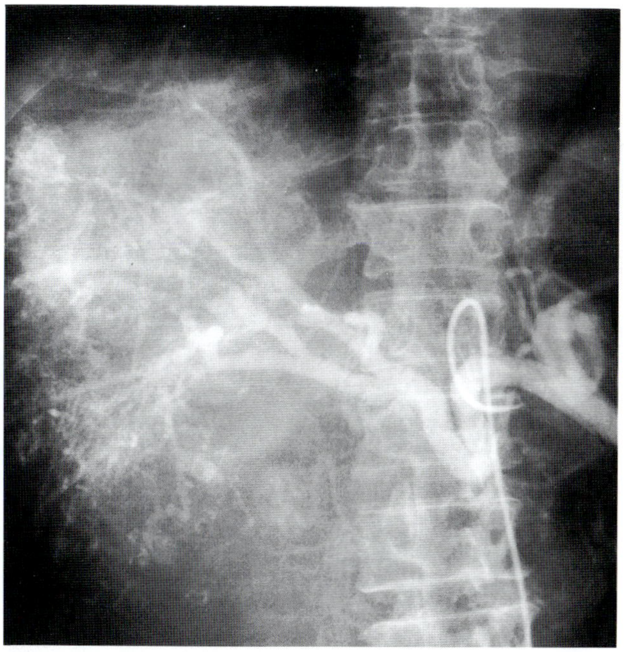

(b) Hepatic arteriogram (arterial phase): many tumor vessels are seen as continuations of the dilated right hepatic artery.

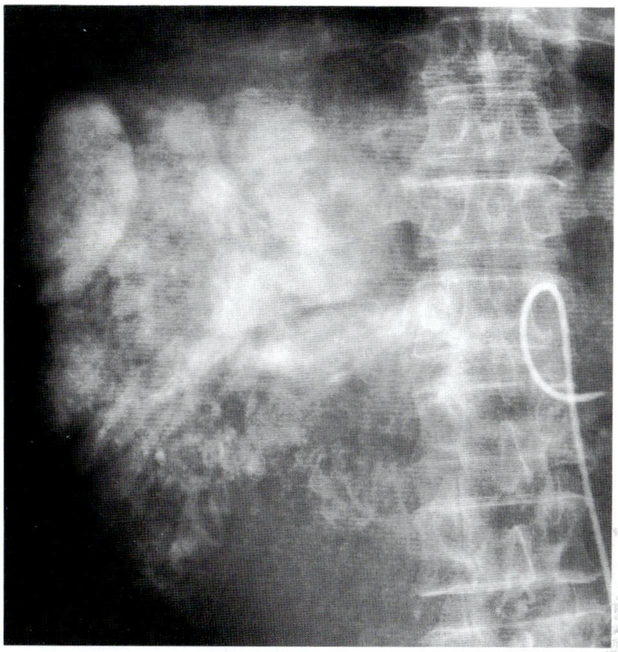

(c) Hepatic arteriogram (parenchymogram): many nodular stains are seen except for the inferior area of the liver.

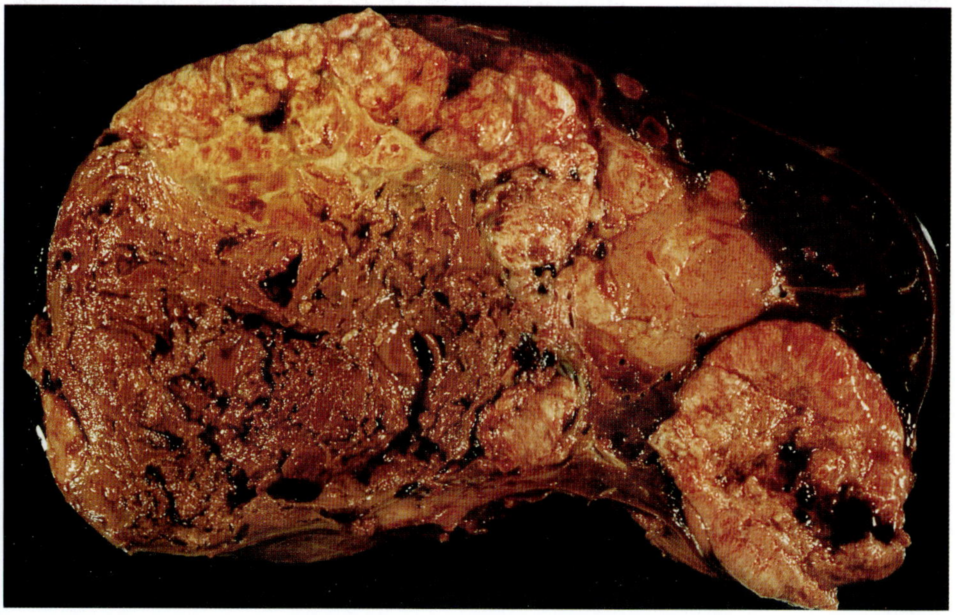

(d) Cut surface of resected specimen: extended right lobectomy was carried out (5500 g). The mass measured 33 × 22 cm. Sagittal section yielded a large amount of brownish fluid coming from the necrotic area that occupied the caudal half of the mass (to the left of the photo). Part of the tumor was covered by a fibrous capsule. The tumor was histologically Edmondson's grade II > III, and the non-cancerous area was normal (same as Case 2, p. 503).

Medium- and large-sized HCC—Case 4: A large nodular HCC with its cranial portion supplied by the right inferior phrenic artery.

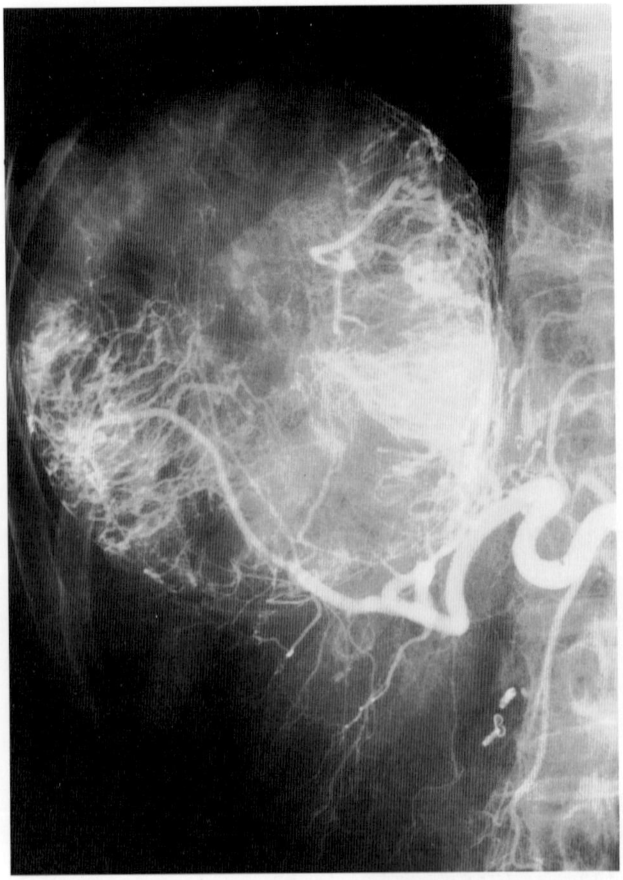

(a) Hepatic arteriogram: three-quarters of the mass is supplied by the hepatic artery, but the cranial quarter was not opacified even in the parenchymal phase.

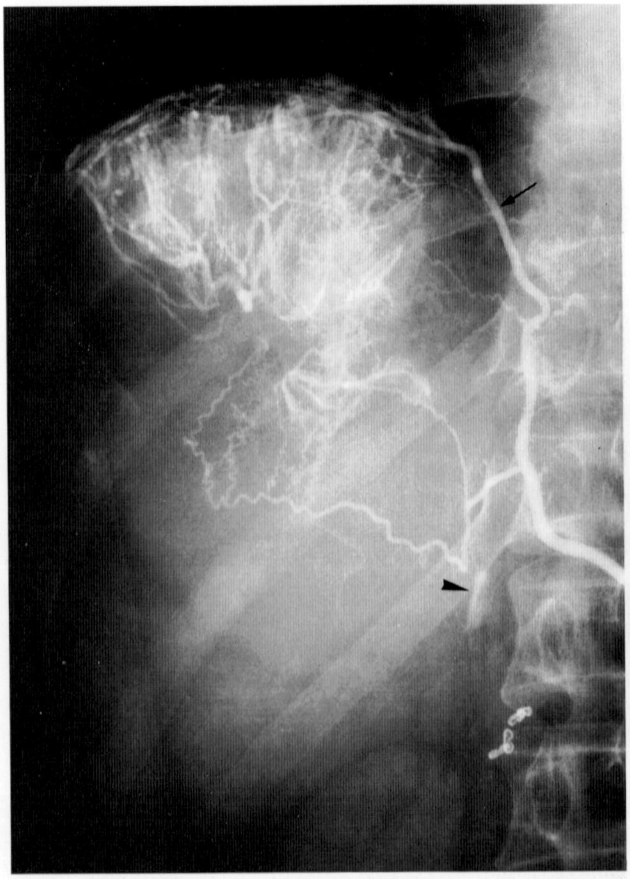

(b) Selective right inferior phrenic arteriography: one-quarter of the mass is supplied by the anterior branch of the inferior phrenic artery (→), and some winding inferior branches are also participating in the supply. The right adrenal in its cranial part (▶) is also opacified through the right suprarenal artery derived from the inferior phrenic artery.

Medium- and large-sized HCC—Case 5: HCC with a stellate high-echo area in the center requiring differential diagnosis from focal nodular hyperplasia.

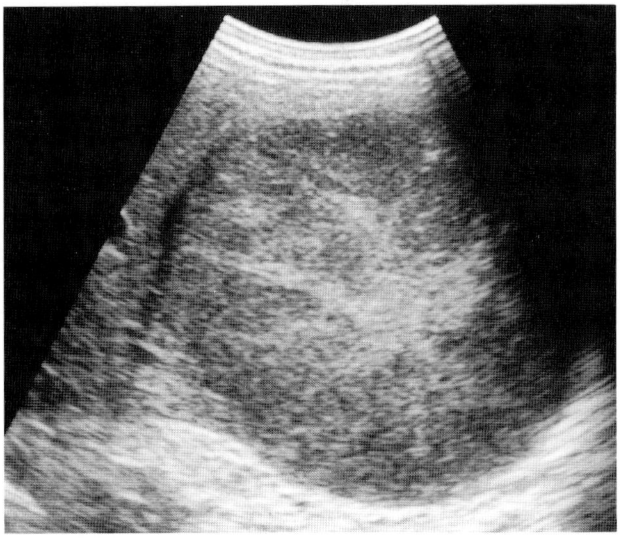

(a) US: the center of the mass with a smooth border found in S^{VI} has a stellate shaped high-echo region. The mass also shows a lateral shadow along the right border.

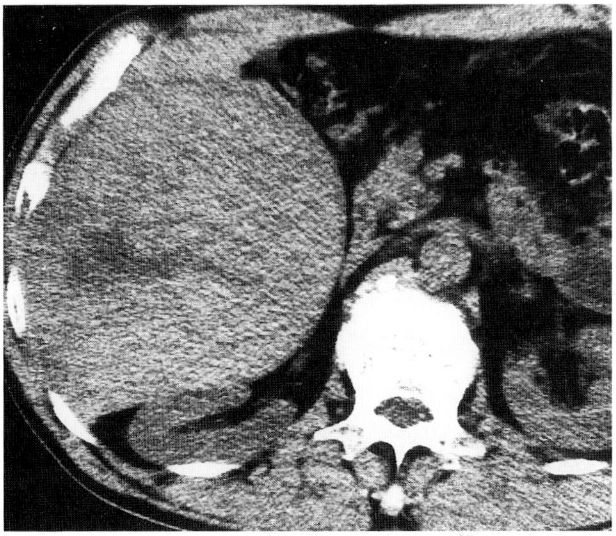

(b) Plain CT: a round mass is seen in S^{VI} that has a homogeneous density with a cord shaped low-density area in the center.

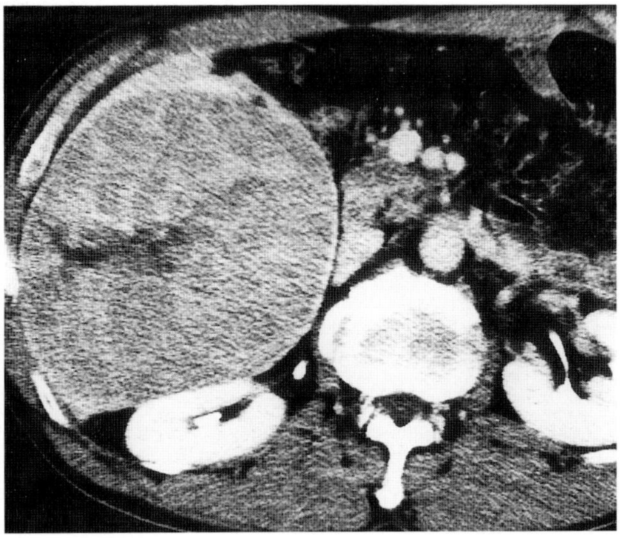

(c) Enhanced CT (late phase): a number of streaks of stain are seen in the interior. With this finding alone the differentiation between HCC and FNH was difficult.

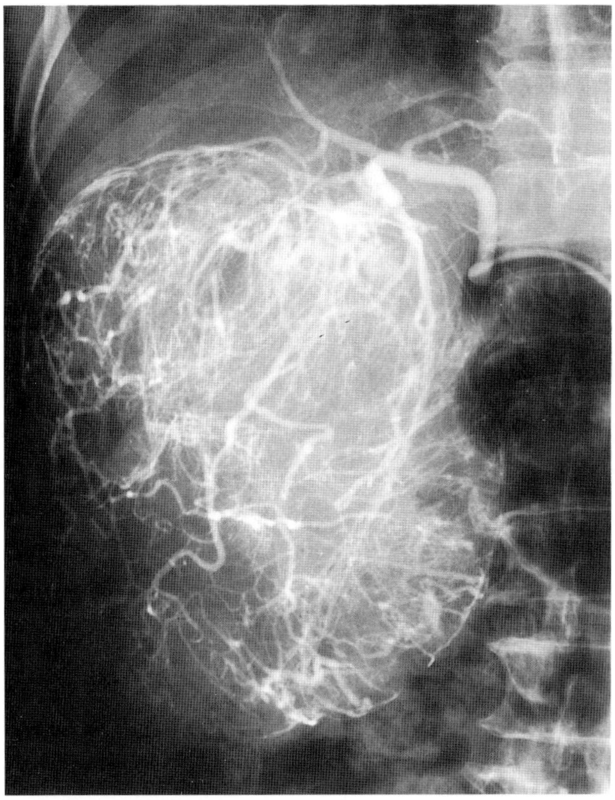

(d) Angiography (arterial phase): many tumor vessels strongly suggest HCC.

Case 5 (contd.)

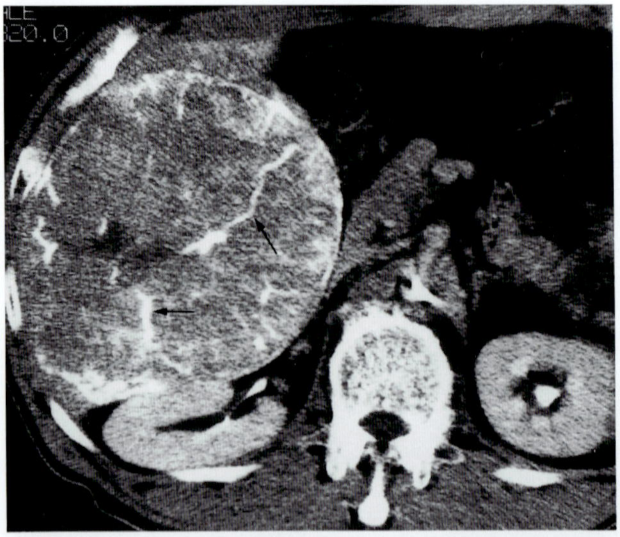

(e) Arterial-CT: arterial-CT followed. The vascular structure of the interior can be assessed from this film, namely, many feeding arteries enter the mass from the periphery. Some are feeding the necrotic interior and others lobular or nodular areas in the periphery.

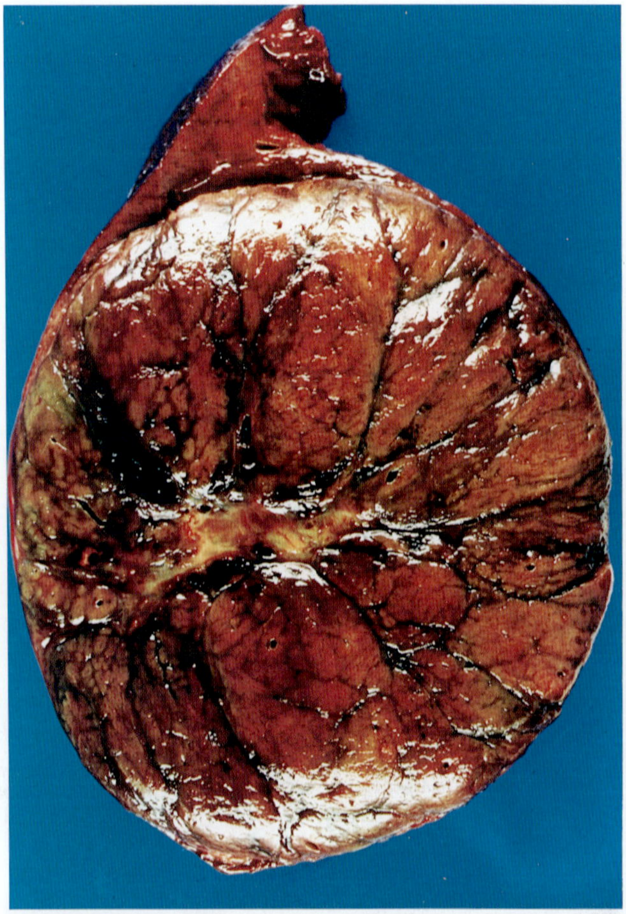

(f) Cut surface of resected specimen: the cut surface bulged, and the mass was divided by fibrous septa in a regular geometric fashion. The center did not bulge and consisted of a coagulative necrotic tissue. Histologically, the tumor was Edmondson's grade II, and III in part. There were tumor thrombi in the right hepatic vein and the posterior segment bile duct (not shown). The non-cancerous parenchyma was normal.

Medium- and large-sized HCC—Case 6: Reduced arterial and increased portal flow to the contralateral lobe in a liver with a huge HCC receiving a large amount of arterial supply.

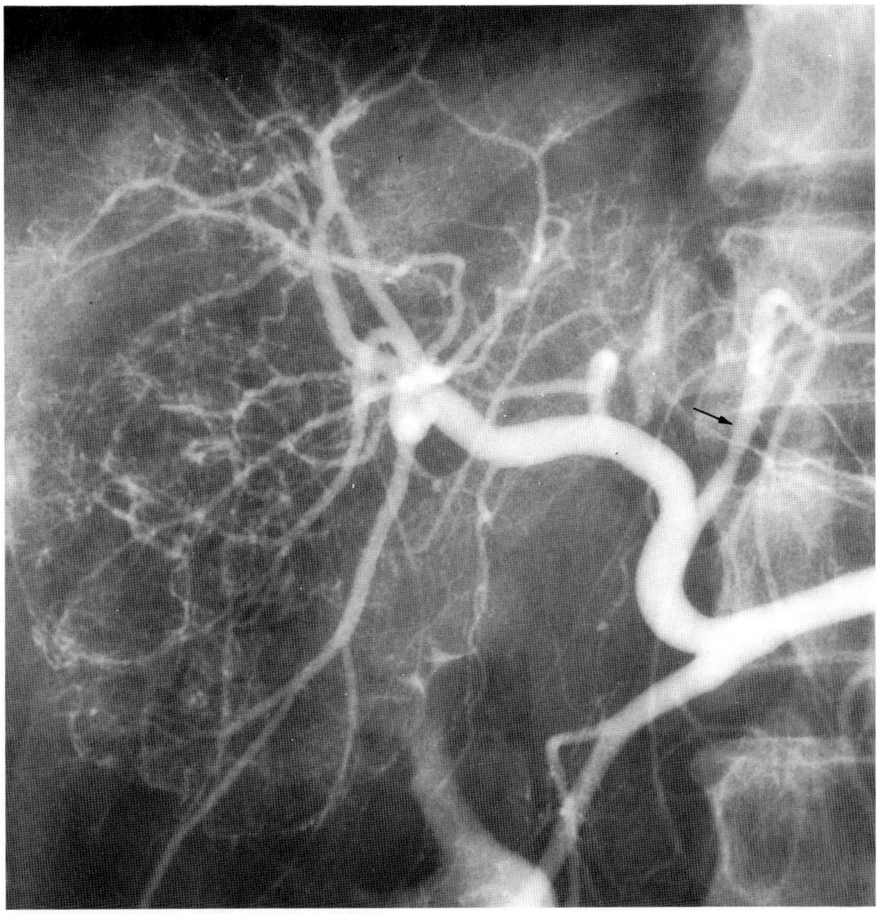

(a) Hepatic arteriography: a huge HCC occupies the right lobe. The bulk of the blood in the common hepatic artery goes into the mass and the flow in the left hepatic artery is proportionally reduced (→).

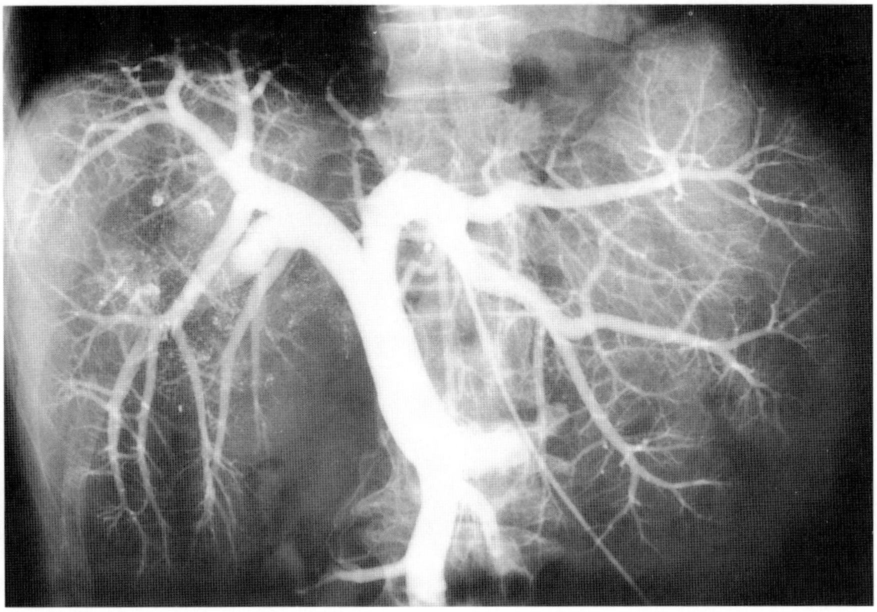

(b) Percutaneous transhepatic portography: the right portal venous flow is reduced due to compression by the mass, and the flow in the left portal vein is increased in compensation for reduced arterial blood flow to this lobe.

Medium- and large-sized HCC—Case 7: Assessment of vascular anatomy in a large nodular HCC by arterial-CT.

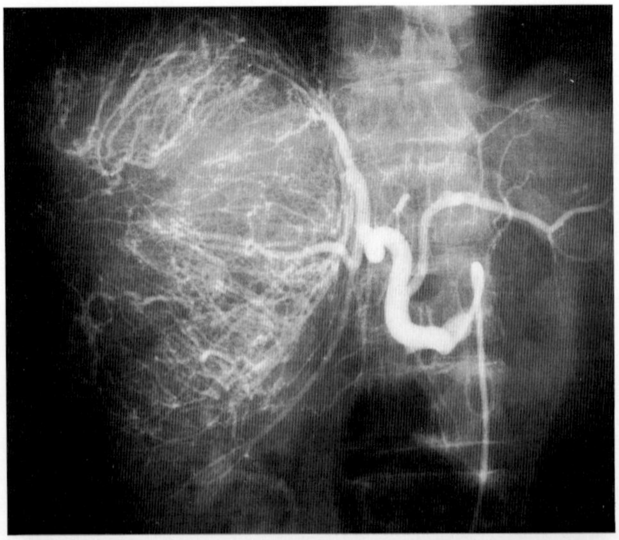

(a) Common hepatic arteriography: a large nodular HCC is seen in the right lobe. The arteriogram demonstrates numerous tumor vessels arising from the tumor periphery and running toward the center.

(b) Sequential changes in arterial-CT (1–4): many dilated tumor vessels are apparent (1). Relatively short feeding vessels in the periphery slowly stain tumor lobules in the periphery (2, 3), some going further toward the center. However, the areas immediately around the vessels are not stained until a late phase (4). As a result, the whole mass is seen as an inhomogeneously stained tumor (4). The feature of tumor vessels running from the periphery toward the center (centrifugal flow) is one of the important characteristics of HCC that contribute to the differentiation from FNH. Behind the main mass are seen several small stains that represent secondaries.

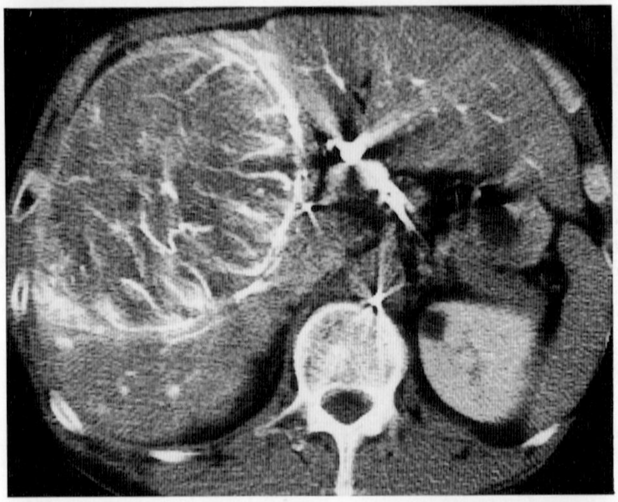

1

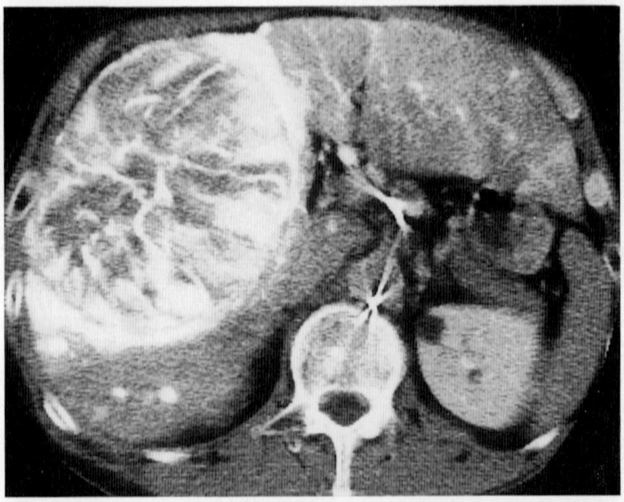

2

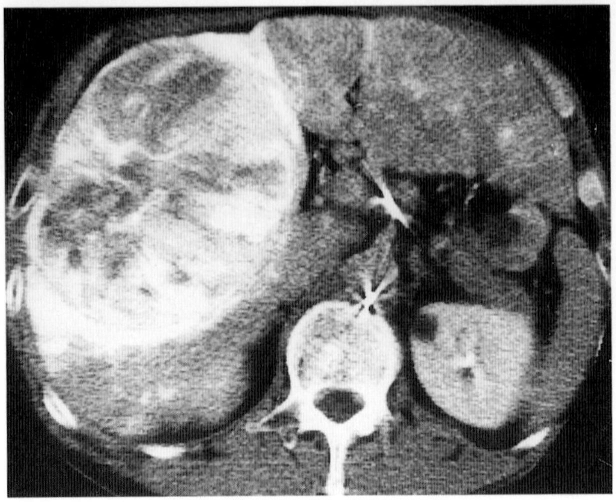

3

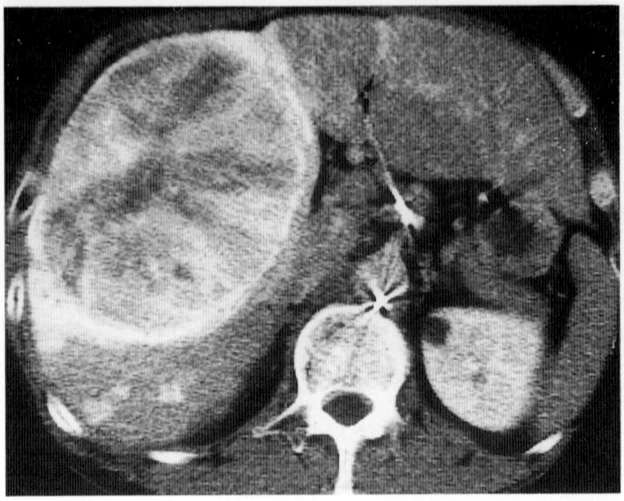

4

Medium- and large-sized HCC—Case 8: Delineation by dynamic CT of a fibrous capsule that surrounds a nodular HCC.

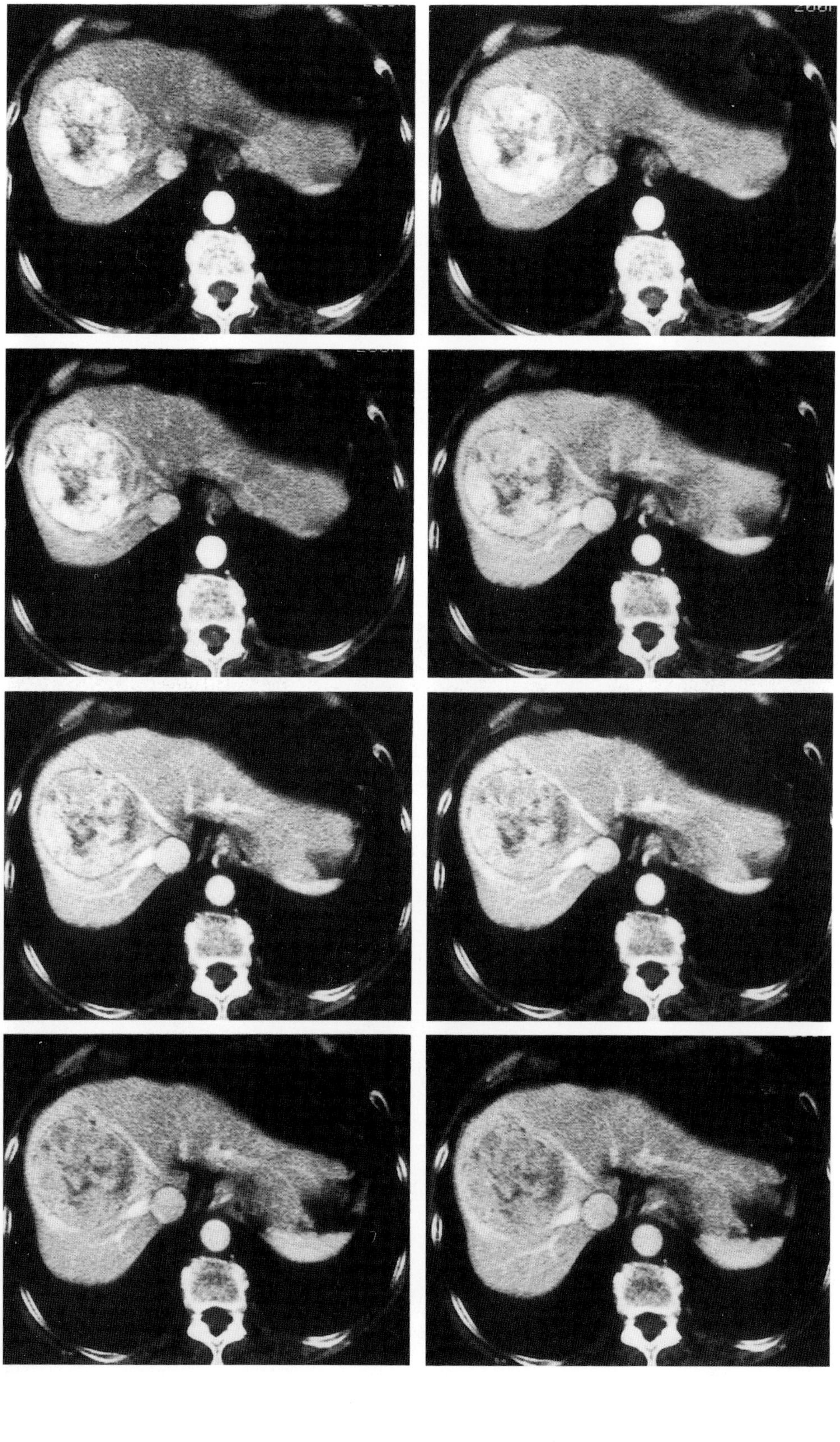

(a) Dynamic CT: changes in CT findings in the cross section of the tumor (imaging started 25 s from contrast injection, 3 ml/s, via the peripheral vein). The density of the capsule changes with time as the density of the mass and of the non-cancerous parenchyma changes. In an early phase (1), the capsule is seen as a thin circular ring of low density which becomes better contrasted as the density of the parenchyma increases (4, 5), and slowly turns to a thicker high-density ring.

1	2
3	4
5	6
7	8

Case 8 (contd.)

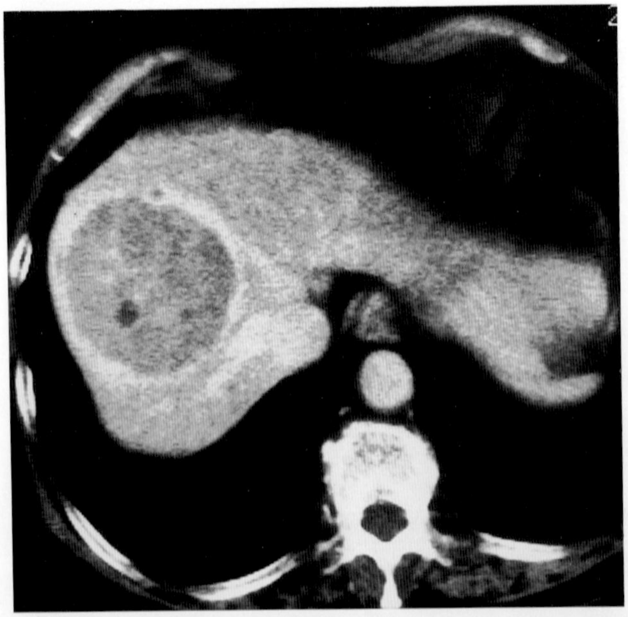

(b) Dynamic CT (late phase, 3 min): the high-density ring becomes more distinct. The thin fibrous capsule is first seen as a low-density ring, and after a lapse of 5 min, the capsule as well as the portion of the parenchyma compressed by the expanding tumor are also stained, to result in increasing the thickness of the stain.

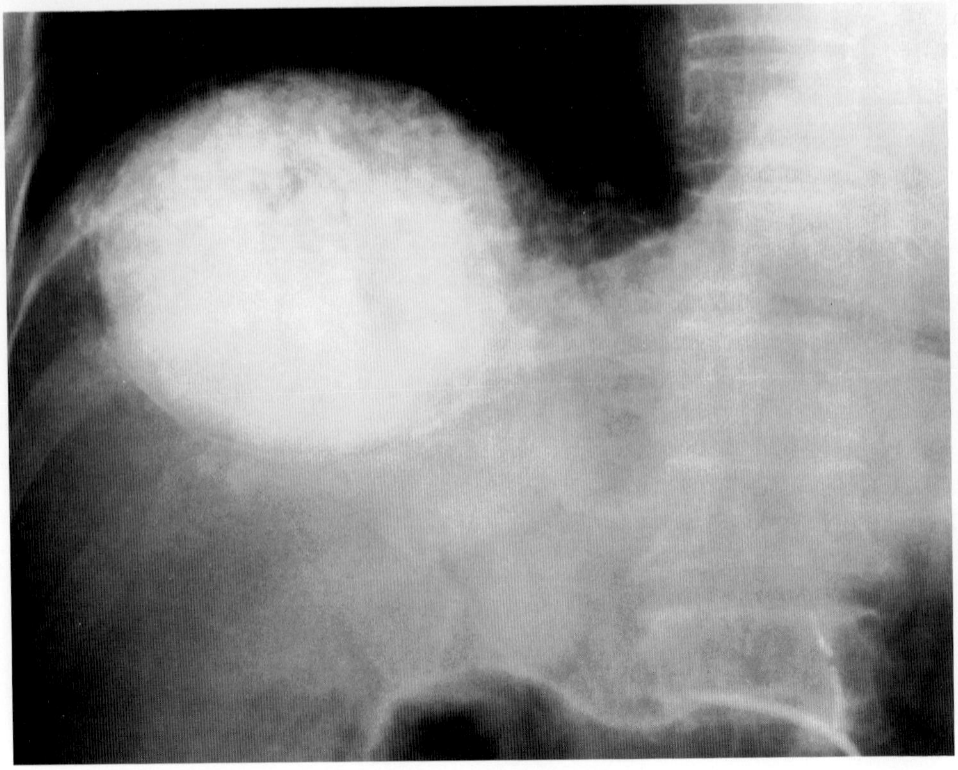

(c) Angiography (late phase, 15 s): a thin translucent ring (seen as a black rim) surrounding the mass and another ring of high density (a white ring) are apparent. This phase of the angiogram may correspond to phases (4) and (5) of dynamic CT.

4.5 Intravascular tumor thrombosis associated with HCC

HCC is known for its frequent vascular invasion, particularly into the portal vein (Okuda *et al.* 1975*b*), hepatic vein (Okuda *et al.* 1977*a*), and henceforth into the inferior vena cava (Okuda 1976*a*), and it less commonly invades the biliary system (Kojiro *et al.* 1982). The frequencies of portal and venous invasion are 62 per cent and 26 per cent in autopsy cases (Liver Cancer Study Group of Japan 1990), and 14 per cent and 5 per cent in resected cases (Liver Cancer Study Group of Japan 1995). Intrabiliary or intraductal invasion is less common. HCC invasion into the portal vein and formation of a tumor thrombus expedite intrahepatic tumor spread, and arterio-portal communications as a result of tumor thrombosis increases portal venous pressure (Fig. 4.5) leading to esophageal varices and encephalopathy.

Classification of tumor thrombosis

Portal tumor thrombosis

Tumor thrombus in the first-order portal branch or portal trunk is readily recognized by US (Subramanyam *et al.* 1984), enhanced CT (Inamoto *et al.* 1981; Mathieu *et al.* 1988), and angiography (Okuda *et al.* 1975*b*) (Case 1). If it is in the first- or second-order portal branch, the area that has lost portal blood supply receives increased arterial blood as a compensation, and a lobar or segmental attenuation difference may be seen on enhanced CT and hepatic arteriography (Matsui *et al.* 1984). Normal liver tissue atrophies in the absence of portal blood flow whereas HCC in the same situation grows faster as it receives increased arterial supply as a compensation; it also expedites growth of portal tumor thrombosis supplied by arteries (Nakashima 1976). If tumor thrombosis extends into the portal trunk, cavenous transformation develops along the pre-existing portal vein to its right through the peribiliary venous plexus (Case 2). It takes only several weeks for cavenous transformation to develop after portal obstruction (Ohnishi *et al.* 1984*b*). With the development of cavenous transformation, the enhanced CT features become complex as a result of communications of intra- and extrahepatic portal veins, and increase in arterial blood flow in compensation for portal obstruction. Color Doppler US is useful in the diagnosis of cavernous transformation (Weltin *et al.* 1985). In some the patients with cavernous transformation, TAE may be feasible despite portal vein occlusion because of sufficient hepatopetal portal blood flow. In patients with tumor thrombosis in the major portal vein, the liver frequently has extensive tumor growth, and identification and size measurement of the primary lesion may be impossible (Case 2).

Angiographic diagnosis of tumor thrombosis is made from the 'thread and streaks' sign (Okuda *et al.* 1975*b*) (Case 3) coined by one of the authors. This feature was first seen during postmortem arteriography and subsequently identified in the actual arteriogram made in patients. On portography, it is seen as a filling defect. Arterial-CT further reveals the detailed internal structure of the tumor thrombus (Case 4). Such large thrombi are supplied by arteries through the portal vein wall (Nakashima 1976), and the blood flows retrogradely toward the hilum (arterio-portal shunt). In the process of tumor thrombus growth, the thrombus receives arterial blood from the main tumor in the early stage, but subsequently from the arteries surrounding the portal vein (periportal artery and vasa vasorum) (Case 5). On enhanced CT, the dilated periportal arteries are seen as lines of heavy stain which look like railway tracks (rail sign) (Mathieu *et al.* 1984), suggesting their role in the sup-

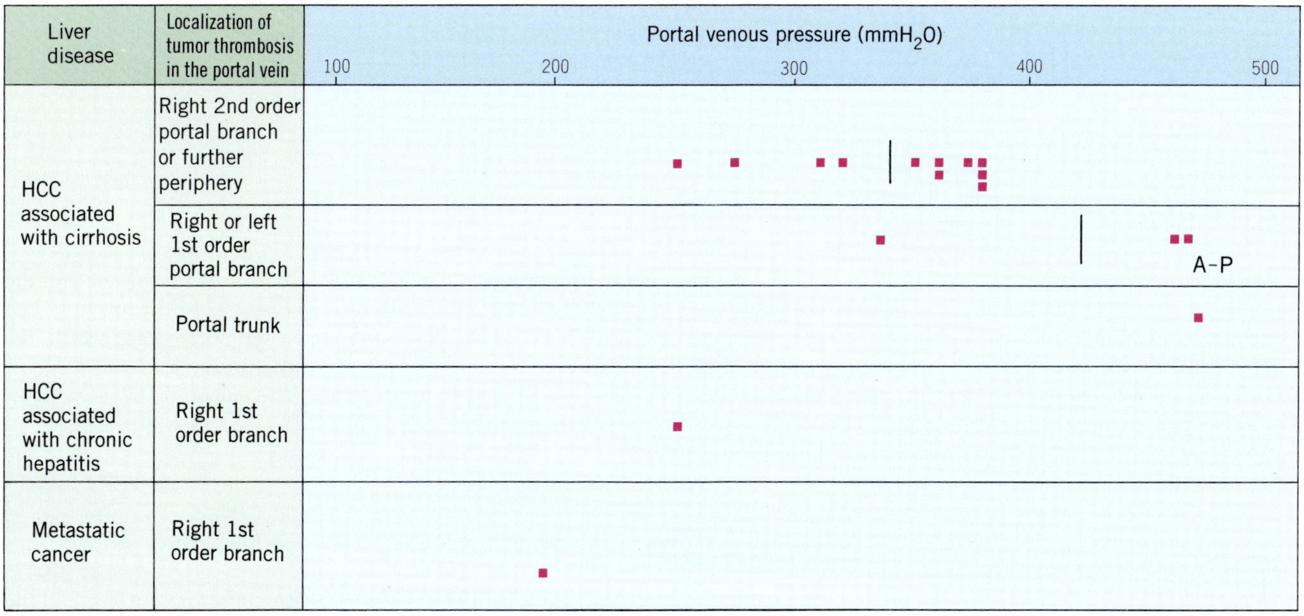

Fig. 4.5 Correlation between portal venous pressure and localization of portal tumor thrombosis in HCC. Portal venous pressure was measured by portal vein catheterization, setting the zero point at 10 cm from the table surface. A-P, portal tumor thrombosis with arterio-portal anastomosis.

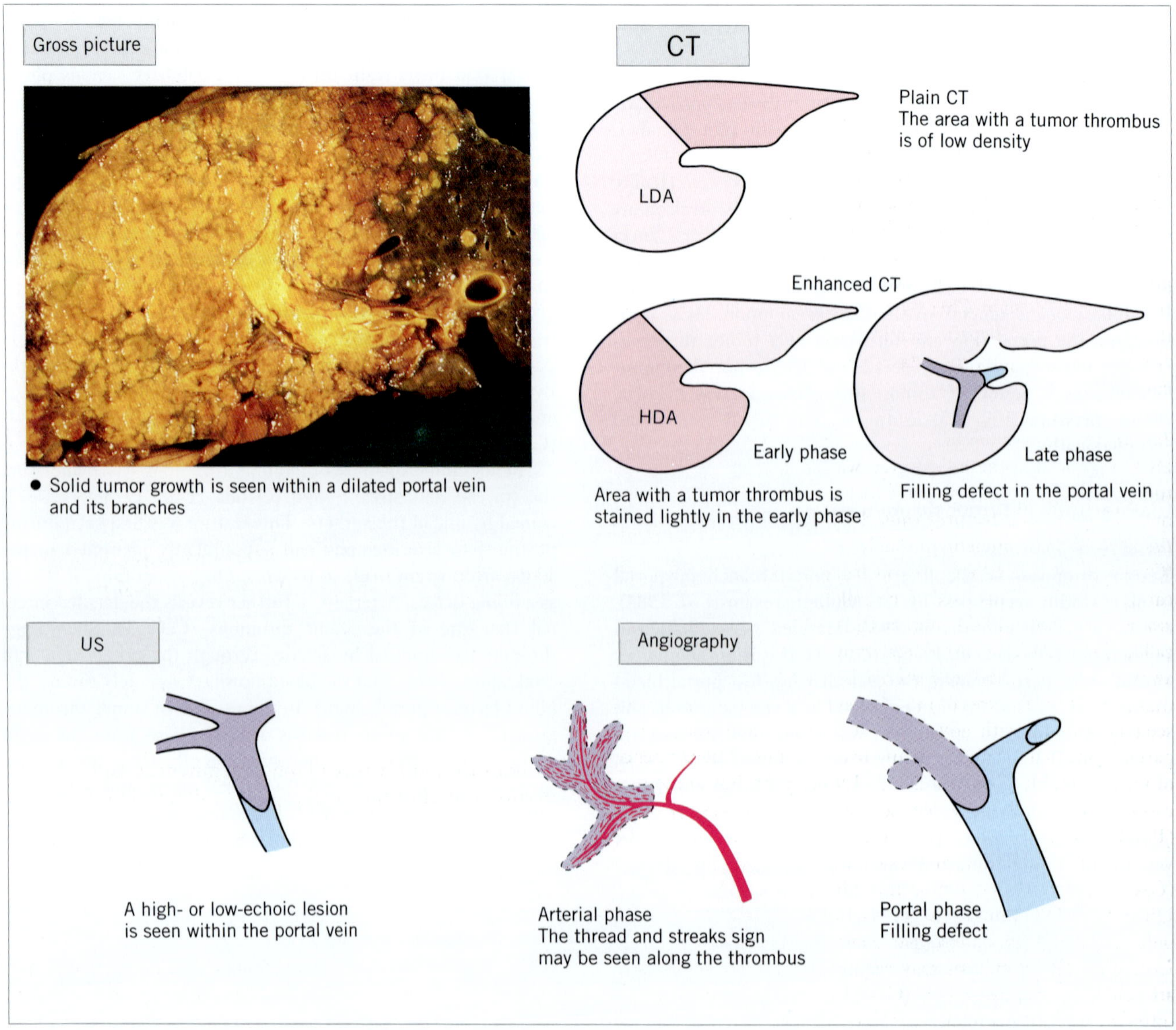

Fig. 4.6 Imaging features of portal tumor thrombosis in HCC.

ply of tumor thrombus (Case 6). Histology of the tumor thrombus varies; it may be a thick firm, tissue lined by a single layer of endothelium, looking like a ballistic missile, or a frail tissue easily crushed resembling 'tofu curd' (necrotic). Nakashima and Kojiro (1987) divided portal tumor thrombi into proliferative, necrotic, mixed proliferative and necrotic, and organized types. The angiographic 'thread and streaks' sign is commonly associated with the solid and proliferative thrombus. The diagnosis of tumor thrombi in the peripheral portal branches is not as easy as a large thrombus (Okuda *et al.* 1977*d*). On portal-CT, a tumor thrombus may produce a fan-shaped low-density area. Some radiologists interpret this as a diagnostic feature of high sensitivity, but similar features may be produced by compression onto a portal vein, and an arterio-portal anastomosis. Careful interpretation is required.

MR imaging may be very diagnostic for portal tumor thrombosis (Ohtomo *et al.* 1985)(Case 7). MR images are not affected by an arterio-portal shunt which they do not delineate, and the identification of the main mass is easier with MR imaging than with CT. Beside these thrombi in the portal vein system, we have seen a tumor thrombus growing within a dilated paraumbilical vein, and in a vein within the omentum adherent to an HCC in the liver surface (Tachimori *et al.* 1988) (Case 8)

Hepatic vein tumor thrombosis

The imaging features of hepatic vein tumor thrombosis are very similar to those of portal tumor thrombosis (Okuda *et al.* 1977*a*; Mathieu *et al.* 1988) (Case 9). If a tumor grows further into the right atrium, sudden heart stoppage may occur as a result of the phenomenon of the tumor ball occluding the heart valves, or the patient may develop dyspnea upon changing the posture.

Transit of broken pieces of the thrombus gives rise to a pulmonary infarct. We have seen at autopsy a large tumor thrombus occluding the pulmonary artery (Okuda 1976). Pulmonary metastases can also be a sequela to transit of HCC cells through the left gastric vein supplying the esophageal varices due to retrograde portal flow (Arakawa *et al.* 1986*b*). Grossly, most venous tumor thrombi are grossly lustrous with a single layer of endothelium (Case 9) growing actively in the vein; occasionally they may look like a bundle of thread or thin noodles (Case 10). If the inferior right hepatic vein is involved, the thrombus grows into the inferior vena cava and occludes its hepatic portion (secondary Budd-Chiari syndrome) (Case 11). In the past, it was thought that hepatic vein invasion almost invariably gives rise to extensive lung metastases, but our experience has not corroborated such a notion.

Intraductal tumor thrombosis

HCC may invade the biliary tree within the liver and form a tumor thrombus, or may cause bleeding into the biliary tract producing imaging features caused by a blood clot or necrotic tissue fragments indistinguishable from a tumor thrombus (Okuda 1976*a*). In either case, obstructive jaundice is the clinical presentation. This used to be called an icteric type of hepatoma (Lin *et al.* 1975), but nowadays it is more commonly called 'HCC with an intraductal growth'. The icterus may go away when the occluding material is expelled into the duodenum, one of the features of intraductal HCC growth, but icterus seen in patients with advanced HCC may simply be due to parenchymal icterus due to failing liver function. The incidence of intraductal HCC growth is 0.7–1.9 per cent, but in autopsy cases it accounted for 9 per cent according to Kojiro *et al.* (1982). Most such cases have advanced HCC having portal and venous tumor invasion, and exact diagnosis may be difficult (Case 12). Intraductal tumor thrombosis may be detected by US and CT (Nakamura *et al.* 1984), but a definitive diagnosis is only possible with endoscopic cholangiography; peripherally located ductal thrombosis may require percutaneous transhepatic cholangiography (PTC) (Case 13). HCC associated with intraductal growth is often hypovascular in our experience, and dilated bile ducts may be recognized near the tumor thrombus calling for differential diagnosis from intrahepatic bile duct carcinoma (Case 14). In such situation, intraductal thrombosis as well as portal tumor thrombosis have to be identified in a direct way.

An intraductal tumor thrombus is generally seen as a hypovascular lesion, but it could occasionally be hypervascular (Case 15); TAE may prove effective as treatment. If early diagnosis of intraductal growth becomes possible, more hepatic resections may be carried out

Others

Portal and intraductal tumor thrombosis can occur in other malignacies, such as metastatic liver cancer. The direction of growth is from the periphery toward the hepatic hilum, as in HCC. Carcinoma arising in the stomach and pancreas sometimes, but rarely, grows into the portal vein in continuity from the primary lesion (Takayasu *et al.* 1989*g*; Araki *et al.* 1990) (Case 16).

Differentiation of portal tumor thrombosis and blood clot

Both a tumor thrombus and a blood clot in the portal vein are seen as an abnormal structure within the lumen (direct finding) on US and CT, and on portography it is seen as a filling defect (indirect finding). Tumor thrombosis is usually associated with (1) signs secondary to enlarged and increased arteries such as thread and streaks on angiography (Okuda *et al.* 1975*a*) and the rail sign on dynamic CT (Mathieu *et al.* 1984), (2) continuity with the primary mass or arterio-portal shunts; (3) dilatation of the portal vein as the mass grows longitudinally as well as sideways seen by CT and US (Cases 1, 5, and 6), and (4) a filling defect looking like a bird's beak (Case 3). By contrast, a blood clot does not expand the diameter of the vein, and no new vasculature develops to supply it; only the venous wall is enhanced (Case 17). Occasionally, however, a portal blood clot may grow sideways (Case 2, p.394; Case 6, p.365) making differential diangosis difficult. Arterial-CT is required in such cases for determining whether or not feeding arteries are present. Doppler US is most useful in differential diagnosis of blood clot and tumor thrombus (Wang *et al.* 1991) and with color Doppler US it has become even easier (Tanaka *et al.* 1990). When an old clot acquires a new one on its tip, the new one may be seen as a high-density mass (Mori *et al.* 1987). In the presence of incomplete occlusion whether due to a clot or tumor, post-stenotic dilatation may ensue as a result of turbulent blood flow (Case 1).

Diagnostic significance of lobar, segmental, and perihilar attenuation differences on dynamic CT

On dynamic CT, one occasionally sees attenuation differences between major lobes, segments, and between the hilum and peripheral areas. Their common causes are:

(1) Portal obstruction as a result of tumor (HCC) thrombosis (Itai *et al.* 1982) (Cases 2, 6) and portal infiltration of bile duct carcinoma (Takayasu *et al.* 1986*c*) (Case 18). More recently, attenuation differences may be produced as a result of portal embolization carried out prior to an operation. The area not receiving portal vein blood is seen in low density on plain CT, and often becomes high density in the early phase of enhancement. It is due to increased arterial supply as a compensatory effort of the liver to maintain a constant blood supply. In a late phase, this phenomenon is no longer recognized as the whole liver becomes of the same density. In the presence of cavernous transformation, the CT findings become more complex depending on the degree of its development (Mathieu *et al.* 1988). If cavernous transformation has developed compensating for the lack of portal blood flow, arterial flow may not increase to such an extent as to show early high density. However, if cavernous transformation has not grown into the depth of the liver toward the periphery and is supplying only the parenchyma in the hilum, attenuation differences are seen between the hilar area and the periphery of the liver (Takayasu *et al.* 1989*b*) (perihilar attenuation difference) (Case 19).

(2) Another cause is arterio-portal shunt that develops in HCC and cirrhosis (Case 20). In such cases, attenuation differ-

ences are seen not on plain CT, but only in the early phase of dynamic CT. It can thus be differentiated from attenuation differences due to portal obstruction. Doppler US may be useful in the diagnosis.

(3) Partial obstruction of hepatic veins, namely one or two major hepatic veins partially occluded (partial Budd-Chiari syndrome), may also cause attenuation differences. HCC is the most common cause (Case 21), but it can also follow bone-marrow transplantation and veno-occlusive disease (VOD) due to drinking bush tea.

Arterio-portal communication associated with HCC

Arterio-portal shunts are seen on angiography in benign disease such as cirrhosis (Case 4, p.363) and hemangioma (Case 16, p.70), but much more often in HCC (Cases 22 and 23). It is an important finding for quality diagnosis. It occurs in more than 60 per cent in advanced HCC (Okuda *et al.* 1977*d*), but in less than 10 per cent in HCC smaller than 5 cm (Takayasu *et al.* 1986*e*). Arterio-portal shunts may be indirectly diagnosed when the portal vein system is opacified in an early phase of dynamic CT (Nakayama *et al.* 1983) (Cases 22 and 23). There are several patterns of arterio-portal shunts. It may vary from a large shunt in which portal vein flows retrogradely toward the hilum on arteriography (Case 22) to a small shunt in which real periphery of the portal branch is opacified through a tumor thrombus (Okuda *et al.* 1977*d*). Arterio-portal shunts are closely associated with intraportal tumor thrombosis, and the periportal artery (vasa vasorum) (Bookstein *et al.* 1982). In some, the arteries that have entered the tumor thrombus transverse longitudinally through it and enter the portal vein lumen (Okuda *et al.* 1975*b*). In others, tumor growth has destroyed the thrombus feeding arteries, and arterial blood freely flows into the portal vein lumen (Nakashima and Kojiro 1987). Usually, as the tumor grows larger the shunts become more extensive, but an HCC as small as 1.5 cm could cause a marked shunt sending contrast medium into a large portal branch in the hilum (Case 22). Sometimes, too much contrast medium regurgitating into the portal vein obscures the location of the main mass or the portal tumor growth. If TAE is carried out in such a patient, the arterio-portal flow ceases making the diagnosis of thrombus location possible (Case 23). Arterio-portal shunts increase the complications of portal tumor thrombosis and intrahepatic spread, aggravate portal hypertension, and increase the chances of variceal bleeding, making the prognosis much worse.

Speed of intraportal tumor growth and prognosis

It is important to know the speed of growth of a tumor thrombus within the portal vein for the selection of treatment modality and prediction of prognosis. It is now possible to identify the tip of the tumor thrombus by a combination of various imaging modalities, follow it, and determine the growth speed. We made such measurements, and calculated the number of days the growth required to move from one branch to a branch larger by one order. As shown in Table 4.8, it took on average 60–80 days. In this table, the tip of the thrombus seen at the major bifurcation (the right and left main portal veins) (1) progressed to the portal trunk in 80.9 ± 78.8 days (n = 16). In (6), there was no tumor thrombus in the second-order branch, but in 160 ± 84.9 days, a tumor thrombus was recognized in the portal trunk. Thus, the speed of growth varies considerably. In one surgical case, it took only 20 days for a tumor thrombus in the second-order branch to reach the first-order branch. In another, a tumor thrombus was recognized in the splenic vein, but there was no progression, and the patient lived 1.5 years (Case 25).

It has been our impression that the tumor thrombus grows faster in patients with good liver function tests compared to those with poor ones. The tumor thrombus does not seem to grow directly or immediately toward the portal trunk from the periphery. Rather it does so after having invaded several more peripheral branches (Case 26). Our analysis of the location of thrombus and prognosis based on non-surgical cases suggests that those with a growth in the first-order branch and the trunk had a poorer prognosis than those who had a growth in the second-order branch. The former had more frequent GI (variceal) bleeding and hepatic failure (Table 4.9). Further analysis may be required.

Table 4.8 Speed of growth of portal tumor thrombus in HCC

(1) Bifurcation → trunk (n = 16)	80.9 ± 78.8 (days)
(2) Trunk → splenic or superior mesenteric vein (n = 5)	71.4 ± 69.6
(3) First order → bifurcation (n = 7)	68.9 ± 33.6
(4) Second order → first order (n = 3)	70.0 ± 26.5
(5) Second order → bifurcation (n = 1)	60
(6) No tumor in second order → bifurcation (n = 2)	160 ± 84.9

Bifurcation = at the junction of the right and left first-order branches; a thrombus is protruding at the junction from one major branch but the other major branch is patent. Parentheses show the number of patients studied. For the numbering of the order of branches see Chapter 1 (Fig. 1.55, p. 00).

Table 4.9 Length of survival from detection of portal tumor thrombosis (n = 26)

Site of tumor thrombus	Survival period (months)
1. Portal trunk (n = 19) (including the splenic or superior mesenteric vein)	4.7 ± 5.4
2. First-order branch (n = 5) (including major bifurcation)	5.7 ± 3.8
3. Second-order branch (n = 2)	11.8 ± 11.7

Parentheses show number of patients studied.

Table 4.10 Causes of death in HCC patients with portal tumor thrombosis

1. Rupture of varices	8 (3)[a]
2. Hepatic failure	8
3. Intraabdominal bleeding	2
4. Respiratory failure	2
5. Cancer death	1
6. Unclear	4

[a] Includes GI bleeding.

Intravascular tumor thrombosis—Case 1: Growth of HCC tumor thrombus could be followed from the primary lesion in the left lateral region up to the hepatic hilum.

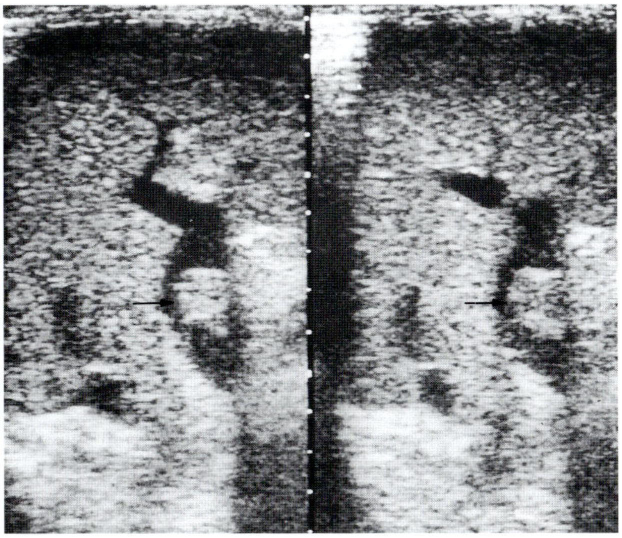

(a) US (right intercostal scan): the first-order branch of the right portal vein is dilated and a cylindrical hyperechoic tumor thrombus is seen growing within it.

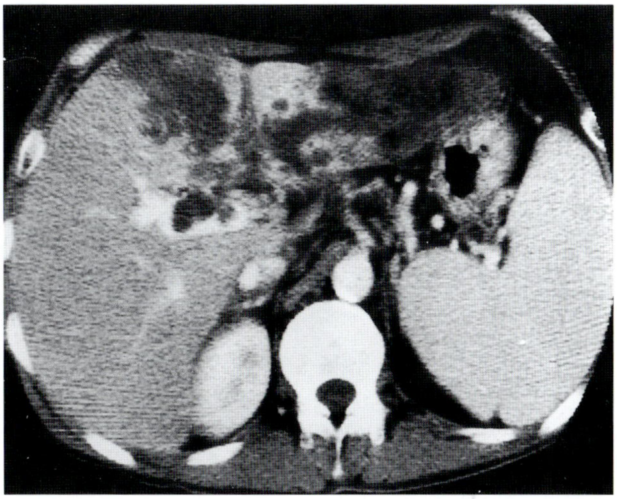

(b) Dynamic CT: in the CT image at the hilar level, a filling defect is seen in the right first-order branch. Another tumor thrombus is seen continuous from the main mass in S^{III} through the left portal vein, P^{III}. The low-density lesion in S^{IV} is metastases continuous from the tumor thrombus.

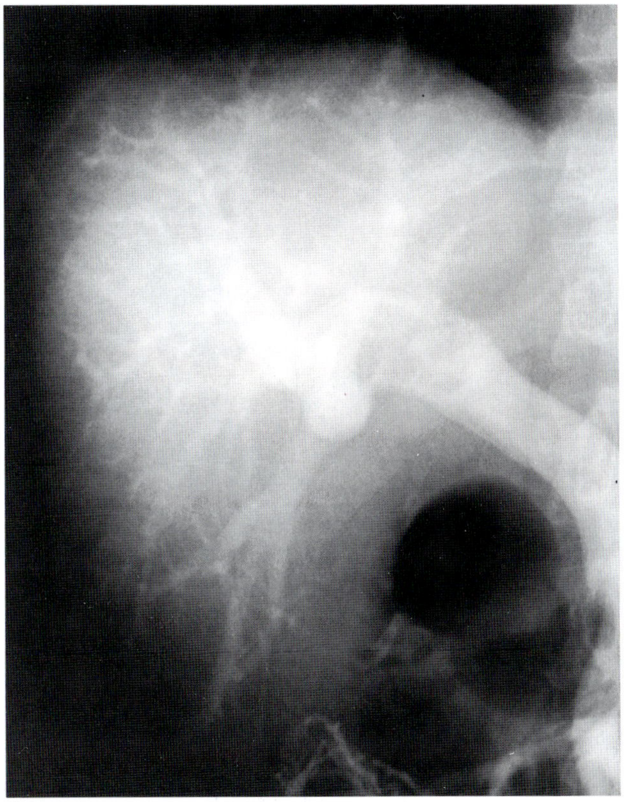

(c) Superior mesenteric arteriographic portogram: the left portal vein is not opacified from its origin. The right first-order branch is dilated (post-stenotic dilatation), and a filling defect in its central part is obvious.

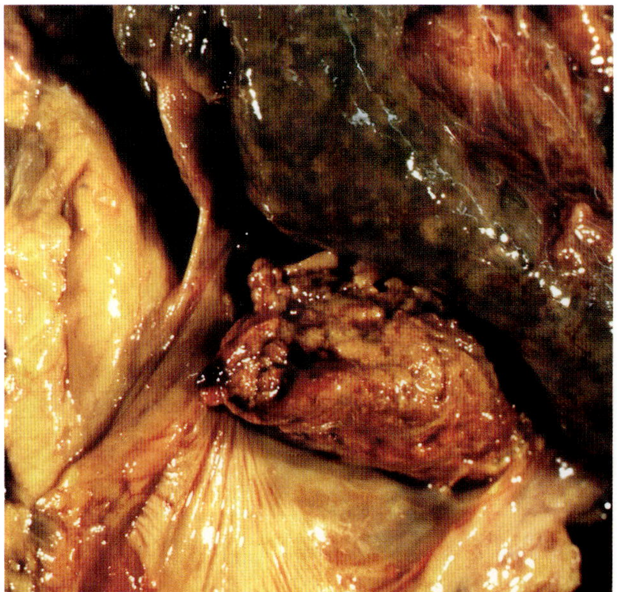

(d) Autopsy findings: a growing tumor thrombus was seen in the portal trunk. The tip of the thrombus was soft and frail.

Intravascular tumor thrombosis—Case 4: The internal structure of a tumor thrombus delineated as thread and streaks by arterial-CT.

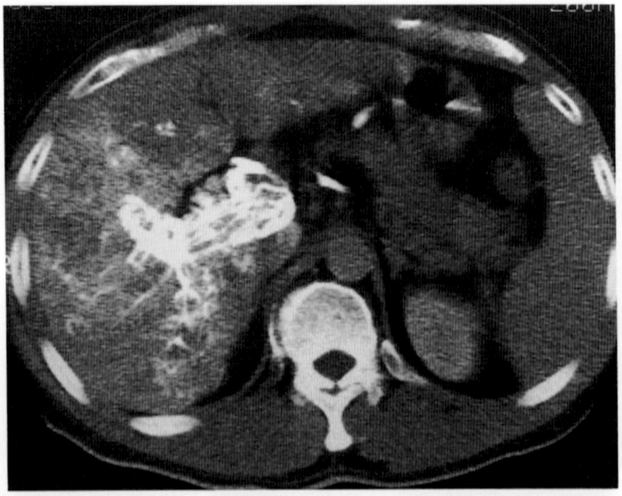

Arterial-CT: arterial-CT carried out at the level of the hilum in a patient with a tumor thrombus revealed numerous feeding arteries in a bundle (thread and streaks sign) within the tumor thrombus (same as Case 2, p. 162).

Intravascular tumor thrombosis—Case 5: Participation of the periportal artery in the feeding of portal tumor thrombi

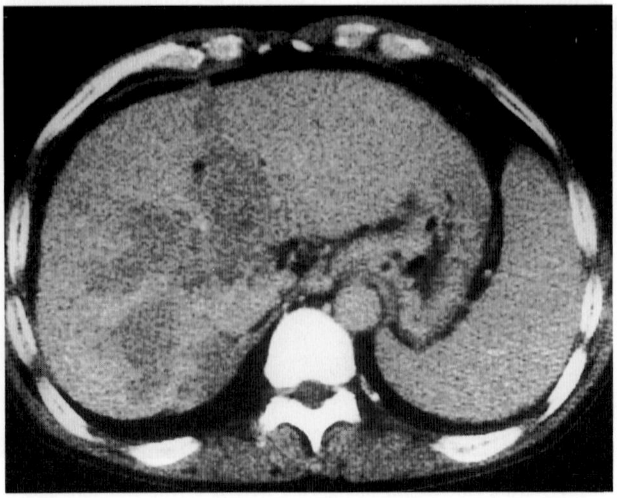

(a) Enhanced CT (late phase): thick portal thrombi of low density are seen in both lobes.

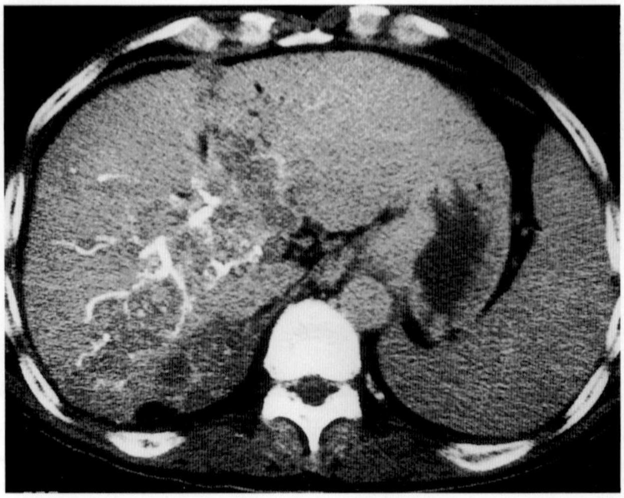

(b) Arterial-CT: enlarged extensive periportal arteries are seen surrounding the tumor thrombi. Some feeding arteries are seen within tumor thrombi whereas arteriography did not demonstrate the thread and streaks sign.

Intravascular tumor thrombosis—Case 6: Dynamic CT of the periportal arteries seen as a 'railway track' along the tumor thrombi.

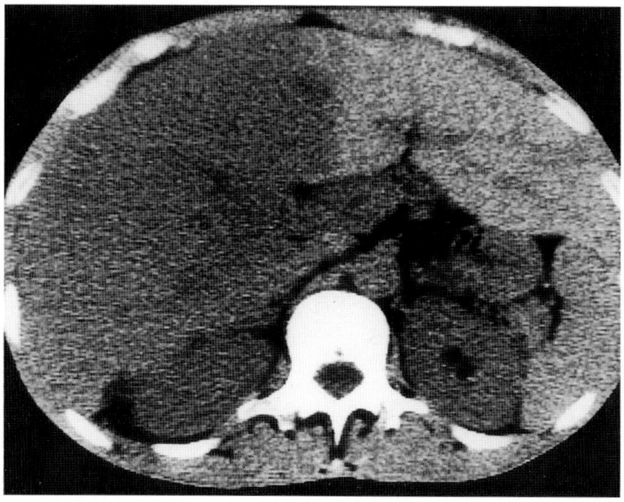

(a) Plain CT: lobar attenuation difference is apparent as a result of portal tumor thrombosis.

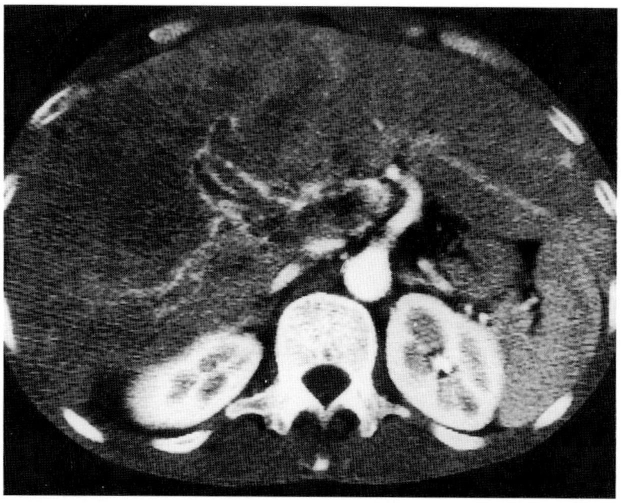

(b) Dynamic CT (early phase): a pair of feeding arteries are seen along tumor thrombi in the right lobe. They may be compared to a railway track (rail sign). It is assumed that these arteries derive from the periportal arteries as seen in Case 5.

Intravascular tumor thrombosis—Case 7: Delineation of portal tumor thrombosis by MR imaging.

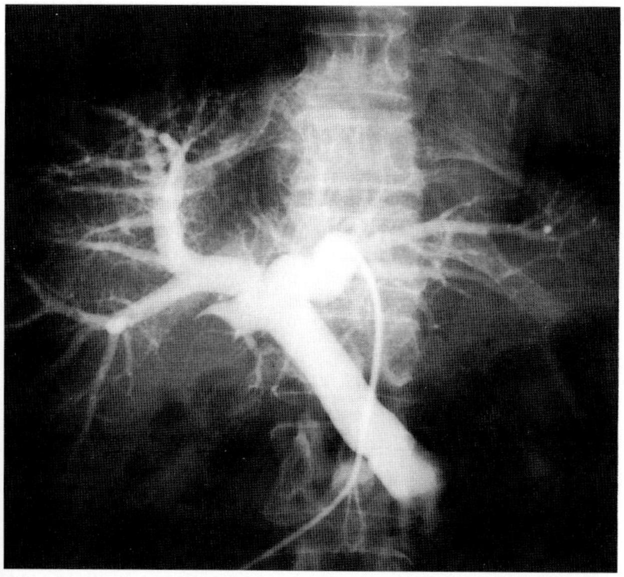

(a) Percutaneous transhepatic portogram: a filling defect looking like a crab's claw is obvious in the right posterior portal branch (P-point), suggesting the presence of tumor thrombi peripheral to this point.

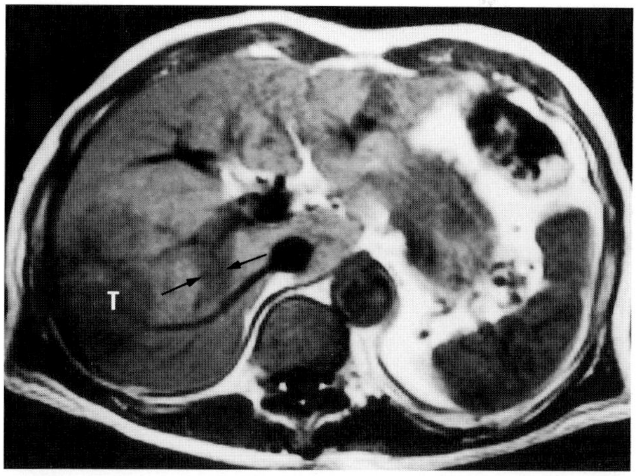

(b) MR imaging (T1-weighted image): in this T1-weighted image, made at the level of the hilum, a thick vascular structure of low intensity (→) is seen. Since an accompanying artery is recognized, this may be diagnosed as a portal tumor thrombus. T, HCC.

Intravascular tumor thrombosis—Case 8: Recurrent HCC showing tumor thrombosis in the omental vein.

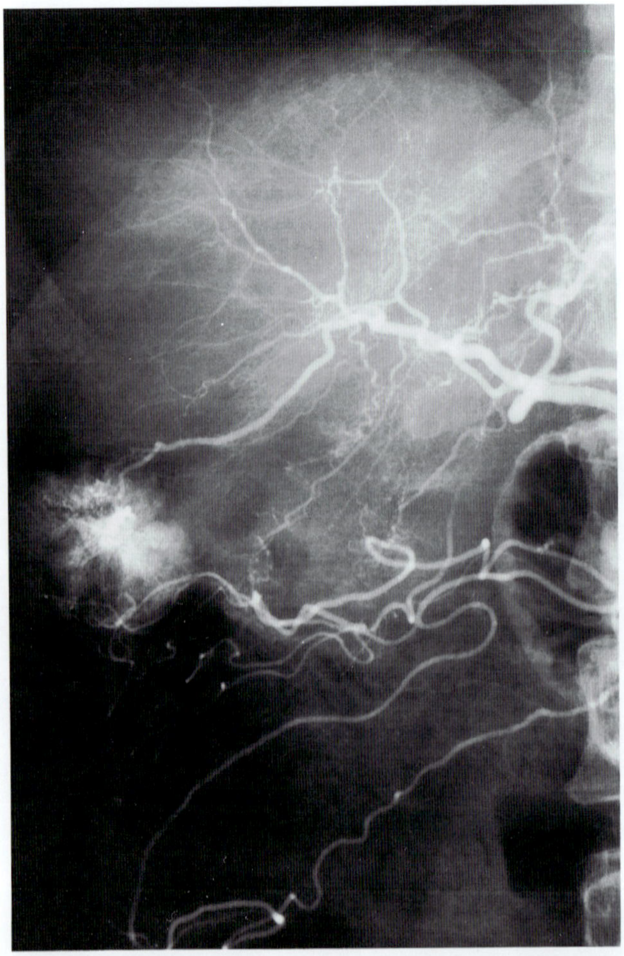

(a) Hepatic arteriography (early phase): a recurrent lesion within the remnant liver supplied by the hepatic artery and a branch of the omental artery are recognized.

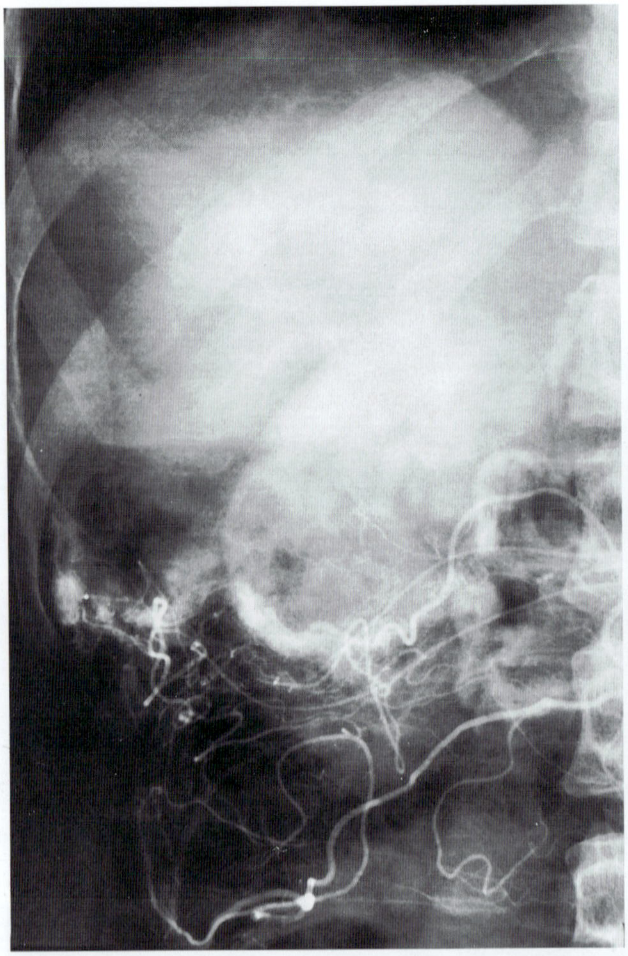

(b) Hepatic arteriography (late phase): a cord-like vessel is opacified along the omental vein.

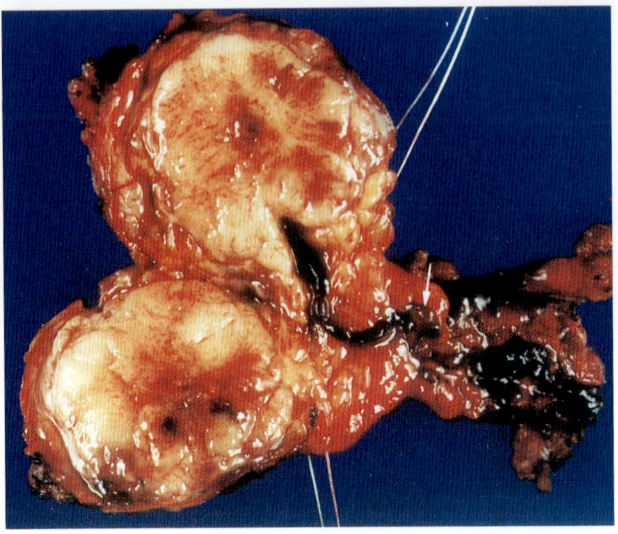

(c) Section of resected specimen: on surgical removal, the recurrent tumor was adherent to the omentum, and in its section, a tumor thrombus (→) was seen growing from the mass toward the omental vein.

Intravascular tumor thrombosis—Case 9: HCC thrombus in the middle and left hepatic veins.

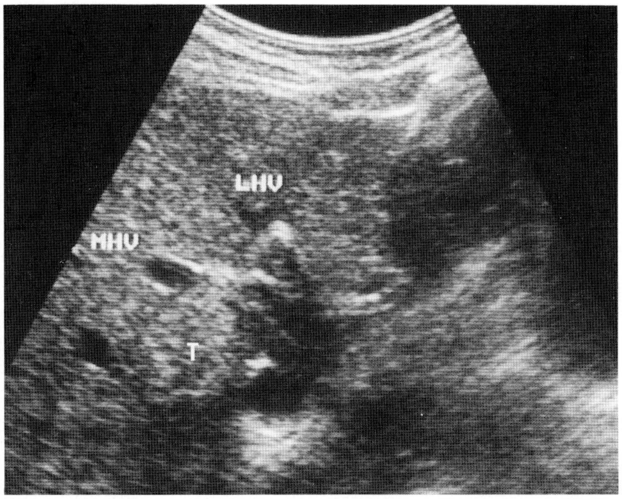

(a) US (transverse scan): at the level slightly cranial from the hilum, a main tumor (T) (in S^{VIII}–S^{I}) and tumor thrombi continuous from it are seen within the middle hepatic (MHV) and left hepatic (LHV) veins as high-echo materials.

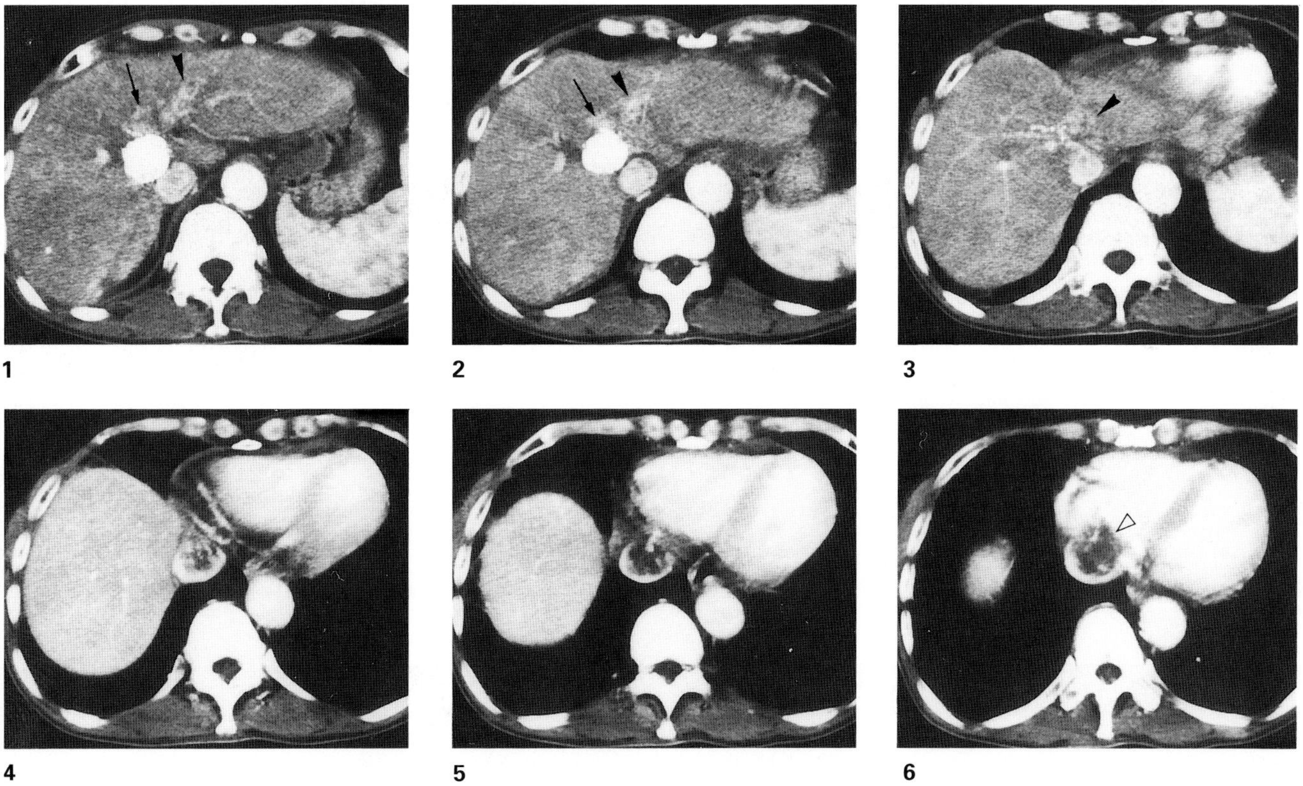

(b) Dynamic CT (shifting the cutting section from the hilum toward the diaphragm: (1–6): incremental CT sectioning. The main mass shows Lipiodol retention. The thread and streaks sign has appeared from the early phase of dynamic CT in the middle (→) and left (▶) hepatic veins. The tip of the tumor thrombus has reached the right atrium (▷) through the inferior vena cava.

Case 9 (contd.)

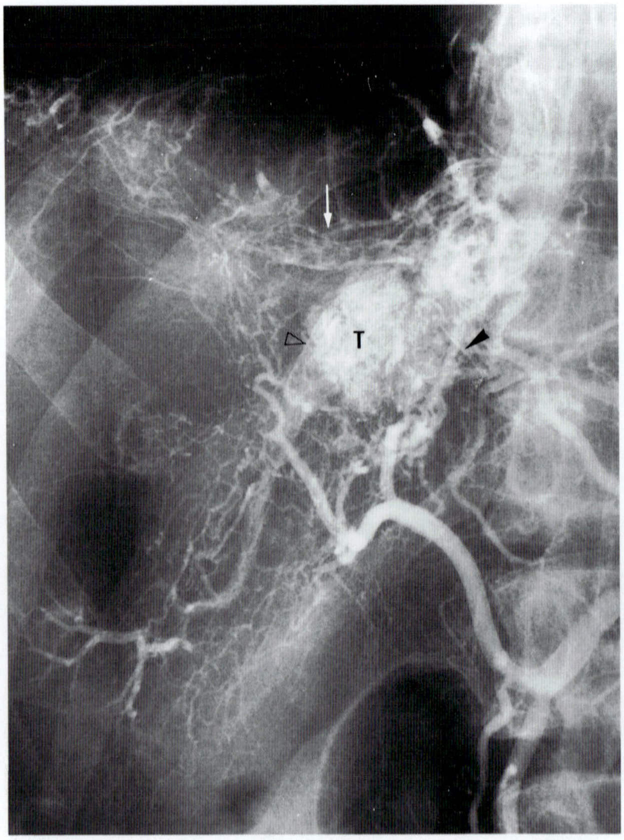

(c) Hepatic arteriography: tumor thrombi (the thread and streaks signs) are seen around the main tumor (T); one in the middle hepatic vein (▷) and another in the left heptic vein (▶) are extending into the right atrium. Another thrombus is seen in a branch of the middle hepatic (→). A small arterio-portal communication is also seen in the periphery of the S^{IV} region.

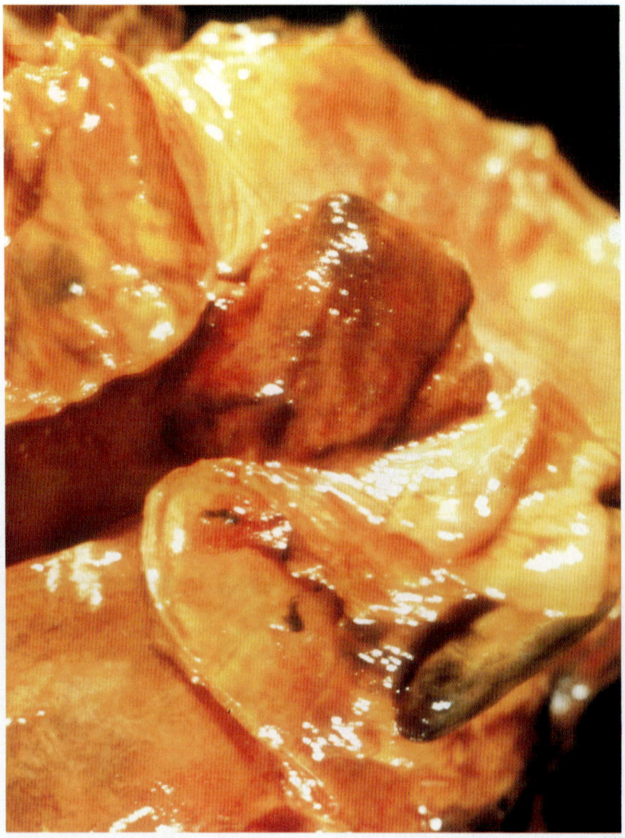

(d) Autopsy finding: a tumor thrombus is protruding into the right atrium through the hepatic vein and inferior vena cava. The surface of the thrombus is lined by a single layer of endothelium and is grossly smooth (different from Case 9).

Intravascular tumor thrombosis—Case 10: Hepatic vein tumor thrombus that has turned into a thread-like material following TAE.

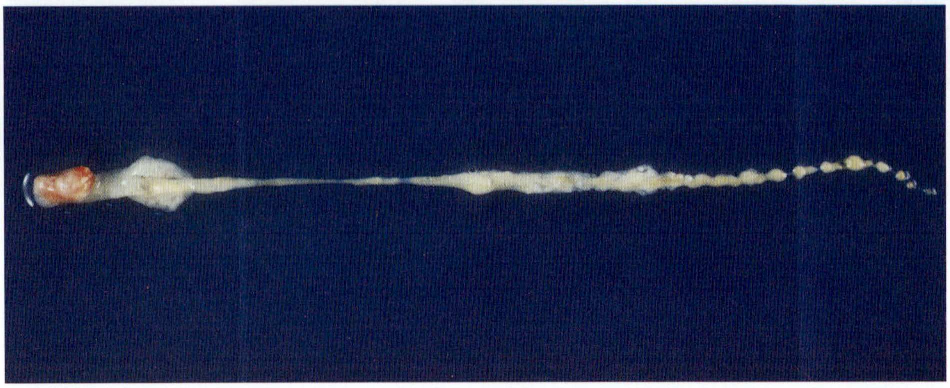

Gross picture on resection: intra-operative US revealed a hyperechoic cord-like material in the hepatic vein. Upon removal from the resected liver, it was found to be a whitish tumor thrombus; the red area is the origin of the thrombus which was histologically thin trabecular HCC of Edmondson's grade II. The whitish side of the thrombus was covered by a layer of endothelium and did not contain cancer cells.

Intravascular tumor thrombosis—Case 11: Tumor thrombus growing in the inferior right hepatic vein.

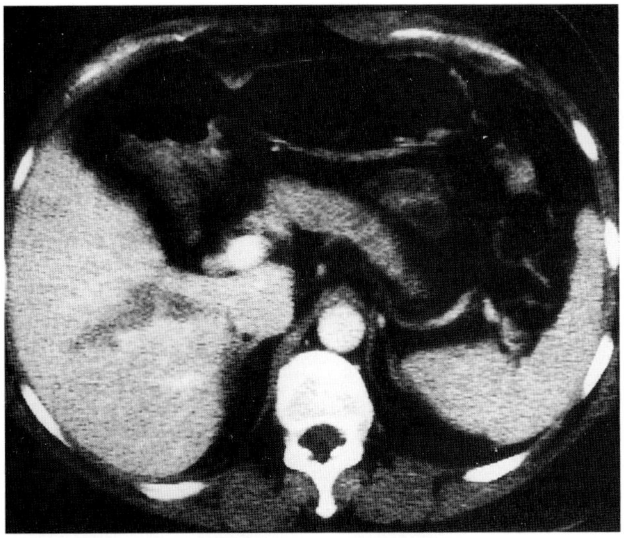

(a) Dynamic CT: a tubular structure of low density is seen in the right lobe inferiorly.

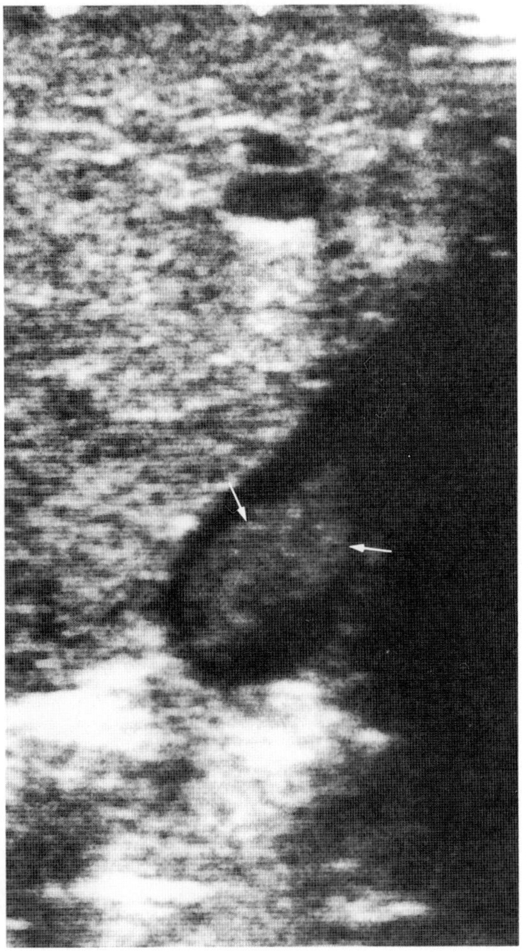

(b) Intraoperative US: a tumor thrombus is seen growing from the inferior right hepatic vein into the inferior vena cava.

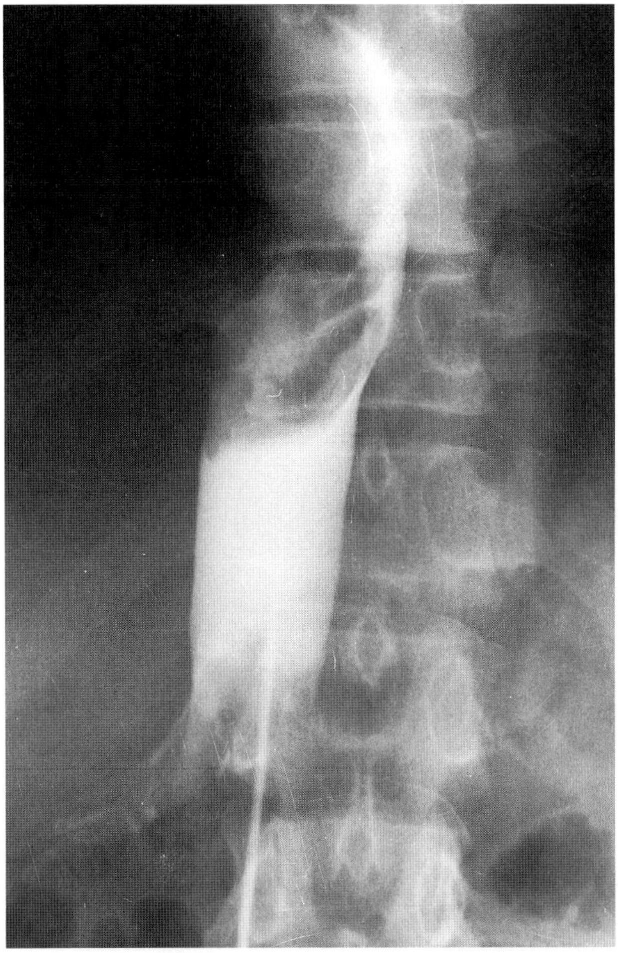

(c) Inferior cavography: subsequent inferior vena cavography demonstrated that the tumor thrombus growing from the inferior right hepatic vein had further grown cranially in the vena cava.

Intravascular tumor thrombosis—Case 12: HCC associated with three types of tumor thrombosis, intraductal, intraportal, and intravenous growths.

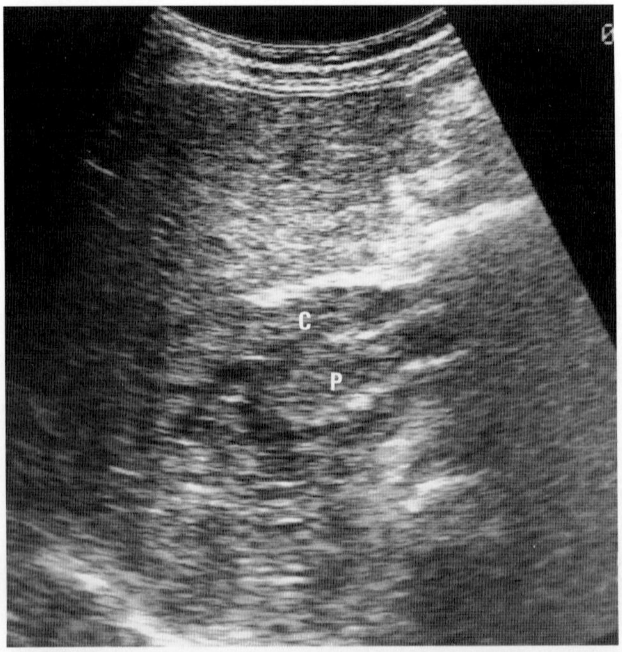

(a) US (sagittal scan at the hilum): an isoechoic tumor thrombus is seen within a dilated common bile duct (C). A dilated portal trunk (P) behind it also contains a tumor thrombus.

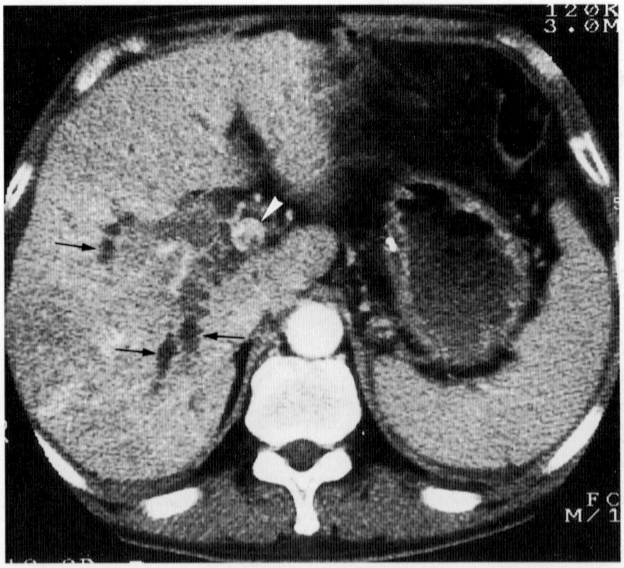

(b) Dynamic CT: the portal vein is opacified minimally (two dots of low density representing the growing tip of the tumor thrombus), but the right anterior and posterior branches are not opacified because of tumor thrombosis. In the periphery, however, there are some dilated vessels or ducts (→) which are assumed to be ducts because they are continuous with the vascular structure containing a low-density material. However, with just one film, differentiation from accompanying portal thrombosis is not feasible. In general, the portal system runs medial to the duct system (cf. Fig. 1.44, p.28).

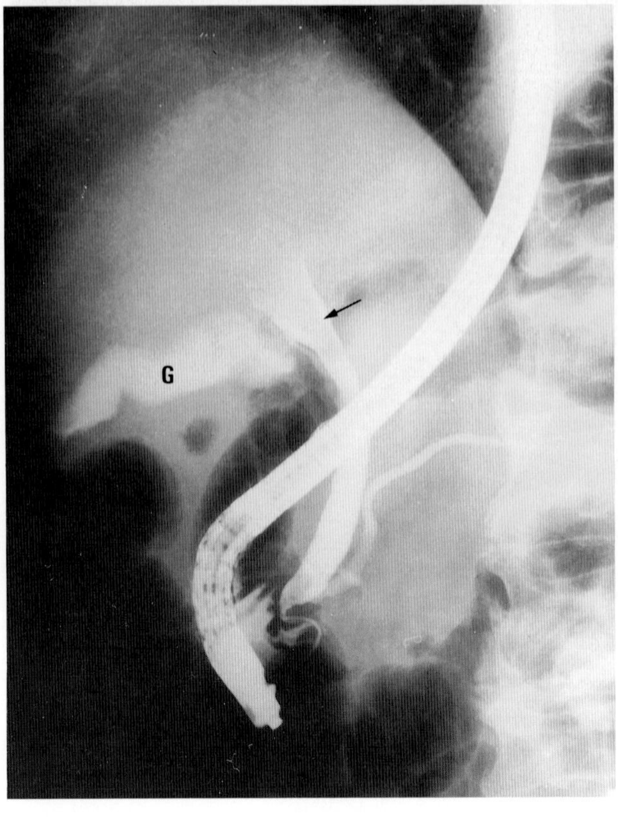

(c) ERC: the common bile duct contains a filling defect with a narrowed tip (→) and the surrounding wall is dilated but smooth. G, gallbladder.

Intravascular tumor thrombosis—Case 13: Ductal tumor thrombus that required differential diagnosis from portal thrombus.

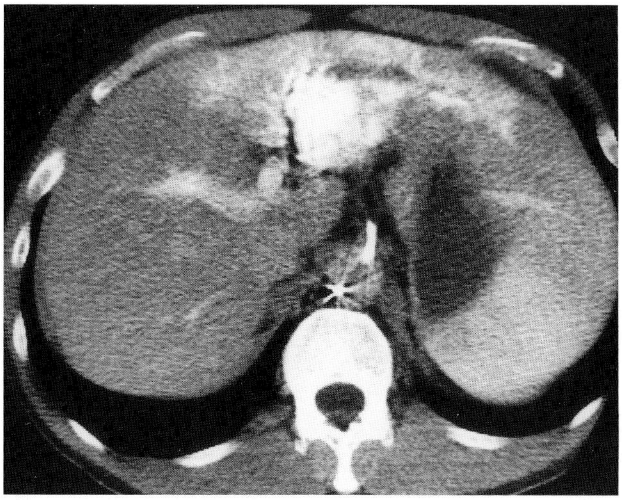

(a) Arterial-CT: conventional enhanced CT demonstrated a 3 cm mass and dilatation of the vessels in the left lobe, and arterial-CT was carried out. In its early phase, a clearly stained main mass in S^{III} and a dilated vessel anterior to it were seen, but there was no thread and streaks sign or rail sign. While the right portal vein was opacified, the left portal vein was not, and there was some density difference between the ventral area ($S^{III}+S^{IV}$) and the other area (S^{II} and right lobe). Therefore, tumor thrombosis in P^{III} and P^{IV} was suspected.

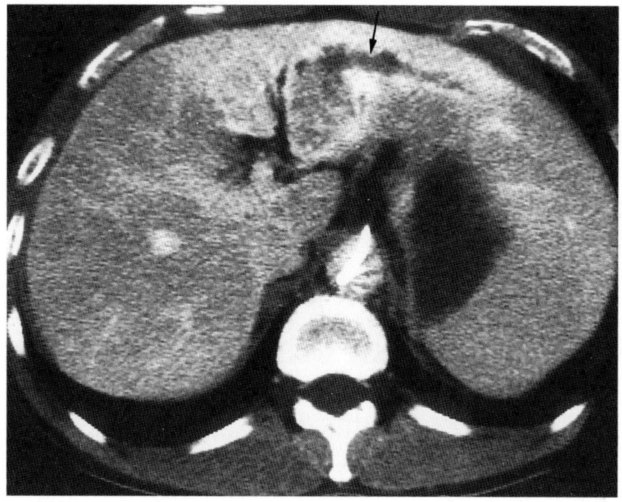

(b) Arterial-CT (late phase): the main mass has become low density and a dilated vessel (→) is seen as its continuation.

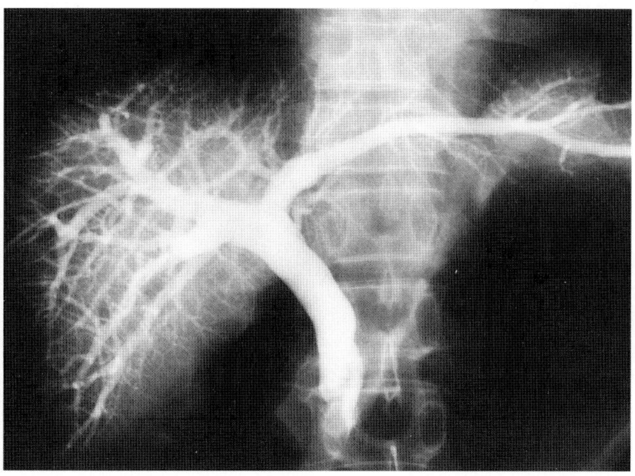

(c) Percutaneous transhepatic portogram: to determine whether tumor thrombosis was intraportal or intraductal, portography was carried out. Portography failed to demonstrate the left lateral inferior branch (P^{III}) in the left lobe. There still was a possibility of ductal thrombosis.

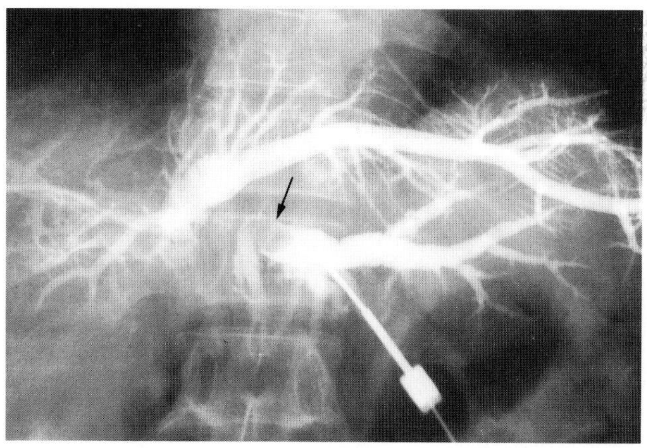

(d) PTC: direct puncture cholangiography was carried out in the left lateral inferior bile duct (B^{III}). It was dilated with a filling defect (→) suggesting bile duct tumor thrombus. Subsegment selective left portal venography demonstrated only P^{II}. Tumor thrombosis both in the portal vein (P^{III} and P^{IV}) and bile duct was the most likely diagnosis.

Intravascular tumor thrombosis—Case 14: HCC with intraductal and portal tumor thrombosis that required differential diagnosis with peripheral bile duct carcinoma.

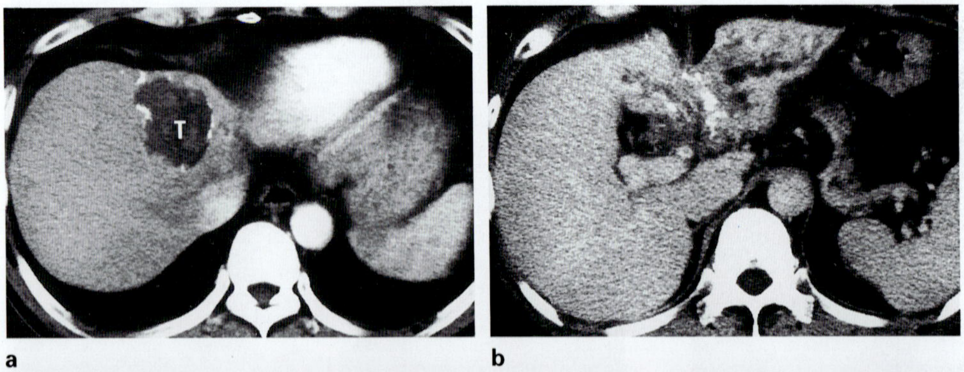

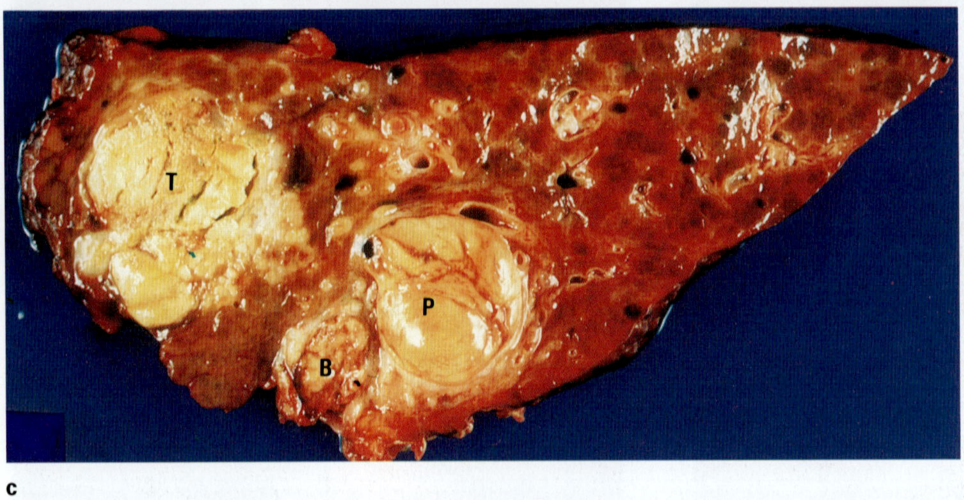

(a) Dynamic CT (early phase): Lipiodol CT was already done at a previous hospital, and minimal Lipiodol retention is seen around the tumor. The main tumor was not stained by dynamic CT.

(b) Enhanced CT (late phase): dilatation of the left lateral bile duct and Lipiodol retention in a tumor thrombus are recognized—from Lipiodol retention vertical to the anterior plain the tumor thrombus was thought to be in the umbilical portion of the portal vein.

(c) Section of resected specimen: 90 per cent of the main mass was necrotic. A tumor thrombus was seen in a markedly dilated portal vein (P) and in a bile duct (B).

Intravascular tumor thrombosis—Case 15: Intraductal tumor thrombus stained by hepatic arteriography.

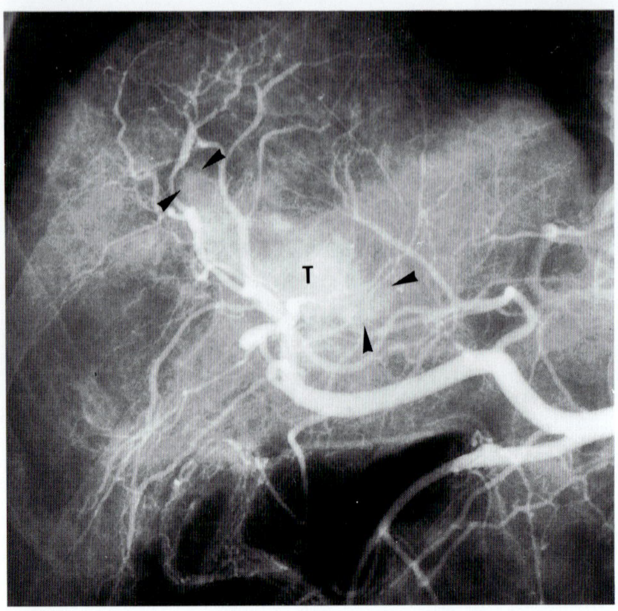

Hepatic arteriography (early phase): a 7 × 2 cm tumor stain is seen mainly in S^{VIII} and in S^{IV} in part. This consists of the main mass (T) and tumor thrombi in the bile duct growing centrally and peripherally (▶). Displacement of A^{VIII} by the mass is recognized. Arteriography may stain intraductal tumor thrombi, and TAE may prove efficacious for such thrombosis.

Intravascular tumor thrombosis—Case 16: Portal tumor thrombosis growing hepatopetally from stomach cancer.

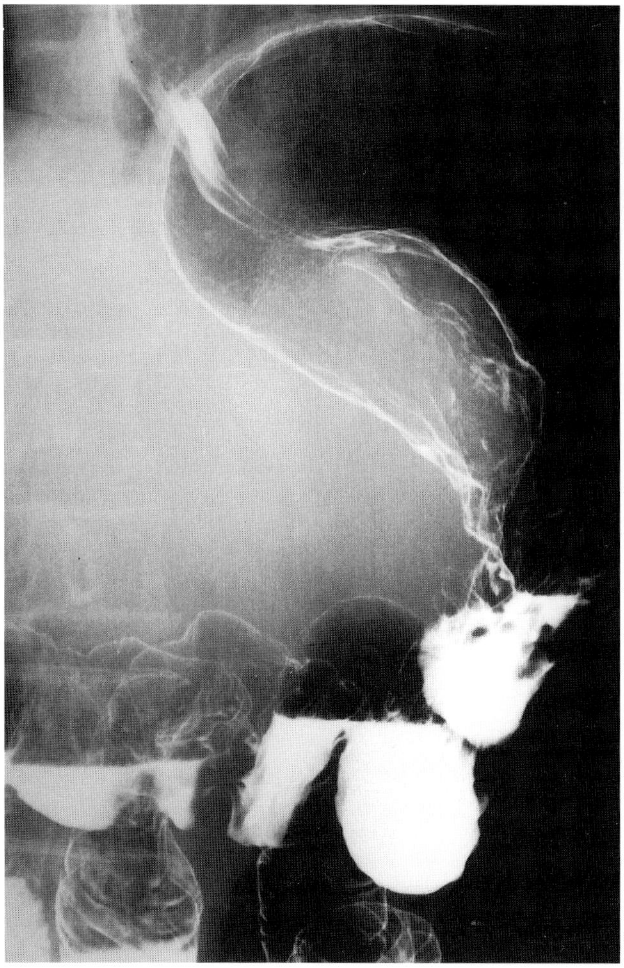

(a) Double contrast barium examination of the stomach in an erect position: a marked compression exerted from an extragastric lesion is seen along the lesser curvature in the body. Muscosal changes are minimal.

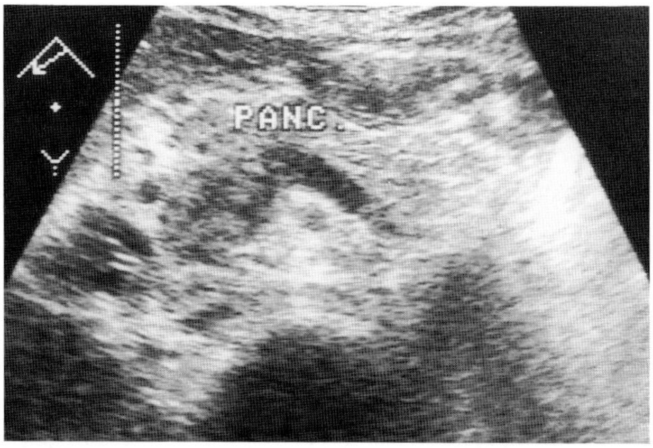

(b) US (transverse scan): a mass-like lesion of inhomogeneous echoes is seen at the junction of the splenic and superior mesenteric veins. There is no dilatation of the pancreatic duct.

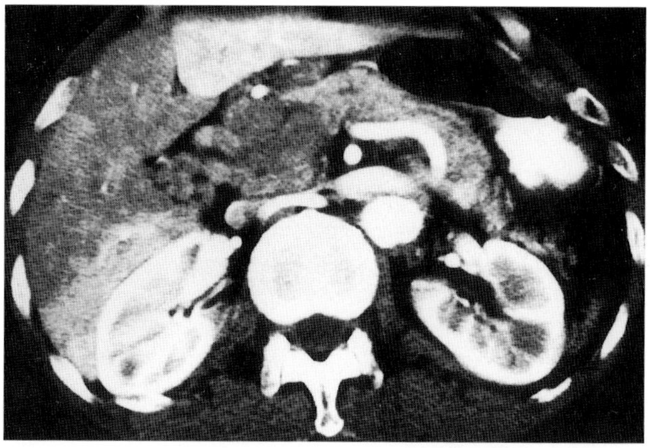

(c) Dynamic CT (early phase): there is a low-density mass lesion posterior to the head of the pancreas. Dilated vessels surrounding it (cavernous transformation) are recognized.

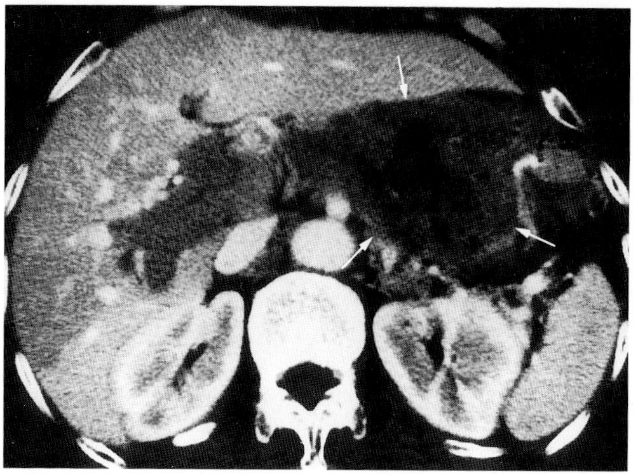

(d) Dynamic CT [slice 3 cm cranial from (c)]: a dilated vascular structure is seen in the hilum and a diagnosis of portal tumor thrombosis was made. The large low-density mass (→) posterior to the left lobe is gastric cancer growing extragastrically. The area supplied with portal venous blood through the cavernous transformation (right anterior and left medial segments) and the area not supplied with portal venous blood (right posterior and left lateral segments) are quite different in staining—the latter is heavily stained as a result of compensatory arterial supply (as remarkably seen in (c)).

Case 16 (contd.)

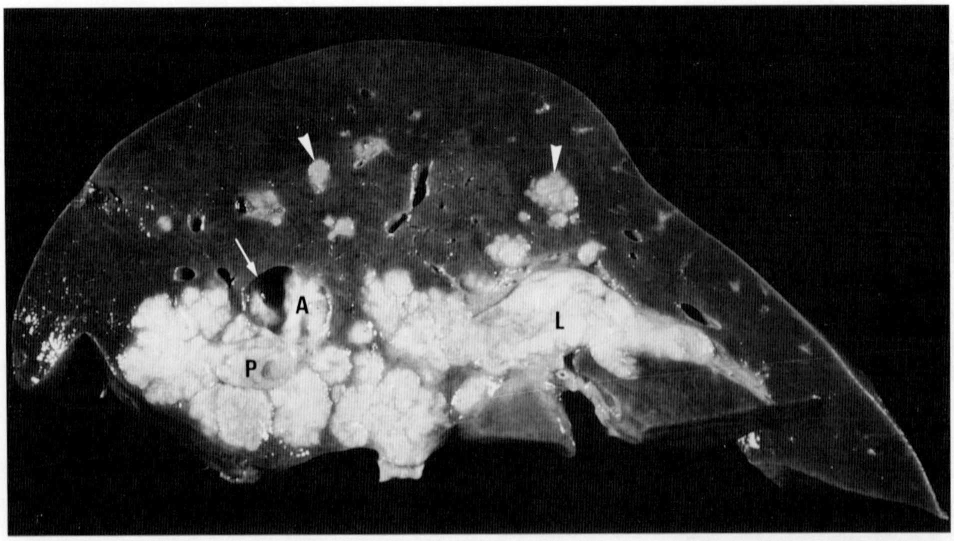

(e) Cut section of autopsy liver: the right and left portal veins are invaded by yellowish white tumor thrombi (P, posterior segment portal vein; A, anterior segment portal vein; L, left portal vein). The tumor thrombus was continuous up to the splenic hilum. (▶) indicates a small intrahepatic metastasis. →, a cyst. The gastric cancer was grossly Borrmann type 3, and histologically moderately differentiated adenocarcinoma.

Intravascular blood clot—Case 17: Thrombosis of the superior mesenteric vein.

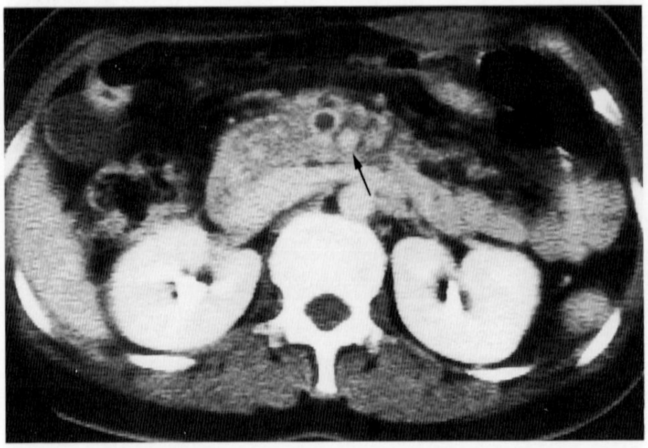

Enhanced CT (late phase): thrombosis of the superior mesenteric vein is seen to the right of the superior mesenteric artery (→) as a vessel structure without opacification of the lumen; the vein wall is seen as a ring.

Attenuation difference—Case 18: Lobar attenuation difference as a result of right portal vein obstruction due to hilar bile duct carcinoma.

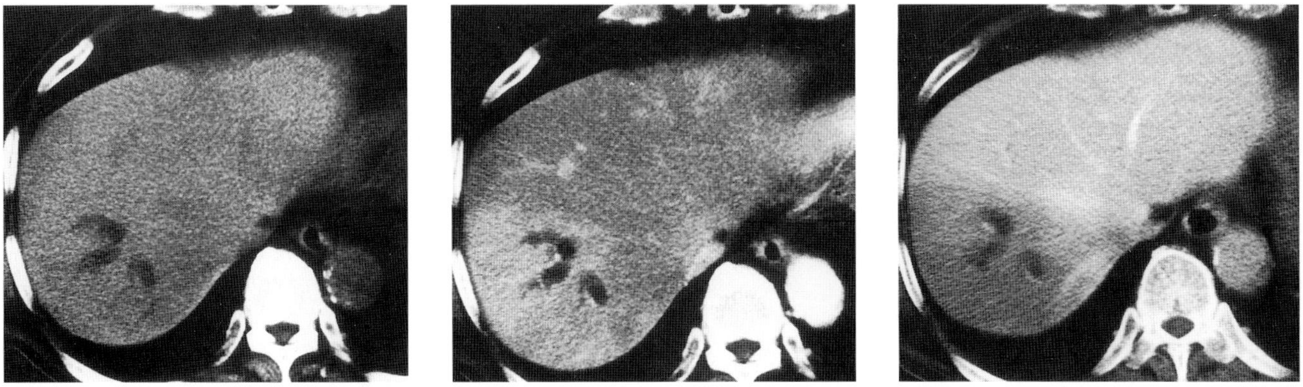

a b c

(a) Plain CT: bile duct (B^{VIII}) in the right lobe is dilated. (b) Enhanced CT (early phase): the right lobe is opacified to a greater extent than the left lobe, producing a difference in density between the two lobes. Obstruction of the right portal vein is suspected. (c) Portal-CT: only the left lobe was opacified, suggesting that the right lobe did not receive portal venous blood.

Attenuation difference—Case 19: Perihilar attenuation difference due to portal vein thrombosis associated with cavernous transformation.

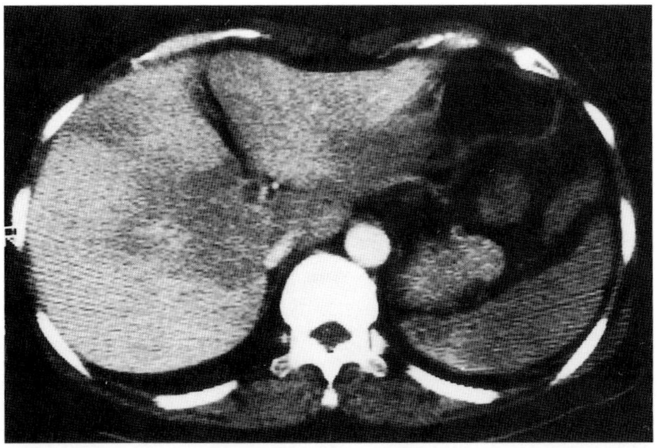

(a) Dynamic CT (early phase): an irregularly shaped low-density area is seen in the hilar area.

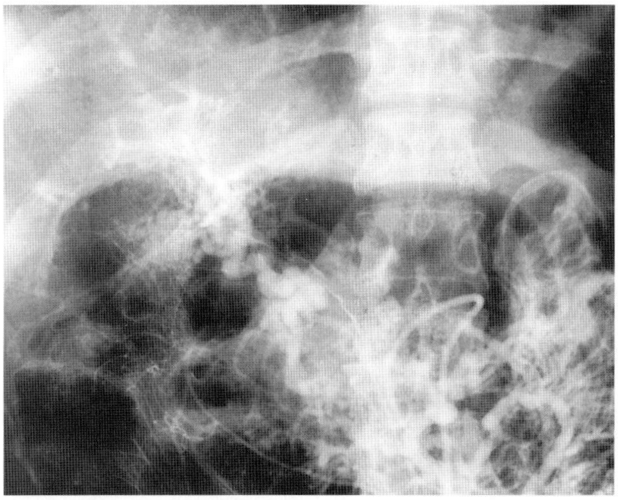

(b) Superior mesenteric arterial portogram: the portal trunk is occluded and cavernous transformation to its right and opacified intrahepatic portal branches as its continuation are seen.

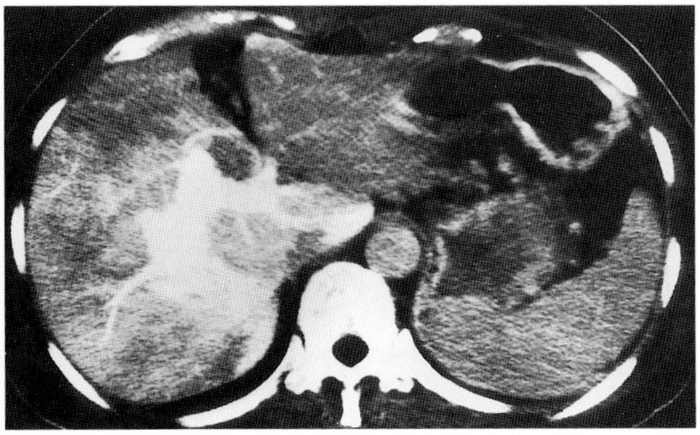

(c) Portal-CT: portal venous blood flows into the area around the hilum through the cavernous transformation, but the flow to the periphery is minimal. It was suggested that the periphery that received little portal blood flow had increased arterial supply as a compensation, producing some attenuation difference between the hilar area of low density and increased density in the periphery as was seen on dynamic CT (a).

Attenuation difference—Case 20: Lobar attenuation difference due to arterio-portal shunting secondary to HCC.

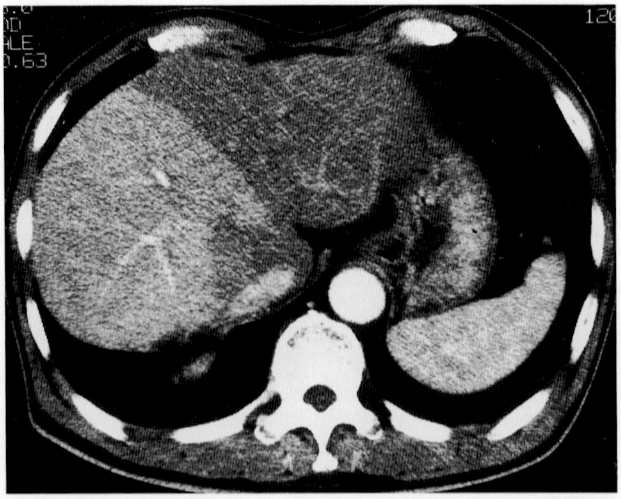

Dynamic CT (early phase): there is a distinct attenuation difference between the right and left lobes with the dividing Cantlie line. A diagnosis of arterio-portal shunting is possible from the discretely delineated portal branches in the right lobe.

Attenuation difference—Case 21: Attenuation difference due to partial obstruction of the hepatic vein (same as Case 9, p.167).

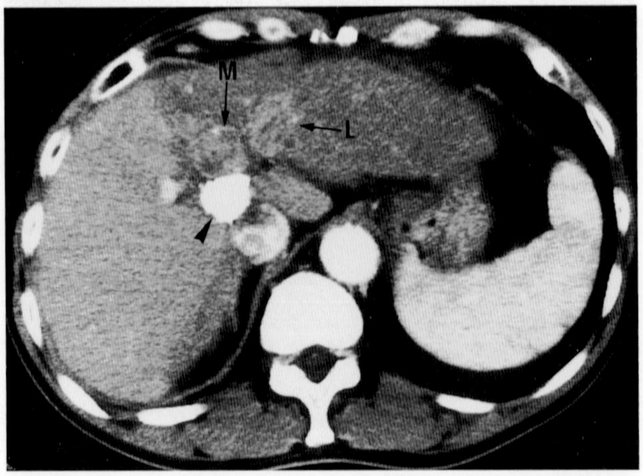

(a) Dynamic CT (early phase): a feature of lobar attenuation difference is recognized. The boundary of difference is not the Cantlie line, but is the middle hepatic vein (→) occluded by a tumor thrombus. The boundary was therefore between the area drained by the middle hepatic vein and one not drained by it. →, tumor thrombus in the middle hepatic (M) and the left hepatic (L) veins. ▶, Lipiodol retention in HCC.

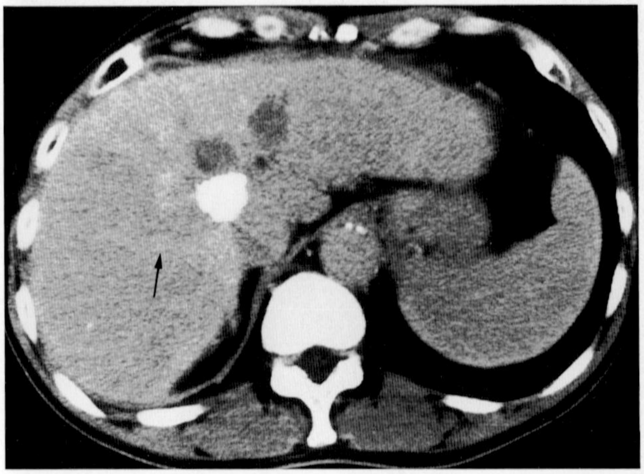

(b) Dynamic CT (late phase): the liver is nearly homogeneous in density, and only the tumor thrombus in the hepatic vein is low in density. →, the faintly opacified right hepatic vein.

Arterio-portal shunt association with HCC—Case 22: Arterio-portal shunt and retrograde contrast flow up to the hilum masking the primary of a small size.

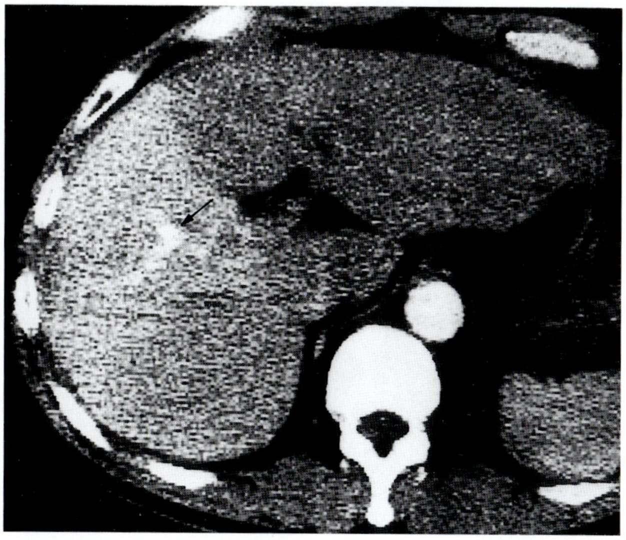

(a) Dynamic CT (early phase): the right anterior portal branch and the area it supplies were opacified early on dynamic CT.

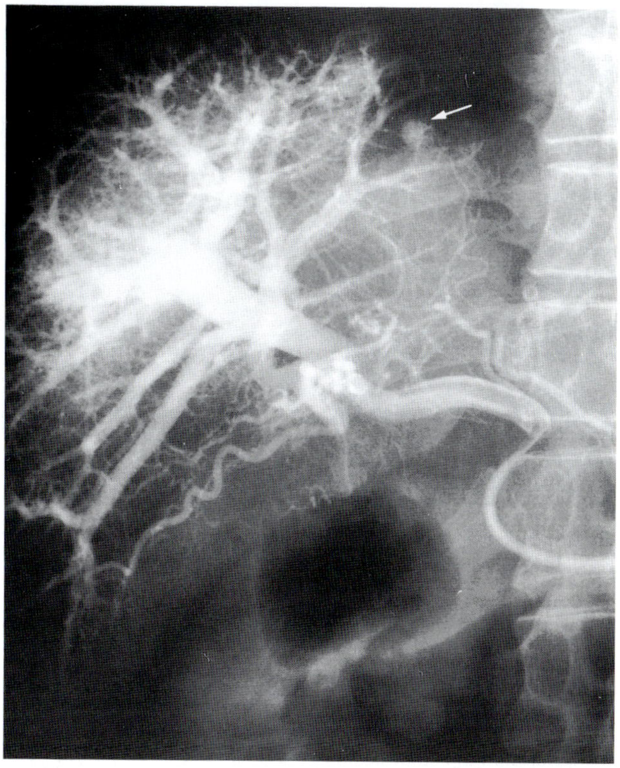

(b) Hepatic arteriography (early phase): a large hepatofugal contrast flow is seen in the portal vein as a result of arterio-portal shunting. The identification of the primary and its localization was difficult. →, a small metastasis of HCC identified by resection (S^{VIII}).

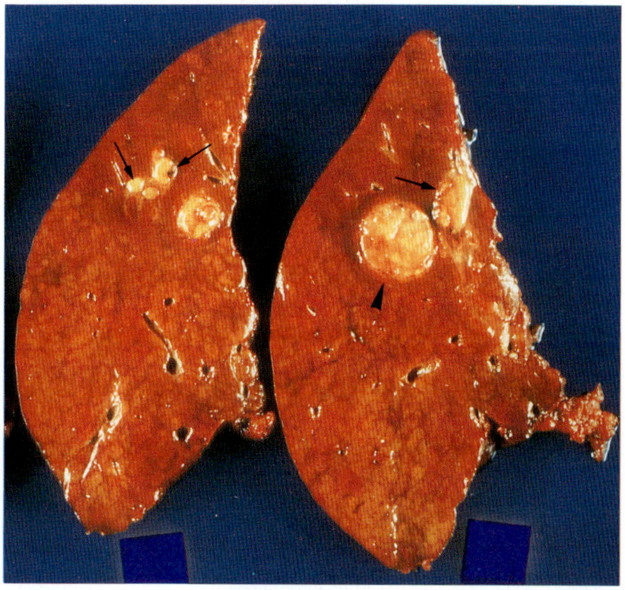

(c) Cut section of resected specimen: a 1.5 cm main tumor (in S^{V}) (▶) and a tumor thrombus continues from it growing in the peripheral portal branches (→) are seen.

Growth pattern of a portal tumor thrombus—Case 26: A case which provided information on the growth pattern of portal thrombosis.

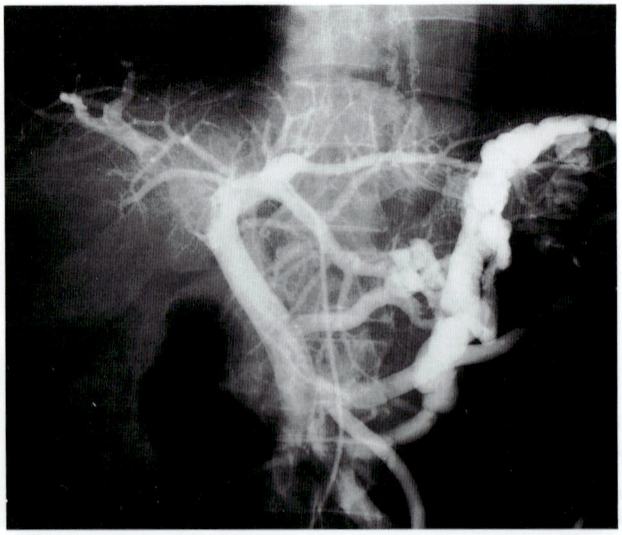

(a) Percutaneous transhepatic portography: PTP made on the 61st hospital day demonstrating lack of opacification of the posterior segment portal branch, and a filling defect due to tumor thrombosis in the anterior segment branch.

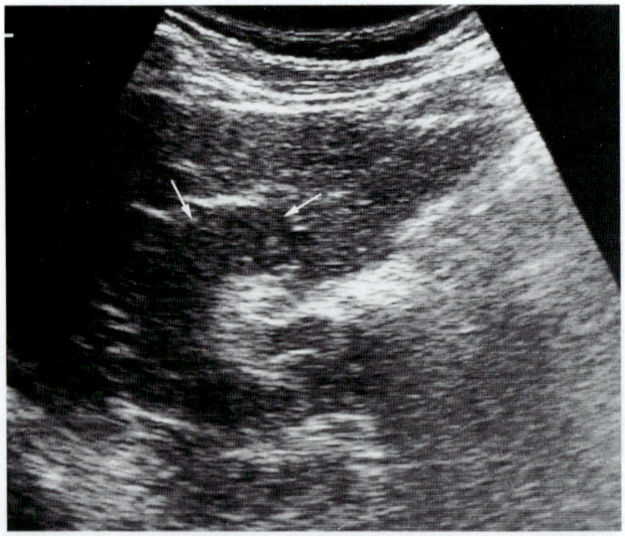

(b) US: US 69 days after PTP showed the tumor thrombus growing further in the transverse portion of the left portal vein (→). The patient died 31 days later from variceal rupture.

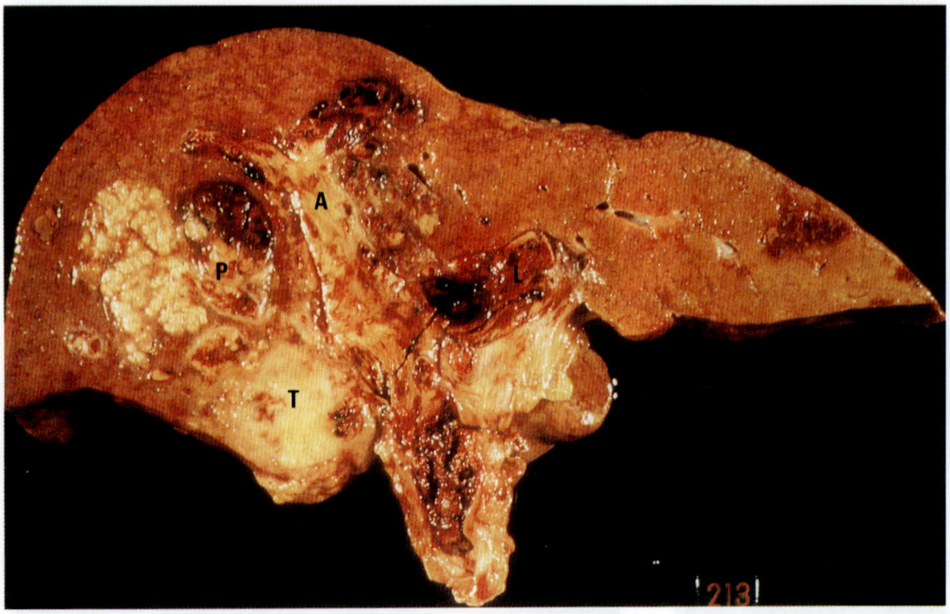

(c) Cut section of the liver at autopsy: tumor thrombosis filling the right and left portal veins and extending into the portal trunk is recognized. T, main mass; P, A, L, tumor thrombi in the posterior, anterior, and left portal branches respectively.

4.6 Uncommon hepatocellular carcinomas

HCC arising in the caudate lobe

The caudate lobe is anatomically in a special location and HCC arising in this lobe is uncommon. At the National Cancer Center Hospital, Tokyo, we have so far seen only 10 cases or so, and the resection rate has been only 0.5 per cent (Takayasu *et al.* 1986*a*; Takayama *et al.* 1991) for the reason given below. This lobe is situated near the hilum. The portal vein runs anterior and the inferior vena cava posterior to it. The branches of the portal vein and the short hepatic vein in the caudate lobe are all short, and intrahepatic spread readily occurs (Case 1). Thus, invasion into the portal vein (Case 2) and inferior vena cava (Case 3) is an early event. For these reasons, the prognosis of HCC occurring in the caudate lobe is usually poor despite its small size. We have seen a patient in whom a metastasis to the orbit lead to the detection of a primary in the caudate lobe which was accompanied by rapid tumor growth in the portal vein (Case 4) (Takayasu *et al.* 1986*a*).

Since a primary HCC in the caudate lobe gives rise to early extensive intrahepatic spread, it may be mistaken for a diffuse type HCC in a late stage. Particular attention should be given to the caudate lobe in studying the liver with diffuse HCC. If the primary in the caudate lobe is small and not superimposed on the digestive tract, irradiation of the primary and tumor thrombus combined with TAE may be worthwhile. One of our patients lived 3 years (Case 1) after such treatment (Takayasu *et al.* 1986*a*).

Extrahepatic growth of HCC

Though infrequent, HCC may grow from the liver surface into the abdominal cavity—generally called 'extrahepatic growth' (Cases 5 and 6). The origin of such growth may be: (1) an accessory lobe, (2) the Riedel lobe; or (3) physiologically or pathologically induced surface protrusion. If the transitional portion between HCC and the non-cancerous liver is wide, it may be called a 'protruding' type, and if it is a pedicle, 'pedunculated' type (Horie *et al.* 1983). Some investigators believe that the latter is derived from an accessory lobe of the liver. Clinically, clear distinction is not always possible. The former usually receives much fewer parasitic arteries while the latter may have many parasitic arteries because of inadequate feeding vessels coming from the liver and which tend to adhere to the surrounding tissues.

Ectopic vs heterotopic origin of HCC

Liver tissue found in a non-hepatic organ or tissue is called 'ectopic liver', and has no continuity with the liver (Collan *et al.* 1978). Heterotopic HCC is a collective term for HCCs believed to have arisen from such tissue (Horiuchi *et al.* 1973)—Case 7 is an HCC thought to have arisen from ectopic liver tissue in the left hemidiaphragm (Takayasu *et al.* 1994*a*). The lesion was supplied by the left inferior phrenic artery with no feeding vessel coming from the liver.

Spontaneous regression of HCC

Spontaneous regression or disappearance of HCC is extremely uncommon although there have been several reports (Lam *et al.* 1982; Gottfried *et al.* 1982; Suzuki *et al.* 1989; Gaffey *et al.* 1990). More commonly regression includes shrinking rather than complete disappearance. The natural course of an HCC can now be followed with certain accuracy by improved imaging techniques, and spontaneous decrease in size has been seen in increasing numbers of patients. In Case 8, the mass shrank without treatment while being followed by CT, a rather uncommon phenomenon for a clinically distinct HCC of a considerable size. Angiography sometimes causes spasm of the hepatic artery or damage to the vascular intima, effecting ischemia in HCC as with TAE. We have seen one patient with HCC in whom complete tumor necrosis was induced by angiography alone (Takayasu *et al.* 1986*b*) (Case 6, p.491). One has to be careful in making the diagnosis of spontaneous regression.

Spontaneous rupture of HCC into the abdominal cavity

The patient may come or be rushed to the hospital because of sudden abdominal pain, abdominal distension, and occasionally a state of shock (Ong and Taw 1972). If a liver mass and bloody ascites are demonstrated, the diagnosis is simple, but there may not be hemorrhagic ascites if the omentum is adherent to the surface of the mass. In the latter case, a localized pool of blood is frequently found near the liver surface by CT and US (Case 9). Tumor rupture is not uncommon in advanced HCC of a large diameter. The prognosis is poor with conservative therapy, and emergency TAE may be carried out to be followed by hepatic resection in patients without complications (Okazaki *et al.* 1991). However, long-term prognosis in such patients with successful management is not favorable because of dissemination of cancer cells in the free abdominal cavity and subsequent peritoneal carcinomatosis that ensues (Case 9, p.208).

Fibrolamellar carcinoma

This is a variant of HCC that occurs in young adults (15–35 years) with a relatively good prognosis if resection is carried out in time. Edmondson first described this type in 1956, and Peters added five cases in 1976 with a name 'eosinophilic HCC with lamellar fibrosis' but later changed it to 'fibrolamellar carcinoma' (Craig *et al.* 1980). Subsequent studies have shown that this type of HCC is not that uncommon among Caucasians with an incidence of 1–2 per cent (Rolfes 1987), and it corresponds to the type of HCC among young adults biochemically characterized by very high serum vitamin B_{12} levels (due to increased transcobalamin I) (Paradinas *et al.* 1982). Serum AFP is seldom elevated and there is no etiologic relationship with contraceptives. Fibrolamellar carcinoma is very rare in the Far East, and only nine cases have been reported in Japan up to 1993 (Hirokawa *et al.* 1993).

Grossly, the periphery of the tumor is irregularly lobular with central fibrosis (Brandt *et al.* 1988) (Case 10). In cut section it resembles FNH, and differential diagnosis is a problem. A nodular structure in the tumor interior is also recognized by

US, and the mass is of low-density on plain CT which demonstrates staining of tumor nodules and a central low-density area on plain CT (Friedman *et al.* 1985). The interior undergoes calcification (Case 11) in more than half of cases. Such features are helpful in differential diagnosis from conventional HCC. Hepatoblastoma may also have calcification within the mass, but the center is rarely fibrosed. Fibrolamellar carcinoma is usually hypervascular on angiography (Friedman *et al.* 1985) (Case 1), and distinction from HCC by angiography alone is not easy; arterio-portal shunting and intravascular tumor invasion is very rare, although neovasculature occurs.

This tumor appears on MR images as a well demarcated and lobulated mass with a central scar. The lesion is seen as isointense relative to liver parenchyma on T1-weighted SE images, and on T2-weighted images it is either iso-, slightly hyper- or hypointense (Titelbaum *et al.* 1988). The central scar is seen as hypointense on both T1- and T2-weighted images, a feature that may be helpful in distinguishing fibrolamellar carcinoma from focal nodular hyperplasia, because the central scar is depicted as hyperintense rather than hypointense in the latter on T2-weighted images (Mattison *et al.* 1987; Lee *et al.* 1991). The difference in intensity of the central scar on T2-weighted images between these two entities is explained as follows: the central scar of fibrolamellar carcinoma is mainly composed of collagen with very little or no vascularity, hence hypointensity on T2-weighted images (Mattison *et al.* 1987; Lee *et al.* 1991), whereas the scar of focal nodular hyperplasia contains blood vessels, bile ducts and collagen (i.e. vascular scar) and is seen as hyperintense (Rummeny *et al.* 1989). Recently, one exceptional case of fibrolamellar carcinoma was reported in which the MR feature closely resembled that of focal nodular hyperplasia (Hamrick-Turner *et al.* 1994).

Sclerosing HCC

This type was first described by Omata *et al.* (1981) as a distinct variant of primary liver cancer which occurs in a non-cirrhotic liver as a whitish firm mass. Histologically, it consists of extensive fibrous tissue containing sparsely distributed cancer cells, and biochemically hypercalcemia (69 per cent) is a common feature. Some cancer cells may be identified as of hepatocellular origin, but in others the cell origin is obscure. Since the gross picture resembles that of cholangiocarcinoma and metastatic adenocarcinoma (Yoshida *et al.* 1992) (Case 12), histological assessment becomes important. Sclerosing HCC in Japan is somewhat different from the report made in the USA in that hypercalcemia is uncommon, HBsAg is frequently positive, not encapsulated and the recurrence rate after resection is low (Iha 1994). The relationship between sclerosing HCC and the scirrhous type of HCC is not clear, and the revised edition of the WHO *Histological Typing of Liver Tumors* (Ishak *et al.* 1994) states that the former does not constitute a distinct histopathological entity.

Small HCC with calcification

Calcification of the tumor was once emphasized as a characteristic feature of HCC for diagnosis, but this has not been our experience in Japan (Case 13). Calcifications in HCC tend to be distributed unevenly, more in one side than in the other whereas calcifications in metastatic colon cancer are seen more often as dots of zonal concentric distribution (Case 8, p.271). By imaging, Lipiodol retention in the tumor may mimic calcification.

Circulatory disturbances caused by compression exerted by an expanding HCC

Dynamic CT sometimes demonstrates a heavily stained zone between the mass and the liver capsule. This was previously thought to be due to arterio-portal shunting, but the continuous heavy stain lasting into the late phase of examination could not be explained. Subsequent studies and experience based on resected material and its section have shown that it corresponds to a yellowish white firm tissue located lateral to an expanding tumor. Histologically, it consists of collapsed liver cells and proliferating bile ducts, a sequela to compression of liver tissue by an expanding HCC with its capsule (Case 14). A similar imaging feature may be produced in an early phase of dynamic CT in the presence of an arterio-portal shunt. The differential diagnosis depends on continuous heavy stain by contrast medium in the late phase on dynamic CT. The mechanism is perhaps the same as that whereby central staining of the mass (such as adenocarcinoma) occurs in the late phase of dynamic CT as a result of contrast uptake by fibrous tissue in the center.

Uncommon HCC—Case 1: Small HCC in the caudate lobe causing early portal invasion and multiple intrahepatic spread. US and CT demonstrated multiple small lesions in the right lobe.

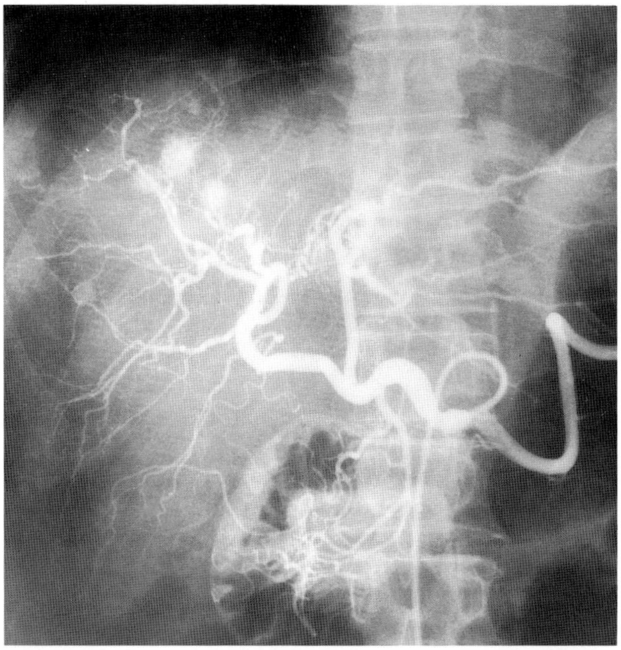

(a) Hepatic arteriography: arteriography demonstrated multiple hypervascular lesions in the right lobe and the superior mesenteric arteriographic portogram failed to delineate the left umbilical portion clearly. The overall picture resembled postoperative recurrence, but there was no such history. The main tumor is obscure.

(b) Plain CT (immediately after arterial injection of Lipiodol; slices from cranial to caudal): multiple Lipiodol-retaining lesions are seen in both lobes (▶), but the largest one was a nodular Lipiodol retention in the left caudale lobe (→); (3) shows Lipiodol retention in the left transverse portion of the portal vein.

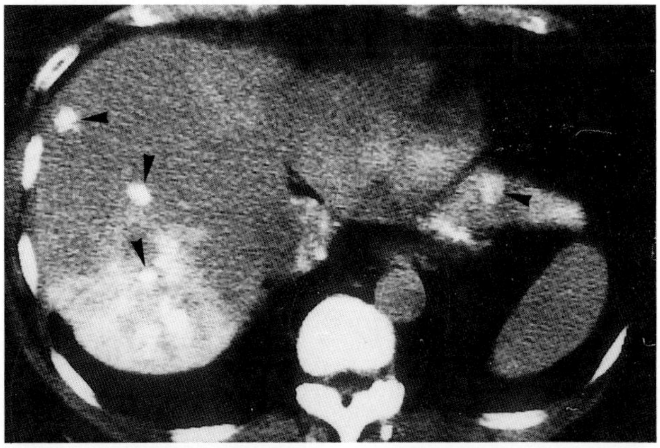

1

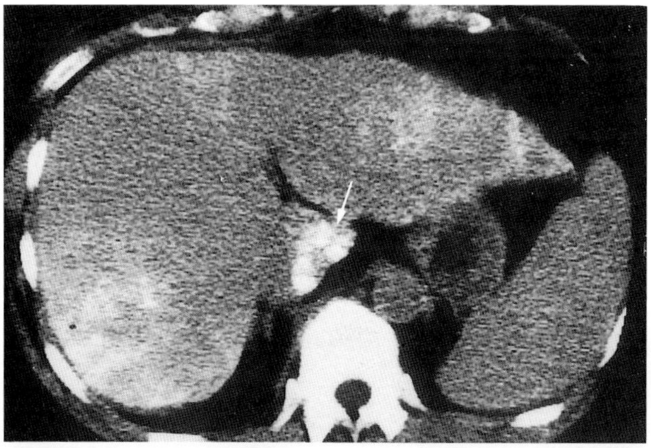

2

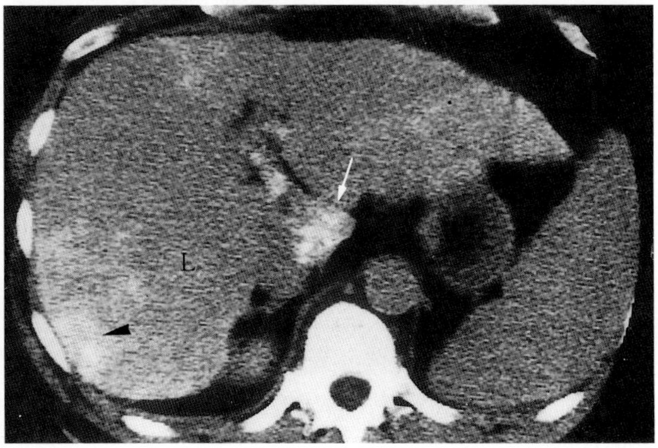

3

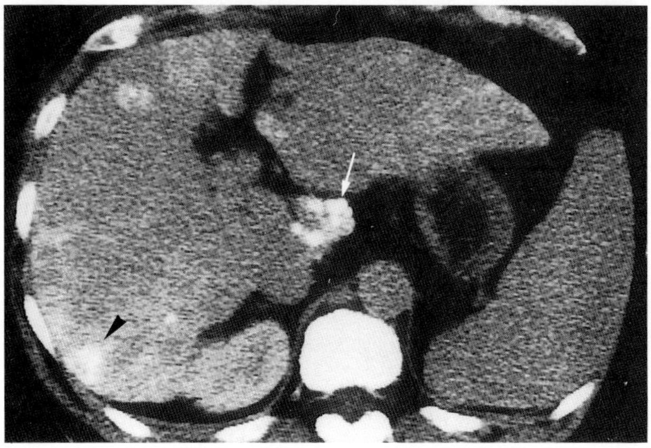

4

Case 1 (contd.)

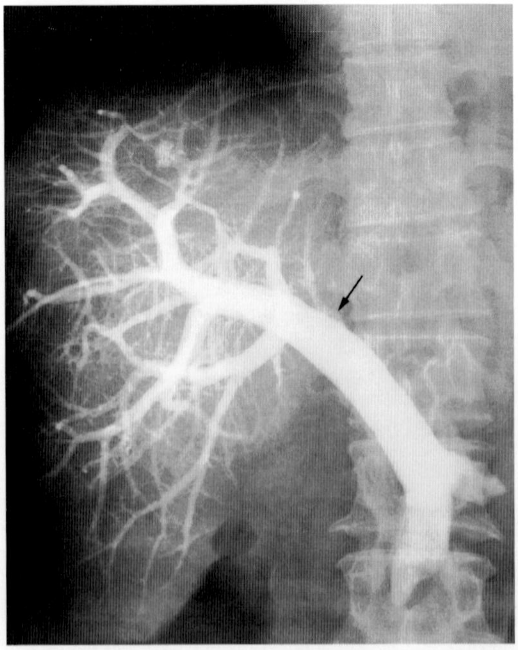

(c) Percutaneous transhepatic portography (6 days after Lipiodol injection): the left portal vein (→) was cut out from the portal trunk.

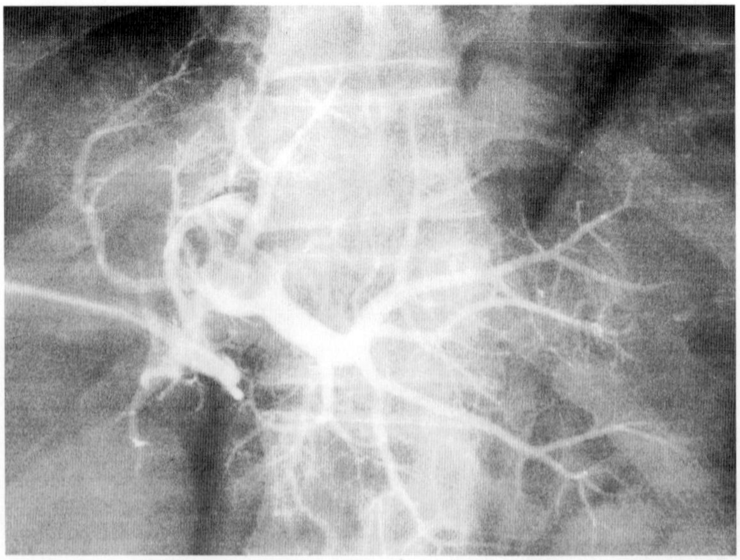

(d) Selective portography: the catheter was pushed into the left portal vein selectively and contrast injected. A filling defect is clearly seen in the umbilical portion extending into the transverse portion making the diagnosis of tumor thrombosis possible. From the periphery of the thrombus the lateral inferior (P^{III}) and medial (P^{IV}) branches were opacified. It was assumed that HCC arising in the left caudate lobe caused early spread through a portal tumor thrombus.

Uncommon HCC—Case 2: HCC in the caudate lobe in which evaluation of tumor thrombosis could be made during follow-up.

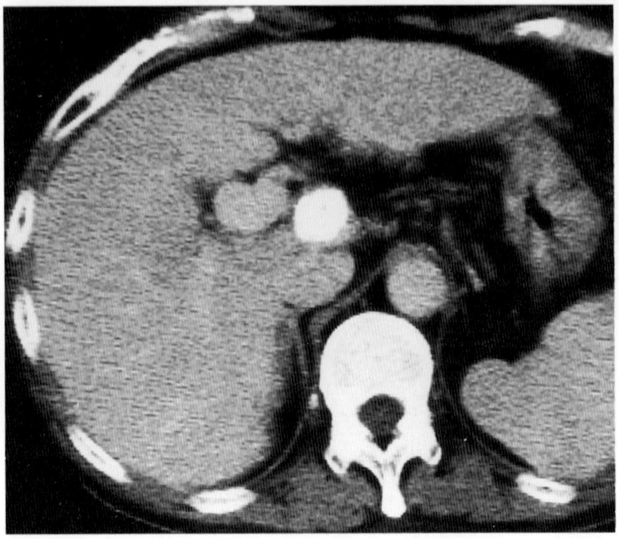

(a) Dynamic CT: a 1.5 cm HCC with Lipiodol retention is seen in the caudate lobe. The portal vein was unremarkable at this time.

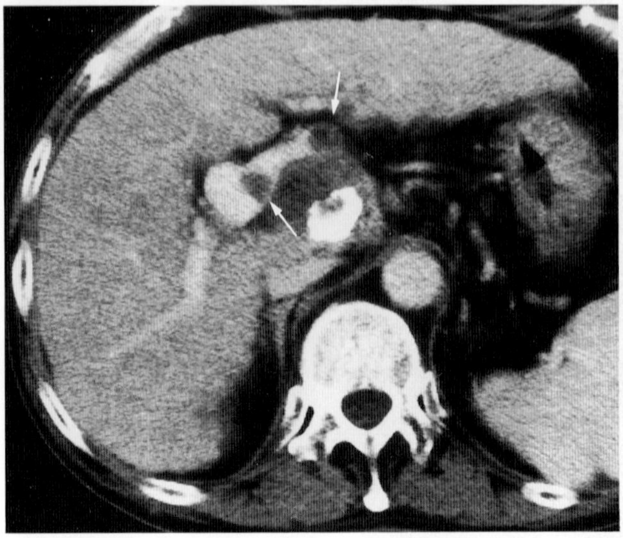

(b) Dynamic CT (2 months later): the tumor expanded to 3 cm compressing the portal vein anteriorly at the hilum. In addition, tumor thrombi are clearly seen in the right and left portal veins (→).

Uncommon HCC—Case 3: HCC in the caudate lobe with extensive tumor thrombosis filling the inferior vena cava and the right atrium.

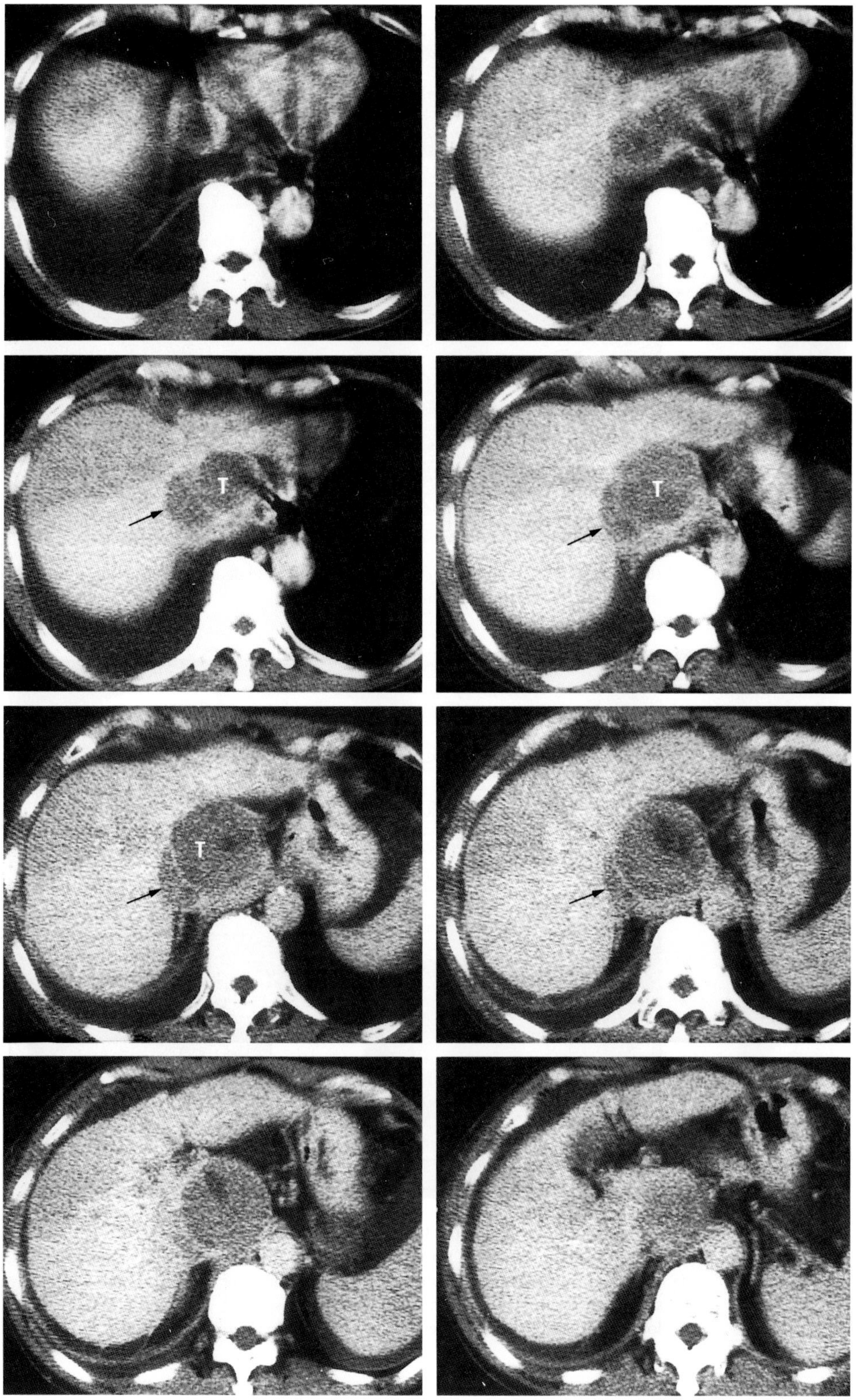

Dynamic CT (from cranial to caudal): in these images, a 6 cm mass (T) and the inferior vena cava seen to its right in a semilunar shape (→) are apparent. The inferior vena cava was not opacified following contrast injection, and the cranial tip of the tumor thrombus was in the right atrium, suggesting extension of the tumor bolus into the right atrium from the vena cava. There was no demonstrable intrahepatic spread or portal tumor thrombosis.

1	2
3	4
5	6
7	8

Uncommon HCC—Case 6: Extrahepatic growth of HCC (pedunculated type).

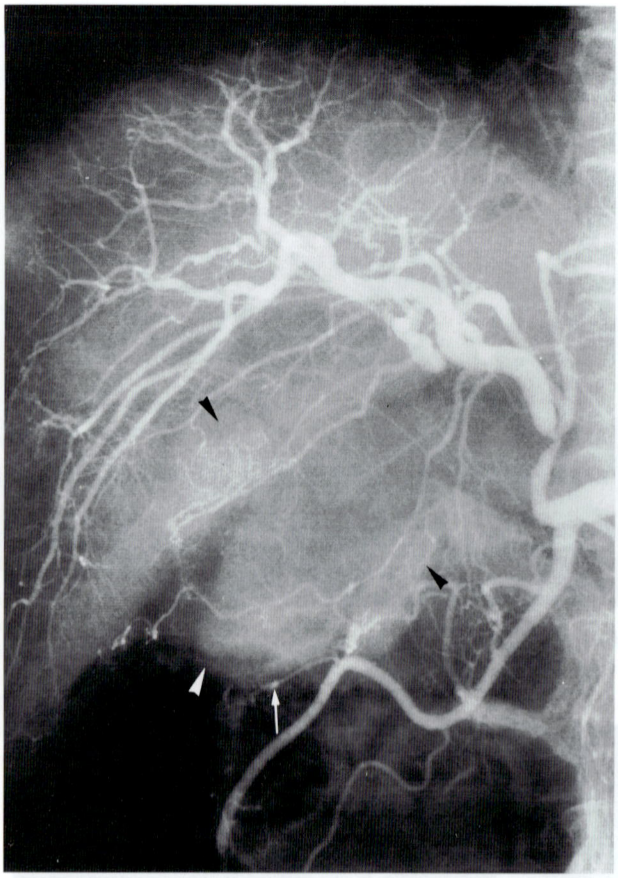

(a) Hepatic arteriography (early phase): a protruding mass is seen in the right posterior region of the liver. It is supplied mainly from intrahepatic arteries, but also from the omental artery in part (→). ▶, periphery of the mass.

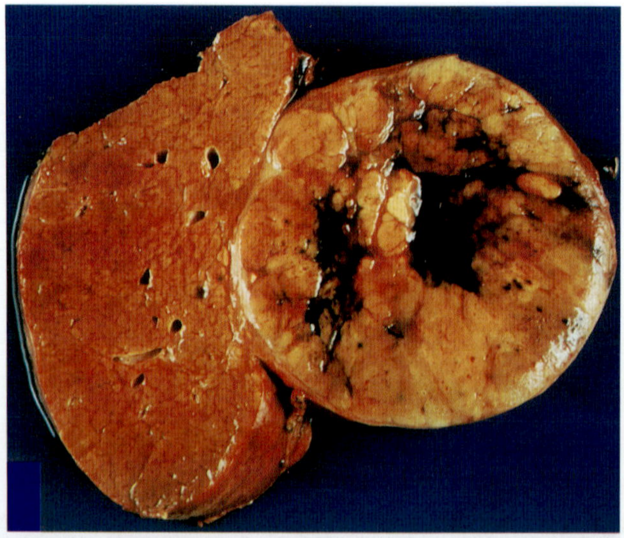

(b) Cut section of resected specimen: the mass and a portion of S^{VI} were resected. The bulk of the mass was growing outside the liver, and a small portion was in continuity with the posterior segment of the liver. There was extensive adhesion between the mass and the lesser omentum, gallbladder, and inferior vena cava, and upon separation, considerable bleeding occurred.

Uncommon HCC—Case 7: Ectopic HCC difficult to differentiate from rhabdomyosarcoma of the left hemidiaphragm. This patient came to the hospital because barium examination of the stomach showed displacement of the fundus by an extragastric force. Serum AFP was 2207 ng/ml and CEA 6.6 ng/ml.

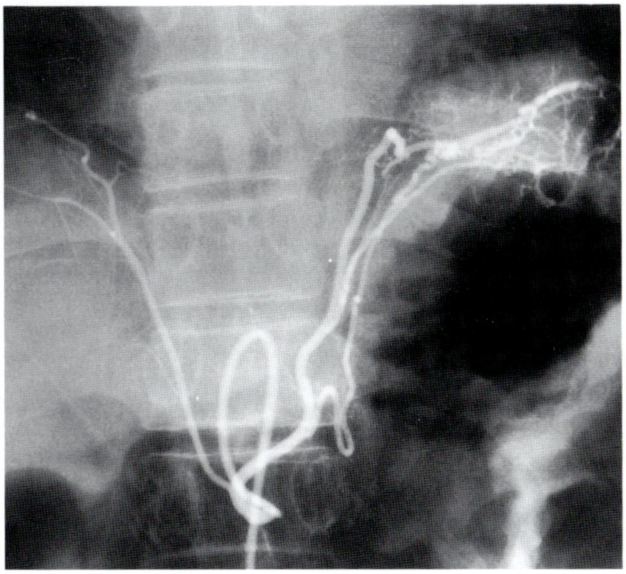

(a) Left inferior phrenic arteriography: left gastric arteriography was carried out for a suspected gastric leiomyosarcoma, but no mass was found in the stomach. Subsequent inferior phrenic arteriography demonstrated marked dilatation of this artery and a hypervascular mass associated with tumor vessels and stains. There was no feeding vessel derived from the liver, nor was there any intrahepatic lesion.

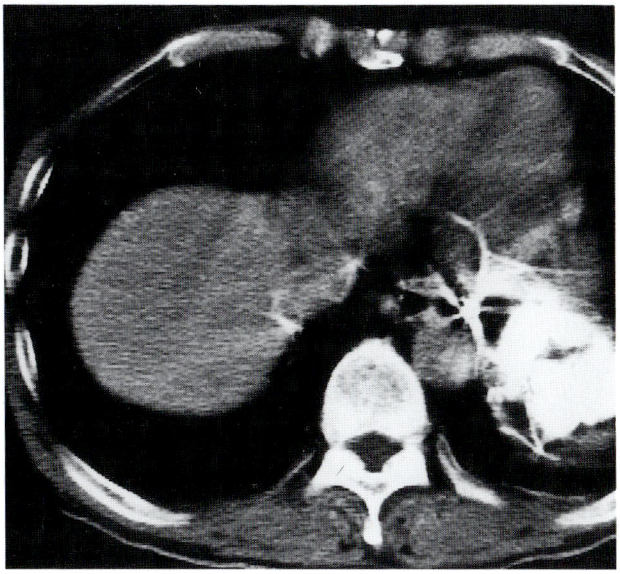

(b) Inferior phrenic arterial-CT: a 5.5 cm mass was identified by this examination. The elevated serum AFP was an enigma since rhabdomyosarcoma arising from the diaphragm was the most likely diagnosis.

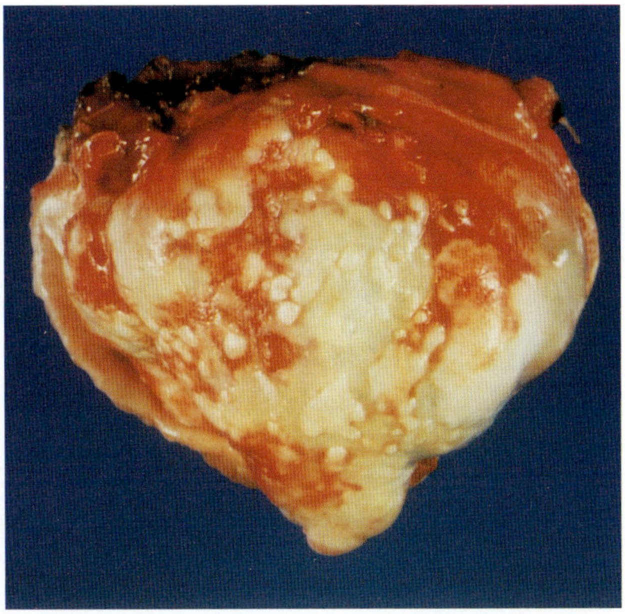

(c) Removed mass seen from the abdominal side: the left diaphragm and the mass were resected. The surface was studded with multiple white nodules. The mass was histologically HCC of Edmondson's grade II. There was no connection between the mass and the left lobe of the liver. Serum AFP levels returned to normal and the diagnosis was HCC arising heterotopically in the diaphragm. The patient is well 5 years postoperatively.

Uncommon HCC—Case 8: Spontaneous regression of HCC without treatment.

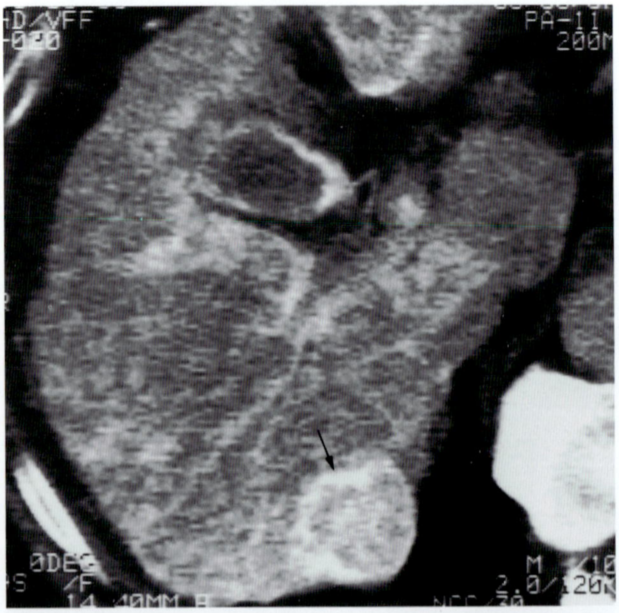

(a) Arterial-CT: a 3 cm hypervascular mass with a strong staining in the periphery is seen in S^{VII} (→). Serum AFP was 2181 ng/ml.

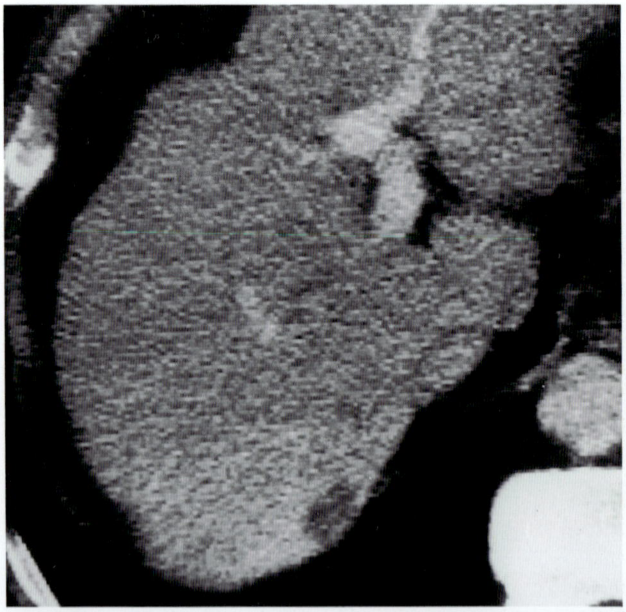

(b) Dynamic CT (5 months later): the S^{VII} lesion is now seen as a low-density mass of 1.5 cm in diameter. Serum AFP level was also decreased to 57 ng/ml, and became normal half a month later. CT was regularly repeated every 6 months, and the lesion completely disappeared 1 year after CT (b).

Uncommon HCC—Case 9: HCC that ruptured into the abdominal cavity. This patient with HCC was on a waiting list for operation. He suddenly developed upper abdominal pain, and emergency Lipiodol-TAE was carried out for suspected tumor rupture.

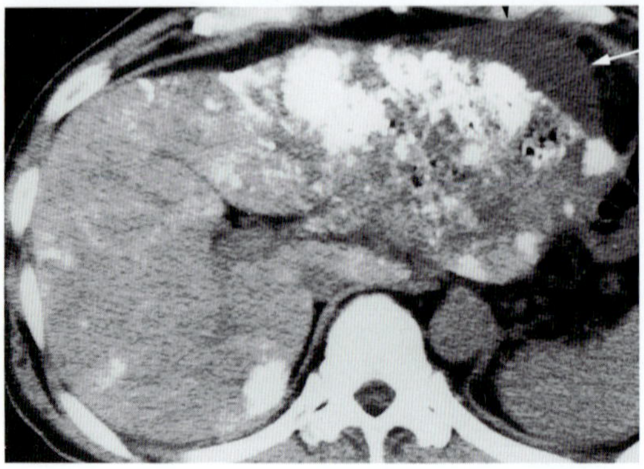

(a) Plain CT: this CT was made 14 days after Lipiodol-TAE, demonstrating a 12 cm mass in the left lobe that contained some gas. There was a semilunar shaped homogeneous low-density area lateral to the mass (→). In view of the absence of ascites, this was diagnosed as extrahepatic bleeding.

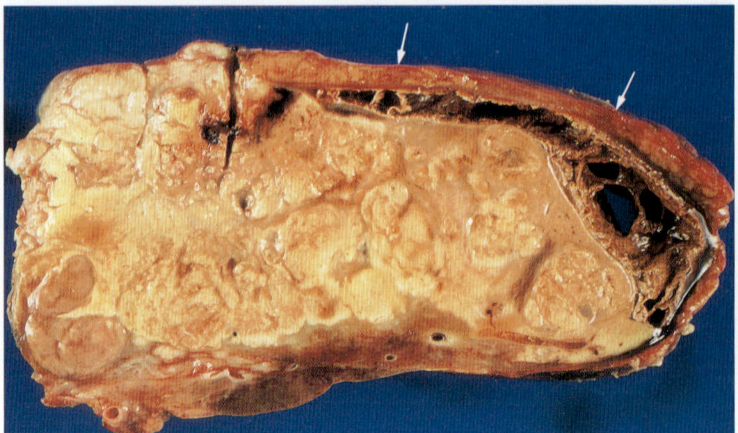

(b) Cut section of the resected left lobe: the cut surface of the resected left lobe ($S^{II, III, IV}$) showed an HCC with extensive necrosis, and a clot transformed into an alveolar structure was seen between the liver surface and the omentum (→).

Uncommon HCC—Case 10: Fibrolamellar carcinoma (courtesy of Dr D. J. Brandt; *A.J.R.* 1988, **151**, 295).

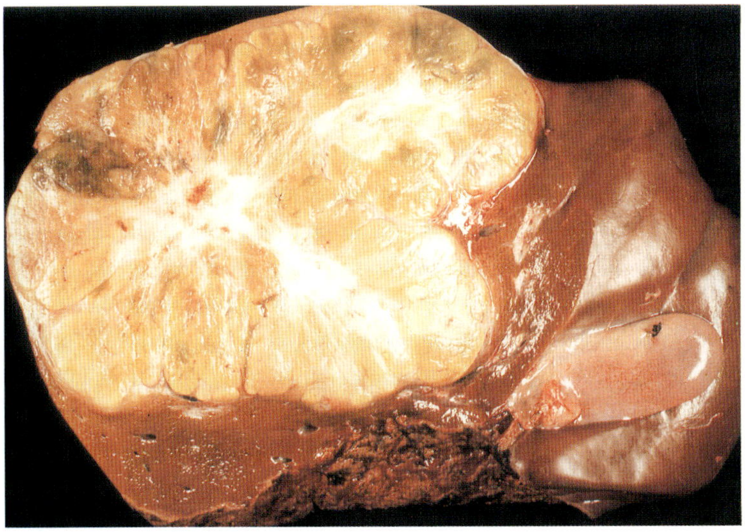

(a) Cut section: fibrolamellar carcinoma itself is very uncommon in Japan, and therefore a gross picture is shown first. The periphery of the mass is smoothly irregular with no fibrous capsule. The mass is lobulated with a whitish fibrosis in the center, but there is no necrosis. Grossly, this looks like FNH and differential diagnosis is not feasible just by gross study. The non-tumor liver is normal.

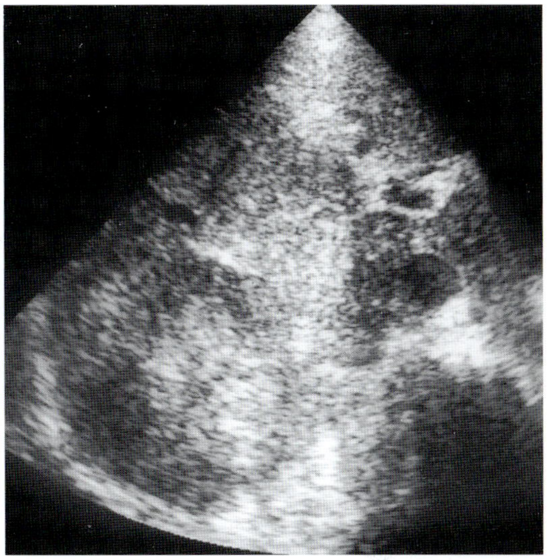

(b) US: the mass is somewhat round and the interior is mosaic with mixed echoes. The boundary is irregular with a lobular contour, but there is no halo or lateral shadow.

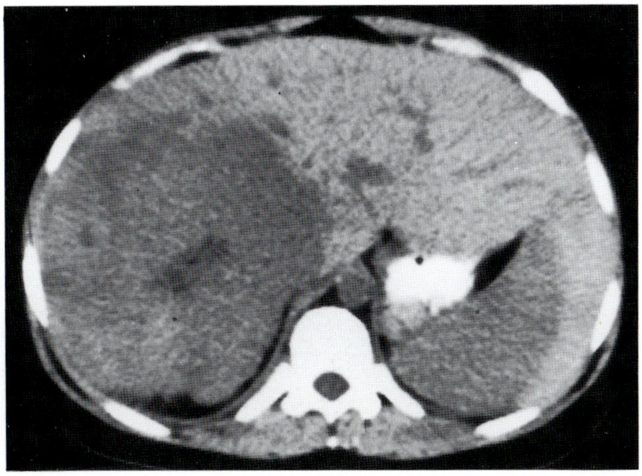

(c) Plain CT: a large low-density mass is seen in the right lobe. The interior contains an area of low density. A posterior portion of the mass has a somewhat higher density.

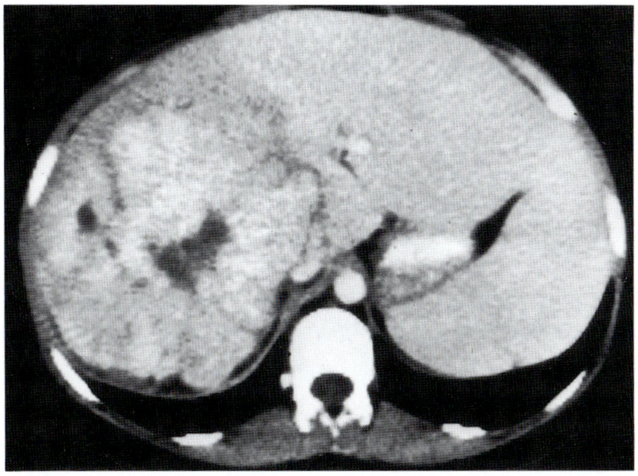

(d) Dynamic CT: the mass was stained well, disclosing an irregular periphery and a lobular structure with some septation in the interior. The unstained center may be interpreted as necrosis or a fibrous tissue. The gross picture (a) and this CT image correspond very well. The low-density area extending from the mass toward the Cantlie line may be an outcome of compression or occlusion of the portal vein branches by the tumor.

Case 10 (contd.)

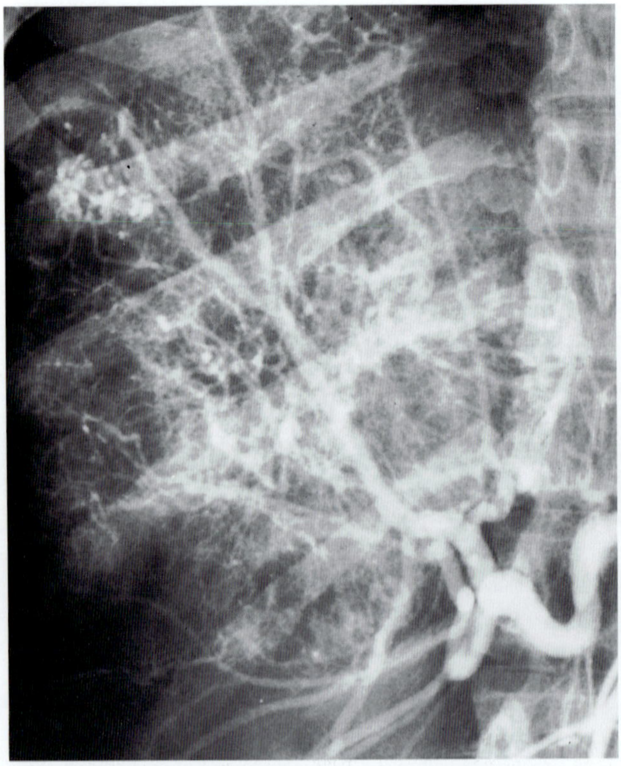

(e) Hepatic arteriography: the right hepatic artery is markedly dilated with numerous tumor vessels in the right hepatic lobe. This picture is quite different from that in FNH, and a malignant mass is strongly suggested. No arterio-portal shunt or tumor thrombus is recognized.

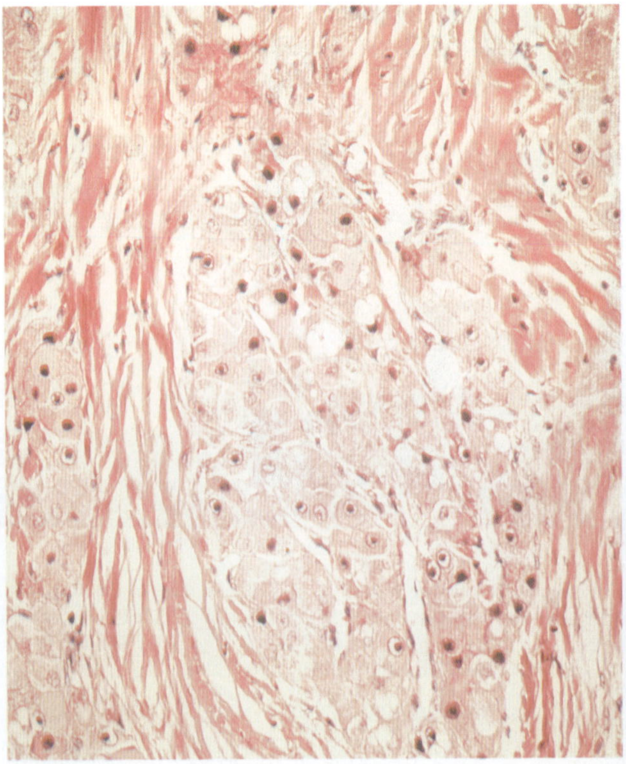

(f) Histopathology: eosinophilic cancer cells are arranged in thin trabeculae surrounded by lamellar fibers, a typical fibrolamellar carcinoma.

Uncommon HCC—Case 11: Fibrolamellar carcinoma with a surface indentation and internal calcification (courtesy of Dr D. J. Brandt; *A.J.R.*, 1988, **151**, 295).

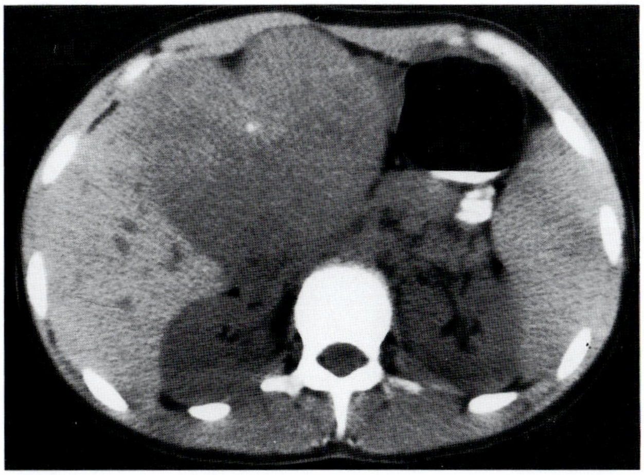

(a) Plain CT: an 11 cm heart-shaped mass with a calcific spot in the center is seen in the medial aspect of the left lobe and the anterior segment of the right lobe.

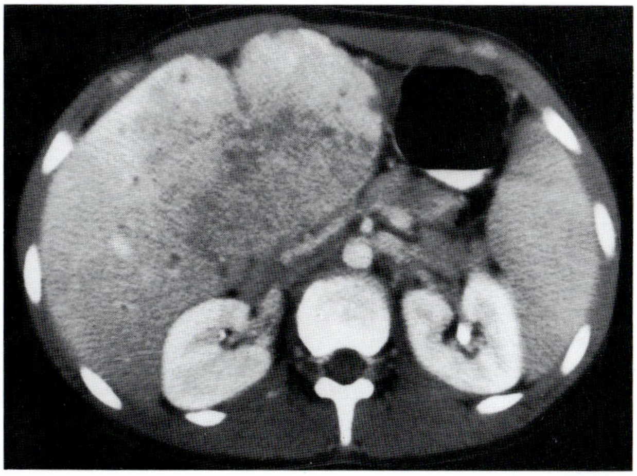

(b) Enhanced CT: the mass was slightly stained, and small low-density spots and low-density strands radiating toward the periphery are recognized.

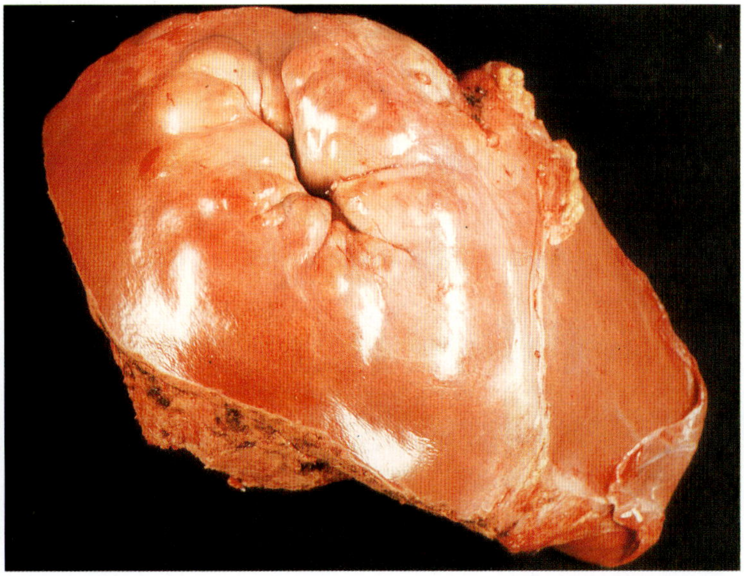

(c) Resected liver: the surface of the mass is bulging with a large indentation, and the individual bulges correspond to lobulated tumor nodules near the surface. The indentation is deep, reaching the tumor center, and this picture closely resembles the CT image. A tumor with calcification in a young adult could also be a hepatoblastoma.

Uncommon HCC—Case 12: Selerosing HCC.

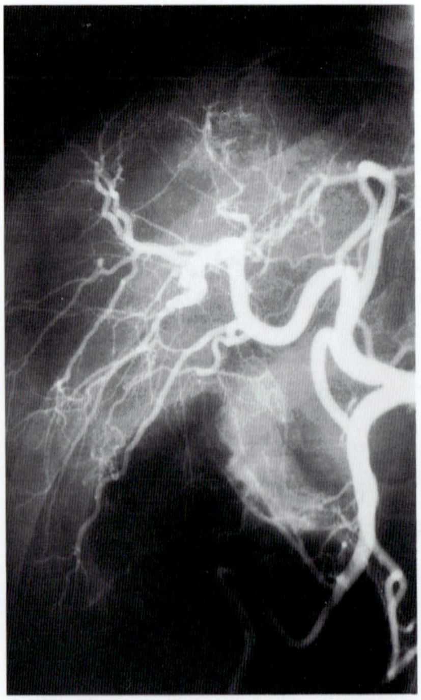

(a) Hepatic arteriography (early phase): tumor vessels are seen in S^{VII}.

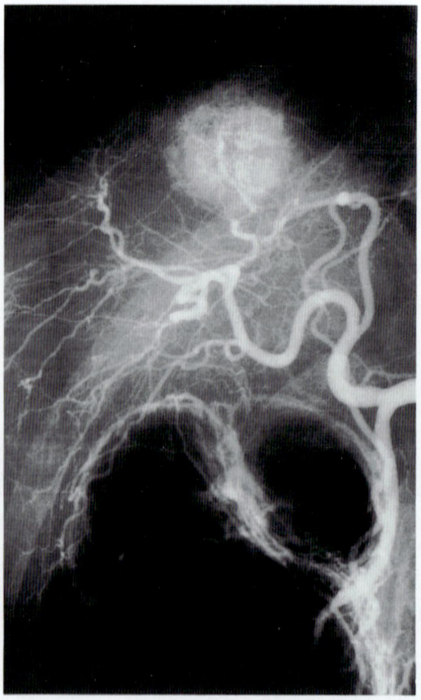

(b) Hepatic arteriography (mid-phase): the mass is slowly stained.

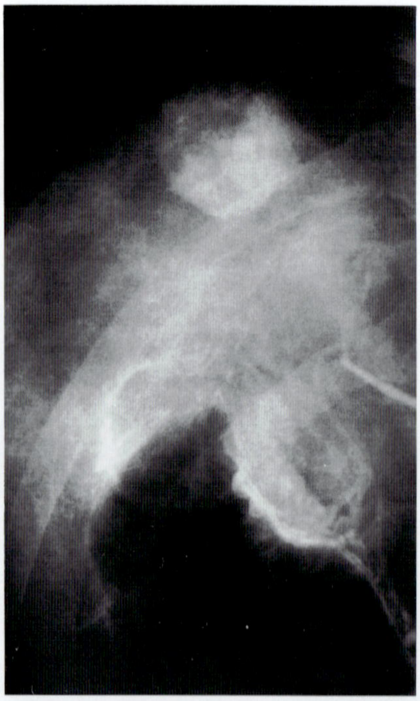

(c) Hepatic arteriography (late phase): a number of nodular stains are seen within the mass, and the whole picture is that of a conventional HCC.

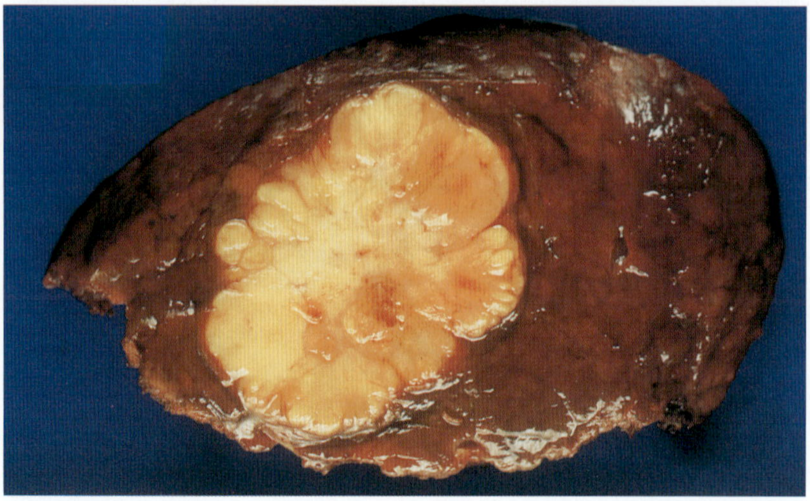

(d) Cut section: the periphery of the mass is undulant and the interior firm and concave, and differentiation from bile duct carcinoma and combined hepatocholangioma is difficult. Histologically, this tumor consisted of cancer cells of the trabecular pattern, and in places of pseudoglandular arrangement. It contained abundant hyalinized stroma showing scirrhous tumor invasion. The non-cancerous liver showed mild chronic hepatitis.

Uncommon HCC—Case 13: Small HCC with calcification.

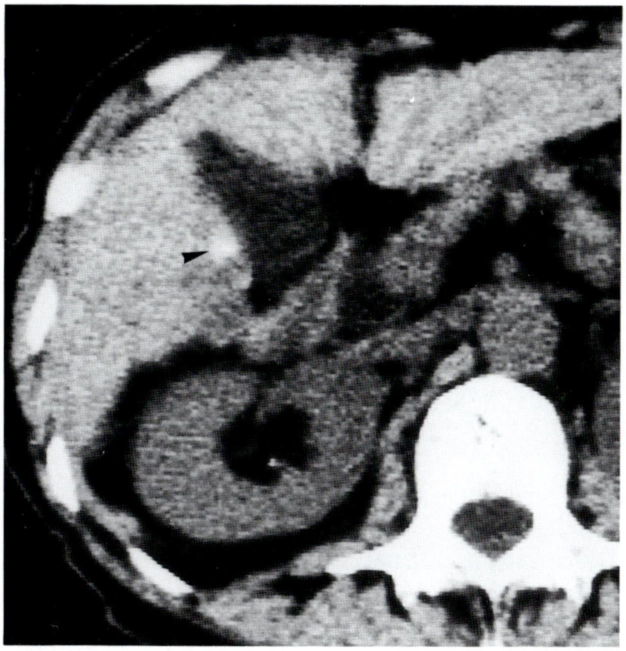

(a) Plain CT: a 7 mm calcific lesion (▶) is seen in S^V near the gallbladder.

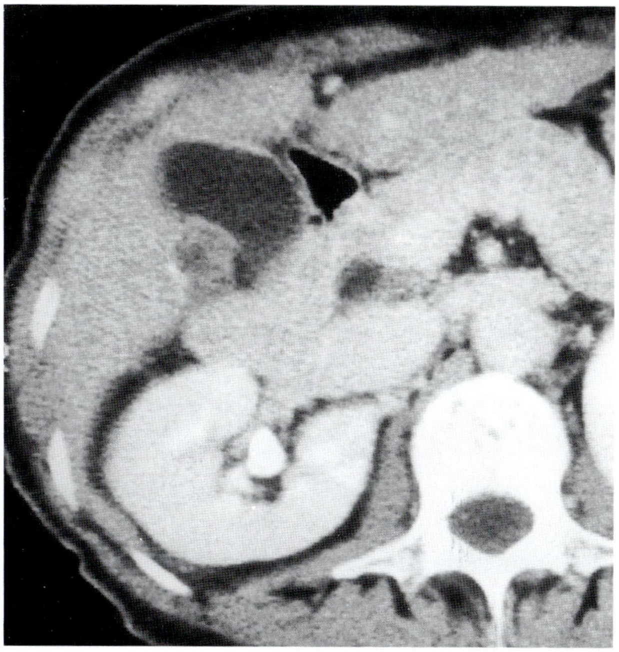

(b) Enhanced CT (late phase): an HCC with internal calcification is seen pushing the wall of the gallbladder.

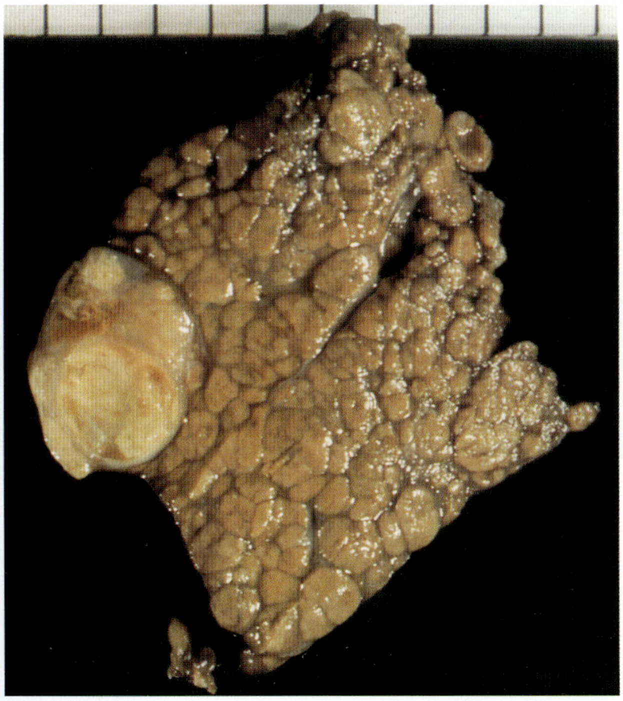

(c) Section of resected specimen: calcification is seen within the tumor. It perhaps developed in a necrotic area along the capsule.

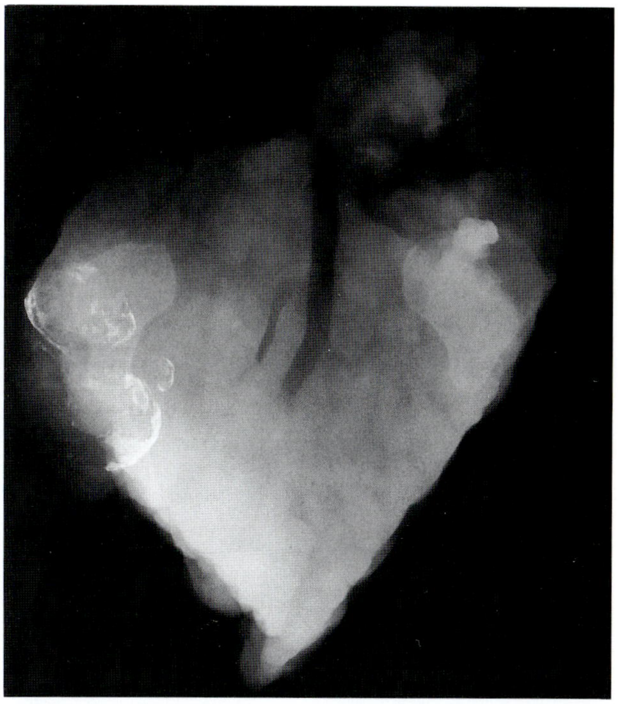

(d) Soft X-ray of resected specimen: calcific rings and plaques are seen in the tumor.

Uncommon HCC—Case 14: HCC producing a fibrosing area with pseudo bile duct proliferation between the liver surface and the mass.

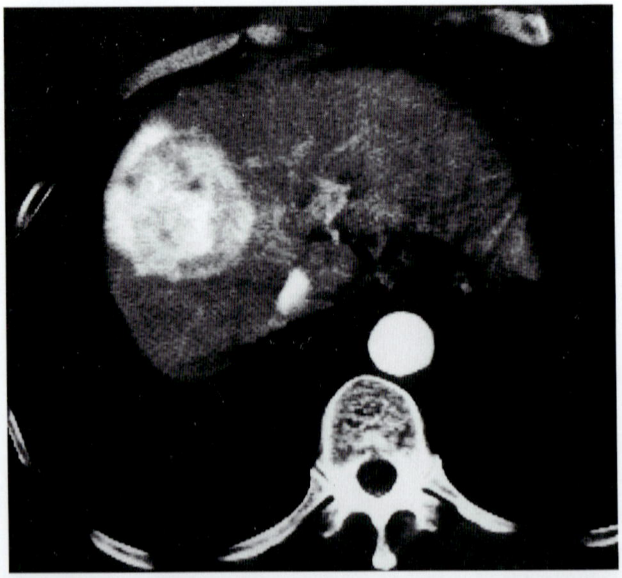

(a) Dynamic CT (early phase): a 4.5 cm strongly stained tumor and a band of tissue also strongly stained are seen in S^{VIII} between the mass and liver capsule.

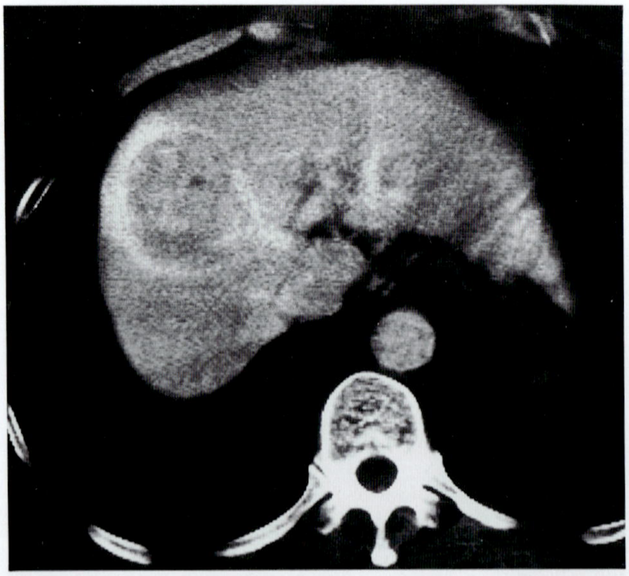

(b) Dynamic CT (25 s later): the interior of the mass has turned iso-dense, but the tumor capsule as well as the subcapsular band area of the liver still remain heavily stained. The appearance of this stain is too late to be produced by an arterio-portal shunt.

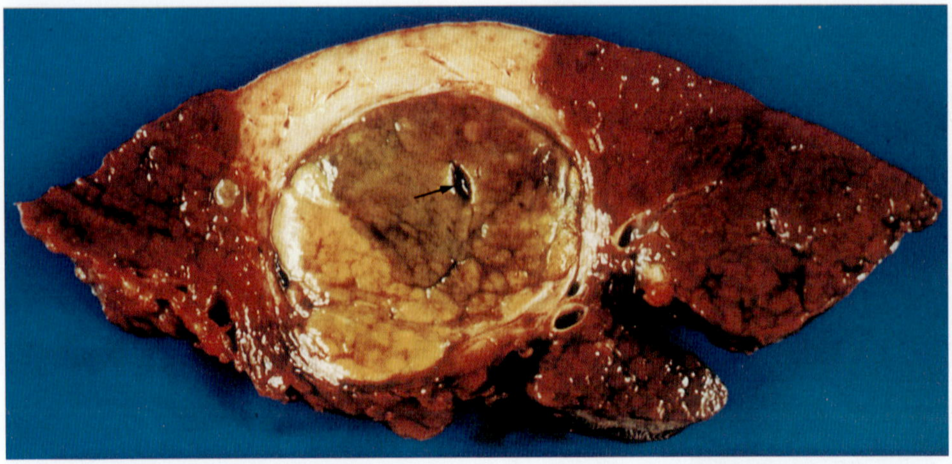

(c) Cut section of resected specimen: a yellowish white tissue is seen toward the liver surface with a slight surface concavity. Histologically, this area consisted of proliferating pseudo bile ducts and increased fibrous tissue. It was assumed that this benign change in this region was due to circulatory disturbances produced by growing and expanding tumor, and a result of reparative reactions to collapse of hepatocytes. →, vascular lake corresponding to low-density spots within the tumor in (a, b).

4.7 Direct invasion of HCC into the surrounding organs

Unlike other cancers, direct invasion into the surrounding organs is very uncommon in HCC.

Invasion into the diaphragm

A large HCC or an HCC arising in the immediate subphrenic region may be supplied by the inferior phrenic artery (Case 1). Resection is usually done for the liver combined with the diaphragm, but direct invasion into the diaphragm is very uncommon when studied histopathologically. The lymph flow going into the thorax through the bare area is scarce (Okuda *et al.* 1976*b*; Magari 1990), and it may perhaps explain such rarity. However, if the immediate subphrenic area of the liver is not opacified by hepatic arteriography, there is a good possibility that the inferior phrenic artery is supplying there (Case 4, p.150).

Invasion into the stomach

The left hepatic lobe and the stomach are anatomically in close proximity, yet direct invasion of HCC of the left lobe into the stomach is very uncommon. If HCC infiltrates into the stomach wall (Case 2), it has to be differentiated from stomach cancer infiltrating into the liver. In the illustrative case in which HCC was resected, the histology was poorly differentiated HCC (Edmondson's grade III-IV) with sarcomatous changes in some part of the mass. The possibility was then discussed that the sarcomatous changes were induced by TAE (Kakizoe *et al.* 1989) and subsequent growth became very invasive.

Others

There are sporadic reports on HCC directly invading into the falciform ligament and gallbladder.

Direct invasion—Case 1: A large HCC in which diaphragmatic invasion was suspected from the tumor supply coming from the inferior phrenic artery.

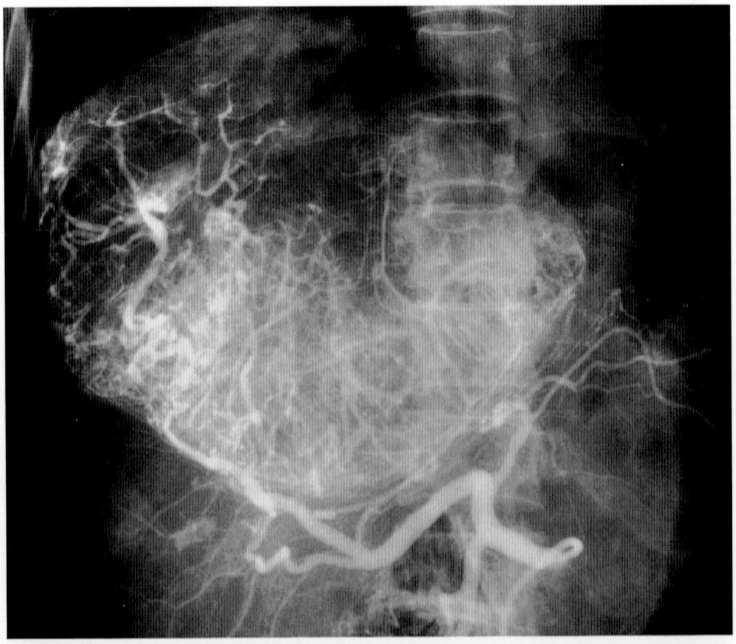

(a) Hepatic arteriography: this huge HCC in its cranial portion was not supplied by the hepatic artery, and it was suspected that the inferior phrenic artery was feeding that area.

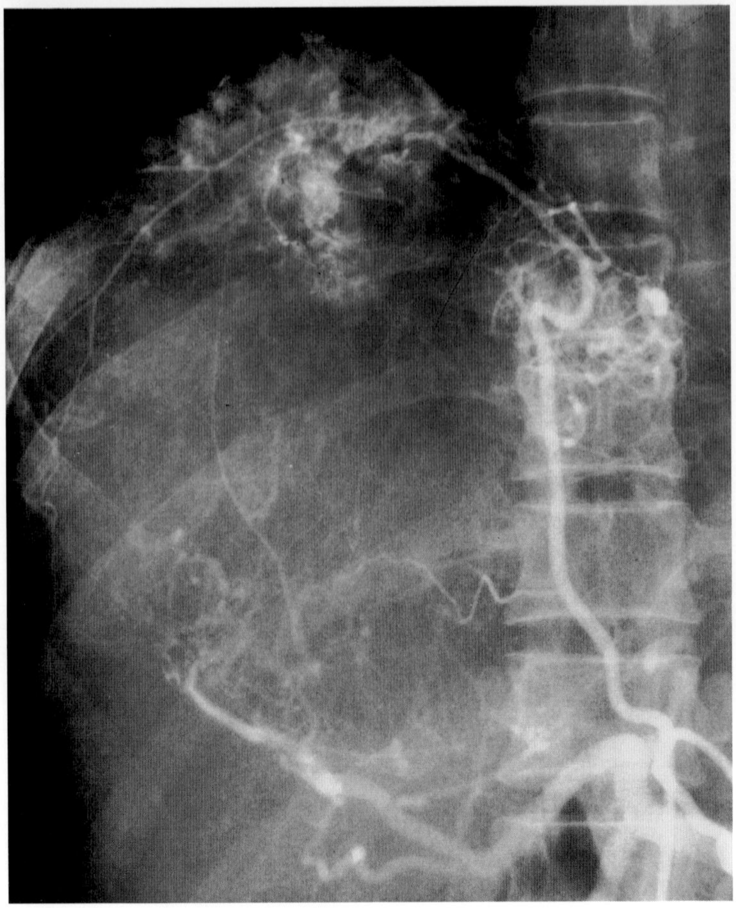

(b) Right inferior phrenic arteriography: the cranial portion of the mass was receiving subphrenic arterial supply, and direct invasion into the diaphragm was suspected. The diaphragm was surgically removed along with the liver, but no direct invasion was recognized on histopathological examination.

Direct invasion—Case 2: Direct invasion of HCC into the stomach wall following repeated TAE. Four sessions of TAE were carried out for an HCC in S^{III}, the left lateral segment. The patient entered the hospital for resection. However, upper GI examination revealed a protruding lesion in the stomach and endoscopy was done.

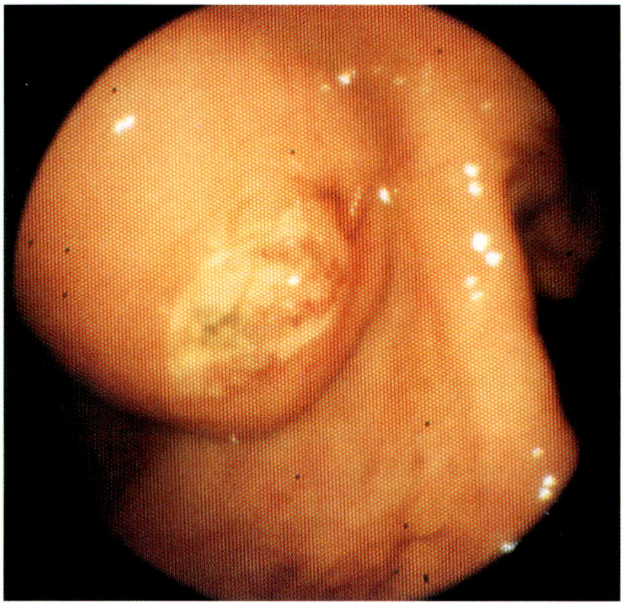

(a) Endoscopy: a protruding submucosal lesion was found in the anterior wall of the antrum; it resembled a submucosal tumor. Biopsy disclosed HCC, and combined left lobectomy and gastrectomy were carried out.

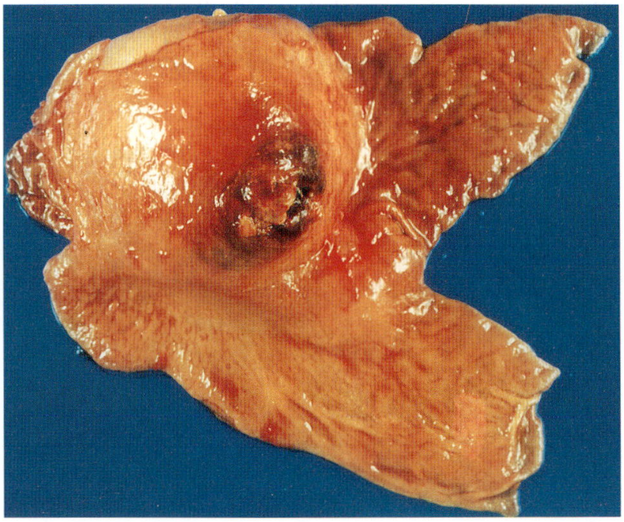

(b) Resected stomach (mucosal surface): tumor is exposed in the center of this protruding lesion.

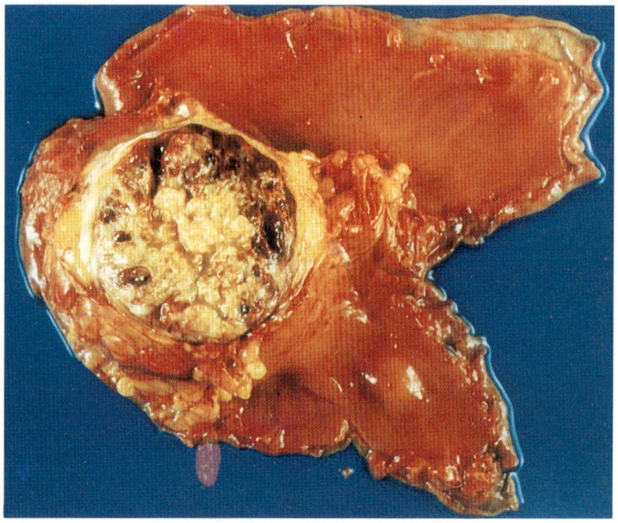

(c) Resected stomach (serosal surface): HCC invasion is seen. TAE had induced necrosis in 75 per cent of the mass.

4.8 Distant metastases of HCC

HCC is one type of cancer in which early lymphatic spread is much less common when compared with stomach and lung cancers. However, in advanced HCC at autopsy, extrahepatic-metastases are seen in 64 per cent, more frequently hematogenous (56 per cent) than lymphatic (27 per cent) (Nakashima *et al.* 1983).

Hematogenous metastasis

In autopsy cases, metastases to the lung, adrenal and bone are common in this decreasing order (Fig. 4.7). Lung metastasis is usually multiple and similar in size (in its early stage) on both sides (coin lesions) (Case 1). Lung metastasis is very frequent in patients with a large HCC, but in those with hepatic vein tumor invasion lung metastasis is much less frequent than expected. Following disappearance of the primary in the liver treated by TAE, the lung lesions spontaneously regress in some reported cases (Itsuji *et al.* 1987), but we have not had such an experience.

Adrenal metastasis in most cases is incidentally discovered at the time of imaging assessment of the primary lesion. It is stained on enhanced CT and angiography as well, like the primary lesion in the liver, showing neovasculature and tumor stain (Takayasu *et al.* 1989*c*) (Case 2). However, in a small adrenal mass of about 2 cm, differential diagnosis from adenomatous hyperplasia of the adrenal is difficult. For the diagnosis, follow-up of the tumor size or CT guided needle biopsy is required. The common site of bone metastases is the spine and rib (Kuhlman *et al.* 1986). Occasional cases may develop a pathologic fracture or a rib pain which will lead to the detection of the primary in the liver (Okazaki *et al.* 1985). Bone lesions may also be found by CT examination done for the assessment of the primary (Case 4). These are osteolytic lesions. When bone metastasis is suspected, ^{99m}Tc-hydroxymethylene diphosphonate bone scintigraphy is recommended as a routine examination.

The other sites of HCC may include the spleen (Case 5) and brain (Case 6).

Lymphatic metastasis

Lymphatic metastasis is relatively uncommon, seen in 27 per cent of autopsy cases (Nakashima *et al.* 1983). This figure is even lower among the patients considered for surgery. The sites of metastasis are in a decreasing order, the hepatic hilum (15 per cent), pancreas head (11 per cent) (Case 7), paraaortic node (8 per cent), etc. and for the diagnosis of mediastinal lymph node metastasis (Case 8), CT excels plain chest x-ray. The node is seen with a discrete peripheral margin (Kakizoe *et al.* 1989), but as the size increases, the interior tends to be necrotized (Araki *et al.* 1988).

Peritoneal dissemination

Unlike adenocarcinoma arising in the abdominal organs, intraabdominal dissemination of HCC is uncommon, and peritoneal carcinomatosis is seldom experienced except in terminal patients. However, growths within the abdominal cavity can occur as a result of spontaneous rupture (Case 9), maneuver during an operation, and needle biopsy in which a cluster of cancer cells has been spread within the free abdominal cavity. Cancer cells settling on the peritoneum lead to tumor growth.

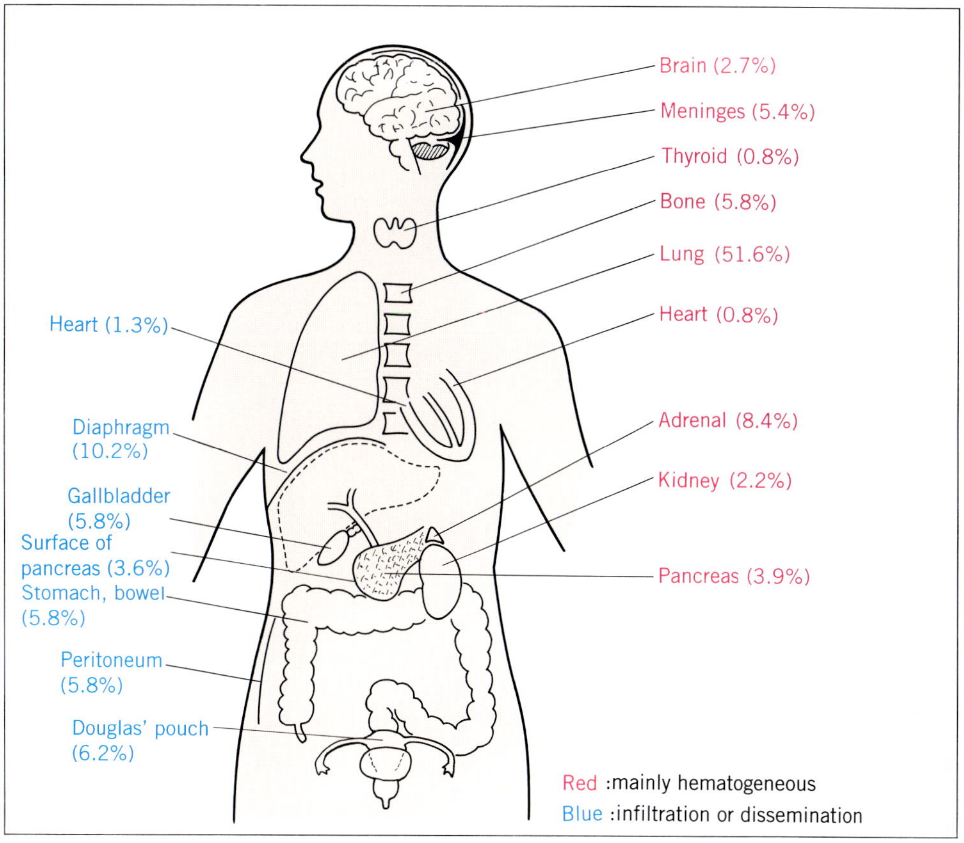

Fig. 4.7 The organs and frequencies with which hematogenous metastases and infiltration or dissemination were seen at autopsy (n = 225) according to Nakashima *et al.* (1983).

Distant metastasis—Case 3: Adenomatous hyperplasia of the adrenal incidentally found in association with HCC.

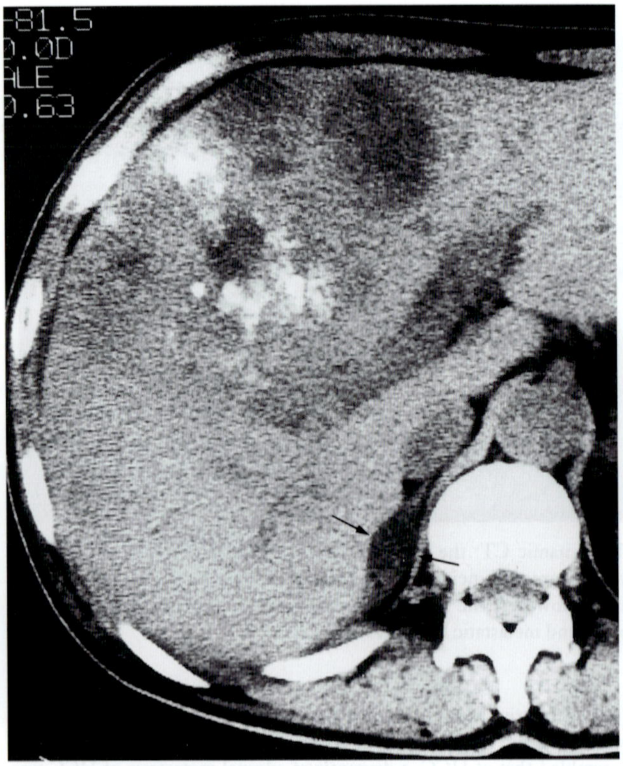

(a) Plain CT: a large HCC with Lipiodol retention is seen occupying both lobes. At the time of imaging examination, a 2 cm adrenal mass (→) was found. The density is much lower than the one in Case 2.

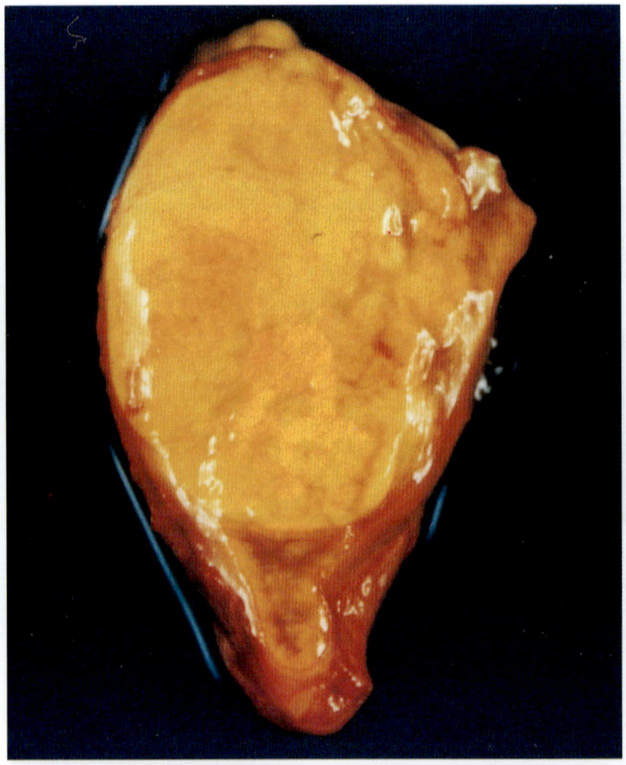

(b) Cut section of the resected adrenal: resection of HCC and the right adrenal was carried out. The cut surface of the adrenal showed a homogeneous tumor growing laterally from the original adrenal gland. Histologically, this was adenomatous hyperplasia without a malignant feature.

Distant metastasis—Case 4: Vertebral metastasis of HCC.

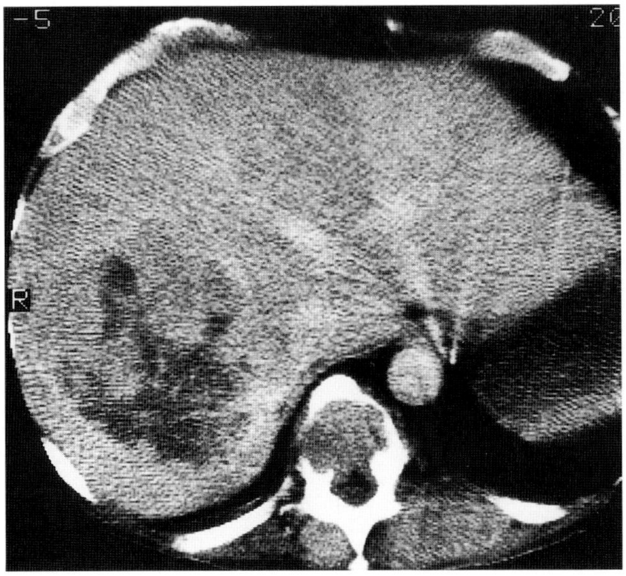

(a) Enhanced CT: an osteolytic lesion was incidentally discovered in the vertebra and the planned operation was called off.

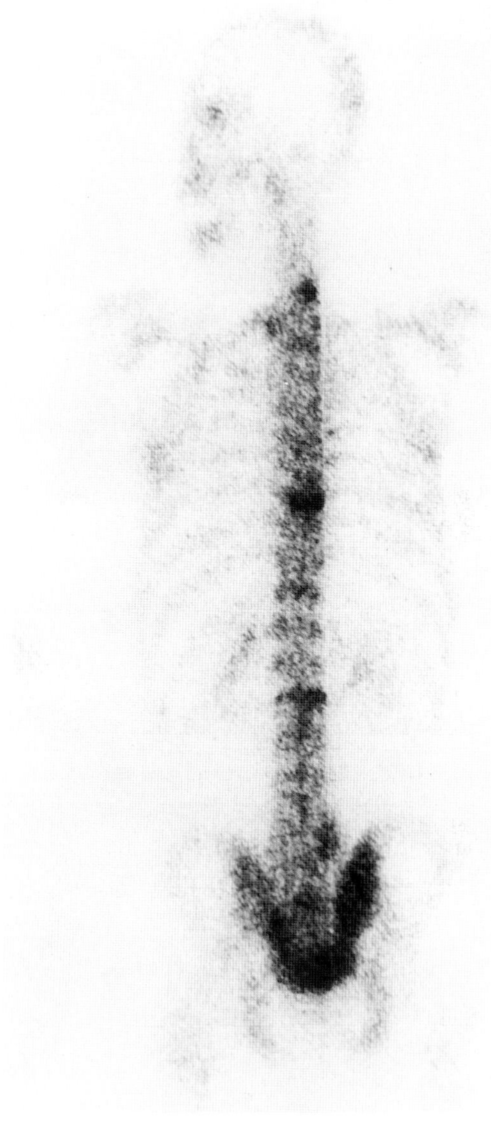

(b) Bone scintiscan: on this bone scan made with ^{99m}Tc-hydroxymethylene diphosphonate (posterior view), multiple accumulations of activities are seen along the vertebral column which were diagnosed as bone metastases (different case from (a)).

Distant metastasis—Case 5: Splenic metastases of HCC.

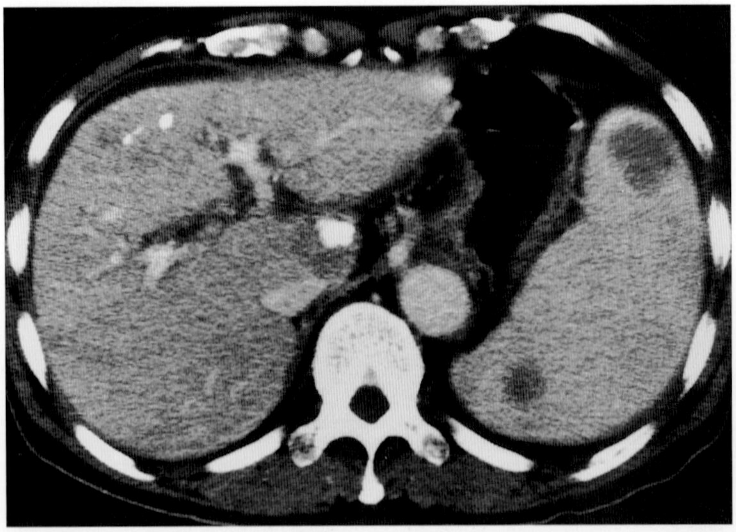

Enhanced CT: during the treatment of primary HCC in the left caudate lobe (a low-density mass with Lipiodol retention in one part), mutiple lesions were found in the spleen. Splenic metastasis of HCC is uncommon, and splenic metastasis rarely causes significant symptoms because of the pre-existing splenomegaly.

Distant metastasis—Case 6: Brain metastasis of HCC.

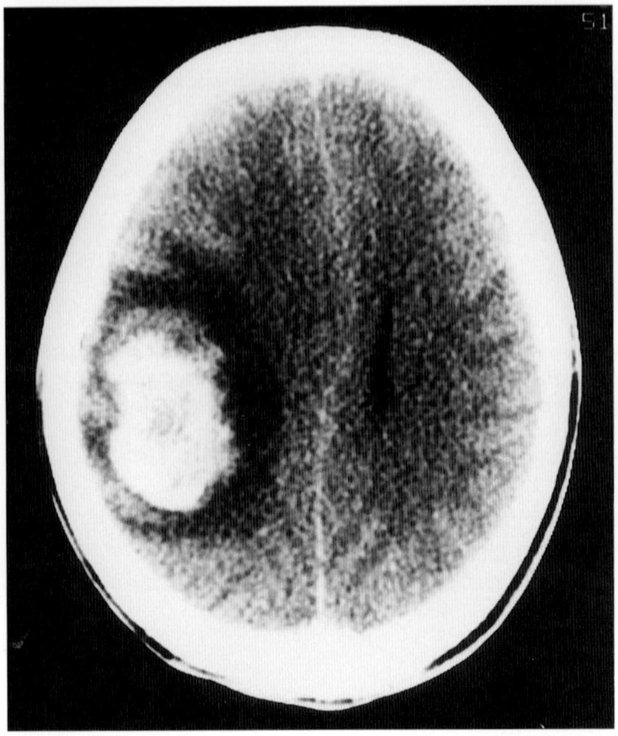

Plain CT of the brain: during the treatment of HCC complicating Budd–Chiari syndrome, the patient suddenly developed left hemiplegia. Plain CT of the head demonstrated a 5 cm high-density mass in the right hemisphere with surrounding edema and deviation of the cerebral falx to the left. It was removed by operation and found to be HCC. There was a large hematoma surrounding the mass. Brain metatasis of HCC is commonly hemorrhagic.

Distant metastasis—Case 7: Survival for more than 3 years after resection of primary HCC in the liver and parapancreatic lymph node metastasis.

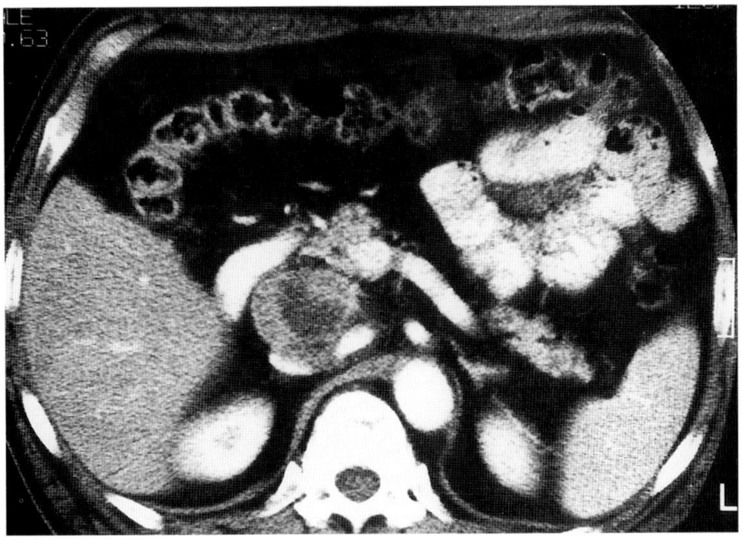

(a) Dynamic CT: on dynamic CT, a 4.5 cm round mass was seen between the pancreas head and inferior vena cava in addition to a 3 cm primary in S^{VI} (not shown). From the smooth boundary with expanding growth and an irregularly shaped low density in the interior, a diagnosis of lymph node metastasis of HCC was made. Both were removed by operation.

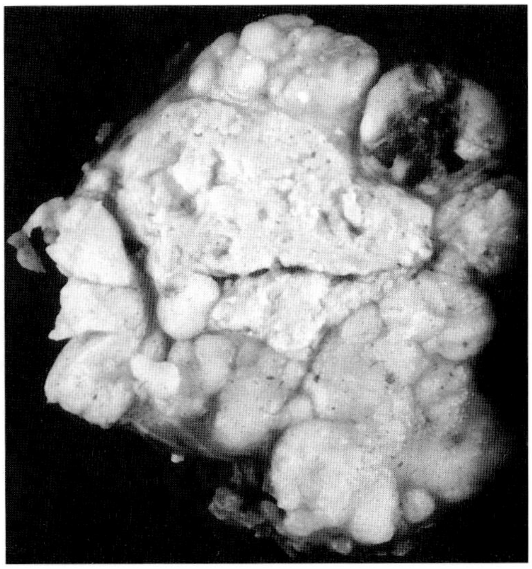

(b) Cut section of the removed lymph node: the primary was necrotic in large part as a result of TAE, and was Edmondson's grade III–IV, poorly differentiated. The tumor in the node was a combined form producing both AFP and CEA. The patient is well after 3 years after the operation.

Distant metastasis—Case 8: Mediastinal metastasis of HCC.

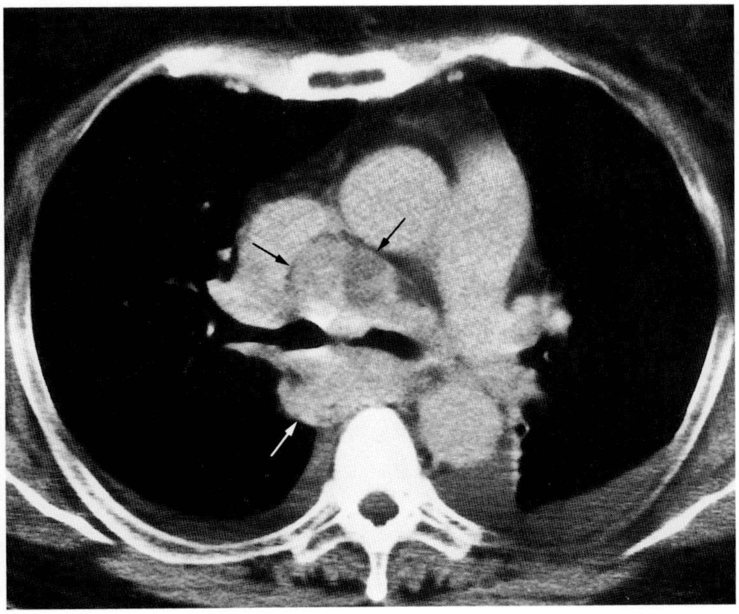

Enhanced CT: the primary in the liver was under control with repeated TAE. During the course, the patient developed an uncontrollable cough, and CT examination of the chest disclosed multiple lymph node metastases (→) behind the ascending aorta compressing upon the trachea. Accumulation of a small amount of pleural fluid is also seen.

Distant metastasis—Case 9: Intraabdominal spread of HCC that followed rupture of the tumor. The primary was resected following spontaneous rupture. The patient came to the hospital 6 months later with a mass in the left abdomen.

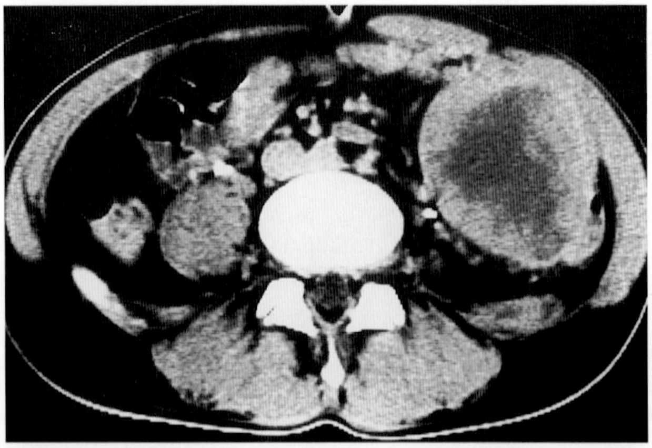

(a) Enhanced CT: an 8 cm stainable mass was found in the left side of the abdomen. The interior is not enhanced because of necrosis.

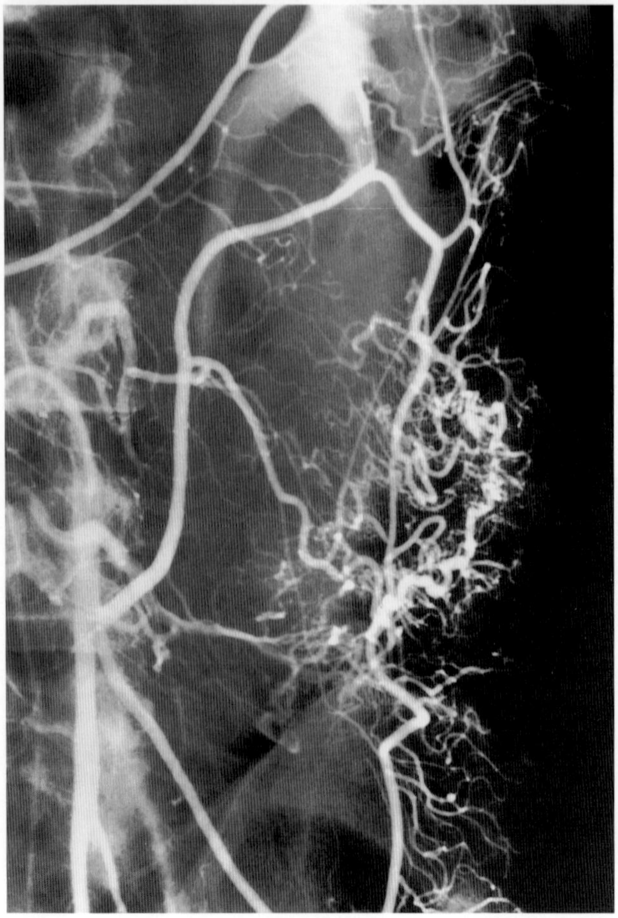

(b) Inferior mesenteric arteriography (early phase): a mass supplied by this artery is recognized. No encasement of the vessel is seen; this is common in the case of alimentary tract cancer.

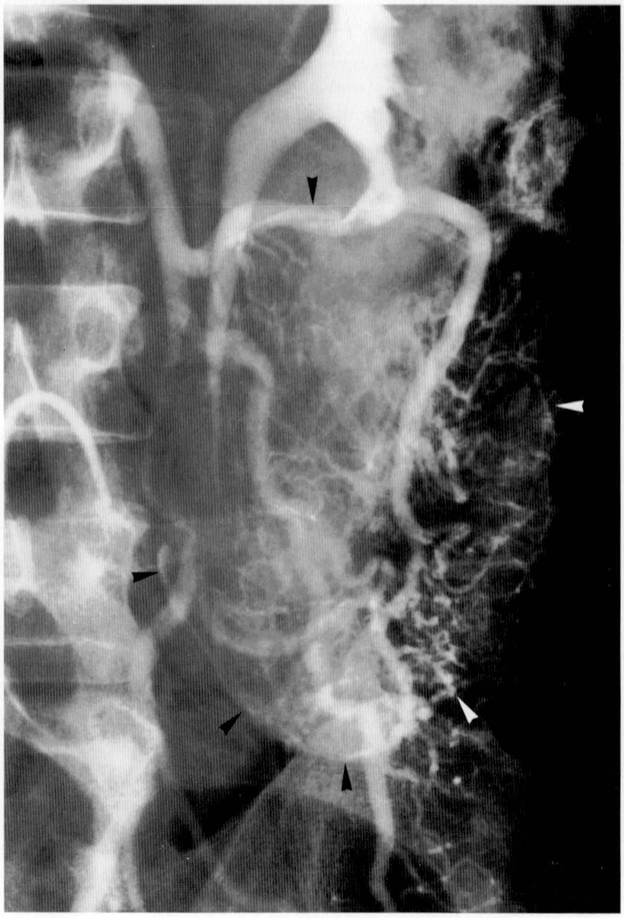

(c) Inferior mesenteric arteriography (late phase): tumor stain and dilated veins were demonstrated, and a further operation was carried out. ▶, tumor silhouette. The mass was diagnosed as an intra-abdominal metastasis.

4.9 Bile duct carcinoma

Bile duct carcinoma is a cancer composed of cells resembling those of biliary epithelium. It is usually divided into 'intrahepatic' and 'extrahepatic' depending on the site of origin. In Japan, the former is defined as a cancer situated further within the liver from the right and left hepatic ducts. In strict anatomical terms, both hepatic ducts and bifurcation are extrahepatic. Intrahepatic bile duct carcinoma is also called cholangio- or cholangiocellular carcinoma (Leevy *et al.* 1976). Some surgeons call extrahepatic bile duct carcinoma 'cholangiocarcinoma', creating a semantic problem. The old term 'cholangioma' coined by Yamagiwa (1911) is no longer used, because it was a counterpart of 'hepatoma' which was a cause of subsequent confusion. In 1965 Klatskin called attention to a bile duct carcinoma which arises at the hilum, causes obstructive jaundice despite its small size, and in which biliary decompression markedly alleviates clinical symptoms. Subsequently hilar carcinoma came to be called 'Klatskin tumor'. Since this cancer spreads along the bile ducts toward the liver parenchyma as well as extrahepatically to form a mass in the hilum, the exact site of origin is seldom determined even by surgery. Therefore, in the clinical setting, separation of hilar carcinoma into intraheptic and extahepatic bile duct carcinomas is difficult. Edmondson and Steiner (1960) included hilar carcinoma in primary liver cancer. For practical reasons, Okuda *et al.* (1977*b*) separated intrahepatic bile duct carcinomas into the peripheral and hilar types, because the clinical presentation and features are quite different. With the recent progress in imaging diagnosis, small cholangiocarcinoma arising in the hepatic duct or a subsegment bile duct has come to be detected (Zeman *et al.* 1980). Cholangiocarcinoma is much less common than HCC, comprising 5 per cent to 10 per cent of primary hepatic malignancies (Sugihara and Kojiro 1987).

Peripheral type cholangiocarcinoma (intrahepatic bile duct carcinoma)

This type of bile duct carcinoma usually shows features characteristic of adenocarcinoma, readily differentiated from HCC or hemangioma by imaging (Fig. 4.8). Histopathologically, however, distinction from metastatic adenocarcinoma is not always easy. In the cut surface, the tumor periphery makes an irregular wavy border with the noncancer parenchyma and bulges somewhat because there are more viable cancer cells. The interior is frequently firm with more fibrous tissue and is slightly depressed from the periphery (Case 1). If the tumor is located near the capsule, cancer umbilication (depression) is commonly recognized. US of the periphery type of cholangiocarcinoma shows an irregular boundary with a thick halo (63 per cent in our experience) and inhomogeneous interior echoes (60 per cent). On plain CT, it is seen as an irregular low-density mass; in the early phase of enhanced CT, the tumor periphery is stained mildly, and in the late phase a peripheral low-density area with a high-density center is seen (Choi *et al.* 1988) just like a metastatic adenocarcinoma (Muramatsu *et al.* 1986). The

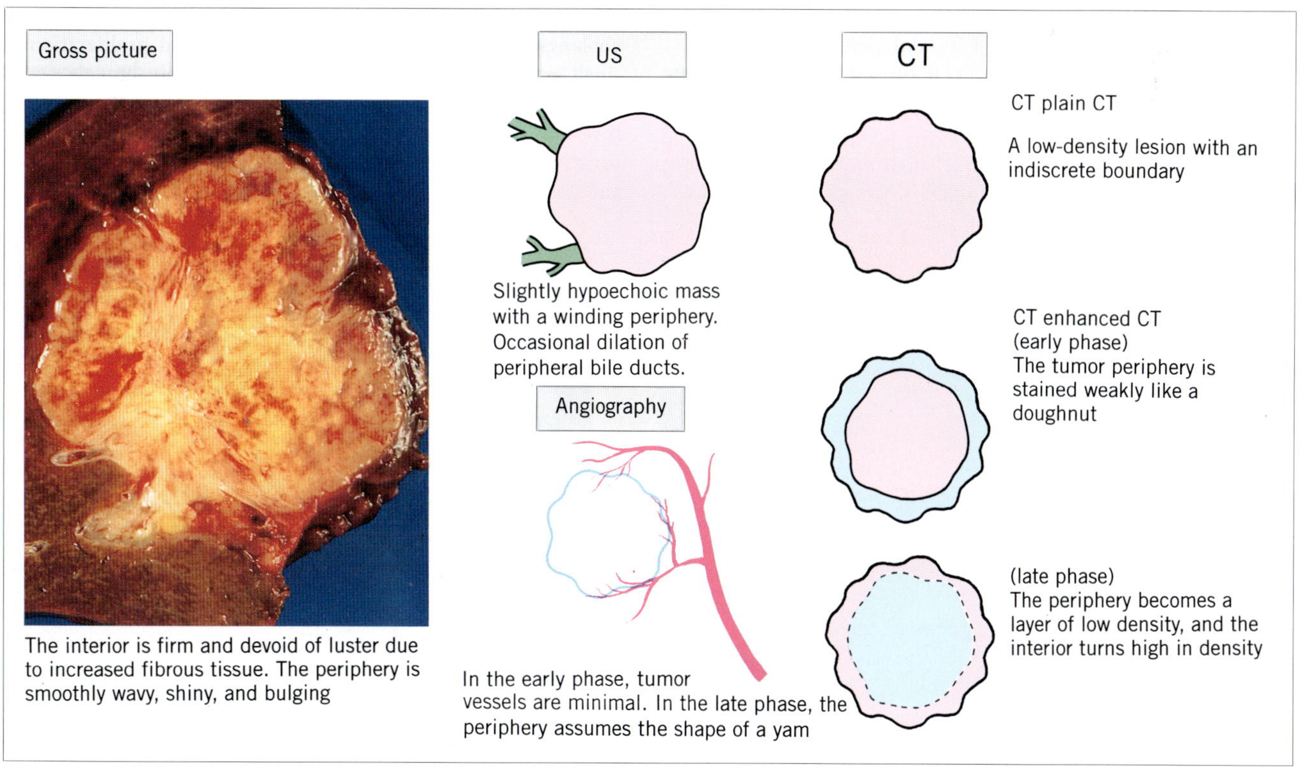

Fig. 4.8 Imaging features of cholangiocarcinoma.

Case 1 (contd.)

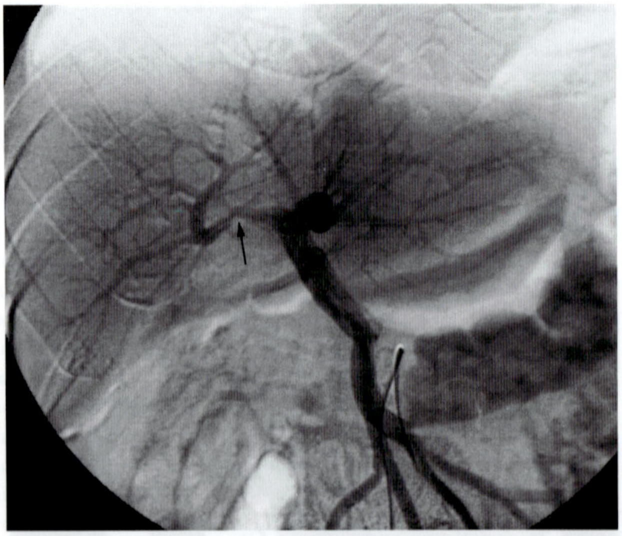

(e) Superior mesenteric arterial portogram: a marked stenosis is seen in the first-order right portal vein and the beginning of the right posterior segment branch is about to close (→). The anterior segment branch is already occluded and not opacified. This kind of infiltrative feature is not seen in HCC, and is characteristic of adenocarcinomas including cholangiocarcinoma.

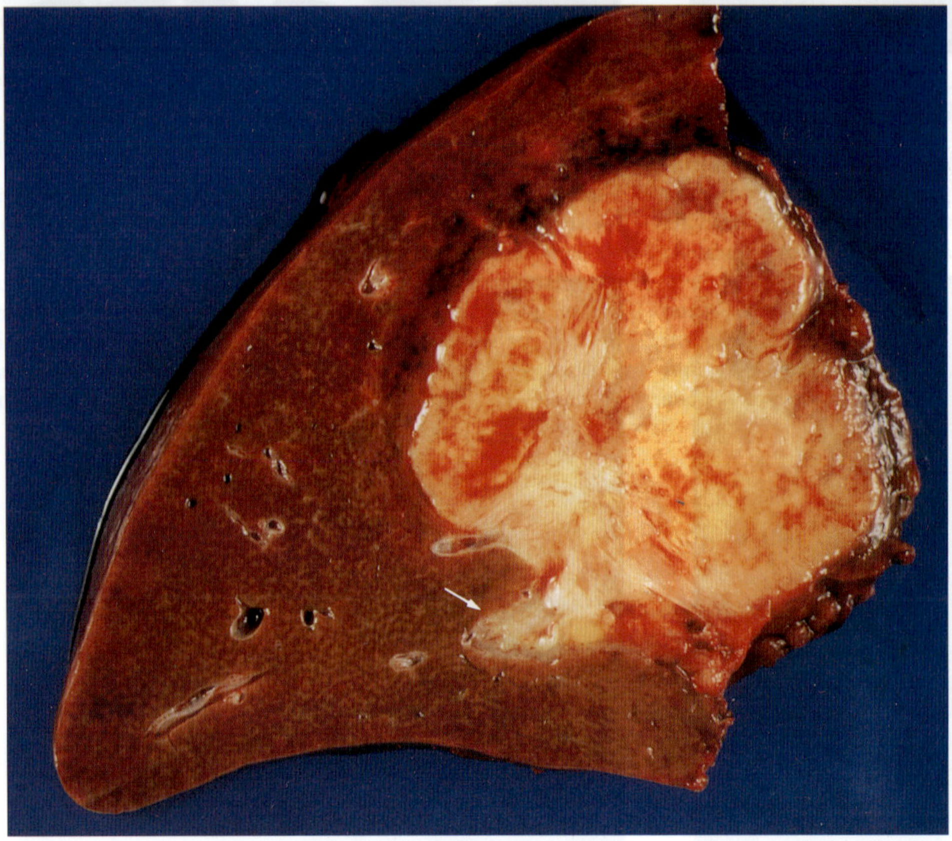

(f) Cut section of resected liver: extended right lobectomy was carried out. The interior of the mass in its section is firm with fibrosis, and the periphery is slightly bulging (with viable cancer cells) and shiny. →, the portal tract going to the right posterior segment. It is occluded by tumor invasion.

Bile duct carcinoma—Case 2: Peripheral type cholangiocarcinoma that showed a peripheral low density on late enhanced CT.

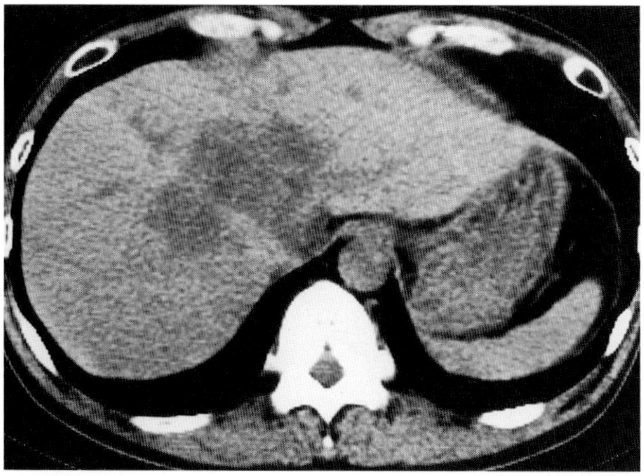

(a) Plain CT: a low-density mass with an irregular border is seen in the middle of the liver.

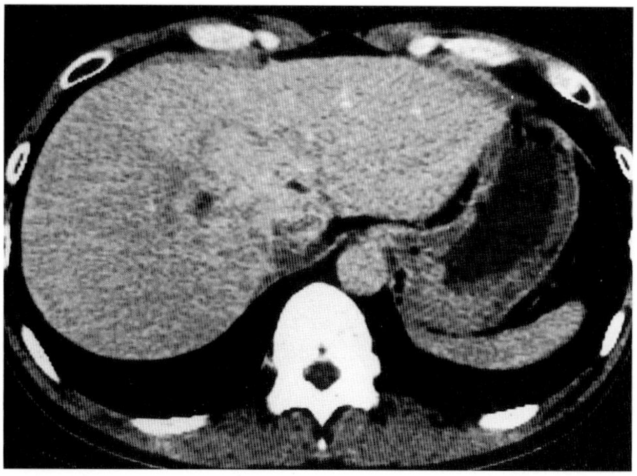

(b) Enhanced CT (late phase): the interior is mildly enhanced and the periphery is seen as a low-density ring. The yam-shaped contour makes a likely diagnosis of adenocarcinoma. Since no primary was found elsewhere, cholangiocarcinoma (peripheral type) was strongly suspected. Needle biopsy showed adenocarcinoma histologically. However, due to invasion of the inferior vena cava and major hepatic veins, surgery was not indicated.

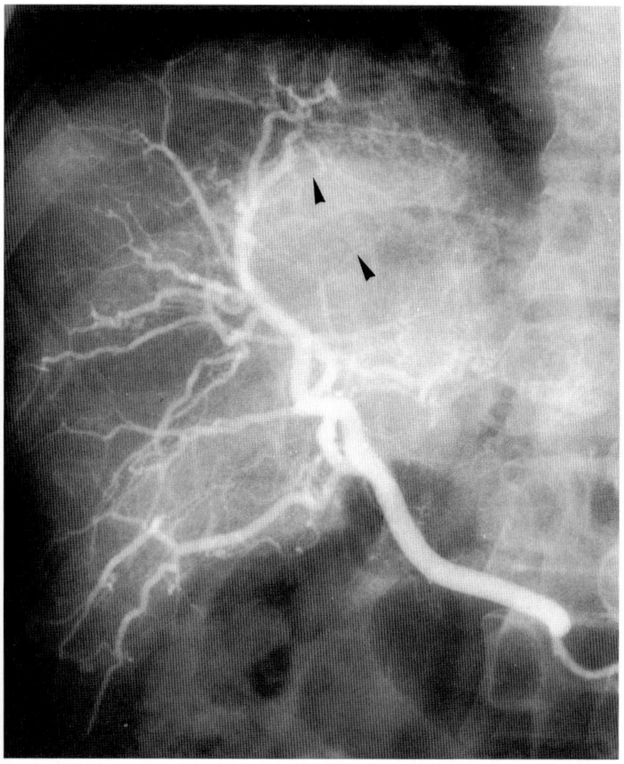

(c) Right hepatic arteriogram: a tumor stain is seen in $S^{VIII}{}_{d}$, to $S^{VII}{}_{b}$, with encasements and interruptions of peripheral arteries (▶).

Bile duct carcinoma—Case 3: Papillary infiltrating cholangiocarcinoma of the peripheral type producing localized dilatation of the peripheral bile duct seen on enhanced CT.

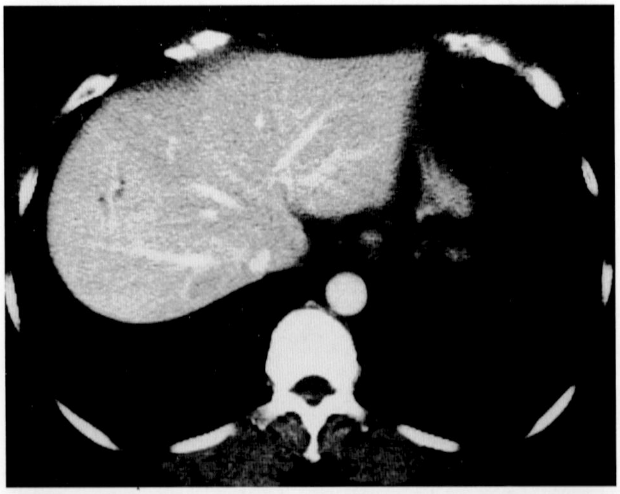

1

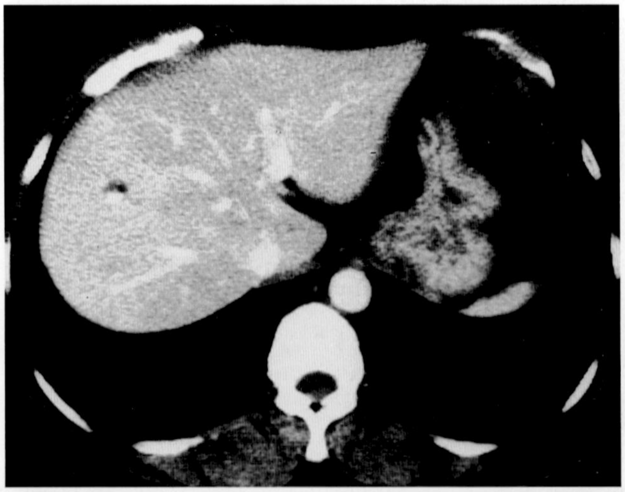

2

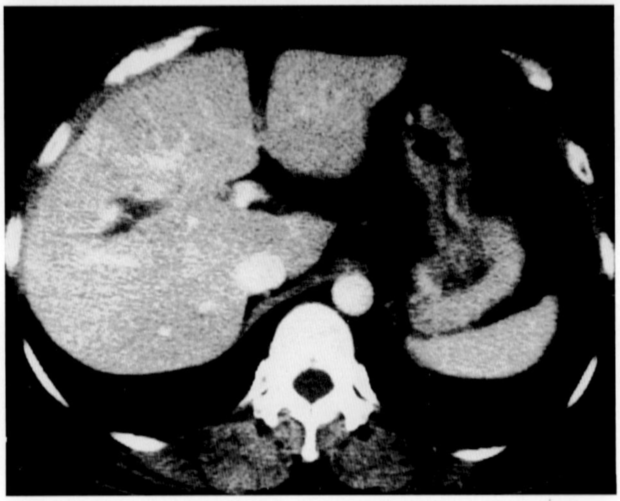

3

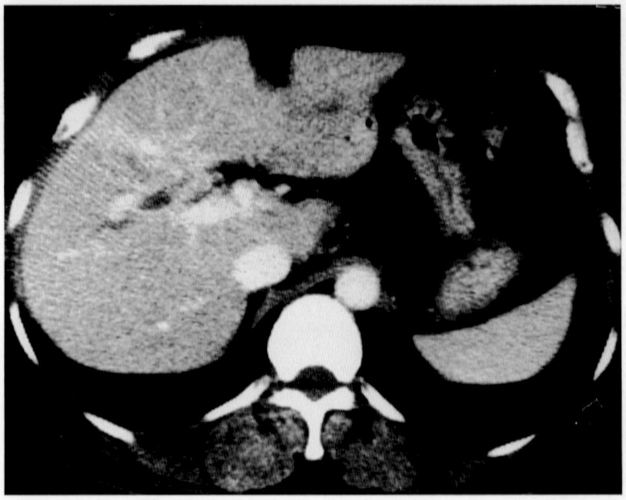

4

a

(a) Dynamic CT (cranial to caudal): dynamic CT was carried out with the table incremental technique demonstrated a localized dilatation of $B^{VIII–V}$ duct. The mass is obscure.

(b) Hepatic arteriogram: tumor vessels are seen along arterial branches, A^{V} (→), but the mass was not delineated.

(c) Opacification of the right hepatic duct by needle puncture cholangiography: a filling defect is seen in the bifurcation and the right hepatic duct. The diagnosis was a protruding lesion with an irregular surface.

(d) Cut section of resected specimen: right lobectomy combined with resection of major bile ducts was carried out. A papillary tumor growing in the right hepatic duct was found. There was periductal invasion along the duct B^{V} (→). They were thought to correspond to angiographic changes.

Case 3 (contd.)

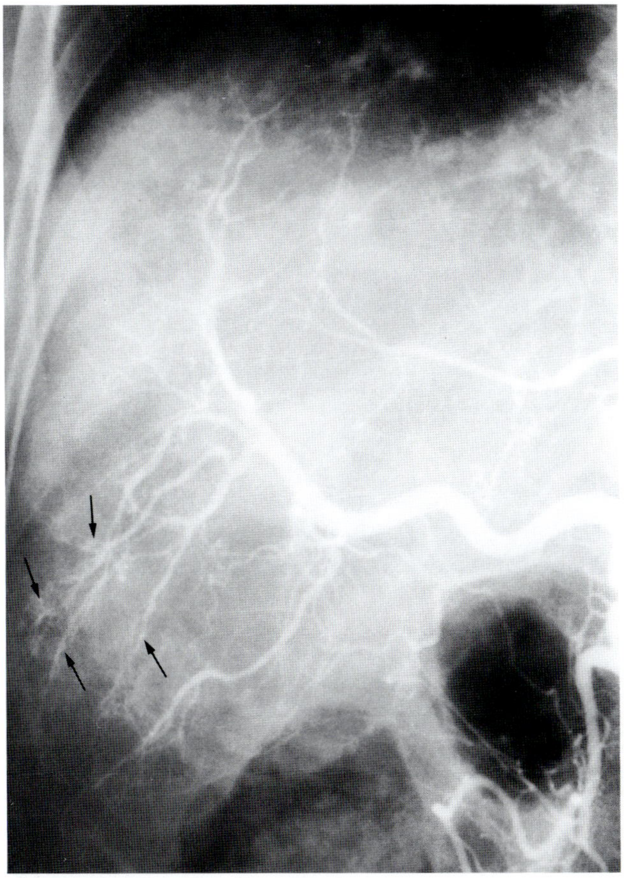

b

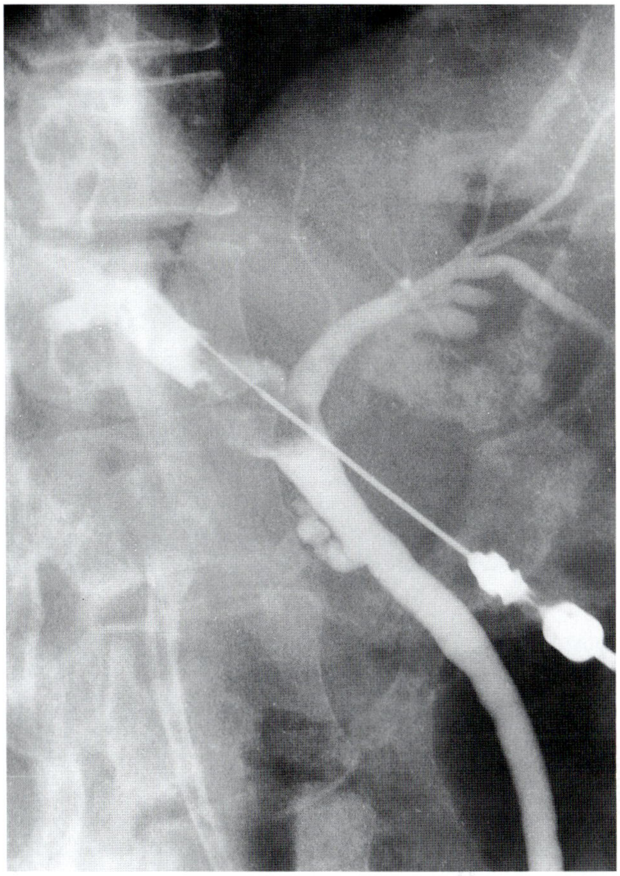

c

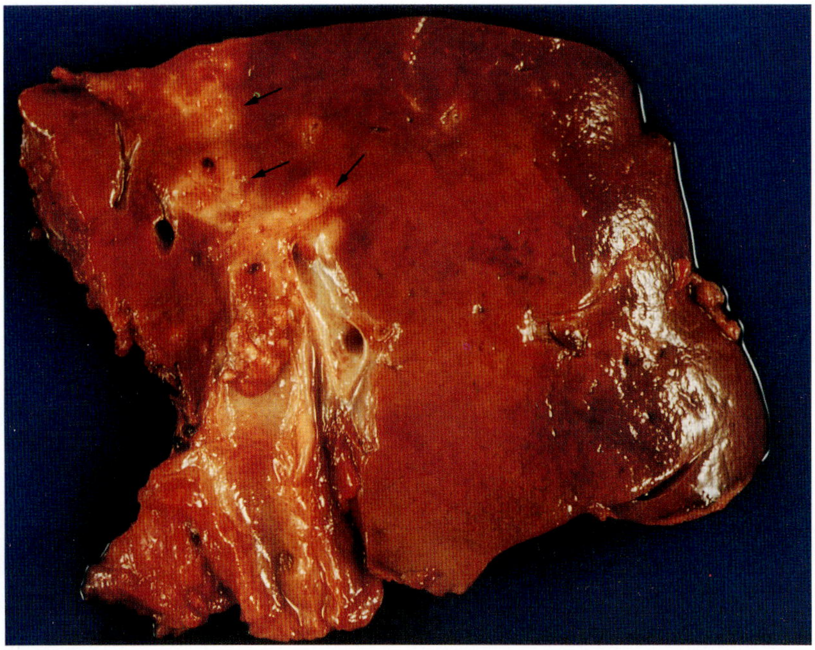

d

Bile duct carcinoma—Case 4: Hilar bile duct carcinoma producing marked atrophy of the right anterior segment.

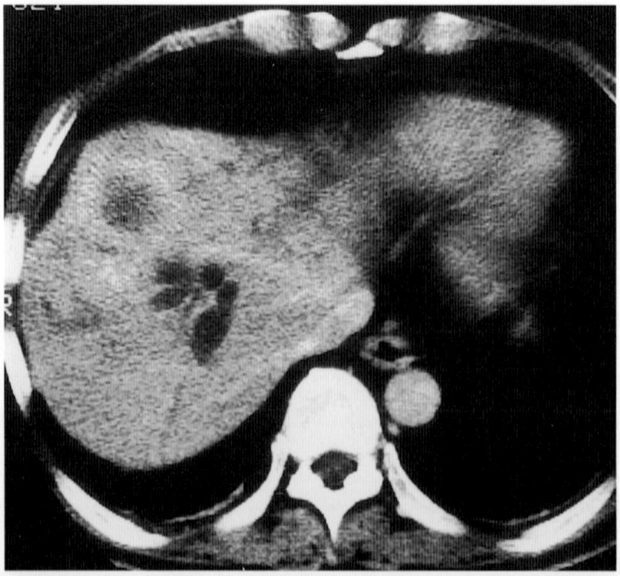

1

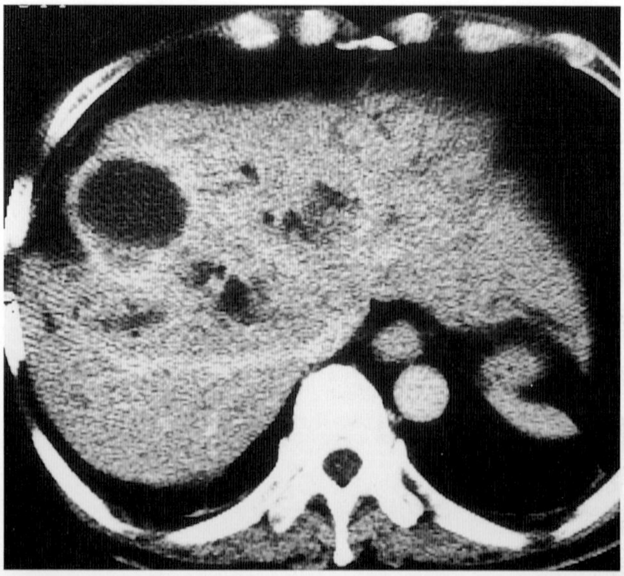

2

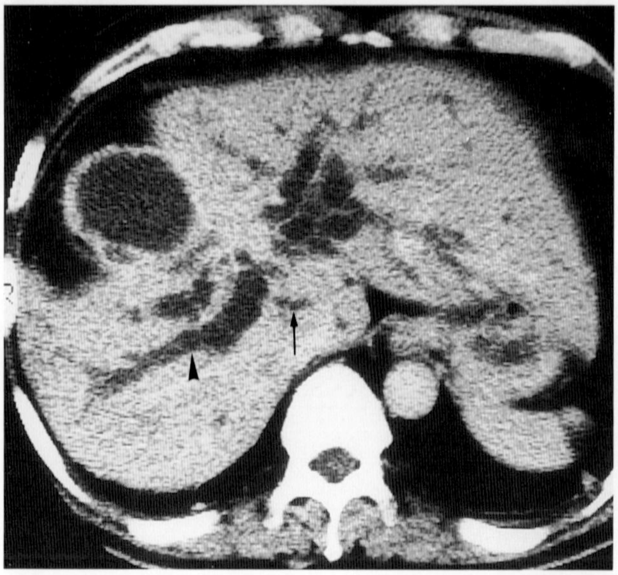

3

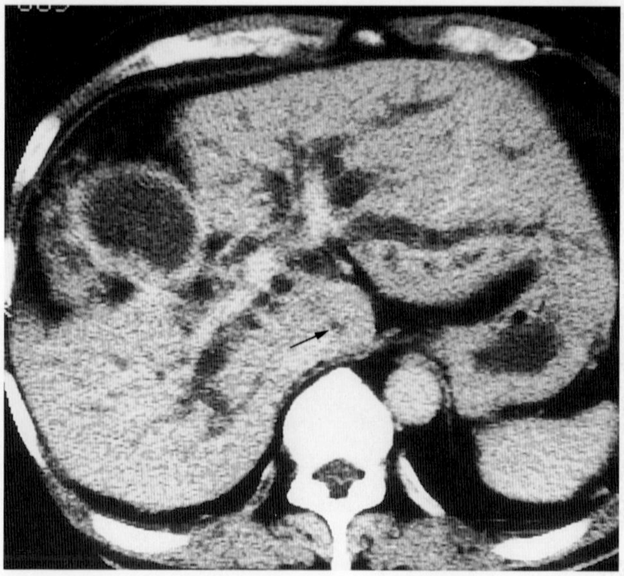

4

(a) Dynamic CT: dynamic CT with the table incremental method demonstrated marked biliary dilatation in both lobes (1–4), and atrophy of the anterior segment, particularly S^{VIII}, with a cranial shift of the gallbladder. Bile duct dilatation in the caudate lobe (→) was also marked. ▶, B^{V}.

Case 4 (contd.)

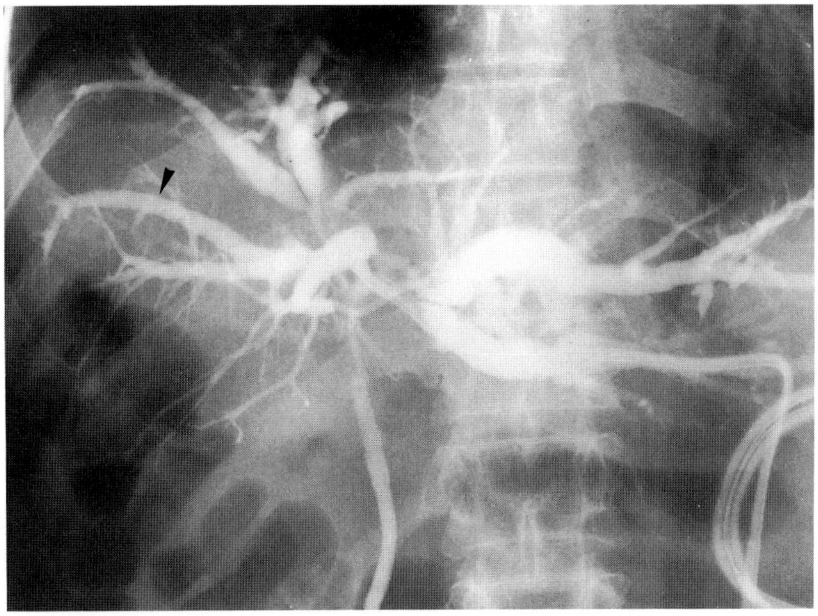

(b) Cholangiography through PTCD tube: the right and left hepatic ducts demonstrated by separated PTCD tubes are almost closed, and the common hepatic duct also stenosed. ▶, B^{V}.

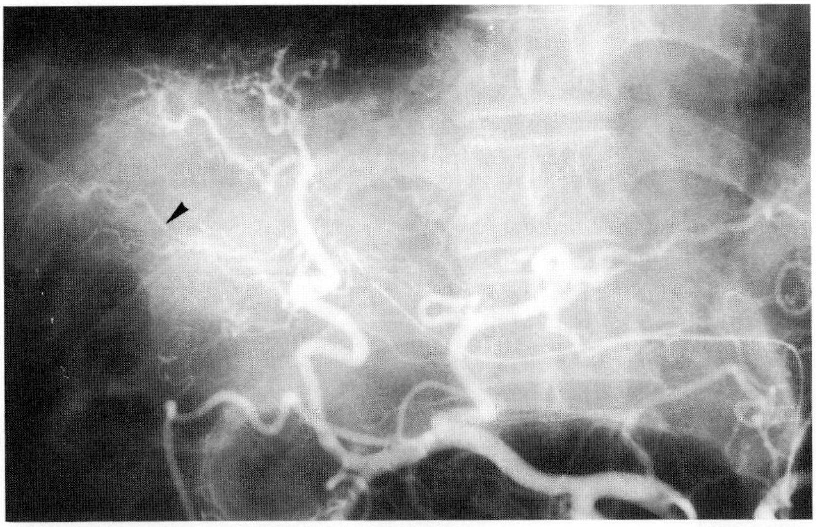

(c) Angiography (arterial phase): an intrahepatic arterial branch runs along the bile duct. ▶, A^{V}.

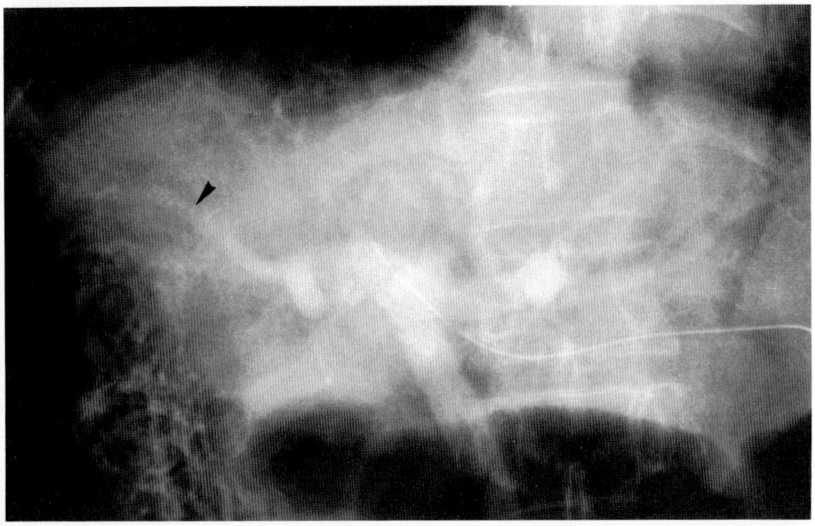

(d) Superior mesenteric arterial portogram: the portal vein supplying S^{VIII} is not opacified due to occlusion. ▶, P^{V}.

On opening the abdomen, the hilum was seen occupied by a cancer mass which could not be removed. The anterior segment of the right lobe was markedly atrophied.

Bile duct carcinoma—Case 5: Anicteric hilar bile duct carcinoma with dilated caudate lobe bile ducts.

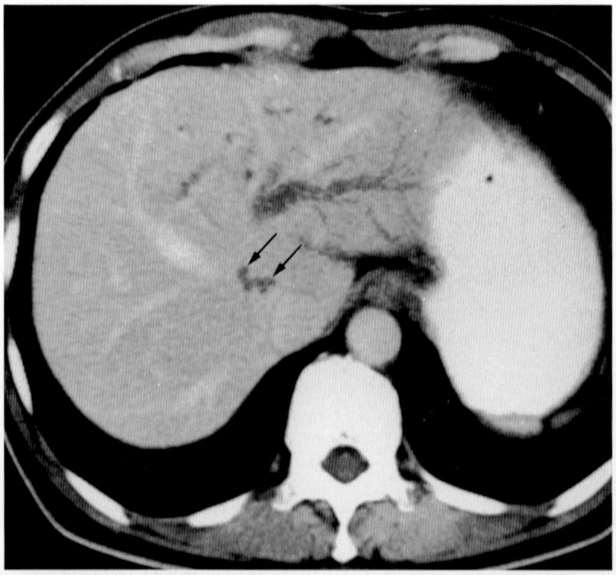

(a) Enhanced CT: dilatation of the bile ducts in the left lobe and of the caudate lobe ducts to the right of the inferior vena cava is recognized.

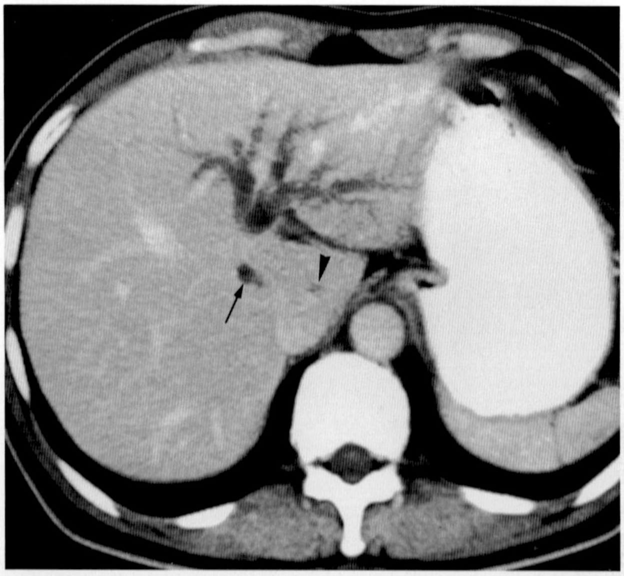

(b) Enhanced CT [slice 1 cm caudal from (a)]: dilated caudate lobe ducts (→) to the right of the inferior vena cava join to form a more dilated duct. A dilated small duct (▶) is also seen in the left caudate lobe. The diagnosis was occlusion of the left hepatic duct central to the confluence of the ducts of the right and left caudate lobes.

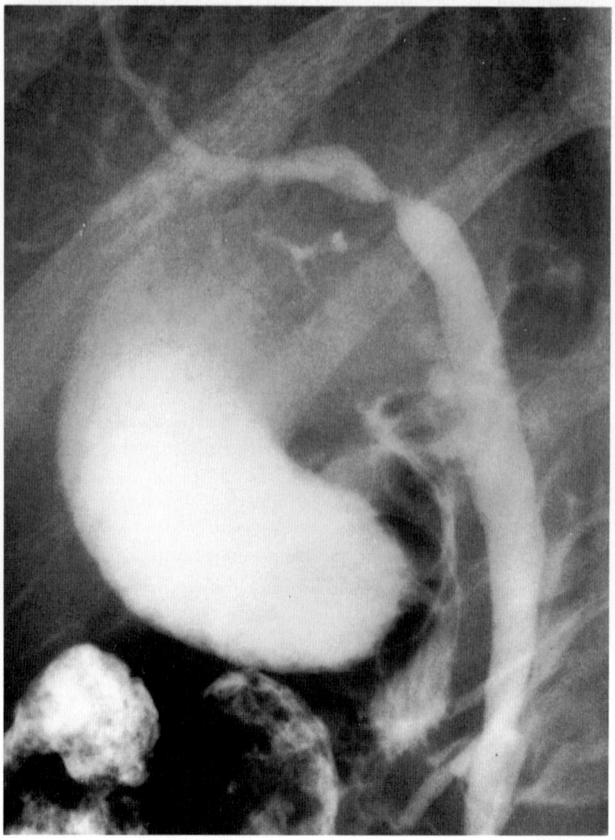

(c) ERC: the left bile duct is not opacified, and a marked stenosis is obvious at the bifurcation.

Considering these findings, there was a strong possibility that caudate lobe bile ducts were branching off the left hepatic duct. However, since the right hepatic duct was also stenosed, occlusion at the opening of the right caudate lobe duct could not be denied. Careful interpretation of enhanced CT images is important in the preoperative assessment as it provides accurate information on caudate lobe bile ducts.

Bile duct carcinoma—Case 6: Hilar bile duct carcinoma causing complete obstruction of the right portal vein and compensatory hypertrophy of the contralateral lobe.

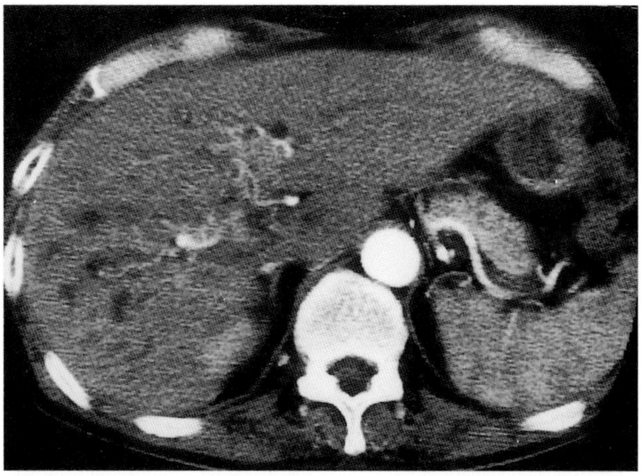

1

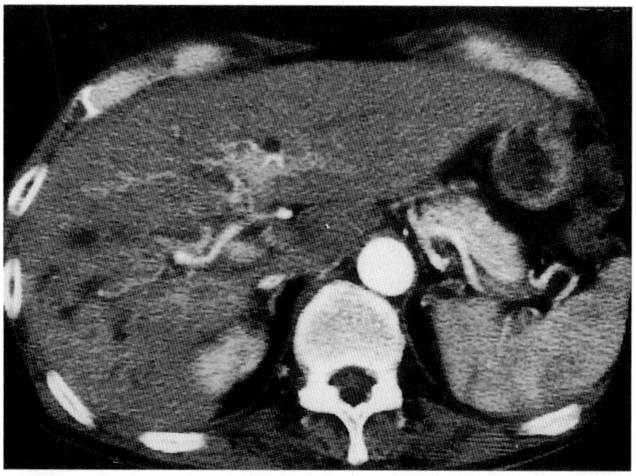

2

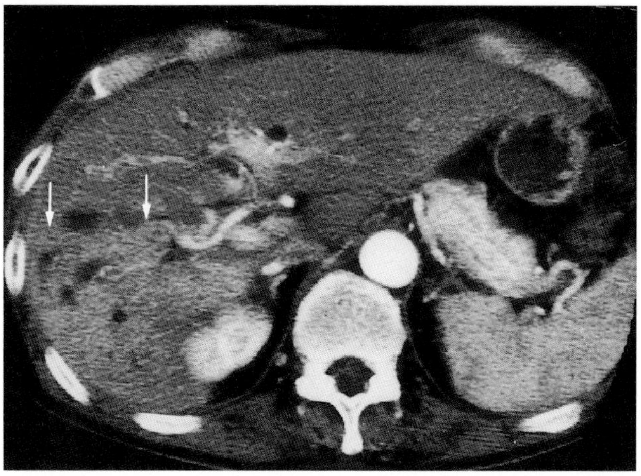

3

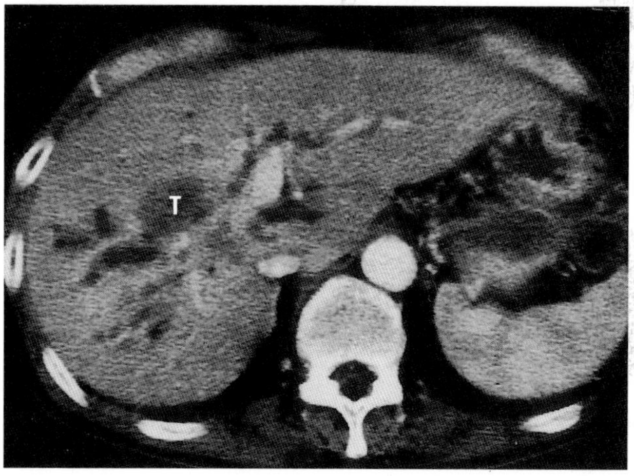

4

(a) Dynamic CT: bile duct dilatation of both lobes and lobar attenuation difference (→) (3) are recognized. The right lobe is atrophied and compensatory hypertrophy of the left lobe is also apparent. A main hypovascular mass (T) (4) is seen to the right of the hilum.

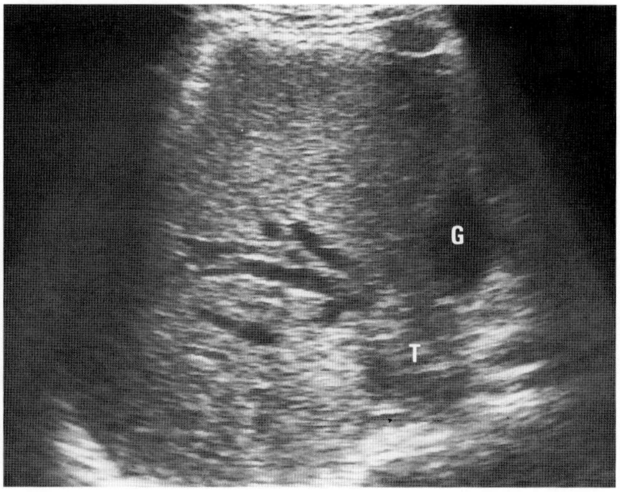

(b) US (right intercostal scan): dilatation of the bile ducts in the right anterior segment and a hypoechoic mass (T) of an irregular periphery is seen central to biliary dilatation. G, gallbladder.

Case 6 (contd.)

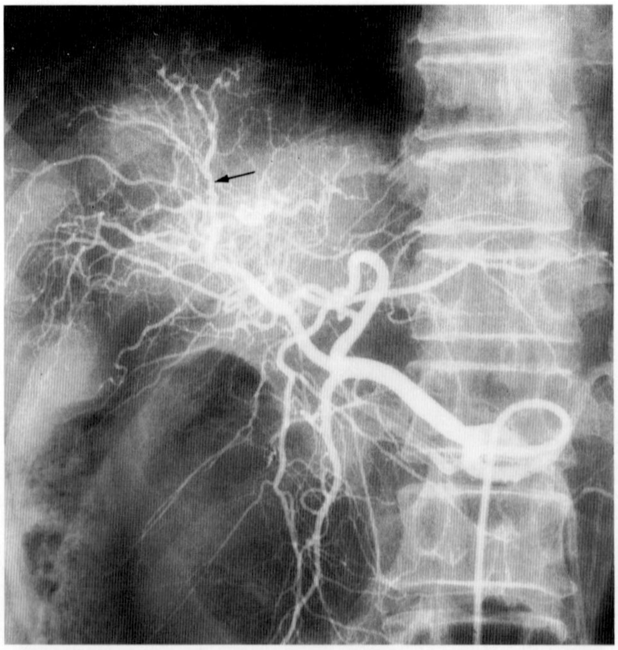

(c) Hepatic arteriogram (early phase): the main arteries in both lobes are free of encasement or interruption, but the wall of A^{VIII} is partly irregular (→). The left lobe is enlarged in compensation.

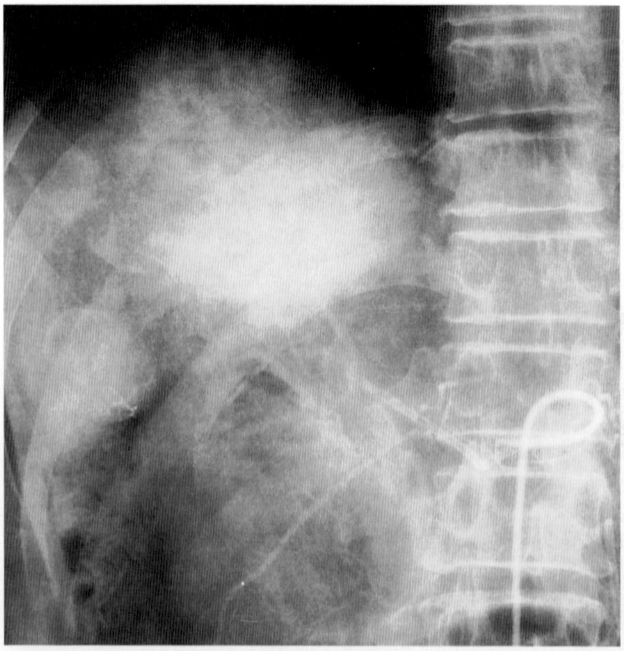

(d) Hepatic arteriogram (late phase): the stain of the right lobe is much stronger than that of the left, and the stain could be mistaken for a tumor stain. This phenomenon is due to increased arterial flow that follows portal vein obstruction.

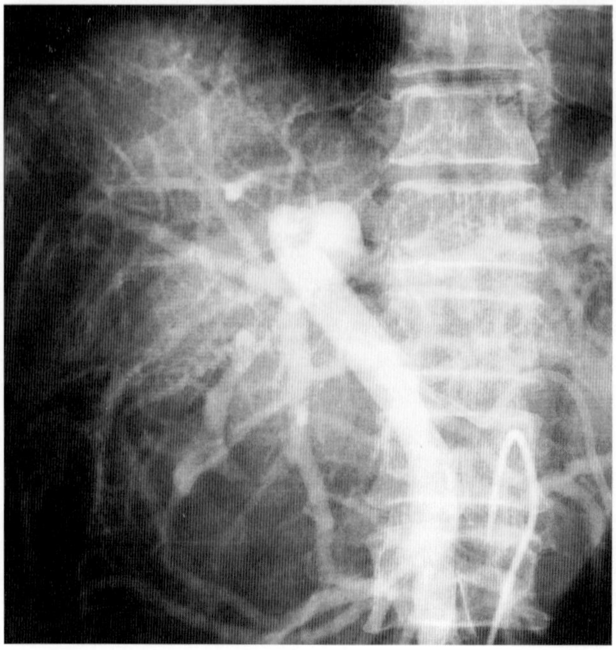

(e) Superior mesenteric arterial portogram: it looks as though all portal vein branches in the right lobe are opacified. However, if each portal branch were examined with reference to the arterial branches (c), it would become clear that all these portal branches are of the left lobe; no portal branch of the right lobe is seen.

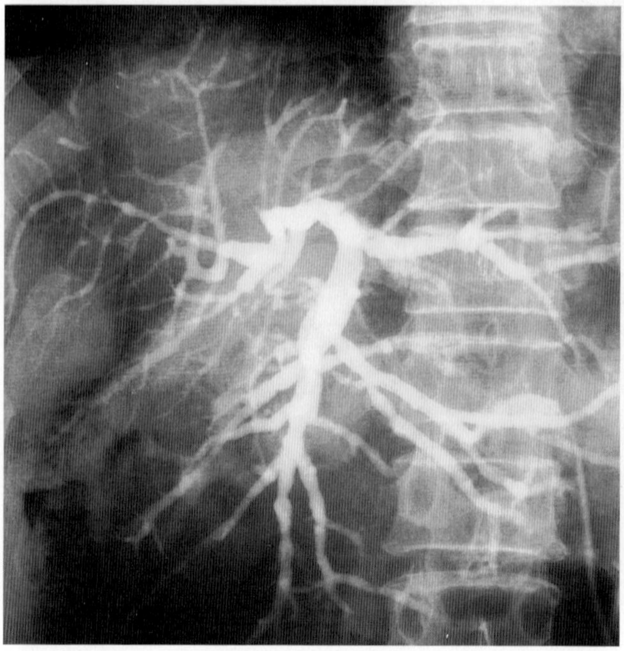

(f) Cholangiogram made through the drainage tube: if compared with the portogram (e), one would readily recognize that these are also of the left lobe. There is no communication with the right lobe bile ducts. Extended right lobectomy was carried out. The main tumor (adenocarcinoma) was located to the right of the hilum infiltrating along the biliary tract up to the periphery.

Bile duct carcinoma—Case 7: Left hepatic duct carcinoma in which late enhanced CT proved useful in differentiating the duct and carcinoma.

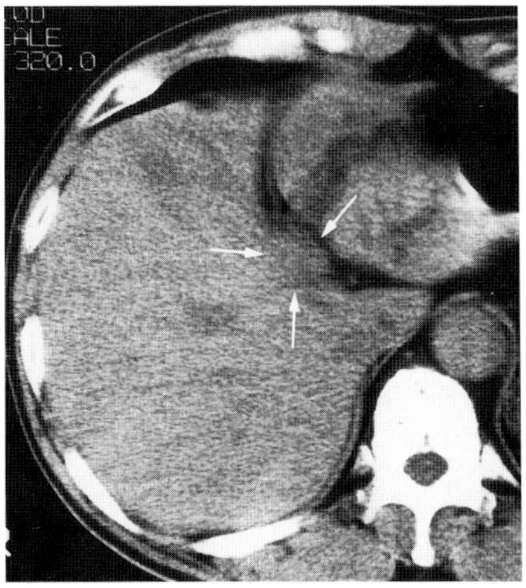

(a) Plain CT: biliary dilatation in the left lobe, particularly in the lateral segment, is seen. A low-density mass (→) is recognized central to it in the left hilar area.

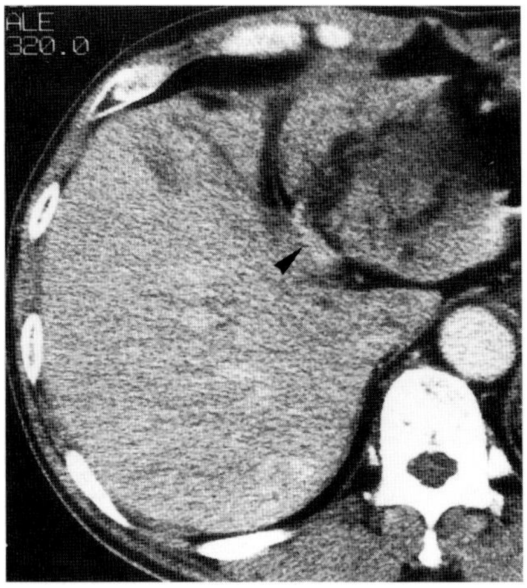

(b) Enhanced CT (early phase): since the left umbilical portion of the portal vein (▶) was opacified within the lesion, the area seen in (a) minus the umbilical portion was thought to be the mass itself.

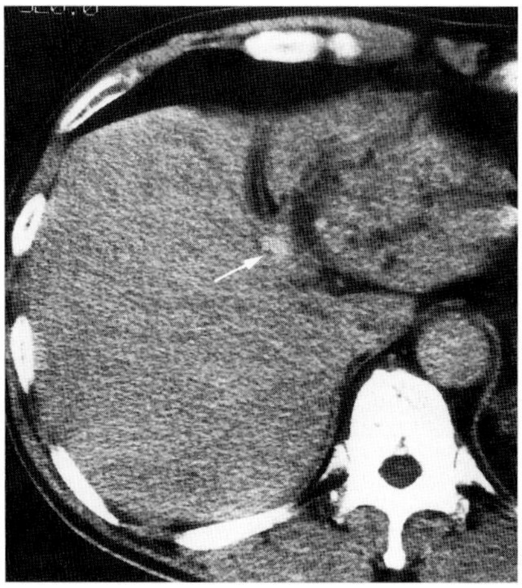

(c) Enhanced CT (late phase): the blood vessels including the portal vein are already isodense at this time. However, the area thought to be the mass is now of high density (→). This suggested that this portion contained abundant fibrous tissue, and in view of its size of 1.2 cm, the imaging diagnosis was bile duct carcinoma of the left hepatic duct.

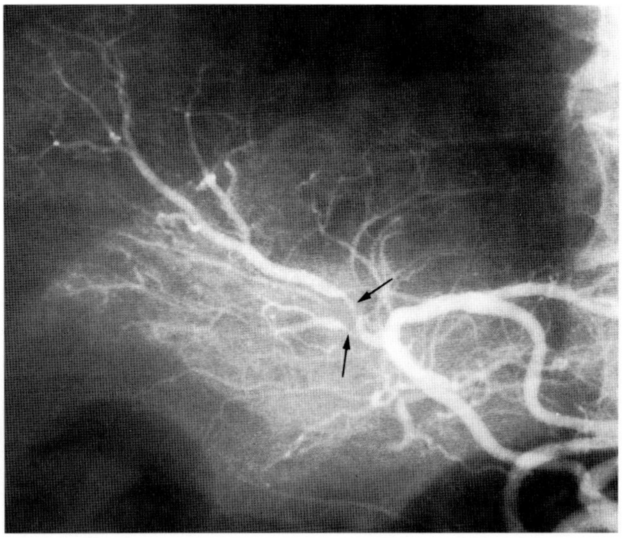

(d) Left hepatic arteriogram: the beginning of the middle hepatic artery was encased (→), and a cancer arising in this region was suspected. The portogram was almost normal. Left heptectomy disclosed a 1.7 × 1.0 cm mass which was very firm.

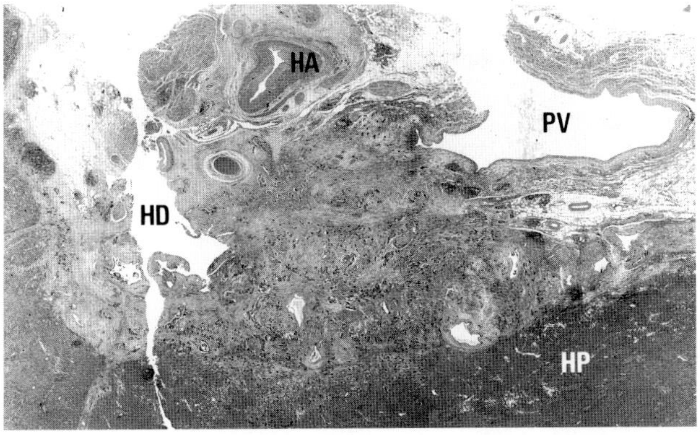

e

(e) Histopathology: the wall of the left hepatic duct (HD) was thickened, and tumor infiltration was confined to the immediate neighboring liver parenchyma (HP) and a small portion of the portal vein (PV). HA, hepatic artery.

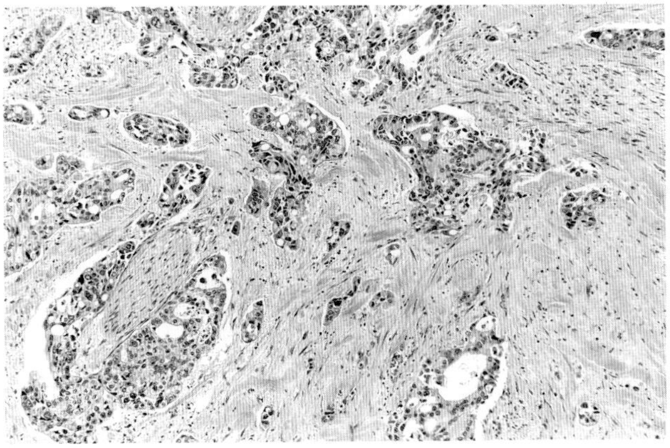

f

(f) Histology [enlargement of (e)]: within the thickened hepatic duct wall there was a moderately differentiated adenocarcinoma with abundant fibrous tissue.

Bile duct carcinoma—Case 8: Common duct carcinoma in which enhanced CT demonstrated thickening and staining of the duct wall.

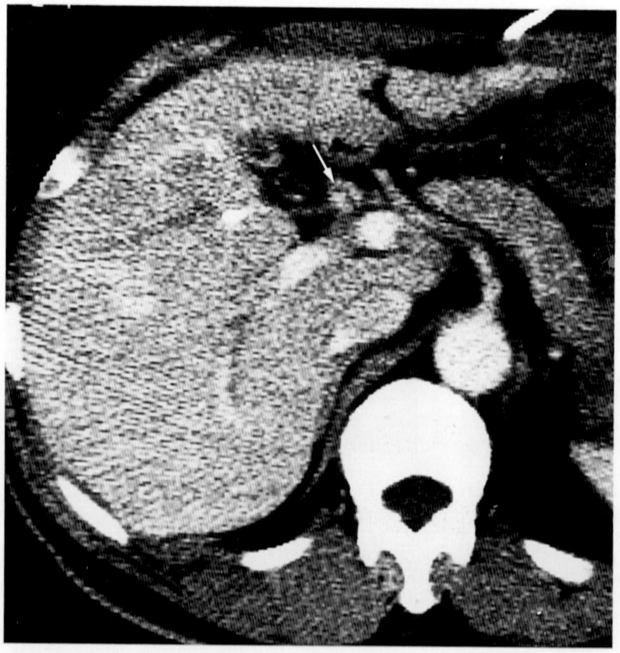

(a) Dynamic CT (early phase): a ring enhancement (→) is seen in the common bile duct near the bifurcation. This area was seen as a low-density mass on plain CT.

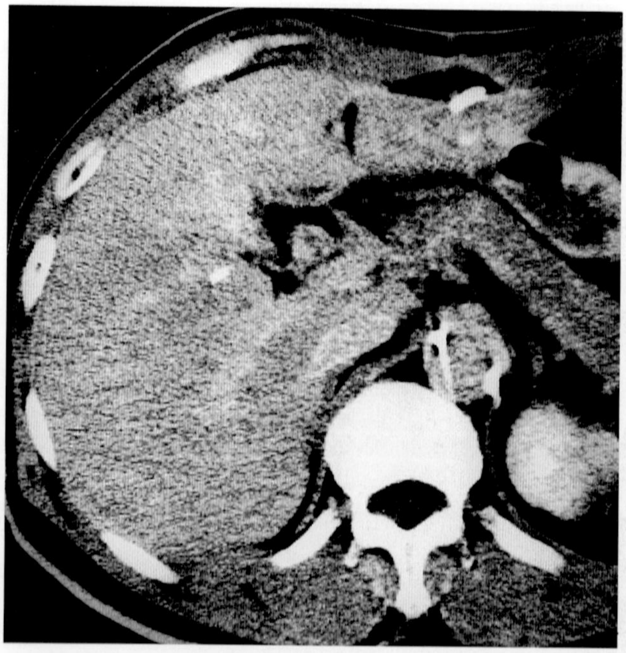

(b) Dynamic CT (late phase): the ring enhancement was still recognized in this area. With a diagnosis of bile duct carcinoma in the hilum, extended right lobectomy was carried out.

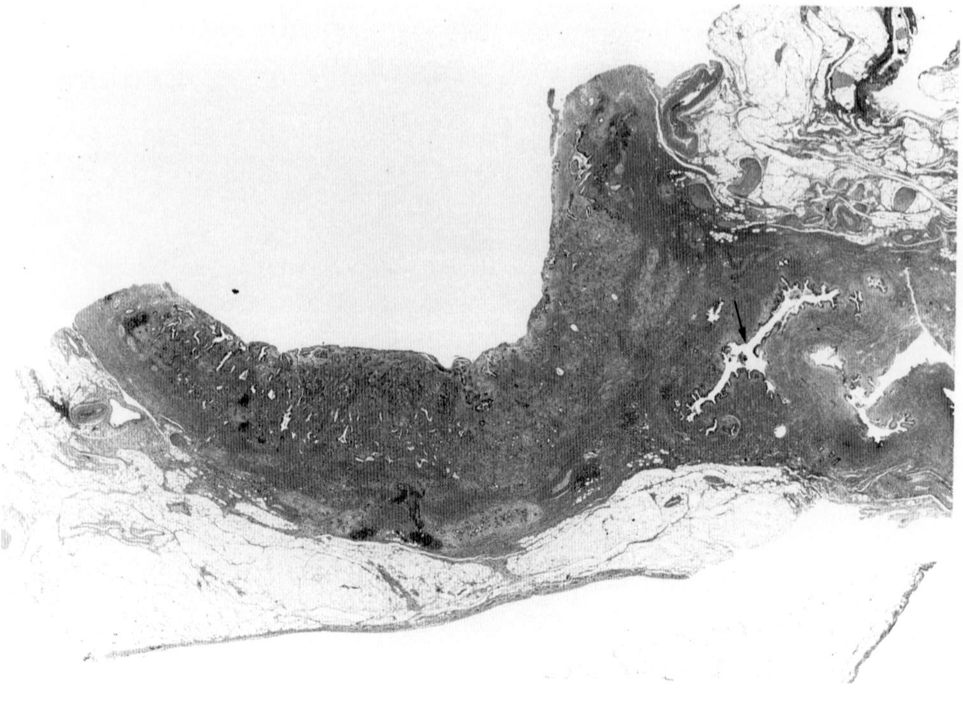

(c) Histopathology: the common bile duct was thickened to 4 mm by circumferential tumor infiltration. It was a well differentiated adenocarcinoma with desmoplasia around it. →, cystic duct.

Bile duct carcinoma—Case 9: Left hilar bile duct carcinoma causing portal flow insufficiency as a result of inadequate PTCD drainage.

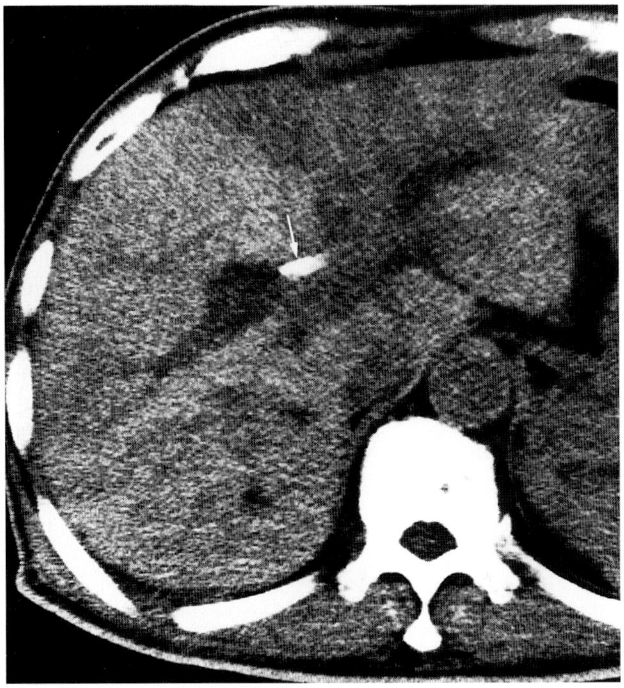

(a) Plain CT: hilar carcinoma of the left lobe with an irregular boundary is seen infiltrating into the bifurcation. →, tip of the drainage tube inserted through the right lobe. Cholangiography indicated inadequate decompression and drainage.

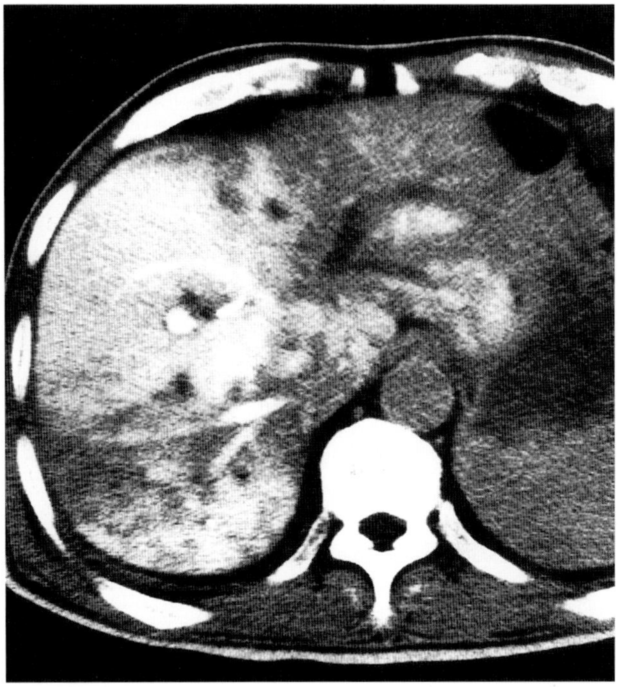

(b) Portal-CT: a superior mesenteric arterial portogram demonstrated patent portal vein branches in the right lobe. However, portal-CT clearly showed uneven portal perfusion in the right lobe which was to be spared by resection. The irregular portal perfusion was perhaps due to portal vein obstructions secondary to cholangitis resulting from inadequate drainage. The patient died 10 months after extended left lobectomy.

4.10 Combined hepatocellular and cholangiocarcinoma

Coexistent HCC and cholangiocarcinoma in the same liver may be divided into the following three subtypes (Allen and Lisa 1949), and the Liver Cancer Study Group of Japan (1989) has adopted this subdivision (Fig. 4.9):

1. Double cancer. Hepatocellular carcinoma and cholangiocarcinoma are present at different sites in the same liver, each composed of a single cell type (Kojiro *et al.* 1982; Wada *et al.* 1986; Takayasu *et al.* 1989*d*). One organ containing more than one type of cancer and two different organs having different primaries are usually distinguished, but combined hepatocellular and cholangiocarcinoma has both features.
2. Combined type. Hepatocellular carcinoma and cholangiocarcinoma are present in close contact, each composed of a different cell type, but becoming intermingled as they collide—collision tumor.
3. Mixed type. This is a mixture of hepatocellular carcinoma and cholangiocarcinoma in the same mass. It seems as though both have developed at the same site.

However, the new edition of WHO Tumor Typing (Ishak *et al.* 1994) treats this cancer as an equivalent of the mixed type. It defines combined hepatocellular and cholangiocarcinoma as 'A rare tumor containing unequivocal elements of both hepatocellular and cholangiocarcinoma that are intimately admixed'. This tumor should be distinguished from separate hepatocellular carcinomas and cholangiocarcinomas arising in the same liver. Such tumors may be widely separated or close to each other (collision tumor). The presence of both bile and mucus should be sought in the combined tumor (Goodman *et al.* 1985). This category should not be used for tumors in which either form of growth is insufficiently differentiated for positive identification. In such cases the tumors should be identified from the recognizable components or classified as an undifferentiated carcinoma.

Double cancer

This may be either synchronous (Case 1) or metachronous (Case 2). In Case 1, two masses were found by imaging preoperatively (Takayasu *et al.* 1989*d*). On the late phase enhanced CT, one lesion had a peripheral low-density area, and the other tumor became homogenously of low-density, suggesting two different types of tumor. Histologically, it was of the double cancer type. Another case (Case 2) developed metachronous double cancers (Takayasu *et al.* 1989*d*). Cholangiocarcinoma was resected first, and HCC developed in the remanant liver 6 years later. The liver parenchyma was compatible with chronic hepatitis at the time of the first operation, and was precirrhotic when HCC was found. The relation between tumor types and underlying liver disease is of interest. This kind of case may also be included in this subtype.

Combined type

This type can occur in the growth process of the previous type and should be included in it. We have not yet experienced this type.

Mixed type

The imaging features depend on the degree of predominance of one of the two types of cancer cells. If a large part of the mass consists of cholangiocarcinoma, the imaging finding is similar to that of cholangiocarcinoma (Case 3) and difficult to differentiate from it. By contrast, if HCC occupies a large part of the mass, differential diagnosis from HCC is not possible. There may be conflicting features (Case 4) and the serum levels of tumor markers such as AFP and CEA do not corroborate imaging diagnosis (Aoki *et al.* 1993).

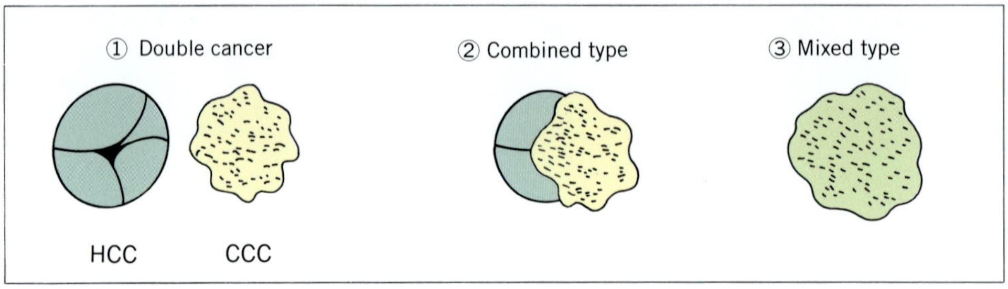

Fig. 4.9 Schematic drawing of the three types of combined hepatocellular and cholangiocarcinoma according to Allen and Lisa (1949).

Combined hepatocellular and cholangiocarcinoma—Case 1: Synchronous double cancer consisting of HCC and cholangiocarcinoma. A 53-year-old man, negative for AFP, CEA, and HBsAg.

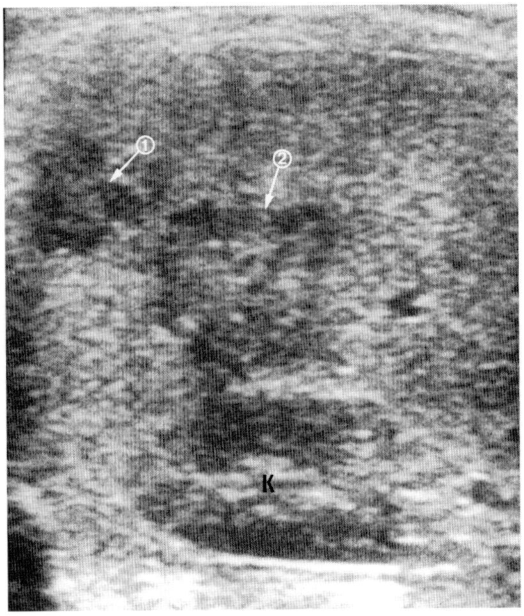

(a) US (right intercostal scan): two lesions are seen in the right lobe. The smaller lesion (1) is located cranially with a hypoechoic interior and a smoothly wavy periphery. The other larger one (2) is square shaped. K, right kidney.

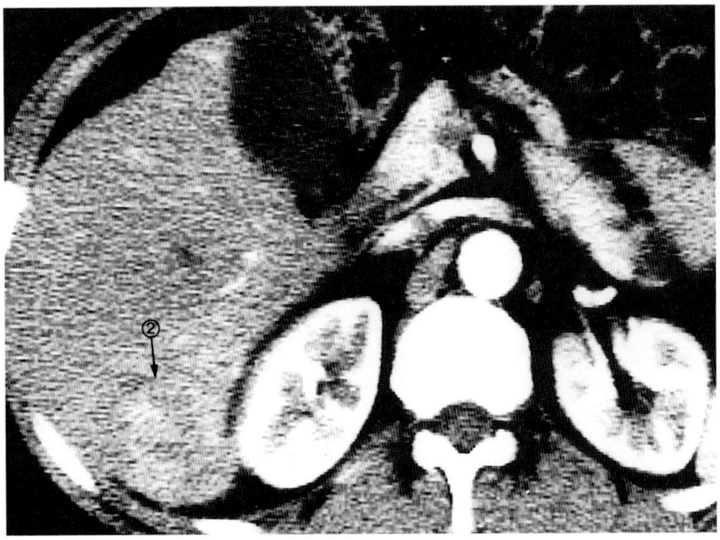

(b) Dynamic CT (early phase): lesion (2) is enhanced inhomogeneously.

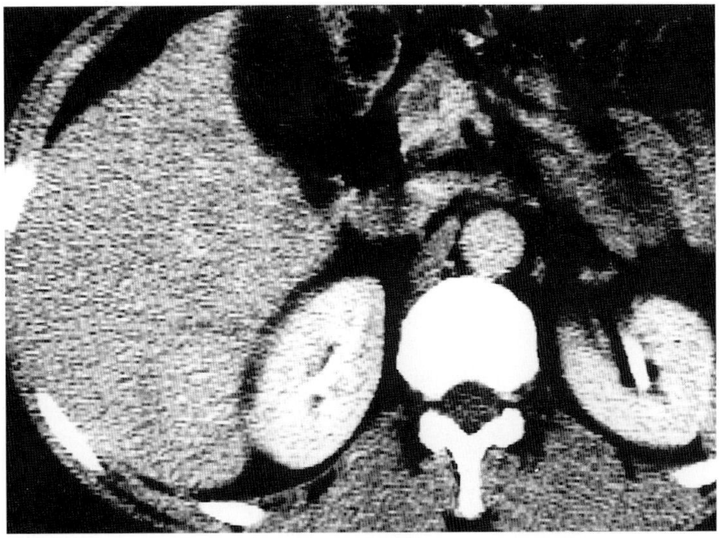

(c) Dynamic CT (late phase): the center of lesion (2) is now of high density and the periphery low density (peripheral low-density area), suggesting adenocarcinoma. Lesion (1) was not sliced in the early phase, but was seen as a low-density mass suggestive of HCC in the late phase (not shown).

Case 1 (contd.)

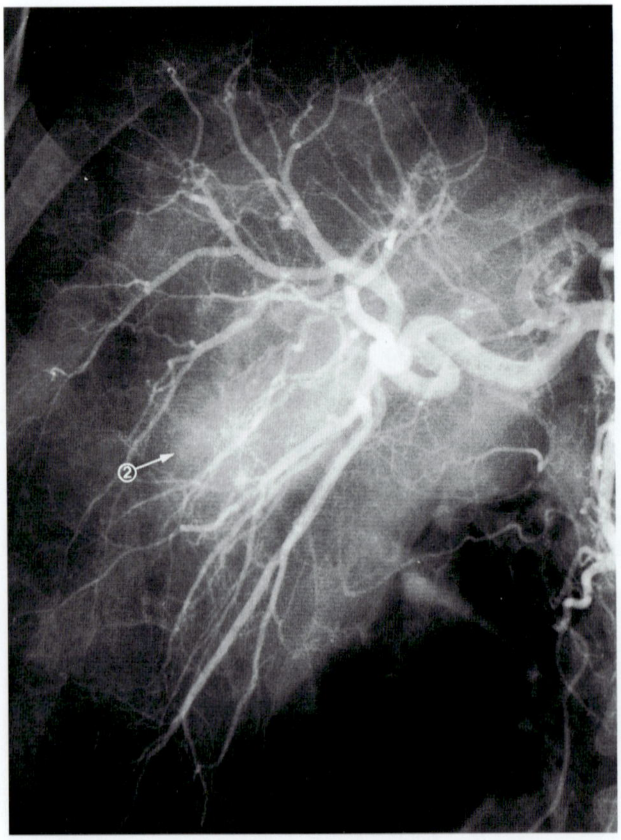

(d) Angiogram (early phase): lesion (2) is seen as a homogeneous tumor stain in S^{VI}.

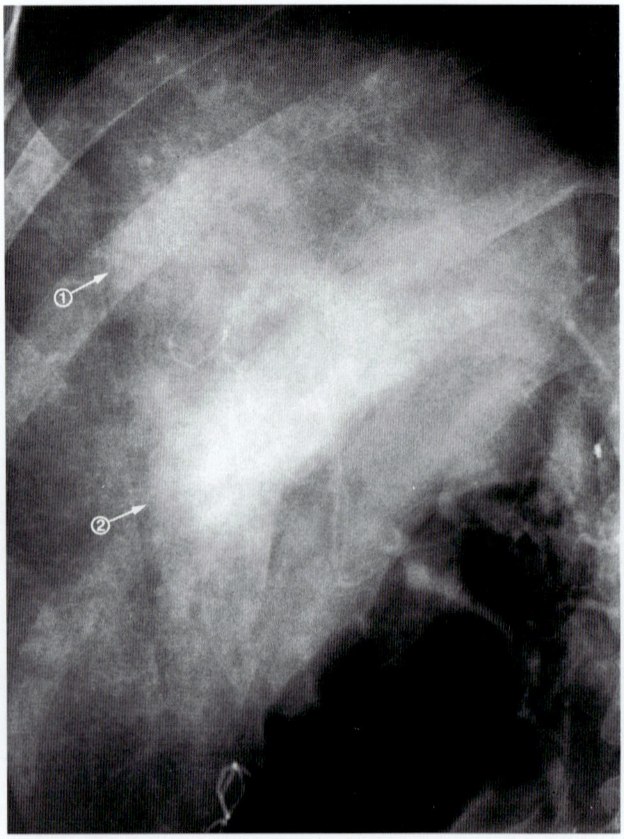

(e) Angiogram (late phase): in addition, lesion (1) is now seen in S^{VIII} as a weak tumor stain.

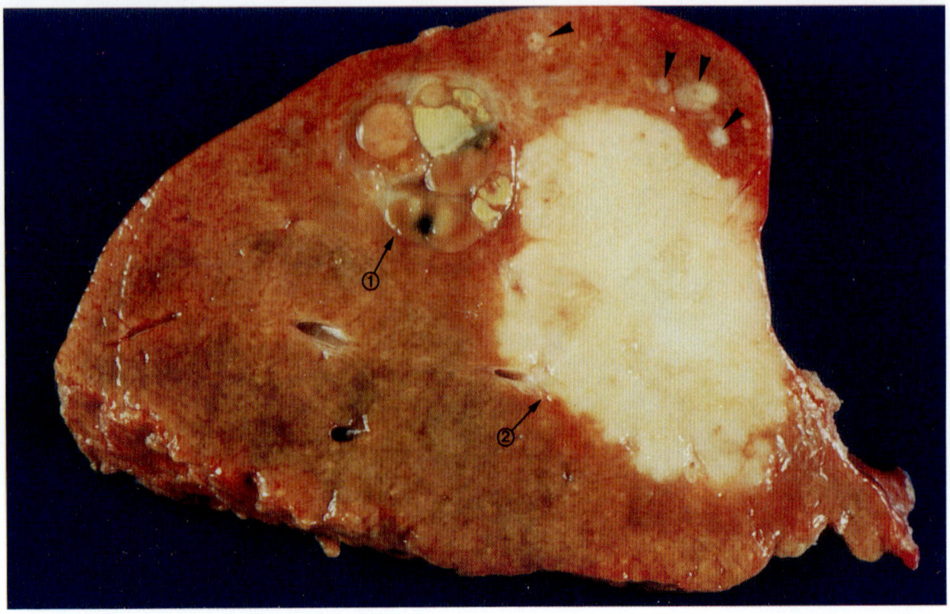

(f) Cut section of resected specimen: a sagittal cut showed the larger mass (2) as a 5.3 × 3.5 cm whitish firm lesion with an irregular margin, and the smaller (2 cm) lesion (1) in its vicinity. The latter may be grossly diagnosed as HCC from its nodule-in-nodule appearance. Lesion (2) was a moderately differentiated adenocarcinoma and the diagnosis was cholangiocarcinoma of the peripheral type. Lesion (1) was Edmondson–Steiner's grade II > I. ▶, intrahepatic spread of cholangiocarcinoma.

Combined hepatocellular and cholangiocarcinoma—Case 2: Metachronous double cancer in which HCC was found 6 years after resection for cholangiocarcinoma.

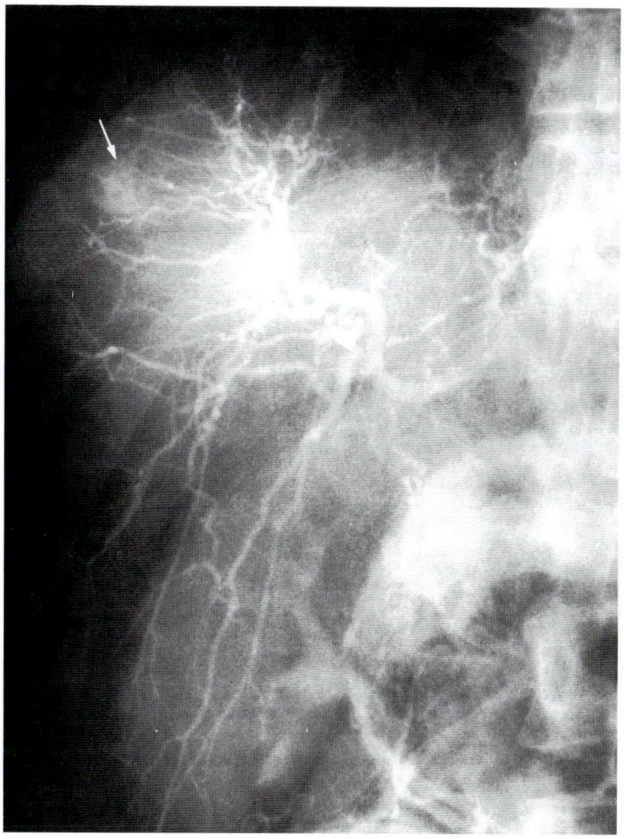

(a) Angiogram: a 2 cm tumor stain (→) seen in S^{VIII} was resected with a diagnosis of HCC.

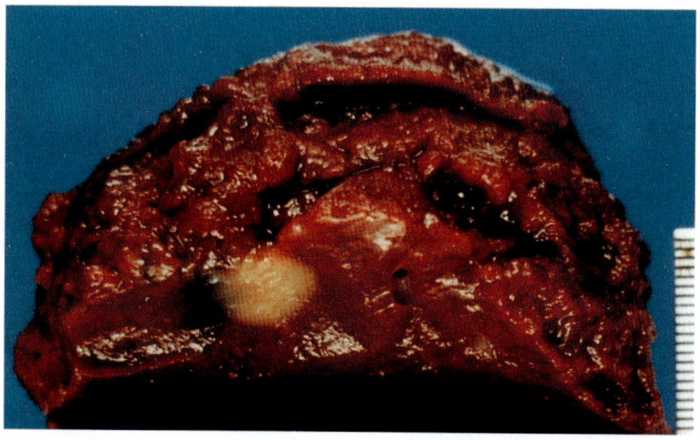

(b) Cut section of resected specimen: the mass was light yellow and firm without a capsule or a mosaic interior. Histological diagnosis was cholangiocarcinoma. The patient had been well for 6 years. Then serum AFP slowly increased to a level of 143 ng/ml and he was admitted for investigation.

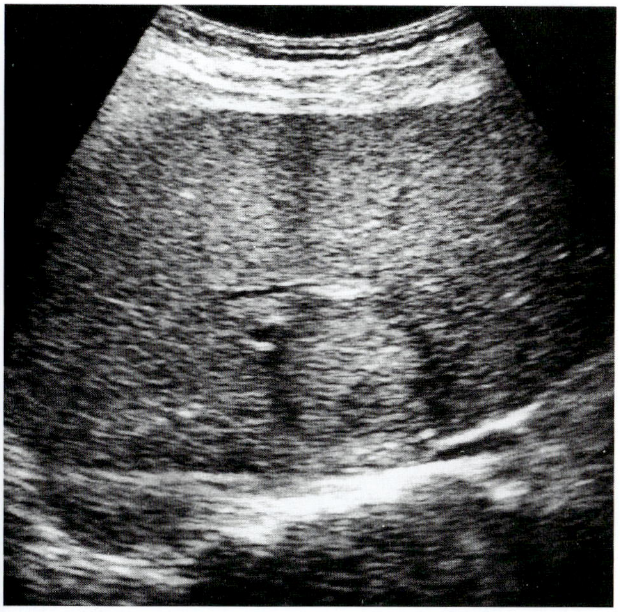

(c) US of the liver 6 years later (right intercostal scan): a mass was found in S^{VIII}. Since the lesion was not multiple and had a mosaic interior surrounded by a halo, the diagnosis was HCC as opposed to possible metastatic cholangiocarcinoma.

Case 2 (contd.)

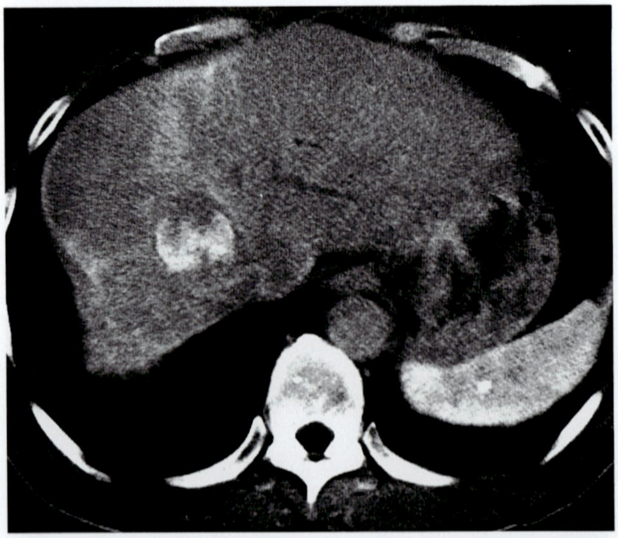

(d) Lipiodol-CT: celiac arteriography was not very successful due to severe arteriosclerosis, and 5 ml of Lipiodol was injected for diagnosis. A mosaic deposition of Lipiodol with a surrounding low-density ring was seen on CT made immediately after injection. The diagnosis was HCC with a fibrous capsule.

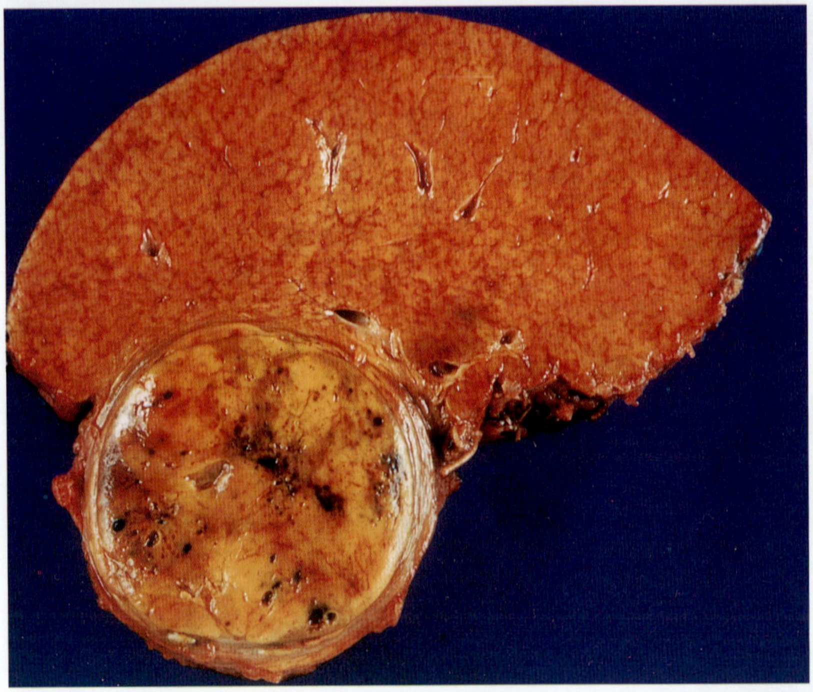

(e) Cut section of resected specimen: typical HCC (Edmondson's grade II) with a fibrous capsule. The non-cancerous liver parenchyma showed early stage cirrhosis, apparent progression from chronic hepatitis 6 years earlier. The metachronous development of two cancers may be related to the changes of liver parenchyma since HCC is known to develop against a background of underlying cirrhosis.

Combined hepatocellular carcinoma and cholangiocarcinoma—Case 3: Mixed type cancer diagnosed as cholangiocarcinoma from the enhancement pattern on dynamic CT. AFP 162 ng/ml, CEA 3.7 ng/ml, HBsAg (+).

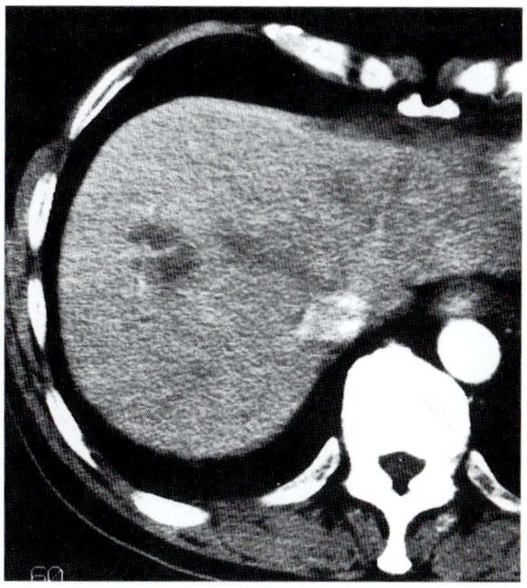

(a) Dynamic CT (early phase): a low-density mass with an enhanced vascular structure in its center is seen in S^{VIII}.

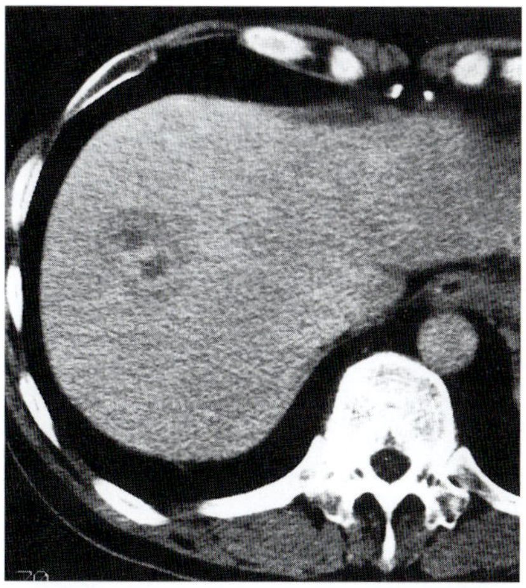

(b) Dynamic CT (late phase, 10 min): the mass consists of a high density area sandwiched between two low-density areas. The tumor is also surrounded by a peripheral low-density ring. No bile duct dilatation is seen peripheral to the mass.

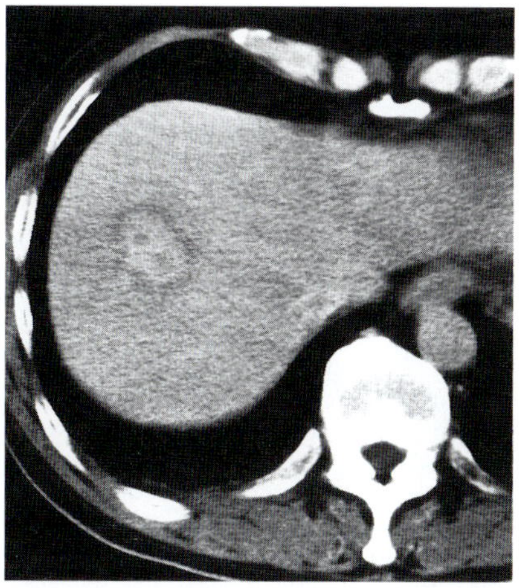

(c) Dynamic CT (late phase, 20 min): the peripheral low-density ring has become more discrete. Since no other primary was found, the diagnosis was cholangiocarcinoma.

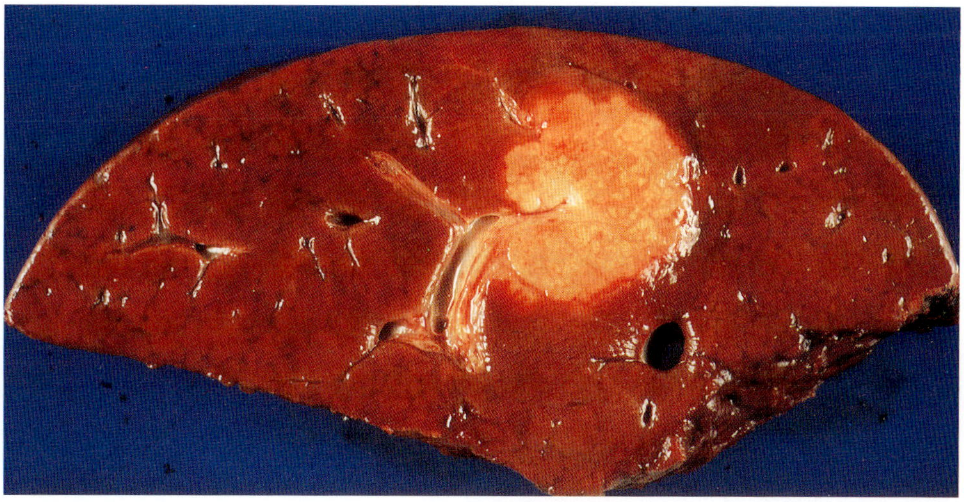

(d) Cut section of resected specimen: extended right anterior subsegmentectomy was carried out. The mass had an irregular boundary and the interior was homogeneous and fibrous. Since one portal tract was seen penetrating the mass, it was thought on gross study that this was cholangiocarcinoma arising from B^{VIII}. Histologically, however, about 5 per cent of the cut surface consisted of HCC cells. The final diagnosis was a mixed type of combined hepatocellular and cholangiocarcinoma. In retrospect, the vascular stain in the early phase of dynamic CT perhaps represented an arterial branch in that particular portal tract.

Combined hepatocellular carcinoma and cholangiocarcinoma—Case 4: Mixed type in which CT and angiography showed conflicting features. AFP (−), CEA 1.9 ng/ml, HBsAg (+).

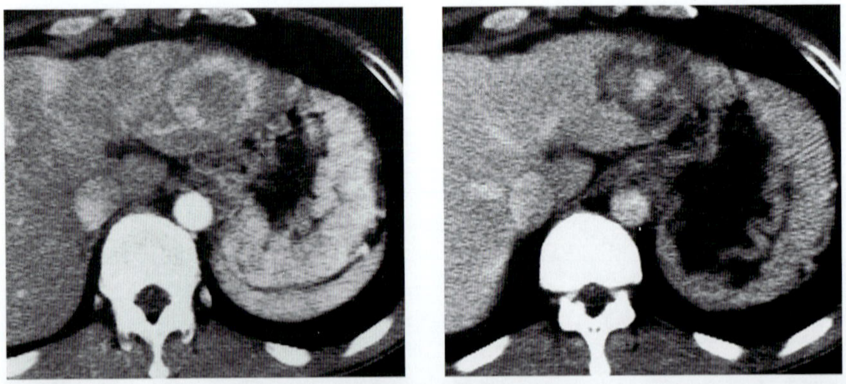

a b

(a) Dynamic CT (early phase): the periphery of this tumor found in the lateral areas of the left lobe (S^{II}) was enhanced.

(b) Dynamic CT (late phase, 15 min): the center of the mass is of high density while the periphery shows a low-density ring with an irregular margin, suggesting adenocarcinoma (cholangiocarcinoma).

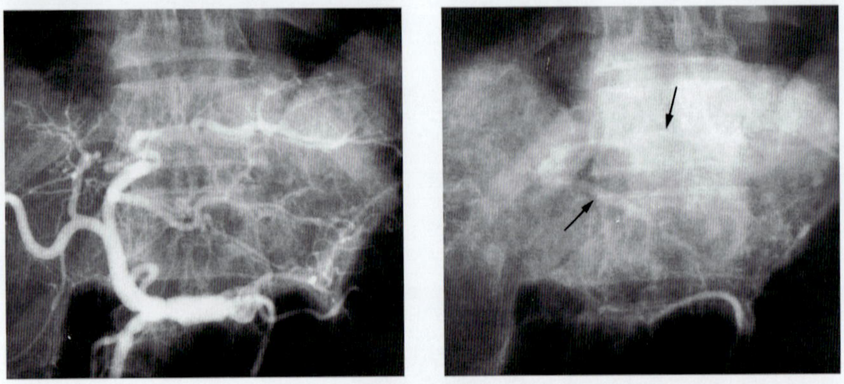

c d

(c) Angiogram (early phase): a weak tumor stain is seen in the periphery of A^{II}. There are no dilated tumor vessels commonly seen in HCC.

(d) Angiogram (late phase): intrahepatic portal branches (P^{II}, P^{III}, P^{IV} in part) (→) are opacified as a result of anterio-portal shunting. Formation of an arterio-portal shunt is very uncommon in cholangiocarcinoma, and the possibility of HCC could not be ruled out.

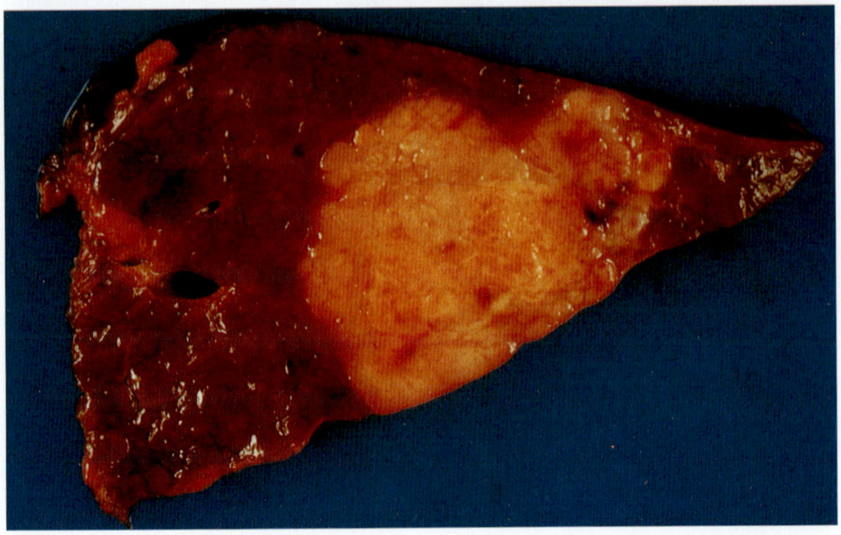

e

(e) Cut section of resected specimen: left lateral resection was carried out. The section demonstrated a tumor with an irregular margin without a capsule. Histological diagnosis was HCC of Edmondson's grade III > II mixed with cholangiocarcinoma cells.

4.11 Intrahepatic bile duct cystadenocarcinoma

Intrahepatic biliary or bile duct cystadenocarcinoma is a malignant cystic tumor lined by mucus secreting epithelium with papillary infoldings. This cancer occurs with an incidence of about 0.5 per cent of primary liver cancer, more commonly in middle aged women. Diagnosis is possible in a typical case from the internal structure of the tumor (Case 1). Namely, US and CT demonstrate multiple cysts containing fluid and papillary neoplastic growths continuous with the cyst wall (Takayasu *et al.* 1988*c*) (Fig. 4.10). The angiogram lacks characteristic features. However, the presence of neovasculature and encasement may be a useful finding for differentiation between cystadenocarcinoma and benign cystadenoma. If the tumor consists mainly of a mass filling the cysts and not having much fluid (Case 2), differentiation from cholangiocarcinoma, well differentiated HCC with little staining, and HCC that has undergone spontaneous necrosis is difficult.

On MR imaging this tumor is seen as a hypointense mass on T1-weighted images and as a hyperintense one on T2-weighted images, unless high density protein or hemorrhage is present. The signal intensity on T1-weighted images varies from hypo- to hyperintensity depending on the content of the cyst. A mural nodule arising from the wall of the cyst and its enhancement by Gd-DTPA strongly suggests malignancy, namely cystadenocarcinoma. A communication between the cyst and the bile duct does not always reflect the malignant nature of the lesion.

This tumor is considered to be a malignant counterpart of cystadenoma of the liver. Differentiation of the both is difficult by imaging (Ishak *et al.* 1977; Choi *et al.* 1989), and the diagnosis necessarily depends on histology. Therefore, a cystic tumor with a papillary growth should be operated on with a suspicion of malignant cystadenocarcinoma. Puncture of the cyst may cause intraabdominal seeding (Imamura *et al.* 1984), and a very careful procedure is required if it is ever done from diagnostic necessity. The cyst content is usually mucoid with high levels of tumor markers such as CEA and CA 19-9, but elevated marker levels do not permit diagnosis of malignancy, and cytological diagnosis is necessary.

Cystadenocarcinoma has to be distinguished from a carcinoma arising in a simple cyst. The latter is highly suspected if one finds emergence of a protruding lesion from the wall of a simple cyst during the follow-up. Just one imaging study is not sufficient for such differential diagnosis (Imamura *et al.* 1984). Cystadenocarcinoma is usually multilocular whereas carcinoma arising from a cyst is unilocular, a difference of diagnostic significance. Histopathological diagnosis requires the study of lining cells of the cyst. Other conditions that require differential diagnosis include cystic dilatation of peripheral bile ducts secondary to occlusion by mucin produced by bile duct carcinoma, and malignant transformation of cystic dilatations of peripheral bile ducts (Caroli disease). The diagnostic value of the demonstration of a communication between the biliary tract and the cyst by ERC and PTC remains to be defined.

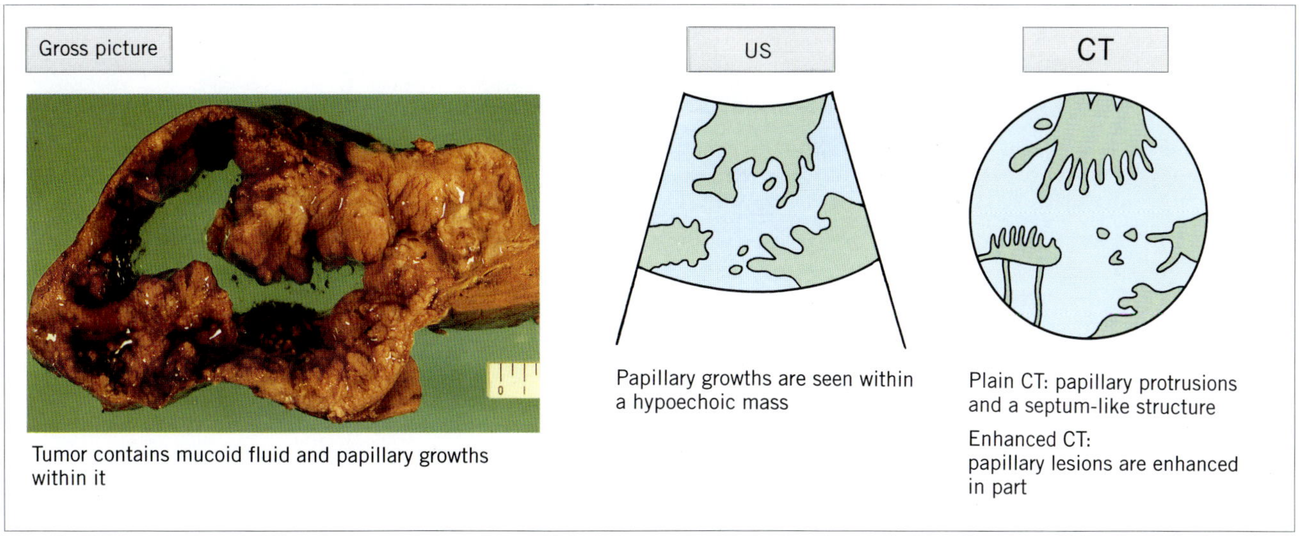

Fig. 4.10 Imaging features of intrahepatic bile duct cystadenocarcinoma.

Intrahepatic bile duct cystadenocarcinoma—Case 1: Large bile duct cystadenocarcinoma demonstrating typical imaging features. A 65-year-old man. A liver mass was incidentally found at the annual medical check-up. AFP (−), CEA (−).

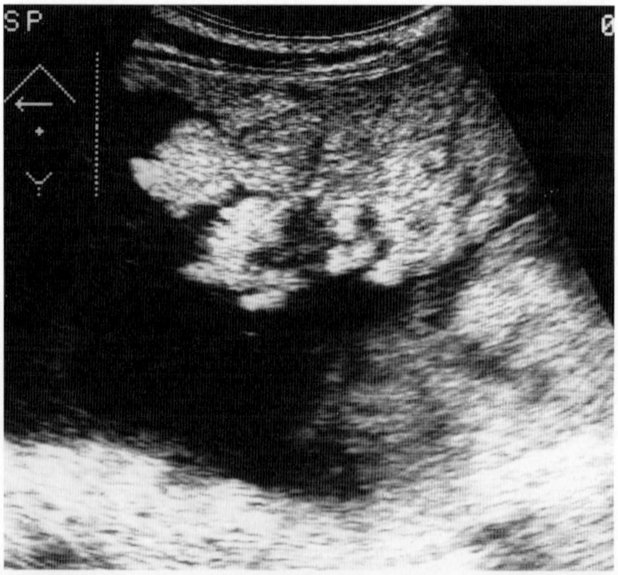

(a) US (transverse scan): a cystic lesion with posterior echo enhancement that has many papillary growths within it.

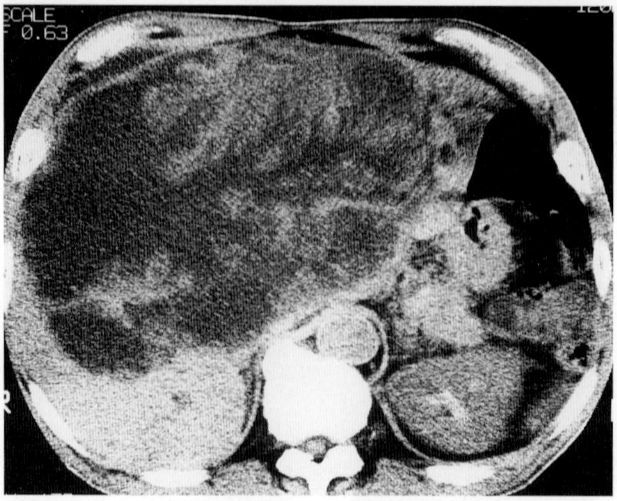

(b) Plain CT: there is a large cystic lesion occupying almost the entire liver. Within the lesion are seen a number of fern-leaf-like elevated papillary growths with a septum-like structure hanging from the wall.

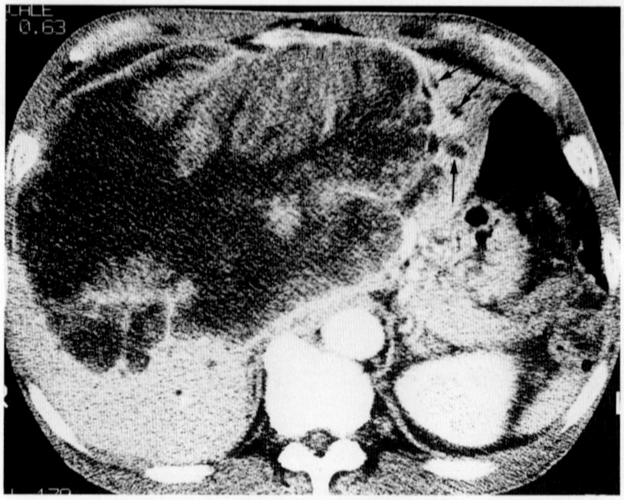

(c) Enhanced CT: the elevated lesions are enhanced, making the picture more distinct than plain CT. Bile duct dilatation (→) due to compression by the tumor is seen to the left of the mass.

Case 1 (contd.)

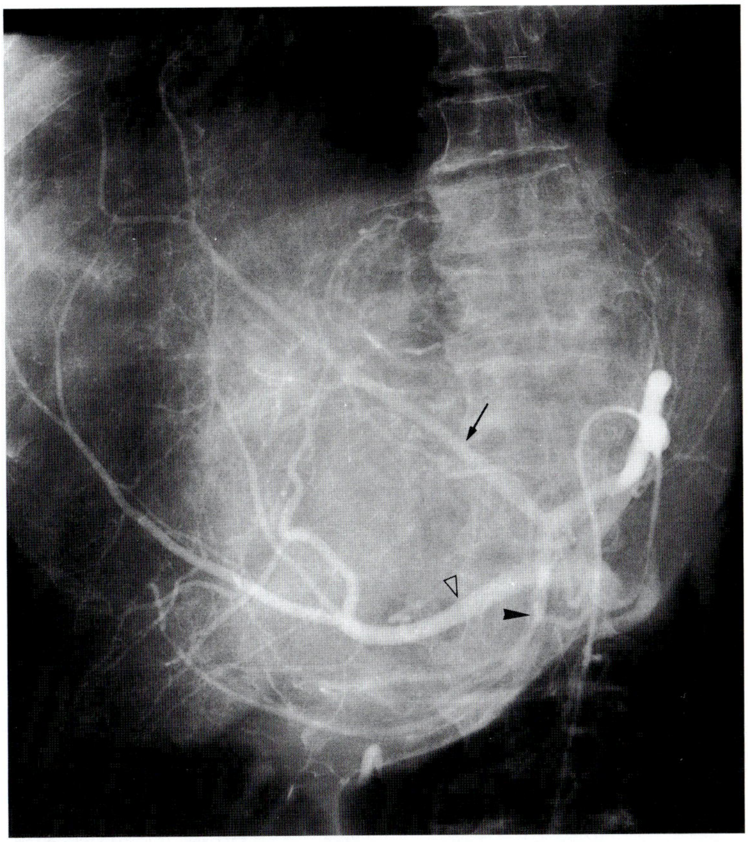

(d) Celiac arteriogram: there is a large hypovascular lesion stretching all the hepatic arterial branches. The medial artery (A^{IV}) shows neovasculature suggesting that this is not a benign mass. →, A^{IV}; ▷, right anterior segment branch; ▶, right posterior segment branch.

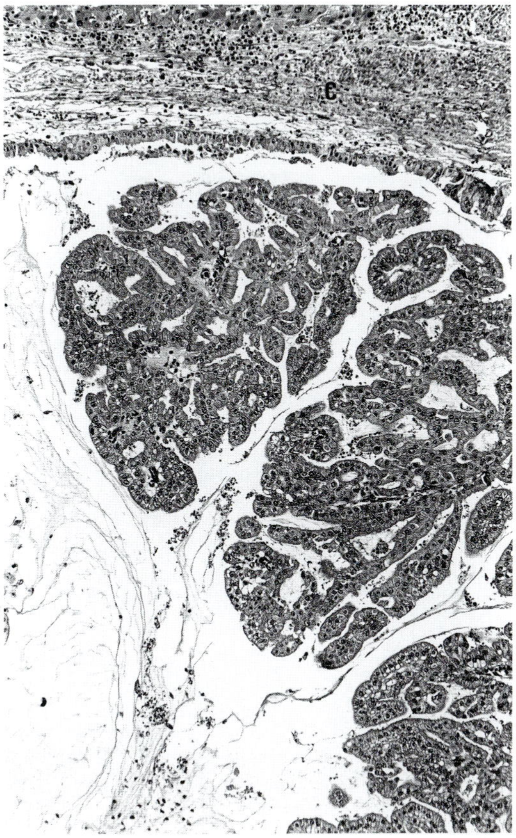

(f) Histopathology: the tumor consisted of cuboid tumor cells growing extensively in a papillary fashion. Infiltration into the stroma was recognized in other sections. The cyst contained a large amount of mucoid fluid and its wall was made up of thin fibrous tissue.

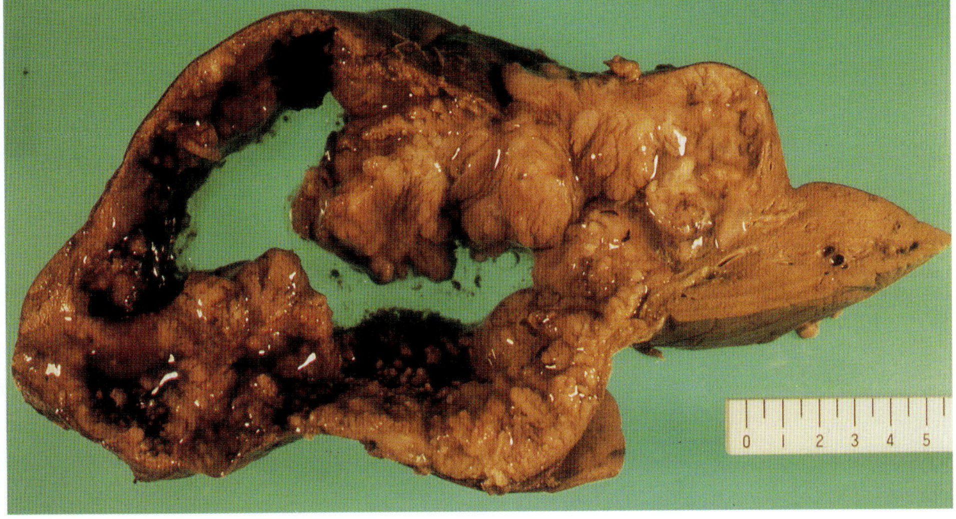

(e) Cut section of resected specimen: left-sided trisegmentectomy combined with left caudate lobectomy was carried out. When cut, a large amount of clear mucoid fluid came out. The mass was multilocular containing protruding papillary growths.

Intrahepatic bile duct cystadenocarcinoma—Case 2: Solid bile duct cystadenocarcinoma difficult to differentiate from peripheral type cholangiocarcinoma and HCC with spontaneous necrosis. A 60-year-old man. A liver mass was incidentally found at the annual medical check-up. AFP, CEA and HBsAg all (−).

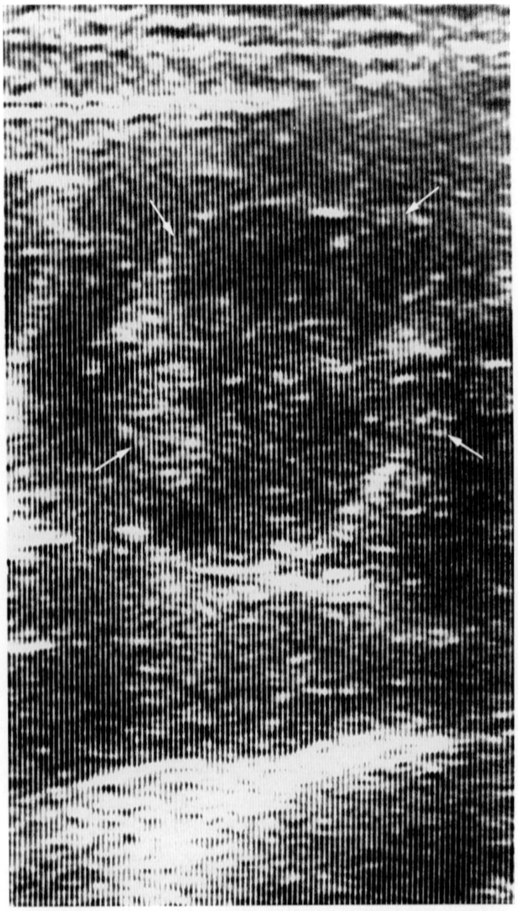

(a) US (transverse scan): a solid mass with mosaic internal echoes is seen in the left lobe (→).

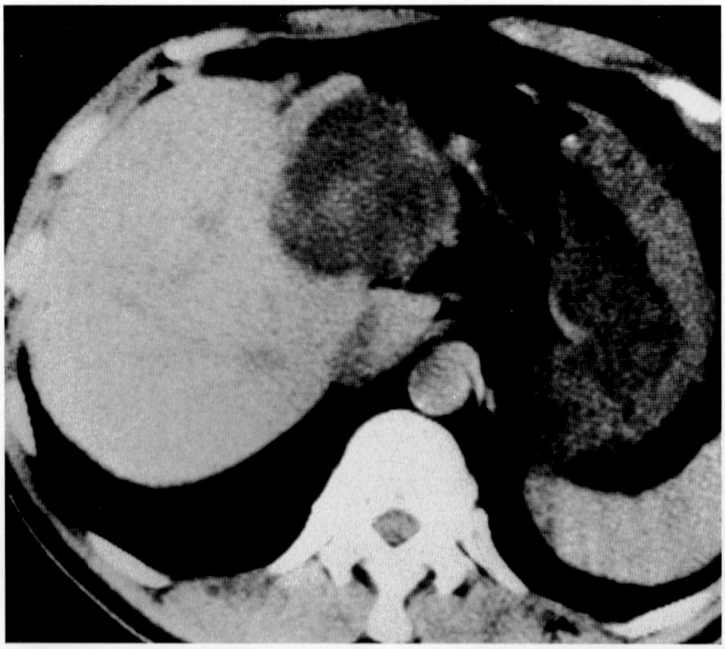

(b) Plain CT: a 7 cm low-density mass is seen in the left lobe laterally.

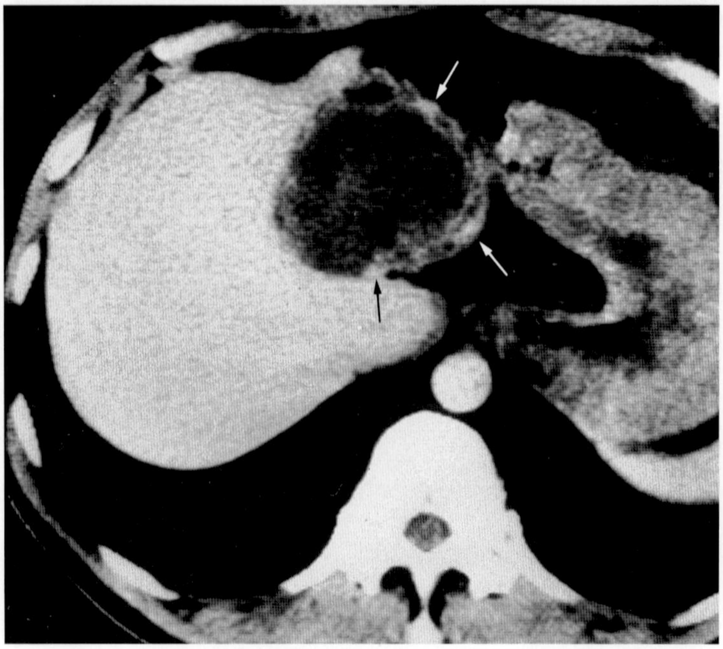

(c) Enhanced CT: the tumor interior was not enhanced, and only the periphery enhanced in places, assuming a dotted appearance (→). These features were compatible with bile duct carcinoma and HCC that has undergone spontaneous necrosis.

Case 2 (contd.)

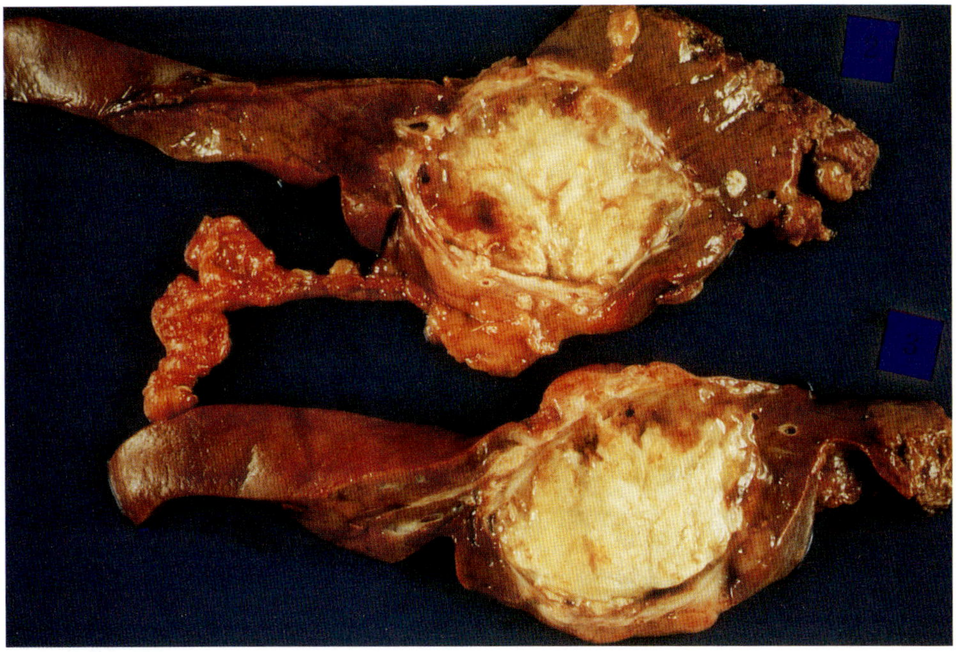

(d) Cut section of resected specimen: left lobectomy was carried out. The interior of the tumor consisted of yellowish white necrotic material and mucin. The tumor periphery contained viable cancer cells in places that were thought to correspond to the stained dotted areas.

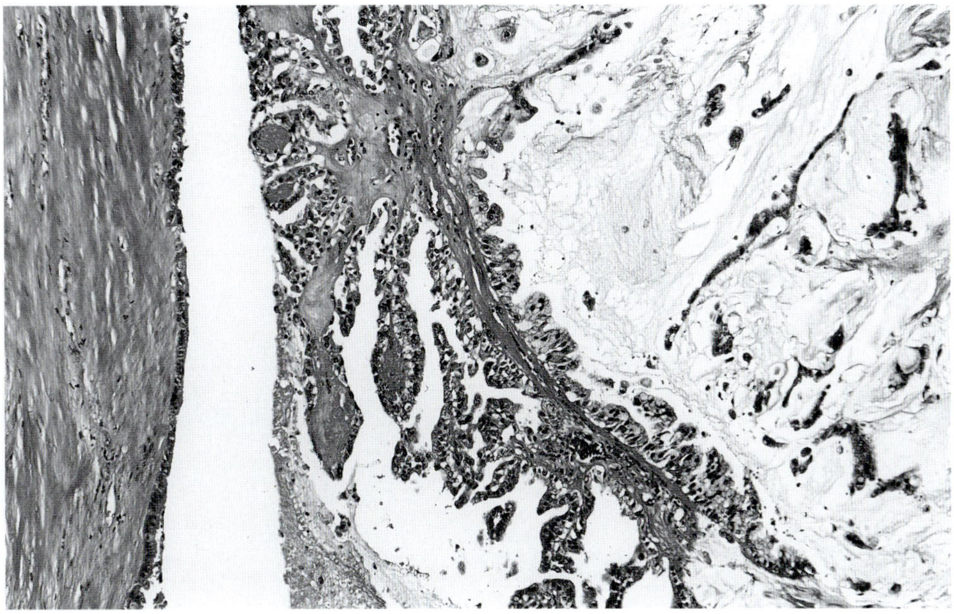

(e) Histopathology: cancer cells supported by thin fibrous tissues were growing in a papillary fashion. The mucoid fluid contained many floating cancer cells.

4.12 Hepatoblastoma

Hepatoblastoma is the most common liver tumor in childhood. It accounts for nearly 45 per cent of all primary liver tumors and tumor-like lesions in children (Stocker and Ishak 1987). Both hepatoblastoma and ordinary (adult type) HCC occur below age 15, but the ratio is approximately 4:1. Hepatoblastoma is most common below age 3, but it can also occur in adults. When one of the authors (KO) surveyed primary liver tumors in Japan in 1968–77 (Okuda *et al.* 1980), there were 69 hepatoblastomas among 4031 primary liver malignancies. Of the 69 cases of hepatoblastoma, 64 were below age 10, but 3 were seen in adults (the oldest case, 70 years). Each year, about 30 new hepatoblastoma cases are registered in Japan. Of the solid tumors of the abdomen in children, neuroblastoma, Wilms tumor and hepatoblastoma are the most common, with a ratio of 4:2:1. Hepatoblastoma is more frequent in males below age 5 (1.75:1), but this difference becomes smaller with advancing age. The presenting symptom in the majority of patients is abdominal enlargement and hepatic mass. This tumor is not relatd to hepatitis B infection nor liver cirrhosis. Serum AFP is-elevated to very high levels in the majority (75–96per cent) (Lack *et al.* 1982; Schmidt *et al.* 1985).

The tumor is composed of cells resembling primitive hepatic parenchymal cells with or without mesenchymal elements. Grossly, it may be divided into massive, diffuse and multinodular forms, but in reality clear categorization of the tumor is difficult. Histologically, epithelial hepatoblastoma and mixed epithelial-mesenchymal hepatoblastoma are separable. Within epithelial hepatoblastoma, the fetal and embryonic types may be separated. Some authors incorporate the small cell variant which Kasai and Watanabe called anaplastic hepatobastoma into the epithelial and mixed types (Stocker and Ishak 1987).

Imaging study is useful in differentiating hepatoblastoma from other liver disorders. CT attenuation values are usually between those of water and normal liver (low density) (Amendola *et al.* 1984), and contrast enhancement is about the same as liver parenchyma (Korobkin *et al.* 1981), but the CT features vary considerably from case to case. The tumor may be seen as a massive tumor consisting of multiple nodules (Cases 1 and 2). Calcifications are seen in about 50 per cent by CT which delineates them better than does plain radiography (Cremin and Nuss 1974; Miller and Greenspan 1985). US displays a solitary mass with nodules of increased inhomogeneous echoes, and punctate or amorphous calcifications which represent mesenchymal osteoid elements. The tumor is well enhanced on dynamic CT, and angiography also reveals ample tumor vessels and tumor stains as in HCC (Case 1).

HCC in children may be mistaken for hepatoblastoma. We have seen an adult type HCC in a 10-year-old boy. Preoperative differentiation between HCC and hepatoblastoma by imaging alone was difficult, but he was positive for HBsAg and the AFP value was 1456 ng/ml, much lower than in most hepatoblastoma patients. The resected liver had a number of tumor nodules and portal invasion. The parenchyma showed a histological feature of chronic hepatitis.

Hepatoblastoma—Case 1: Massive hepatoblastoma seen as coalescent multiple nodules. A 15-year-old girl. AFP 59 100 ng/ml, HBsAg (−), anti-HBs (−).

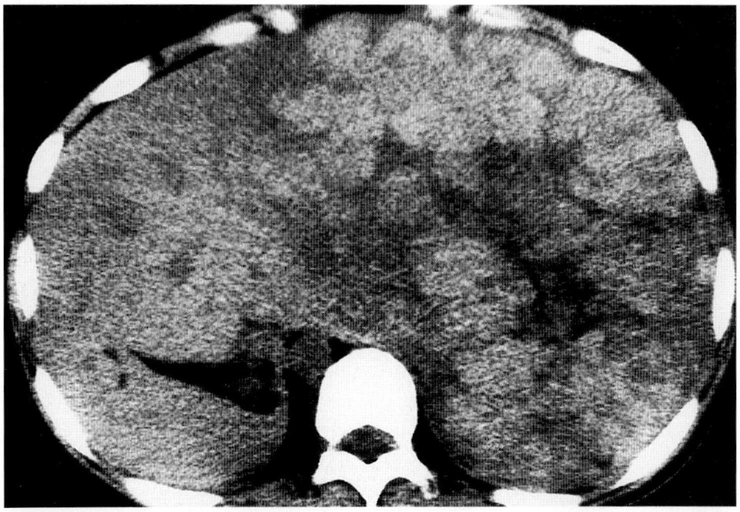

(a) Plain CT: a massive tumor consisting of confluent multiple nodules occupies the entire right lobe. The tumor periphery is of iso- or high density and the interior low density.

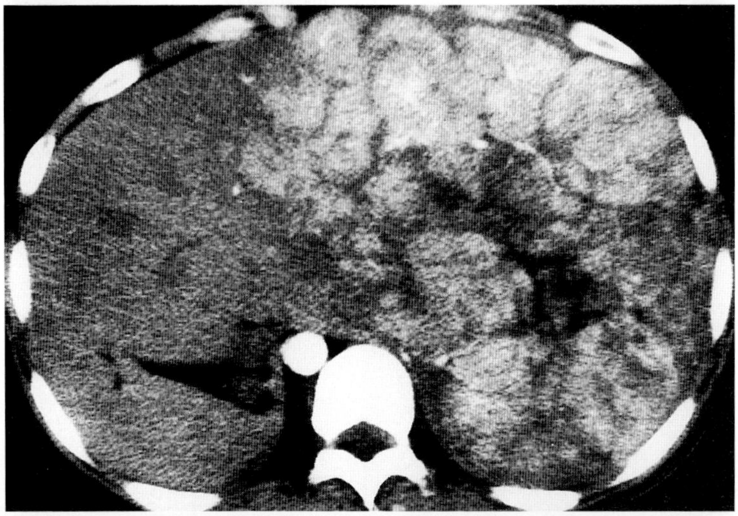

(b) Dynamic CT (early phase): the individual nodules were enhanced and some tumor vessels were also delineated (contrast medium: 80 ml/2 ml/s).

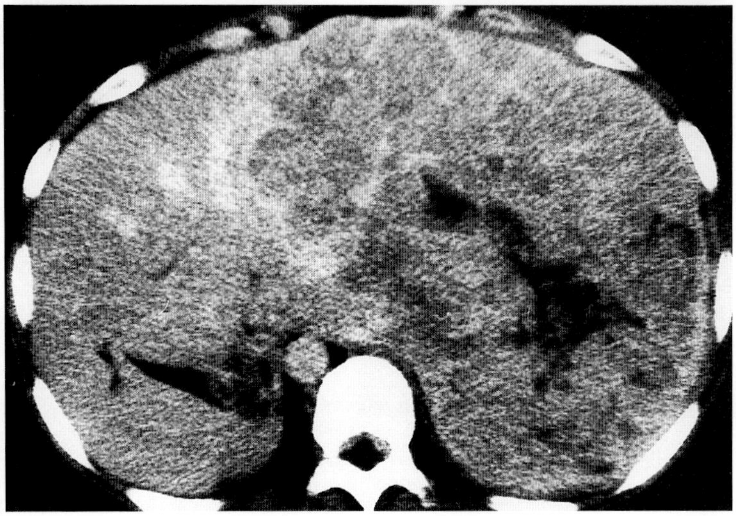

(c) Dynamic CT (late phase, 3 min): the tumor as a whole has turned to a low-density mass. The interior shows a stellate area of very low density, suggestive of necrosis.

Case 1 (contd.)

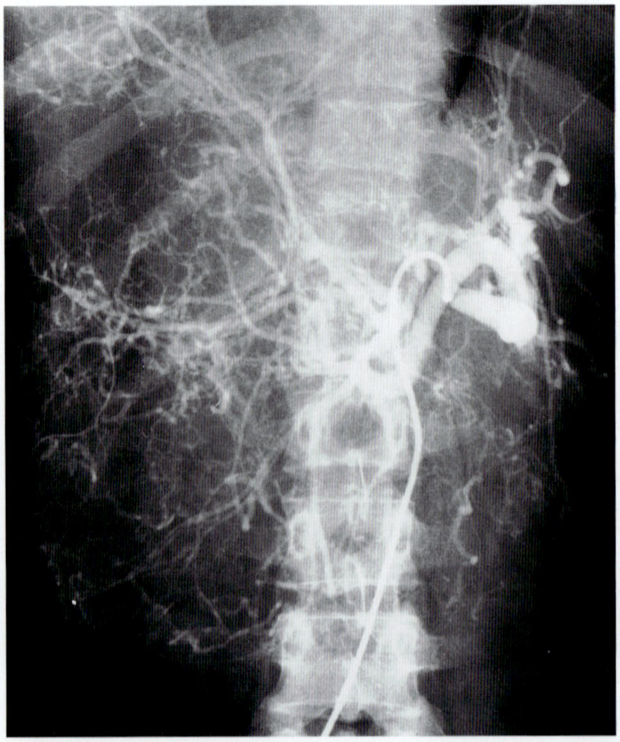

(d) Celiac arteriogram (early phase): many tumor vessels are seen, mainly in the right lobe.

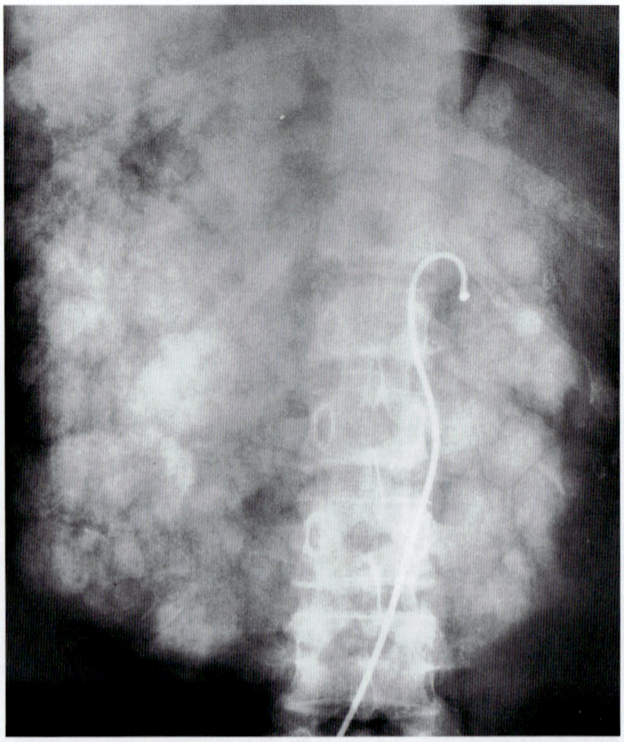

(e) Celiac arteriogram (late phase): many nodular tumor stains similar to the CT images are seen.

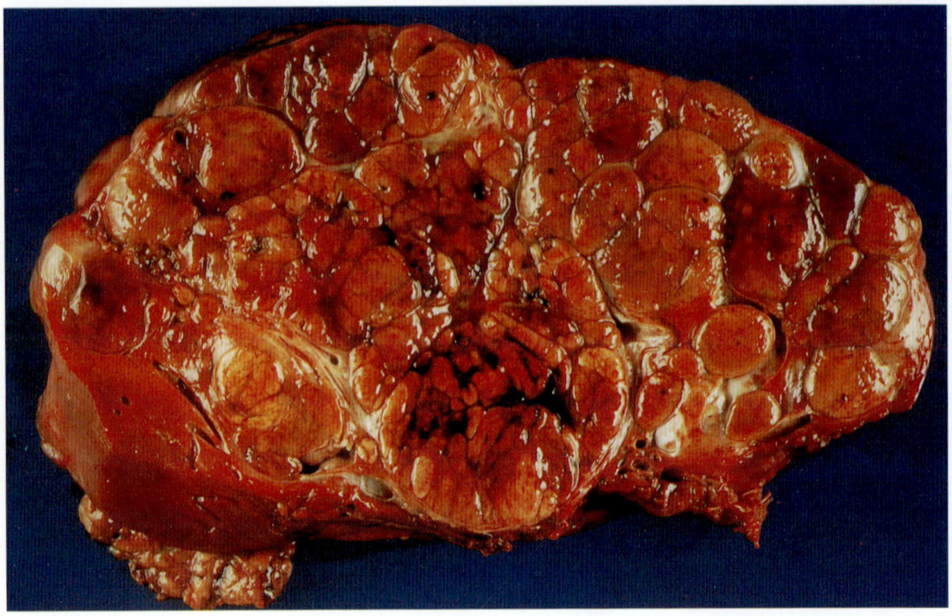

(f) Cut section of resected specimen: extended right lobectomy was carried out (3500 g). As seen by imaging, multiple tumor nodules were confluent forming a large mass (20×11 cm). A fibrous capsule was recognized in places. Grossly, no portal invasion or intrahepatic metastasis was seen, and histologically, it consisted of well differentiated epithelial cells (fetal type) not containing mesenchymal elements.

Hepatoblastoma—Case 2: Hepatoblastoma seen like a stone pavement by ultrasound. A 3-year-old boy. AFP 23 990 ng/ml, HBsAg (−), anti-HBs (−).

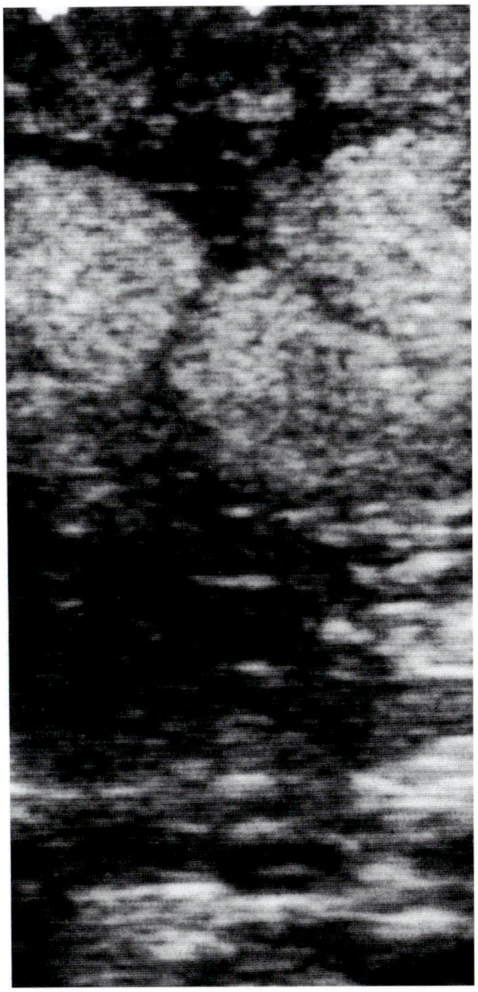

(a) Intraoperative US: hyperechoic and hypoechoic nodules are confluent, looking like a stone pavement.

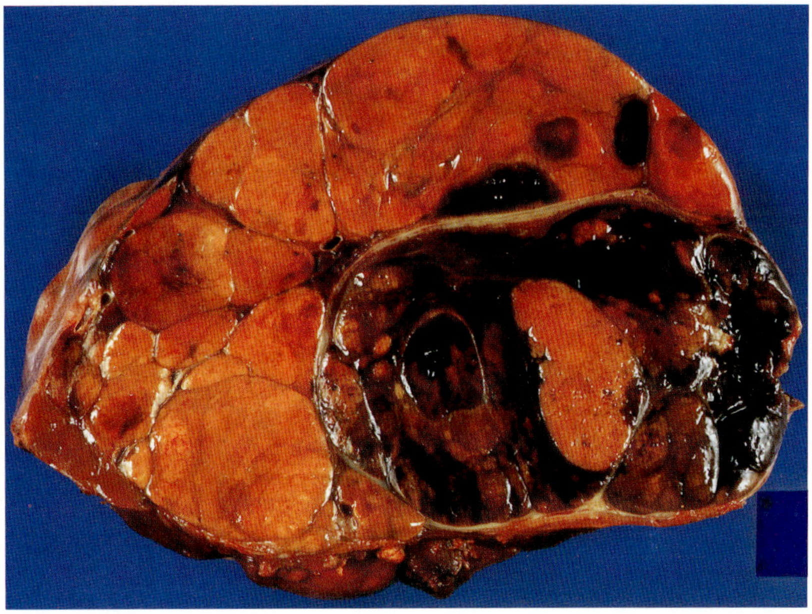

(b) Cut section of resected specimen: right trisegmentectomy was carried out. This was a massive hepatoblastoma (11.5×8 cm) consisting of a medially situated encapsulated dark reddish (due to bleeding) portion and a reddish yellow area made up of coalescent nodules lateral to it. These lesions were further divided by fibrous thin septa. Histologically, it was well differentiated epithelial hepatoblastoma of the fetal type. Tumor cells showed bile stasis, fatty changes, and clear cell changes in places which accounted for the variegated colors.

Hepatoblastoma—Case 3: Hepatoblastoma containing calcifications. A 1-year-old girl. AFP 226 ng/ml, HBsAg (−), anti-HBs (−).

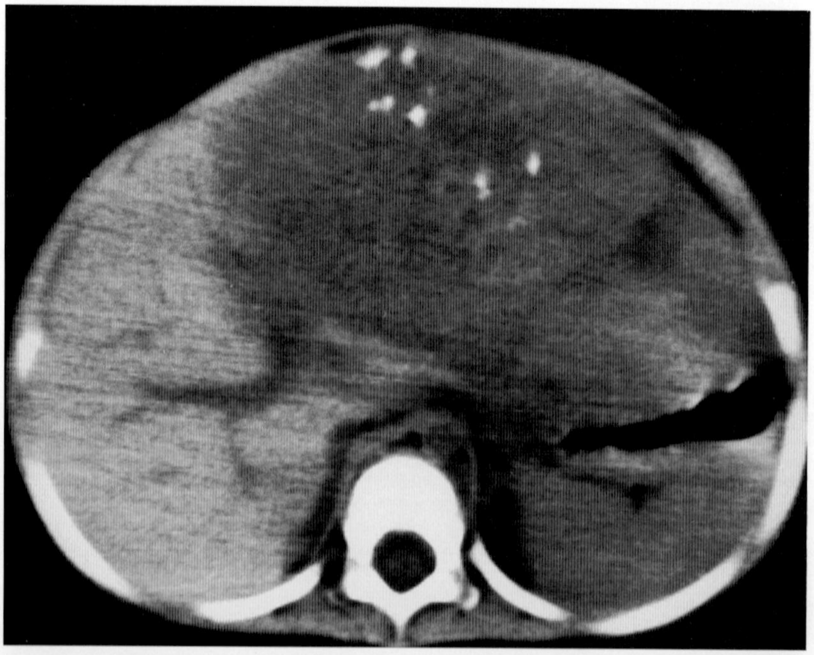

a

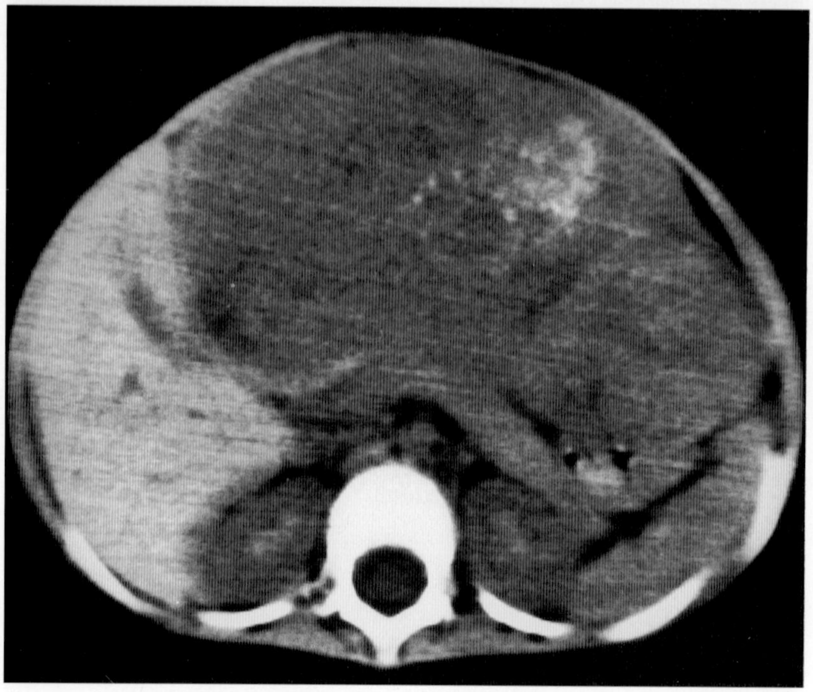

b

(a), (b) Plain CT: the left lope is occupied by a large low-density mass that contains calcifications of varying sizes and shapes. In slice (a), relatively large calcific lesions are scattered, and in slice (b), calcifications are small and densely scattered assuming a ground-glass appearance. Histologically, this was a well-differentiated epithelial hepatoblastoma of the fetal type which was studded by osteoid tissue.

4.13 Primary hepatic carcinoid tumor

Carcinoid tumor metastatic to the liver is not rare, but primary hepatic carcinoid tumor is very uncommon (Edmondson 1958; Andreola *et al.* 1990; Miura, Shirasawa 1988). Only 27 cases were found in the English literature up to 1992 (Takayasu *et al.* 1992*c*). In the review of 2837 carcinoid tumors at the National Cancer Institute, USA in 1974, none was primary to the liver (Godwin 1975). This tumor is thought to derive from the Kulchitsky cell, a type of neuroendocrine cell. We have seen two female cases, 30 and 74 years of age. In the younger case, a hepatic mass was incidentally found by US, and the older patient came to the hospital because of abdominal symptoms. They did not have the carcinoid syndrome such as flushing and wheezing. There was no characteristic imaging feature. The mass was seen as a hypervascular tumor on dynamic CT and angiography (Case 1). Formation of neovasculature was not recognized. The tumor periphery was smooth and wavy without ring enhancement or a translucent rim, which suggests no encapsulation. In both cases, small cystic lesions were seen by US and CT within the mass, perhaps resulting from bleeding. On MR imaging, the mass was of low-intensity in T1-weighted images and high-intensity in the T2-weighted. The cysts with bleeding were seen as high intensity lesions by both imaging modalities (Case 2).

The cut surface of the mass resembled that of metastatic carcinoid tumor. Therefore, to make a diagnosis of primary carcinoid tumor, one has to carefully exclude a primary in the gut and the lung.

Primary hepatic carcinoid tumor—Case 1: Primary hepatic carcinoid tumor difficult to differentiate from hepatocellular adenoma. A 74-year-old woman.

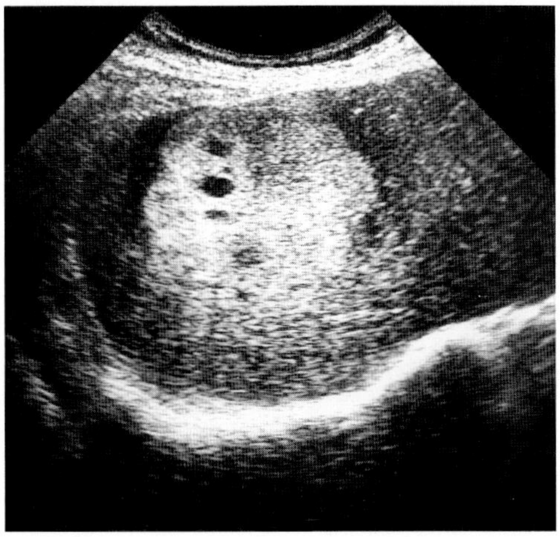

(a) US (subcostal scan): an 8×7 cm discrete hyperechoic mass was seen in S^{VIII}. The interior had several cystic lesions, but there was no halo, and hemangioma was suspected.

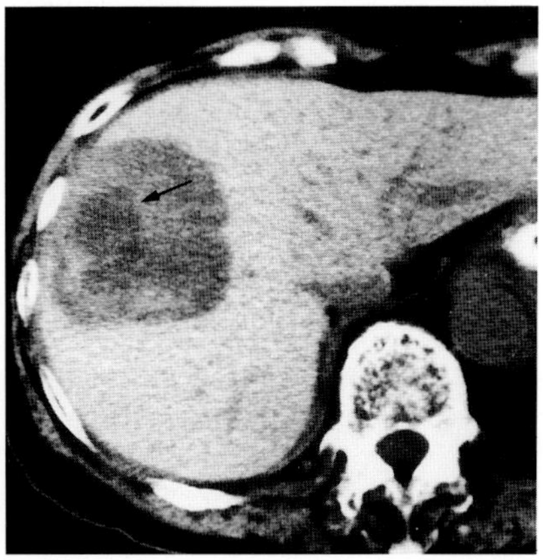

(b) Plain CT: there is a low-density mass in the anterior segment of the right lobe with a smooth but wavy margin. The interior has an area of lower density (→) and is surrounded by denser areas.

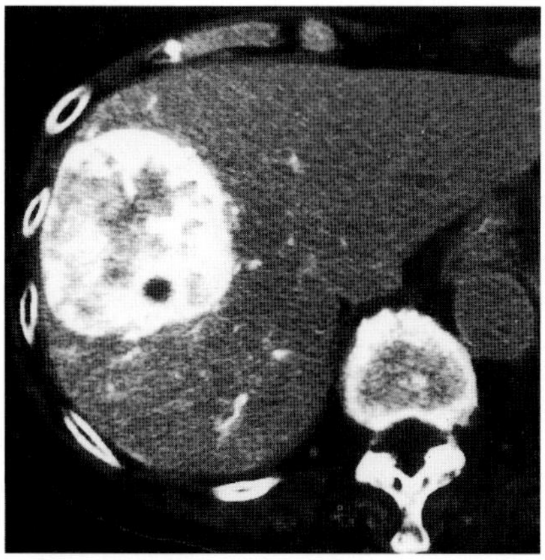

(c) Arterial-CT (early phase): the mass was enhanced from the periphery toward the center.

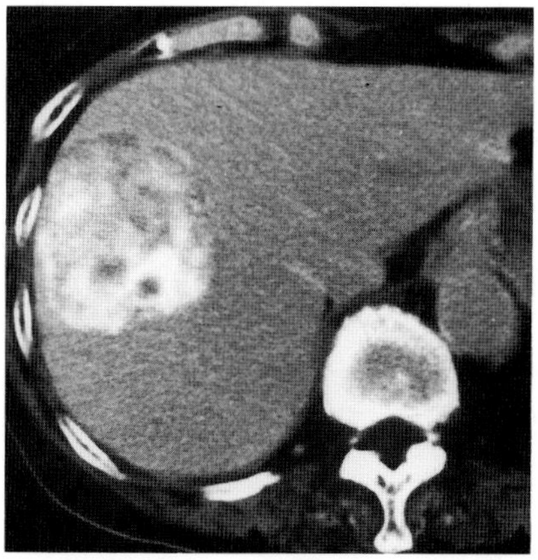

(d) Arterial-CT (late phase, 10 min): considerable pooling of contrast medium within the mass was recognized. However, peripheral low density commonly seen in adenocarcinoma was not seen.

Case 1 (contd.)

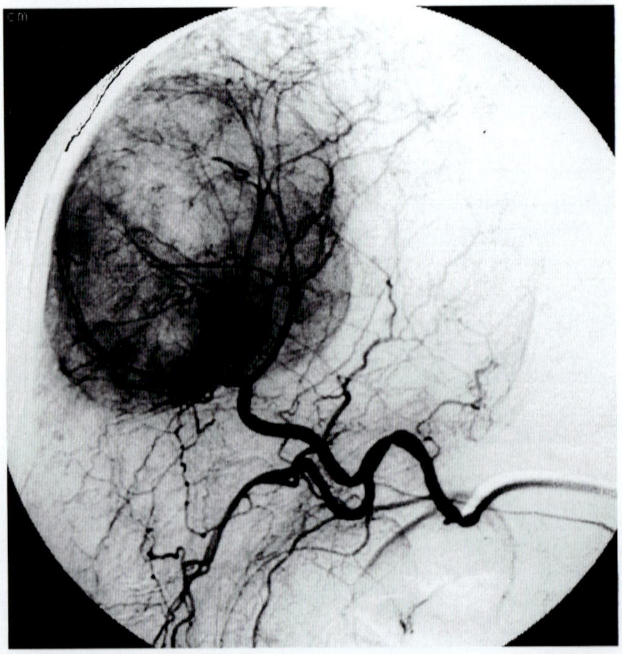

(e) Hepatic arteriogram (early phase): slight dilatation of arterial branch A^{VIII} with a distinct tumor stain is seen, but there is no tumor vessel formation or arterio-portal shunting.

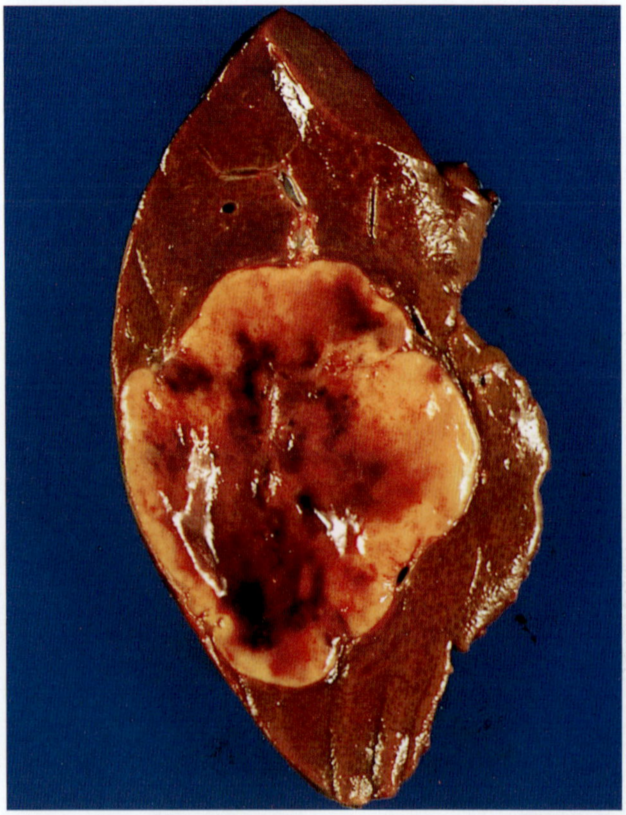

(f) Cut surface of resected specimen: the tumor was yellowish red with a smooth and wavy margin, and extensive bleeding in the center. There was no capsule formation. With conventional and immunochemical histological examinations the diagnosis of carcinoid tumor was made. The liver parenchyma was normal.

Primary hepatic carcinoid tumor—Case 2: Primary hepatic carcinoid tumor difficult to differentiate from FNH, hepatocellular adenoma and other benign tumors. A 30-year-old woman.

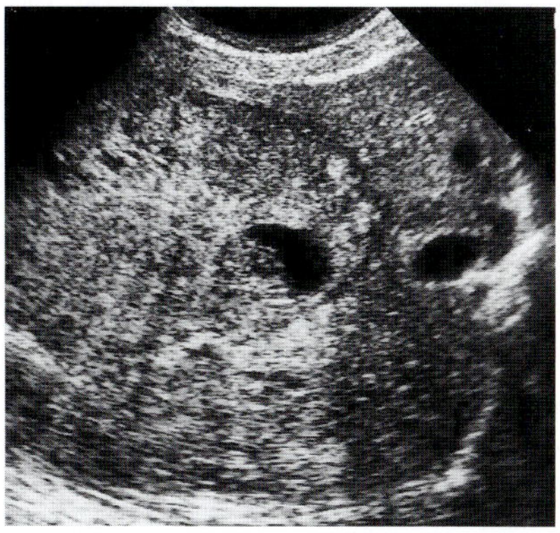

(a) US (subcostal scan): an ovoid, hyperechoic 14×7 cm mass is seen in S^{VIII-V}. The interior has a high-echo cord structure, and cystic lesions of varying sizes in the periphery. FNH was suspected.

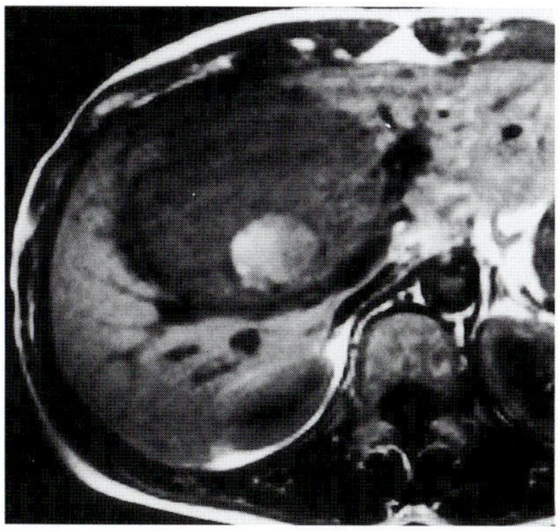

(b) MR imaging (T1-weighted SE, 500/15): a 12 cm low-intensity mass having no ovoid high-intensity area is seen in the right lobe.

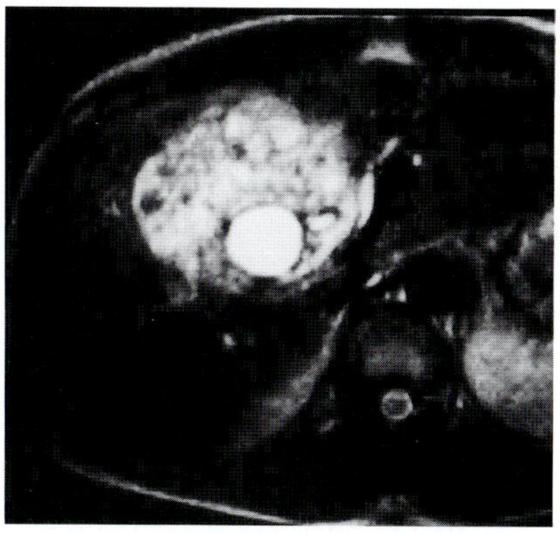

(c) MR imaging (T2-weighted SE, 2400/80): most of the mass is of high intensity consisting of confluent multiple nodules. The ovoid high-intensity lesion seen in the T1-weighted image became higher in intensity.

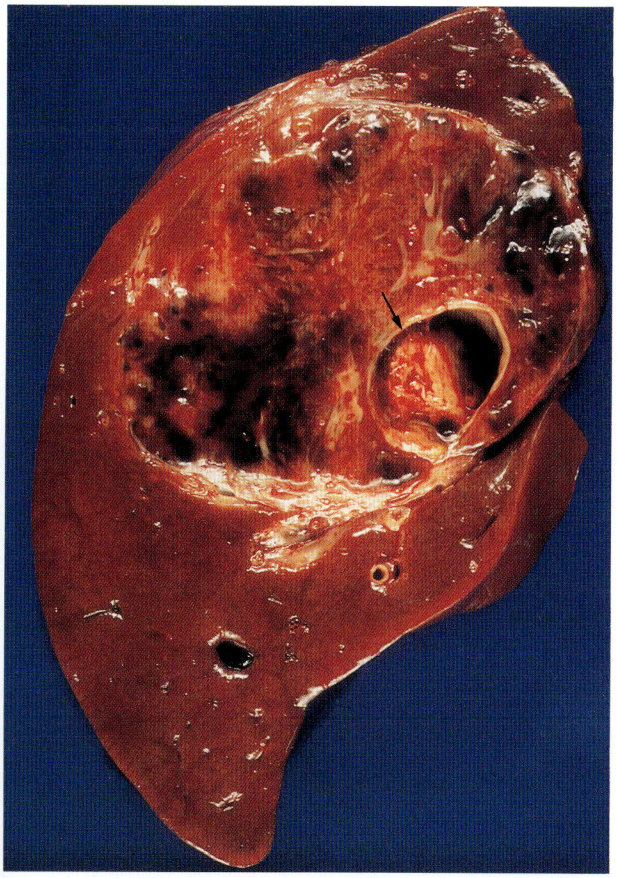

(d) Cut section of resected specimen: right trisegmentectomy was carried out. Unlike the previous case, there was a nodule-in-nodule appearance, and it grossly resembled HCC. There was bleeding and necrosis in the periphery, and capsule formation was recognized in some parts of the mass. It had a 3 cm cyst (→) containing blood, necrotic material, and exudate. Immunohistochemical study showed this to be carcinoid tumor.

4.14 Undifferentiated (mesenchymal) sarcoma

This is a malignant tumor occurring primarily in children. It is composed of primitive spindle cells with myxoid stroma without recognizable sarcomatous differentiation. This tumor has also been referred to as embryonal sarcoma (WHO 1979) and malignant mesenchymoma. The incidence varies with the report from 1 per cent (Craig *et al.* 1989) to 5 per cent (Stanley *et al.* 1973; Dehner 1978) of primary malignant hepatic tumors. By the time the diagnosis is made, the tumor is already large with internal bleeding. Grossly, it is divided by fibrous bands into cystic compartments, and on imaging, it looks like a cystic tumor. The prognosis is very poor with an average survival time of less than 1 year. The benign counterpart of this tumor may be mesenchymal hamartoma of the liver (MHL) which is difficult to differentiate from undifferentiated sarcoma preoperatively. Patients with MHL are usually younger than 5 years whereas undifferentiated sarcoma is more common in children about 10 years of age.

Undifferentiated sarcoma of the liver—Case 1: Undifferentiated sarcoma of the liver with massive internal bleeding and necrosis that looked like an hepatic cyst on CT. A 10-year-old boy with a complaint of abdominal distension. AFP 0.1 ng/ml, HBsAg (−).

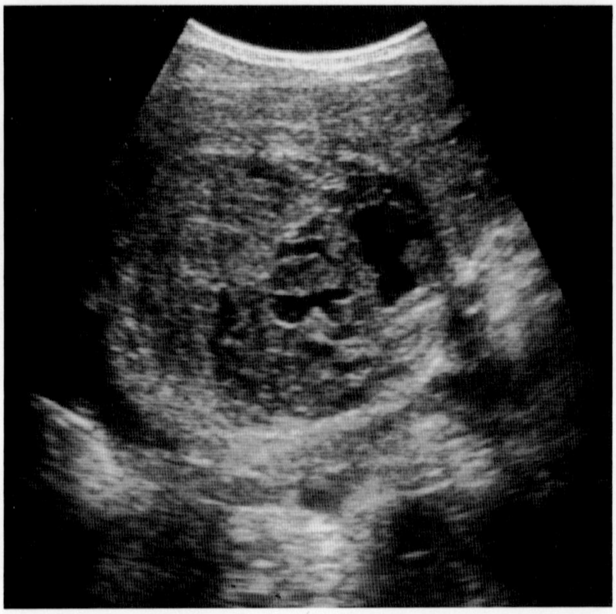

(a) US (transverse scan): there is a round discrete mass in the right lobe. The internal echoes are homogenously isoechoic mixed with several cystic lesions, looking like a honeycomb.

Case 1 (contd.)

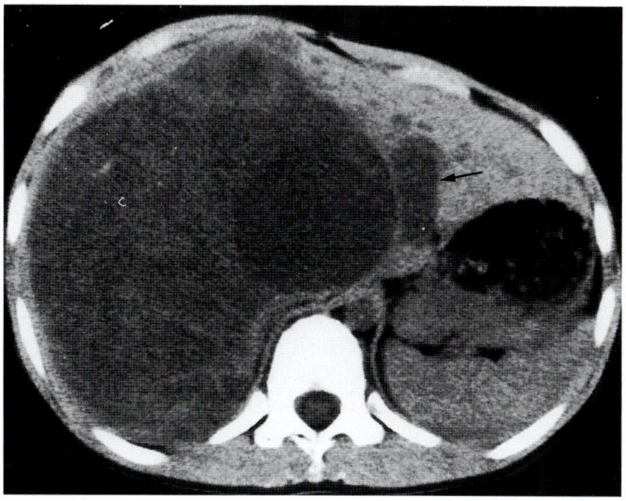

(b) Plain CT: the right love is occupied by a large low-density mass. The area anterior to the vertebral column is even lower in density. The other area of the mass has band structures. A tube-like low-density area adjacent to the mass (→) may be a metastatic lesion.

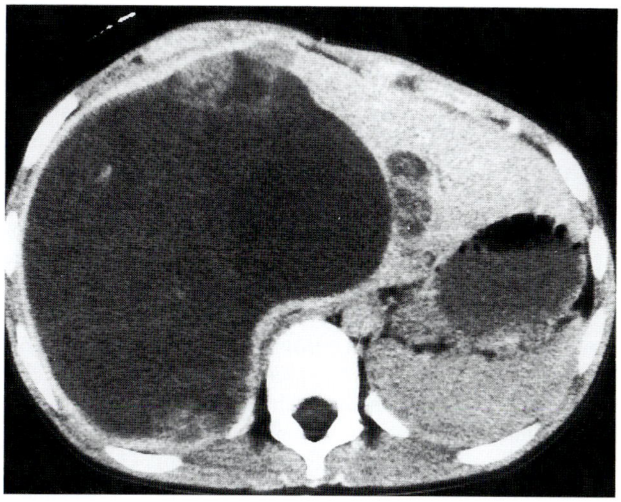

(c) Enhanced CT (late phase, 13 min): the mass was not enhanced except for small areas located anteriorly and posteriorly, and coagulative or liquefied necrosis was suspected. A cystic mass in childhood is usually mesenchymal hamartoma or its malignant counterpart, and considering the patient's age, the latter was a likely diagnosis.

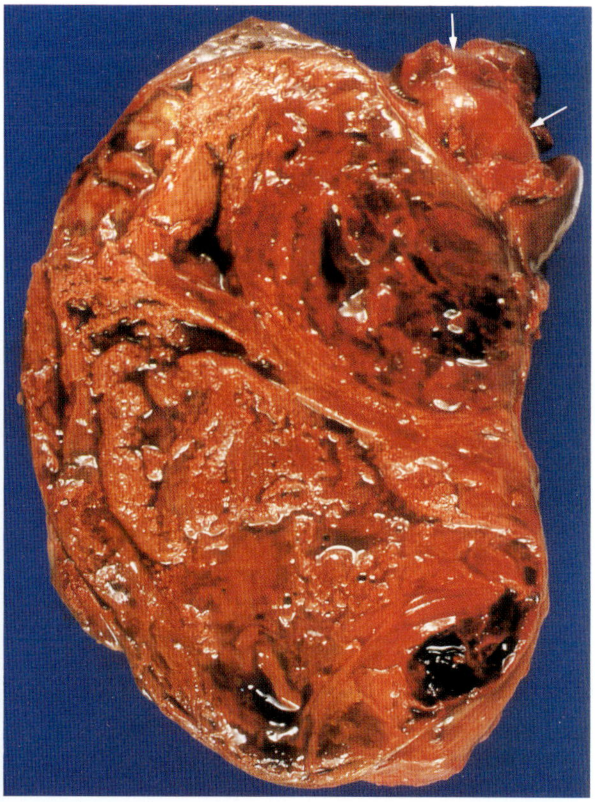

(d) Cut section of resected specimen: right trisegmentectomy was carried out (2010 g). There was a fibrous capsule surrounding the tumor. Bleeding and necrosis accounted for about 90 per cent of the mass. Histologically, spindle-shaped cells with pleomorphic nuclei and frequent mitoses were proliferating in bundles. The area shown by an arrow (→) in (b) was in continuity with the main tumor, and considered to represent a budding growth. The non-tumor portion was normal.

4.15 Hepatic angiosarcoma

This is a malignant tumor derived from the endothelial lining cell occurring in adults (Locker *et al.* 1979) in asssociation with certain chemicals (vinyl chloride monomer, arsenical, etc.) (Falk *et al.* 1974) and radiation (Throtrast, radium implant) (Brady *et al.* 1977). The prognosis is very poor, and most patients die within six months of diagnosis. Although hepatic angiosarcoma is rare, it is one of the most common malignant mesenchymal tumors of the liver. The male:female ratio is 3 to 1 and the average age is 53 years (Locker *et al.* 1979). Childhood angiosarcoma is very rare with fewer than 12 patients reported before 1984 (Falk *et al.* 1981; Nornha and Gonzalez-Crussi 1984). Clinical presentations include hepatomegaly, ascites (25 per cent), jaundice (25 per cent), thrombocytopenia (50 per cent) and rupture (15 per cent) (Ishak 1976).

The tumor usually contains multiple bleedings that produce cystic changes with blood and coagulum. Therefore, when seen by US, it consists of solid and cystic portions. On enhanced CT, it shows the fill-in pattern as in cavernous hemangioma (Itai and Teraoka 1989), but the enhancement is much stronger. The internal structure of angiosarcoma in CT images is much more complex, making differential diagnosis possible. Angiosarcoma is seen as a hypointense mass on T1-weighted MR images and a hyperintense one on T2-weighted images (Ohtomo *et al.* 1992; Buetow *et al.* 1994). As it frequently has hemorrhage, the intensity of the lesion on T1-weighted images varies from hypo- to hyperintensity. The pattern of enhancement with Gd-DTPA is similar to that of hemangioma, because both tumors contain a large number of blood-filled vascular spaces. However, angiosarcoma is more inhomogeneous with a dilated neovasculature. As a benign hemangioma enlarges, the low density interior becomes even lower in density (hyalinization) and is not stained by contrast medium even in the late phase of enhanced CT (cf. Case 2 of hemangioma, p.56). However, hemangioma is generally less complex in the interior and has no complicated hemodynamics. On angiography, there are many tumor vessels in angiosarcoma showing a marked tumor stain in the late phase. There may be artrio-portal shunts and spread within the liver and spleen (Kishikawa *et al.* 1977).

Hepatic angiosarcoma—Case 1: Hepatic angiosarcoma displaying marked tumor stain on angiography while resembling hemangioma on dynamic CT (courtesy of Dr H. Ohkado).

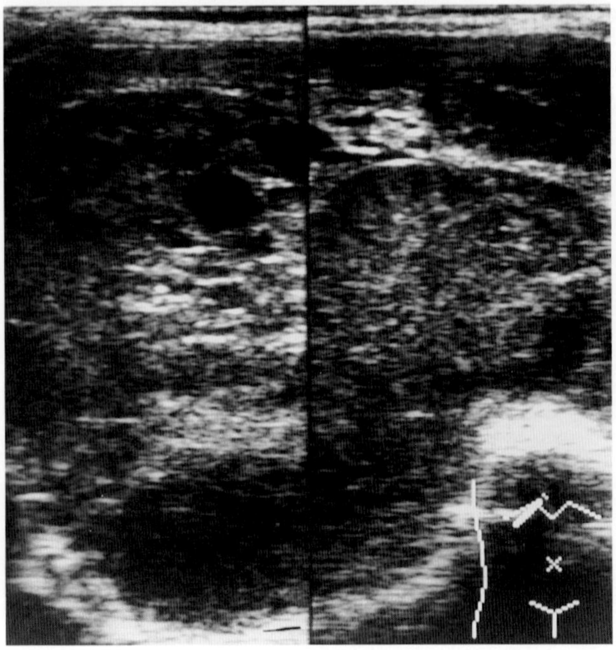

(a) US: a large mass is seen occupying the right lobe. A number of cystic lesions are seen anteriorly.

Case 1 (contd.)

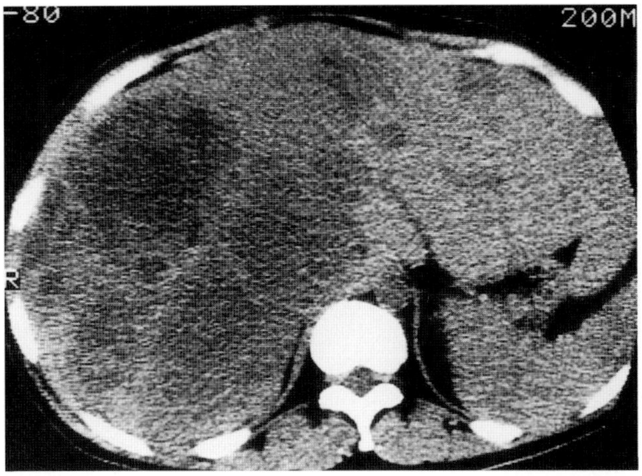

(b) Plain CT: a large low-density tumor occupies the right lobe and the medial part of the left lobe. The interior demonstrates an uneven density and a complex structure.

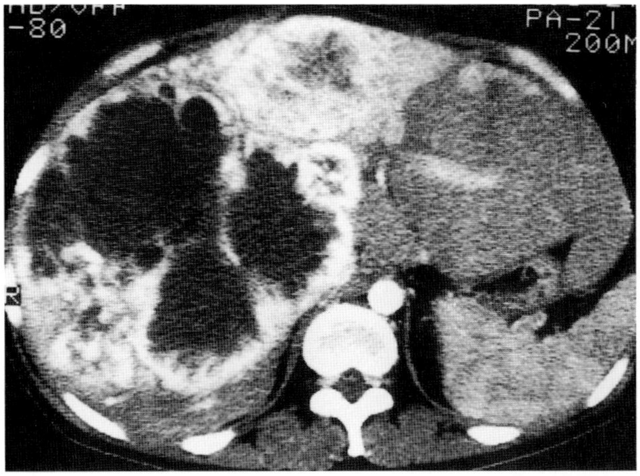

(c) Enhanced CT (early phase): the periphery was strongly enhanced and the interior showed a septal structure. The main mass was sandwiched by secondaries, one to the right and another to the left.

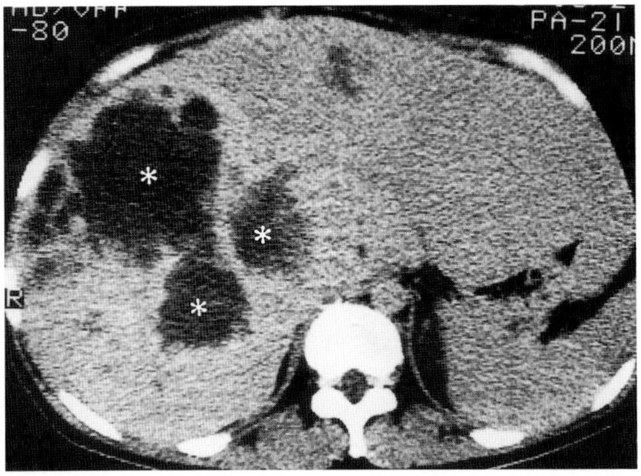

(d) Enhanced CT (late phase): the enhancement somewhat increased toward the center (fill-in), and the whole mass except the cystic areas (*) showed a homogeneous stain. The secondaries turned isodense.

Case 1 (contd.)

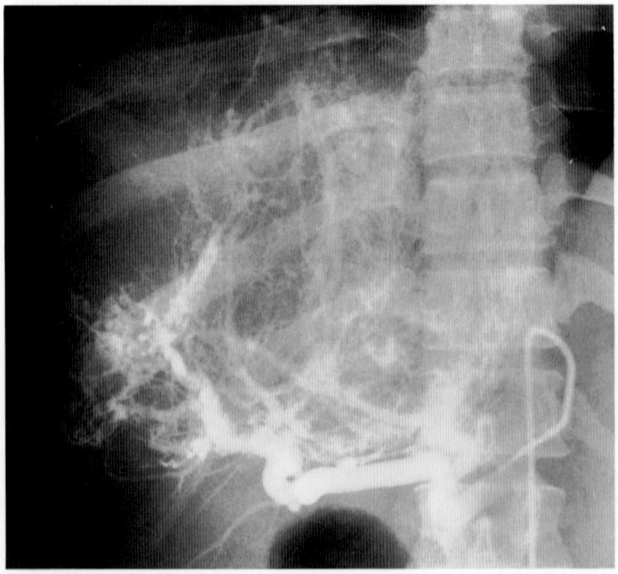

(e) Angiography (early phase): numerous tumor vessels are seen coming off the enlarged right and medial hepatic arteries.

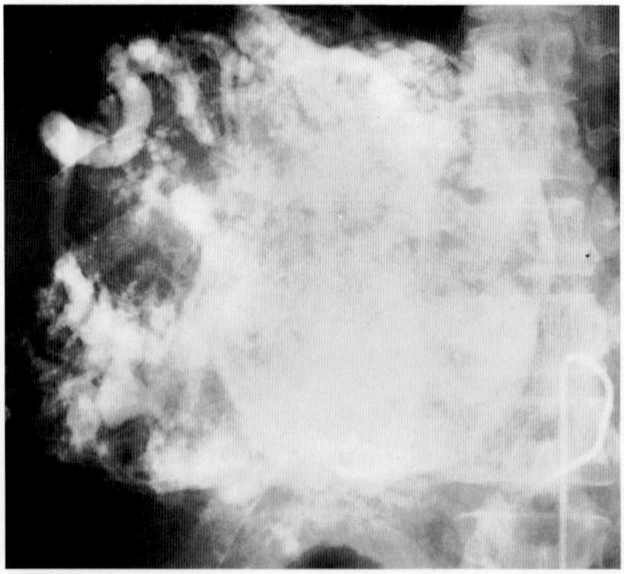

(f) Angiography (late phase): marked tumor stains and accompanying tortuous large vessels are apparent. There are many intrahepatic secondaries.

4.16 Epithelioid hemangioendothelioma

The term 'epithelioid hemangioendothelioma' (EHE) coined by Weiss and Enzinger (1982) does not reflect its malignant nature and should perhaps be called malignant EHE (Craig *et al.* 1989). It is a slowly growing tumor composed of epithelioid cells, abundant sclerosis, and myxoid stroma (Ishak *et al.* 1984). It arises in soft tissue (epithelioid hemangioendothelioma of soft tissue) (Dail *et al.* 1975), lung (intravascular bronchioloalveolar tumor, IVBAT) (Ellis and Kratichvil 1986) and liver. Liver EHE is rare and is thought to derive from the endothelium that forms the sinusoid. The lesion is usually located beneath the hepatic capsule with a capsular retraction in the center of the mass. The epithelioid cells consist of elongated cells with vacuolated cytoplasm called dendritic cells and plump pleomorphic epithelioid cells. They grow into sinusoids in a papillary fashion. The factor VIII stain by immunoperoxidase confirms the vascular origin of these cells. It is a firm tumor with occasional calcifications. If it evolves in the liver, it is usually multiple and grows slowly, and metastasis to distant organs is not very common. Thus, this is a tumor of low malignancy, and while 20 per cent of patients die in two years, another 20 per cent live 5–28 years (Ishak *et al.* 1984). It occurs in adults of all ages, and 66 per cent of patients are women (Radin *et al.* 1988).

CT findings suggest that the tumor begins as multiple nodules that grow and coalesce, forming large confluent masses, preferentially involving the liver periphery. The tumor interior is hypoechoic on US and low in density in CT study, and it may appear like an arrow target (Noguchi *et al.* 1987; Furui *et al.* 1989) (Case 1). In our patient, arterial-CT demonstrated a three-layer structure, the center never being stained while the low-density outermost layer slowly enhanced. On angiography, there was no neovasculature in the early phase, and multiple target-like hypovascular lesions were seen in the late phase. On MR imaging, the tumor signal is hypointense on T1-weighted images and hyperintense on T2-weighted images with a halo of hypointensity (Miller *et al.* 1993). According to Van Beers *et al.* (1992), however, the lesions were composed of a hyperintense rim and central concentric low- or high-intensity areas on T2-weighted images. The hyperintense peripheral area histopathologically corresponded to viable tumor and the central zone of high intensity to loose and edematous connective tissue; the central zone of hypointensity contained mainly coagulation necrosis, calcifications, and scattered hemorrhages. More information is needed to settle the inconsistency.

As long as there is no extrahepatic metastasis, liver transplantation may be considered, and in fact good results have been reported in 10 cases (Kelleher *et al.* 1989). As regards the origin of multiple tumors, both intrahepatic spread and multifocal evolution are possible, but as these nodules are similar in size without an apparent large primary mass, the latter seems more likely. The imaging features of EHE may be distinguishable from those of hepatic vascular tumors such as angiosarcoma, hemangioma, and infantile hemangioendothelioma. Infantile hemangioendothelioma spontaneously regresses, as already discussed. The major difficulty in imaging diagnosis is differentiation from metastatic hypovascular tumors. The prognosis varies with the reports (Radin *et al.* 1988).

Hepatic epithelioid hemangioendothelioma—Case 1: Epithelioid hemangioendothelioma difficult to differentiate from metastic tumors. A 19-year-old man. Multiple liver masses were incidentally discovered by US.

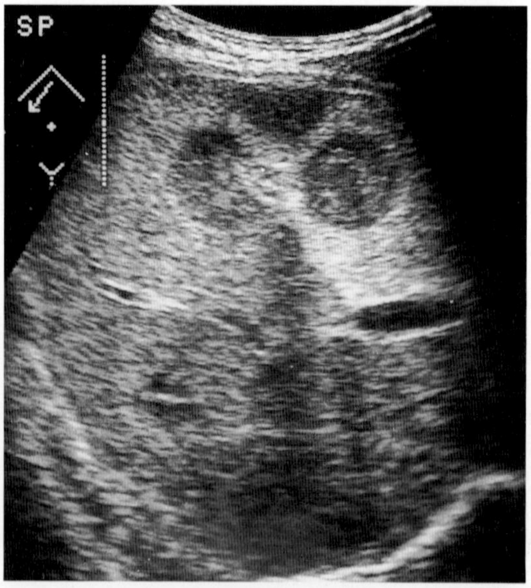

(a) US (transverse scan): many 2 cm size hypoechoic masses are recognized. The boundary between the tumor and parenchyma is discrete. A three-layer structure is discerned with a low-echo center, an isoechoic middle zone, and an outermost hypoechoic layer; it looks like an arrow target.

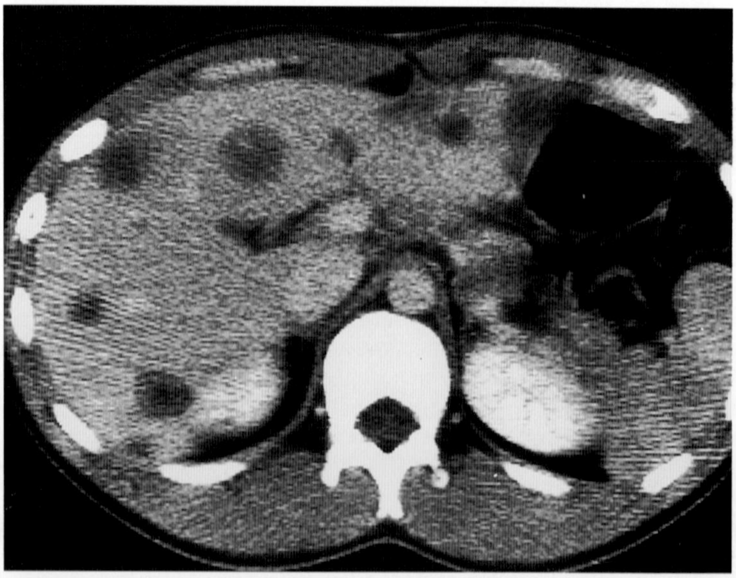

(b) Enhanced CT: plain CT displayed multiple, somewhat ill-demarcated, low-density lesions (not shown). These lesions were not enhanced at all, making the contrast with the surrounding liver parenchyma stronger in the late phase. Metastatic cancer was the most likely diagnosis, but no extrahepatic primary was detected.

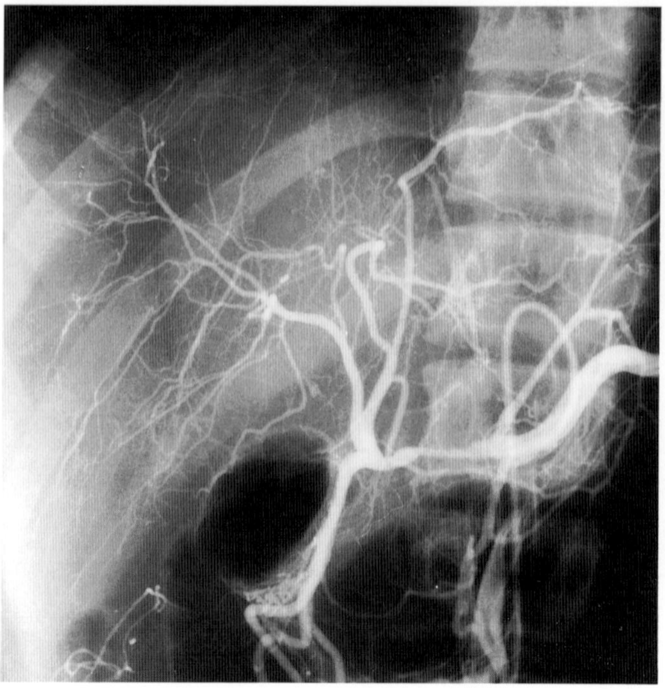

(c) Hepatic arteriogram (early phase): there is no tumor stain.

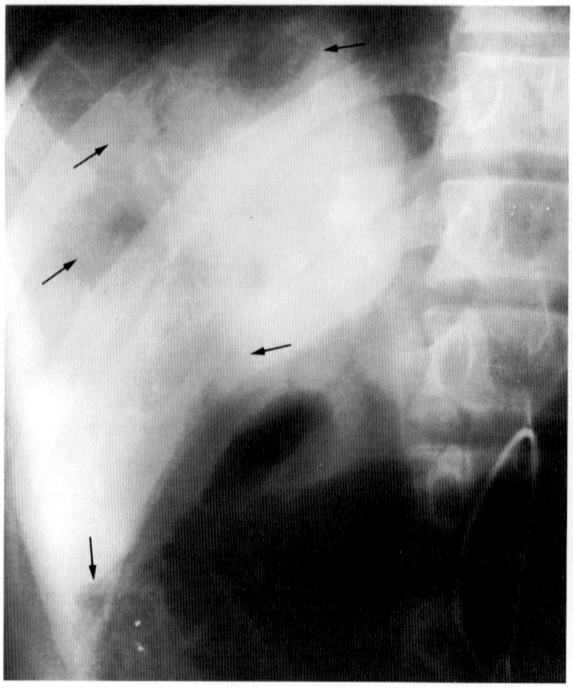

(d) Superior mesenteric arterial portogram: the portal vein is intact and many filling defects (→) are discerned in the parenchymal phase.

Case 1 (contd.)

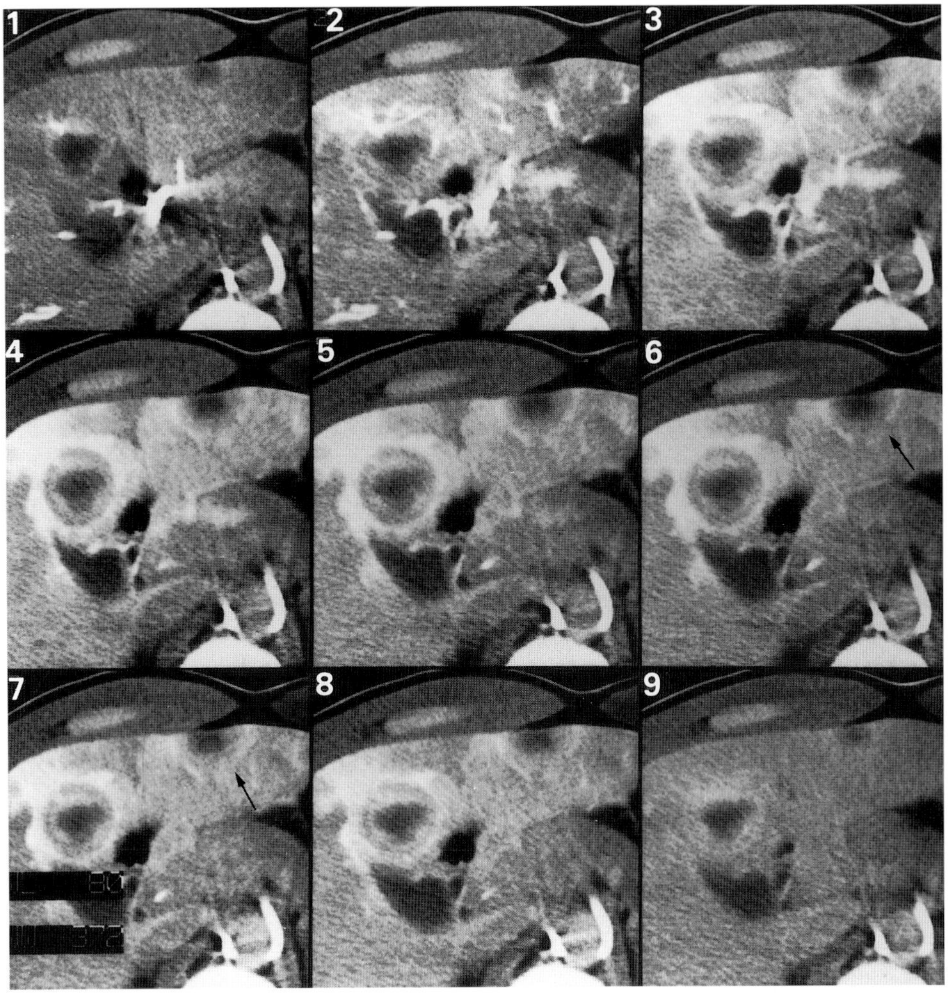

(e) Arterial-CT: temporal changes that occurred in one lesion in S^{IV} on arterial-CT are displayed here (1–9). The center remained unenhanced throughout. The midzone was enhanced from an early phase while the peripheral zone was enhanced less rapidly, and the enhancement seemed to come through the midzone. At 5 min (9), both the midzone and peripheral zone remained enhanced. It was thought that the extratumoral enhancement occurred through portal invasion in the tumor periphery, or compensatory increase of arterial flow in the periphery as a result of portal occlusion. Some of the tumors near the liver surface (→) showed cancer umbilication.

Case 1 (contd.)

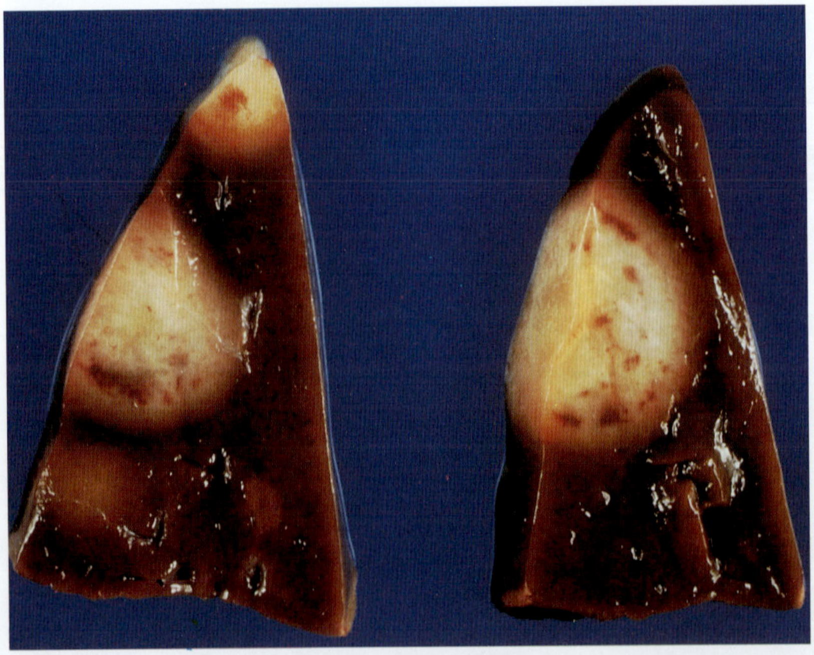

(f) Cut surface of resected specimen: exploratory resection of the lateral portion of the left lobe was carried out. The tumor–parenchyma border showed a gradual transition and the advancing tumor head seemed blurred. There were several sites of bleeding along the inner aspect of the peripheral zone. The midzone was white and the center yellow. There was a cancer umbilication on the liver surface. Histopathologically, in the peripheral zone tumor cells were growing in a papillary fashion into sinusoids and medium-sized blood vessels (perhaps portal). Immunohistochemically these cells were positive for factor VIII, making the diagnosis of EHE possible. Liver parenchyma was normal.

4.17 Primary hepatic lymphoma

Primary hepatic lymphoma is a malignant tumor with lymphoid markers and is confined to the liver without a primary lesion in the lymph node or extrahepatic tissue. Hodgkin's disease and non-Hodgkin lymphoma metastatic to the liver are common, being seen in 15 and 25 per cent respectively of the patients with these diseases at our hospital. At the autopsy table, they are more frequent. However, primary hepatic lymphoma is very rare. There were 28 documented cases in the world literature up to 1985 (Osborne *et al.* 1985; Gaulard *et al.* 1986; DeMent *et al.* 1987), and only 4 cases reported in Japan. Bechtold *et al.* (1985) observed delayed enhancement of the mass in an enhanced CT study, and suggested this to be characteristic of hepatic lymphoma. Our experience has been different. In our case (Case 1), the CT feature resembled that of HCC except for the tumor periphery which was indented in places. Gazelle *et al.* (1994) failed to find characteristic imaging features to differentiate primary from secondary lymphoma except for the findings that the former had a single well-defined lesion and the latter multiple or diffusely infiltrating lesions.

Primary hepatic lymphoma—Case 1: Primary hepatic lymphoma (courtesy of Dr D. J. Brandt). A 68-year-old white man with weight loss and night sweating.

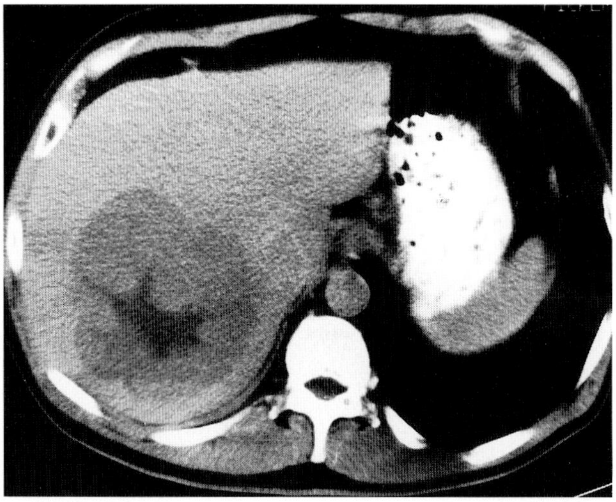

(a) Drip infusion enhanced CT (i.v. infusion, late phase): a large mass is seen in the right lobe. The periphery is smooth but wavy. The interior has a low-density stellate area.

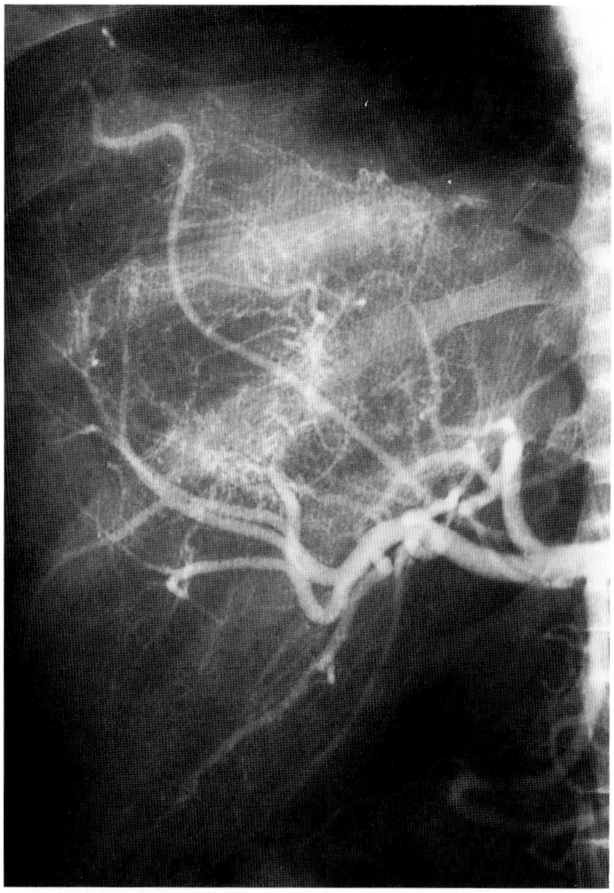

(b) Celiac arteriogram: many thin tumor vessels are seen, but no encasement. Laparotomy was carried out, but radical operation was not possible because of infiltration into the diaphragm and major hepatic veins. Only the hepatic mass was removed which was histologically diagnosed as histiocytic lymphoma.

4.18 Other malignant hepatic tumors

Other primary malignant hepatic tumors include leiomyosarcoma (Fong and Ruebner 1974; Boulstein 1978), rhabdomyosarcoma (Horowitz *et al.* 1987; Davis *et al.* 1969), fibrosarcoma (Ishak 1976; Gen *et al.* 1983), squamous cell carcinoma (Song *et al.* 1984; Craig *et al.* 1989), malignant schwannoma (Sordillo *et al.* 1981; Lederman *et al.* 1987), osteosarcoma (Sumiyoshi and Niho 1971; von Hochstetter *et al.* 1987), malignant fibrous histiocytoma (Conran and Stocker 1985; Alberti-Flor *et al.* 1985), and a few others.

4.19 Primary liver cancer and cancers in other organs

With improved imaging techniques, increasing numbers of patients with HCC are found to have other cancers developing synchronously or metachronously, creating new problems in differential diagnosis and therapy. Multiple cancers primary to different tissues and site-pairings are to be distinguished (Cook 1966). At the National Cancer Center Hospital, Tokyo, 33 of 393 cases (8.4 per cent) of HCC had another cancer elsewhere. Of these 65 per cent were metachronous, mostly developing prior to HCC detection (Fig. 4.11). They consisted of carcinomas of the stomach (31 per cent), colorectum (16 per cent), larynx (13 per cent), tongue (6 per cent), etc. One-third ware synchronous and two-thirds metachronous (Case 1) (Takayasu *et al.* 1992*a*). The incidence of multiple cancers seems to be increasing, perhaps due to prolonged survival of patients.

The main clinical problems with multiple primary cancers are firstly accurate diagnosis of whether the discovered liver tumor is primary or secondary. To achieve it, one must be familiar with the differences in imaging features between HCC and metastatic tumors, and interpret the findings without a preformed idea. Secondly it is important to know that there is a 10 per cent possibility of a secondary and even a tertiary cancer developing after complete cure of the first cancer. One should not immediately assume a tumor found in the liver to be metastatic if the patient has an extrahepatic primary. When we analyzed patients with multiple primary cancers in whom hepatic resection was carried out, preoperative quality diagnosis was made by angiography in 91.3 per cent, CT in 79.3 per cent and US in 78.6 per cent. In patients with a primary liver cancer, combined hepatocellular and cholangiocarcinoma (Case 1, p.261) and intrahepatic bile duct carcinoma were difficult to differentiate from metastatic cancer.

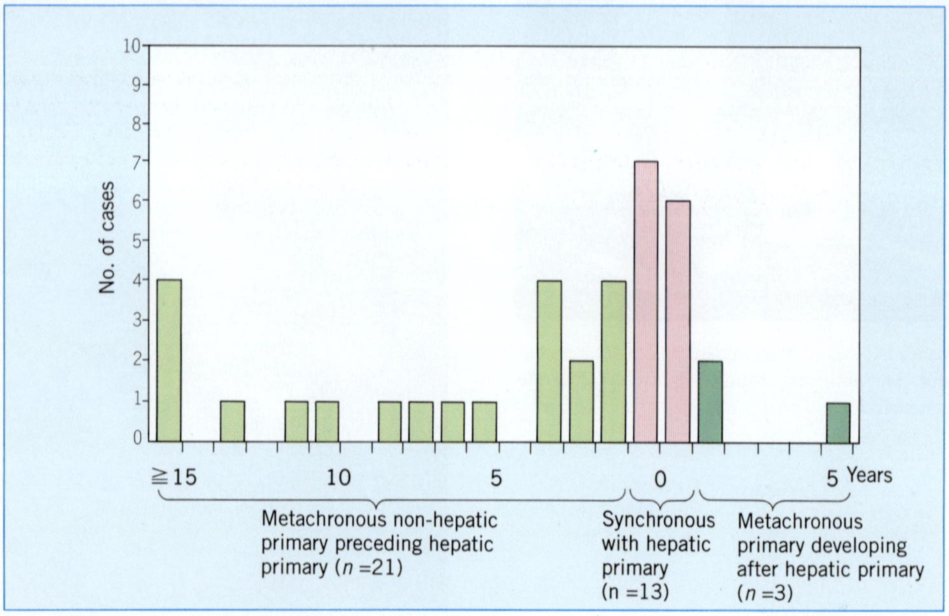

Fig. 4.11 Interval between the development of primary hepatic cancer and of another primary. Analysis of 37 cases (including 4 triple cancers) for the interval between hepatic and non-hepatic primary cancers. Non-hepatic primaries detected within 1 year of hepatic resection were considered synchronous.

Primary liver cancer and cancers in other organs—Case 1: Metachronous colon cancer and HCC. A 73-year-old man who underwent sigmoidectomy for sigmoid colon cancer 2.5 years earlier. Elevation of AFP (170 ng/ml) lead to the detection of hepatic tumor by US.

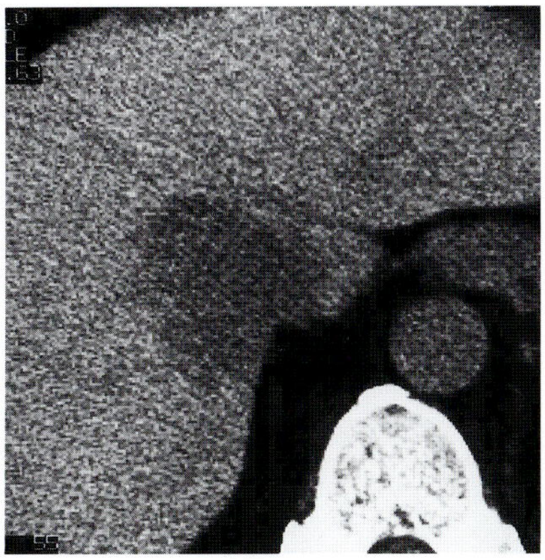

(a) Plain CT: a 3.5 cm low-density mass with an irregular margin was found in the right lobe.

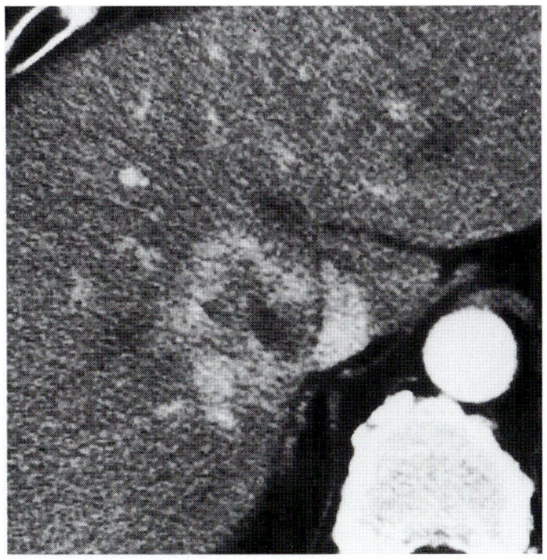

(b) Dynamic CT (early phase): the periphery of the mass was enhanced in a nodular pattern in close proximity to the inferior vena cava. The tumor lies in S^{VIII}, S^{VII} and the right caudate lobe (S^{I}_{r}). In this particular situation, operability depends on quality diagnosis, because if it is an adenocarcinoma separation of the tumor and the inferior vena cava is difficult, whereas if HCC, it may be possible.

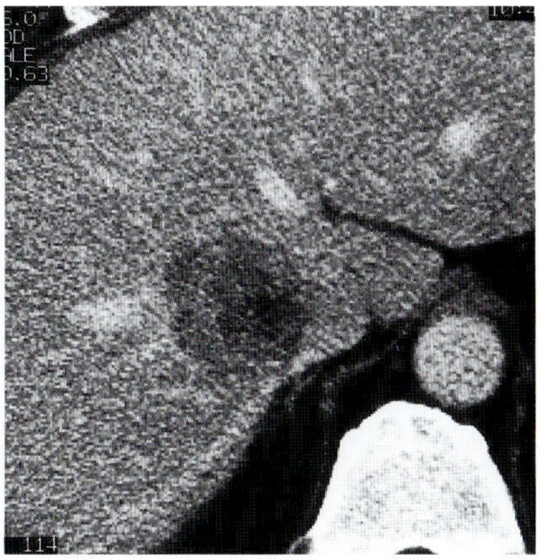

(c) Dynamic CT (late phase, 5 min): the mass turned low in density, but there was no ring enhancement or peripheral low-density area. Since the margin was irregular, unencapsulated HCC or combined hepatocellular and cholangiocarcinoma was the likely diagnosis.

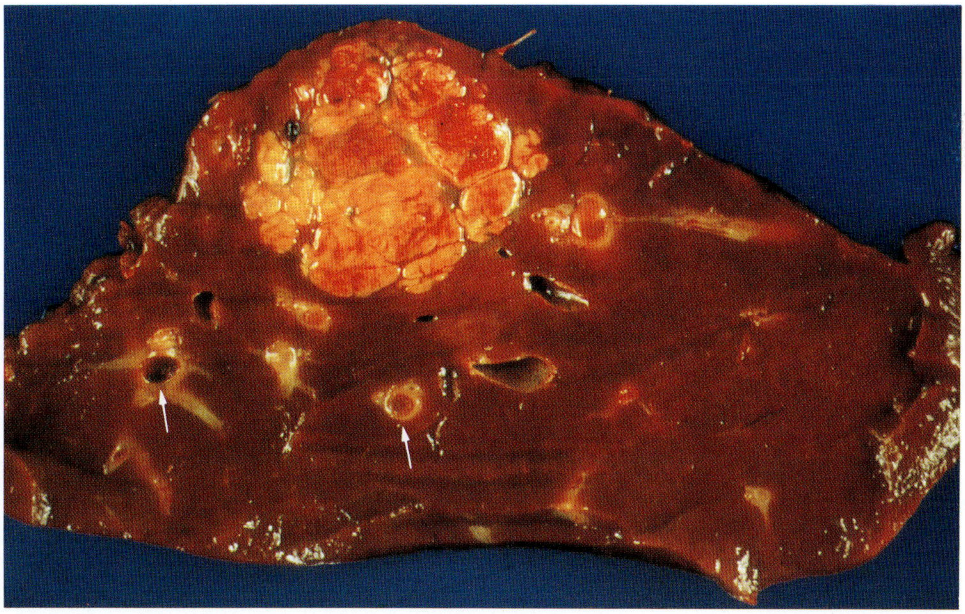

(f) Cut section of resected specimen: there was no infiltration to the inferior vena cava, and right lobectomy was carried out. Grossly, the tumor was of the confluent multinodular type (type 3) without encapsulation. Histologically, it was Edmondson's grade III. The blood clot in a portal vein branch (→) was due to preoperative portal vein embolization.

Primary liver cancer and cancers in other organs—Case 2: Metachronous gastric cancer (Borrmann type IV) and HCC. A 61-year-old man. One year after the start of chemotherapy for advanced gastric cancer, a liver tumor was found.

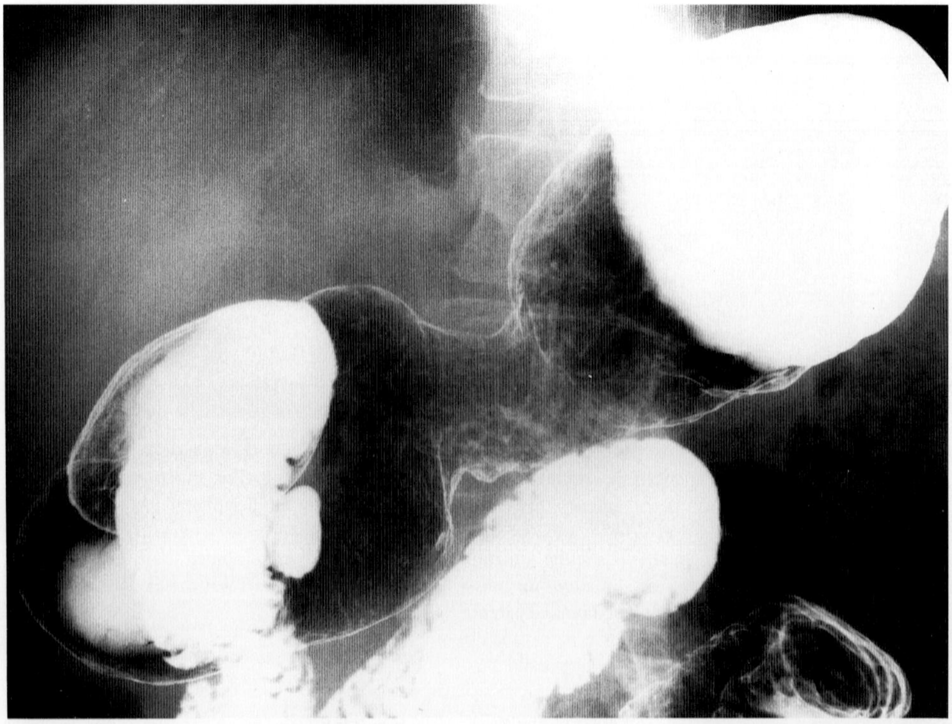

(a) Double contrast barium examination of the stomach: the middle portion of the body is rigid with little extendibility, and the mucosa is irregular. The diagnosis was advanced Borrmann type IV cancer. Systemic chemotherapy was started with Mitomycin C and Tegafur.

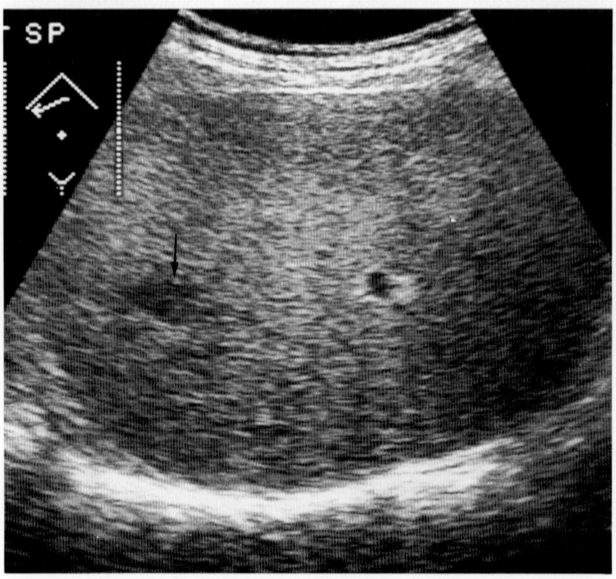

(b) US: at the time of gastric cancer detection, US examination of the liver was unremarkable (not shown). One year later, a 1.4 cm low-echo lesion (→) was found which was thought to be metastatic.

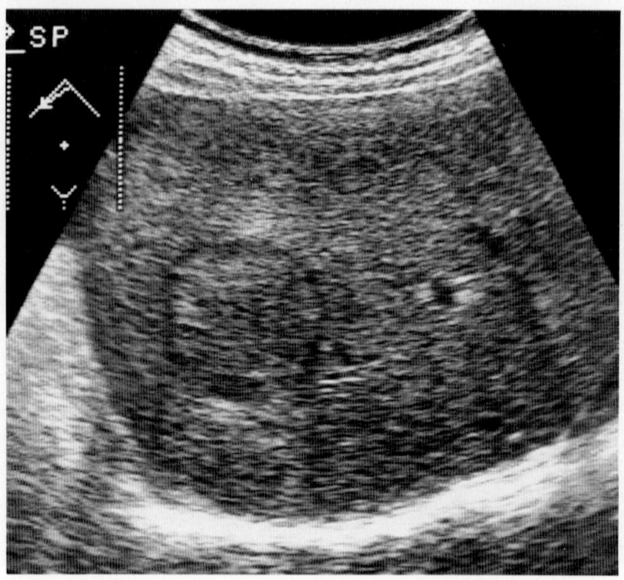

(c) US: the mass slowly enlarged (4×3 cm). Lateral shadowing and a halo, typical of HCC, are now recognizable. Subsequent needle biopsy proved this to be HCC.

4.20 Metastatic hepatic tumors

In the past, metastatic liver cancer was not considered for surgery due to delayed diagnosis. This attitude of surgeons has changed and currently early detection and early operation are common practice owing to improved imaging diagnosis. For that reason, determination of whether the found mass is really a metastasis to the liver, primary liver cancer incidentally discovered (multiple primaries) (Case 1), or an incidental benign hepatic tumor, is important. To screen patients for metastatic liver cancer, various tumor markers, mostly organ specific, should be determined at regular intervals along with US and/or CT examination (Fig. 4.12).

Clinical pathology

The route of hepatic metastasis may be either hematogenous (via the portal vein or hepatic artery), direct invasion from a neighboring tissue, or intraabdominal dissemination. In medical books it is generally stated that hepatic metastasis is a late event occurring mostly in stage IV cancer (cancer of the stomach, colon, breast, etc.). However, prognosis varies considerably with the site of the primary as these cancers differ in biological properties, response to chemotherapy, and mode of metastasis. Some patients with breast cancer can live for more than 10 years while bearing the cancer whereas patients with pancreatic cancer live for only a short period. In hematogenous metastasis to

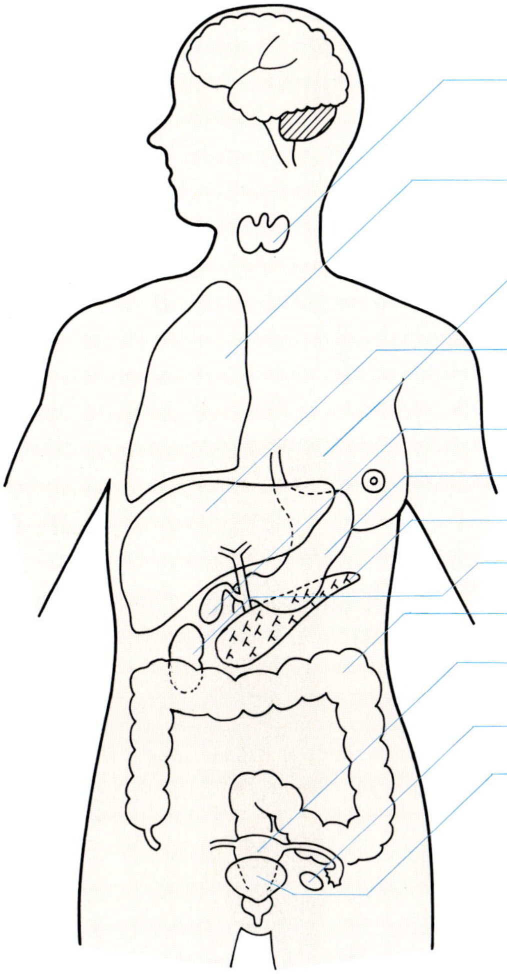

Tumor	Tumor marker	Positivity rate (%)
Medullary thyroid ca	Calcitonin CEA	90 90
Lung cancer: Squamous cell ca Adenoca Small cell ca Oat cell ca	SCC CEA NSA ACTH	40–60 50 65–75
Breast cancer		35–50
HCC Cholangiocarcinoma	AFP PIVKA-II CA 19–9 CEA	80 50 70 50
Gallbladder, bile duct cancer	CA 19–9, CA50 or Span-1	80
Stomach cancer	CA 924 or STn	50
Pancreas cancer	CA 19–9 or Span-1	80–90
Renal cancer	BFP	50
Colorectal cancer	CEA or CA 19–9	60
Uterine, cervical cancer Body cancer	SCC CA 125	60 60
Ovarian cancer	CA 125	80–85
Prostate cancer	PAP, PSA, or γ-SM	70
Choriocarcinoma	hCG PL-ALP	100 80
Endocrine tumor	Individual hormone	90

CEA, carcinoembryonic antigen; SCC, squamous cell carcinoma antigen; NSE, neuron specific enolase; CA 19–9, carbohydrate 19–9; AFP, alpha-fetoprotein; PIVKA-II, protein induced by vitamin K absence or antagonist II, BFP, basic fetoprotein; PAP, prostatic acid phosphatase; PSA, prostatic cancer specific antigen; gamma-SM, gamma-seminoprotein; hCG, human chorionic gonadotropin; PL-ALP, placenta alkaline phosphatase; STn, sialylated Tn antigen.

Fig. 4.12 Tumor markers with relatively high organ specificity and positivity.

the liver, therapy and prognosis vary with the route that transported the cancer cells. If the route was arterial, extahepatic metastases should be expected, and if portal, metastasis may be limited to the liver (e.g. colon cancer); it depends on the site of primary.

Frequencies of hepatic metastases in autopsies

Our analysis of 392 autopsies for extrahepatic primary malignancies showed hepatic metastases in 55 per cent of the cases (Table 4.11). The types (organs) of cancers causing hepatic metastasis in decreasing order were skin cancer (100 per cent), colon cancer (93.3 per cent), breast cancer (87.5 per cent), ovarian tumor (87.5 per cent), etc. Metastases from pancreatic cancer and gallbladder cancer were also frequent. Although the incidence of skin cancer is low in Japan, widespread metastases including the liver are commonly seen at the time of death because patients live quite a long time. The same may be said of breast cancer. Primaries in certain organs are biologically very malignant and kill patients early before distant metastasis occurs, making the frequency of hepatic metastasis low.

Although much disputed, many reports have suggsted that metastatic cancer is uncommon in cirrhotic liver (Lisa *et al.* 1942; Gall 1960; Ruebner *et al.* 1961), and a cancer found in a cirrhotic liver is more likely to be HCC, particular in the Orient. In our case control study on 529 cirrhotic and 529 noncirrhotic livers autopsied, there were only 22 metastatic liver cancers in the former and 395 cancers in the latter (Melato *et al.* 1989).

Table 4.11 Frequencies of hepatic metastases in relation to the sites of primaries based on autopsy cases (Jan. 1985–Feb. 1987)

Site of primary	No. of autopsies	No. of cases with hepatic metastasis (%)	Order
Lung	75	38 (51.4)	
Stomach	57	31 (54.4)	
Breast	32	28 (87.5)	3
Oral cavity, pharynx	27	7 (25.9)	
Esophagus	21	7 (33.3)	
Malignant lymphoma	21	11 (52.4)	
Pancreas	19	15 (78.9)	6
Leukemia	16	8 (50.0)	
Colon	15	14 (93.3)	2
Uterus	13	8 (61.5)	
Upper respiratory tract	11	0	
Kidney	9	7 (77.8)	7
Gallbladder	8	6 (75.0)	8
Rectum	8	5 (62.5)	
Ovary	8	7 (87.5)	3
Bone, soft tissue	8	3 (37.5)	
Prostate	7	2 (28.6)	
Urinary bladder	7	5 (71.4)	9
Skin	6	6 (100)	1
Thyroid	6	3 (50.0)	
Peritoneum, retroperitoneum	5	4 (80)	5
Nervous system	4	0	
Eye	3	0	
Adrenal	2	1 (50.0)	
Small bowel	1	0	
Vagina	1	0	
Unclear	3	1 (33.3)	
Total	392	217 (55.4)	

Imaging diagnosis

Metastatic hepatic cancers generally have low neovasculature and only the periphery of the mass is enhanced on dynamic CT and angiography to assume a doughnut shape.

(1) Leiomyosarcima (Case 3), paraganglioma (Case 4) and adrenal carcinoma (Case 5) are highly vascularized and may mimic HCC. Differential diagnosis is made from the structure of the interior and periphery, and if the mass is smaller than 2 cm, enhance pattern of tumor (hemodynamics) should be analyzed.

(2) Metastatic adenocarcinoma such as colon cancer, stomach cancer (Case 6) and breast cancer (Case 7) has an irregular periphery which often looks like ripple and bulges, and appears shiny on cutting. The center of the mass commonly contains much fibrous tissue. Histopathologically there are more viable cancer cells in the periphery, and necrosis and fibrosis increase in the center. For these reasons, dynamic CT demonstrates early enhancement in the periphery which turns low-density (peripheral low-density area, LDA) after 10 min (late enhanced CT) (Muramatsu *et al.* 1986). Conversely, the tumor center which is not enhanced and appears low in density in the early phase turns high density in the late phase. These imaging features are important for differential diagnosis. On angiography, the time for exposure is short and the late films do not display peripheral LDA, although in its early phase peripheral enhancement may be discerned. Solitary metastatic cancer which resembles HCC (Case 8) can be differentiated from HCC from the enhancement pattern and calcifications. Cholangiocarcinoma is adenocarcinoma and shows the imaging features of adenocarcinoma (peripheral LDA in 50 per cent); differentiation from metastatic adenocarcinoma is difficult.

(3) Occasional adenocarcinoma cases show as much enhancement in the center as the liver parenchyma. If the tumor has a very narrow peripheral zone of viable cancer cells, peripheral LDA may not be recognized. The fill-in phenomenon typical of cavernous hemangioma may also be seen in some adenocarcinomas (Case 9) calling for careful interpretation.

(4) Mucinous adenocarcinoma (Case 10) displays increased echoes on US, and peripheral LDA is seldom rcognized.

(5) Calcifications within the mass are frequently seen in metastatic colon cancer, and are suggestive of its colon origin (Bernardino 1979). It may be seen by US as a hyperechoic mass with acoustic shadowing (Case 11).

(6) Adenocarcinoma metastasizing to an area immediately beneath the liver capsule may form a cancer umbilication which is also recognized by imaging. One should look for such irregularity in the hepatic surface countour.

(7) Metastatic leiomyosarcoma (Cases 12 and 13), chondrosarcoma (Case 14), and carcinoid tumor (Case 15) are usu-

ally spherical with a smooth convex tumor surface. They are hypervascular on angiography, and hepatic veins may be opacified early (early venous return). Intratumor bleeding may produce a septal structure following fibrin clot formation.

(8) Most tumors derived from endocrine organs such as insulinoma, gastrinoma (Case 16), and thyroid cancer (Case 17), and from exocrine glands (lacrimal gland carcinoma, Case 18) metastasizing to the liver are hypervascular. Hydatidiform mole metastatic to the liver is also rich in tumor vessels.

(9) Meningioma metastatic to the liver (Case 19) is rare, and the one we experienced was also hypervascular.

(10) Squamous cell carcinoma especially well-differentiated (Case 20: esophagus, lung, cervix, etc.), metastatic to the liver, may become cystic as the interior is necrotized extensively and liquefies. It should be distinguished from a simple cyst.

(11) As far as our experience is concerned, malignant melanoma (Case 21) metastatic to the liver was hypovascular unlike its metastases outside the liver which are hypervascular (Charnsangavej *et al.* 1982).

(12) Portal tumor thrombosis (Case 22) caused by metastatic liver cancer is uncommon. Its incidence has been 6 per cent when studied by intraoperative US (Kikuchi *et al.* 1987). We have also seen intraductal tumor growth in metastatic liver cancer (Case 23), but it is more uncommon.

Preoperative examination

For multiple secondaries in both lobes (stage H3) hepatic resection is not indicated. However, when conventional enhanced CT and US have found sufficient liver tissue devoid of cancer, the patient may be scheduled for operation. It then requires a more extensive investigation that may include portal-CT which is more diagnostic for small lesions that dynamic CT fails to find (Case 24). Portal-CT has the additional merit of providing information necessary for segment diagnosis (Matsui *et al.* 1987*b*).

Our analysis of resected metastatic liver cancers suggests that of the various imaging modalities, portal-CT is most diagnostic. This study can be carried out following hepatic angiography without withdrawing the catheter, and is therefore practical as well. However, it demonstrates all lesions as low-density masses, not contributing to quality diagnosis. To make up for this demerit, it should be preceded by conventional CT and US examination for quality diagnosis. Lipiodol-CT developed for detecting small HCC is not commonly done in metastatic cancer, because most metatatic cancers considered for resection are hypovascular; not enough Lipiodol remains in the mass, and the results have been poorer than expected (Case 25). We no longer use Lipiodol in metastatic liver cancer.

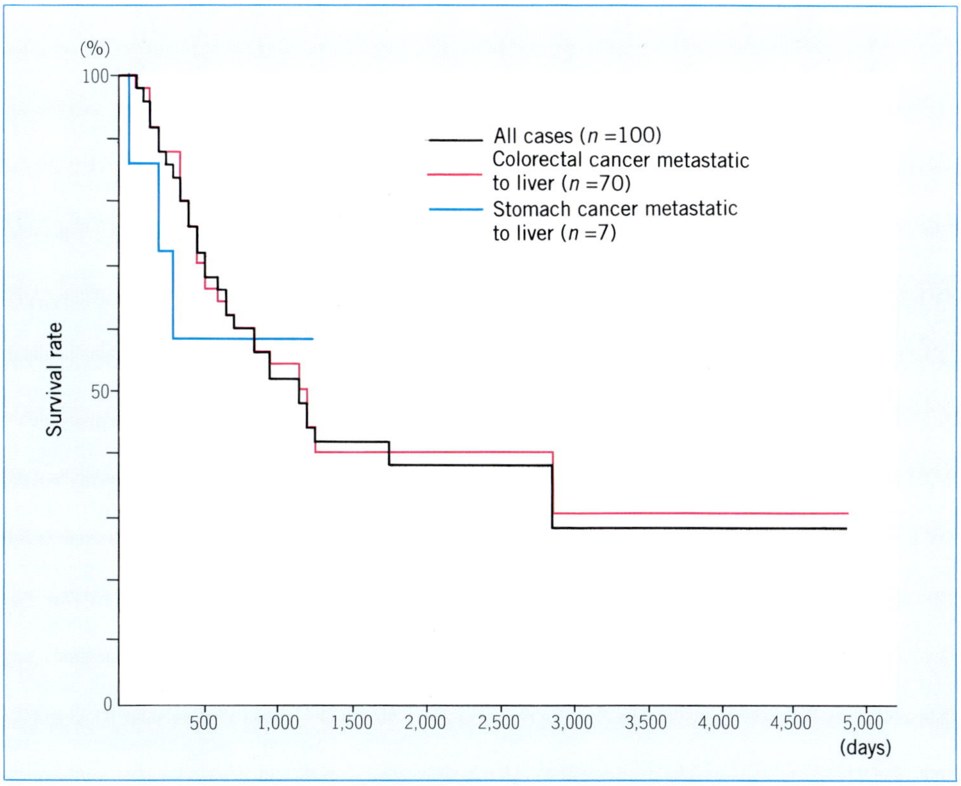

Fig. 4.13 Operative results in patients with metastatic liver cancer.

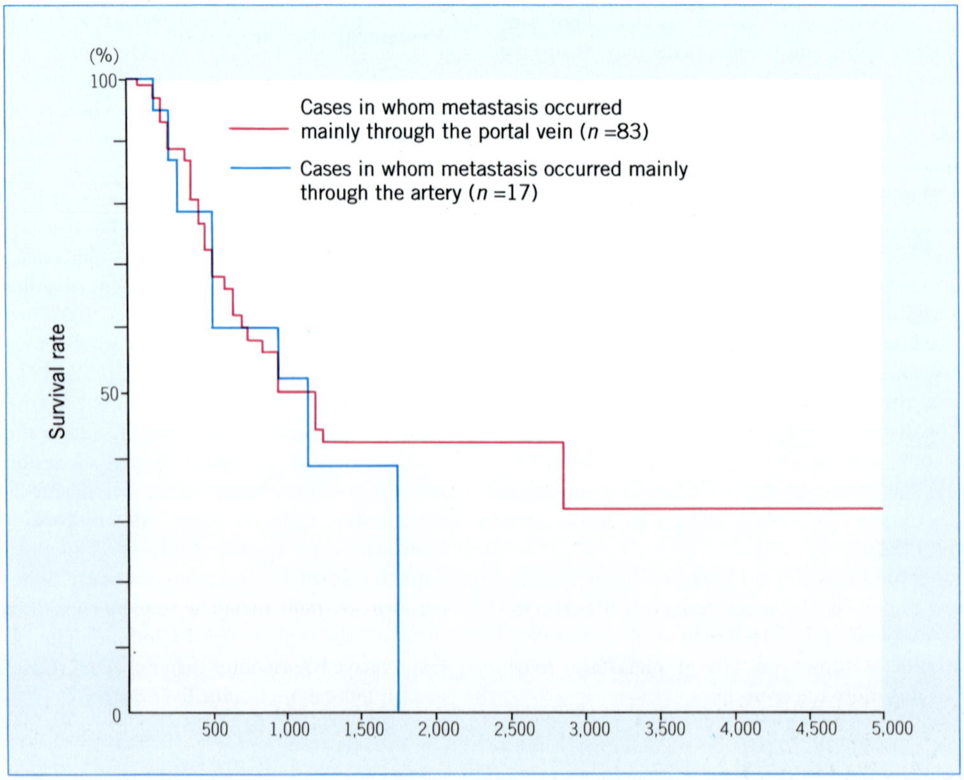

Fig. 4.14 Operative results comparing patients with metastasis via the portal vein and those via the hepatic artery.

Therapy

There are five possible treatments : (1) operation, (2) catheterization of the hepatic artery and administration of anticancer drugs, (3) TAE, (4) systemic chemotherapy, and (5) combination of some of these as a multidisciplinary treatment. The surgical techniques for hepatic resection and postoperative care of patients have been vastly improved along with operative results in recent years, and currently surgery is positively considered in patients with localized secondaries.

Operation
Indications for metastatic liver cancer are:

1. The extrahepatic primary can be completely removed (synchronous hepatic metastasis) or it has already been successfully resected (metachronous).
2. No other extrahepatic organ has metastasis (one organ metastasis).
3. At least one segment of the liver is free of metastatic lesions.
4. There is sufficient functional reserve to tolerate the operation.

It is to be remembered that small lesions which were overlooked in the past are now detectable by intraoperative US and resected. The liver is seldom cirrhotic (Melato *et al.* 1989) in metastatic liver cancer, and intraoperative US is particularly diagnostic. When compared with HCC, the function of the remnant liver after resection is much better, and operation is easier in the absene of portal hypertension. A number of patients with metastases to both the liver and lung have recently been resected, and indication of resection for metastatic liver cancer is expanding.

There are several possibilities at the time of detection of metastatic liver cancer. Namely, simultanous resection of the primary and liver metastasis (synchronous) , and liver metastasis is found and resected after the primary was resected (metachronous). In the case of colon cancer, the postoperative prognosis is said to be better for metachronous metastasis than synchronous metastasis. There were 100 cases of metastatic liver cancer which were resected up to December 1987 at the Cancer Center Hospital, Tokyo. About 80 per cent of them were colon cancer metastasizing to the liver via the portal vein. Transarterial metastasis such as carcinoid tumor of the lung and breast cancer constituted only about 20 per cent, because most such patients already had metastases to other sites.

Figure 4.13 represents the operative results in these two groups of patients. The 10-year survival rate for the whole group (n = 100) was 28.0 per cent. All 38 patients who had colon cancer with hepatic metastases died in 2 years without treatment according to Bengmark and Hafstrom (1969), and our results are very encouraging. When the routes of cancer cell transport were compared between the portal vein and hepatic artery (Fig. 4.14), all arterial metastasis cases died in 4.7 years whereas portal vein metastasis cases had a 31.3 per cent survival at 13 years. The poorer results with arterial metastasis were due to subsequent metastases to other organs resulting in early death.

Transcatheter arterial embolization (TAE)

The liver function is usually well preserved in metastatic liver cancer and operation is frequently carried out, and therefore TAE is usually indicated in patients with multiple lesions (H3). Colon and stomach cancer metastases to the liver are usually hypovascular, but occasional hypervascular cases may respond to TAE as illustrated with Case 26 in whom complete necrosis was induced. In other words, TAE may be considered in patients with hypervascular secondaries. Nevertheless, without resection of the primary site, treatment is difficult, and no long survivor has been experienced as continual new metastatic lesions develop in the liver.

Metastatic hepatic tumor—double cancer—Case 1: Synchronous esophageal cancer and combined primary liver cancer in which late enhanced CT proved useful. In this patient with carcinoma of the lower esophagus (squamous cell carcinoma) preoperative CT found a mass in the liver. Differential diagnosis was the problem. AFP (−), CEA (−), HBsAg (−), and anti-HBs (−).

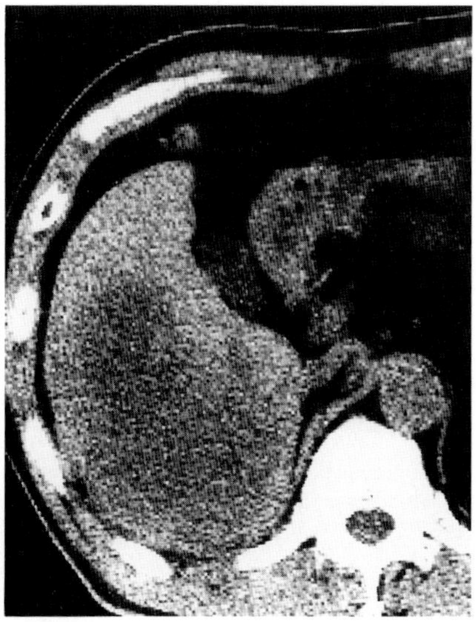

(a) Plain CT: a solitary low-density mass with an irregular margin was found in the right lobe.

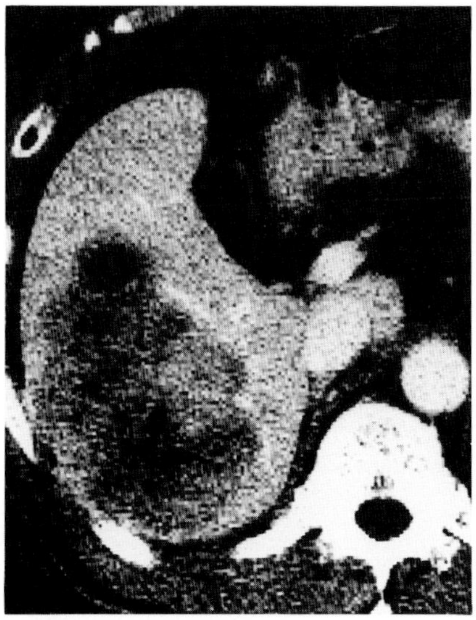

(b) Enhanced CT (early phase): the tumor periphery and some parts of the interior are enhanced.

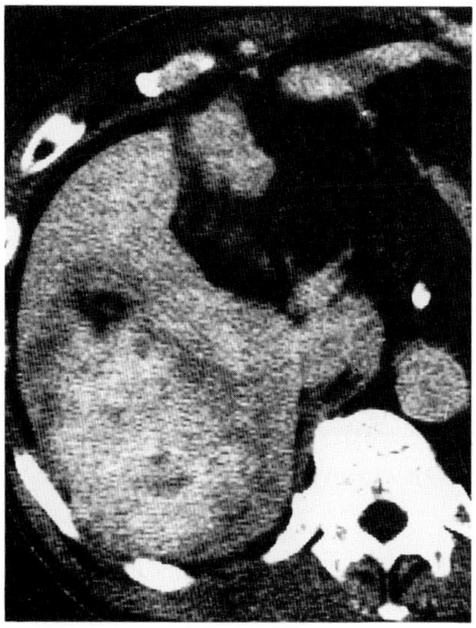

(c) Enhanced CT (late phase, 10 min): enhancement is now reversed with an enhanced interior and a low-density area in the periphery, a finding compatible with adenocarcinoma. In view of these imaging features that conflict with the diagnosis of squamous cell carcinoma, a synchronous double cancer should have been suspected. This patient was seen in 1984 when our knowledge and experience in imaging were limited, and esophageal cancer metastatic to the liver was the diagnosis.

Case 1 (contd.)

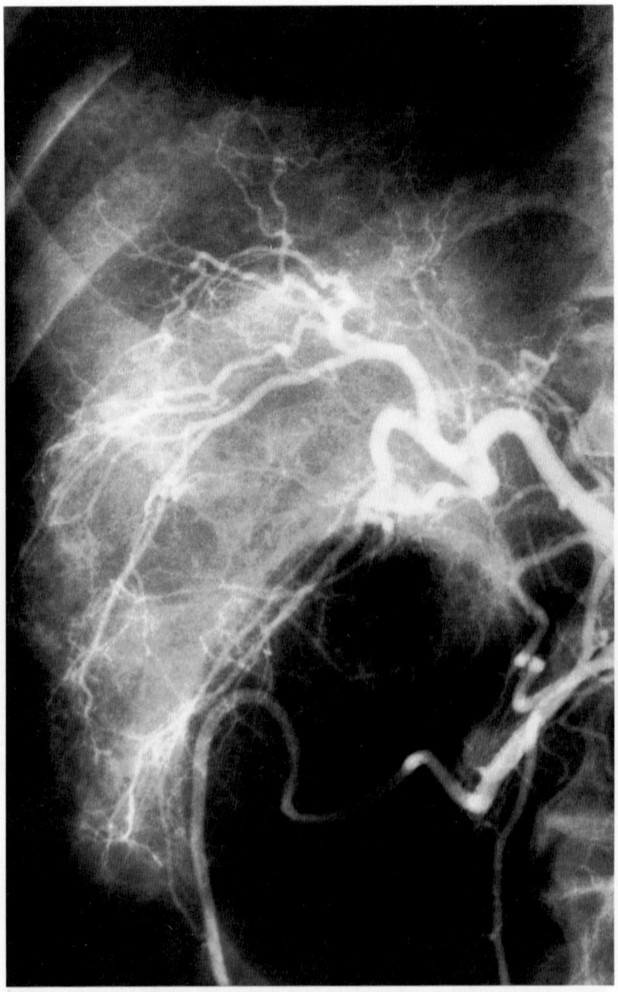

(d) Angiogram (early phase): many fine tumor vessels are evident.

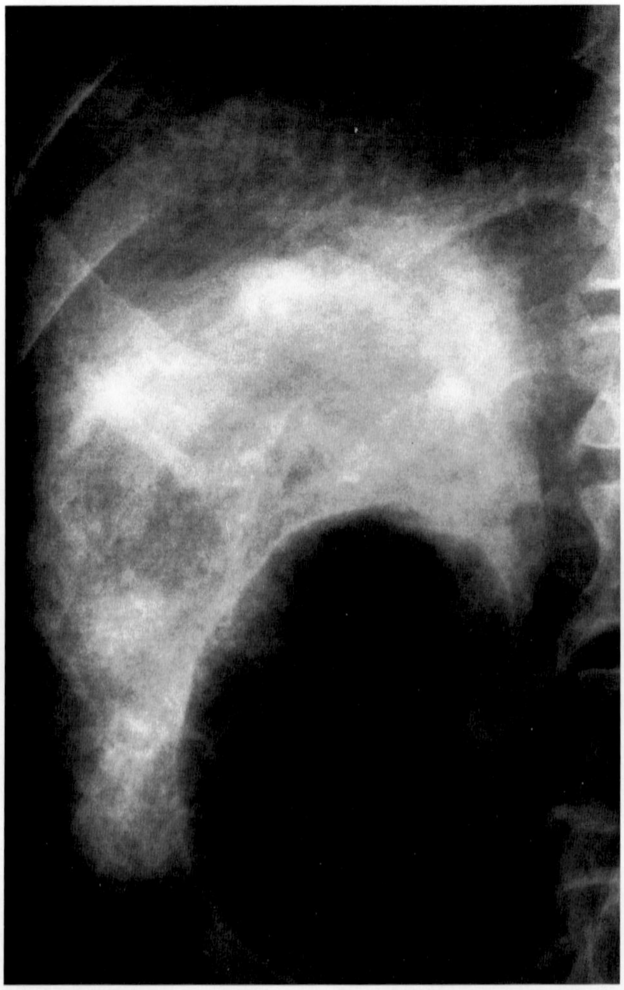

(e) Angiogram (late phase): the tumor periphery is stained like a doughnut. This feature excluded HCC, but was compatible with metastatic esophageal cancer at that time.

Case 1 (contd.)

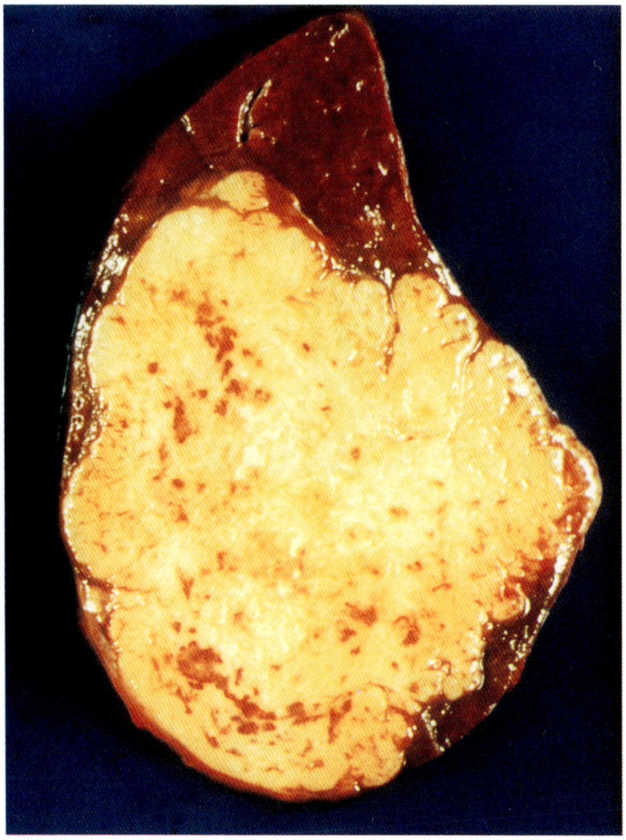

(f) Cut section of the resected specimen: simultaneous resection of the esophageal cancer and hepatic tumor was carried out. The hepatic mass was combined hepatocellular and cholangiocarcinoma, and the liver was histologically normal.

Metastatic hepatic tumor—Case 2: Colon cancer metastatic to a liver having a hemangioma and a cyst. A 58-year-old woman. She underwent colon cancer resection 1.5 years earlier. During the follow-up, serum CEA was elevated and US revealed three lesions, one in the left lobe laterally ($S^{II–III}$) and two in the right lobe (S^{VIII}, S^{VI}).

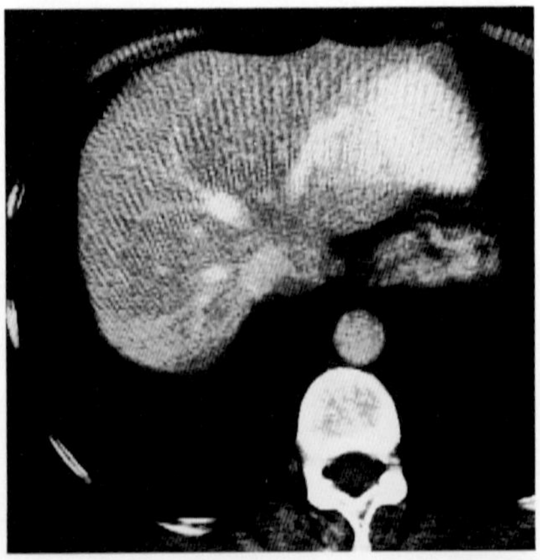

(a) Enhanced CT: the mass in $S^{II–III}$ was strongly enhanced turning isodense in the late phase, and was diagnosed as hemangioma.

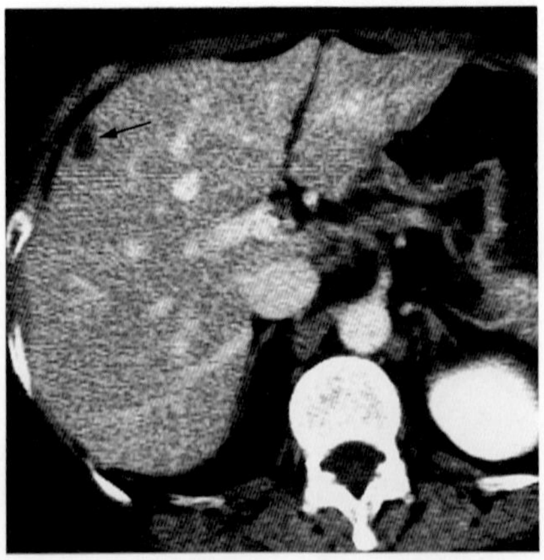

(b) Enhanced CT: the S^{VIII} lesion was not enhanced throughout, and the periphery was clearly demarcated; this was a cyst (→).

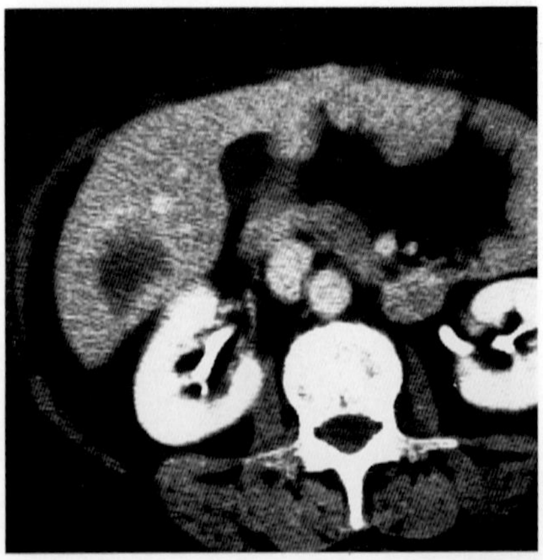

(c) Enhanced CT: the S^{VI} lesion was low in density in the interior and the periphery mildly enhanced, and metastatic colon cancer was suspected.

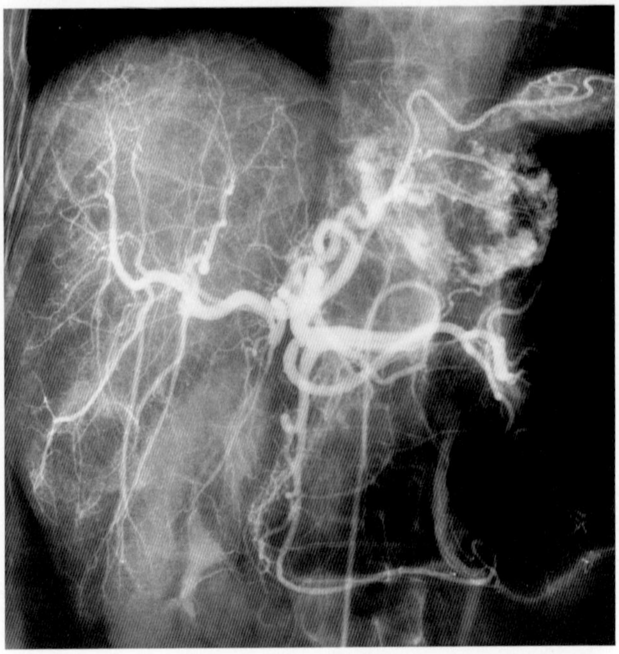

(d) Angiogram (early phase): the lesion in the left lobe was a typical hemangioma. The S^{VI} lesion showed a ring-shaped stain in the periphery, a finding compatible with colon cancer metastasis.

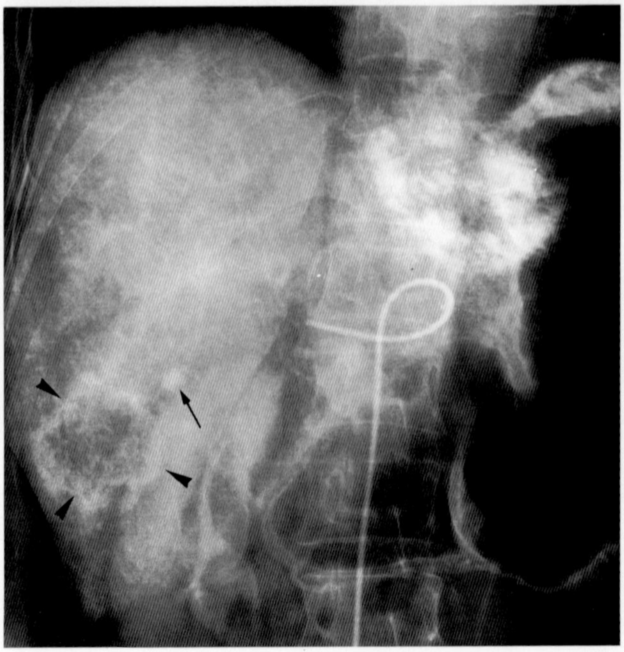

(e) Angiogram (late phase): another small hemangioma was found in S^{VI} (→). A solitary metastic colon cancer (▶) was resected.

Metastatic hepatic tumor—Case 3: Uterine leiomyosarcoma metastatic to the liver demonstrating a centripetal neovasculature. A 47-year-old woman who came to the hospital because of lower abdominal discomfort.

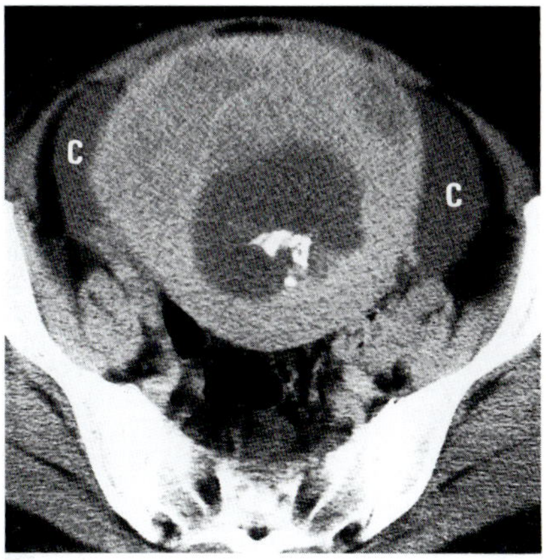

(a) Pelvic CT: a 12 cm uterine leiomyosarcoma with calcification is seen. The low-density areas on both sides of the mass are compressed ovarian cysts (c).

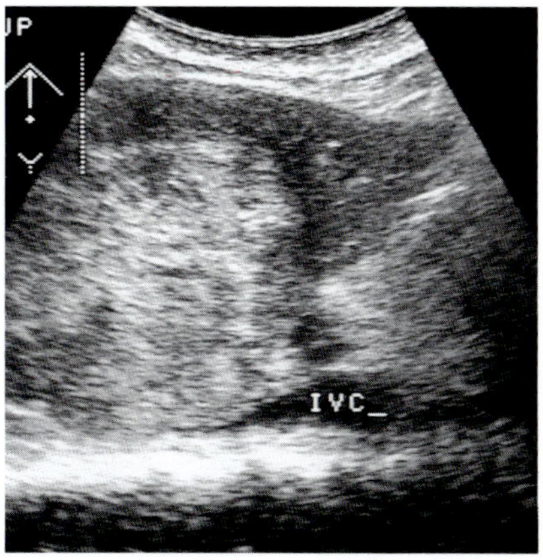

(b) US: a large echogenic mass occupying the right lobe.

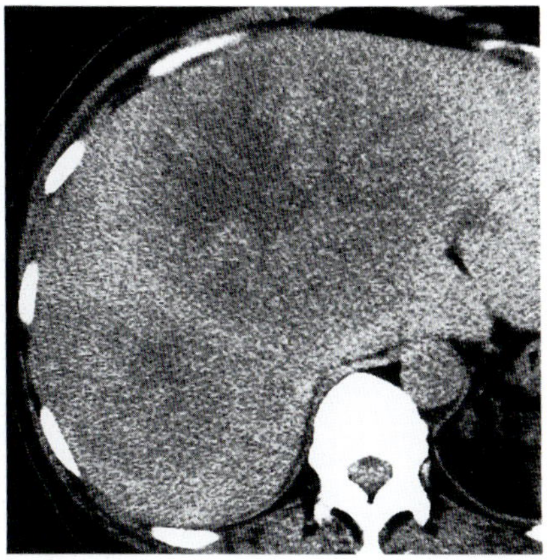

(c) Plain CT: two spherical masses are seen, and the large one has a stellate low-density area in the center.

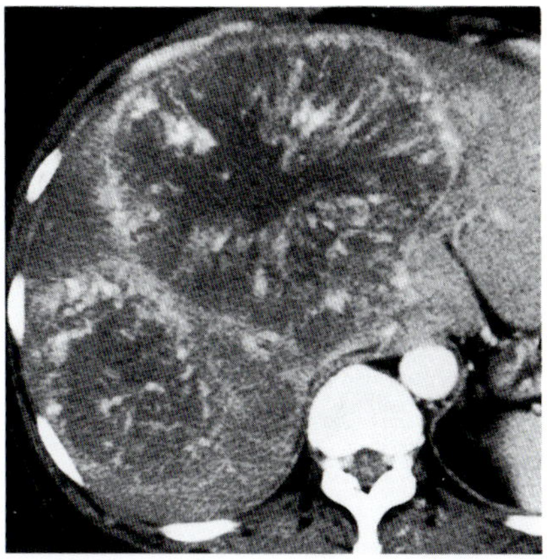

(d) Enhanced CT (early phase): many tumor vessels are seen running from the periphery toward the center (centripetal).

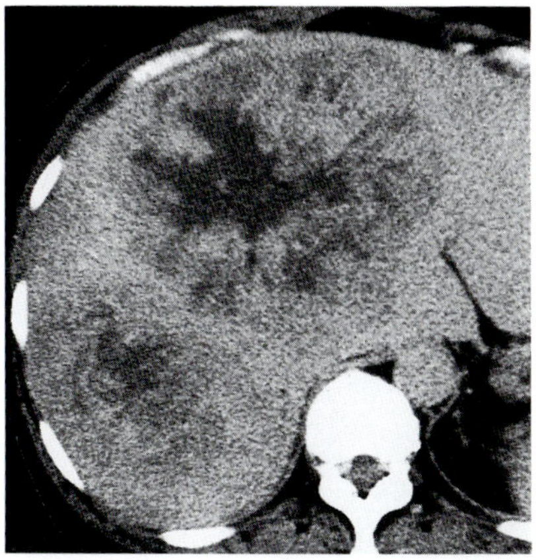

(e) Late enhanced CT: the centrally located stellate area of low density has become more discrete.

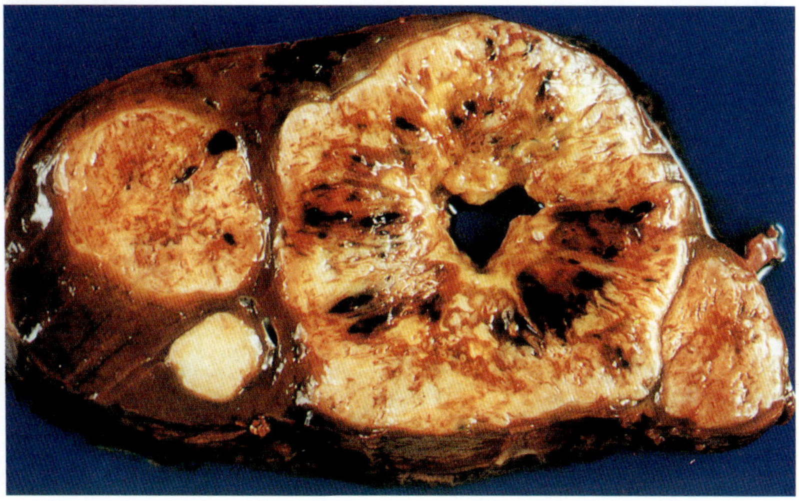

(f) Cut section of resected specimen: extended right lobectomy was carried out. There were four metastases. The largest one had liquefied central necrosis and large dilated tumor vessels. Histological diagnosis: metastases of uterine leiomyosarcoma.

Metastatic hepatic tumor—Case 4: Metastatic paraganglioma seen by angiography as a large hypervascular mass posing a problem for quality diagnosis. A 25-year-old man. Paraganglioma near the right kidney was removed 7 years earlier. A large hepatic mass was found.

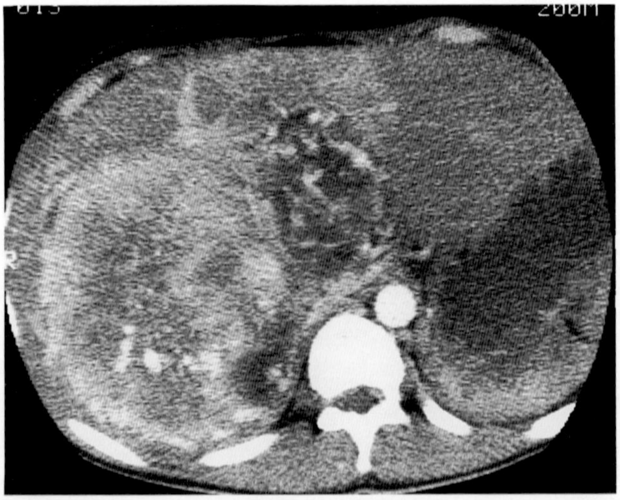

(a) Dynamic CT (early phase): the mass was well enhanced disclosing large tumor vessels in the interior.

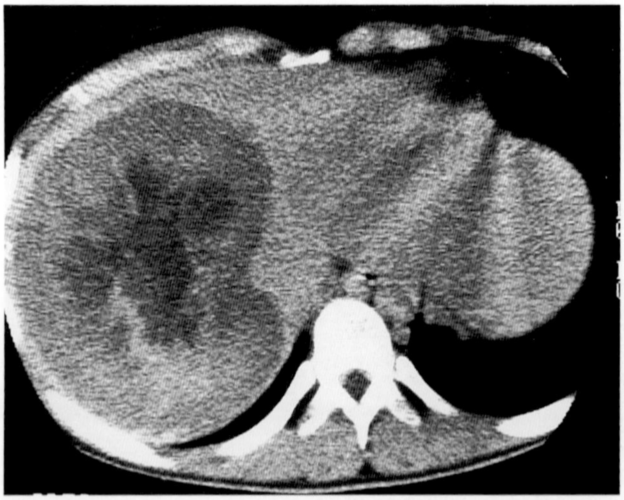

(b) Dynamic CT (late phase): the mass now shows a discrete, smooth and round low-density margin. The central area is lower in density.

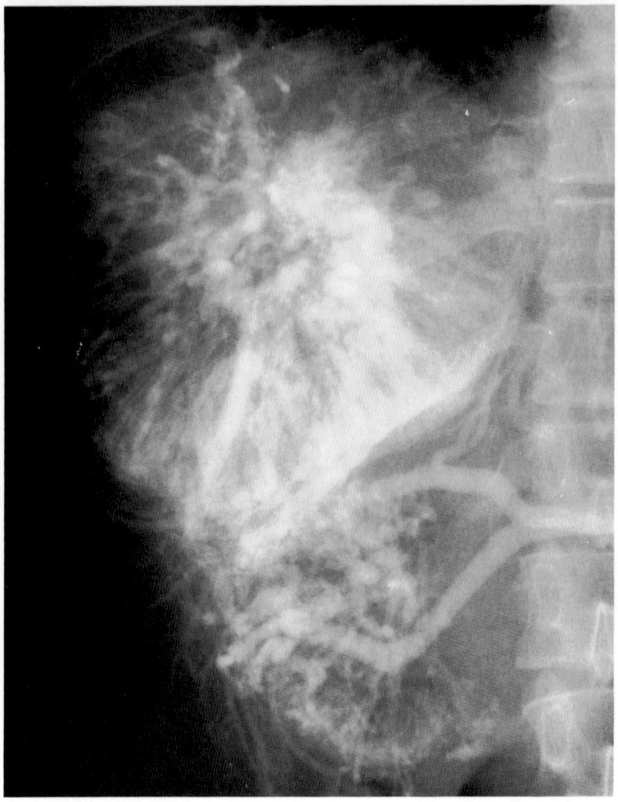

(c) Hepatic arteriogram (early): the large mass is supplied by a dilated right hepatic artery. Many tumor vessels are seen running from the periphery toward the center.

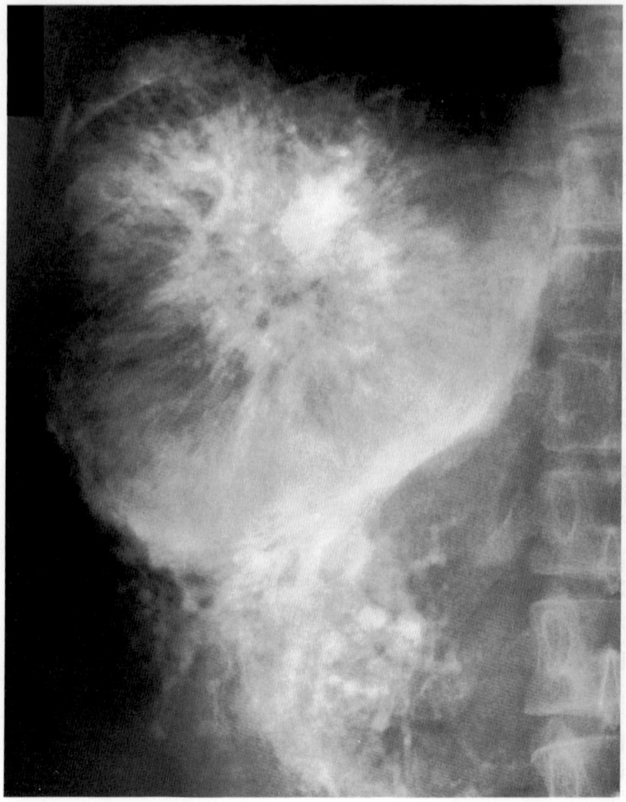

(d) Hepatic arteriogram (delayed phase): in a slightly delayed phase, the center looks like a fire-ball as a result of centripetal inflow of contrast medium.

Case 4 (contd.)

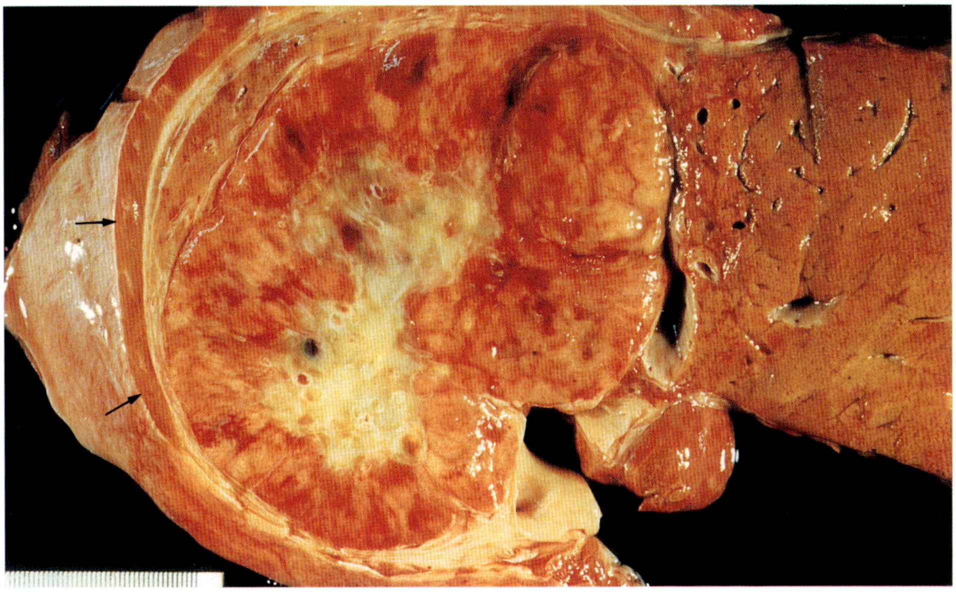

(e) Section of the liver at autopsy: autopsy revealed a yellow red mass occupying the right lobe. It was lobulated in part. Blood vessels traversed toward the fibrous center. Histological diagnosis: liver metastasis of paraganglioma.

Metastatic hepatic tumor—Case 5: Metastatic adrenal cancer resembling HCC by imaging and gross study. A 48-year-old Indonesian man. AFP, CEA normal. He had left adrenalectomy for an adrenal cancer 6 years earlier in Singapore.

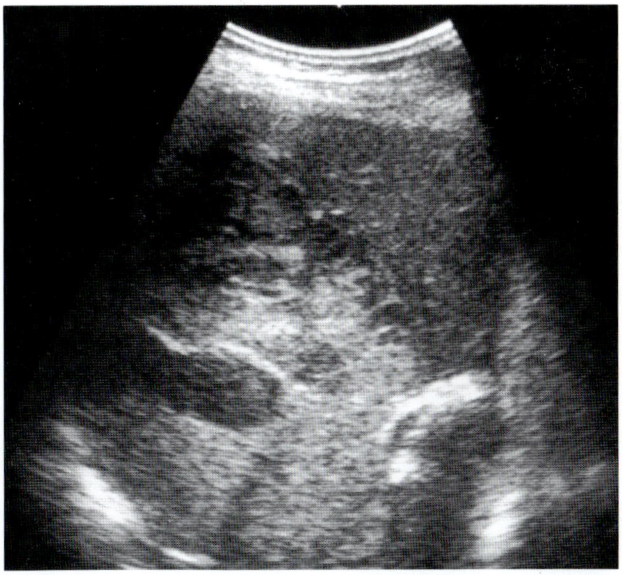

(a) US: during the follow-up, a 7.5 cm hyperechoic mass was found in $S^{VIII-IV}$. The interior was somewhat mosaic.

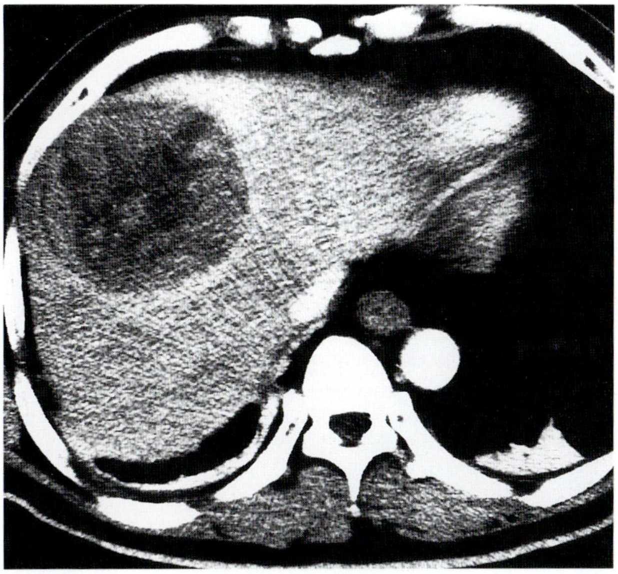

(b) Enhanced CT (early phase): the tumor periphery is stained like a ring, and the interior shows a stellate low-density area with a nodule-in-nodule appearance. The overall stain of the mass is low.

Case 5 (contd.)

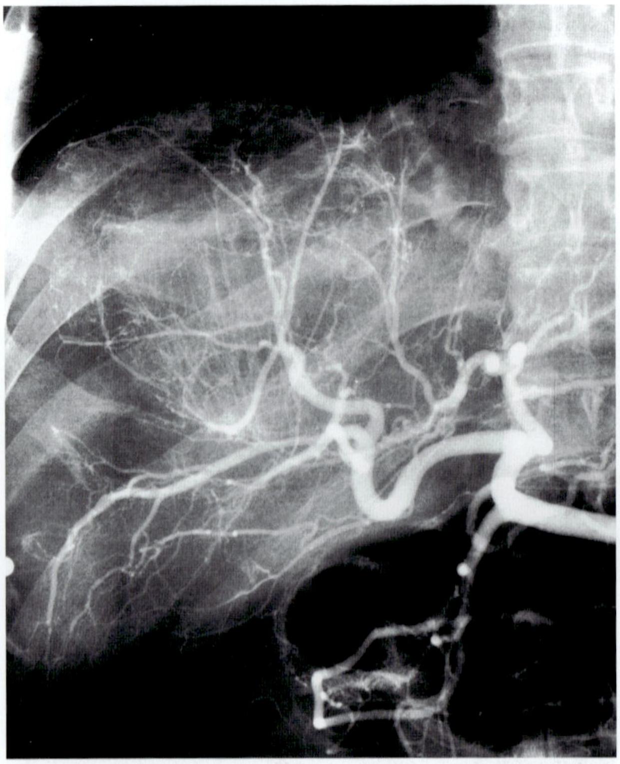

(c) Angiogram (early phase): many thin straight tumor vessels are seen in this mass in $S^{VIII-IV}$.

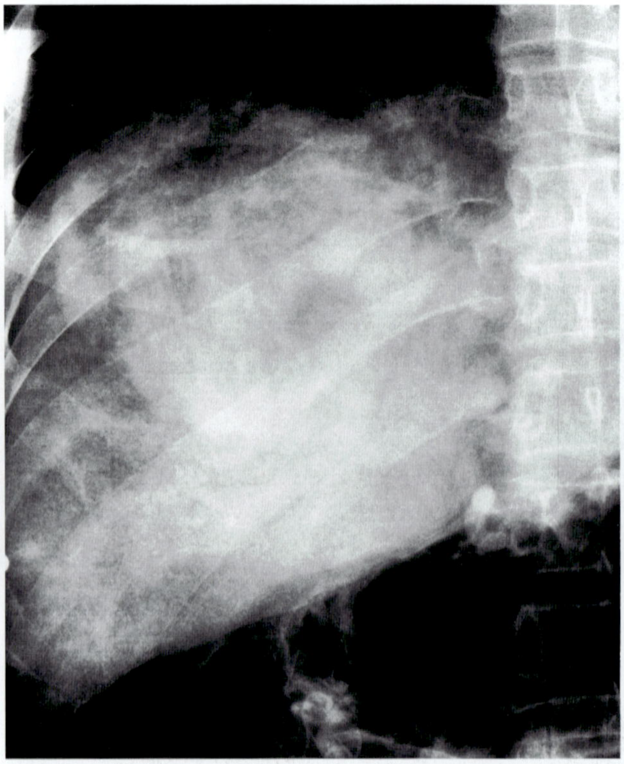

(d) Angiogram (late phase): the mass is stained homogeneously.

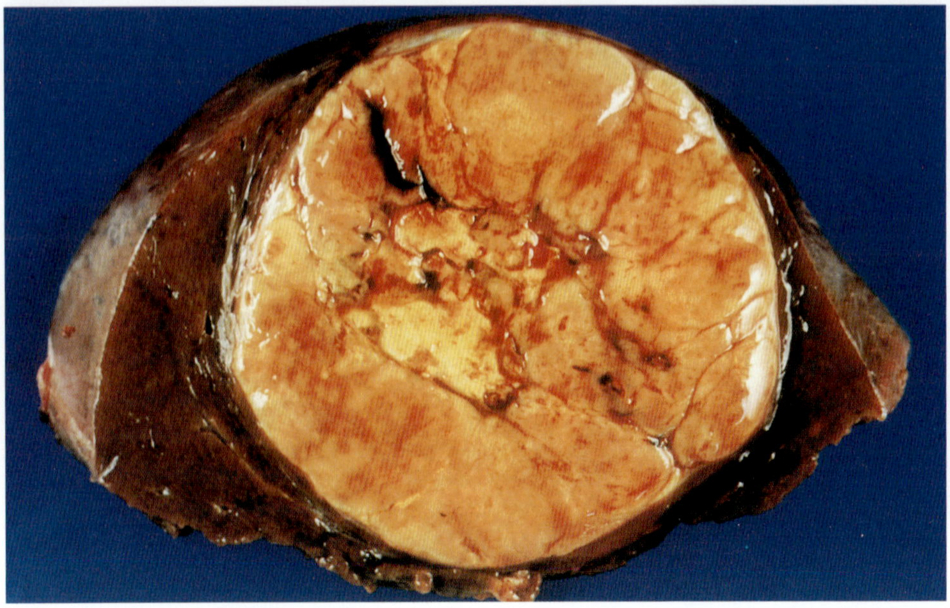

(e) Cut section of resected specimen: resection was carried out with a suspicion of HCC. The tumor was elastic, showing an expanding growth. The interior had nodular elements arranged in a mosaic pattern with yellowish necroses. Grossly, this mass resembled HCC. Histologically, it was a well differentiated epithelial tumor with no bile production. Immunochemical stain for keratin which is usually strongly positive with hepatocytes was negative, and a diagnosis of adrenal cancer metastatic to the liver was made. Although the mass had a well demarcated boundary, there was no capsule formation. The non-cancer portion was normal.

Metastatic hepatic tumor—Case 6: Stomach cancer metastic to the liver—usefulness of late enhanced CT. A 52-year-old woman underwent gastrectomy for an advanced stomach cancer 1 year and 4 months earlier. During the follow-up, serum CEA was elevated (146 ng/ml).

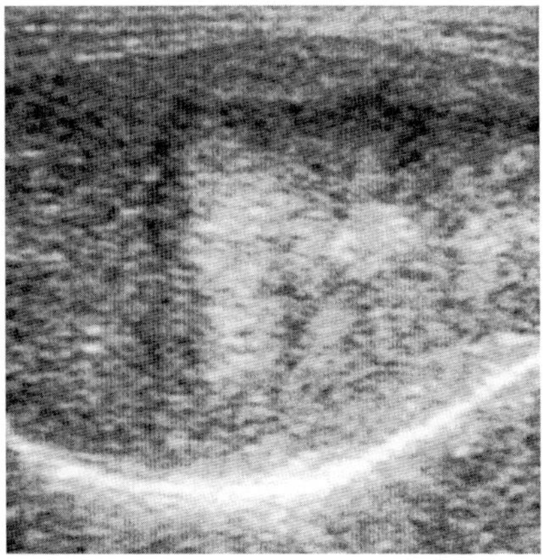

(a) US: a lesion with an irregular hypoechoic periphery and a hyperechoic interior is seen.

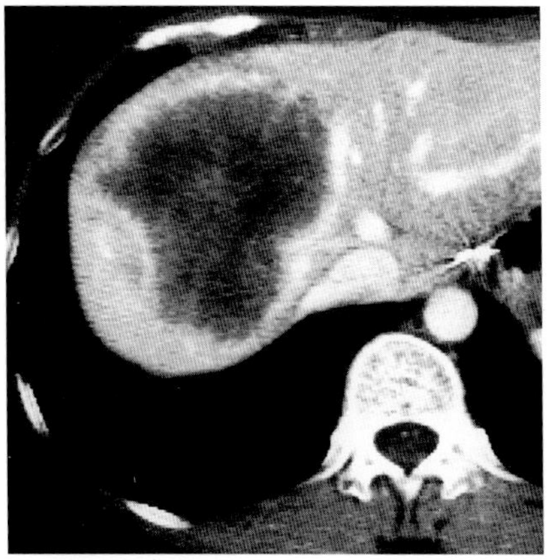

(b) Enhanced CT (early phase): the periphery is enhanced like a doughnut.

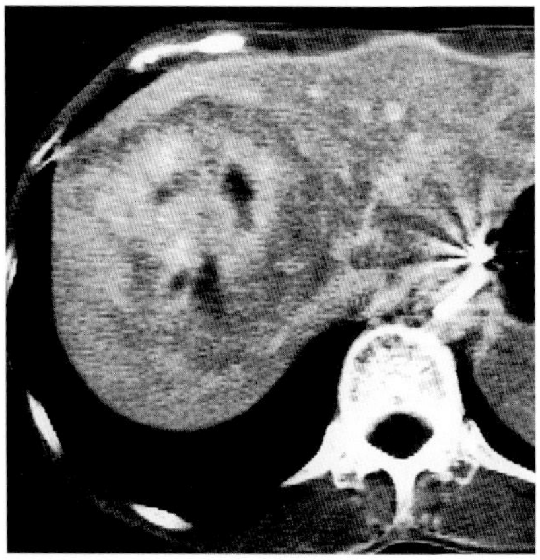

(c) Enhanced CT (late phase, 10 min): the interior has turned high in density and the periphery a low-density ring, a typical feature of adenocarcinoma in which the enhancement pattern reverses with time between the periphery and interior.

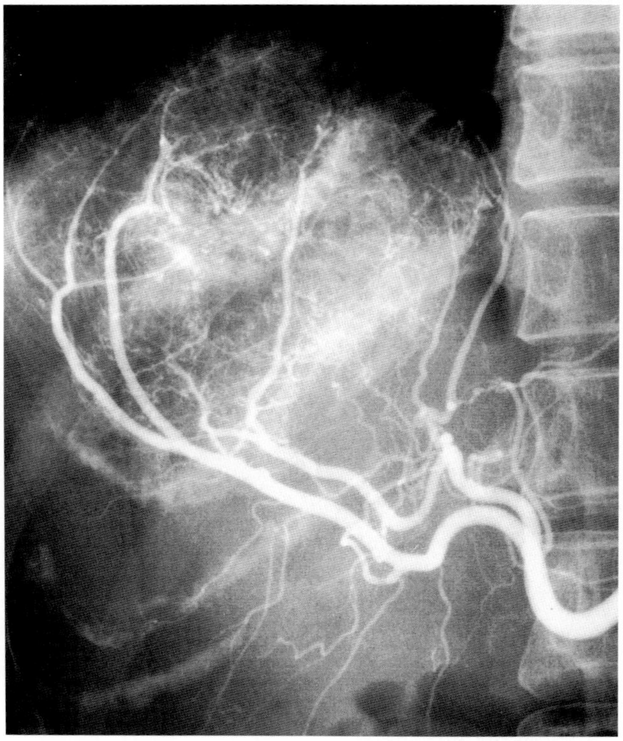

(d) Hepatic arteriogram (early phase): many fine tumor vessels are seen.

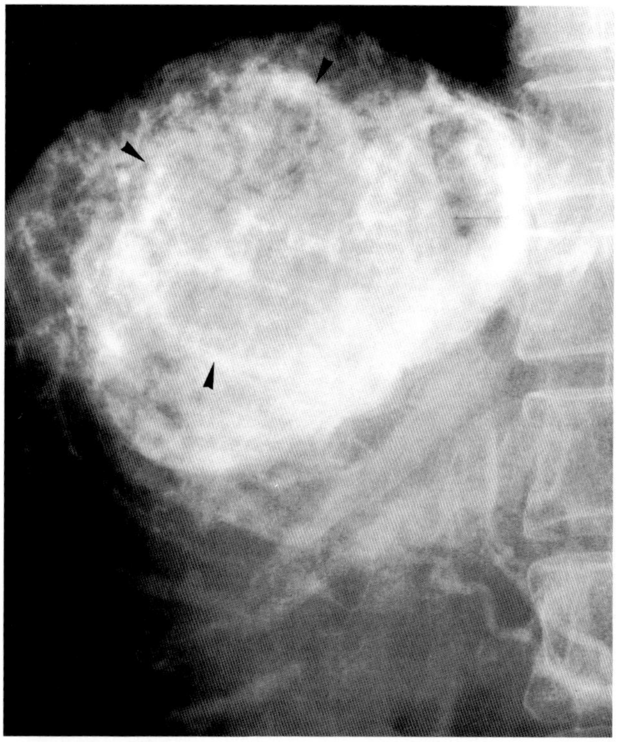

(e) Hepatic arteriogram (late phase): the periperhy is stained like a doughnut as seen on CT. The double rings (▶) are due to a protruding lesion in the posterior aspect of the main mass.

Case 6 (contd.)

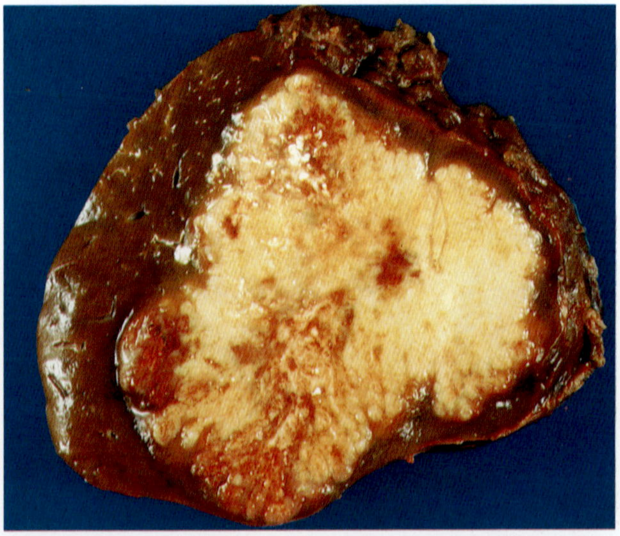

(f) Cut section of resected specimen: hepatic resection was done. The cut surface is closely reflected on CT images. The periphery is irregular with ripple-like small protrusions mimicking Rias coast. The white spots in the mass is the barium used in microangiography.

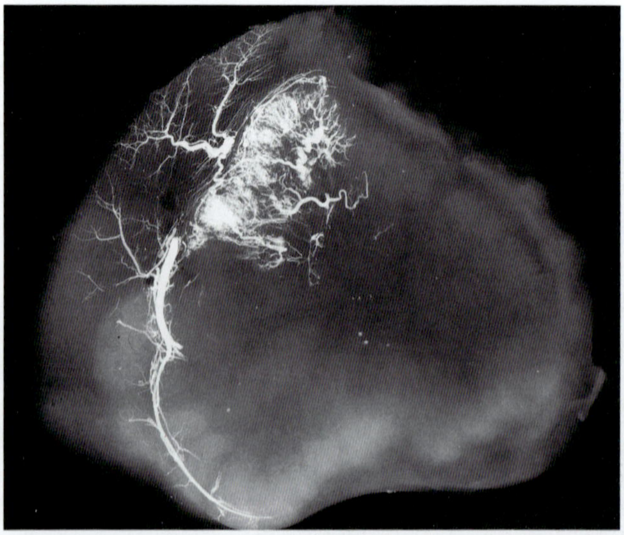

(g) Microangiogram made in the specimen: fine tumor vessels are seen arising in the periphery and feeding the interior.

Metastatic hepatic tumor—Case 7: Multiple hepatic metastases from breast cancer. A 43-year-old woman. She underwent left mastectomy for medullary adenocarcinoma 7 years earlier. Metastases were subsequently found in the stomach and liver. CEA 12 ng/ml.

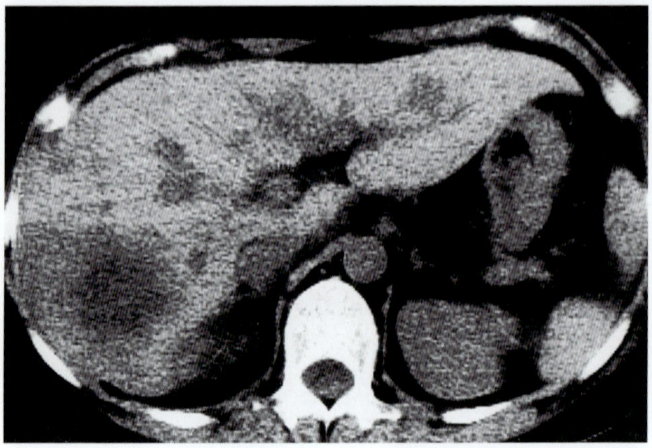

(a) Plain CT: multiple low-density lesions in both lobes.

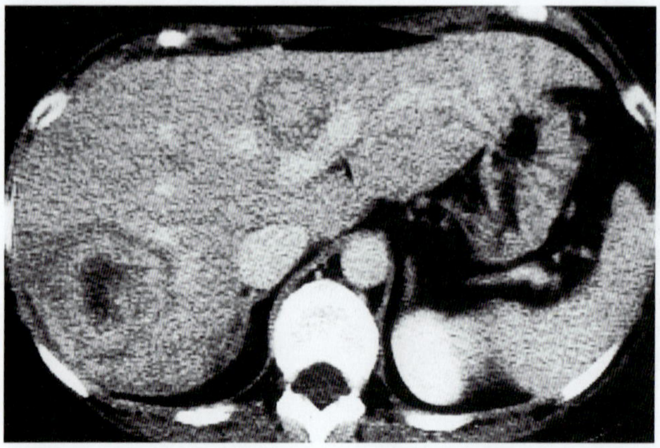

(b) Enhanced CT (3 min): peripheral low-density area was recognized both in large and small lesions. The center of the largest lesion was not enhanced even in a very late phase, although small lesions were enhanced in the center. It was assumed that the center was fibrosed or hyalinized with little blood flow. These features are compatible with adenocarcinoma, hence metastases of breast cancer.

Metastatic hepatic tumor—Case 8: Solitary colon cancer metastasis to the liver containing small calcifications. A 46-year-old woman. Colon cancer (Borrmann type II, moderately differentiated) and a hepatic metastasis were found at the same time.

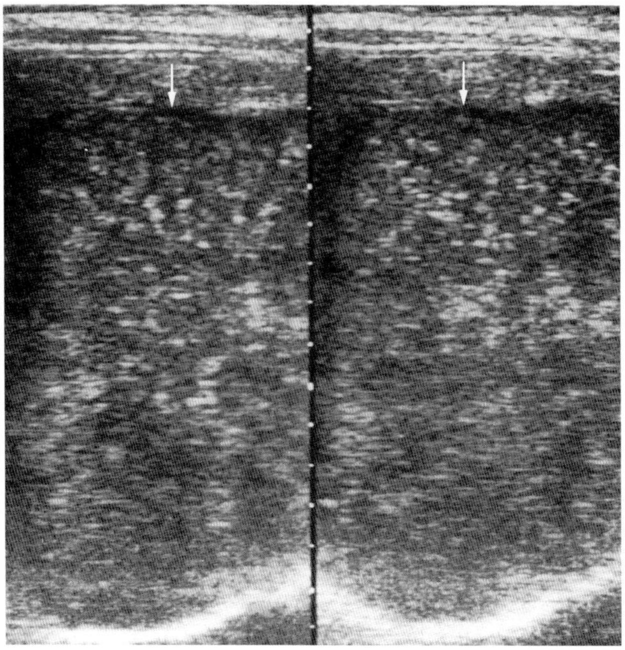

(a) US: a huge hypoechoic mass containing multiple spotty high echoes is seen in the right lobe. The boundary (→) is relatively smooth.

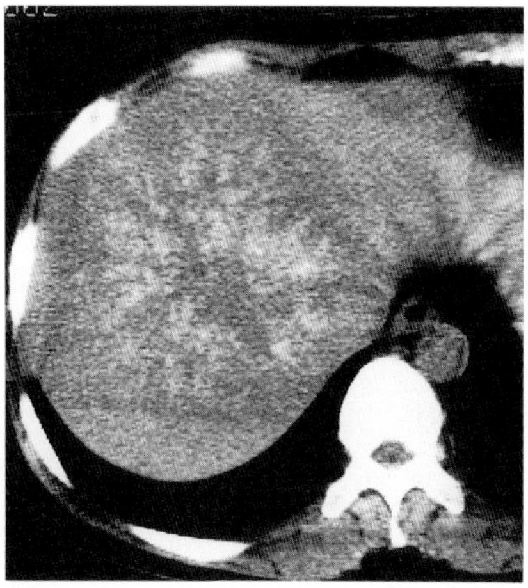

(b) Plain CT: in the midzone of the mass radiating calcific lesions are seen.

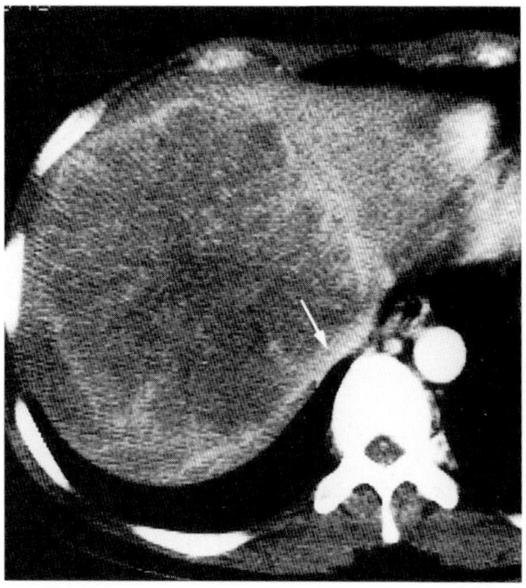

(c) Enhanced CT (early phase): the periphery is enhanced like a thin ring.

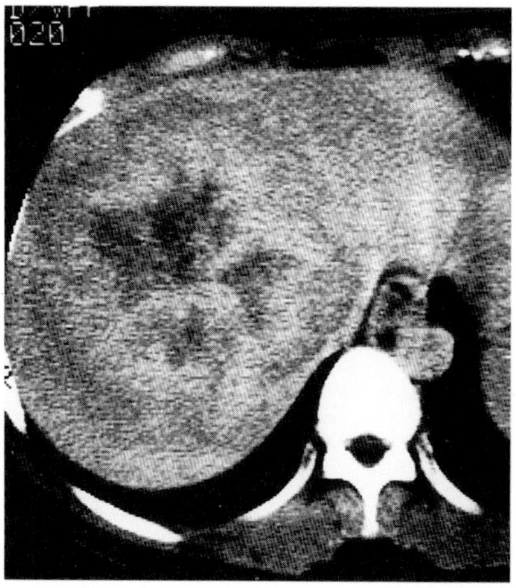

(d) Enhanced CT (late phase): from the peripheral LDA, this is a typical adenocarcinoma, and calcification strongly suggests colon cancer metastatic to the liver. The finding of compressed vena cava [→ in (c)] suggested infiltration into the caval wall, and the contemplated operation was called off.

Metastatic hepatic tumor—Case 9: Metastatic lung cancer displaying the fill-in phenomenon. A 66-year-old man underwent right upper lobectomy for lung cancer 5 years ago. CEA 170 ng/ml.

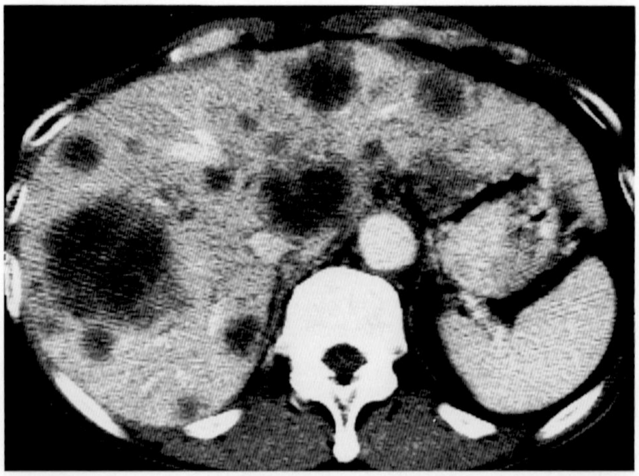

(a) Enhanced CT (early phase): multiple low-density lesions are seen in both lobes.

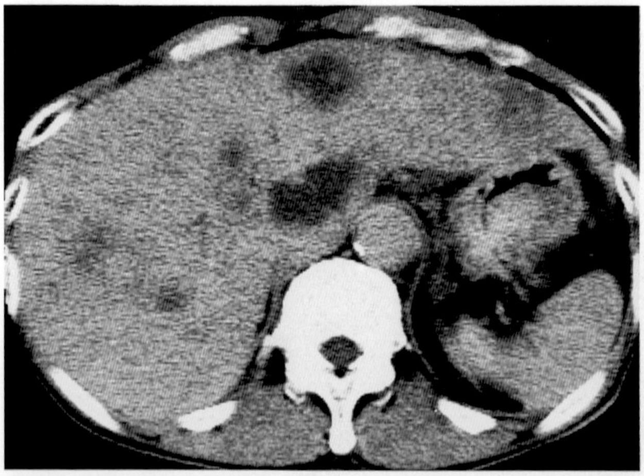

(b) Enhanced CT (late phase, 16 min): many lesions are isodense as contrast medium is retained in the tumor, interfering with accurate evaluation. In a late phase of enhanced CT, the fill-in phenomenon may be seen as in hemangioma, and therefore, interpretation of early phase images in dynamic CT study is important for diagnosis. In this particular case, peripheral LDA was not demonstrated, although it was a poorly differentiated adenocarcinoma histologically.

Metastatic hepatic tumor—Case 10: Hepatic metastasis of mucinous carcinoma primary to the sigmoid colon, displaying minimal enhancement. A 32-year-old woman. Because of continual lower abdominal pain, barium examination of the colon was carried out, and a mucinous carcinoma of Bormann type I was found. At the same time US detected hepatic masses. CEA 322 ng/ml, high.

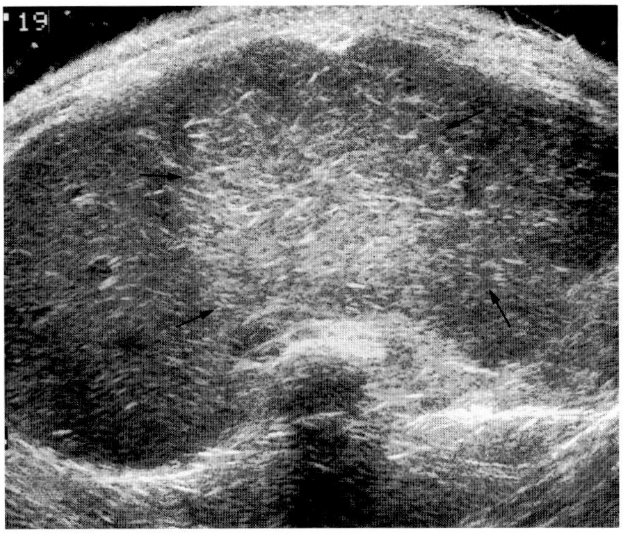

(a) US (Octoson type): a high-echo lesion (→) is seen in the left lobe.

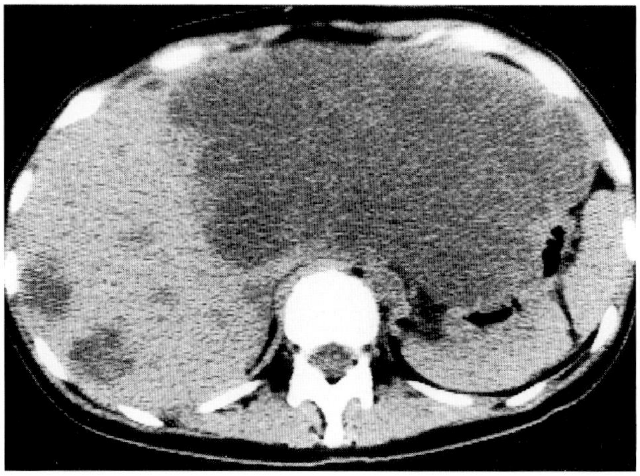

(b) Plain CT: there is a large low-density lesion replacing the whole left lobe and several small lesions in the right lobe.

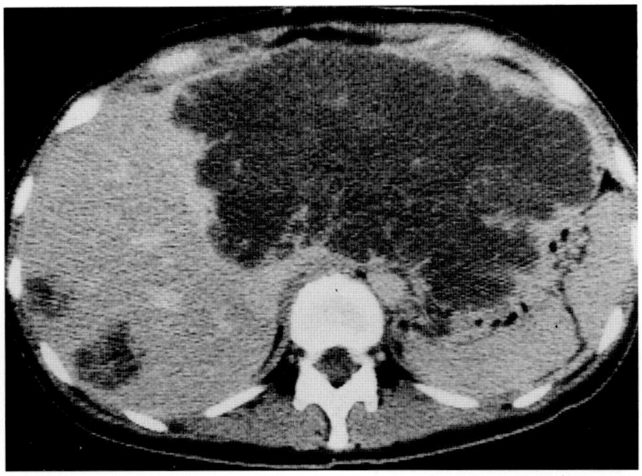

(c) Enhanced CT (late phase): there was no peripheral enhancement as seen in typical adenocarcinoma, except for mild enhancement of the margin, nor was the interior enhanced.

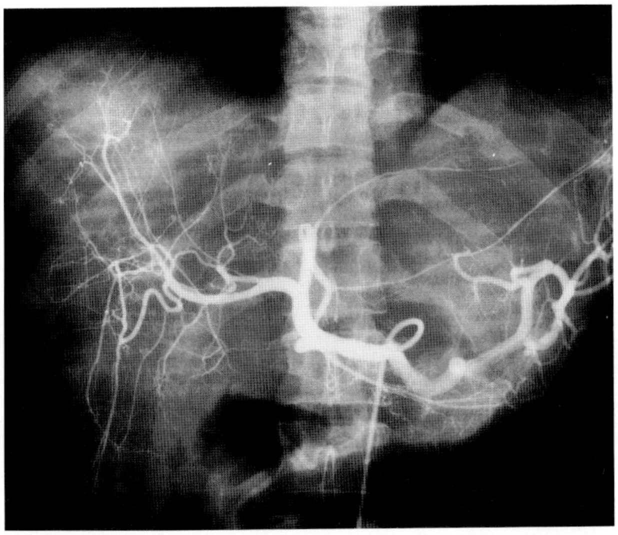

(d) Angiogram: there is no tumor vessel and the arteries in the left lobe are markedly stretched.

Metastatic hepatic tumor—Case 11: Colon cancer metastatic to the liver which was calcified *in toto*. A 52-year-old man. The ascending colon was resected for colon cancer 4 years earlier. Serum CEA slowly increased thereafter (4790 ng/ml) and a hepatic mass was found by US.

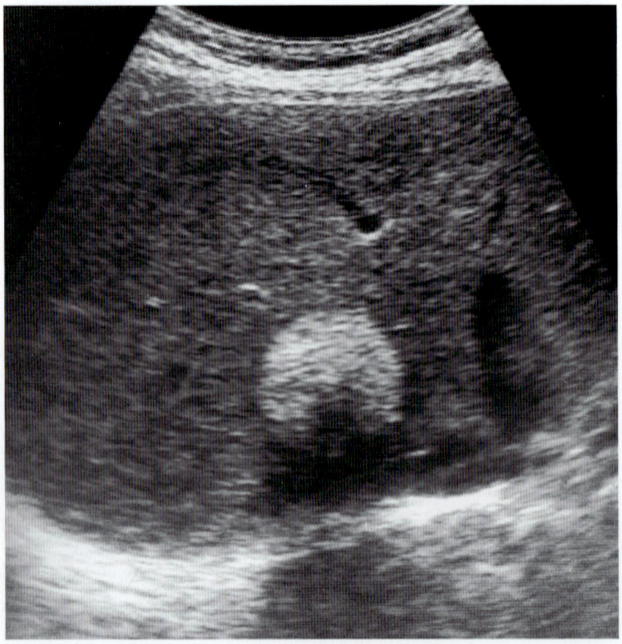

(a) US: a solitary hyperechoic mass is seen in S^{VIII}. From the posterior acoustic shadow, a calcified secondary was suspected.

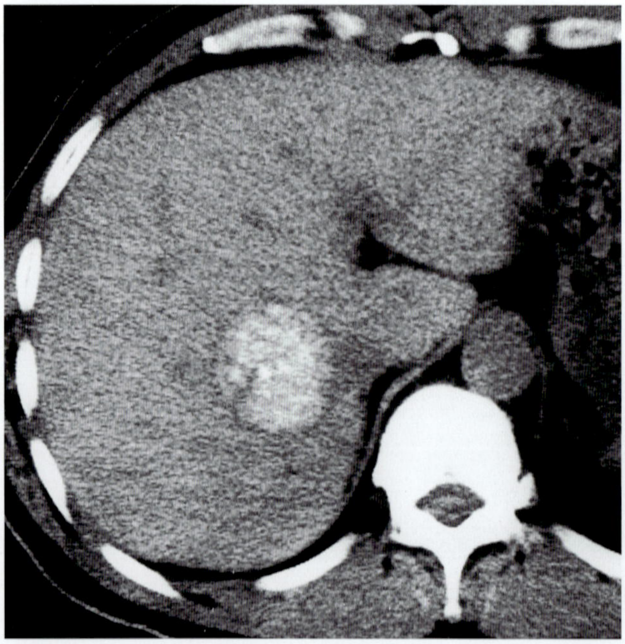

(b) Plain CT: like the US study, the whole mass is calcific.

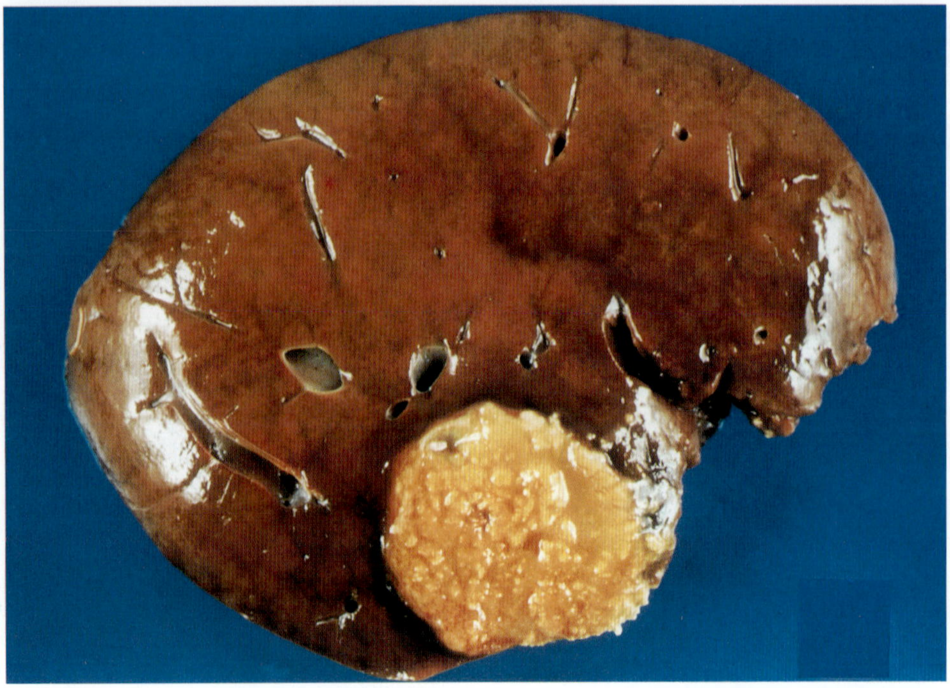

(c) Cut section of resected specimen: except for the periphery, most part of the mass was necrotic containing numerous small calcifications.

Metastatic hepatic tumor—Case 12: Hepatic metastasis of leiomyosarcoma of the stomach with internal bleeding. A 63-year-old man. He felt a mass in the upper abdomen by himself and visited a physician who found a mass in the stomach and the liver. AFP and CEA normal.

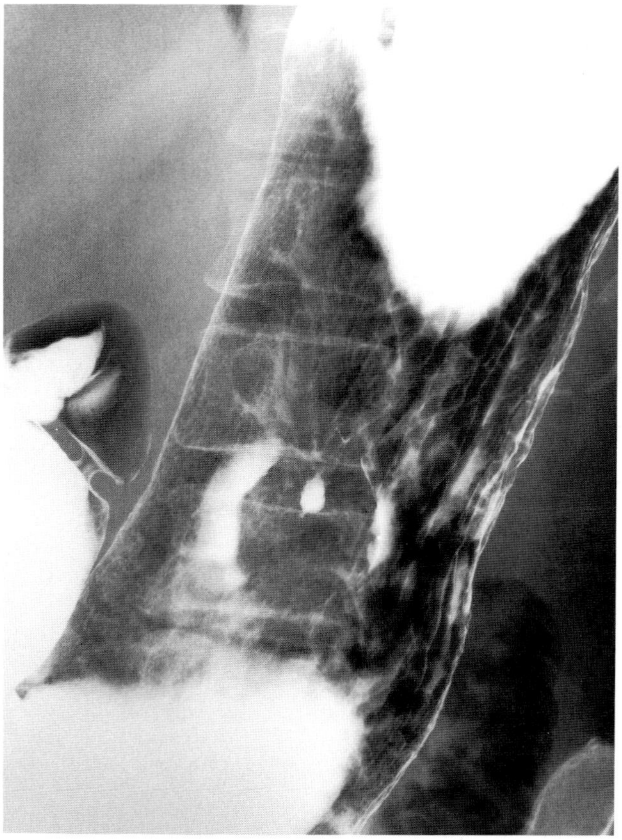

(a) Double contrast barium study of the stomach: a 5 cm submucosal mass with a central concavity and a smooth surface was found. From its large size, leiomyosarcoma was suspected.

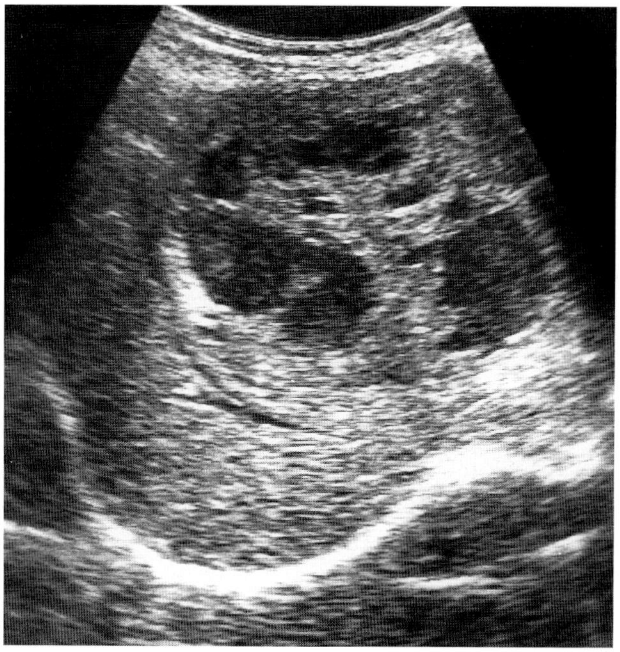

(b) US: a well demarcated cystic lesion containing septal structures of varying thickness are seen.

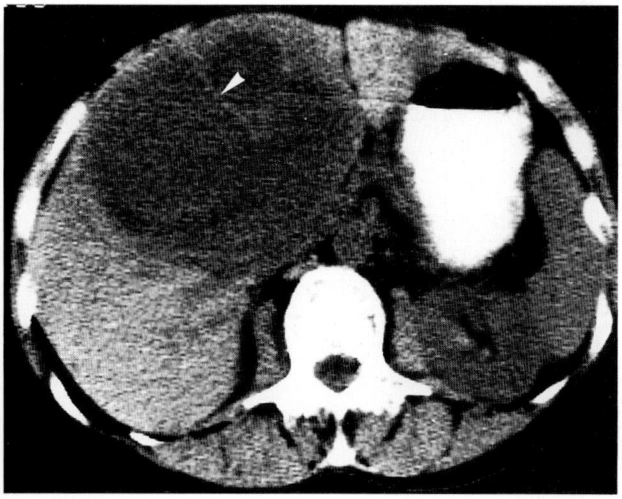

(c) Plain CT: the low-density mass occupies $S^{IV-VIII-V}$. A thin septum-like structure (▶) is seen in it.

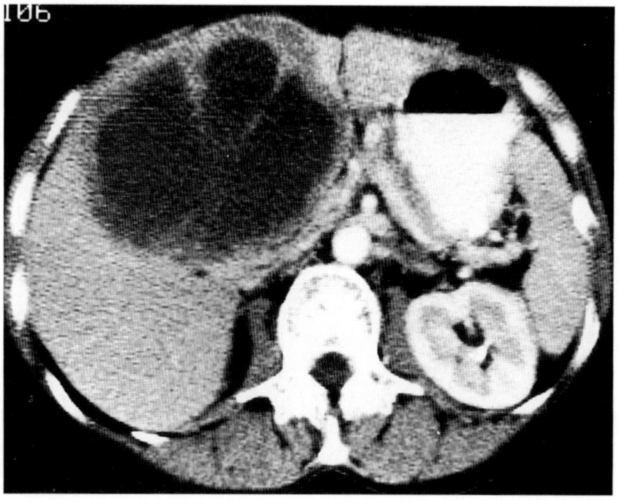

(d) Enhanced CT (early phase): the periphery is weakly enhanced and the thick septal structure has become clearer.

Case 12 (contd.)

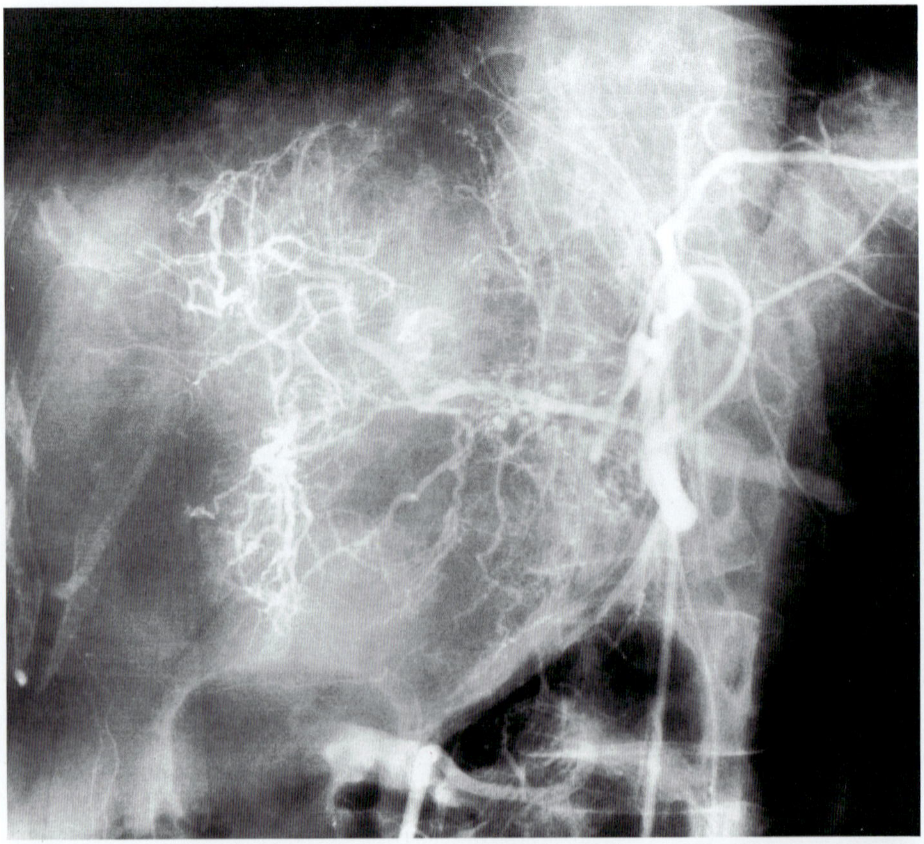

(e) Left hepatic arteriogram: many tumor vessels are seen supplying the ventral aspect of the mass.

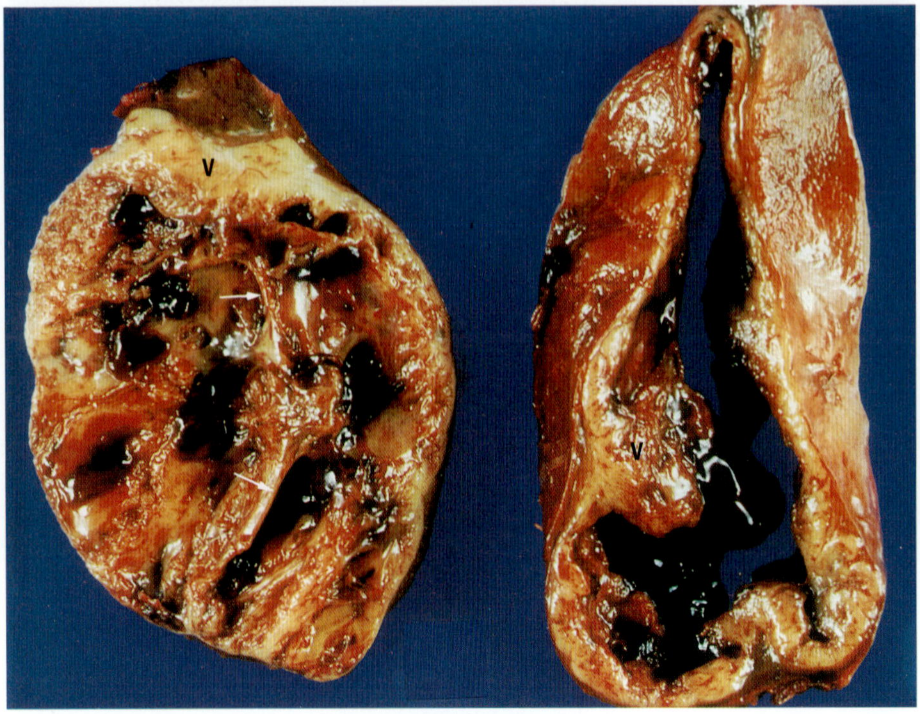

(f) Cut section of resected specimen: the tumor produced brownish fluid on cutting, and the cut surface was largely occupied by old blood clots. It also contained septa (→) consisting of granulation tissue and clots. The periphery that was enhanced contained viable leiomyosarcoma cells (V).

Metastatic hepatic tumor—Case 13: Leiomyosarcoma of the lung metastatic to the liver that displayed hypervascularity. A 58-year-old female. The middle lobe of the right lung was removed for primary leiomyosarcoma 2 years earlier. Subsequently, she developed right upper quadrant pain that led to the discovery of a hepatic tumor. CEA normal.

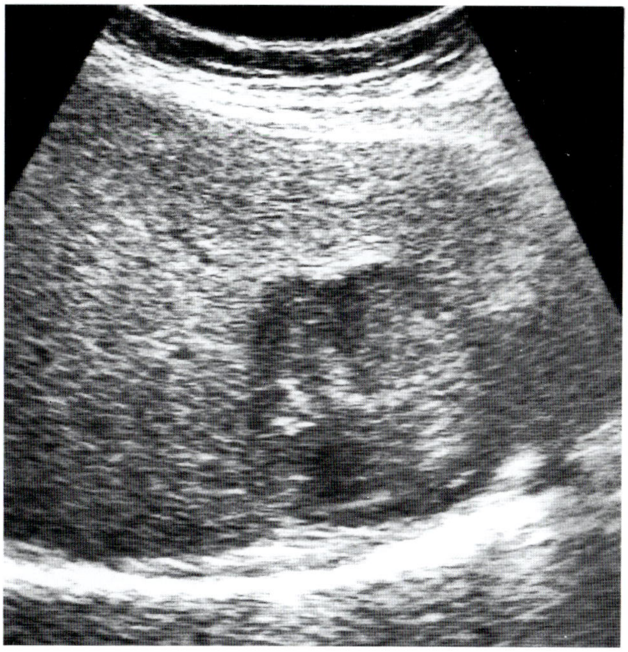

(a) US: a 7 cm mass with a wavy margin and mixed echoes is seen in S^{VIII}.

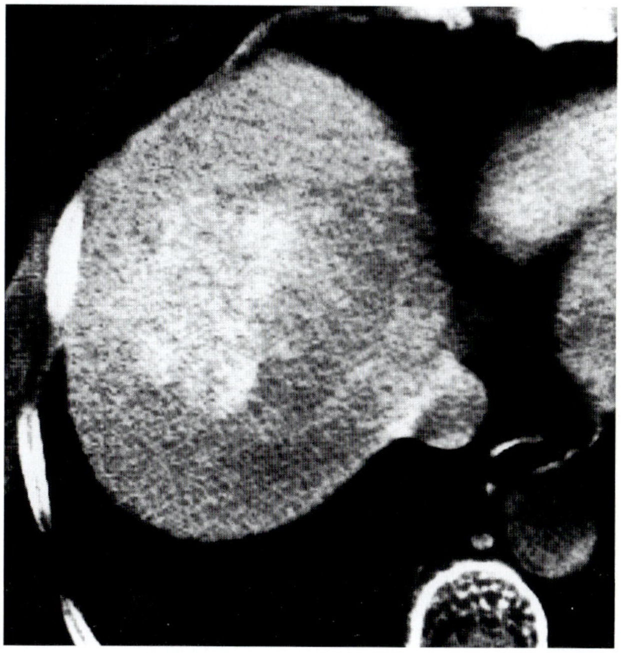

(b) Enhanced CT (late phase, 15 min): distinct contrast retention is seen in the right half of the mass.

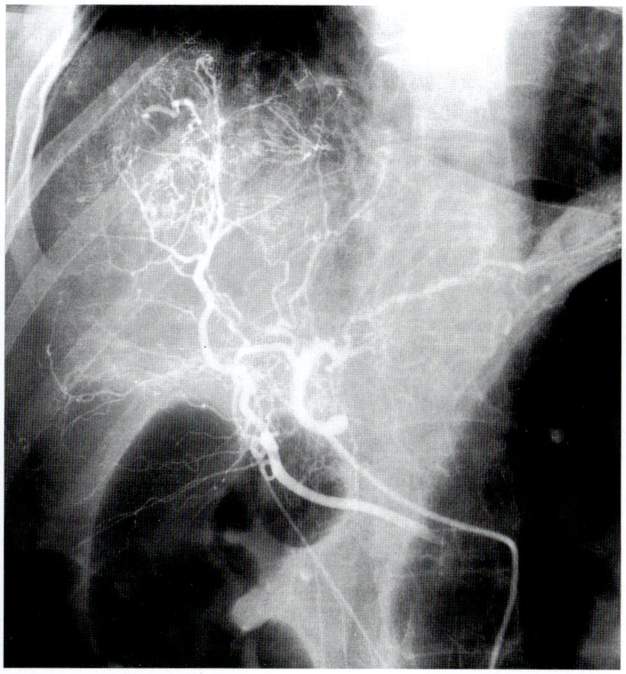

(c) Hepatic arteriogram: a hypervascular tumor with marked neovasculature is seen in S^{VIII}.

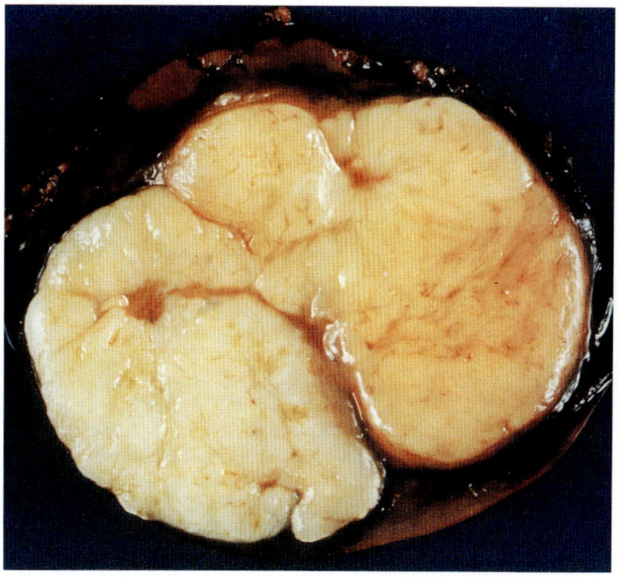

(d) Cut section of resected specimen. The tumor was light yellow, firm, and the margin smooth and wavy. There was a deep indentation into the mass. Histologically, it was leiomyosarcoma with crisscrossing spindle-shaped sarcoma cells closely resembling the resected primary.

Metastatic hepatic tumor—Case 14: Chondrosarcoma of the pelvis metastasizing to the liver. A 33-year-old woman. The right half of the pelvis was removed because of a large chondrosarcoma. 3.5 years later, CT study detected an hepatic mass.

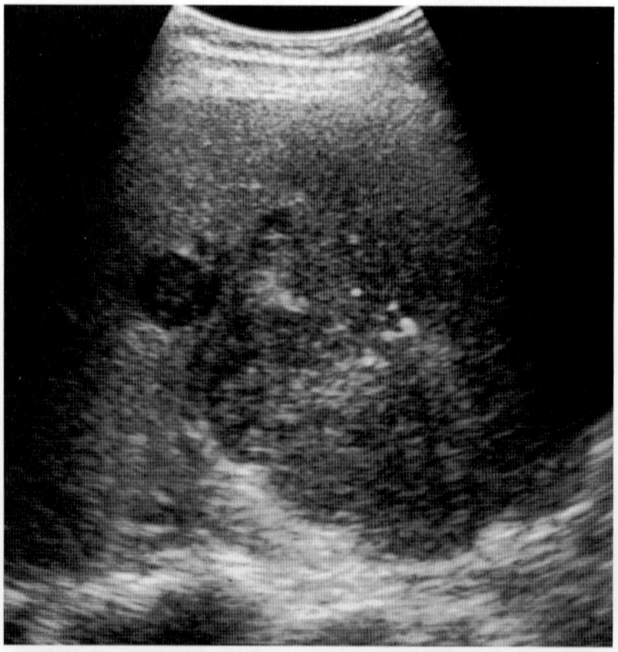

(a) US: a 9 cm hypoechoic lesion is seen in S^{III-IV}. The margin is petal shaped and the center contains high-echo spots with posterior shadowing. Chondrosarcoma with calcific elements was suspected.

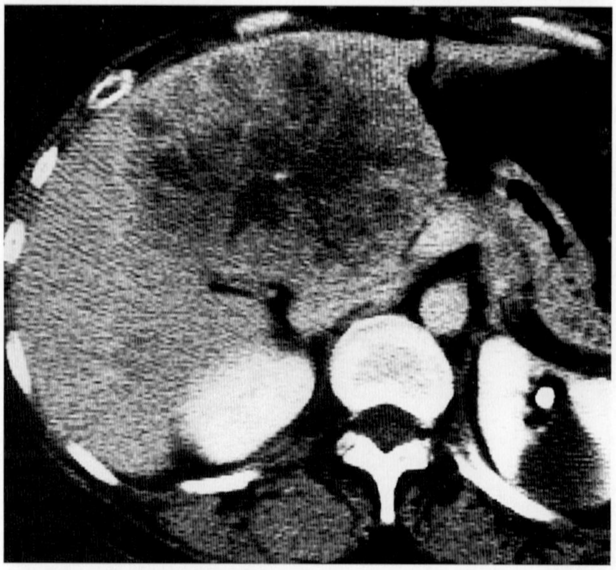

(b) Enhanced CT (early phase): the tumor periphery is slightly enhanced and the interior not enhanced. There is a calcific spot in the center.

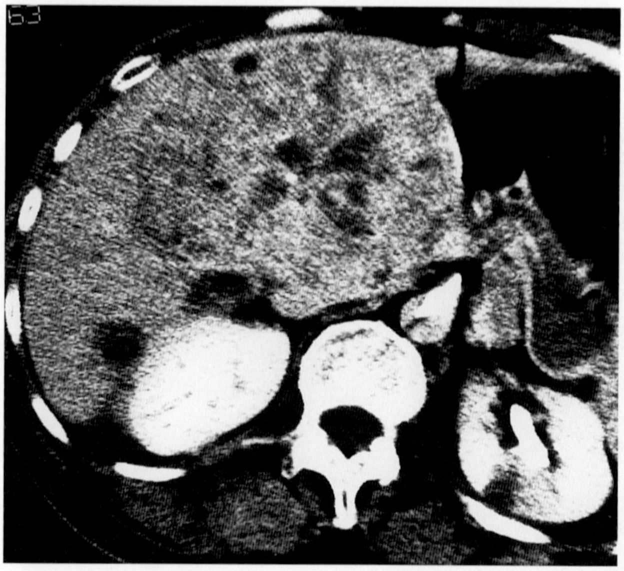

(c) Enhanced CT (late phase): the mass is now enhanced except for radiating low-density areas in the center. The periphery to the right shows a low-density ring.

Case 14 (contd.)

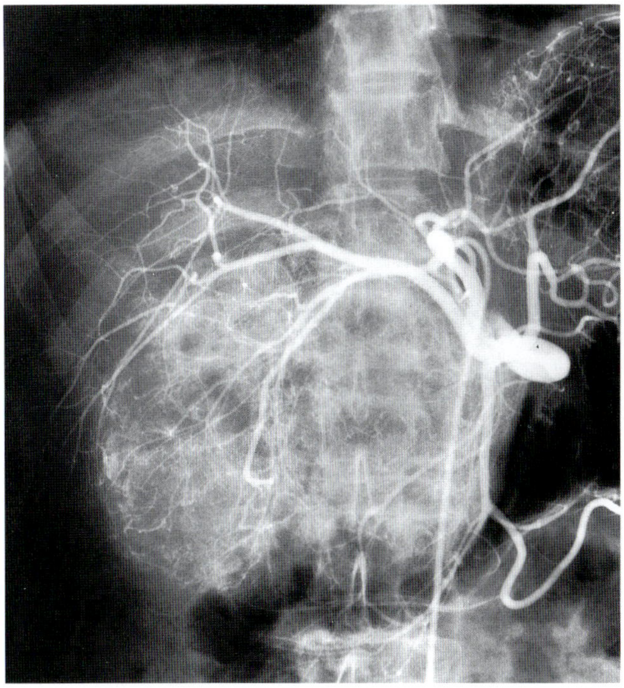

(d) Hepatic arteriogram (early phase): there is a 14 cm mass occupying the S^{IV} area and hanging from the liver. It is hypervascular with fine feeding vessels.

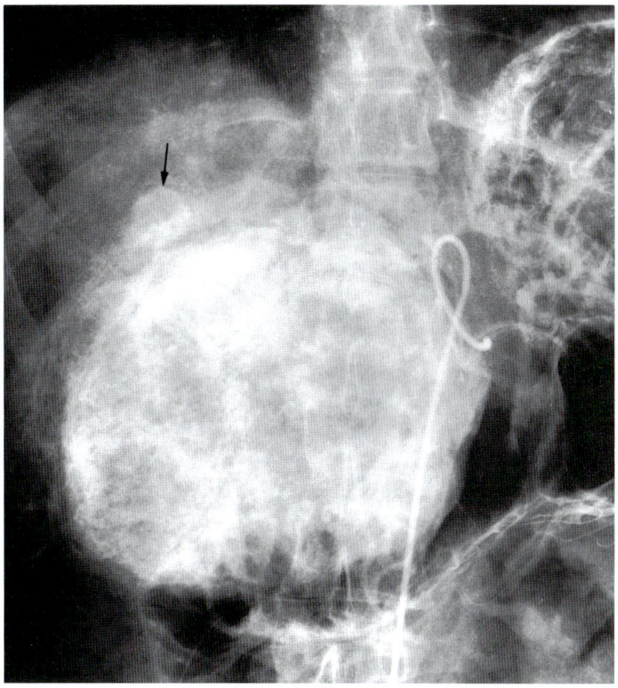

(e) Hepatic arteriogram (late phase): the mass is now stained. A small secondary (→) is seen in S^{VIII}.

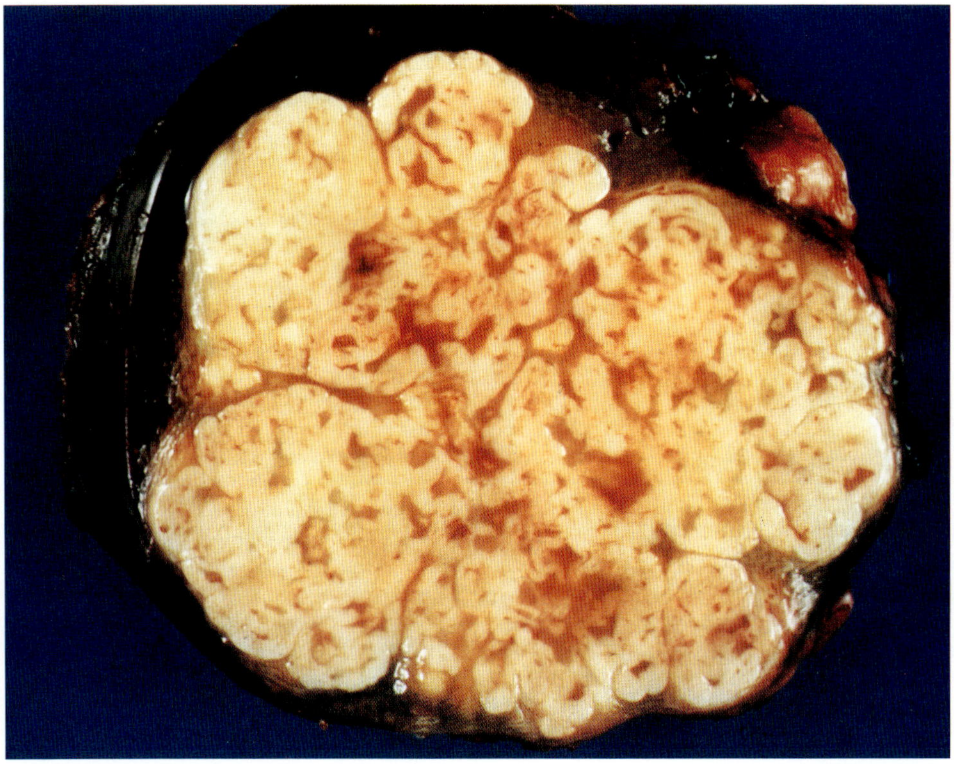

(f) Cut section of resected specimen: enucleation of the mass was done. It was a solid yellowish brown tumor with a lobulated structure assuming an arabesque figure. The periphery was growing in a protruding fashion and almost the entire periphery was fibrously encapsulated. Histopathologically, it was a chondrosarcoma consisting of small spindle-shaped sarcoma cells. Calcific lesions seen by CT and US could not be identified.

Metastatic hepatic tumor—Case 15: Stomach carcinoid tumor metastatic to the liver seen as a honeycomb by US. A 67-year-old female. Gastrectomy was carried out 5 years earlier for a carcinoid tumor. She developed the carcinoid syndrome such as flushing, palpitation, and diarrhea. An hepatic tumor was found by US.

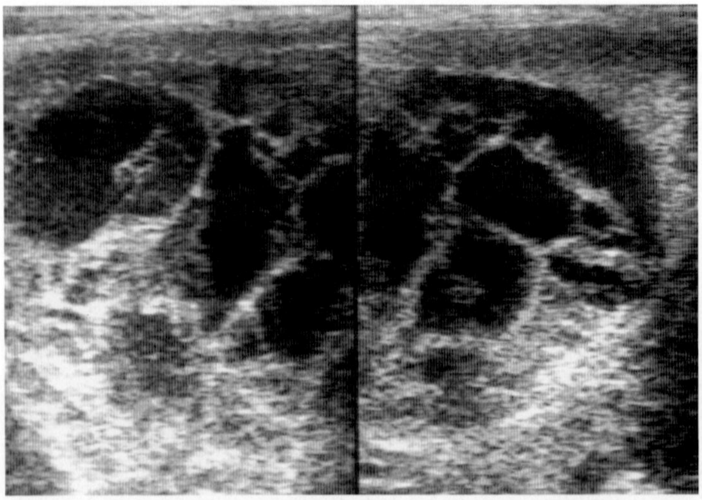

(a) US: a 12 cm lesion with a smooth margin is seen in the right lobe. The interior is a honeycomb structure, suggesting bleeding.

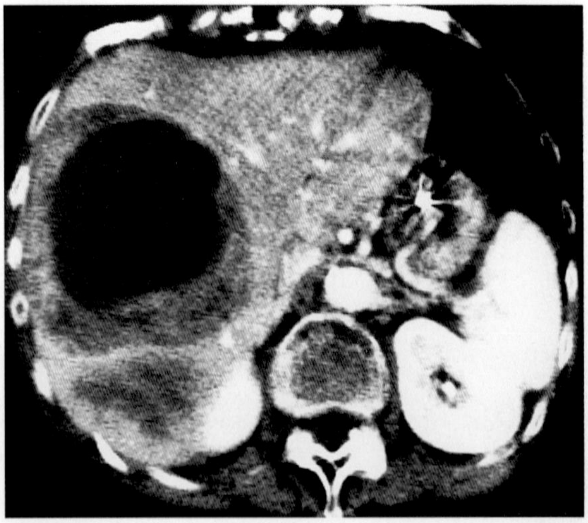

(b) Enhanced CT: the lesion is cystic in the interior surrounded by a single layer of low-density area. Considering her symptoms and the fact that carcinoid tumor readily bleeds, metastatic carcinoid tumor was the most likely diagnosis. However, histological confirmation could not be made.

Metastatic hepatic tumor—Case 16: Pancreatic gastrinoma metastatic to the liver demonstrating a distinct tumor stain. A 50-year-old female. She had undergone gastric resection three times for recurrent ulcers in 7 years. At the time of the last gastrectomy, a mass was found in the head of the pancreas.

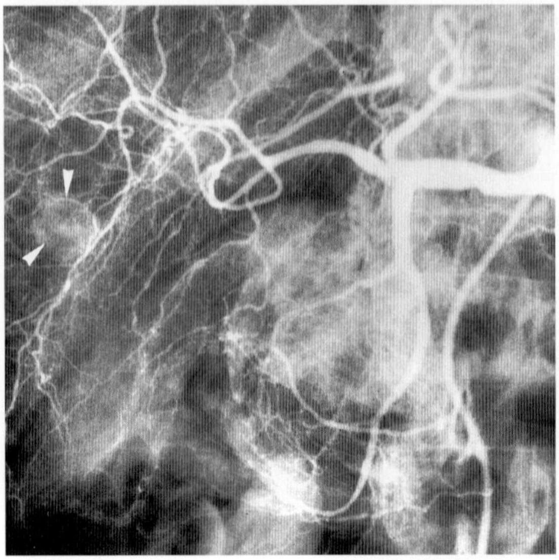

(a) Celiac arteriogram: a 5 cm hypervascular lesion is seen in the area that corresponds to the head of the pancreas and a 1.5 cm tumor stain (▶) in S^{VI} of the right lobe of the liver. An operation was carried out. The diagnosis was malignant gastrinoma arising in the head of the pancreas and its hepatic metastasis.

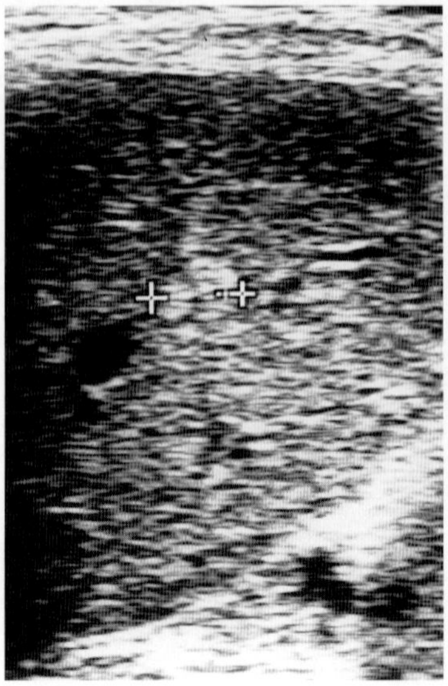

(b) US: there is a hyperechoic 1.4 cm tumor marked by (+) in S^{VI}.

Metastatic hepatic tumor—Case 17: Medullary thyroid carcinoma metastatic to the liver. A 50-year-old male. Total thyroidectomy was carried out for medullary carcinoma of the thyroid. Subsequent elevation of CEA (30.2 ng/ml) led to the detection of hepatic tumor.

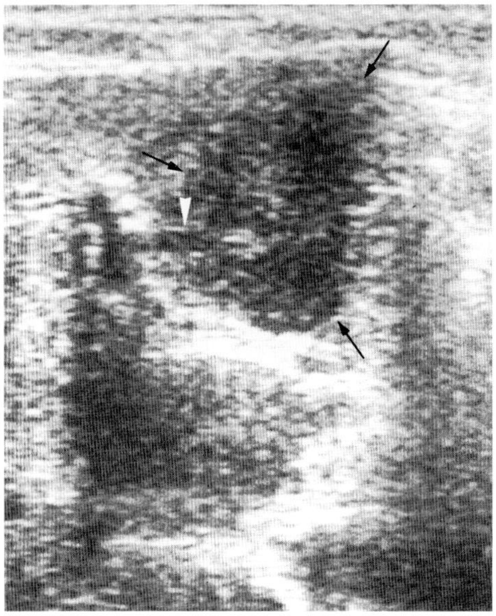

(a) US (transverse scan): a 5.0×4.5 cm hypoechoic mass (→) is seen in S^{II-III}. A portion of portal branch P^{III} (▶) is seen within this mass.

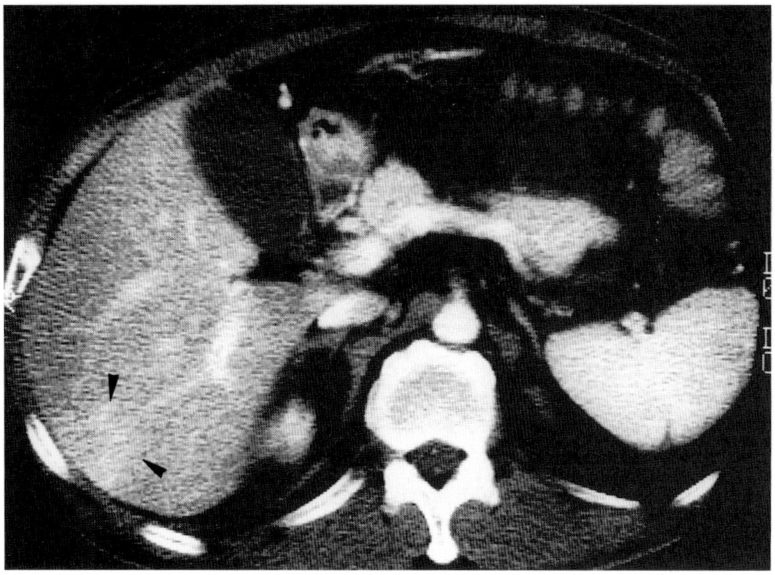

(b) Enhanced CT: another 2 cm hypervascular ill-defined mass (▶) is seen in S^{VI}.

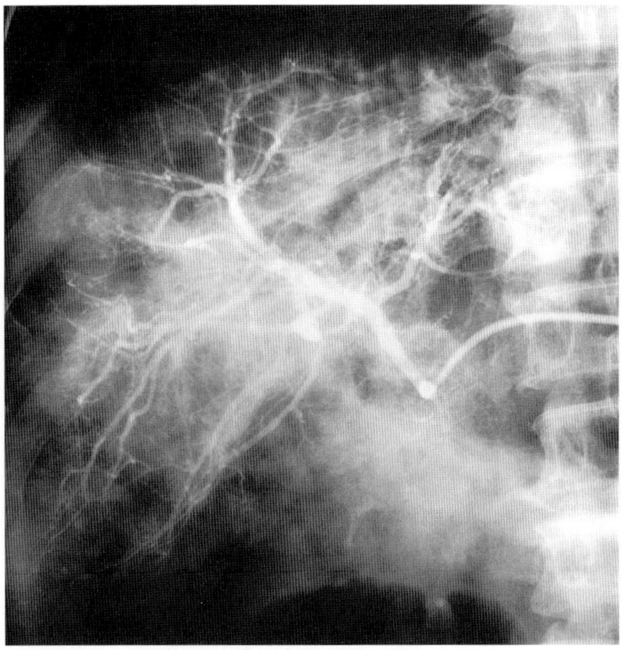

(c) Heptic arteriogram (early phase): a number of hypervascular tumors are seen in both lobes, but neovasculature is not very marked.

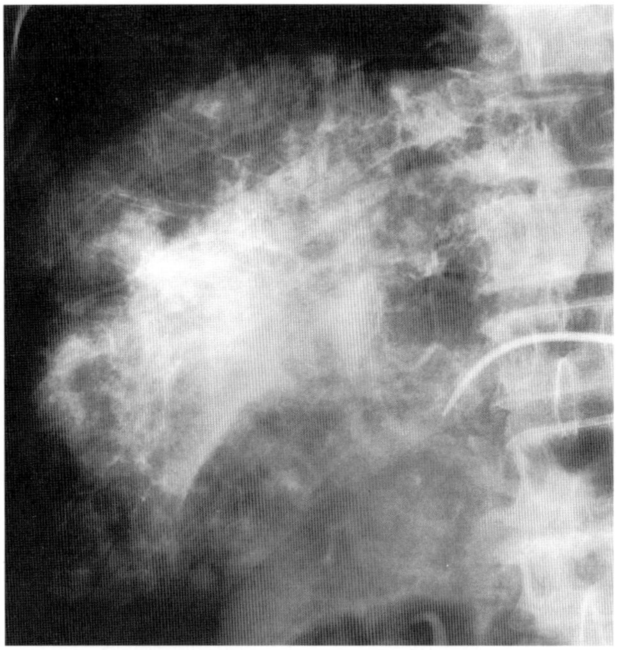

(d) Hepatic arteriogram (late phase): tumors are seen as ill-demarcated stains.

Case 17 (contd.)

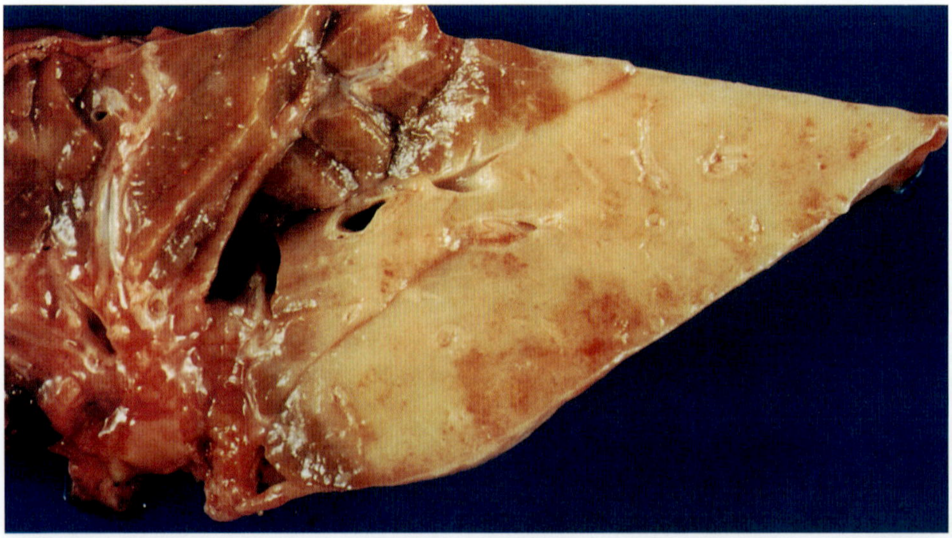

(e) Cut section of resected specimen: upon opening the abdomen, many tumors were seen in the liver, and only the left lobe was resected. The specimen showed a white tumor diffusely occupying the S^{II-III} region. It was a medullary carcinoma, the same as the resected thyroid carcinoma, which contained many portal tracts within it. There were many tumor thrombi within the portal vein, and the tumor also contained some amyloid substance and hyalinized tissue.

Metastatic hepatic tumor—Case 18: Lacrimal gland carcinoma metastatic to the liver recognized as a hypervascular lesion. A 52-year-old male. He underwent enucleation of the right lobe for an anaplastic cancer of the lacrimal gland. Six months later metastases were found in the lung and liver.

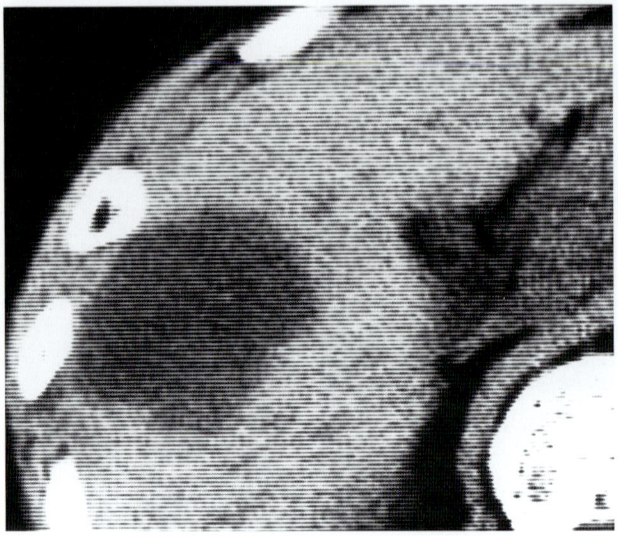

(a) Plain CT: an irregularly margined 4.5 cm low-density lesion is seen in S^{VI-V}.

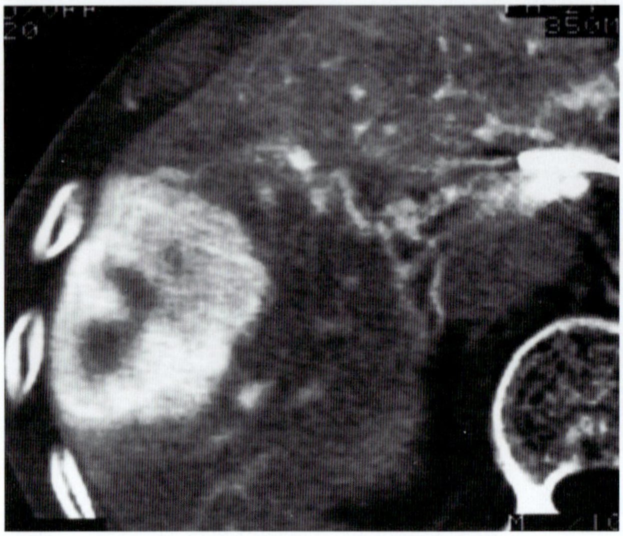

(b) Arterial-CT: the mass was enhanced but the center was not stained in the early phase.

Case 18 (contd.)

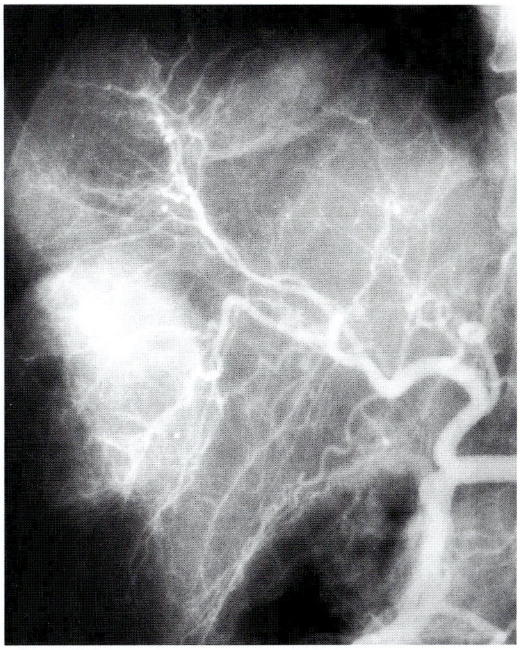

(c) Hepatic arteriogram: a spherical tumor stain and dilated feeding arteries are seen in S^{VI}.

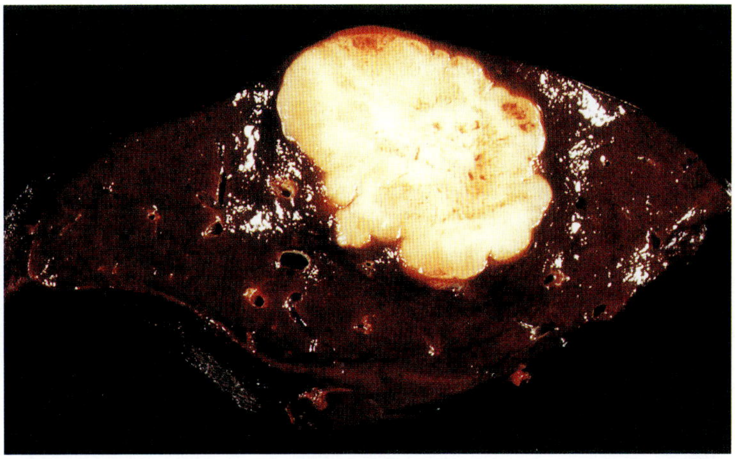

(d) Cut section of resected specimen: the mass was yellow and firm with a smooth and wavy bulging periphery. Histologically, this was adenoid cystic carcinoma with a cellular structure and intrasinusoidal invasion. The center of the mass was hyalinized showing mucoid degeneration.

Metastatic hepatic tumor—Case 19: Intracranial tumor (meningioma) metastasizing to the liver. A 33-year-old male. He underwent resection of cerebral angioblastic meningioma 6 years earlier. He came to the hospital because of right upper quadrant pain.

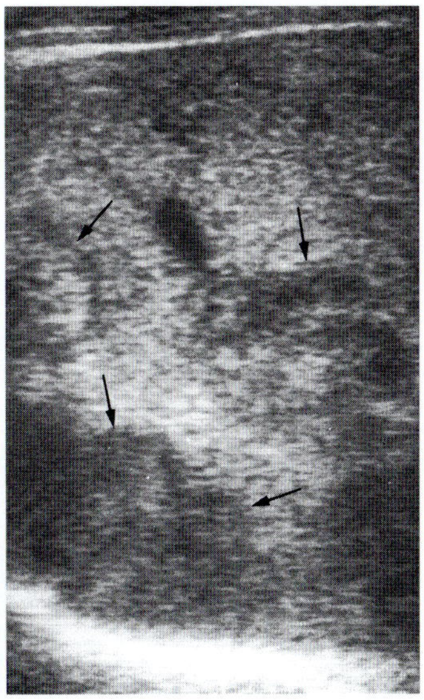

(a) US: a number of hypochoic lesions and isoechoic ones with a halo are seen in the right liver (→).

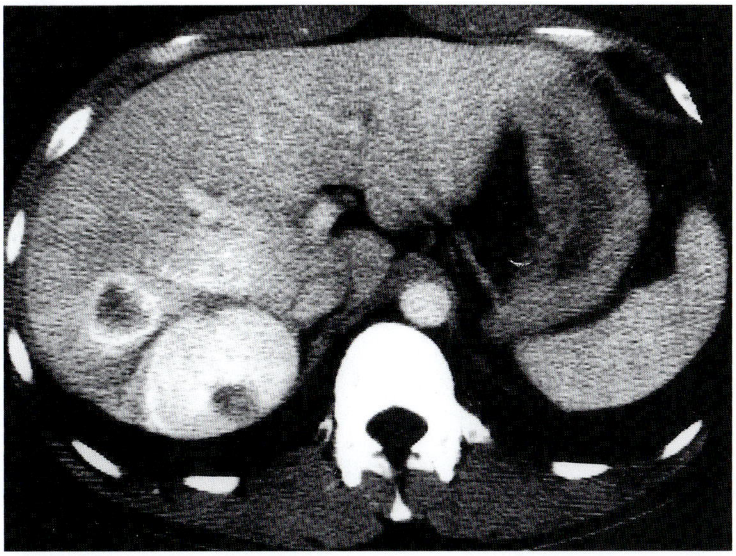

(b) Enhanced CT (early phase): the masses are generally well enhanced. Some have an unenhanced center.

Case 19 (contd.)

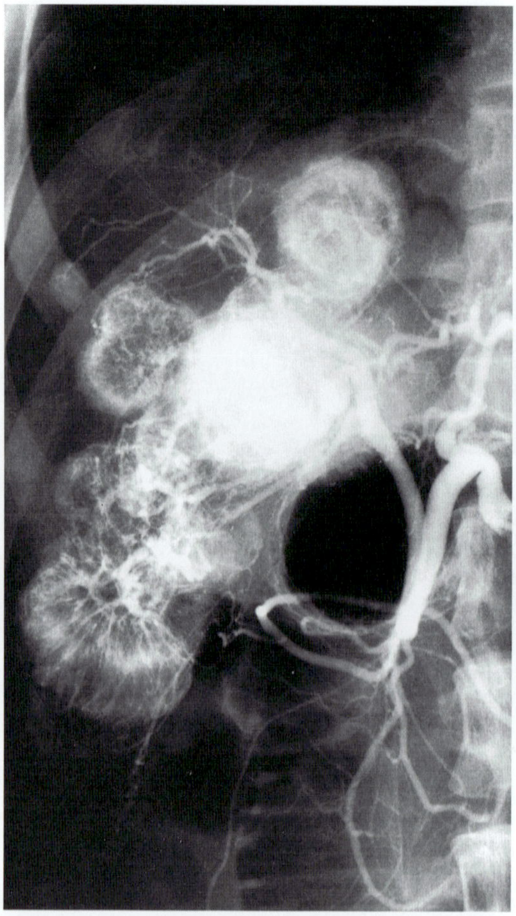

(c) Angiogram: a number of hypervascular lesions are seen mainly in the right lobe. Distinct tumor vessels and subsequent strong tumor stains suggested a non-hormone producing pancreatic tumor, leiomyosarcoma, or carcinoid tumor metastasizing to the liver. Resection was carried out without identification of the primary.

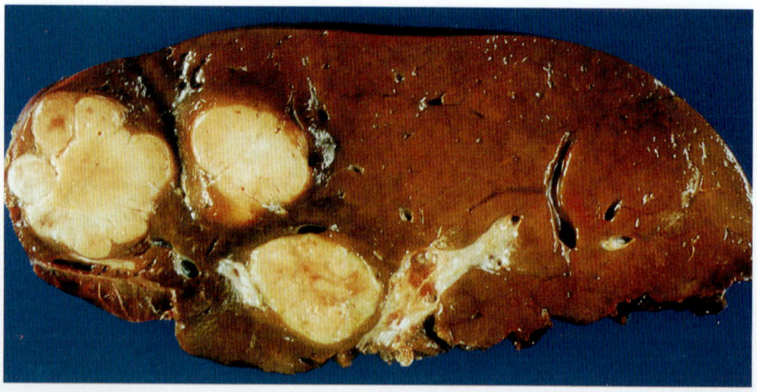

(d) Cut section of resected specimen: a number of grayish white elastic tumors were seen. The margins were wavy in some and smooth in others.

Extracranial metastasis of meningioma is rather uncommon, and successfully resected meningioma metastasis in the liver is very rare.

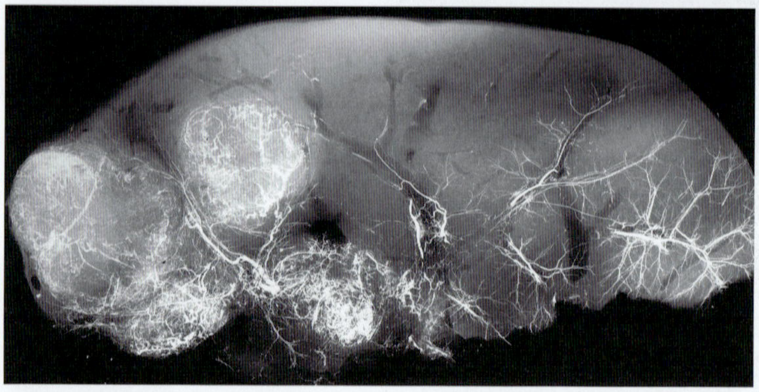

(e) Microangiogram: this is the same slice as (d). Many fine winding and dilated tumor vessels are seen within the tumors.

Metastatic hepatic tumor—Case 20: Cystic hepatic metastasis of esophagus cancer in which US proved useful for differential diagnosis. A 51-year-old male. Total resection of the esophagus was done for carcinoma of the midportion of the esophagus.

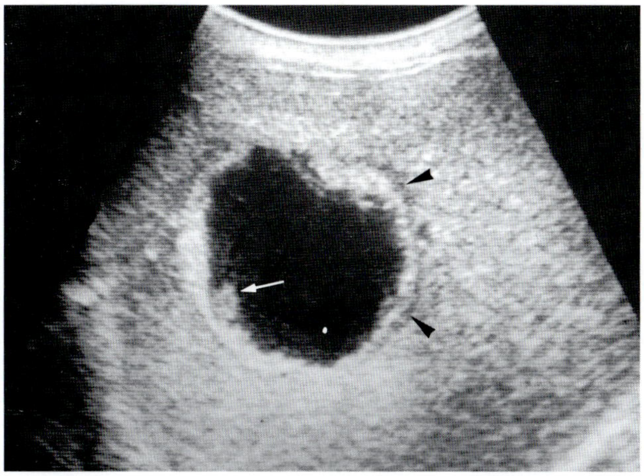

(a) US: during the follow-up, US detected a cystic 5 cm tumor in S^{VIII}. The tumor interior is cystic with posterior echo enhancement. However, the tumor periphery consists of one hyperechoic layer surrounded partially by a thin low-echoic ring (▶), and there is a papillary protrusion (→).

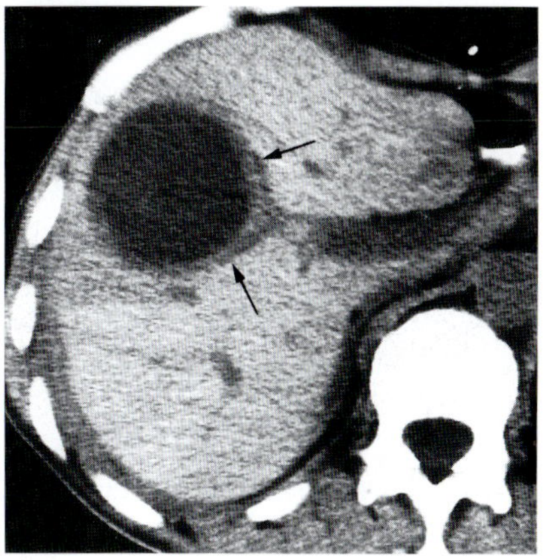

(b) Plain CT: this image may be diagnosed as a simple cyst. However, a low-density layer (→) is seen along the periphery.

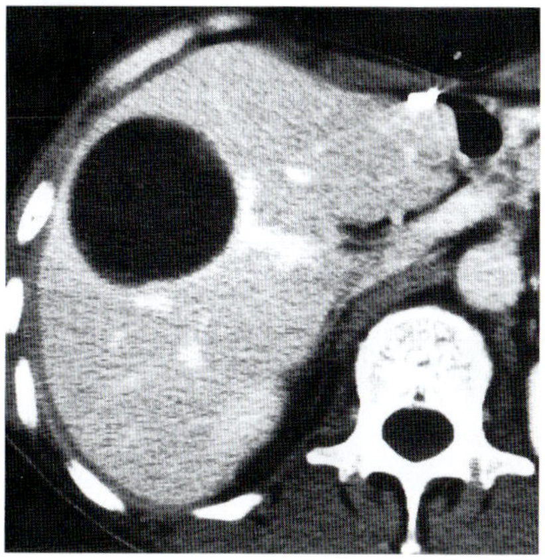

(c) Enhanced CT (early phase): no enhancement is seen in the periphery nor in the center of the mass.

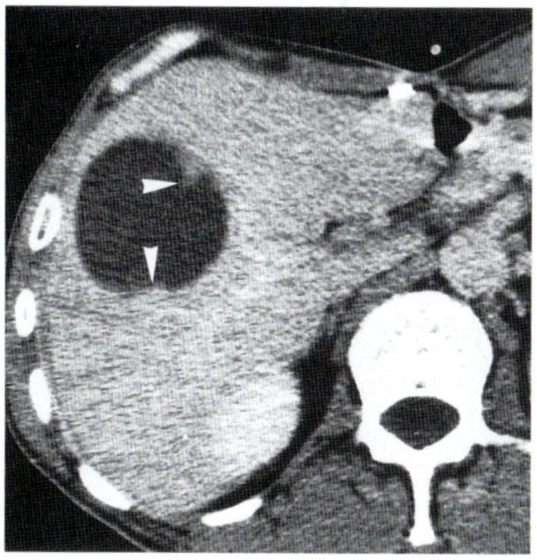

(d) Enhanced CT (late phase): a papillary structure (▶) is seen enhanced within the mass.

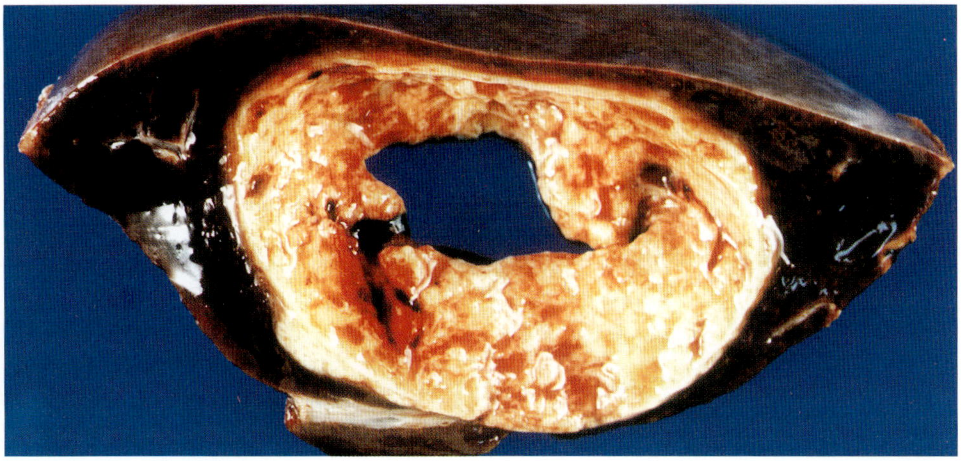

(e) Cut section of resected specimen: Resection was carried out. The tumor produced light brown serous fluid upon cutting. This cut section is near the end of the mass, demonstrating necrotic tissue in the wall of the tumor. Histologically, it was well differentiated squamous cell carcinoma with marked keratinization and stratified differentiation.

Metasatic hepatic tumor—Case 21: Malignant melanoma metastic to the liver. An 81-year-old woman. Malignant melanoma in the external genitalia was resected 2 years earlier, and then a hepatic mass found.

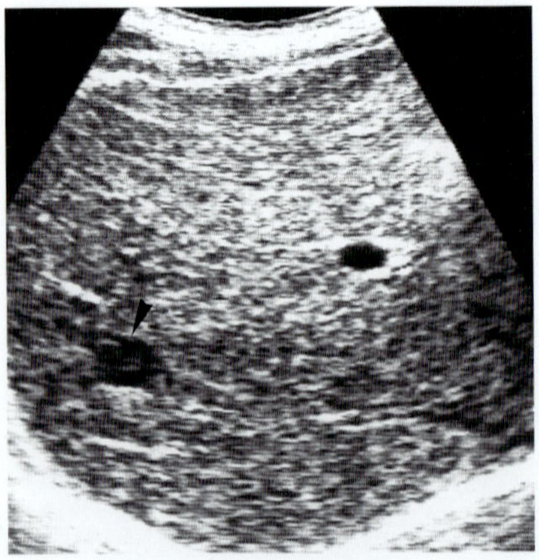

(a) US: a round 1 cm low-echo mass (▶) is seen in S^{VI}. Angiography failed to disclose this lesion.

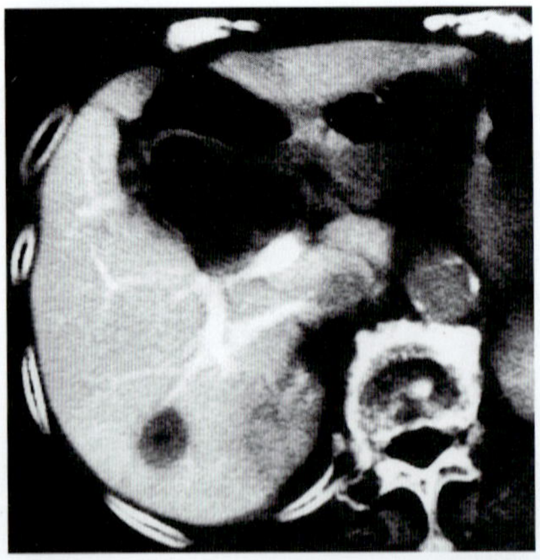

(b) Portal-CT (early phase): this 1.5 cm lesion has a small low-density area in the center.

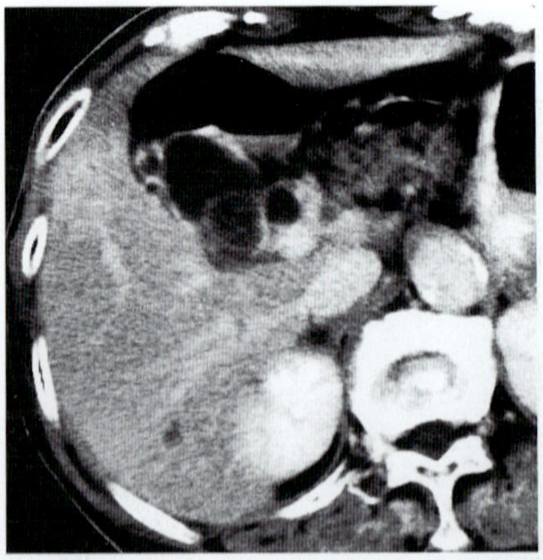

(c) Portal-CT (late phase): most of the tumor has turned isodense, leaving the center as an unenhanced spot.

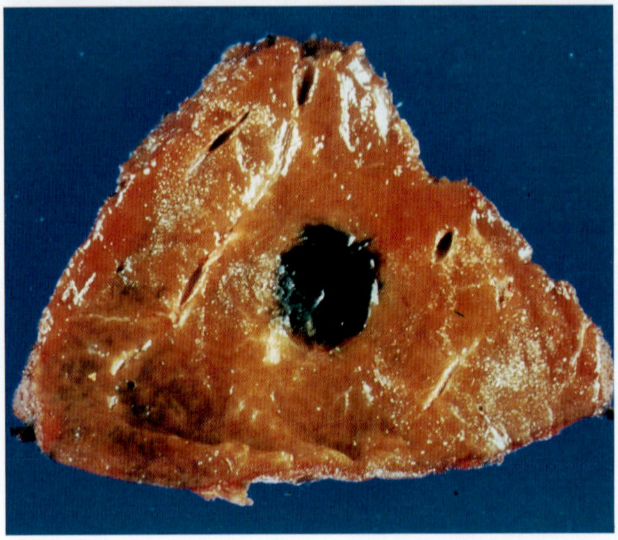

(d) Cut section of resected specimen: a typical black malignant melanoma metastatic to the liver. The boundary between the mass and parenchyma is discrete, but there is no capsule, indicating that the tumor was infiltrating into the surrounding tissue. The center was necrotic with infiltrating melanophages. The non-cancer portion was normal.

Metastatic hepatic tumor—Case 22: Hepatic metastasis of medullary carcinoma of the colon in which portal vein invasion continuous from the mass was seen. A 54-year-old man.

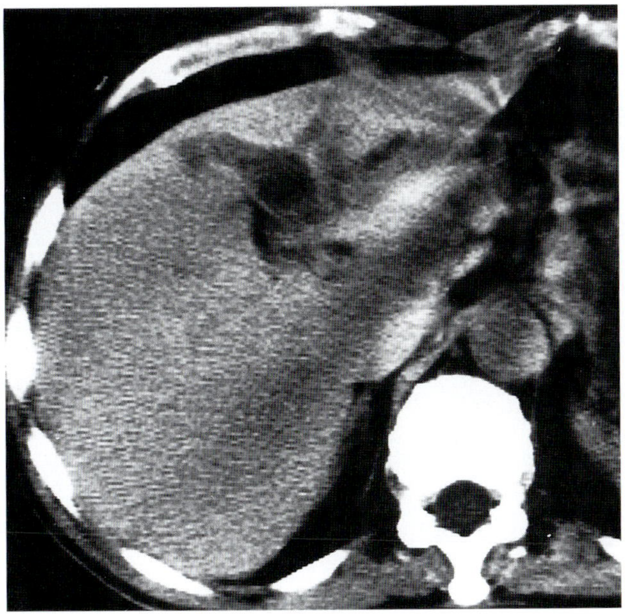

(a) Enhanced CT (late phase): a 12 cm metastatic mass was seen in the left lobe. This caudal slice displays tree branch-shaped low-density areas in S^{IV}.

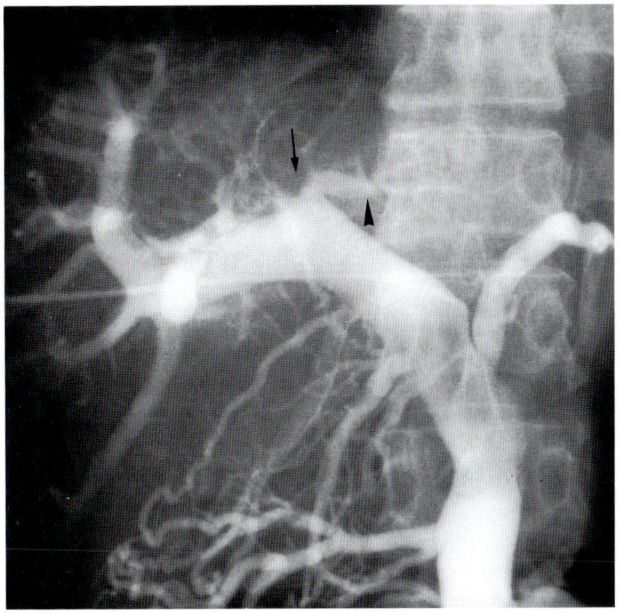

(b) PTP: there is a filling defect at the beginning of the left portal vein (→), and only the left caudal branch (▶) is opacified. The decreased opacity in the portal trunk is due to compression by the tumor anterior to it.

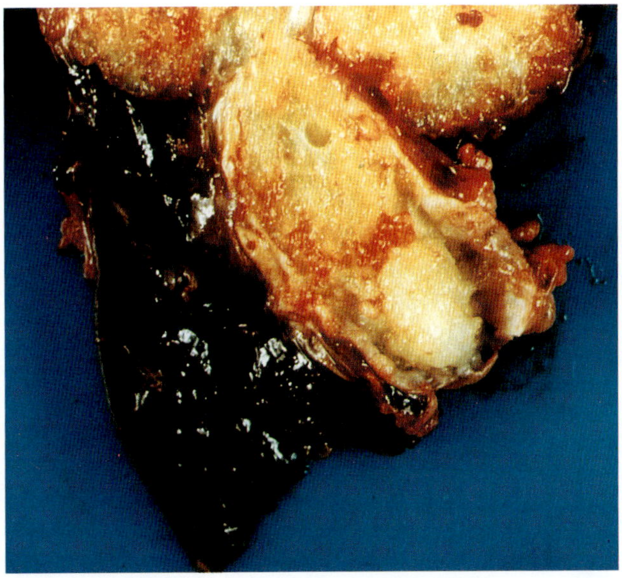

(c) Cut section of resected specimen: this cut surface demonstrates tumor growth in the portal vein with its head reaching the left portal vein.

Metastaic hepatic tumor—Case 23: Moderately differentiated colon cancer metastic to the liver, producing intraductal tumor growth. A 47-year-old man. He underwent resection of carcinoma of the ascending colon 1 year earlier. During the follow-up, multiple metastases were found in the liver by CT, and right lobectomy combined with left lateral segmentectomy was carried out.

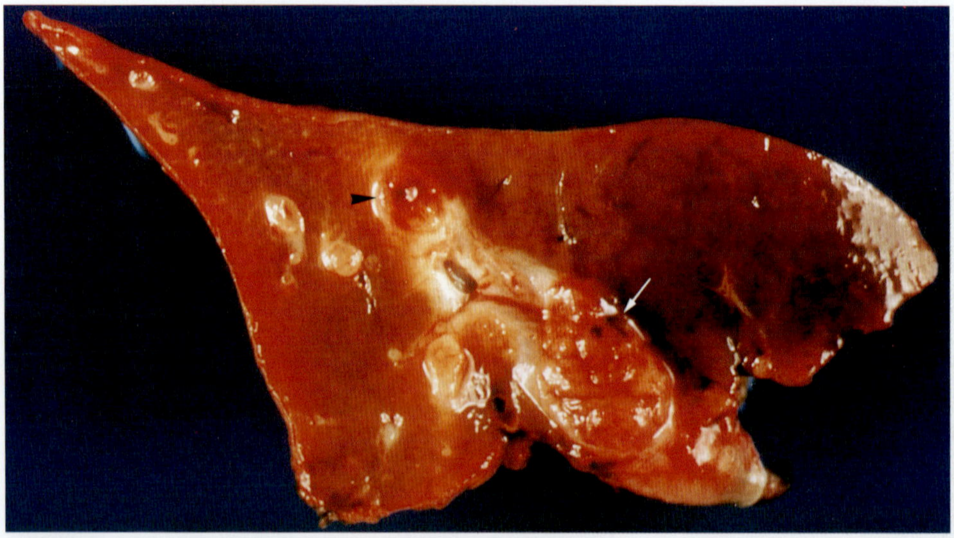

Cut section of resected specimen: in this cut section of the left lateral segment, a 5 mm metastasis (▶) and an intraductal tumor thrombus (→) are seen. Histologically, the tumor thrombus was lined by a single layer of bile duct epithelium. Multiple portal vein tumor thrombi coexisted.

Metastatic hepatic tumor—Case 24: Usefulness of portal-CT in metastatic hepatic tumor.

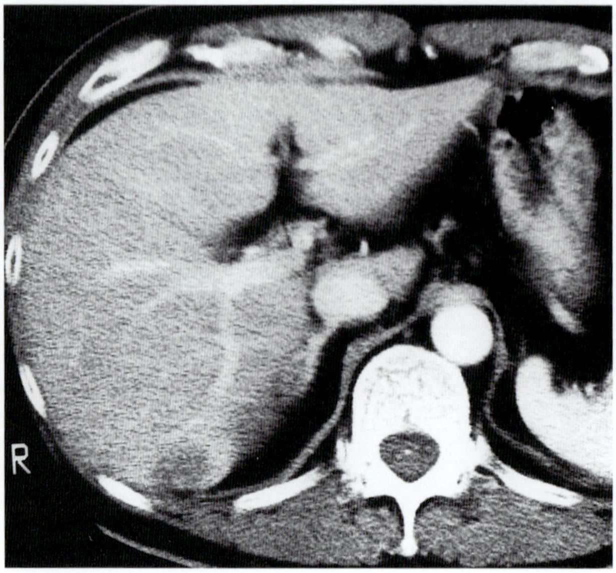

(a) Dynamic CT: in this slice of dynamic CT scan made by the table incremental method, one lesion is seen in S^{VI-VII}.

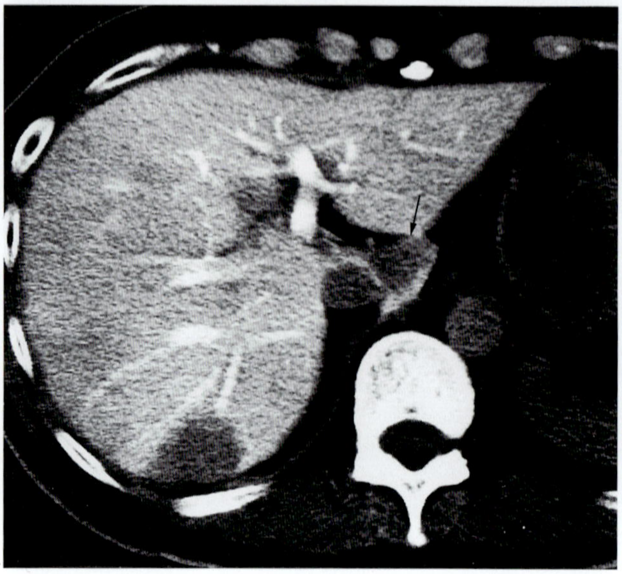

(b) Portal-CT: another metastasis (→) was found by portal-CT.

Metastatic hepatic tumor—Case 25: Demerit of Lipiodol-CT in the study of metastatic liver cancer.

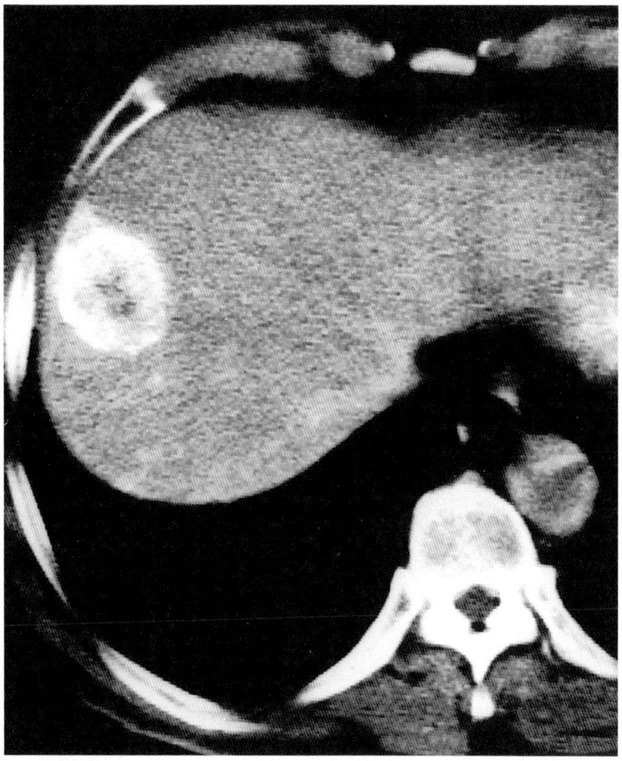

(a) Lipiodol-CT: this CT scan was made immediately after injection of Lipiodol into the proper hepatic artery. A 3 cm lesion is seen in S^{VIII} retaining Lipiodol.

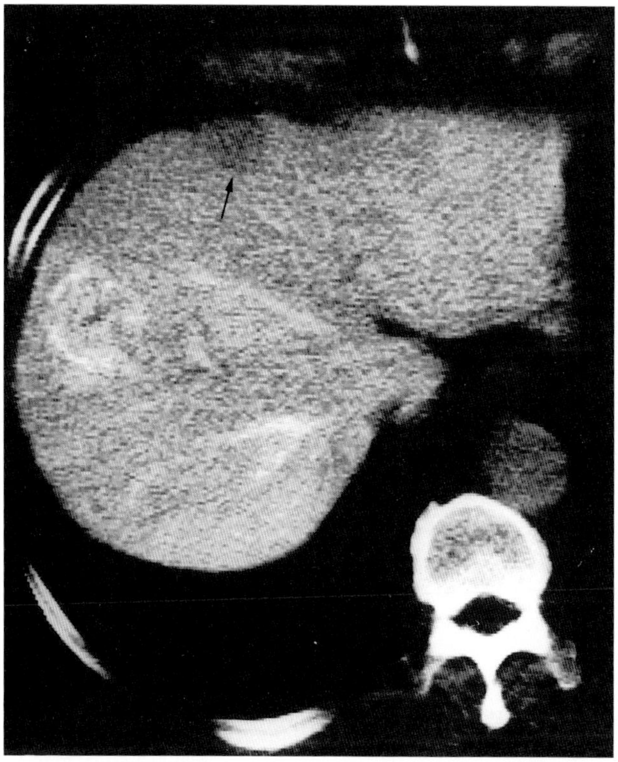

(b) Portal-CT: in addition to the Lipiodol-enhanced lesion, there is another metastasis in S^{IV} (→). By operation, they were both metasatic colon carcinomas. In general, portal-CT is more diagnostic than Lipiodol-CT in hypovascular hepatic metastases. Furthermore, portal-CT clearly delineates the diagnosis.

Metastatic hepatic tumor—Case 26: Hypervascular gastric cancer metastatic to the liver for which TAE was effective.

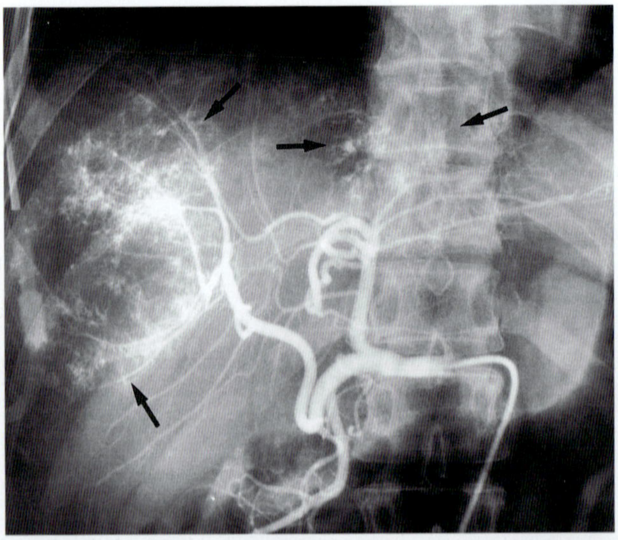

(a) Hepatic arteriogram: the right and the left lobe each has a hypervascular metastasis (→). Since catheterization was easy only for the left lobe, the left lobe alone was embolized with gelfoam particles (TAE).

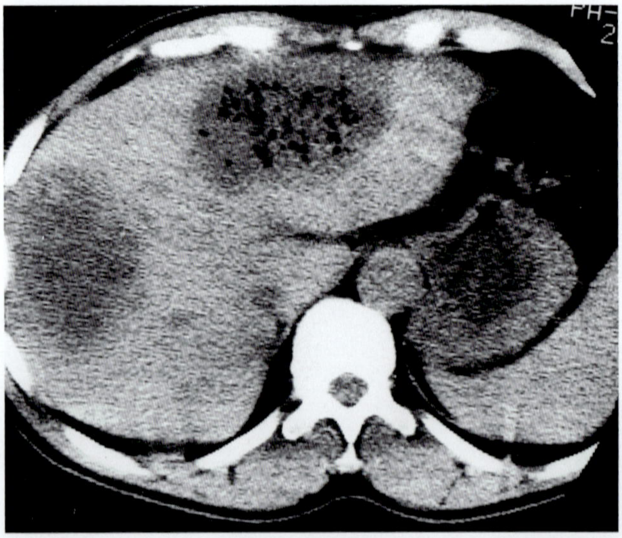

(b) 7 days after TAE: only the embolized lesion produced gas bubbles.

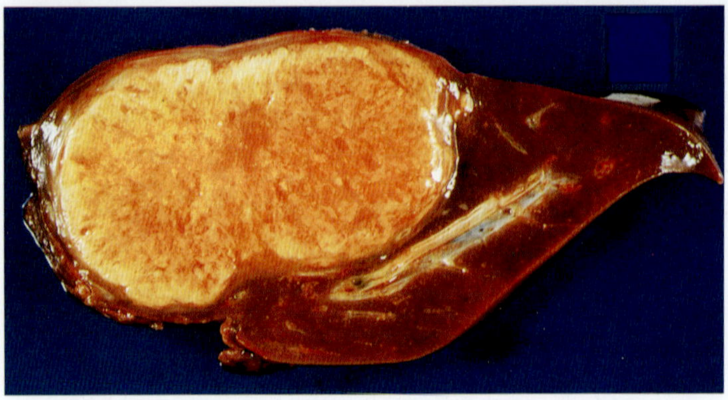

(c) Cut section of the embolized lesion: the tumor is smoothly round and the interior is homogeneous due to necrosis.

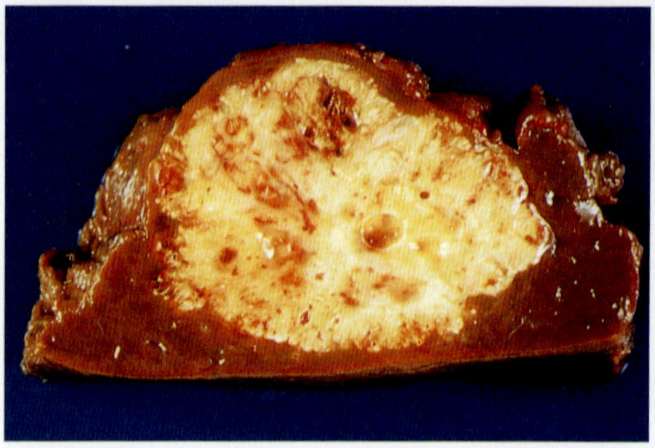

(d) Cut section of the untreated lesion: the mass is grossly typical of viable adenocarcinoma with no necrosis in the interior.

4.21 Extrahepatic tumors that require differentiation from intrahepatic tumors

In imaging diagnosis of hepatic tumors, one may encounter cases in which the origin of the tumor cannot be determined, whether intrahepatic or extrahepatic (Fig. 4.15). Tumors that arise extrahepatically and grow compressing the liver are divided into those arising in the abdominal cavity and those arising extraabdominally.

Intraabdominal tumors include those originating in organs in close proximity to the liver, and those caused by intraabdominal dissemination and producing compression onto the liver or its deformity (Case 1), the latter being more frequent. In Case 2, the lesion appeared as if it were a pedunculated HCC of the left lobe by CT, but it turned out to be an intraabdominal metastasis from an ovarian carcinoma primary to the lesser omentum; many disseminated lesions were seen on opening the abdomen (Lundstedt *et al.* 1992). Operation is indicated for intrahepatic tumors but not for peritoneal dissemination, and preoperative diagnosis is most important because it may prevent an unnecessary operation. Accurate distinction betwen intra- and extrahepatic location of the tumor is thus crucial.

To determine the site of origin, angiography is of importance, but it does not always provide the necessary information. In that case, the artery that could possibly be feeding the tumor should be catheterized and arterial-CT done for more information (Case 3).

Of the tumors primary to the peritoneum, malignant mesothelioma is an important one, because it is reported to be etiologically associated with asbestos (Borow *et al.* 1973). Although not very common, it may arise from the pleura and creep into the abdomen (Whitley *et al.* 1982; Reuter *et al.* 1983). Malignant mesothelioma produces irregular thickenings of the omentum and mesentery during its growth. If it extends to the inferior surface of the diaphragm, it produces diffuse extrahepatic compressions on the liver surface (Cases 4, 5). Differential diagnosis between peritoneal carcinomatosis (Walkey *et al.* 1988) and malignant mesothelioma is not always easy, and a primary in the GI tract or the ovary has to be excluded by various radiological examinations. Pseudomyxoma peritonei is yet another neoplastic disorder that affects the peritoneum (Mayes *et al.* 1981) (Case 6).

Extraabdominal tumors also include malignancies derived from the abdominal wall (Case 7) and the pleural cavity (Case 8). For the diagnosis of the latter, arterial-CT done with a catheter inserted into the inferior phrenic artery is useful because it can determine the location of the diaphragm and the origin of the tumor from their anatomical relation. MR imaging (Case 8) may also prove very diagnostic because it permits sectioning of the mass in any sagittal and coronal direction.

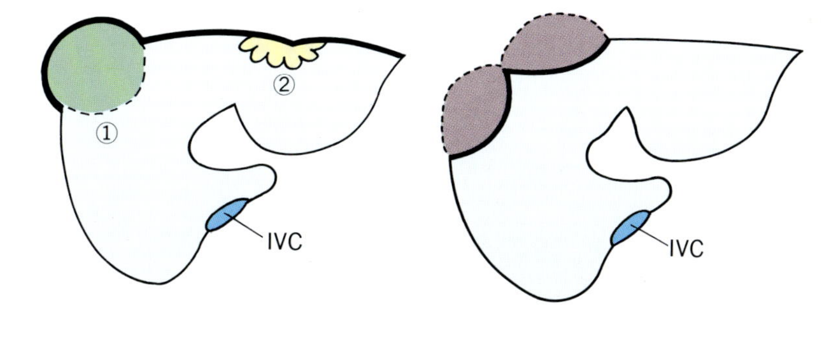

Intrahepatic tumor: intrahepatic tumor growing in an expanding fashion (1) produces a convex protrusion in the liver surface, and an infiltrating intrahepatic tumor (2) produces some surface concavity as it causes cancer umbilication

Extrahepatic tumor: when the liver is compressed by an expanding extrahepatic tumor, the liver surface shows a lens-shaped concavity

Fig. 4.15 CT characteristics of intrahepatic and extrahepatic tumors.

Extrahepatic malignancy—Case 1: Peritoneal dissemination of ovarian carcinoma (serous cystadenocarcinoma). On opening the abdomen, peritoneal dissemination of ovarian carcinoma and localized ascites collection was recognized, and resection of only the bilateral ovaries and the omentum was carried out.

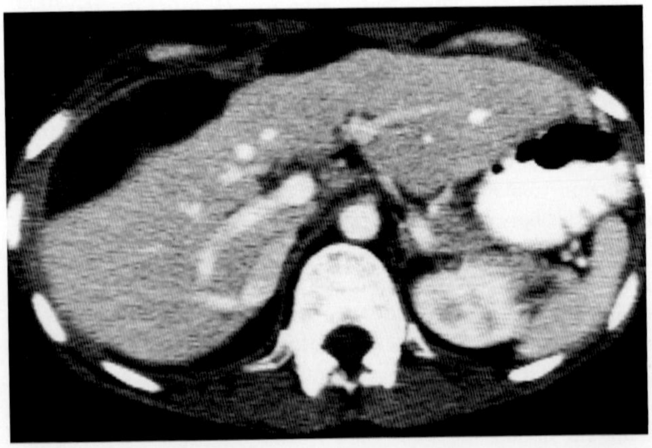

(a) Enhanced CT (6 months postoperative): localized fluid collection as a result of peritoneal adhesion that followed operation, and compression deformity of the liver surface are recognized.

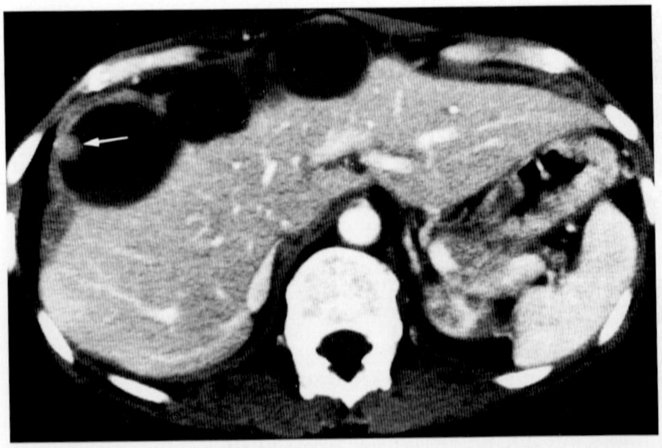

(b) Enhanced CT (10 months postoperative): the localized fluid collections have increased in volume, producing marked surface compressions. A peritoneal dissemination (→) is discernible within the ascites.

Extrahepatic malignancy—Case 2: Peritoneal dissemination of ovarian carcinoma difficult to differentiate from HCC of the left lobe. A 37-year-old woman. Resection of the ovary was carried out 1 year earlier for ovarian carcinoma (poorly differentiated adenocarcinoma) and a metastasis in S^{II} was resected at the same time. During the follow-up, a metastasis in the left lobe was suspected by CT.

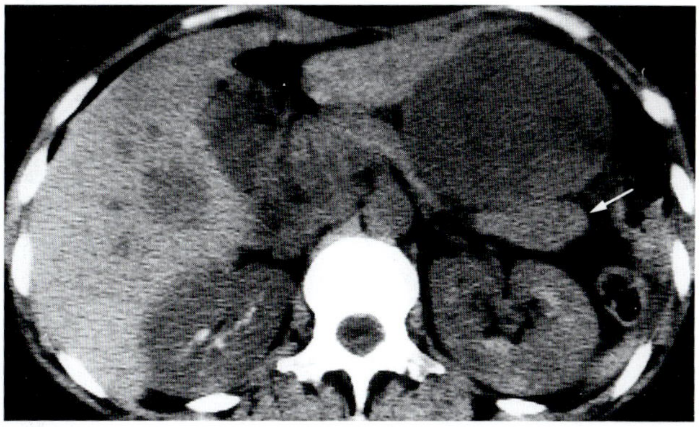

a

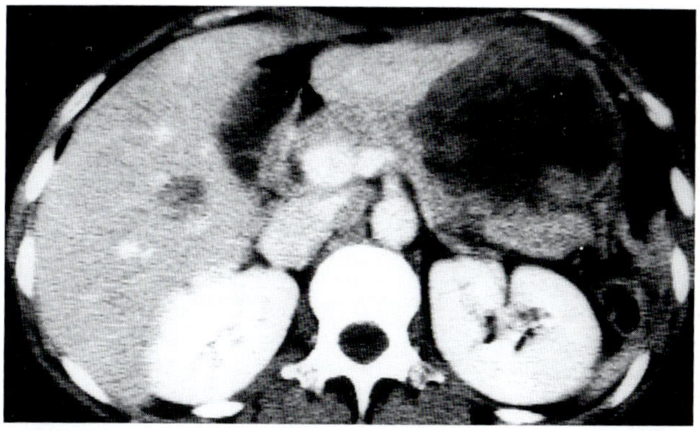

b

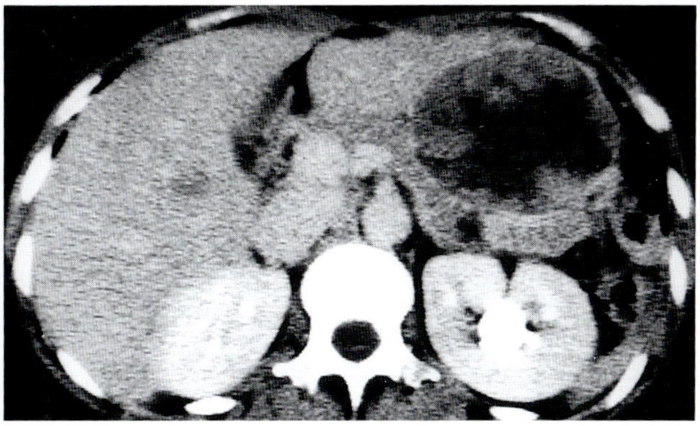

c

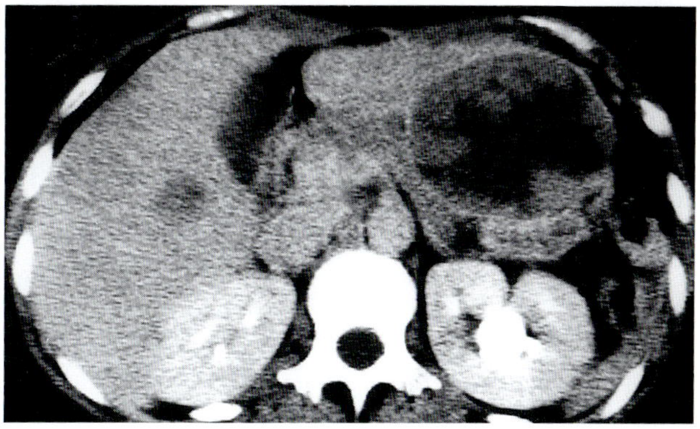

d

(a) Plain CT: a 5 cm mass is seen between the left hepatic lobe and the stomach. →, compressed stomach.
(b)–(d) Dynamic CT: these are dynamic CT images of the same slice as (a). Nodular enhancements and a central stellate low-density area are recognized. From the nodular stains, it was diagnosed as hepatic metastasis of ovarian carcinoma. When the abdomen was opened, it was not in the liver; a seeded secondary in the omentum was adherent to the inferior surface of the left lobe.

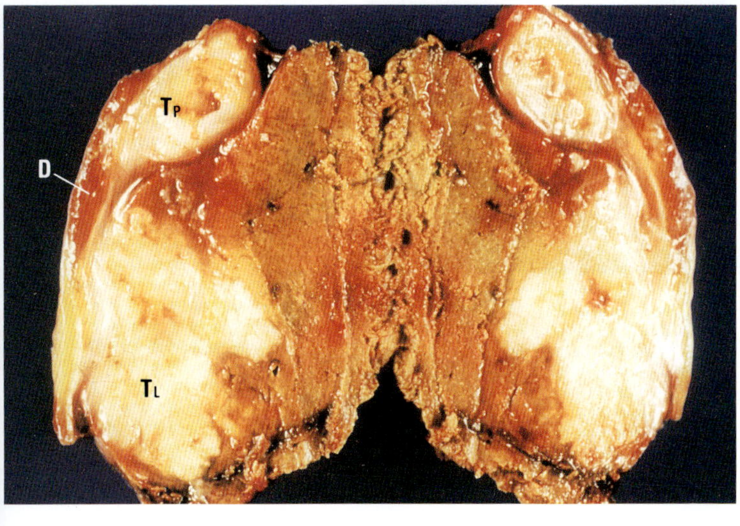

(e) Cut section of resected specimen: the resected specimen was divided and opened (this is another lesion immediately below the diaphragm). The opened liver parenchyma and two masses adherent to the diaphragm (D) are seen. The tumor metastatic to the peritoneum (T_P) was compressing the liver extrahepatically, while the mass mainly occupying the liver appeared to be an intrahepatic metastasis (T_L). However, this also could have been a metastasis infiltrating in both directions, toward the diaphragm and the liver. In ovarian carcinoma with a hepatic tumor, distinction between peritoneal dissemination and hepatic metastasis is often difficult, even with histological examination.

Extrahepatic malignancy—Case 3: Useful artrial-CT in determining the primary site.

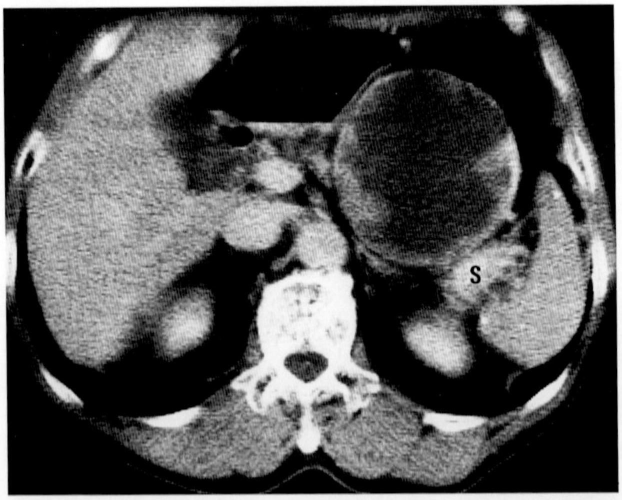

(a) Enhanced CT (late phase): a round 6 cm mass is seen anterior to the stomach (S). Most of this mass is not enhanced except for the periphery. Slices cranial to this CT scan suggested that this might be hanging as a pedunculated mass of the left hepatic lobe. Identification of the primary site was difficult.

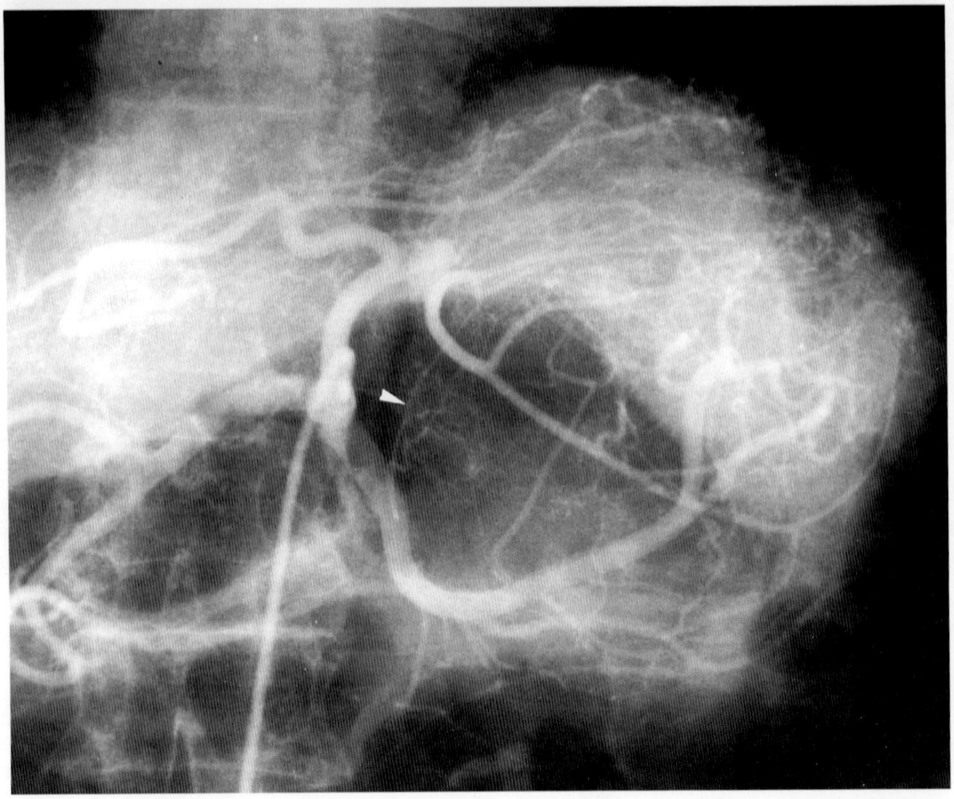

(b) Celiac arteriogram: the mass has tumor vessels derived from the left gastric artery (▶).

Case 3 (contd.)

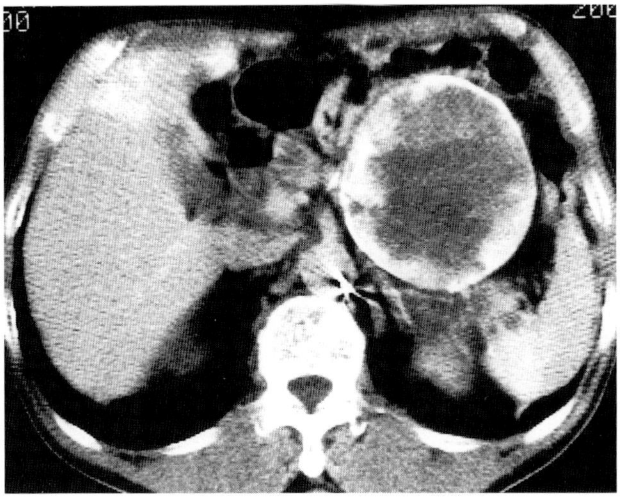

(c) Arterial-CT: to confirm the arteriographic finding, the left gastric artery was catheterized and arterial-CT was carried out. The mass was selectively enhanced, and the site of tumor origin was determined as the stomach. Since a large part of the interior was necrotic, a diagnosis of leiomyosarcoma was made. Histological study of the resected tumor confirmed it.

Extraheptatic malignancy—Case 4: Malignant mesothelioma (epithelioid type). A 62-year-old woman came to the hospital for right upper quadrant pain.

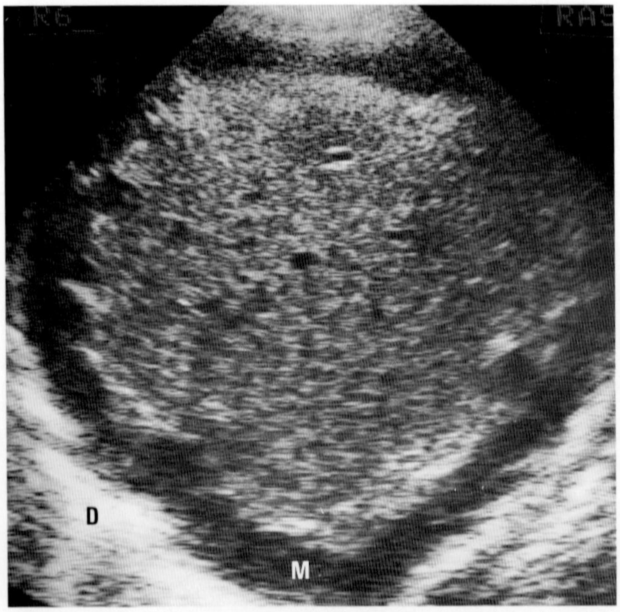

US: the surface of the liver is irregular and a hypoechoic mass (M) surrounding the liver is seen between the right diaphragm and the liver. D, diaphragm.

Extrahepatic malignancy—Case 5: Malignant mesothelioma primary to the omentum. A 11-year-old boy.

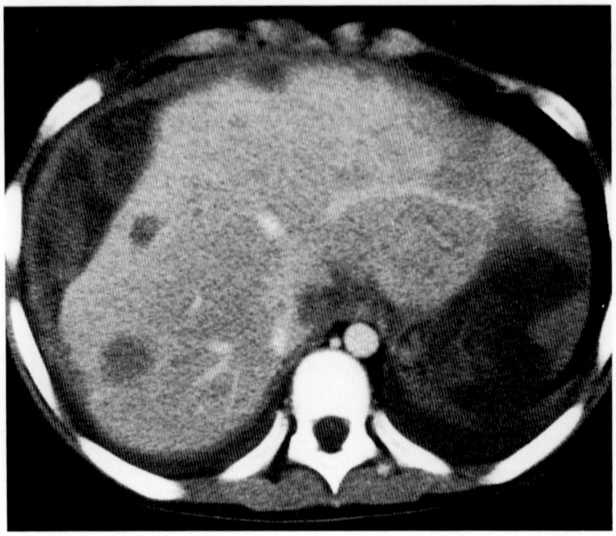

Enhanced CT: the right lobe is markedly compressed by mesothelioma that has developed in the abdominal cavity. The liver has many secondaries. Paraaortic lymph node metastases, ascites, and pleural effusion were also found.

Extrahepatic malignancy—Case 6: Pseudomxyoma peritonei.

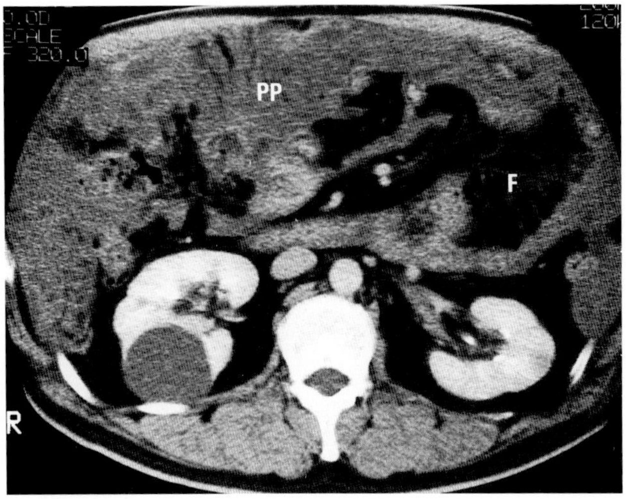

Enhanced CT: a pseudomxyoma peritonei (PP) is seen occupying nearly the entire abdominal cavity. This mass is higher in density than the ordinary fat tissue (F). There is no contraction of the mesentery nor the bowel pull-in phenomenon. Compression over the liver is usually mild with this type of tumor, and the diagnosis is not very difficult.

Extrahepatic malignancy—Case 7: CT in the diagnosis of extrahepatic tumor. A 61-year-old man.

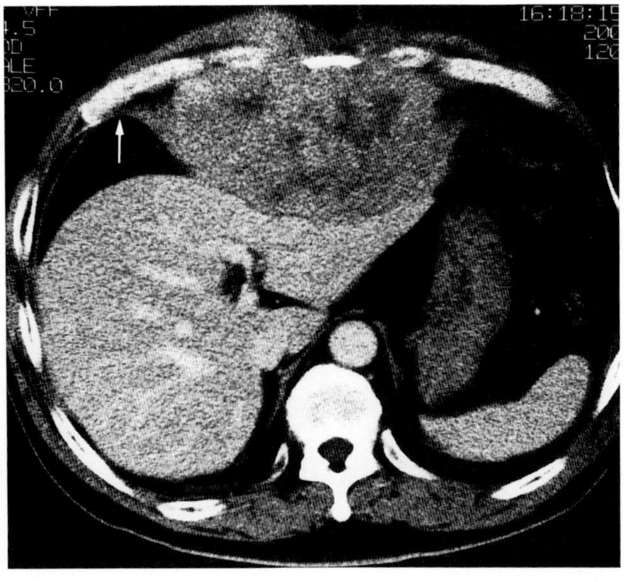

Enhanced CT: the liver is compressed posteriorly by a huge tumor Merkal cell carcinoma metastatic to the rectus abdominis muscle. The mass is covered by the parietal peritoneum (→), and diagnosis of a mass within the abdominal wall is possible. US could not delineate the relationship between the mass and the liver, and the US diagnosis was hepatic metastasis.

Extrahepatic malignancy—Case 8: MR imaging that delineated the spatial relation between the liver and an extrahepatic mass, and diagnosed it as an intrathoracic tumor. A 63-year-old man. Abnormal liver function tests were found at the annual medical examination, and subsequent CT examination disclosed an hepatic tumor and a large mass behind it. The question was the relationship between these two lesions.

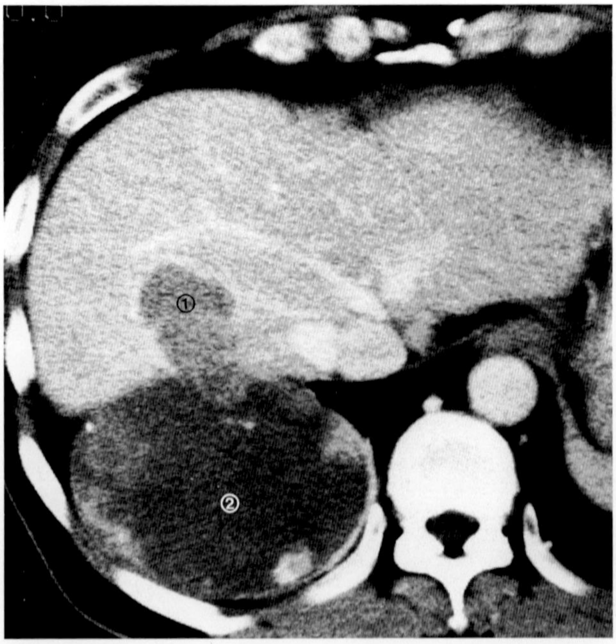

(a) Enhanced CT (early phase): an oblong low-density mass (1) in $S^{VII-VIII}$ and a 10 cm oval mass (2) are seen. There seems to be a connection between the two lesions, but the mutual relation is unclear.

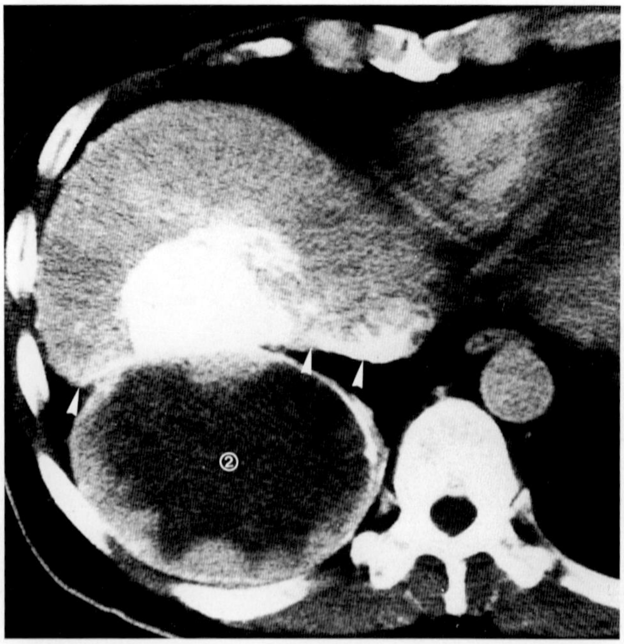

(b) Right inferior phrenic arterial-CT: the mass (2) is lateral to the markedly enhanced diaphragm (▶) suggesting its location to be within the pleural cavity. Since mass (2) is closely adherent to the diaphragm, it is partially supplied by the inferior phrenic artery. Tumor (1) retained Lipiodol injected through the hepatic artery.

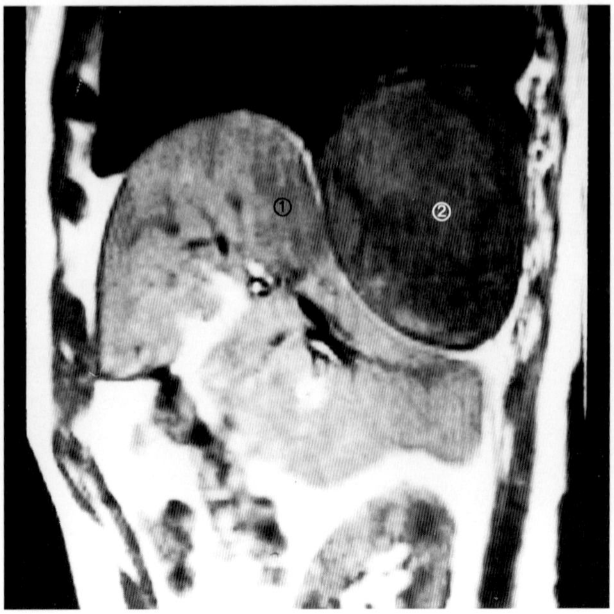

(c) MR imaging (T1-weighted, sagittal scan): tumor (2) is located cranial to the diaphragm (supraphrenic tumor), and the diagnosis is intrathoracic tumor. Tumor (1) was resected, and found to be Edmondson's grade II–III HCC. The intrathoracic mass was diagnosed as tuberculoma preoperatively and not resected. No major changes have been seen for 1.5 years postoperatively.

5

Inflammatory and parasitic diseases of the liver

From the point of view of imaging diagnosis, inflammatory diseases of the liver are important because they often require differential diagnosis from neoplastic diseases, particularly hepatic malignancies. In making imaging diagnosis of inflammatory diseases, special attention should be paid to the patient's place of residence (endemic parasitic disease), and personal history, including past history and clinical course. In inflammatory disease such as hepatic abscess, previous radiologic studies, if available, have to be compared with the current findings because there may be changes within a short period of time.

Liver abscess

Diagnosis of liver abscess is not difficult in patients presenting with fever and leukocytosis, but in their absence, incidentally found asymptomatic liver abscess may pose problems because of the lack of typical imaging features. In tropical and subtropical regions of the world, amebic liver abscess is endemic, but in developed countries, liver abscess is mostly idiopathic occurring without demonstrable source of infection.

In practice, liver abscess is more commonly found by US as an ill defined hypoechoic lesion in the liver, but before liquefaction of the interior it may resemble a neoplastic lesion with mixed low and high echoes. Some abscesses do not assume a round shape. The plain CT findings in conventional full-blown liver abscess include a low-density interior, a low-density peripheral ring and an intermediary zone of high-density ring between these two layers (Mathieu *et al.* 1985) (Case 1). If one sees gas spots and an air-fluid or a fluid-debris level, the diagnosis is easy. Enhancement of the priphery of the lesion in enhanced CT study increases the possibility of abscess (Case 1). Shrinking of the lesion with administration of antibiotics further supports the diagnosis. Imaging at just one time point may not prove very diagnostic (Case 2). In the chronic stage that follows the acute phase, contrast enhancement is minimal and the enhanced CT may not distinguish it from HCC that are not enhanced and cholangiocarcinoma.

Metastatic liver malignancies with a necrotic interior such as leiomyosarcoma, carcinoid tumor, squamous cell carcinoma, ovarian carcinoma, etc. may require differential diagnosis. Fungal infections of *Candida* and *Aspergillus*, and opportunistic infections of *Yersinia enterocolitica* (Leyman *et al.* 1989), etc. are more often small and multiple.

Inflammatory pseudotumor

Also called inflammatory myofibroblastic tumor (Craig *et al.* 1989) or plasma cell granuloma, this is a localized mass in the liver composed exclusively of inflammatory cells, plasma cells, fibrosis, macrophages, and parenchymal elements (Anthony and Telesinghe 1986). It is thought to be a healing process of liver abscess with bile leakage (Goodman 1987). The size could vary considerably, and can be very large. On angiography and enhanced CT, the mass is frequently enhanced (Imazato *et al.* 1990) and differentiation from HCC becomes necessary.

Echinococcosis (hydatid cyst)

Infection with the cestodes *Echinococcus granulosa* and *E. multilocularis* occurs through food contaminated with animal feces (mostly that of domestic dogs) containing the embryonated infectious eggs. Man and cattle are intermediate hosts. The disease caused by *E. multilocularis* behaves like a malignant disease, keeps spreading, and may eventually prove fatal. US readily demonstrates a solitary cyst or multilocular cysts. They may be distinguished from simple liver cysts by the presence of the brood sticking out from the cyst wall into the lumen. Calcification of the wall is a common feature. However, the alveolar form of echinococcosis which is uncommon in the liver presents different imaging features (Didier *et al.* 1985 ; Kalovidouris *et al.* 1986) (Case 3). Demonstration of peripheral calcification of the lesion by CT and a septum-like inner structure by US will assist diagnosis. Otherwise, differential diagnosis from necrotizing metastatic carcinoma is difficult. The birth place and personal history of the patient may provide a clue to diagnosis.

Schistosomiasis

Humans acquire this disease through the skin from penetrating cercariae. *Schistosoma japonicum* does more harm to the liver than *S. mansoni* because the former lays 20 times as many ova as does the latter. The ova produced in the peripheral veins within the abdomen are transported to the liver where they first produce inflammation which is then followed by fibrosis and calcification (Hamada *et al.* 1982) (Case 4). As hepatic schistosomiasis advances, S^{V} and S^{VI} undergo atrophy perhaps due to greater deposition of ova in the area supplied by the right inferior portal branch due to the effect of gravity. Shrinking of the right inferior region of the liver ensues, and the whole liver in the anterior projection (scintiscan) looks like an inverted triangle (Okuda *et al.* 1970; Iio *et al.* 1971). The liver surface shows grooves and grossly may simulate a turtle shell. The section of the liver demonstrates thick fibrosis of large portal tracts which is called 'pipe stem' fibrosis. Hepatic fibrosis due to schistosomasis, however severe, should not be confused with cirrhosis; schistosomiasis alone does not produce cirrhosis, although the patients who have coinfection of hepatitis B or C may develop cirrhosis, and even HCC (Nakashima *et al.* 1975).

Calcification largely depends on the number of deposited ova and time since infection (Okuda *et al.* 1975*a*).

Clonorchiasis

Clonorchis sinensis and *Opisthorchis viverrini* are the two common trematodes that invade the intrahepatic biliary tree. Both are known for their etiologic association with cholangiocarcinoma (Hou 1956; Parkin *et al.* 1993). The infected liver shows dilatation of the biliary tract only within the liver (Choi *et al.* 1988) recognized by CT, and flukes are identified individually by direct cholangiography (Okuda *et al.* 1973*a*).

Inflammatory/parasitic disease—Case 1: Liver abscess that took up ^{67}GTa-citrate and shrank when followed by CT. A 44-year-old man came to the hospital because of continuous high fever (39 °C); leukocyte count 18 600 and alkaline phosphate elevated to 64 U (normal 2.6–10).

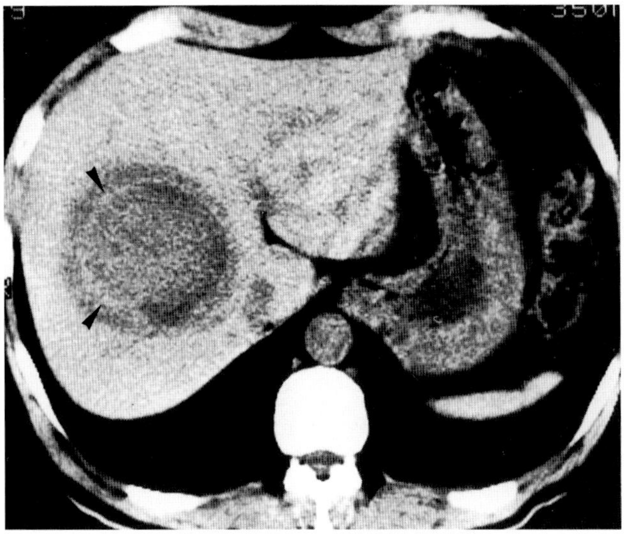

(a) Plain CT: an 8 cm round low-density lesion is seen in the right lobe. It is well demarcated and a high-density ring (▶) is seen near the margin.

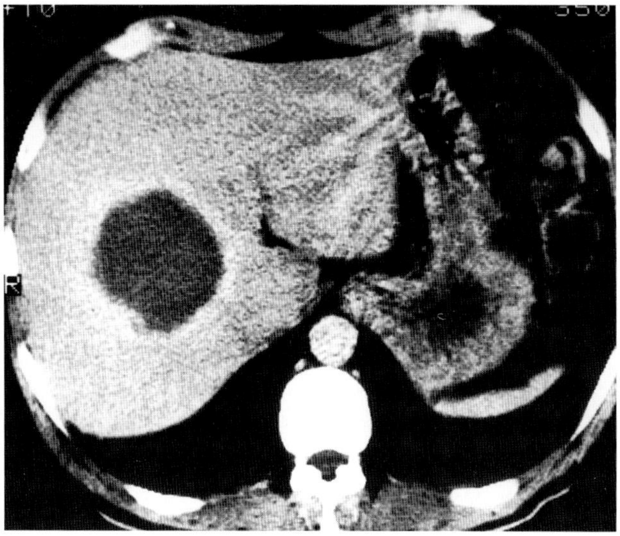

(b) Enhanced CT (late phase): the area along the periphery between the high-density ring in (a) and the margin has turned to a thick high-density area.

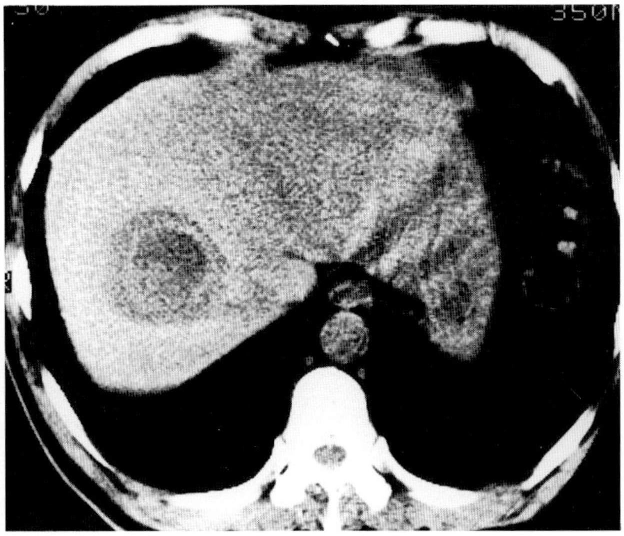

(c) Plain CT (15 days later): antibiotics were given, and the lesion has shrunk to 6 cm. The internal low-density area is now smaller, but the basic CT feature is the same as before.

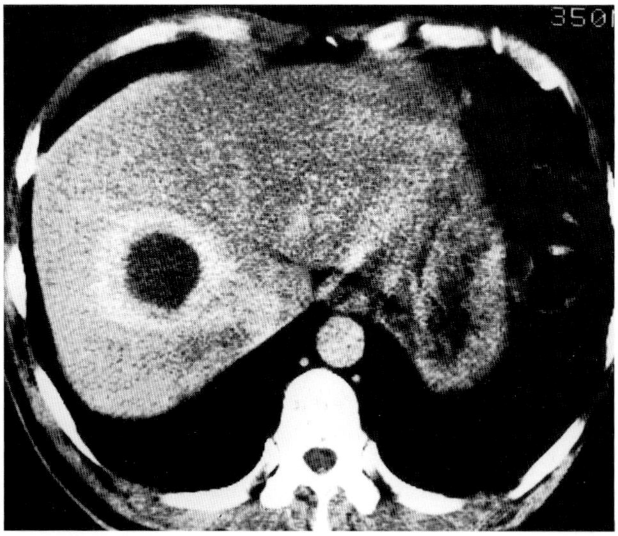

(d) Enhanced CT (15 days later): the periphery of the lesion is enhanced, but the enhanced ring is thicker than before, suggesting proliferating capillaries in the process of healing of inflammation. The abscess completely disappeared 3 months later.

Case 1 (contd.)

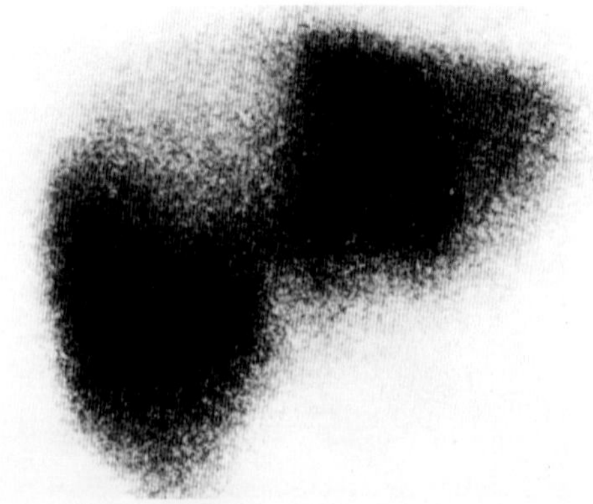

e

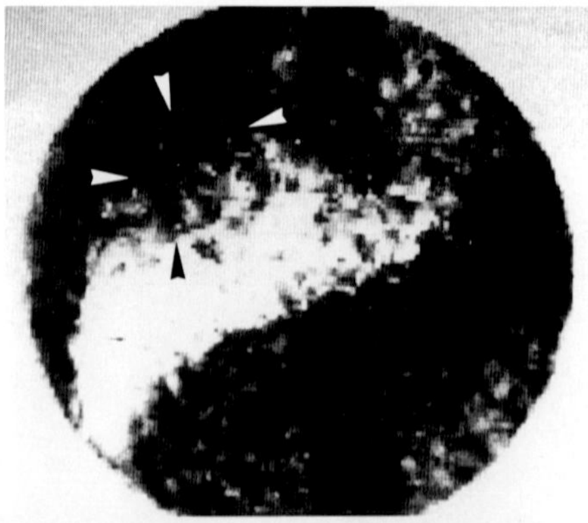

f

(e), (f) Scintigram: ^{99m}Tc-phytate scan (e) was subtracted from the ^{67} Ga-citrate scan (f), and an uptake of the latter (▶) was discerned in the right lobe below the diaphragm. This subtraction scan alone mimics HCC.

Inflammatory/parasitic disease—Case 2: Liver abscess that shrank as followed by CT. This patient underwent a CT study for right upper quadrant pain, and a mass lesion was found in S^{VI}. There was no fever, and CRP (−).

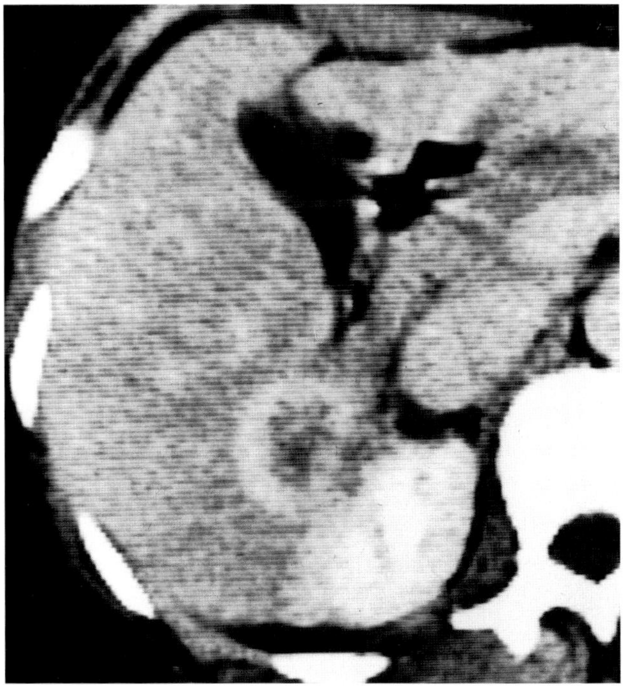

(a) Enhanced CT: a 3 cm lesion in S^{VI} was enhanced in its periphery forming a thick ring that encompassed a stellate low-density area.

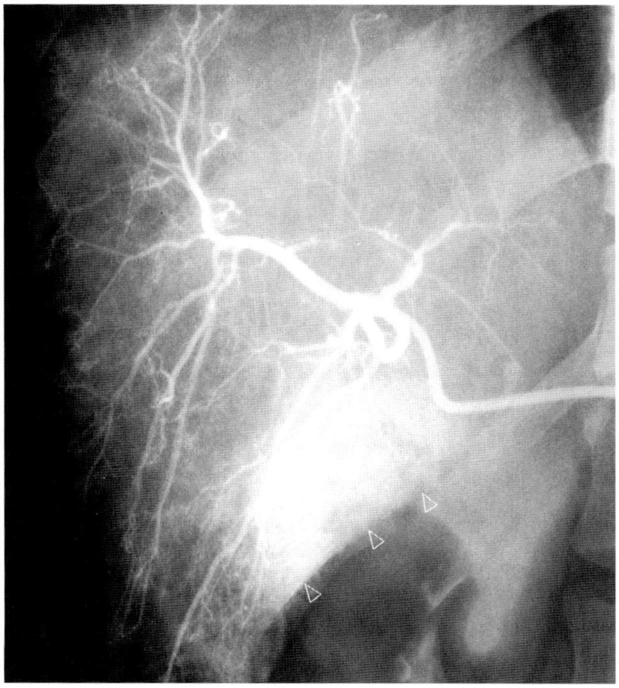

(b) Hepatic arteriogram: a triangular stain is seen where the CT lesion was located. Neovascularization is not recognized. The internal stain is not strong as in the CT finding. The surface of the liver near the stained lesion is smooth (▷), and a growing neoplasm seems unlikely.

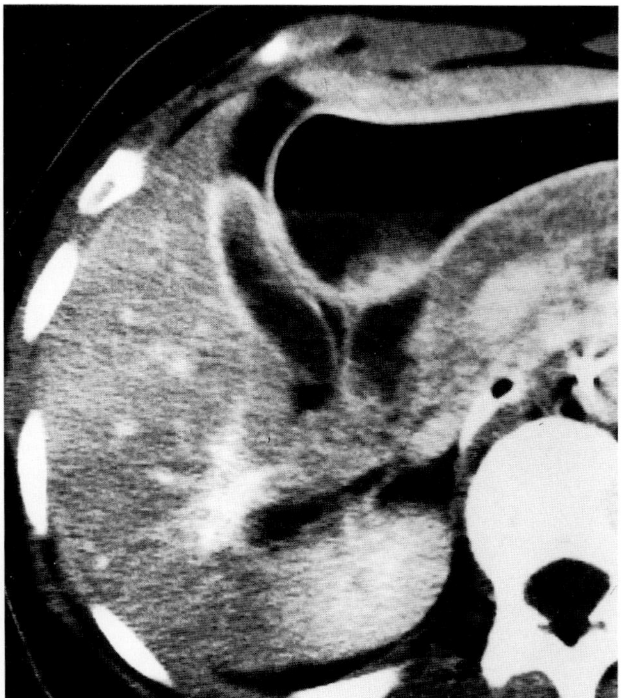

(c) Arterial-CT: angiography 4 months later failed to demonstrate the same lesion (not shown). Subsequently an arterial-CT study was done. The lesion in S^{VI} has markedly shrunk with enhanced spiky protrusions. The internal low-density area was no longer recognized.

Inflammatory/parasitic disease—Case 3: Echinococcosis difficult to differentiate from metastatic liver cancer. A 35-year-old woman. She underwent US examination because of low-grade fever, and multiple lesions were found in the liver.

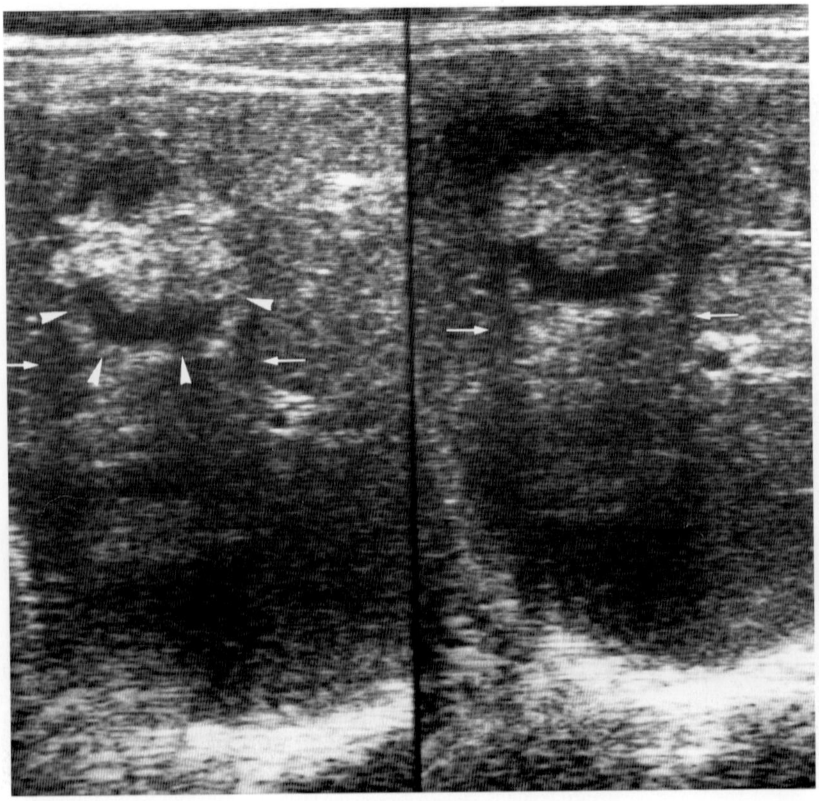

(a) US: the mass lesion has a hyperechoic and partially hypoechoic interior. The periphery has a layer of hyperechoic structure (▶) that resembles a capsule. Lateral shadowing and posterior echo enhancement are also evident.

Case 3 (contd.)

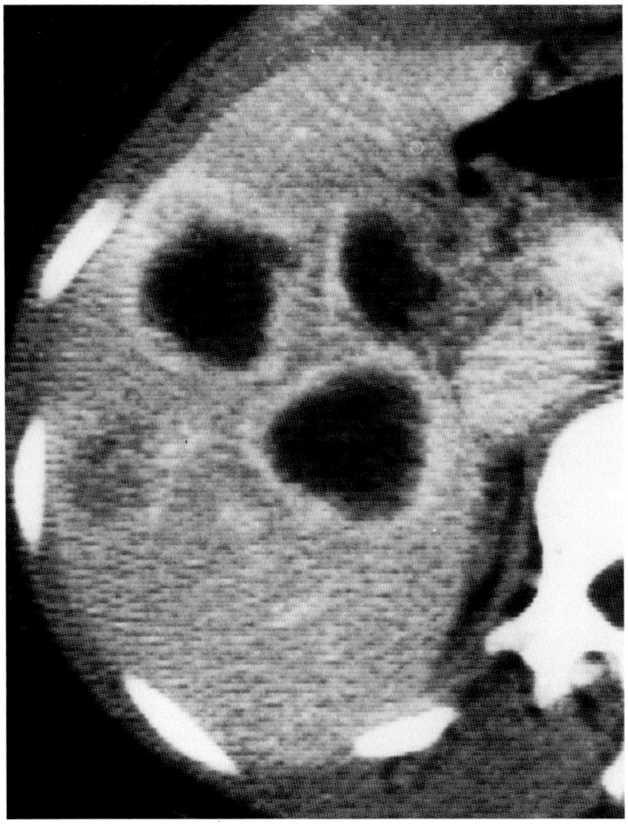

b

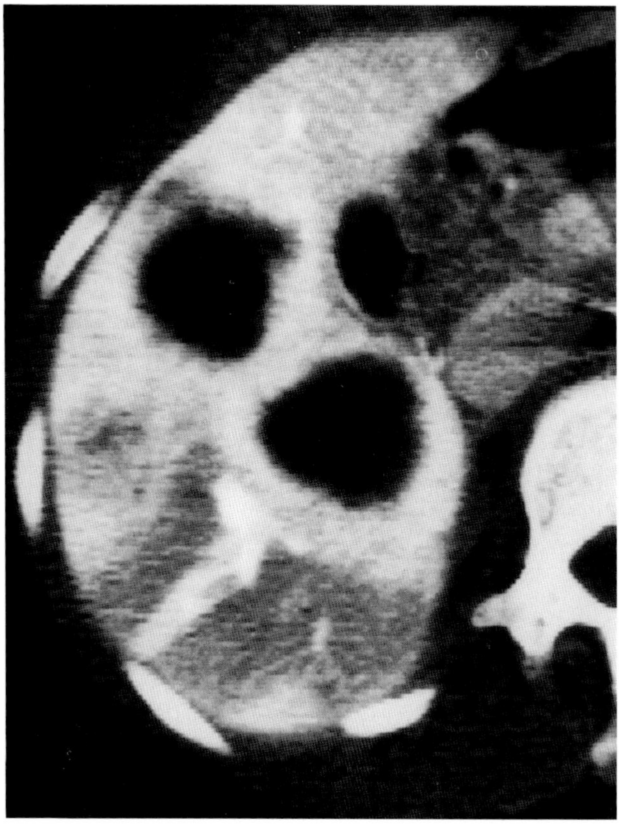

c

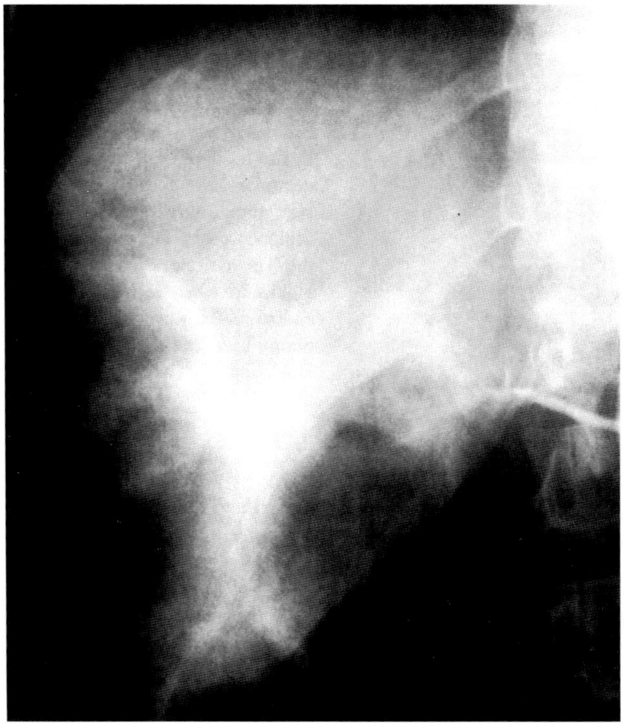

d

(b) Enhanced CT (late phase): the interior of the round or oval lesions was not enhanced and only the periphery enhanced.

(c) Arterial-CT: only the periphery was enhanced and the interior not enhanced at all.

(d) Hepatic arteriogram (late phase): no neovasculature or encasement was seen in the early phase, and only the periphery was stained in the late phase.

6

Vascular disorders of the liver

Various disorders occur to the hepatic vasculature, and a knowledge of some of them may be necessary in differential diagnosis from neoplastic disease. Most such disorders are associated with portal hypertension and are discussed in Chapter 11 on portal hypertension. Therefore, in this chapter only the vascular disorders not associated with HCC will be discussed.

Intrahepatic arterio-portal shunt

Diagnosis is made from early opacification of the portal vein on dynamic CT and subsequent enhancement of the area supplied by that portal vein branch (Takayasu *et al.* 1985*a*) (cf. Case 4, p.363). Only one cut section of the opacified portal vein may simulate a hemangioma or HCC, and for the diagnosis study of several sections caudal and cranial to the one being studied is necessary.

Hepatic aneurysm-portal shunt

Hepatic artery aneurysm is uncommon, and an aneurysm-portal shunt in which arterial blood flows into the portal vein is more uncommon (Takayasu *et al.* 1985*a*). In the past, the diagnosis depended on angiography, but with modern imaging such as enhanced CT and color Doppler a rare vascular disorder can now be diagnosed with relative ease (cf. Case 3, p.362).

Intrahepatic portal aneurysm-hepatic vein shunt

This rather uncommon vascular disorder may be found in a patient who has no particular complaint (Takayasu *et al.* 1984*d*) (cf. Case 27, p.385). The exact etiology of this disorder is not known. Although both congenital (malformation) and acquired etiologies are possible, the one we experienced was associated with portal hypertension.

Intrahepatic collateral vein

A markedly dilated paraumbilical vein may mimic an hepatic tumor on its section (cf. Case 20, p.378). The diagnosis becomes definite if dynamic CT is done with the table incremental method or by spiral CT, because the structure in question is shown as part of a continuous vessel.

Peliosis hepatis

This is defined as multiple blood filled spaces usually not lined by endothelium. The size varies from microscopic up to several centimeters. Some may develop from irregular focal sinusoidal dilations, as produced by prolonged administration of anabolic or contraceptive steroids (Zafrani *et al.* 1983). It may occur in a variety of diseases including granulomatosis due to tuberculosis and other infections, or constitute a reaction to noxious substances such as vinyl chloride and Thorotrast for which peliosis is a pre-malignant lesion of chemical induced angiosarcoma (Okuda *et al.* 1981*c*). The detailed imaging features are not known because of its rarity. In the report made by Tsukamoto *et al.* (1984), a 4 cm peliotic lesion was homogeneously enhanced on dynamic CT, and on angiography it was seen as a tumor stain without tumor vessels. In the case we have seen (Okuda *et al.* 1981c), small multiple-contrast poolings were seen on angiography. More information may be gained in the future.

7

Deformity of the liver

Deformity of the liver is either congenital or acquired. Variations of liver form have been well documented in textbooks of anatomy (Anson 1963). Some are said to be congenital, but a considerable proportion of them are acquired after birth as a result of compression exerted from outside to the liver, such as corset liver or oriental furrows (Okuda and Iio 1976) and diaphragmatic grooves (Netter 1967) , and decreased portal perfusion which causes a marked atrophy, hence gross deformity, of the liver. Reduction of portal vein blood flow results from thrombosis and stenosis or occlusion of the portal vein. The former may occur when inflammation creeps onto the portal vein from cholangitis, therapeutic portal vein embolization, infection, and other causes, and the latter is frequently caused by neoplasms. Parenchymal atrophy is also caused by radiation which leads to gross deformity of the liver. With advancing age, the incidence of partial eventration of the right diaphragm increases, and the right lobe is sometimes displaced into the thoracic cage; the liver on the scintigram simulates a Napoleonic cap (Okuda *et al.* 1979).

Atrophy or absence of the hepatic lobe

Atrophy or absence of one lobe has come to be found by imaging in increasing numbers (Demaerel *et al.* 1989). However, distinction of absence and marked atrophy is very difficult. More often, a seemingly absent liver lobe may be found to be secondary. One typical example is Case 1, in which the right lobe was thought to be absent first, but subsequent study showed this patient to have idiopathic portal hypertension which is known to develop secondary portal vein thrombosis; if it occurs in a large portal vein, the area supplied by that particular portal vein undergoes atrophy, and the liver appears to lack one lobe (Okuda *et al.* 1982*c*). Whatever the cause, there will be compensatory hypertrophy of the contralateral lobe as well as the caudate lobe.

According to Radin *et al.* (1987), the literature contained fewer than 24 cases of presumable congential absence of the right lobe; many cases had biliary tract disease and portal hypertension suggesting secondary atrophy.

The absence of the left lobe has also been reported (Belton and Van Zandt 1983; Yamamoto *et al.* 1988), but the left portal vein is continuous from the umbilical vein in the fetus, and it is known to be thrombosed as a result of omphalitis. Most such cases perhaps represent atrophy rather than congenital agenesis.

Riedel lobe

The right lobe extending further caudally like a tongue is called the 'Riedel lobe'. In text books, it is depicted as an accessory tongue shaped lobe continuous from the liver surface near the gallbladder (Reitemeier *et al.* 1958). It is said to be more common in females and may be mistaken for a tumor on palpation, but we have not yet seen a typical Riedel lobe.

Protrusion, indentation and furrow in a normal liver

As in cirrhotic liver, a normal liver occasionally has localized deformity like protrusions (Case 4), indentations or furrows (Case 5). A protrusion can be the site of origin of HCC (cf. Cases 5 and 6, pp.187–8). Most commonly furrows are seen on the cranial surface of the liver in so called corset liver (Okuda and Iio 1976).

Cirrhosis

In advanced cirrhosis, surface irregularity caused by nodules and atrophy of the right lobe with compensatory enlargement of the left lobe (Torres *et al.* 1986) are common (Case 6). It seems that the latter is particularly common in the Far East. Unlike alcoholic cirrhosis, cirrhosis caused by hepatitis virus (posthepatitic) often shows atrophy of the right lobe and hypertrophy of the left lobe (Okuda and Iio 1976). This deformity is currently troubling radiologists attempting to carry out transjugular intrahepatic portosystemic shunt (TIPS) because of the changes in the spatial relation of the hepatic and portal veins. Large protrusions are not terribly uncommon in cirrhosis, particularly in postnecrotic cirrhosis. Some of them need differentiation from HCC (Cases 7 and 8). HCC could also arise in such a protruding area. As cirrhosis progresses, the hepatic vein and the portal vein systems in the liver undergo morphologic changes and become more difficult to delineate by US and enhanced CT. The spatial relation of the right and left lobes is altered in such a way that the right anterior and posterior segments shift cranially and caudally, respectively, with little overlapping area in the anterior projection. The shrinkage of the right lobe invites the colon to be lodged between the diaphragm and the liver (Chilaiditi syndrome). The caudate lobe is generally enlarged in cirrhosis (Harbin *et al.* 1980) (Case 7), but the degree is greater in alcoholic cirrhosis than in the posthepatitic cirrhosis we see in Japan. The most remarkable enlargement of the caudate lobe occurs in Budd-Chiari syndrome when the right and left hepatic veins are occluded; the caudate lobe is enlarged in compensation and receives more blood to return it into the inferior vena cava.

Regenerative nodules in a cirrhotic liver may be divided into those with and without significant hemosiderin deposition. Regenerative nodules with hemosiderin are demonstrated as low intensity nodules on both T2-weighted SE and gradient echo images appears a little larger than those recognized on T2-weighted SE images because the presence of iron causes increased magnetic susceptibility (Murakami *et al.* 1992). Gradient echo is more sensitive in detecting siderotic nodules than T2-weighted SE imaging. By contrast, regenerative nodules without significant hemosiderin deposit are much more frequently encountered in the routine study of MR imaging, seen on T2-weighted SE images and not detected by gradient echo imaging (Murakami *et al.* 1992). T1-weighted SE images less distinctly demonstrate regenerative nodules than do T2-weighted SE or gradient echo images. Siderotic regenerative nodules are recognized as high-density nodules or heterogeneous regions in the hepatic parenchyma on unenhanced CT (Murakami *et al.* 1992).

Histopathologically it has been found that iron accumulative macroregenerative nodules in a cirrhotic liver are frequently associated with hyperplastic hepatocellular foci and should be included among precancerous lesions (Terada and Nakanuma 1989*a*), and that once transformed to malignant lesions, iron is no longer stainable (Terada and Nakanuma 1989*b*). It is a very delicate situation requiring more extensive investigation. In fact, Mitchell *et al.* (1991) found development of HCC from a siderotic regenerative nodule on MR images as the nodule-in-nodule sign.

Hepatic fibrosis and macronodular scarring liver (potato liver)

Following extensive necrosis (submassive liver necrosis) mostly caused by viral hepatitis and vigorous liver cell regeneration, large regenerative nodules ('potatoes') evolve within collapsed liver parenchyma (Itai *et al.* 1988 ; Ishikawa *et al.* 1989) (Case 9). They may grossly simulate metastatic liver carcinoma. On T2-weighted images, the collapsed fibrosed scar is seen as hyperintense as the spleen (Itai *et al.* 1988). Thus, confluent fibrotic changes of the liver appear as regions of lower signal intensity relative to adjacent liver parenchyma on T1-weighted SE images and of higher intensity on T2-weighted images (Ohtomo *et al.* 1993). Possible cause of high signal intensity of fibrous changes on T2-weighted images are edema, increased numbers of vascular spaces, and inflammatory cells. With improved instrumentation for US and MR imaging, some cirrhotic nodules are now vaguely discerned.

Deformity that follows portal vein obstruction or stenosis secondary to tumor and hepatolithiasis

When the first-order portal vein of either side is occluded by hilar carcinoma, ipsilateral lobar atrophy is commonly seen (Takayasu *et al.* 1986*c*). A similar atrophy may follow therapeutic embolization of the portal vein (PTPE). If intrahepatic stones persist and cause chronic recurrent cholangitis and dilatation of bile ducts, the accompanying portal vein may undergo narrowing with reduced portal blood flow, hence atrophy, of the area supplied by that particular portal vein (Case 10).

Deformity due to radiation

External irradiation is one of the treatment modalities for primary liver cancer, and the number of patients with liver deformity is increasing with frequent radiotherapies. On plain CT, a band-shaped area of low-density is seen (Kolbenstvedt *et al.* 1980; Jeffrey *et al.* 1980), and this area is strongly enhanced for a prolonged period on enhanced CT (Ungar *et al.* 1987; Cutillo et al 1989) (Case 11). Such features are more distinctly seen 2–6 weeks after irradiation, but doses of less than 35 Gy do not cause such CT changes (Ingold *et al.* 1965). Histologically, acute radiation damage to the liver includes centrilobular hemorrhage and sinusoidal congestion, and late effects include more hepatic cellular damage, fatty changes, and changes of the central vein walls and occlusion (Ingold *et al.* 1965; Lansing *et al.* 1968). These changes mimic those seen in Budd–Chiari syndrome. As Kupffer cells drop out, the irradiated area no longer takes up colloids on radionuclide scintigraphy, and the irradiated area is seen as a cold region on colloid scintigraphy (Johnson *et al.* 1967). Recovery takes 3–5 months, but larger doses of radiation may produce lasting atrophy and deformity (Case 12). In proton therapy, only focused hepatic damage occurs in the depth because of its Bragg peak (Okumura *et al.* 1994).

Deformity due to hepatic resection

Large resection of the liver, namely lobectomy and extended lobectomy, produces a compensatory hypertrophy of the contralateral lobe (particularly the left lateral segment) and the caudate lobe (Letourneau *et al.* 1988) (Case 13).

Others

Injury to the liver, such as needle biopsy may cause subcapsular bleeding which is usually semilunar in shape (Case 14), and spontaneous bleeding of an HCC can also cause localized bleeding extrahepatically (cf. Case 9, p.190).

Liver deformity—Case 1: Atrophy of the right lobe simulating agenesis (courtesy of Dr D. J. Brandt).

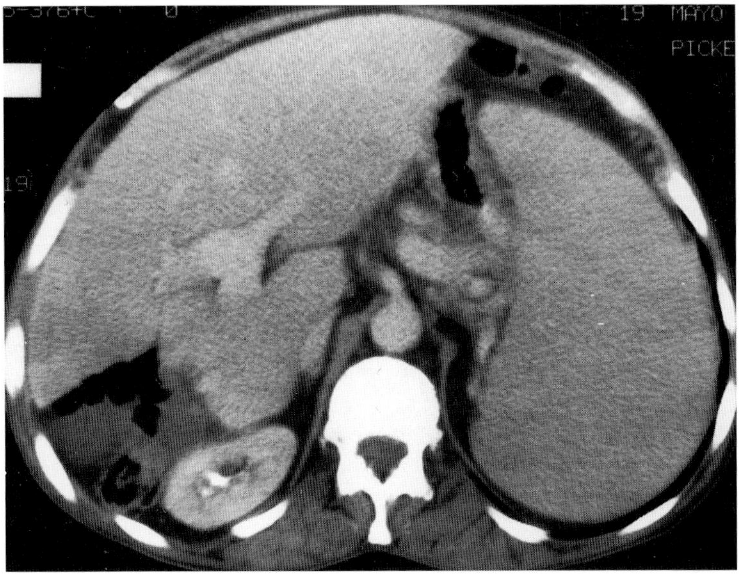

Enhanced CT: hypertrophy of the left and caudate lobes is apparent, and the right lobe seems to be missing. The whole picture resembles a liver after right lobectomy. The spleen is markedly enlarged, and the portal and splenic veins dilated, suggesting portal hypertension. This deformity is most likely caused by thrombotic occlusion of the right posterior portal vein followed by atrophy of the posterior segment of the liver. Such marked atrophy of one lobe is not uncommon in idiopathic portal hypertension (IPH) (Okuda *et al.* 1982*c*).

Liver deformity—Case 2: Congenital agenesis of the right lobe (courtesy of Dr D. J. Brandt).

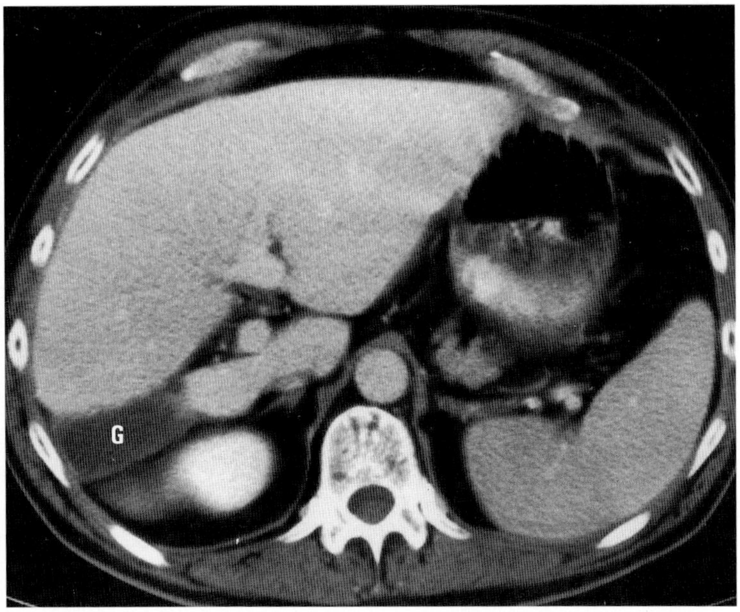

Enhanced CT: the left lobe is enlarged and the gallbladder (G) is seen adjacent to the posterior end of the liver. The caudate lobe enlargement is not distinct, but the right and left portions of the caudate lobe are seen on both sides of the inferior vena cava. This anatomical feature of the caudate lobe may be related to the fetal development of this lobe. Posterior displacement of the gallbladder is one of the diagnostic features of right lobe agenesis.

Liver deformity—Case 3: ?Riedel lobe.

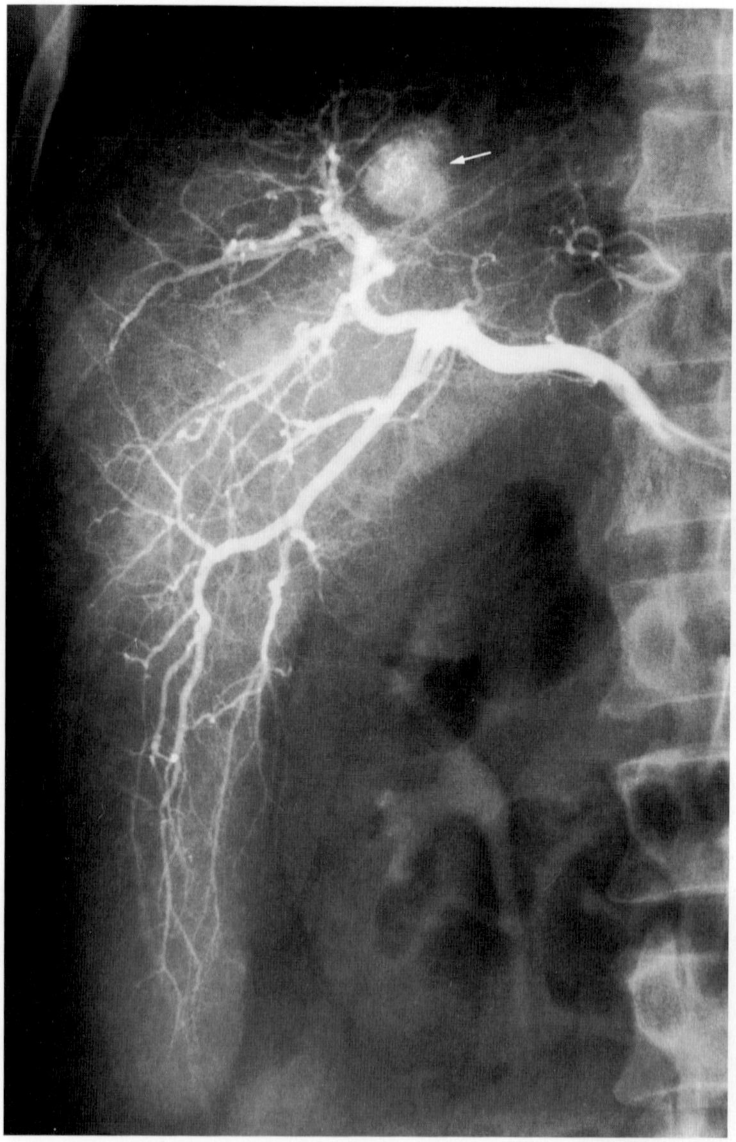

Hepatic arteriogram: the right posterior segment, S^{VI}, is enlarged, simulating a tongue. The left lobe is small. This deformity poses no clinical problem, but for a CT study of the whole liver one has to cut more slices because of its longer vertical span. →, HCC.

Liver deformity—Case 4: Localized protrusion from a normal liver.

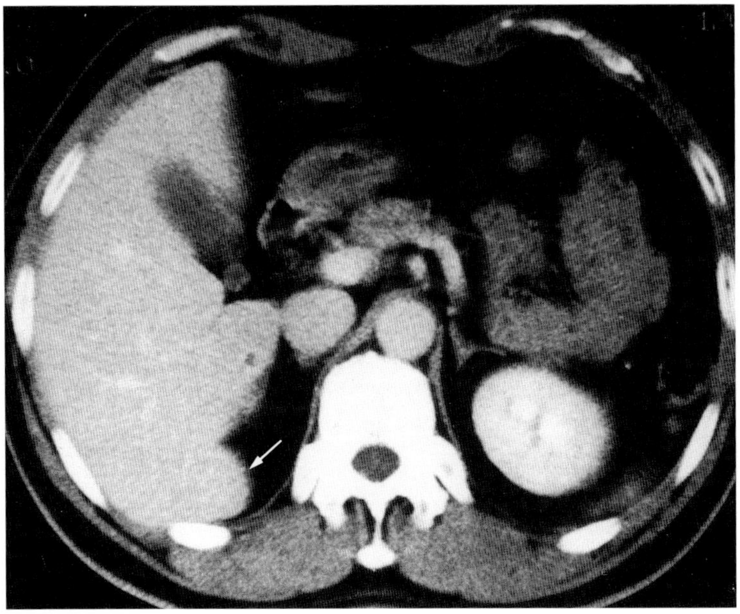

Enhanced CT: a 2 cm protrusion (→) is seen in the right posterior segment (S^{VI}). Earlier US study suggested a possible tumor of the upper pole of the right kidney (normal liver function tests).

Liver deformity—Case 5: Deep indentation in a normal liver.

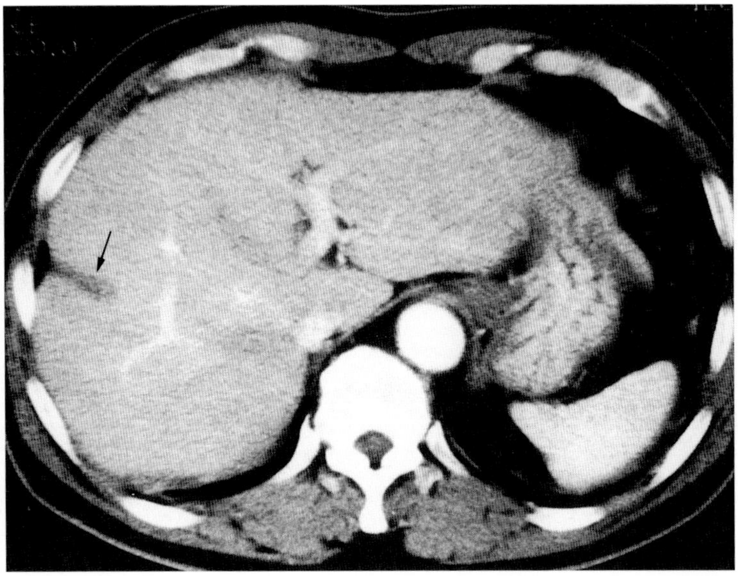

Enhanced CT: in the anterior area of the right lobe, there is a deep indentation (→) extending several centimeters from this slice cranially and caudally. Similar indentation may follow hepatic infarction resulting from TAE, and healing of an abscess, but this patient had normal liver function test with no history of hepatic injury, inflammation, or TAE.

Liver deformity—Case 6: Gross changes of cirrhotic liver.

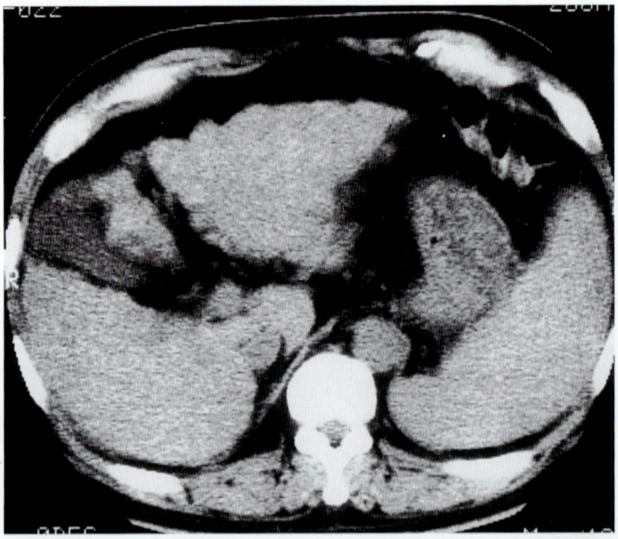

(a) Plain CT: surface irregularity is marked, particularly in the left lobe. The left lateral region has undergone compensatory hypertrophy, and the left medidal area is atrophied. Together with splenomegaly, these findings are the typical features of cirrhosis.

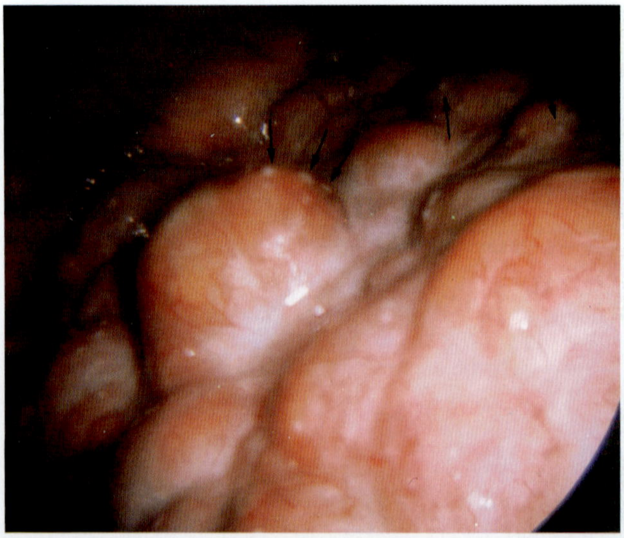

(b) Laparoscopic view: the surface is irregular with regenerative nodules of 0.5–1.5 cm in size. The surface of the nodule is studded with white lymphocysts (→) and many proliferating capillaries.

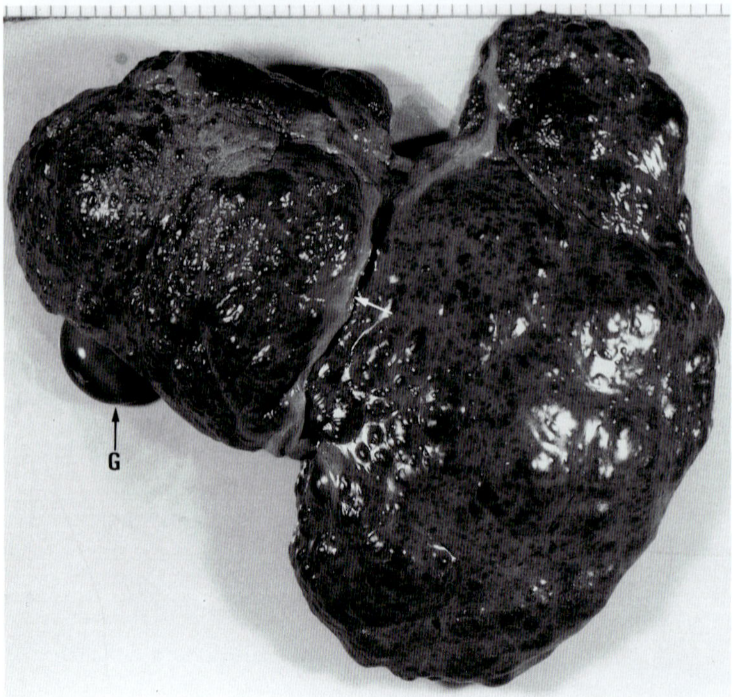

(c) Autopsy: the liver shows advanced cirrhosis. Judging from the location of the falciform ligament attachment (→) and the gallbladder (G), there is a marked hypertrophy of the left lobe and atrophy of the right lobe (this is not the same liver shown in (a) and (b)).

Liver deformity—Case 7: Gross changes of cirrhotic liver.

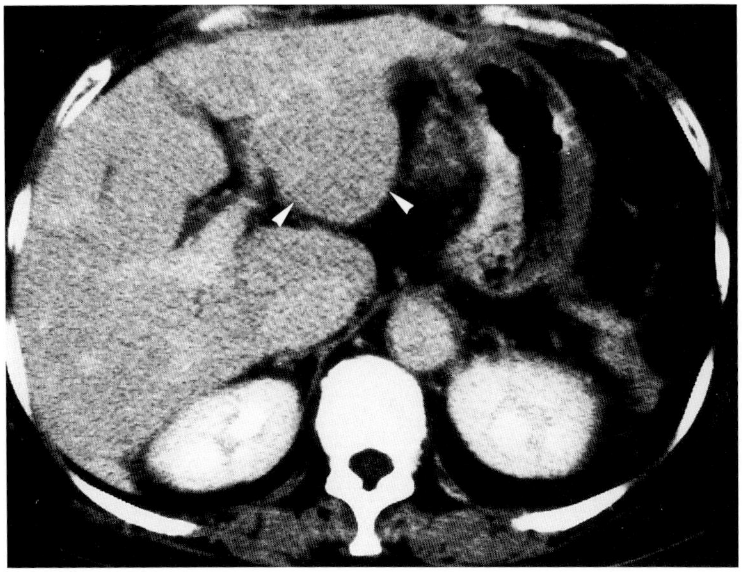

Dynamic CT: a mass hanging from the lateral inferior surface (▶) was found by US. This mass showed the same density as that of the parenchyma throughout the early and late phases of dynamic CT, and the possibility of tumor was denied. If this were an HCC, it could be called a protruding or pedunculated HCC.

Liver deformity—Case 8: Localized mass-like lesion in a cirrhotic liver difficult to differentiate from tumor.

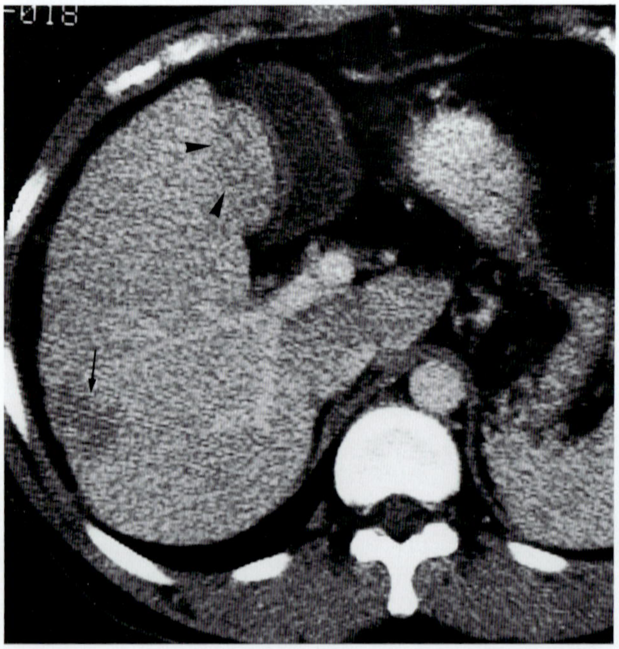

(a) Dynamic CT (late arterial phase): a protruding mass-like lesion (▶) is seen pushing the gallbladder to the left. This image was made in a late arterial phase of dynamic CT, and the mass in question is slightly low in density. Another low-density tumor (→) in S^{V} was eventually diagnosed as HCC.

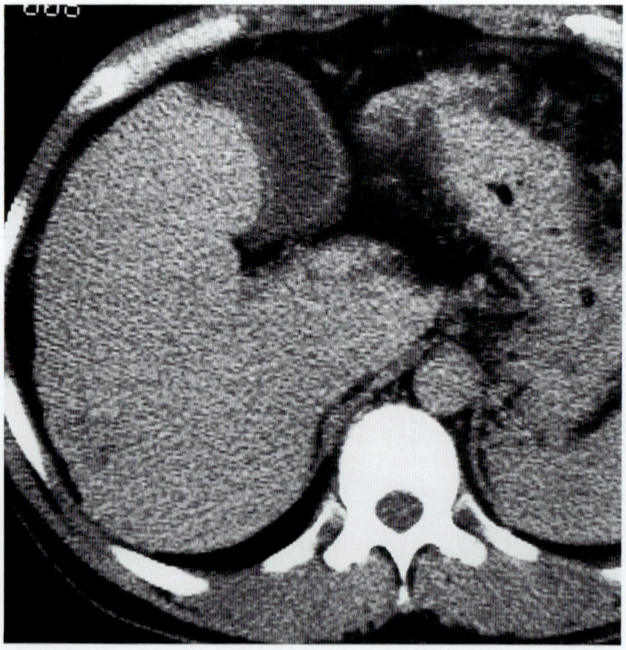

(b) Dynamic CT (late phase): the protruding lesion has turned isodense.

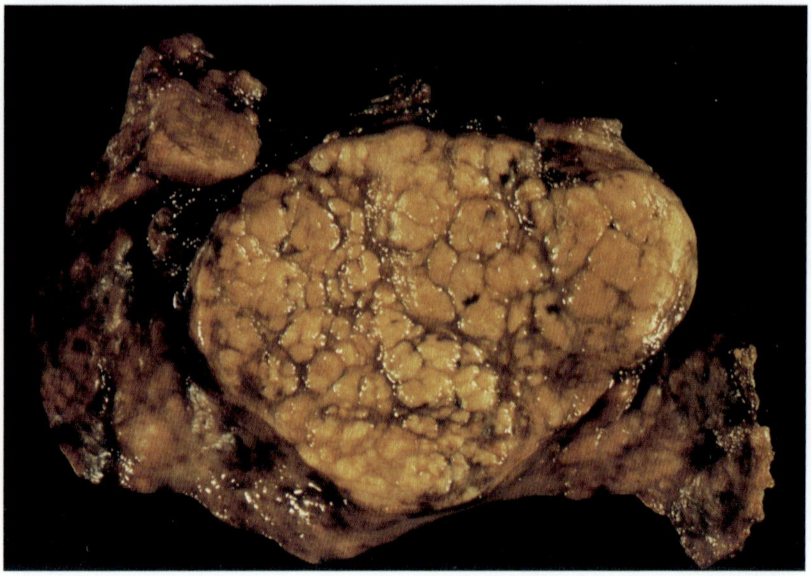

(c) Cut section of resected specimen: at the time of resection for the S^{V} tumor, the lesion in question was also removed. Histologically, it was a regenerative nodule with no malignant feature.

Liver deformity—Case 9: Macronodular scarring liver (potato liver).

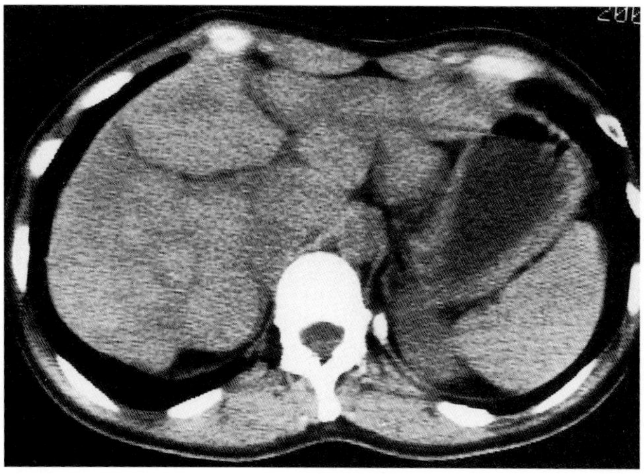

(a) Plain CT: a number of 1.5–4 cm nodular lesions (65 HU) are seen in both lobes. They are surrounded by low-density areas (50 HU) producing a net-like appearance.

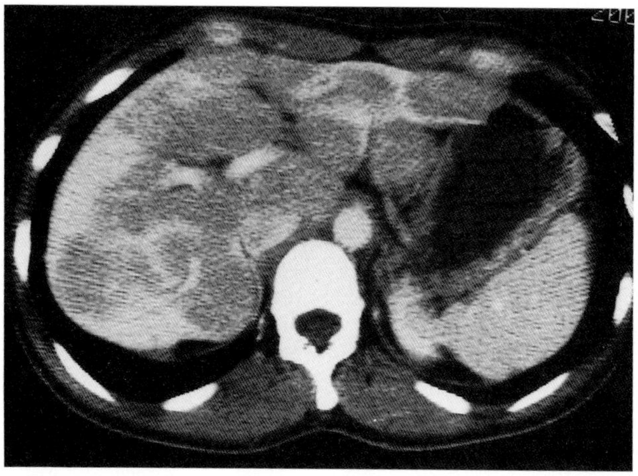

(b) Dynamic CT (portal phase): the nodules were mildly enhanced (106 HU) but the internodular, previously low-density areas, were markedly enhanced (140 HU), reversing the relation of low and high densities. Subsequently, liver biopsy was carried out under laparoscopic view. The nodule showed normal liver histology whereas the net-like region was a scar tissue with fibrosis. The marked internodular enhancement may have been due to proliferating fibrous tissue and congested blood flow.

Liver deformity—Case 10: Deformity and atrophy of the liver as a result of portal vein obstruction secondary to hepatolithiasis.

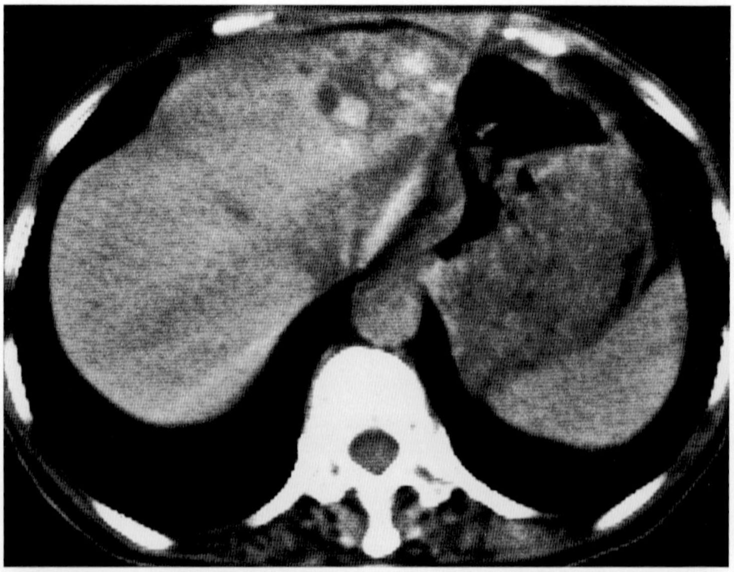

(a) Plain CT: calcific lesions are seen localized in the left lobe laterally.

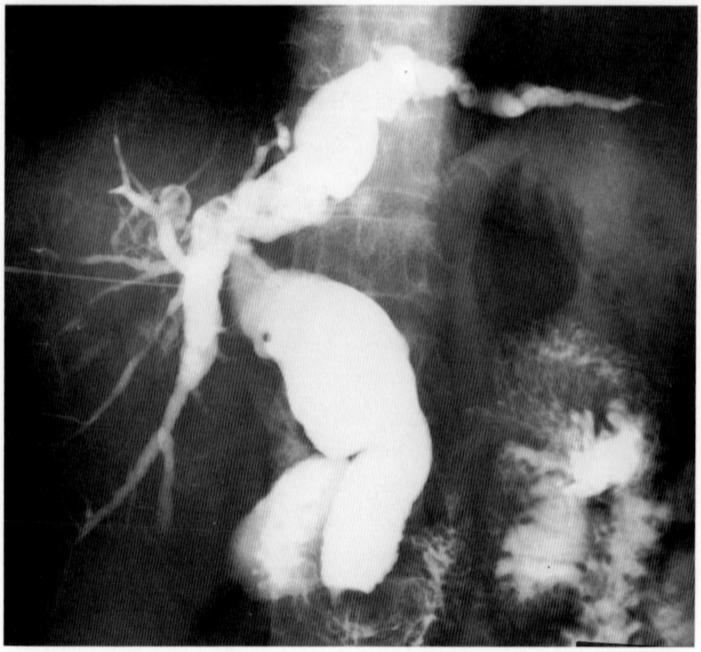

(b) PTC: dilatation of intrahepatic bile ducts mainly in the left side and many stones in the ducts are seen. The extrahepatic bile duct is also markedly dilated.

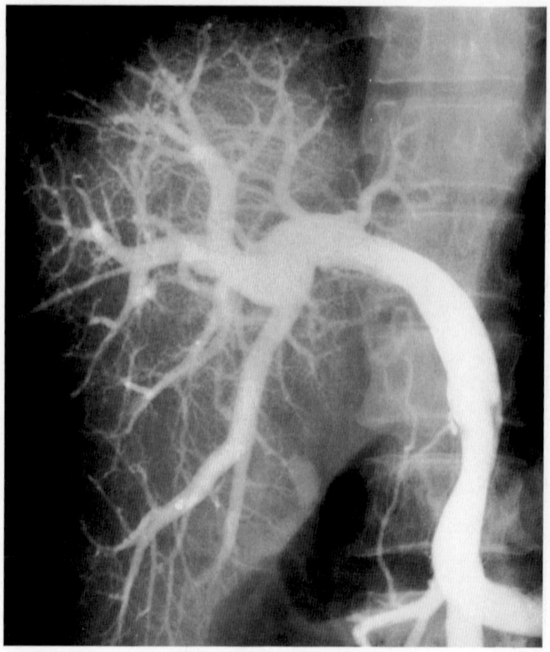

(c) PTP: the left portal vein was not opacified at all, not even the proximal part, except for the left caudate lobe branches. Compensatory hypertrophy of the right lobe is apparent.

Liver deformity—Case 11: Uneven enhancement of the liver on enhanced CT as a result of irradiation. Bidirectional external irradiation (from the abdominal and the right sides at a right angle) was carried out for HCC with a total dose of 60 Gy. This CT was made 4 months later.

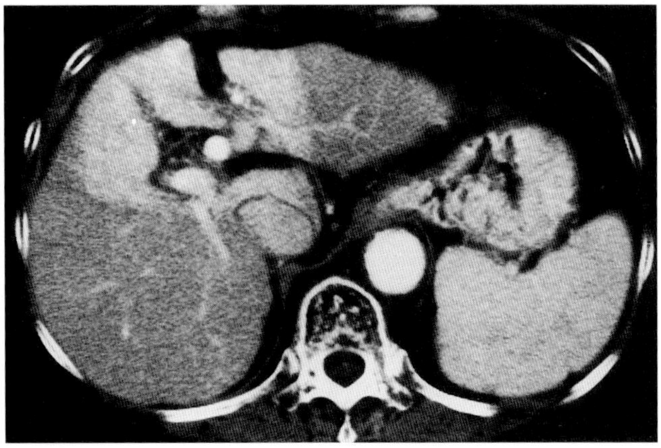

(a) Dynamic CT (early phase): clearly demarcated high enhancement with a geometric shape is seen in the left lateral to right anterior area of the liver.

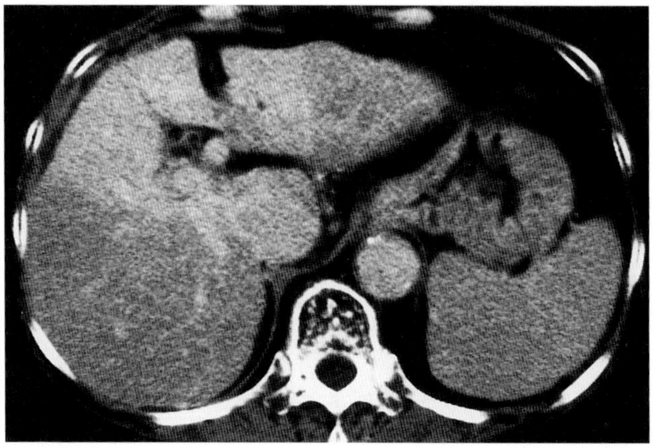

(b) Dynamic CT (late phase, 8 min): the high density still remains in the same area.

Liver deformity—Case 12: Deformity due to radiation. Two HCCs were found, one (2 cm) in S^{VI} and another in S^{III}, and the S^{VI} tumor was irradiated with a total dose of 70 Gy.

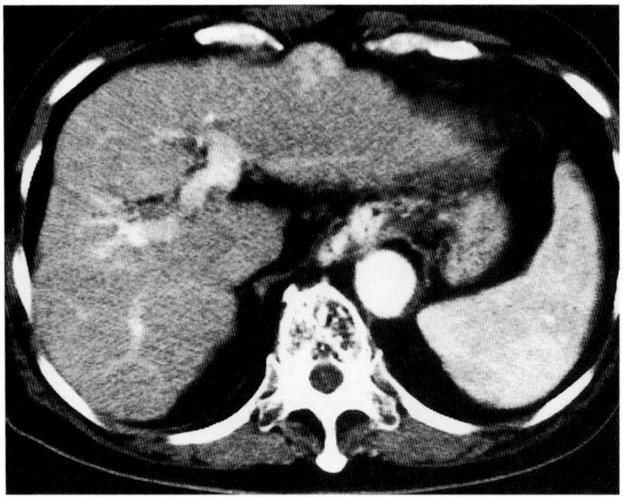

(a) Enhanced CT: this CT was made 3 months later. The S^{VI} lesion is no longer enhanced, but the right lobe was slightly atrophied already.

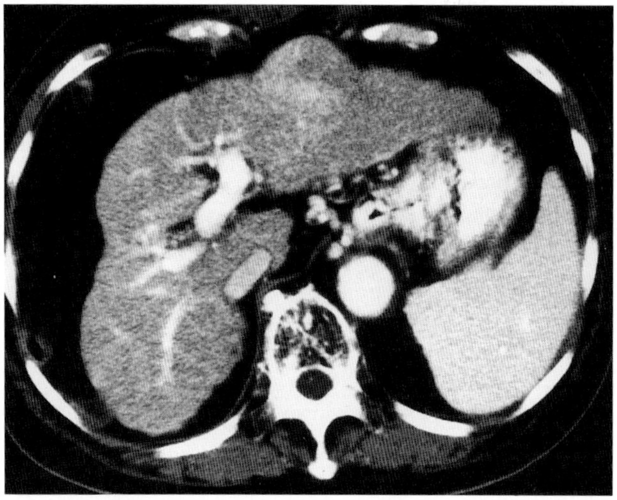

(b) Enhanced CT (9 months after (a)): the S^{VI} lesion disappeared with a considerable atrophy of the right lobe. The S^{III} lesion has grown as it was not treated.

Liver deformity—Case 13: Hypertrophy of the remnant liver after hepatic resection.

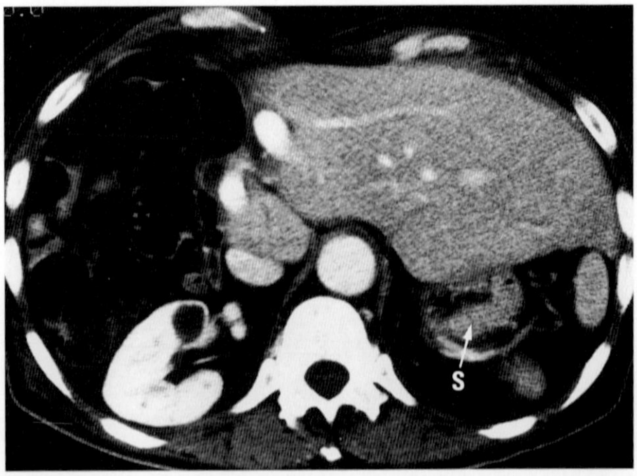

Enhanced CT: right trisegmentectomy was carried out for HCC in the right lobe 2.5 years earlier. By follow-up CT, compensatory hypertrophy was found in the left lobe and the left caudate lobe. The marked hypertrophy of the lateral left lobe is compressing the stomach (s) posteriorly.

Liver deformity—Case 14: Liver deformity due to spontaneous subcapsular bleeding. The patient came to the hospital because of fever and jaundice.

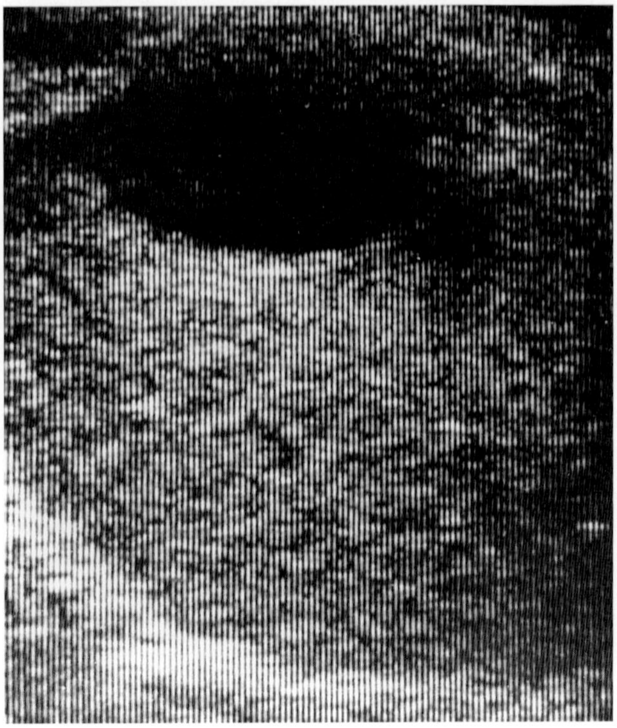

US (right intercostal scan): a 4×2.5 cm lens-shaped echolucent area was found in the right lobe. To distinguish this from liver abscess, US-guided puncture was carried out. The obtained fluid consistent with old bleeding was negative for culture. The diagnosis was relatively old subcapsular bleeding. There was no physical injury to the liver, and the cause of bleeding was not determined.

8

Other disorders

8.1 Fatty liver

Fatty changes are either diffuse throughout the liver (Cases 1 and 2), localized in one segment or subsegment in S^{IV} near the falciform ligament (Kawashima *et al.* 1986; Yoshikawa *et al.* 1987) (Cases 4 and 5), or inhomogeneous with areas of differing degree of steatosis. In some cases, a normal liver area lies within diffusely fatty liver (focal spared area in fatty liver) (Sauerbrei and Lopez 1986; Marchal *et al.* 1986; Arai *et al.* 1988) (Case 3) (Fig. 8.1).

A localized fatty or spared area poses a problem in imaging diagnosis, particularly in differential diagnosis from a neoplasm (Yates and Streight 1986) (cf. Case 8, p.337). The important differentiating features are the presence of a portal or hepatic vein running through it, and an irregular margin or a geometric pattern of the area. Another diagnostic feature is a change in shape during the follow up (Halvorsen *et al.* 1982; Clain *et al.* 1984). The sensivity of individual modalities in diagnosis varies; US is more sensitive than CT. Mild to moderate fatty infiltration of the liver is not demonstrable on conventional MR imaging; it appears normal on T2-weighted MR images, and with slightly increased signal intensity on T1-weighted images. However, these findings are of low conspicuity. The most effective technique to detect regions of steatosis is chemical shift opposed phase (Mitchell *et al.* 1991). While most tissues appear similar on both in phase and opposed phase images, fatty liver has lower signal intensity on opposed phase images. Lack of mass effect, and the presence of normal vascular structure are helpful in differentiating focal fatty liver or focally spared liver from a mass lesion.

Fatty liver is generally defined as a triglyceride content greater than 5 per cent of liver weight, and hepatocytes come to contain so much fat that it is seen as intracellular droplets. Many factors cause fatty liver, such as excessive alcohol intake, diabetes mellitus, obesity, intravenous hyperalimentation (Case 1), drugs such as steroids and tetracycline, ileal bypass, etc. Tetracycline-induced fatty liver is characterized by microvesicular fat deposition within the liver cell cytoplasm. The CT attenuation value decreases by 1.6 HU for every 1 mg of triglyceride deposited per 1 g of liver (Ducommun *et al.* 1979). Normal liver CT is 7–8 HU higher in density than the spleen (Piekarski *et al.* 1980), but fat deposition reverses this relationship, and the liver becomes low in attenuation. As the attenuation decreases, hepatic vasculature comes to be clearly discerned without contrast enhancement.

Fatty liver—Case 3: Focal spared liver that required differentiation from metastatic colon cancer. A 33-year-old obese man with juvenile diabetes. During the follow-up, US detected an hepatic tumor.

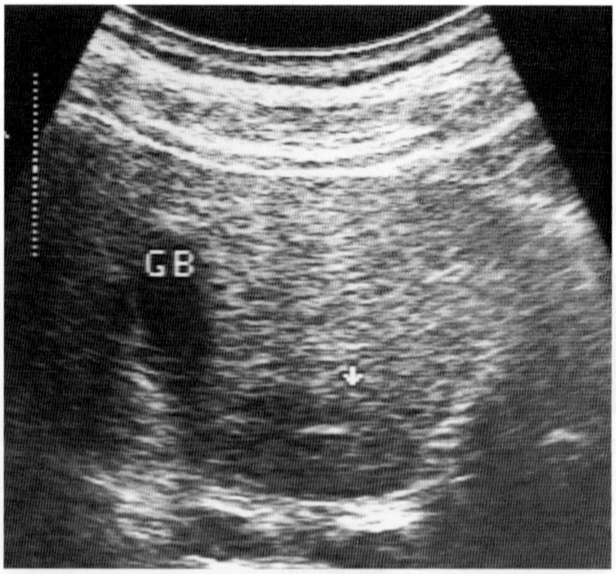

(a) US: an oblong low-echo lesion (→) was found in S^{IV}. The whole liver is bright. GB, gallbladder.

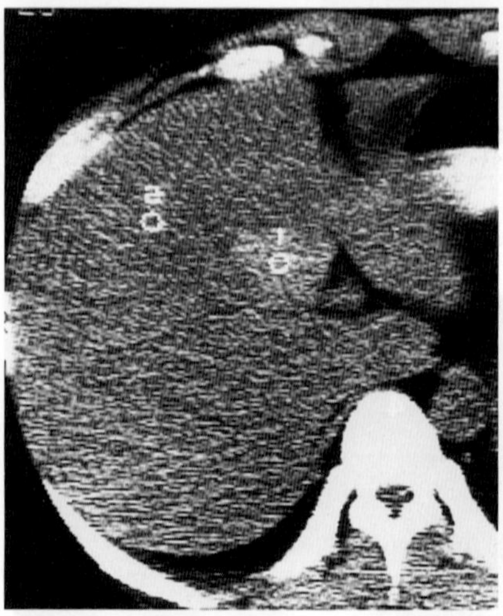

(b) Plain CT: a small area in S^{IV} has a high CT number (#1, 76 HU) contrasted by the whole liver which is lower in density (53 HU). It was diagnosed as a focally spared area.

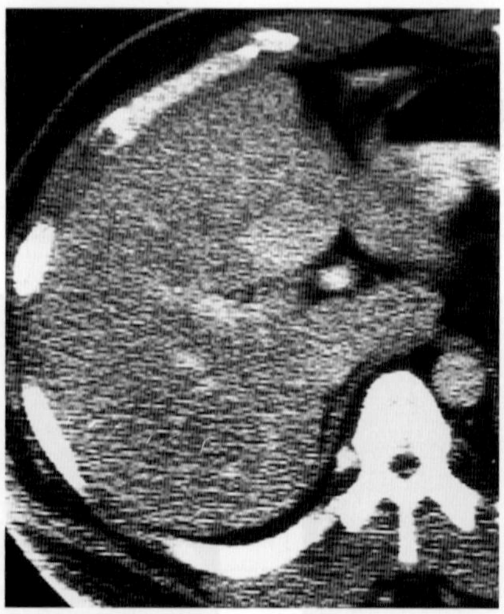

(c) Enhanced CT (early phase): this lesion is still higher in density than liver parenchyma and has an irregular boundary. Since S^{IV} is the most common site for focally spared liver, the diagnosis was a focally spared area within a fatty liver.

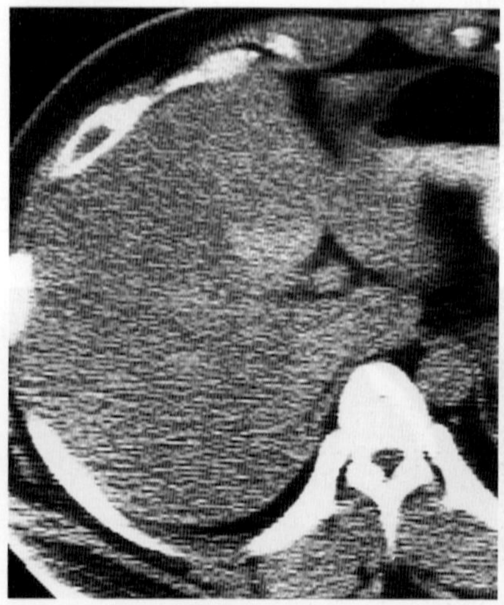

(d) Enhanced CT (late phase, 9 min): this is similar to the early phase CT.

Fatty liver—Case 4: Focal fatty liver requiring differential diagnosis from hemangioma. A 63-year-old woman. She came to the hospital because of an hepatic mass incidentally found in S^{IV-V} by US examination.

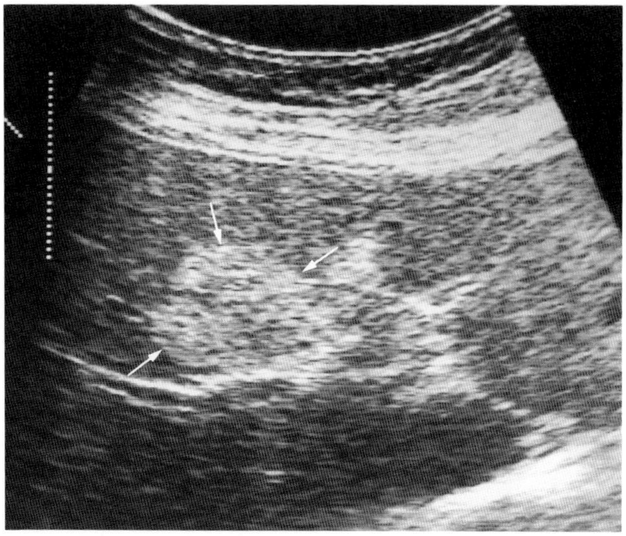

(a) US: an irregularly bordered high-echo mass (→) was found.

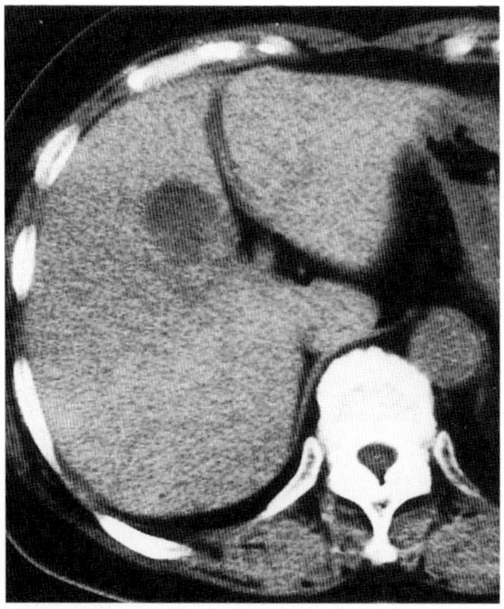

(b) Plain CT: the same area is seen as a low-density lesion. There is also a fan-shaped, wide low-density area to its right. The gallbladder was identified 2 cm caudad to this slice.

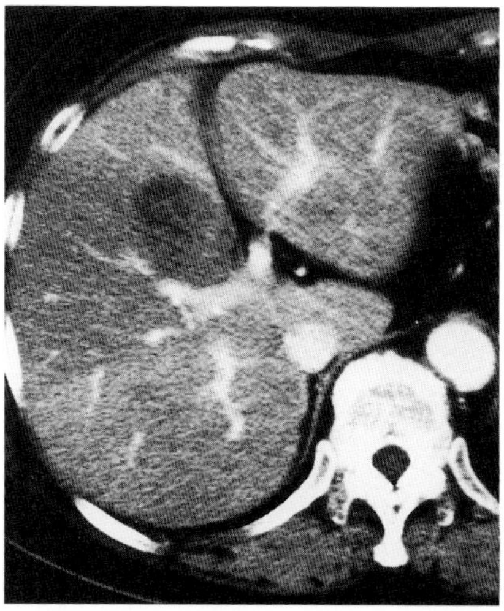

(c) Dynamic CT: in the early phase of dynamic CT, this lesion was not enhanced, and subsequent angiography failed to show any abnormality.

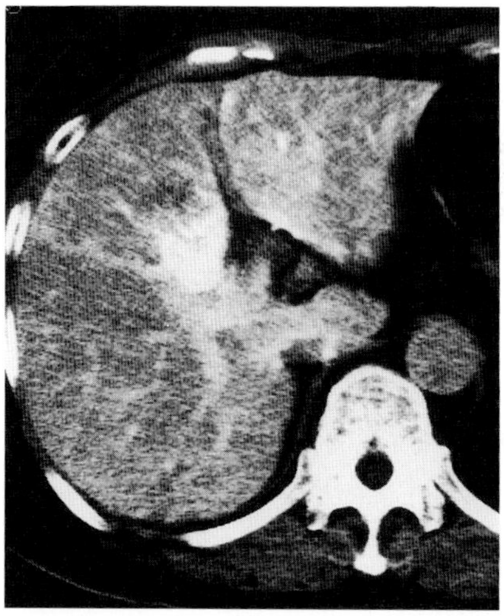

(d) Arterial-CT (late phase): the lesion in question, except for a small abdominal side, was strongly enhanced. As blood vessels were seen running through it, focal fatty liver was most likely. She was followed for 1.5 years when this lesion spontaneously disappeared. It is of interest that most of this focal fatty area had a predominantly arterial supply.

Fatty liver—Case 5: Focal fatty liver which was preoperatively suspected to be a metastasis from gallbladder carcinoma. This patient entered the hospital for suspected gallbladder carcinoma.

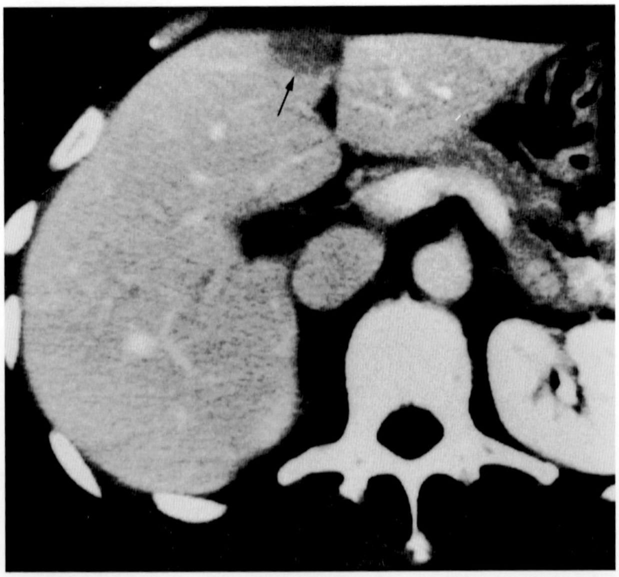

(a) Enhanced CT (early phase): a 2 cm low-density area (→) is seen in S^{IV}.

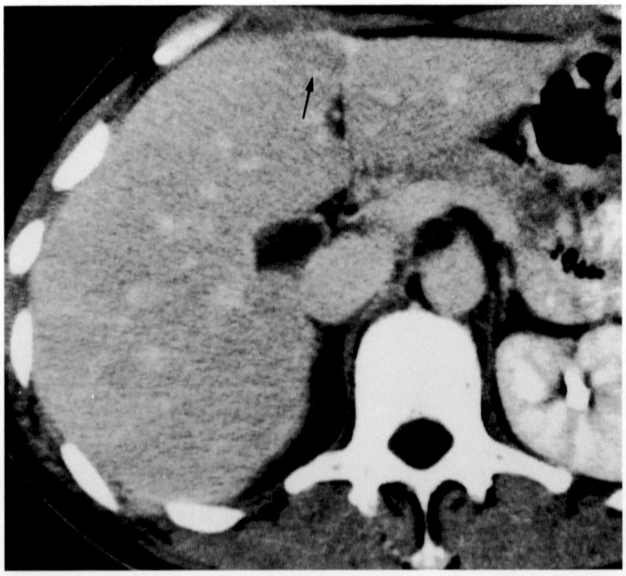

(b) Enhanced CT (late phase): in the late phase, this lesion has turned almost isodense. A small blood vessel (→) was seen within it, and the diagnosis was focal fatty liver. Cholecystectomy was carried out. An exploratory resection of this area in question was done. The section of the resected specimen showed a yellowish tissue and histologically it was localized steatosis.

8.2 Hemochromatosis and Wilson's disease

Hemochromatosis is a condition in which excess iron is deposited in the body, particularly in the liver, pancreas, spleen, and lymph nodes. It is usually divided into hereditary or genetic hemochromatosis, secondary hemochromatosis, and parenteral iron overload. Iron overload is caused either by increased intestinal absorption or repeated blood transfusions. Many patients with iron overload are asymptomatic, but excessive iron deposition causes liver damage of varying severity. With CT examination, some asymptomatic cases may be diagnosed. With large amounts of iron deposited in the liver, parenchymal density increases (75–132 HU) (Mills *et al.* 1977; Goldberg 1980) and the venous systems are visualized as black vessels (Case 1) with a reversed contrast from fatty liver in which vessels are white within a black parenchymal background. On MR imaging, the liver and spleen containing large amounts of iron are seen as low-intensity areas on both T1- and T2- weighted images due to the paramagnetic effect of iron (Brasch *et al.* 1984) (Case 1).

Hemochromatosis is known to be frequently associated with HCC. With improved management of diabetes, the major complication of hemochromatosis, patients are now kept alive for a longer period, and as a result have a greater risk of developing HCC. The previous incidence of HCC among hemochromatosis cases was 7.7–8.2 per cent (Mallory 1932; MacDonald 1957), but since 1975 it has been more than 30 per cent (Niederau *et al.* 1985).

Wilson's disease, also known as hepatolenticular degeneration, has a characteristic pathology of copper accumulation in the liver, brain, and cornea due to impaired biliary excretion of copper. At MR imaging, no corresponding signal intensity changes are recognized due to the non-ferromagnetic effect of copper. If the liver becomes cirrhotic, the imaging features are those of cirrhosis in general.

Hemochromatosis—Case 1: Parenteral iron overload. More than 100 units of blood were transfused for acute myelogenous leukemia.

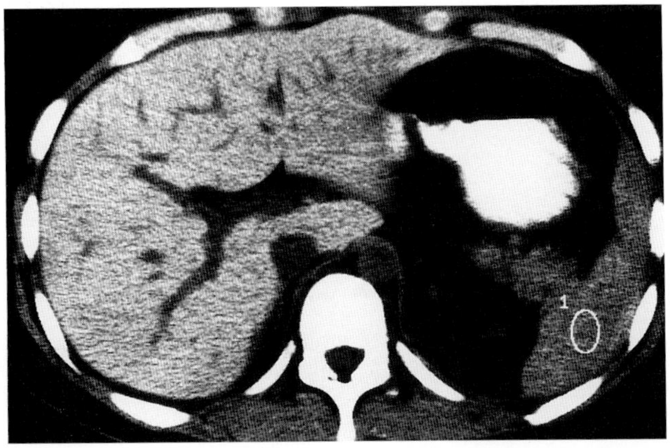

(a) Plain CT: liver parenchyma is of high density due to excessive iron deposition (130 HU) and blood vessels are black.

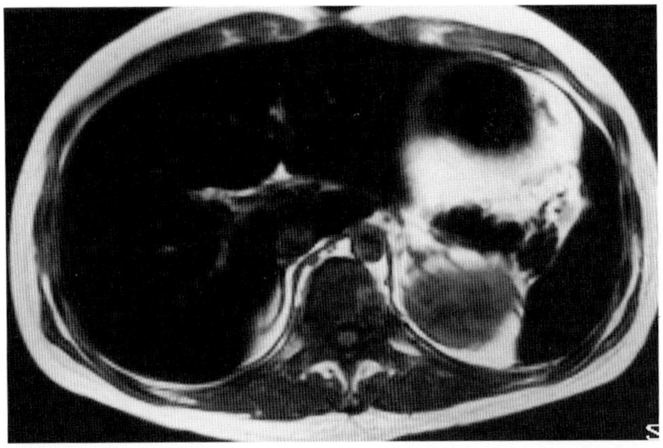

(b) MR imaging (T1-weighted, 600/15): the liver and spleen are black (low intensity), the density being reversed from the CT image, and large vessels are white. The diagnosis is secondary iron overload due to blood transfusions.

8.3 Thorotrast liver disease

Thorotrast is a colloidal preparation of thorium dioxide and was used for angiography during World War II. It emits alpha-rays of a very long half-life (200–400 years) and, once injected intravenously, more than 70 per cent is taken up by the reticuloendothelial system (Looney 1960). It is distributed diffusely within the liver shortly after administration, but slowly undergoes redistribution because of its release by the Kupffer cells and transport by the lymphatic system, and eventually produces a reticular distribution pattern when seen by X-ray. It is also transported toward the pancreas. Due to its large atomic size, nearly twice that of iodine, lymph node deposition simulates calcification and may be mistaken for pancreatic stones (Okuda *et al.* 1976*a*). The spleen slowly undergoes atrophy due to alpha radiation and may be shrunk to a size as small as several grams. The portal tract undergoes fibrosis, and the liver may be deformed to some extent. Malignancies, particularly cholangiocarcinoma, angiosarcoma, and HCC, are the most common late complications. A national study in Japan followed 200 ex-soldiers who were given Thorotrast during World War II, and about 60 per cent of the deaths during the follow up were due to hepatic malignancies. Another autopsy study in Japan involved 102 Thorotrast cases who died from liver tumors: 43 per cent had cholangiocarcinoma, 38 per cent angiosarcoma, 16 per cent HCC, and 3 per cent double cancers (Ito *et al.* 1988). On a plain roentgenogram, the liver may or may not show a typical reticular density, but the spleen stands out as an oblong structure with multiple small high-density dots (Case 1). Even though the liver does not show the reticular density, the lymph nodes in the hilar and pancreatic areas are clearly seen (Okuda and Iio 1976). CT is more sensitive than X-rays in detecting density differences, and will detect Thorotrast deposition which X-rays cannot demonstrate (Rao *et al.* 1986).

Thorotrast liver disease—Case 1: Thorotrast deposition in the liver, spleen, and lymph nodes.

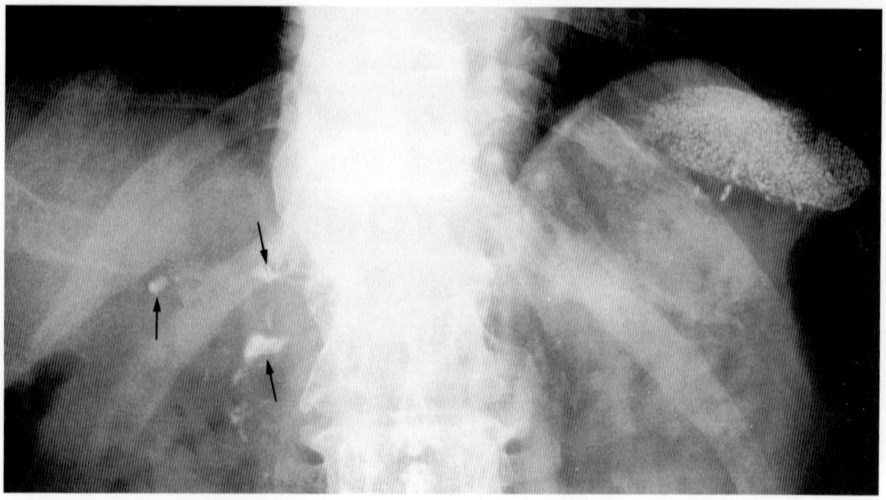

(a) Plain roentgenogram of the abdomen: the spleen is atrophied and seen as a conglomerate of small high-density dots. Lymph node depositions are also noted (→), but there is no visible deposition in the liver.

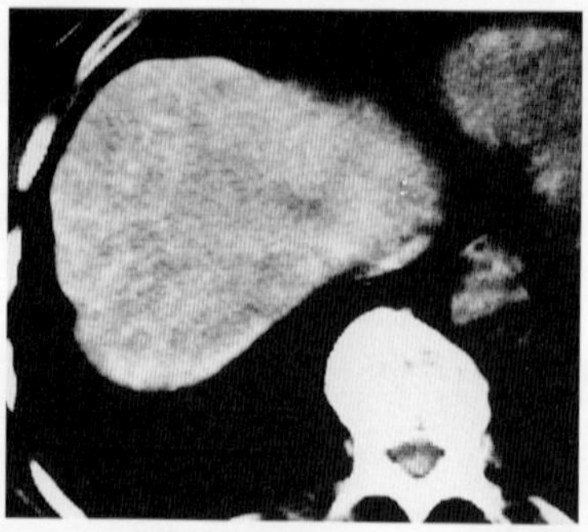

(b) Plain CT: many dots of Thorotrast deposition are seen in the liver. The distribution is uneven, and is denser near the capsule. The strands of low-density areas may correspond to fibrosed area. If an area devoid of Thorotrast develops within the parenchyma which has diffuse Thorotrast deposition, it is most likely a malignancy.

9

Gallbladder carcinoma

Currently a major effort is being made to diagnose early carcinoma of the gallbladder and make quality diagnosis of lesions protruding into the bladder lumen, namely the differential diagnosis of benign and malignant lesions. As with gastric cancer, some early gallbladder carcinomas are confined in the mucosa and are flat, not producing an elevated lesion (like type IIb gastric cancer) or infiltrating within the wall (like scirrhous gastric cancer). These characteristics are attracting the attention of gastroenterologists (Tsuchiya 1991).

US is most suitable for detecting a gallbladder pathology, and quality diagnosis may be possible with US alone for cholesterol polyp and adenomyomatosis (Fig. 9.1). CT is useful in determining the extent of malignant infiltration into the liver bed and an adjacent organ within the abdominal cavity, and in identifying lymph node metastasis (Itai *et al.* 1980*a*). Angiography may prove diagnostic in differentiating between inflammatory mural thickening and infiltrating carcinoma, and for the diagnosis of malignant infiltration into neighboring organs. It is also necessary for drawing a vascular map when an operation is contemplated. Additional diagnostic modalities include cholangio-CT, a combination of intravenous cholangiography and CT, endoscopic US carried out from the duodenum, direct puncture of the gallbladder under US guidance (opacification, cytology, and tumor marker measurement in bile), and gall-

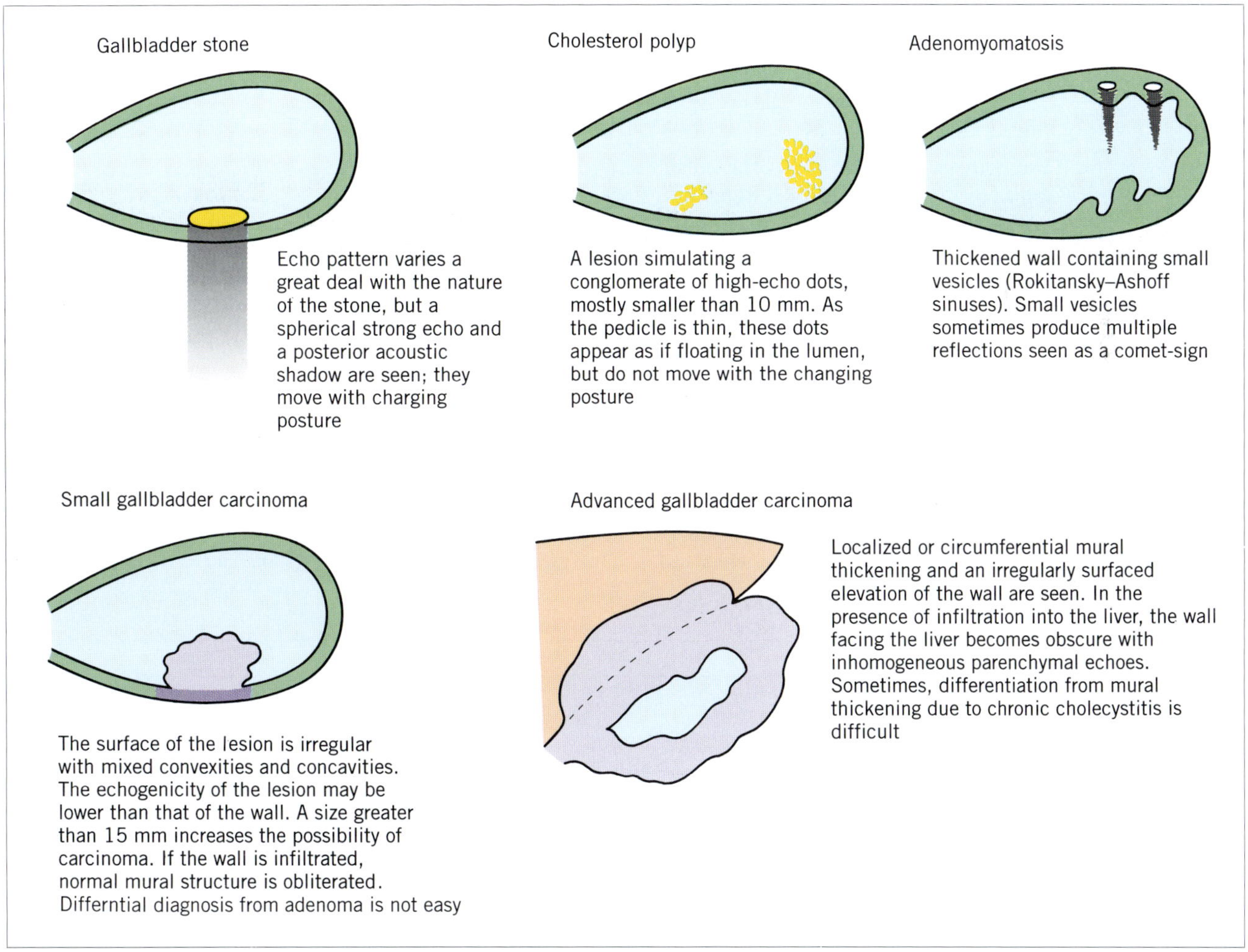

Fig. 9.1 US characteristics of elevated lesions of the gallbladder.

bladder endoscopy preceded by gallbladder puncture. These procedures are contributing significantly to more definitive diagnosis.

Many patients with gallbladder disease have coexisting stones, and for differential diagnosis one has to change the posture of the patient to see if the lesion moves or not. CT may not detect a stone with a low calcium content, which US can pick up (Suzuki *et al.* 1982). It is desirable to do US and CT study early in the morning after overnight fasting. In the General Rules for the Clinical and Surgical Studies on Cancer of Biliary Tract (3rd ed.) (Japanese Society of Biliary Surgery 1993), the gallbladder is anatomically divided evenly along the longitudial axis into three parts, fundus, body, and neck, and the cystic duct lies between the gallbladder and the extrahepatic bile duct (cf. Fig. 10.1, p.345).

Differential diagnosis of elevated lesions of the gallbladder

To make quality diagnosis of elevated lesions of the gallbladder, the shape and size are the important factors to consider, along with assessment of the thickness and structure of the wall, and demonstration of mural infiltration.

Differential diagnosis based on the shape

Cholesterol polyps (Case 1) are usually detected by chance during abdominal US examination. The characteristic features are:

(1) hyperechoic dots;
(2) multiple, and diameter around 5 mm;
(3) thin pedicle (polyp may appear separated from wall by US);
(4) as it enlarges, it simulates a mulberry.

The diagnosis is not very difficult if these features are present. They may be delineated by intravenous cholecystography (Case 2), but US has a much higher sensitivity. It is to be remembered that some cholesterol polyps are large, occasionally exceeding 20 mm in size (Case 3). By contrast, adenoma and fibrous polyp show echoes compatible with solid tissue (Case 4), the former being pedunculated (Case 4) and the latter enhanced on enhanced CT (Case 5). Adenomyomatosis is seen by US as an elevated lesion or mural thickening (Case 6), and differential diagnosis from carcinoma is sometimes difficult. Adenomyomatosis in the fundus may be diagnosed by cholangio-CT carried out with the patient in a prone position (Case 6).

Differential diagnosis of elevated lesions based on size

When we analyzed elevated gallbladder lesions in relation to their sizes (Table 9.1), it became clear that a distinction between benign and malignant lesions is possible from the size. The majority of cholesterol polyps were smaller than 15 mm, except for one which measured 25 mm (Case 3). Adenomas and adenomyomatosis lesions were also smaller than 15 mm. Two fibrous polyps were greater than 15 mm, but they were enhanced in the late phase of enhanced CT, and had a relatively smooth surface; we are of the opinion that they can be differentiated from carcinoma by these features. All 12 carcinomas were larger than 15 mm; two of them were carcinoma in adenoma, but as studied by US the gallbladder wall was clearly discerned, although the sizes of adenomas were large (38 × 35 mm; 45 × 40 mm). Both were early gallbladder carcinoma (Case 7). Except for cholesterol polyp, a solid and broad-based tumor smaller than 15 mm could well be malignant, and it is important that the size be measured by US at regular intervals (Koga *et al.* 1988).

Early carcinoma of the gallbladder

Most institutes call a carcinoma confined to the mucosa (m) or the muscle layer (pm) 'early' carcinoma, and in the UICC classification, stage 1 is defined as T_1, N_0 and M_0. To improve prognosis, early detection is the only possibility (Nevin *et al.* 1976), and US is the major diagnostic procedure to that end because it is much better than other modalities in delineating the lumen and the wall. It has been reported that when gallbladders removed because of stones are studied histopathologically, flat surfaced early carcinoma similar to IIb (flat) gastric cancer is found frequently. However, in the clincal setting, detectable early lesions are mostly elevated (Tsuchiya 1991). At the National Cancer Center Hospital Tokyo, the relative frequency of early carcinoma among all gallbladder cancers has been 13

Table 9.1

Histological diagnosis	No. of lesions
Cholesterol polyp	11
Adenoma	3
Adenomyomatosis	3
Fibrous polyp	2
Carcinoma	12

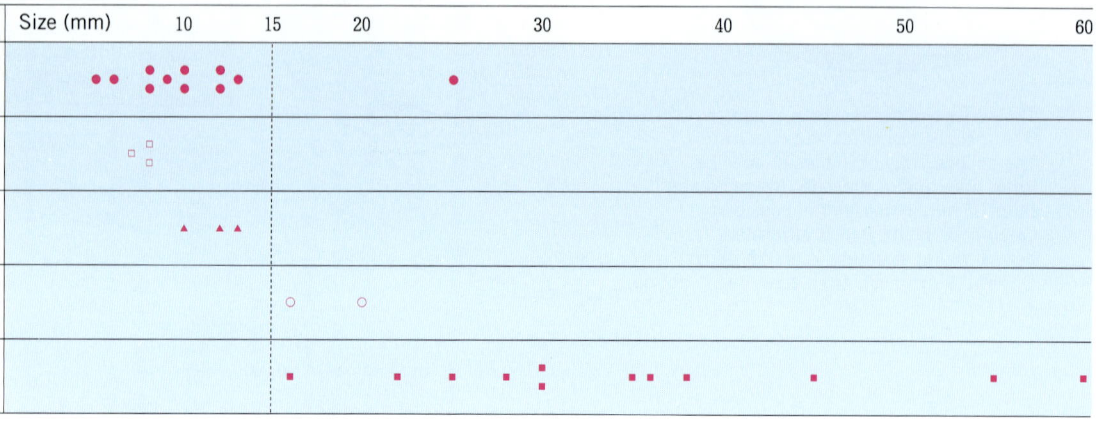

per cent (6/45), and most of them were elevated. They were not recognized by CT or angiography. Histologically, the majority were well differentiated tubular adenocarcinoma.

Advanced carcinoma of the gallbladder

A localized and elevated gallbladder carcinoma (Case 8) is seen by US and CT as an irregularly surfaced solid lesion protruding into the lumen. It is also seen as an encasement on the angiogram. A carcinoma of the thickened wall type is difficult to differentiate from chronic cholecystitis (Duber *et al.* 1984; Thorsen *et al.* 1984) (Case 9). As carcinoma advances, it penetrates the serosa and infiltrates into the liver bed (Case 11), and further into the adjacent organs such as the transverse colon and duodenum. A very hypervascular carcinoma returns a large amount of venous blood into the liver parencyma, and may simulate parenchyma infiltration (Matsui *et al.* 1987*a*) (Case 10). US and MR imaging are required for an accurate diagnosis in such cases (Sagoh *et al.* 1990). Gallbladder carcinoma is a very common complication of anomalous pancreaticobiliary ductal union (Kimura *et al.* 1985), and entry of regurgitating pancreatic juice into the gallbladder is a suggested etiological mechanism (Case 10). If the gallbladder is filled up with carcinoma, it may look like an HCC (Case 12).

Intrahepatic metastases are recognized as multiple lesions, often of similar sizes, and if a peripheral low-density area is seen in a late phase of enhanced CT, the possibility of gallbladder carcinoma becomes stronger (Case 13). Sarcomas of the gallbladder are uncommon, but among them leiomyosarcoma is the most frequent (Case 14).

Gallbladder carcinoma—Case 1: Multiple cholesterol polyps.

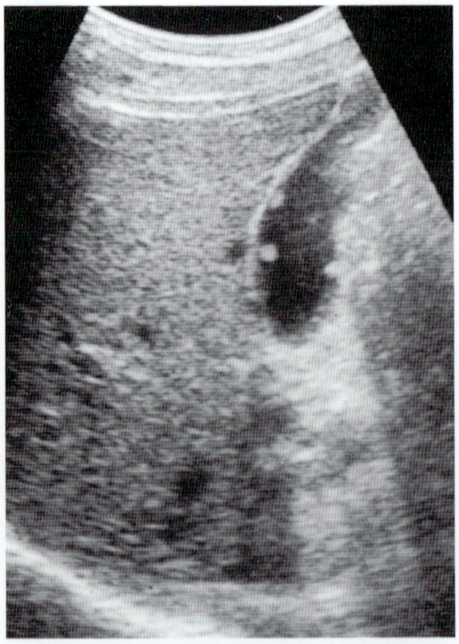

(a) US (right intercostal scan): a number of small elevated lesions are seen in the lumen. They are spherical, and hyperechoic. Pedunculated cholesterol polyps may change in size and shape with different postures, but they never move away.

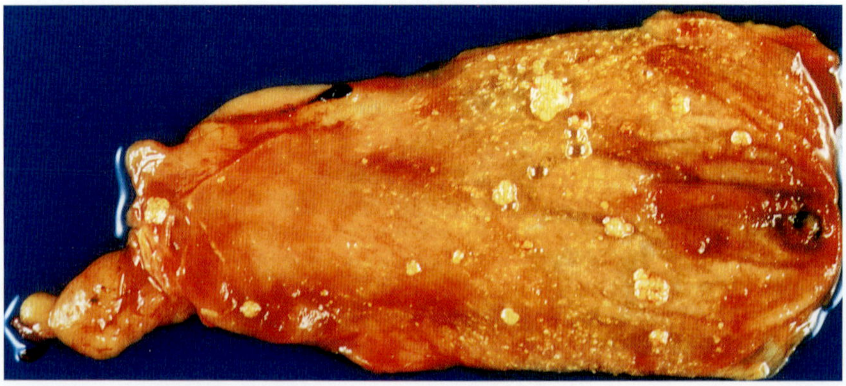

(b) Removed gallbladder (mucosal surface): there are many yellow mulberry-shaped cholesterol polyps, 1–6 mm in size. At the time of operation, some polyps may be freed, suggesting a rather frail attachment to the wall.

Gallbladder carcinoma—Case 2: Drip infusion cholangiogram and CT findings in cholesterol polyp.

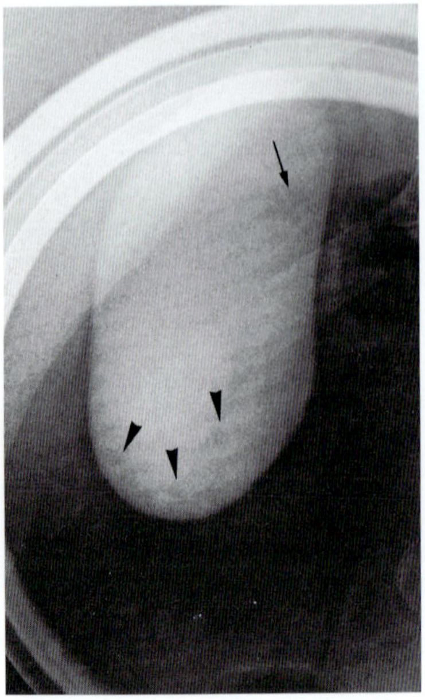

(a) Dripinfusion cholangiogram: when the gallbladder is compressed, cholesterol polyps are seen as filling defects. Delineation of a mulberry-shaped and irregularly surfaced lesion makes the diagnosis of cholesterol polyp most likely.

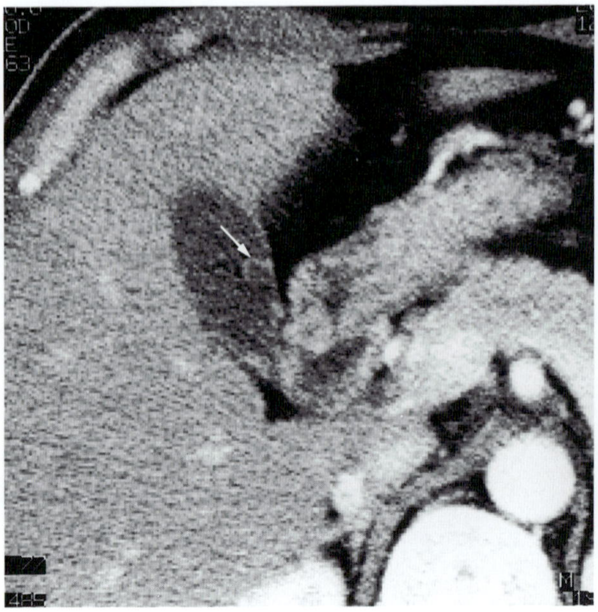

(b) Enhanced CT: a cholesterol polyp plain CT did not delineate may be found by enhanced CT (5 mm slices) as a thread-like protrusion (→).

Gallbladder carcinoma—Case 3: 25 mm cholesterol polyp difficult to differentiate from carcinoma.

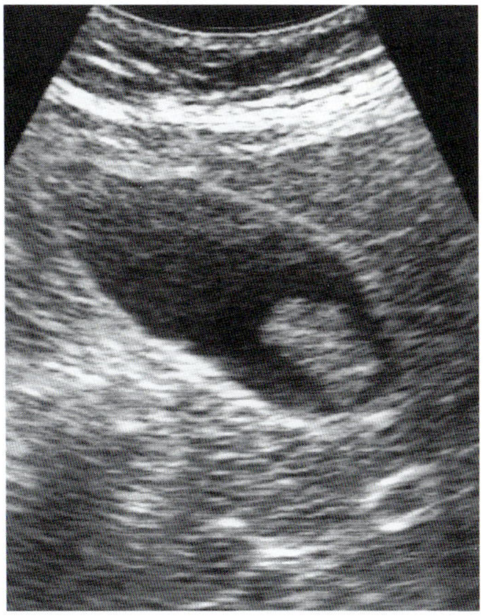

(a) US (right subcostal scan): a 25 mm long protruding lesion showing echoes similar to those of liver parenchyma is seen toward the neck of the gallbladder. The surface is irregular, but the lesion lacks bright echoes seen in ordinary cholesterol polyps. Since no discernible attachment to the wall is recognized, it was thought to be an elevated lesion with a thin pedicle, but the possibility of malignancy could not be denied, and cholecystectomy was done.

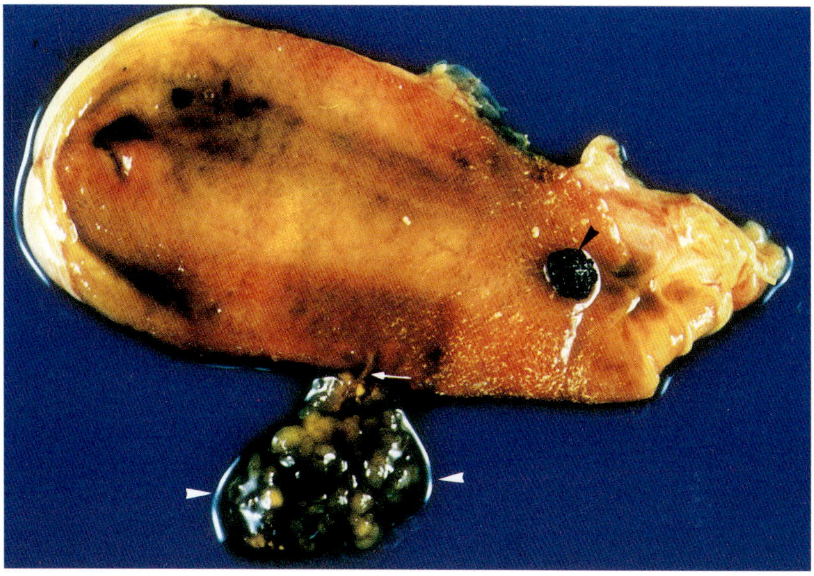

(b) Gallbladder lumen: a 25 mm pedunculated cholesterol polyp was found (→: thread-like pedicle). The whole mass was a soft gelatinous material containing yellow mulberry-like cholesterol polyps (▷). There was a concomitant stone (▶) in the neck.

Gallbladder carcinoma—Case 4: Elevated lesion of the gallbladder mucosa (adenoma).

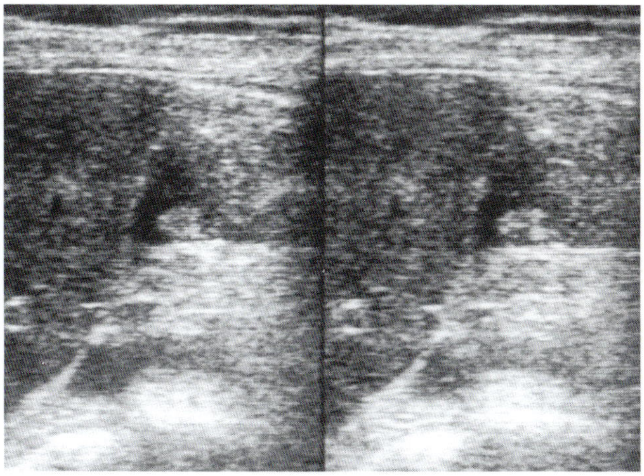

(a) US (right intercostal scan): a 10×9 mm protruding lesion is seen in the center of the gallbladder. It is pedunculated, generally hyperechoic and hypoechoic in part. The size of the lesion did not change for 9 months of follow-up, but cholecystectomy was carried out at the patient's request.

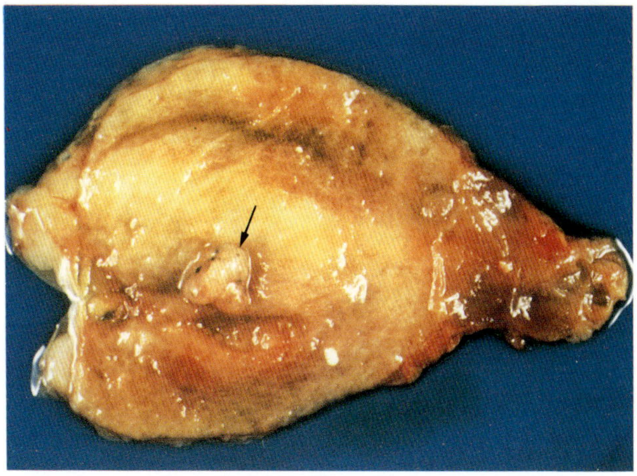

(b) Removed gallbladder (mucosal surface): the mucosa was like velvet and had a 7×6 mm, irregularly surfaced pedunculated polyp (→). Histologically, it was adenoma, but there was a localized area of atypical cells.

Gallbladder carcinoma—Case 5: Fibrous polyp of the gallbladder stained on enhanced CT.

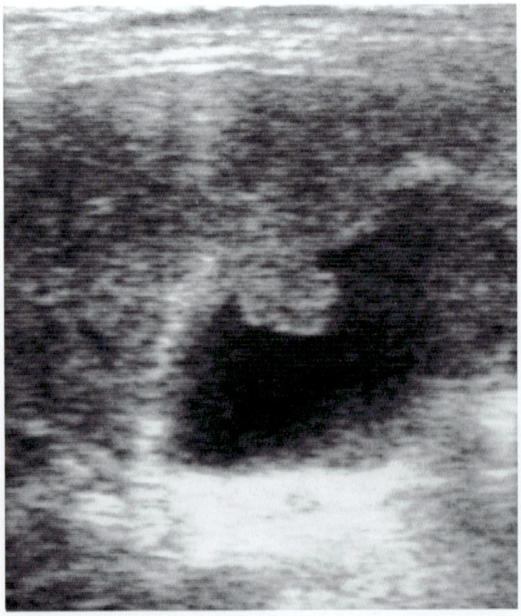

(a) US: a 15 mm isoechoic elevated lesion is seen in the body of the gallbladder. The surface is irregular and it looks as though it was attached to the gallbladder wall with a broad pedicle. Distinction from carcinoma is not easy.

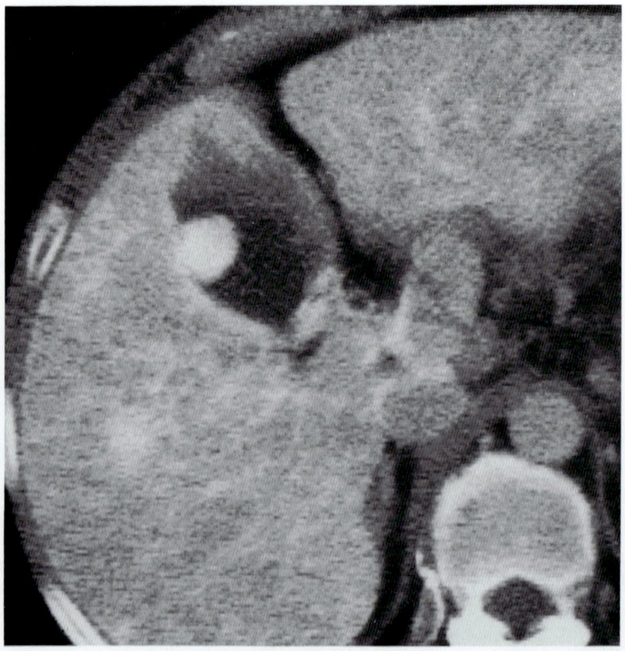

(b) Enhanced CT (late phase): this lesion is now seen as a high-density mass. In general, carcinoma of the gallbladder is not enhanced this much.

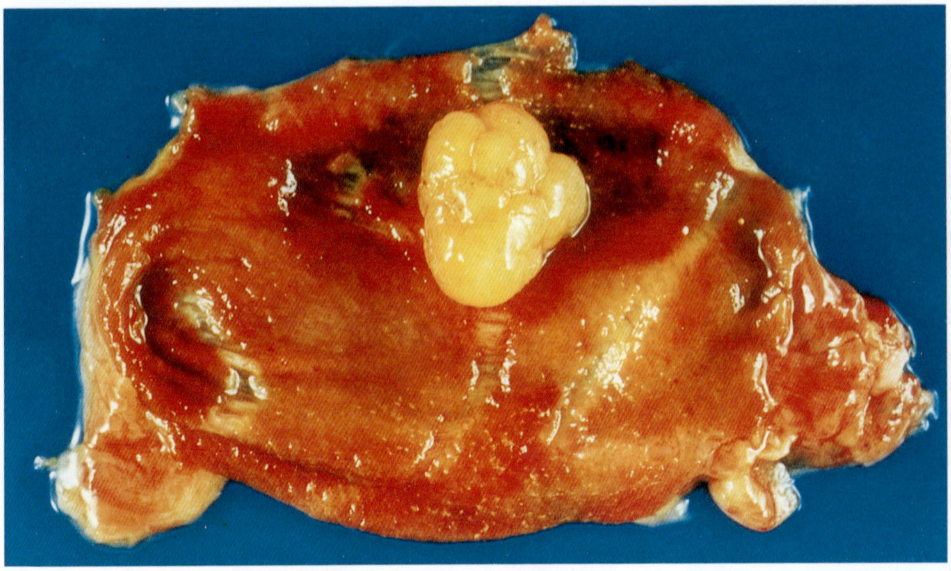

(c) Removed gallbladder (mucosal surface): a yellowish tumor with a nodular surface was found. Histologically, it was a fibrous polyp consisting mainly of collagen fibers. The attachment to the wall was so small that it came off during the operation. There was no recognizable pedicle.

Gallbladder carcinoma—Case 6: Differential diagnosis between adenomyomatosis and gallbladder carcinoma expedited by prone cholangio-CT.

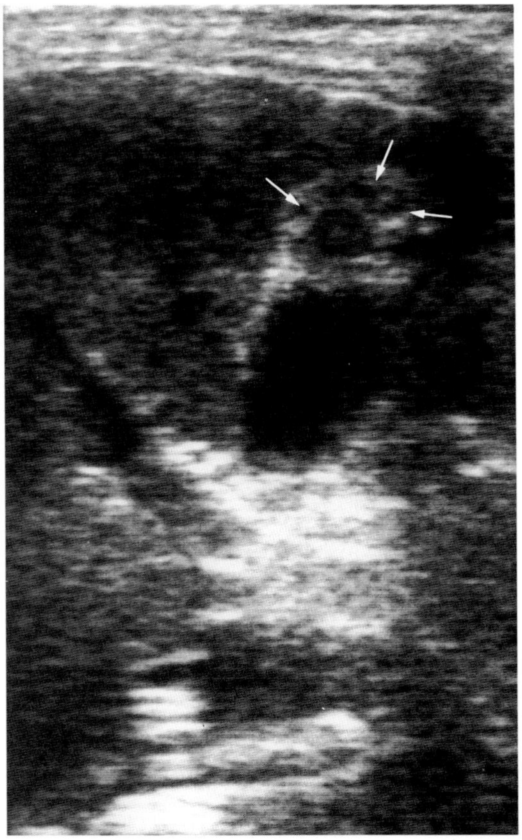

(a) US (right intercostal scan): thickening of the wall is localized to the fundus which contains cystic lesions (→).

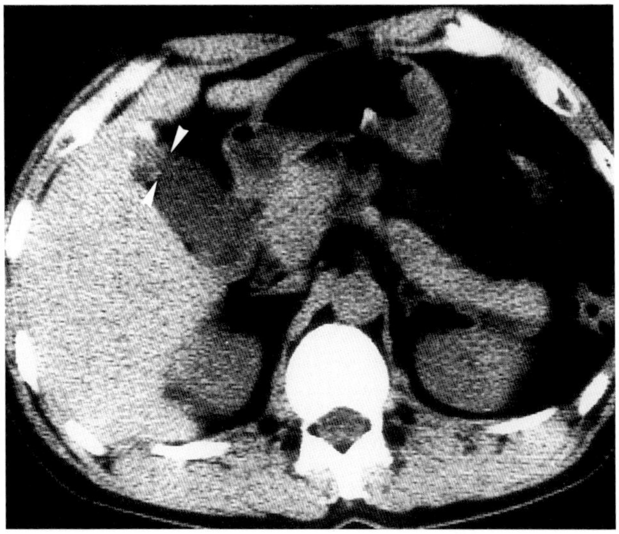

(b) Plain CT: there is a narrowing (▶) between the body and fundus of the gallbladder. The fundus is of higher density and has a small calcification.

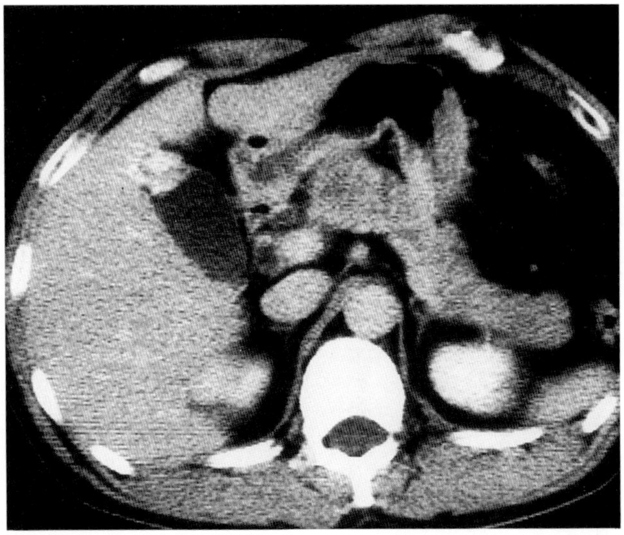

(c) Enhanced CT (late phase): inhomogeneous enhancement is seen confined to the fundus. Since liver parenchyma was unremarkable, localized adenomyomatosis was strongly suspected.

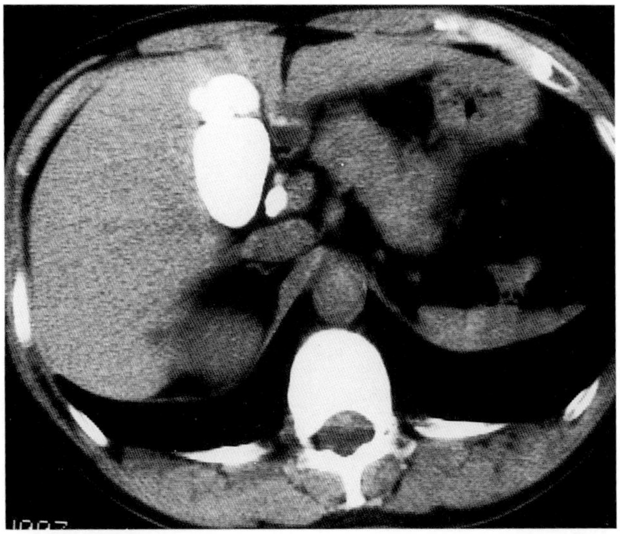

(d) CT made in a prone position during drip infusion cholecysto-cholangiography (40 min after i.v. injection of contrast medium): the fundus has received sufficient contrast medium, disclosing the narrowing clearly. As long as it had no filling defect, the diagnosis was adeno-

Gallbladder carcinoma—Case 7: Early carcinoma (carcinoma in adenoma).

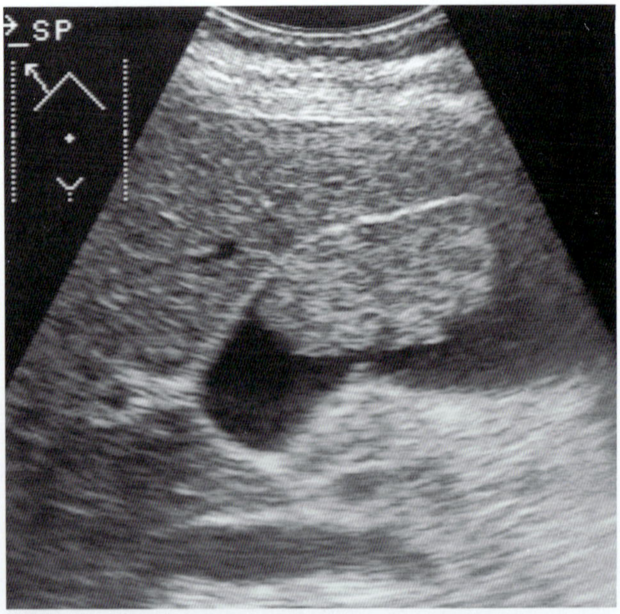

(a) US: an elevated lesion measuring 45 mm in length with a mildly irregular surface is seen in the gallbladder along its liver bed. Since the gallbladder wall and liver parenchyma were clearly visualized with no abnormality, it was assumed that there was no invasion to the gallbladder wall or liver parenchyma.

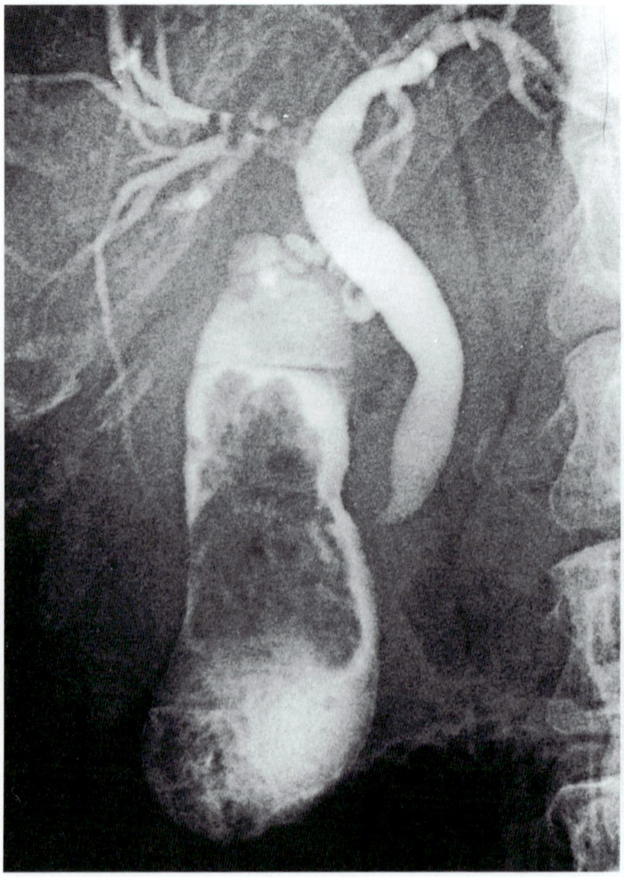

(b) ERC: a filling defect with an irregular surface was recognized in the body and partly in the fundus. From its shape and size, a diagnosis of gallbladder carcinoma was made.

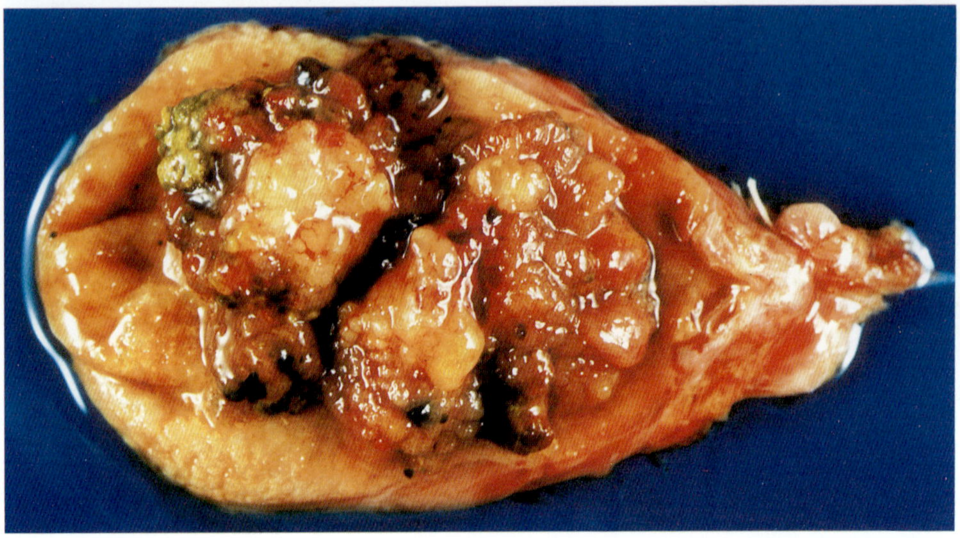

(c) Removed gallbladder (mucosal surface): it was an irregularly surfaced elevated mass containing blood clots. Histologically, it was adenoma that contained several small areas of well differentiated adenocarcinoma considered as early carcinoma. The liver parenchyma along the bed and the serosa of the gallbladder were normal.

Gallbladder carcinoma—Case 8: Focally spared liver suspected of having multiple hepatic metastases associated with gallbladder carcinoma (localized elevated type). A 67-year-old man. Gallbladder carcinoma and fatty liver.

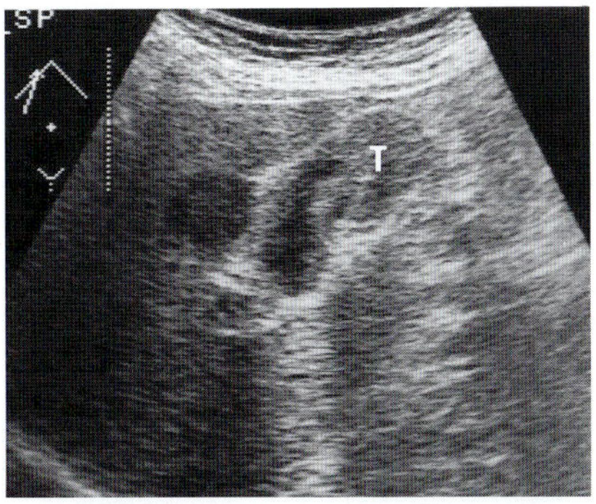

a

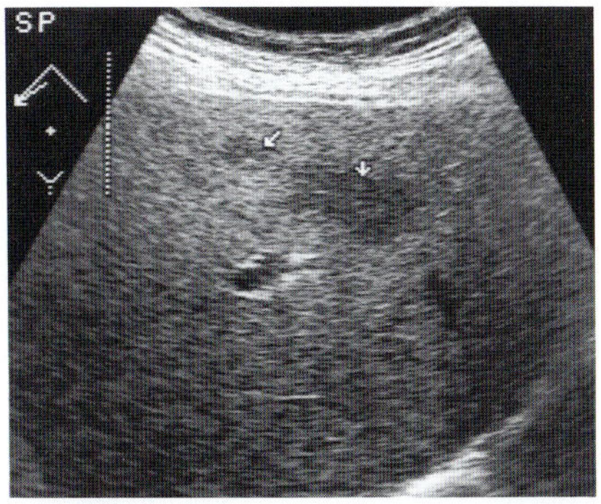

b

(a) US (right subcostal scan): a localized elevated lesion (T) is seen in the fundus.

(b) US (right subcostal scan): one round lesion is seen in S^{V} and two more (→) in S^{IV} near the fundus.

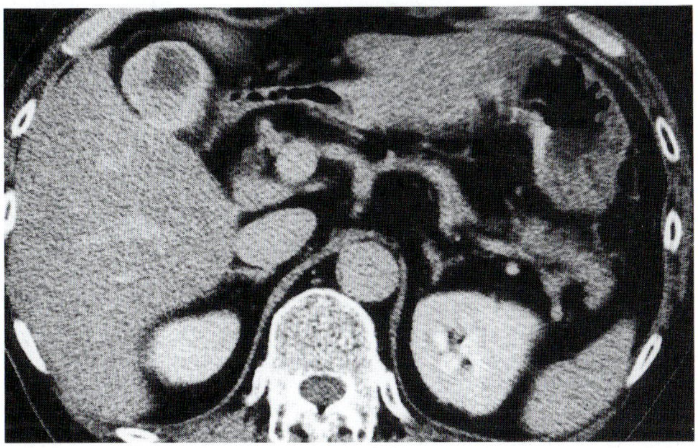

(c) Enhanced CT (late phase, 8 min): An elevated lesion of the same density as that of liver parenchyma is seen in the fundus toward the liver. A diagnosis of gallbladder carcinoma of the elevated type was made. No intrahepatic secondary was recognized. Plain CT showed fatty liver.

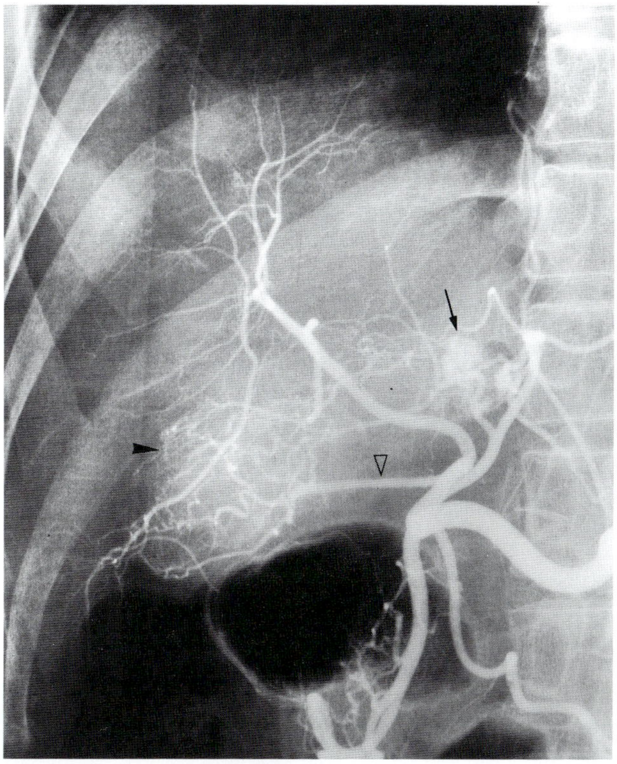

(d) Hepatic arteriogram: dilated cystic artery (▷) is encased in the body/fundus area near the liver bed (▶). A 23 mm hemangioma is seen in S^{IV} (→). Based on these imaging findings, a diagnosis of gallbladder carcinoma associated with hemangioma (the large lesion in S^{IV}) plus focally spared liver (the small lesions in S^{IV} and in S^{V}) was made. Cholecystectomy was done.

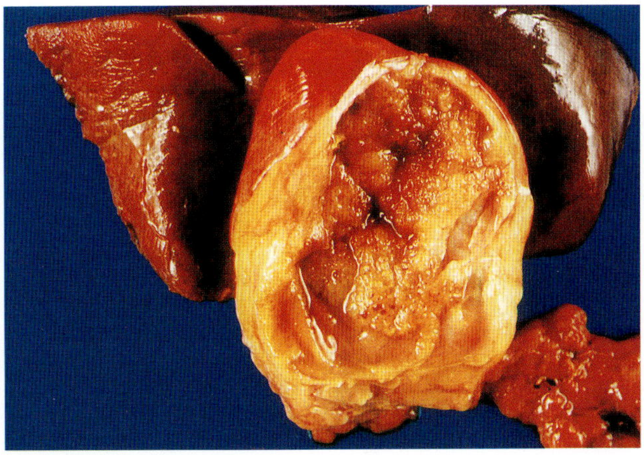

(e) Interior of the removed gallbladder: cholecystectomy combined with partial resection of S^{V} and S^{IV} was carried out. Most of the gallbladder lumen was occupied by an irregularly surfaced cancer (well differentiated adenocarcinoma) with mural thickening (nodular infiltration). However, there was no metastasis into the liver or lymph nodes in the vicinity.

Gallbladder carcinoma—Case 9: Elevated gallbladder lesion (gallbladder carcinoma of the mural thickening type).

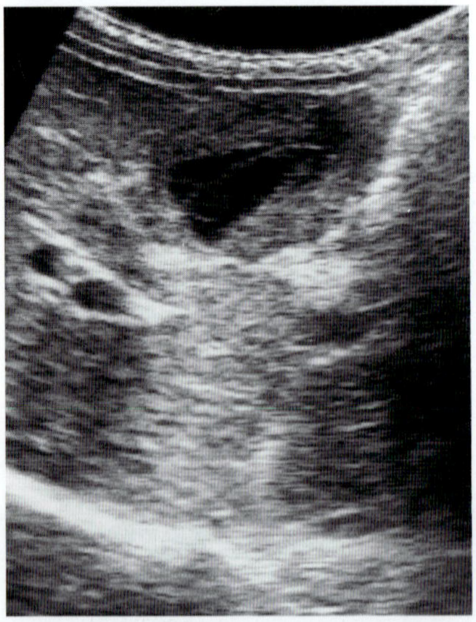

(a) US: diffuse thickening of the wall (10 mm) is seen in the fundus/body region.

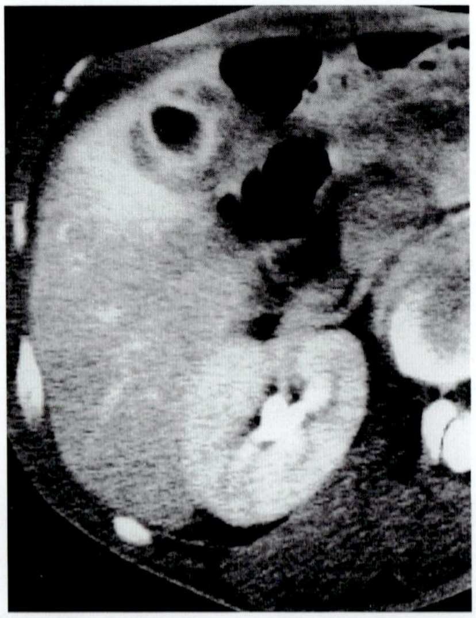

(b) Arterial-CT (early phase): the mucosa and the liver surrounding the gallbladder are enhanced, and the gallbladder wall is seen as a low-density area.

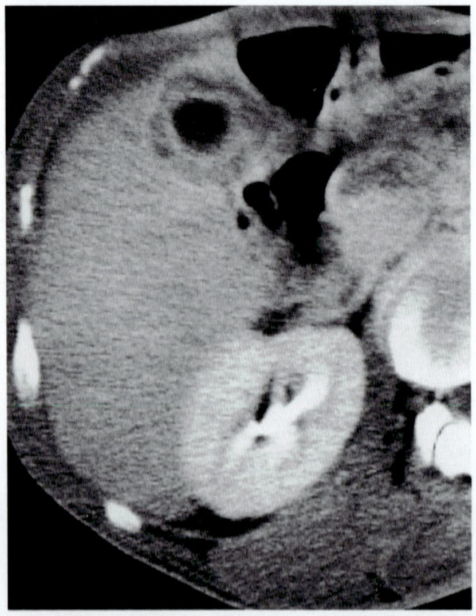

(c) Arterial-CT (late phase, 20 min): the thickened gallbladder wall has remained low in density. No decision was made as to whether this was benign or malignant.

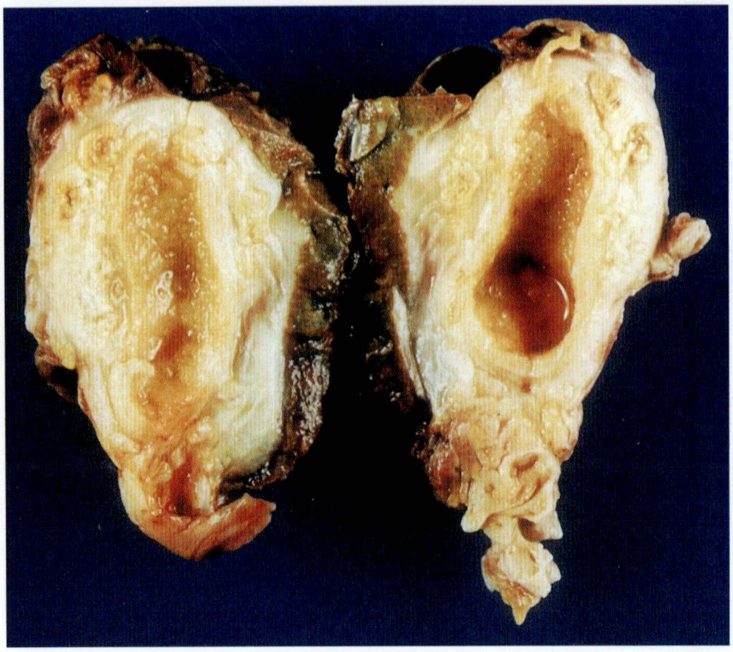

(d) Removed gallbladder: as the gallbladder adhesion to the hepatic bed was very strong, cholecystectomy combined with partial resection of S^{V} was carried out. The gallbladder was thickened and firm. Histologically, this was a well differentiated adenocarcinoma. The origin and the main mass was in the neck. The much thickened area in the body/fundus contained numerous histiocytes phagocytizing fat (xanthogranulomatosis) but no cancer cells. The xanthogranulomatous changes would explain the lack of enhancement. The cancer was infiltrating subserosally, and metastases were present in the lymph nodes of the hilum and near the head of the pancreas.

Gallbladder carcinoma—Case 10: Advanced gallbladder carcinoma (associated with anomalous union of the pancreatic and biliary tracts) in which hepatic infiltration was suspected by dynamic CT, but not proven by operation.

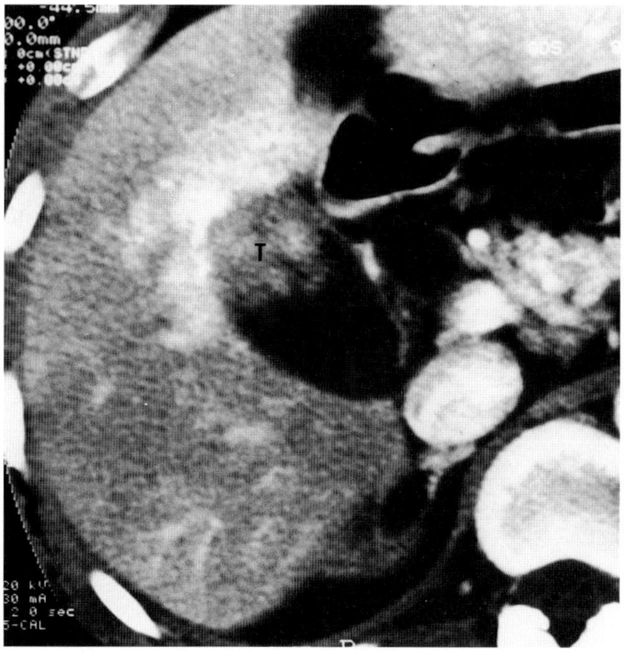

(a) Dynamic CT (early phase): a 50×40 mm enhanced tumor (T) was seen in the body of the gallbladder near the liver bed. An irregular enhanced area was also seen in S^{IV}–S^{V} continuous from it. In the late phase, the enhanced area turned isodense, becoming the same as liver parenchyma in density.

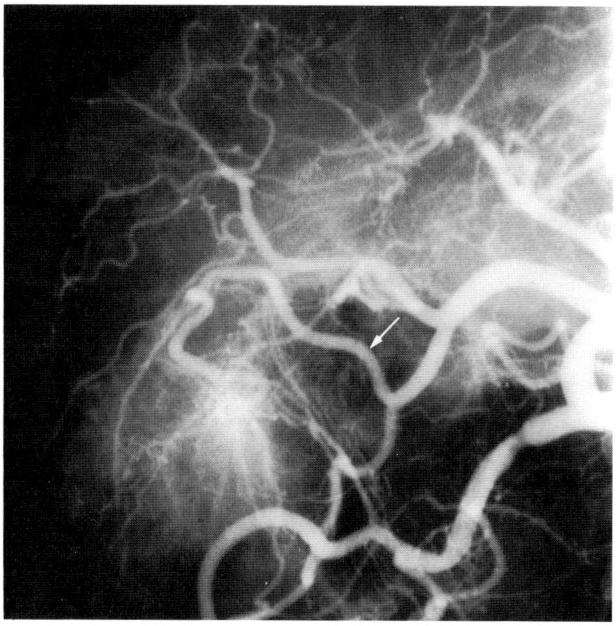

(b) Angiogram (early phase): the cystic artery is dilated (→) and there is a tumor stain.

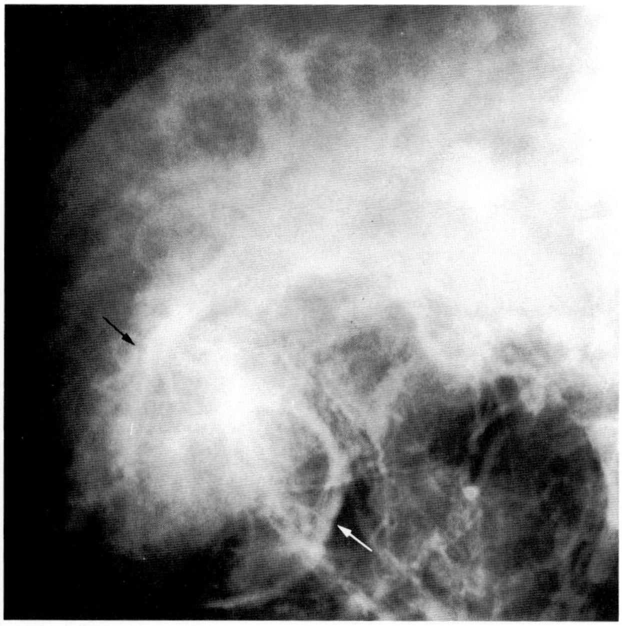

(c) Angiogram (late phase): a dilated cystic vein (→) along the cystic artery is returning blood into the liver bed.

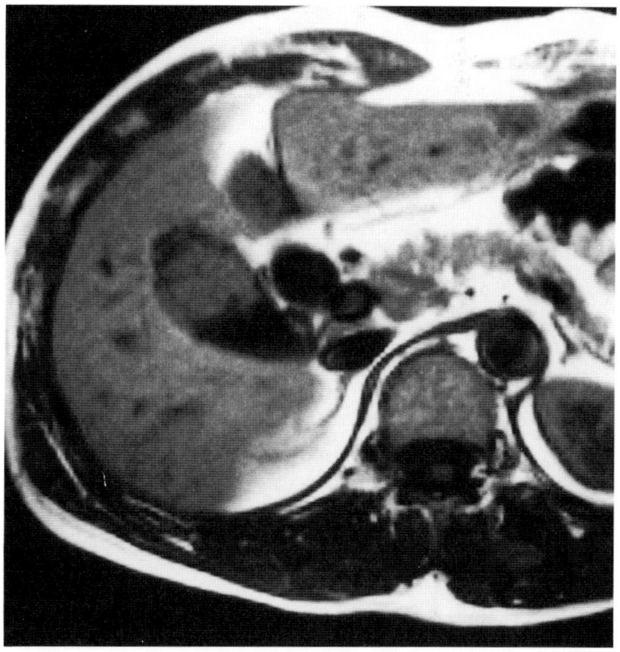

(d) MR imaging (T1-weighted, 600/15): only the gallbladder is delineated with no invasion into the liver.

Case 10 (contd.)

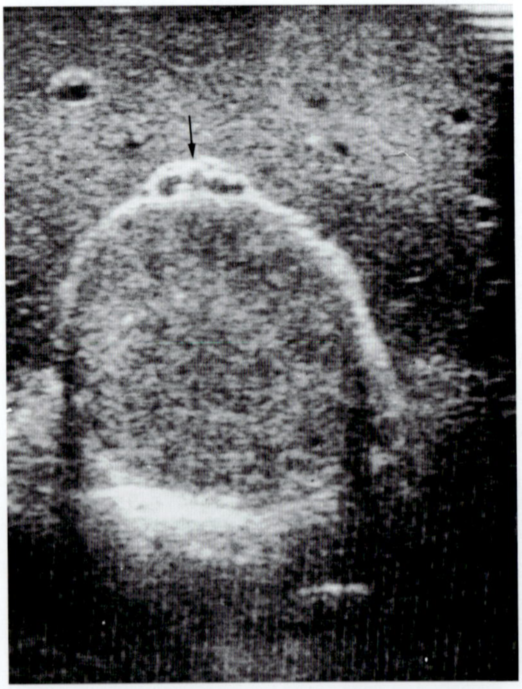

e

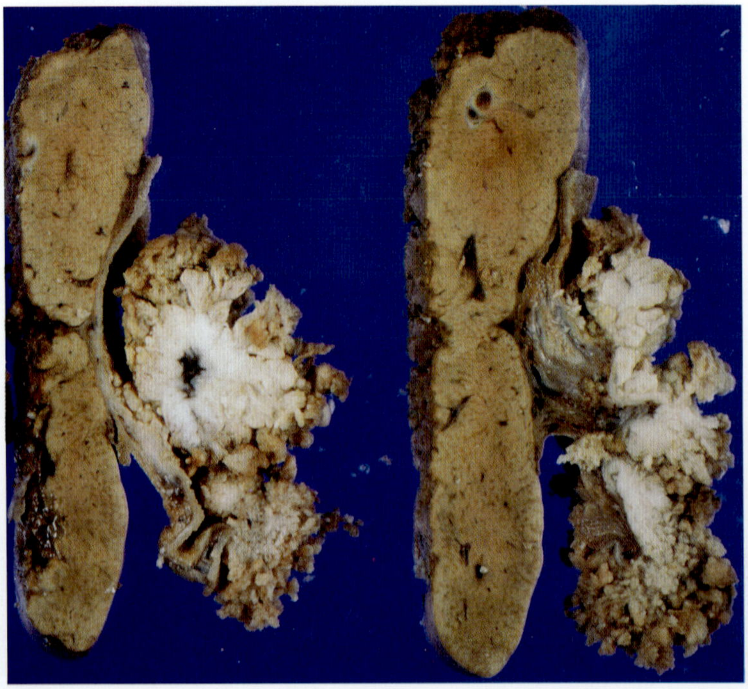

f

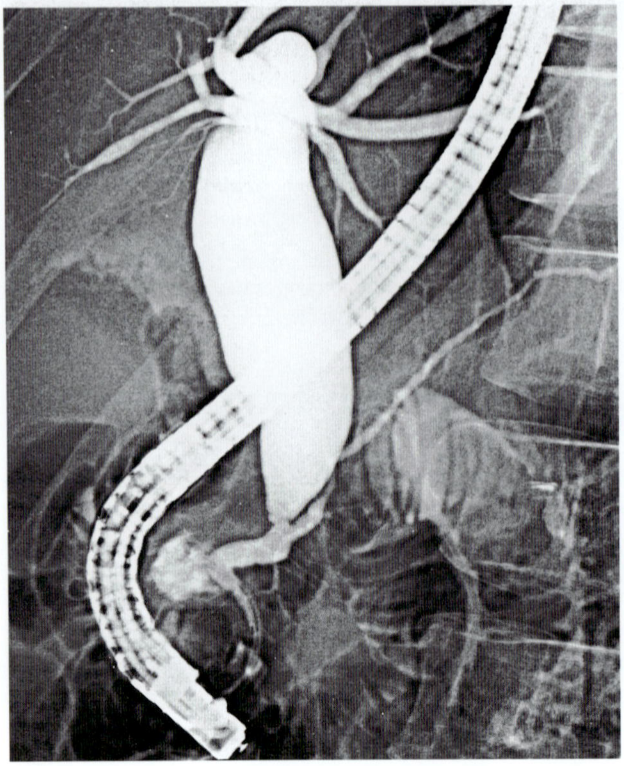

g

(e) Intraoperative US: the entire gallbladder is occupied by a tumor, but no invasion into the liver is recognized. Dilated vessels (→) are seen between the gallbladder and liver bed; they were thought to represent the cystic artery and vein.

(f) Cut section of resected specimen: cholecystectomy combined with resection of S^{IV}–S^{V} was carried out. In the section, no invasion into the liver was seen. Histopathologically, it was a well differentiated papillary adenocarcinoma, mostly confined within the muscle layer. A small invasion was seen beyond the muscle layer. In retrospect, the enhancement of liver parenchyma on dynamic CT (a) suggesting cancer invasion resulted from increased entry of contrast medium into the liver parenchyma due to increased cystic venous flow.

(g) ERCP: there was an anomalous union of the pancreatic duct and the biliary tract with a formation of a long common channel (common bile duct joining the main pancreatic duct in the head of the pancreas).

Gallbladder carcinoma—Case 11: Advanced gallbladder carcinoma infiltrating into the liver bed.

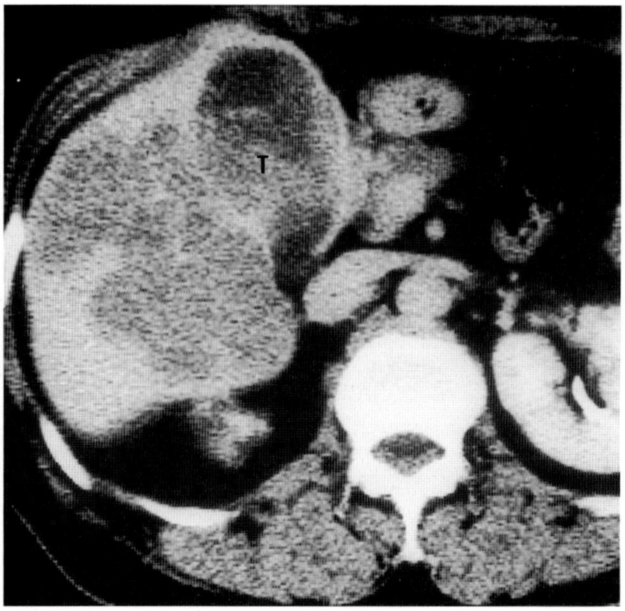

(a) Enhanced CT (late phase): an enlarged gallbladder containing a protruding mass (T) is seen. An irregularly bordered low-density mass is also seen continuous from the gallbladder. The diagnosis would be gallbladder carcinoma infiltrating into the liver bed.

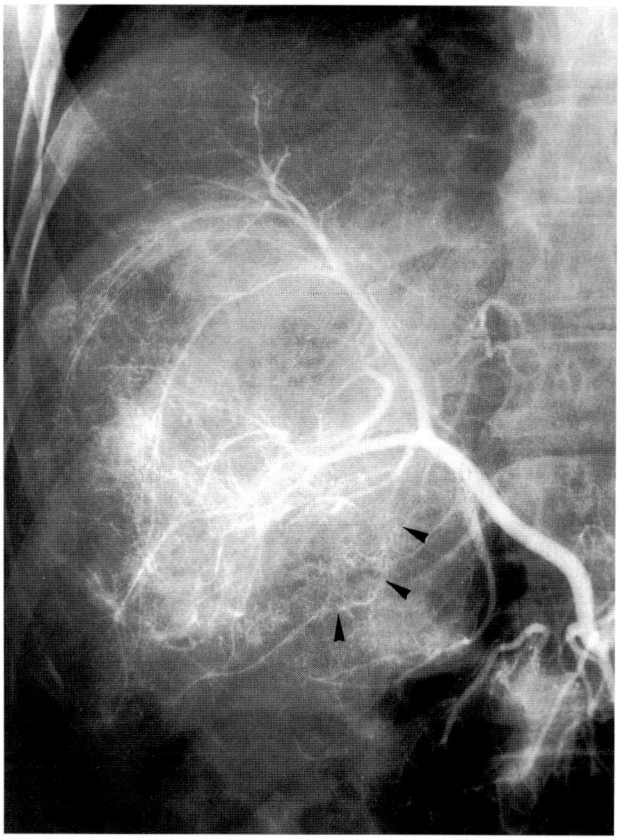

(b) Angiogram: a dilated cystic artery and encasement (▶) of its branches are recognized. Many tumor vessels and displacement of the preexisting hepatic arteries (particularly A^V) are apparent.

Gallbladder carcinoma—Case 12: Gallbladder carcinoma difficult to differentiate from HCC. A 76-year-old woman came to the hospital because of elevated AFP (3765 ng/ml). CEA was normal.

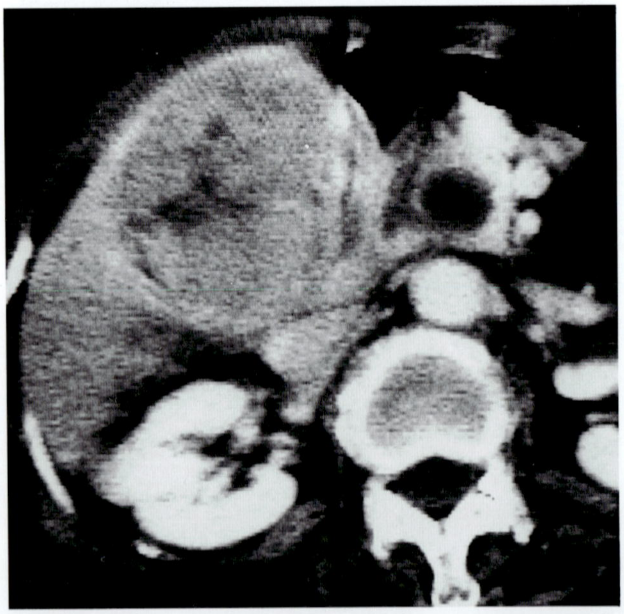

(a) Enhanced CT (early phase): a 60 mm round tumor is seen in the right lobe. The center has a stellate low-density area.

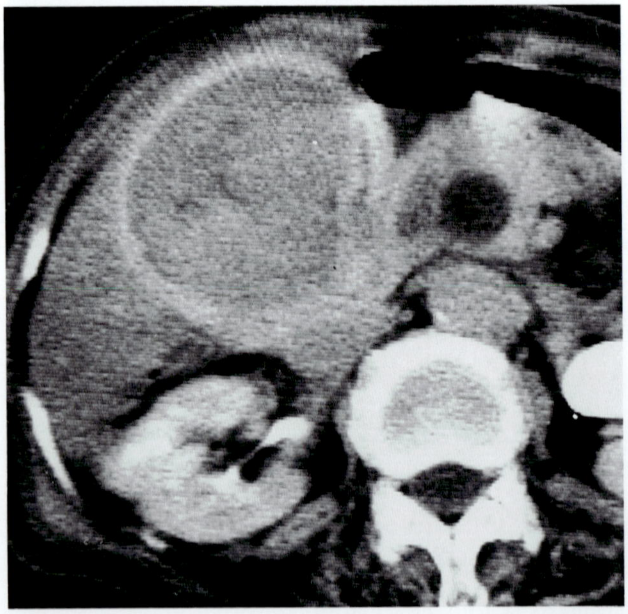

(b) Enhanced CT (late phase): the periphery of the mass was enhanced as a high-density ring. Summing up all the imaging findings, a diagnosis of HCC was made. The common bile duct was dilated to 1.5 cm, but the gallbladder could not be identified.

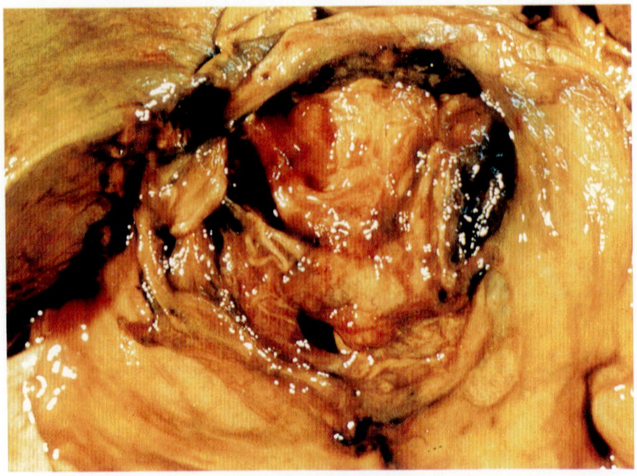

(c) The gallbladder at autopsy: the patient died shortly after admission with abdominal pain. On autopsy, there was a fist-sized cavity filled with necrotic tumor tissue in the gallbladder fossa opening into the transverse colon. Histologically, it contained columnar cell adnocarcinoma. In this patient, gallbladder carcinoma penetrated into the transverse colon, and the purulent necrotizing cholecystitis and peritonitis that ensued were the cause of death. There were many lymph node metastases, and a cholesterol stone at the end of the common bile duct.

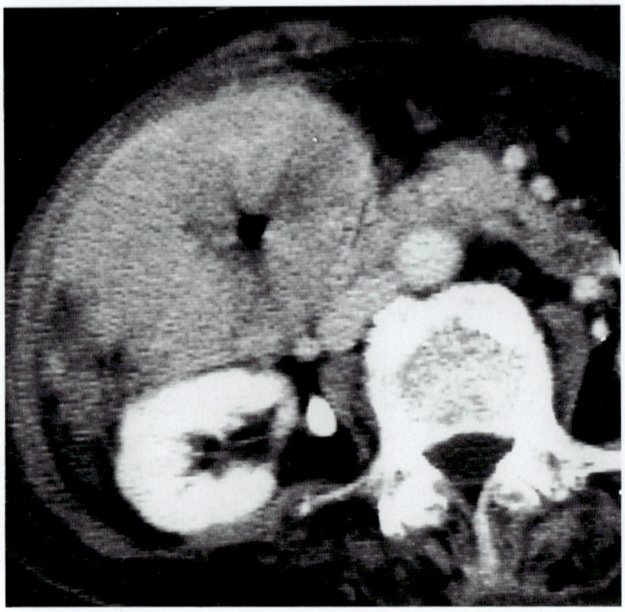

(d) Enhanced CT (4 cm caudal from (a)): retrospective study of the CT film identified gas within the mass, and perforation into the transverse colon was suspected. An enhanced gallbladder wall was misinterpreted as a ring enhancement of HCC. They were the reason for the misdiagnosis.

Gallbladder carcinoma—Case 13: Multiple liver metastases from advanced gallbladder carcinoma displaying periperal low-density rings on late enhanced CT.

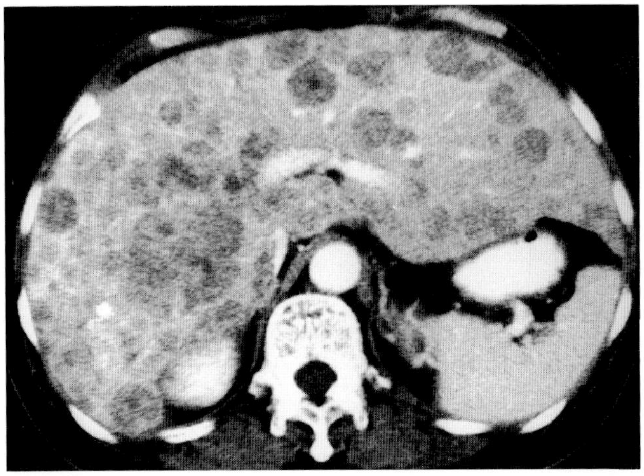

(a) Dynamic CT (early phase): multiple low-density lesions are seen in both lobes.

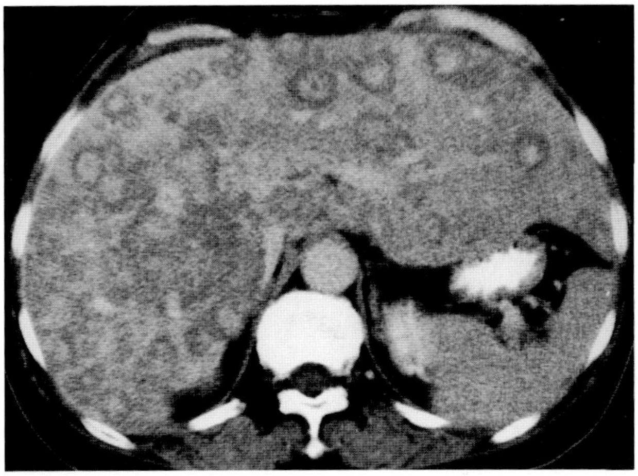

(b) Dynamic CT (late phase, after 10 min): the multiple lesions now demonstrate a low-density ring with a high-density center; the findings are compatible with adenocarcinoma.

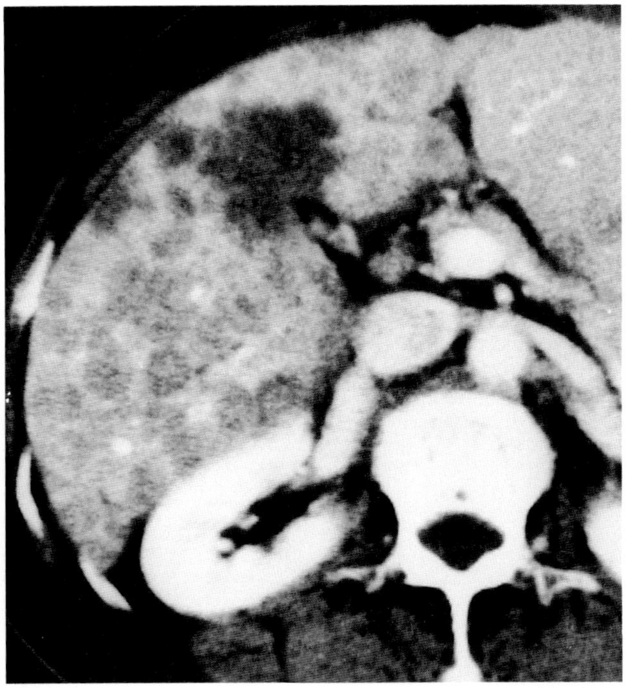

(c) Dynamic CT [slice 3 cm caudal to slice (a)]: an irregularly bounded poorly enhanced mass is seen in the gallbladder fossa. The diagnosis was multiple metastases from gallbladder carcinoma; needle biopsy showed adenocarcinoma.

Gallbladder carcinoma—Case 14: Leiomyosarcoma of the gallbladder. A 76-year-old woman came to the hospital because of a mass felt in the abdomen.

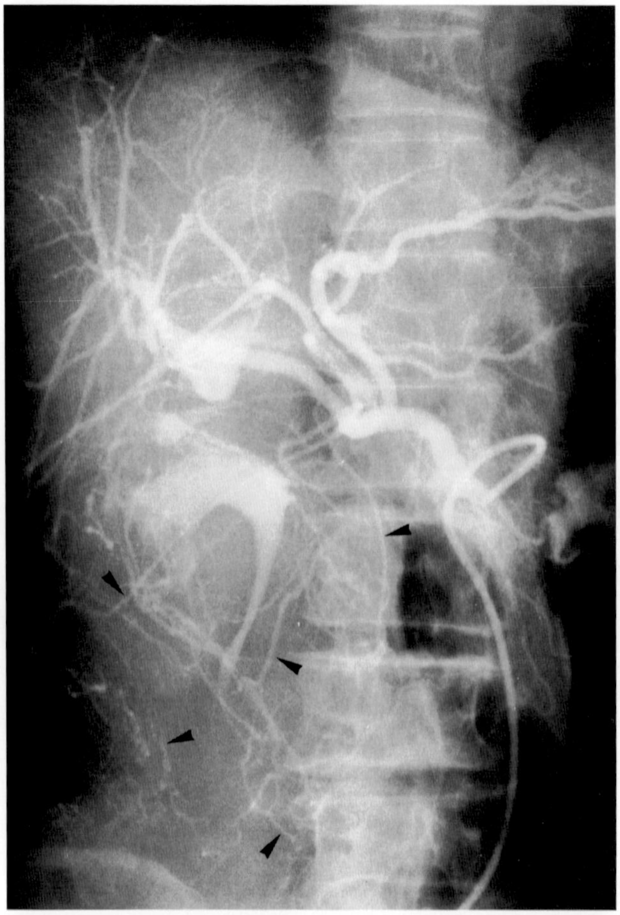

(a) Hepatic arteriogram (early phase): a 15×13 cm oblong tumor with many tumor vessels is seen caudal to the liver. The mass is supplied mainly by the cystic artery, and in part by the gastroduodenal artery. Winding tumor vessels (▶) reach and supply the tumor periphery.

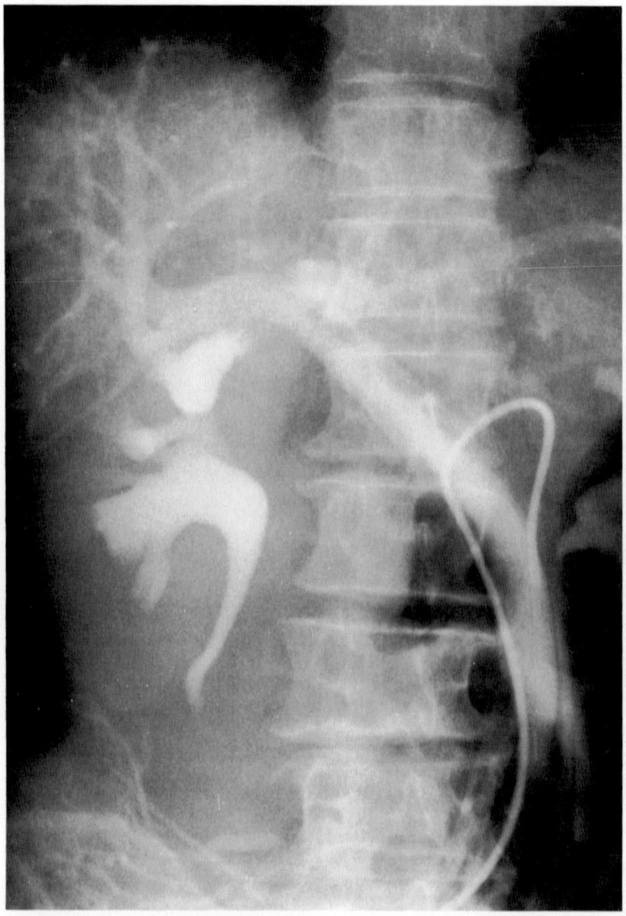

(b) Hepatic arteriogram (late phase): despite its large size, there was no encasement or portal invasion of the portal vein. The mass was compressing onto neighboring organs. Autopsy found this to be a leiomyosarcoma primary to the gallbladder. There was no lymph node metastasis.

10

Carcinoma of the extrahepatic bile duct

Carcinoma of the extrahepatic biliary system is slightly more common in males than in females with the peak age in the 70s. It has been one of the malignancies with a very poor prognosis, because of the difficulty in early diagnosis, proximity of the extrahepatic biliary system to the portal vein and hepatic artery that invites early vascular invasion, and the tendency of carcinoma to spread longitudinally along the extramural lymphatic and nervous tissue. The most common site of origin of extrahepatic bile duct carcinoma is the hilum that includes the upper common hepatic duct and the left and right hepatic ducts, and such carcinomas are collectively called 'hilar carcinoma'. These constitute about 56–58 per cent of all extrahepatic bile duct carcinomas, excluding carcinoma of the papilla (Tompkins *et al.* 1990; Reding *et al.* 1991). The details of hilar carcinoma have already been discussed in Section 4.9, p.210. Extrahepatic bile duct carcinoma includes those carcinomas that arise along the biliary system outside the liver excluding the cystic duct and gallbladder. The extrahepatic bile duct encompasses the bifurcation of the hepatic ducts, common hepatic duct, and the choledochus up to the papilla of the duodenum.

According to the General Rules for the Clinical and Surgical Studies of Carcinoma of Biliary Tract, (3rd ed) (Japanese Society of Biliary Surgery 1993), the bile duct between the bifurcation and the pancreas is divided evenly into the superior (Bs) and the middle bile duct (Bm), and the remaining portion from the cranial border of the pancreas to the papilla called the inferior bile duct (Bi) (Fig. 10.1). The level of the junction of the bile duct and cystic duct (three-duct junction) varies with the individual, and is not the same as the border of the Bs and Bm. Grossly, bile duct carcinomas are divided into six types, papillary, nodular, papillary infiltrating, nodular infiltrating, infiltrating, and special types (Fig. 10.2).

The lymph nodes involved in bile duct carcinoma include those situated toward the liver from the bifurcation (12h), and those caudal to the bifurcation which are further divided into those along the biliary tree (12b), along the portal vein (12p), along the hepatic artery (12a), and along the cystic dyct (12c); they are further subdivided in relation to Bs and Bm, such as 12a1 and 12a2. Bile duct carcinoma metastasizes more commonly to the lymph nodes within the hepatoduodenal ligament and to the suprapancreatic nodes. Hepatic metastasis and peri-

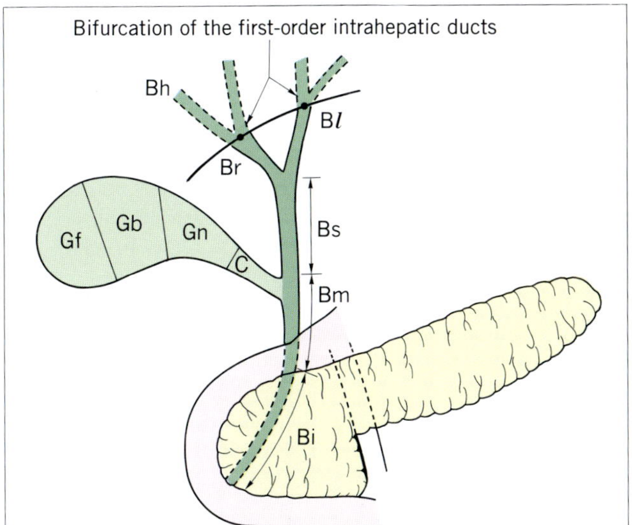

Fig. 10.1 Division of the extrahepatic biliary system. (From *General Rules for the Clinical and Surgical Studies of Carcinoma of Biliary Tract*,

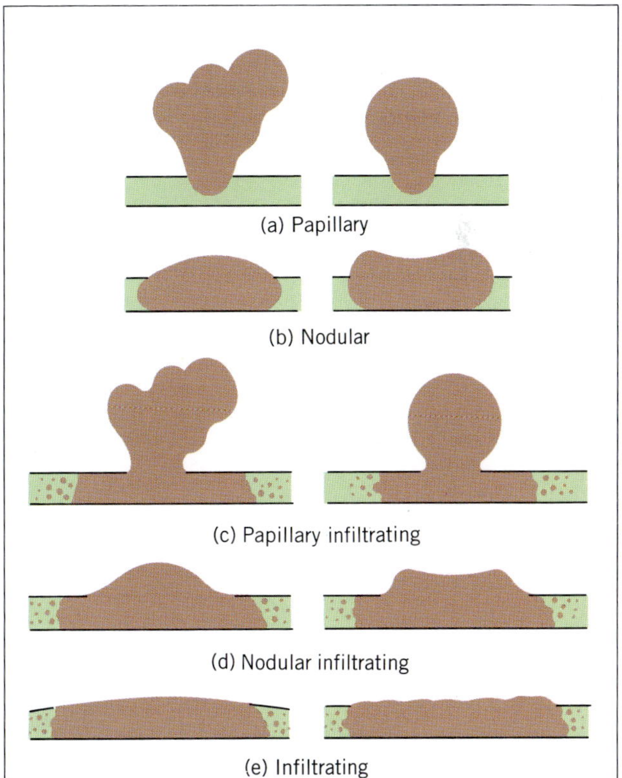

Fig. 10.2 Gross types of bile duct carcinoma. (From *General Rules for the Clinical and Surgical Studies of Carcinoma of Biliary Tract*, Japanese

toneal dissemination are rather uncommon, except in the late stage. However, in more than half of advanced cases are seen metastases to the liver, lymph nodes and pancreas, or infiltration into these tissues. Hilar carcinoma tends to infiltrate along the intrahepatic bile ducts in a radiating fashion.

Diagnosis

Diagnosis of existence and degree of extension

For the early diagnosis of bile duct carcinoma before the onset of jaundice, measurements of serum biliary enzymes such as alkaline phosphatase and γ-glutamyl transpeptidase, tumor markers such as CEA and CA19 9, and US examination are thought to be most effective. With such a policy, increasing numbers of anicteric bile duct carcinoma cases are now being found.

In jaundiced patients, icterus due to mechanical obstruction and parenchymal icterus have to be distinguished by US and CT studies. In the former, the approximate level of obstruction may be determined by CT (Thorsen *et al.* 1984) and US (Okuda and Tsuchiya 1982), but for an exact diagnosis of longitudinal tumor invasion and differential diagnosis from inflammatory stenosis, direct cholangiography, PTC, or ERC, is required. According to Nimura (1988), about 10 per cent of the cases show a continuous or skipping superficial extension, and percutaneous transhepatic cholangioscopy (PTCS) which permits direct vision biopsy becomes necessary (Gazzangia *et al.* 1989; Kamiya *et al.* 1992).

Although CT and US are the useful means for delineating extramural infiltration and invasion into the surrounding organs, angiography proves more diagnostic for invasion onto the portal vein and the hepatic artery which is a critical factor for the determination of operability (Case 1). Angiography also provides information for the vascular map in patients being investigated for operation. For the study of lymph nodes, CT is more useful than US because it is not interfered by duodenal gas. However, its diagnostic accuracy is limited because it cannot distinguish between a dilated and winding cystic or bile duct, and a lymph node. We, in such a case, attempt to improve diagnosis by combining dynamic CT while the biliary tract is opacified through the PTCD tube (Case 2). If a conglomerate of lymph nodes is seen, lymph node metastases are most likely, but a solitary node may be either a reactively swollen node or a metastasis, difficult to distinguish.

Differential diagnosis

The names of diseases that cause biliary tract stenosis and obstruction are listed in Table 10.1. The majority of malignant obstructions are bile duct carcinomas, histologically adenocarcinoma in most of them (Case 3), but there are occasional cases of malignant lymphoma (Tartar and Balfe 1990; Kosuge *et al.* 1991) (Case 4) and leiomyosarcoma. It has recently been shown that choledochal cyst is frequently complicated by bile duct carcinoma (Todani *et al.* 1985; Yoshida *et al.* 1989*a*). Direct metastasis to the bile duct from other primaries is very uncommon; more often one sees infiltration onto the bile duct from a primary arising in an adjacent organ, or from a metastasis to a periductal lymph nodes (Case 5).

Table 10.1 Diseases that cause obstruction/stenosis of the extrahepatic bile duct

1. Malignant bile duct obstructions/stenosis
   (a) Primary bile duct carcinoma
   (b) Metastatic bile duct carcinoma
   (c) Infiltration and compression from carcinoma arising in an adjoining organ (gallbladder carcinoma, pancreatic cancer, etc.) and/or lymph nodes
2. Benign bile duct obstruction/ stenosis
   (a) Common bile duct stone
   (b) Postoperative stenosis
   (c) Mirizzi syndrome
   (d) Sclerosing cholangitis–primary (PSC), secondary
   (e) Inflammation originating in periductal organs and encroaching onto bile ducts
   (f) Parasite (round worm, liver fluke, etc.)

Bile duct carcinoma originates from the mucosa as does gastric cancer, and in the latter double-contrast examination of the mucosal surface is important. However, the bile duct is so small (normal diameter, 8 mm), and has no direct opening to the outside, that a double-contrast study using barium is not possible. We therefore use a water soluble contrast medium to fill up the duct for detecting filling defects. This does not permit diagnosis of superficial extension and depth of intramural invasion. For these reasons, the task of cholangiography is to detect the morphological alterations of the diseased wall, deviation of the wall from the longidutinal axis, irregularities, and sclerotic changes. It is necessary to change the patient's posture for more accurate interpretation. More recently, endoscopic US has come to be used for the same purpose (Mukai *et al.* 1992).

A non-epithelial tumor originating in the submucosal tissue of the bile duct and an infiltration from an adjoining organ leave the mucosal surface smooth for some time without protruding into the ductal lumen. However, if advanced, the mucosal surface is also affected and differential diagnosis from bile duct carcinoma becomes difficult.

Benign stenosis and obstruction of the bile duct is most frequently caused by bile duct stones (Case 6). It can be differentiated from carcinoma because, when studied by US, it is mobile, and the duct wall is clearly delineated. If it is calcified, CT can readily diagnose it. However, Mirizzi syndrome, in which the common bile duct is stenosed by inflammation due to stone impaction in the gallbladder neck and resulting compression, and the same syndrome associated with a gallbladder–bile duct fistula may require differential diagnosis from carcinoma (Becker *et al.* 1984) (Case 7). Postoperative common bile duct stenosis at the level of the cystic–common duct junction which was common in the past has decreased in recent years. Benign tumors such as neuroma arising at the division margin have been reported.

Primary sclerosing cholangitis (PSC) is one of the diseases characterized by bile duct inflammation and stenosis/obstruction due to fibrous tissue proliferation. It poses a diagnostic problem as it resembles scirrhous type bile duct carcinoma (Teefey *et al.* 1988), because the site of involvement can be at any site along the intra and extrahepatic biliary system with variable lengths of involvement, segmental or diffuse.

Bile duct carcinoma arises in patients with PSC during a long follow up (MacCarty *et al.* 1985). However, the incidence of PSC-associated bile duct carcinoma is far less in the Far East than in Western countries. Secondary sclerosing cholangitis has been increasing because of frequent long-standing hepatic artery catheterization for intraarterial injection of anticancer drugs (Botet *et al.* 1985; Pien *et al.* 1985). It commonly occurs in the hepatic ducts and in further peripheral ducts. The diagnosis is not difficult from the history of catheterization (cholangitis may also follow TAE). Bile duct stenosis due to a localized cholangitis can occur (Case 9). Differential diagnosis is difficult. Bile duct stenosis secondary to chronic pancreatitis may be diagnosed from medial displacement of the caudal portion of the common bile duct, smooth mucosal surface, a strangling feature of ductal stenosis, pancreatic duct sclerosis suggestive of inflammation, and absence of pancreatic tumor.

Therapy

Therapy for extrahepatic bile duct carcinoma includes surgery, biliary drainage (PTCD), intraductal irradiation using a small sealed source of radiation (^{192}Ir) (Akine *et al.* 1988), external irradiation (Todoroki *et al.* 1980), hyperthermia, and systemic chemotherapy. The only possible radical treatment is surgery. The results of resection for carcinomas of the midportion of the bile duct is generally good. For advanced bile duct carcinoma, biliary drainage by PTCD (Nakayama *et al.* 1978) and the use of a tube stent for internal fistulization (Lammer and Neumayer 1986) are yielding results comparable to those by surgery. There was a time when it was hoped that internal radiation through the PTCD drainage tube would be a hopeful non-invasive method, but it turned out to be otherwise, and is no longer widely used.

Extrahepatic bile duct carcinoma—Case 1: Carcinoma of the midportion of the bile duct causing portal vein stenosis (not operated).

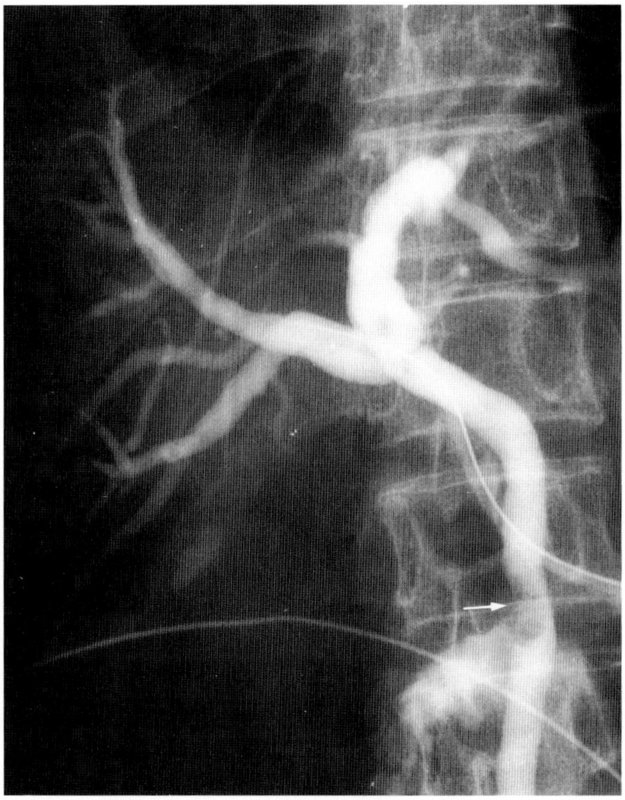

(a) Cholangiography through the PTCD tube: a 1.5 cm filling defect in the midportion of the bile duct and mild dilatation of the peripheral bile ducts are seen. From the linear sclerotic change along the duct wall (→) at the attachment of the mass, invasion across the muscle layer is expected. CT showed a 1.5 cm lymph node in the hilum, but no portal invasion was discerned.

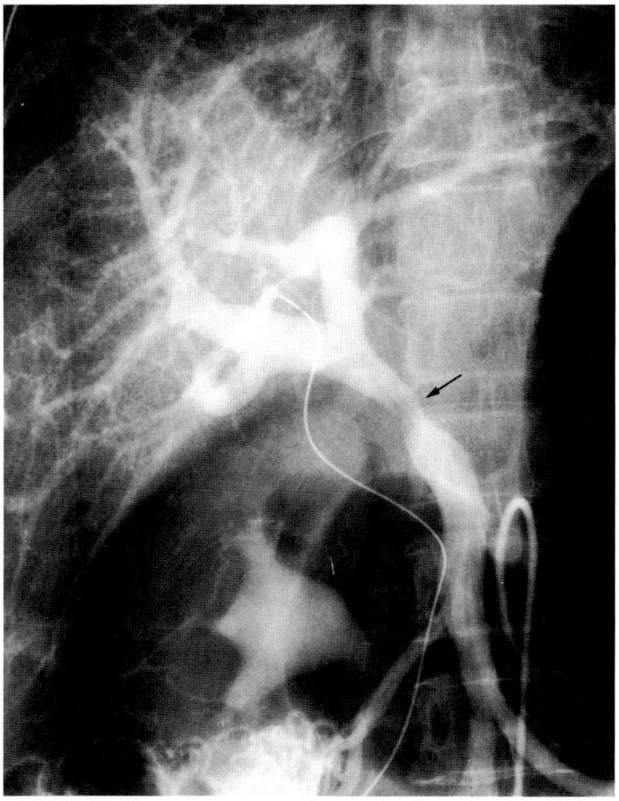

(b) Superior mesenteric arterial portogram: a circumferential stenosis (→) of the portal vein is evident. Compared with the cholangiogram, the portal vein stenosis is further cranial from the bile duct lesion for a distance of one vertebra, suggesting a widespread extramural invasion. The operation was called off. Autopsy disclosed a tumor mass involving the hepatic hilum, pancreas, duodenum, and stomach. Histologically, this was a poorly to moderately differentiated papillary adenocarcinoma.

Extrahepatic bile duct carcinoma—Case 2: Carcinoma of the middle to upper bile duct in which cholangio-CT and dynamic CT proved diagnostic differentiating carcinoma and a lymph node.

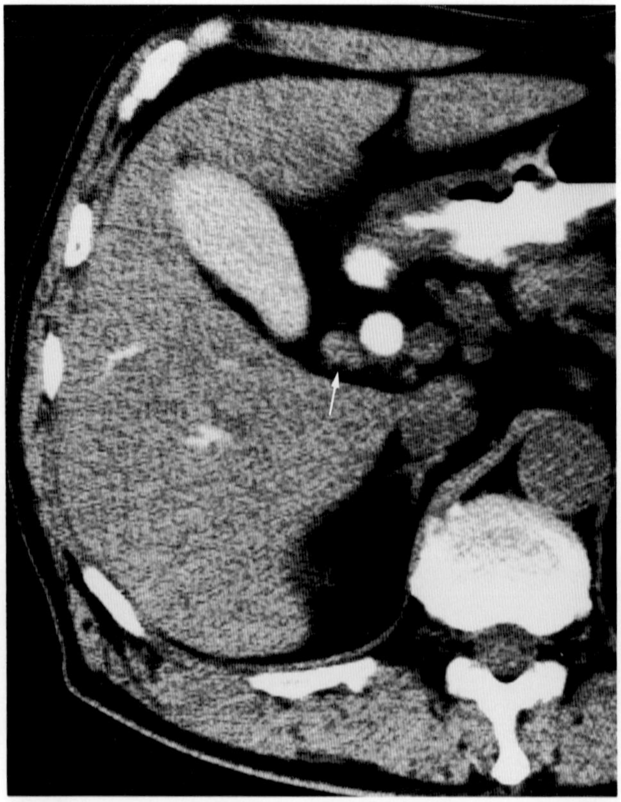

(a) Cholangio-CT through the PTCD tube: determination of the level of occlusion and identification of the gallbladder and cystic duct were possible, but quality diagnosis of a nodular structure (→) adjacent to the bile duct was difficult.

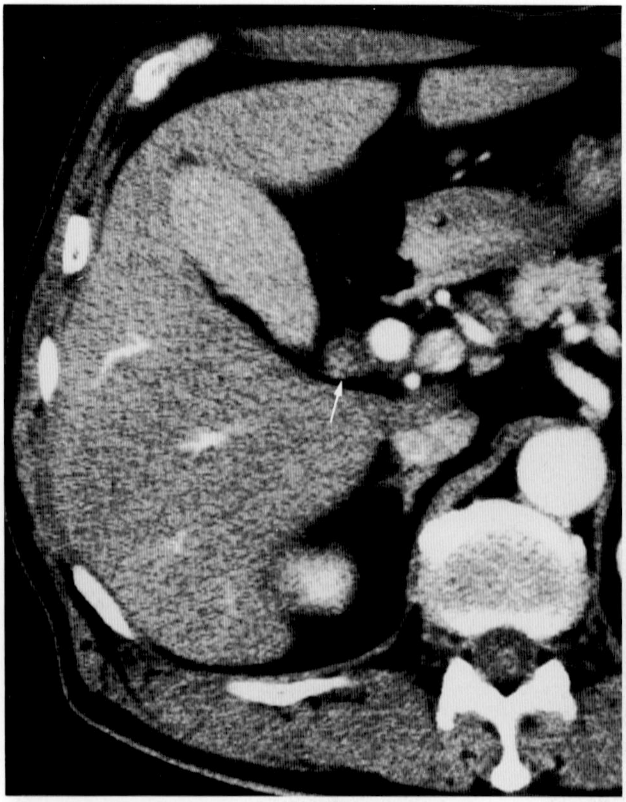

(b) Dynamic CT: cholangiography through the PTCD tube combined with dynamic CT was carried out. It identified not only the hepatic artery and portal vein, but also the nodule to the right of the bile duct as a swollen lymph node. During the operation, a swollen lymph node was found and taken out, but it did not contain cancer cells.

Extrahepatic bile duct carcinoma—Case 3: Carcinoma of the midportion of the bile duct detected in the absence of jaundice. A 72-year-old man. Abdominal pain led to the detection of bile duct stenosis by US and ERCP.

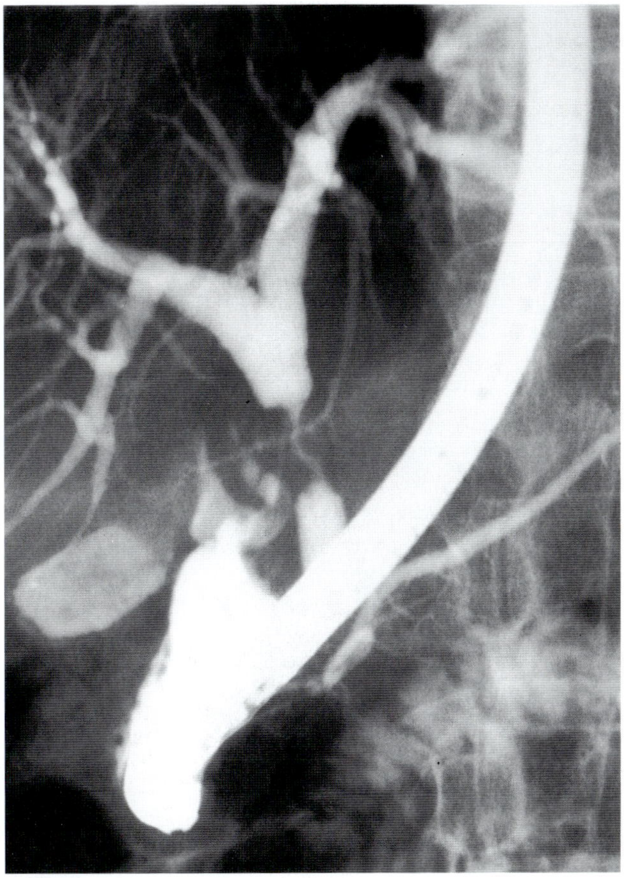

(a) ERCP: a 2 cm circumferential narrowing is seen in the midportion of the bile duct. This is a sharply elevated lesion with an irregular surface, and a diagnosis of carcinoma is possible. CT and angiography demonstrated no abnormalities.

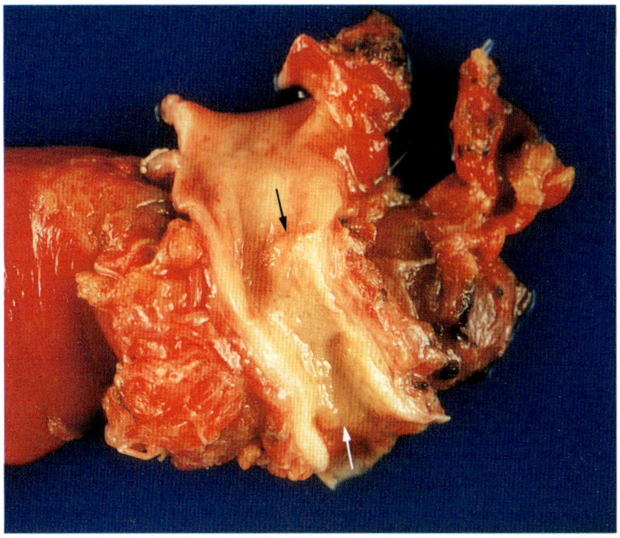

(b) Resected specimen: subtotal resection of the extrahepatic bile duct and cholecystectomy were carried out. There was a nodular infiltration spanning a length of 2.5 cm (→), which was a moderately to well differentiated adenocarcinoma. Part of the cystic duct was involved with serosal infiltration (s_2), but there was no lymph node metastasis. The patient is well 6 years postoperatively.

Extrahepatic bile duct carcinoma—Case 4: Malignant lymphoma primary to the bile duct. A 68-year-old woman presented with jaundice. The jaundice was alleviated by endoscopic retrograde biliary drainage (ERBD), and the drainage tube was extracted; she was doing well without jaundice.

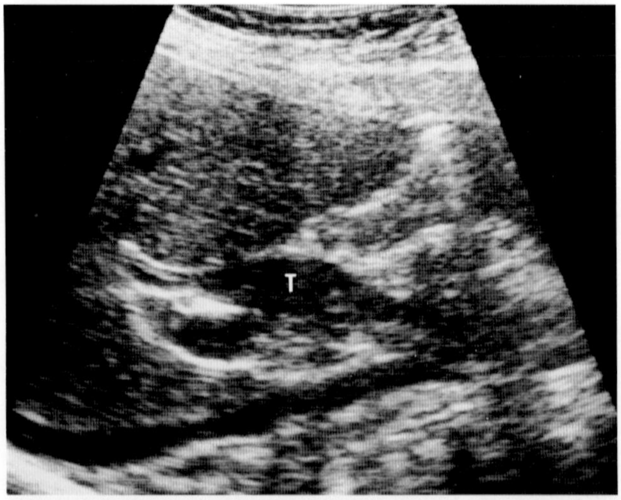

(a) US: a hypoechoic fusiform lesion (T) was seen as the bile duct wall disappeared while the transducer was slowly shifted from the hilum toward the duodenum along the bile duct. There was no dilatation of the peripheral ducts.

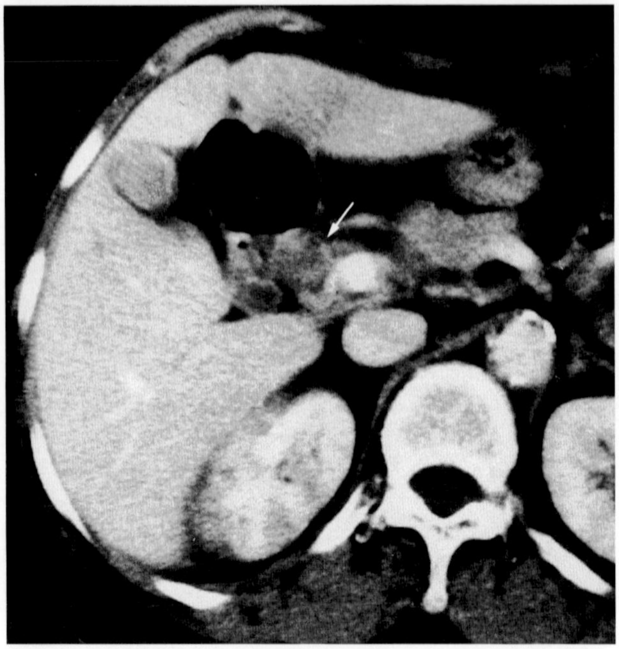

(b) Enhanced CT: a dilated bile duct is seen to the right of the portal vein. The gallbladder has shrunk.

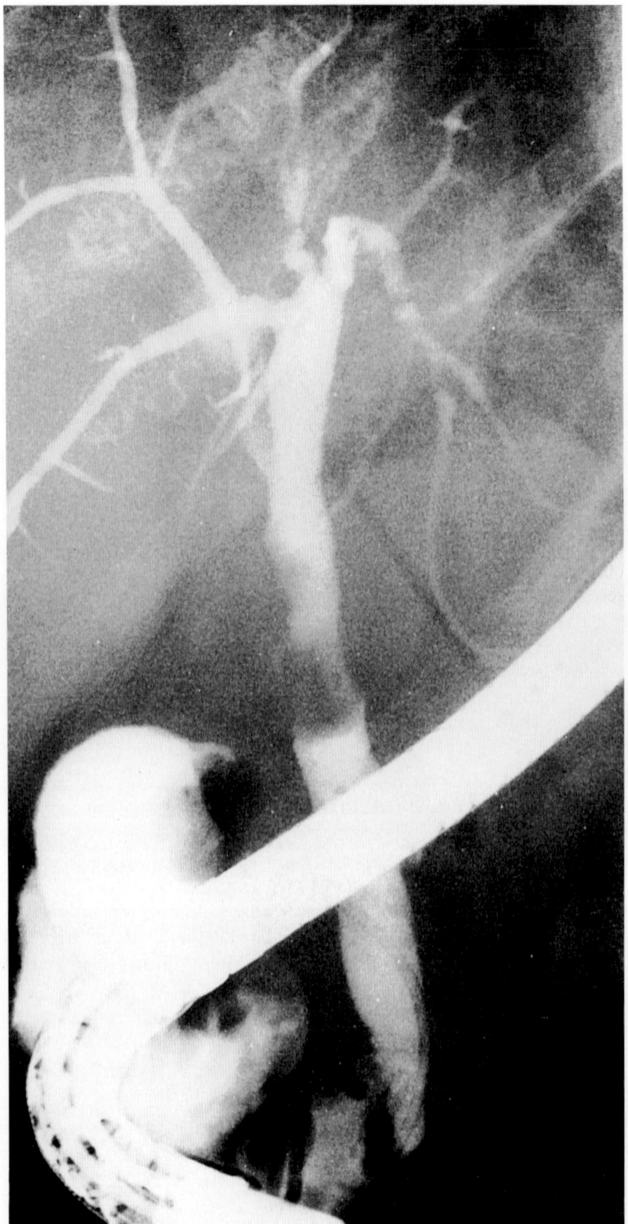

(c) ERC: a 1.2 cm circumferential filling defect is seen in the midportion of the bile duct. Angiography demonstrated no abnormality along the hepatic artery and portal vein. Cholecystectomy was carried out. A nodular lesion was protruding into the common bile duct, and occluding the lumen (2.5 cm). Histological study disclosed this to be a malignant B-cell lymphoma infiltrating onto the serosa.

Extrahepatic bile duct carcinoma—Case 5: Obstructive jaundice due to lymph node metastasis near the head of the pancreas after resection of gastric cancer.

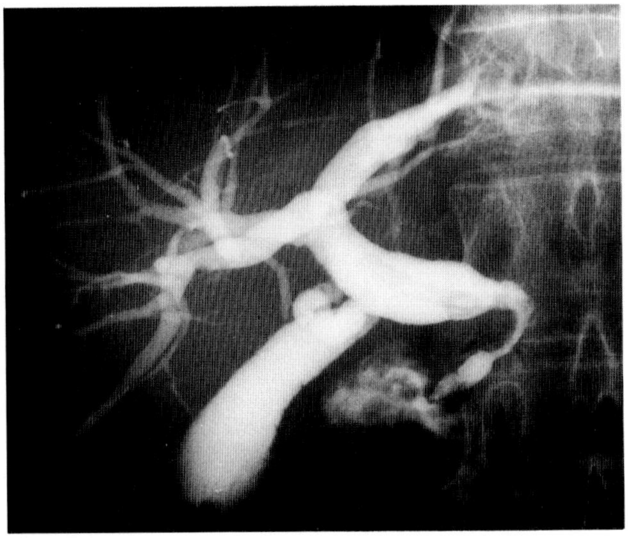

(a) Cholangiography made through PTCD tube: a marked stenosis is seen in the lower bile duct which is displaced to the left.

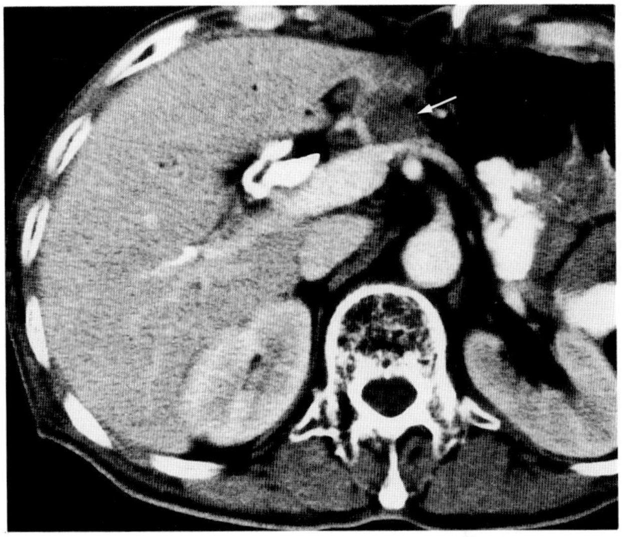

(b) Combined cholangiography through PTCD tube and dynamic CT: a stenosed common bile duct and an enlarged lymph node (→) near the duodenum are recognized. Further slices caudal to this section displayed a 4 cm conglomerate of lymph nodes.

Extrahepatic bile duct carcinoma—Case 6: Common bile duct stone.

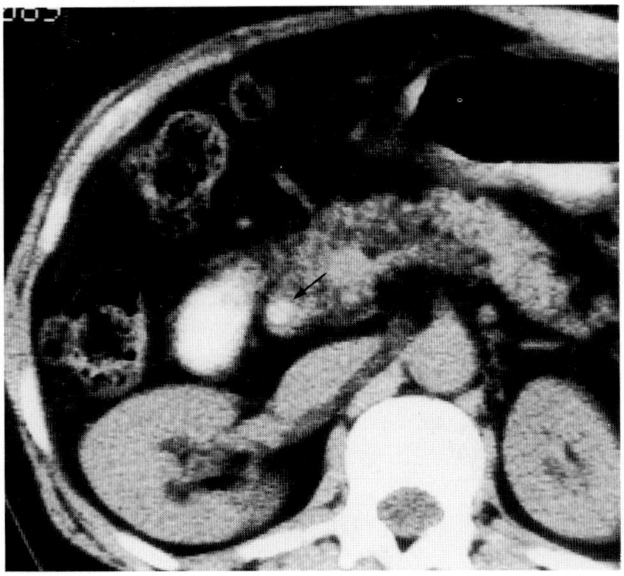

(a) Plain CT: a 1.5 cm calcific lesion (→) is seen at the end of the common bile duct near the duodenum. Mild dilatation of the intrahepatic bile ducts was recognized in the cranial slices. From the continuity of this lesion with the dilated choledochus, this was diagnosed as a choledochal stone.

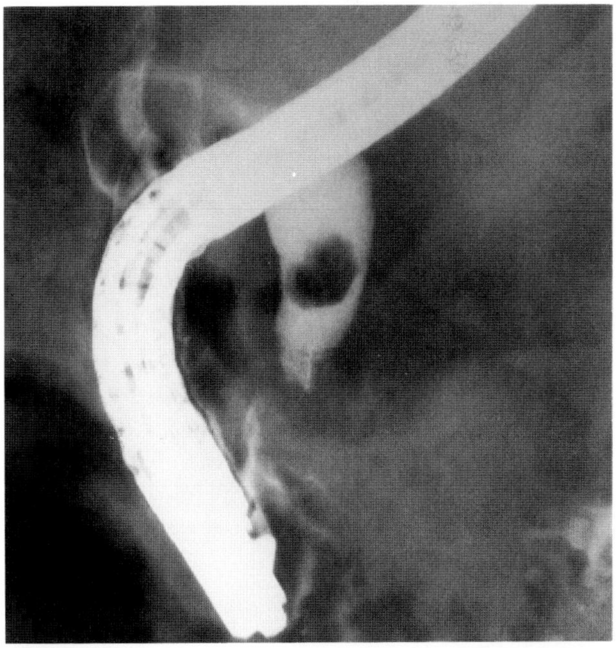

(b) ERC: a stone was demonstrated near the end of the common bile duct, and it was extracted following endoscopic papillotomy.

Extrahepatic bile duct carcinoma—Case 7: Mirizzi syndrome difficult to differentiate from bile duct carcinoma. A 64-year-old woman came to the hospital because of jaundice.

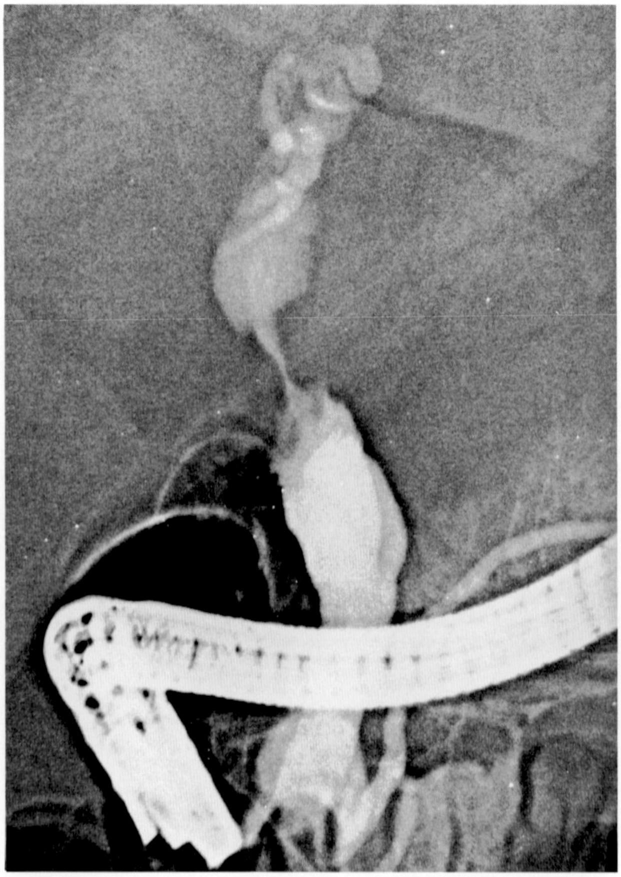

(a) ERC: a marked stenosis with an irregular filling defect is seen in the common bile duct.

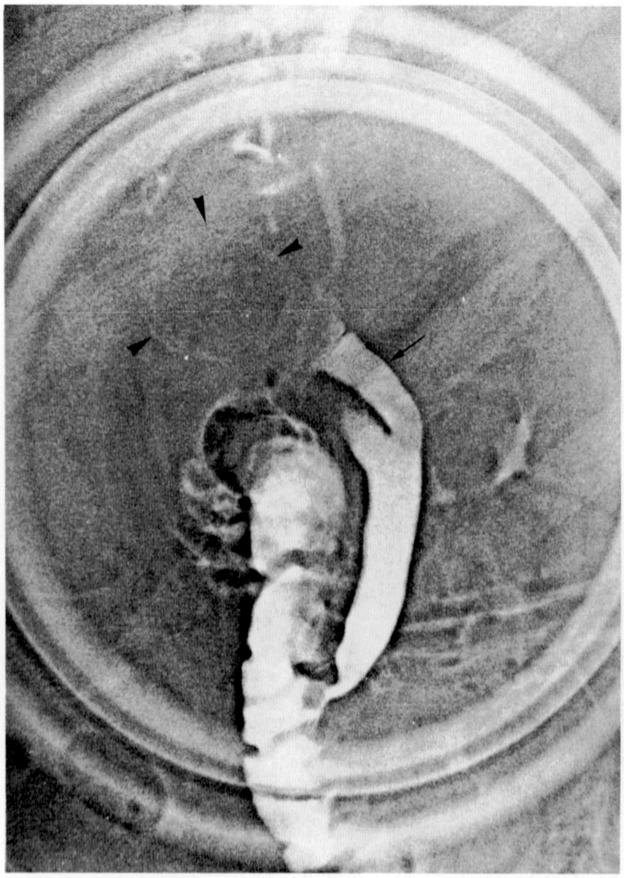

(b) ERC: in a different posture of the patient, the cystic duct →) and a faintly outlined gallbladder (▶) in its continuity are recognized. A diagnosis of associated gallstone disease was made.

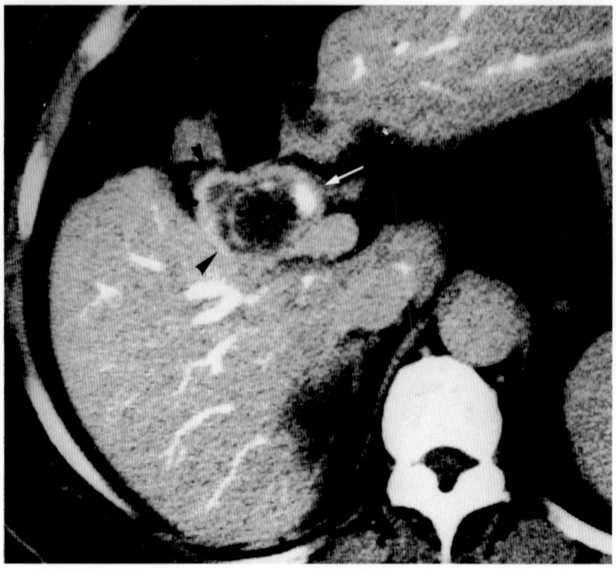

(c) Cholangiography through PTCD tube combined with enhanced CT: the gallbladder contains a radiolucent stone within a thickened wall (▶). The common bile duct (→) running in parallel with the stone is also identified. From the ERC findings, a bile duct carcinoma associated with cholecystolithiasis was strongly suspected.

At operation, the site of the stenosed bile duct was free of tumor invasion. There was a biliobiliary fistula between the atrophied gallbladder and the bile duct, and a stone was incarcerated in the cystic duct. The final diagnosis was Mirizzi syndrome.

Extrahepatic bile duct carcinoma—Case 8: Suspected primary sclerosing cholangitis. A 39-year-old man with jaundice

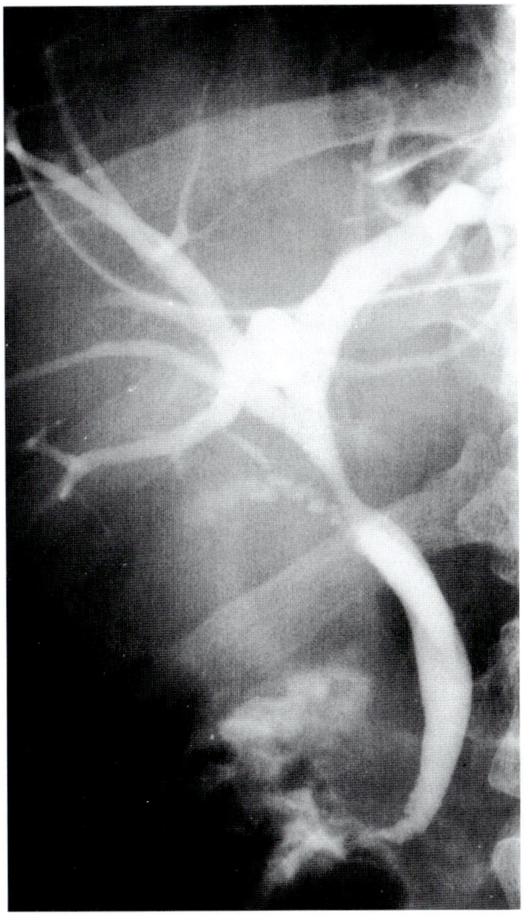

(a) Cholangiography through PTCD tube: there is a 3 cm stenosis involving the common hepatic and the right and left hepatic ducts. The duct wall is smooth with no recognizable filling defect. Angiography and CT were unremarkable. Partial resection of the liver and bile duct was carried out.

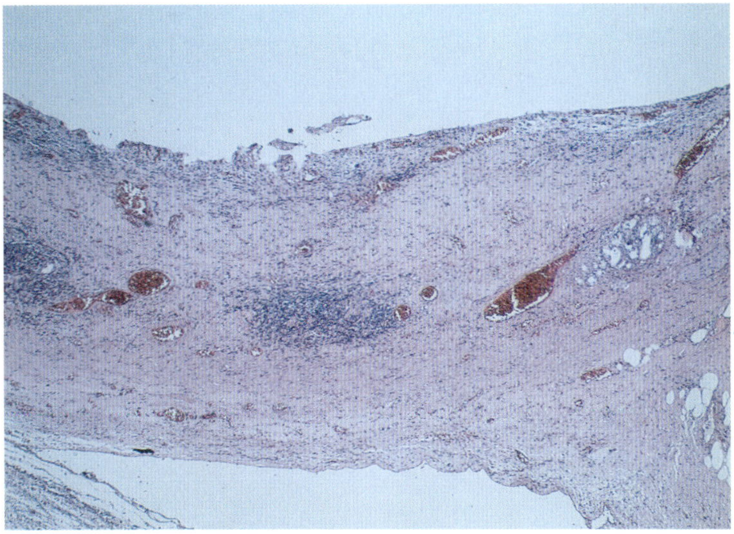

(b) Histopathology: the common hepatic duct and both hepatic ducts were stenosed with submucosally proliferating fibrous tissue and mild to moderate inflammatory cell infiltration. There were no cancer cells, and a diagnosis of probably primary sclerosing cholangitis was made. The patient had no associated ulcerative colitis.

Extrahepatic bile duct carcinoma—Case 9: Benign biliary stonosis difficult to differentiate from compression/stenosis due to lymph node metastasis from breast cancer. A 59-year-old woman. She underwent mastectomy 2 years earlier, and came to the hospital because of jaundice.

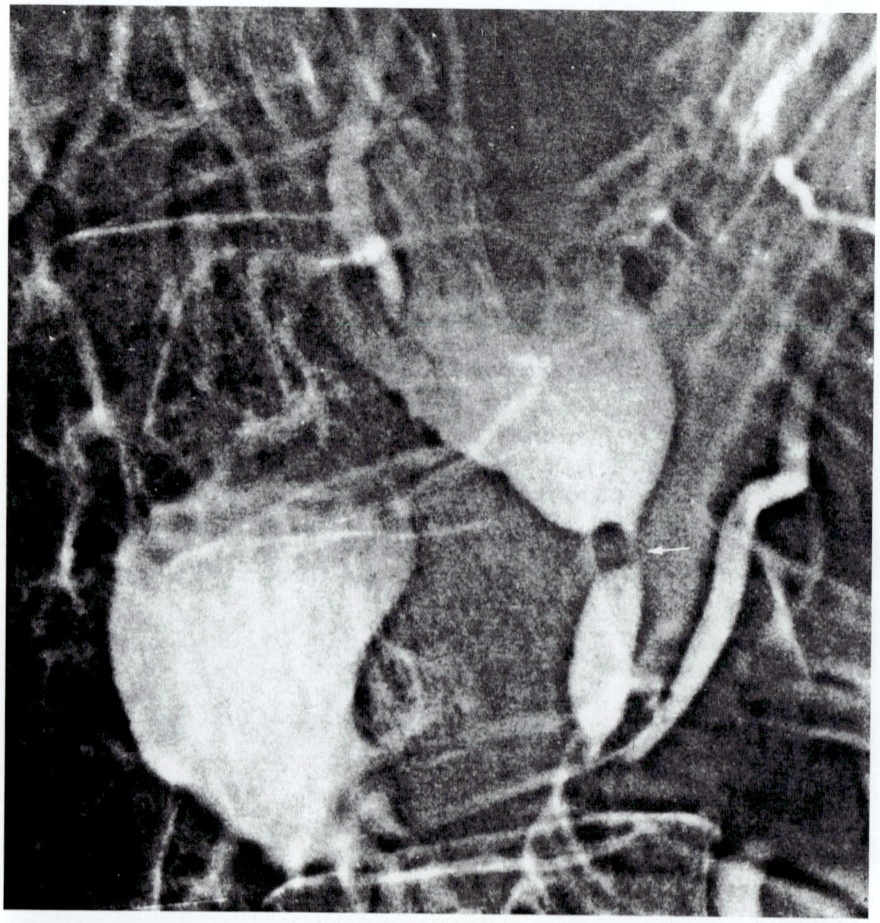

(a) ERCP: the common bile duct is markedly stenosed for a length of 5 mm (→) at a site 2 cm from its end. Since the pancreatic duct was normal, and judging from the smoothness of the stenosed wall, a compression exerted by a metastatic lymph node was suspected. CT, US, and angiography failed to demonstrate abnormalities suggestive of malignancy.

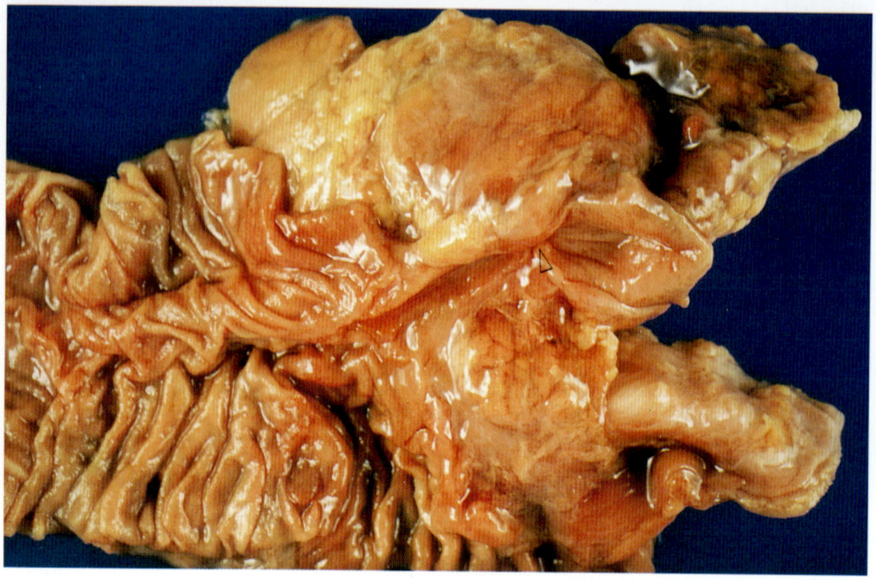

(b) Resected specimen: bile duct carcinoma could not be excluded, and pancreaticoduodenectomy was carried out. However, there were no malignant cells when studied histologically. The stenosed region of the bile duct was fibrosed with inflammation (▷). The patient is doing well without recurrence at 1.5 years postoperatively.

11

Portal hypertension

Portal hypertension encompasses a variety of disorders characterized by elevated portal venous pressure with altered portal hemodynamics. Table 11.1 lists various disorders that cause portal hypertension of which liver cirrhosis is the most frequent. Since more than 80 per cent of patients with HCC have underlying cirrhosis, one has to fully understand the pathophysiology of portal hypertension in order to determine the best treatment and to predict the prognosis. The evaluation of the velocity of portal venous flow, flow volume, and flow direction can now be made non-invasively by Doppler flowmetry along with the imaging delineation of portal systemic collateral routes.

The portal venous pressure in healthy adults is between 100 and 150 mmH_2O (setting the zero point at 10 cm from the posterior body surface). It increases as the resistance along the portal vein branches increases, and many institutes define portal hypertension as a pressure exceeding 200 mmH_2O. The flow volume in normal adults is estimated at 1000–1200 ml/min, whereas the measurement made by Doppler US was 889 ± 284 ml/min and flow velocity 15.3 ± 4.0 cm/s among the Japanese adults according to Moriyasu *et al.* (1983).

Table 11.1 Classification of portal hypertension based on etiology

Classification	Etiology, disease
1. Arterio-portal shunt	
Extrahepatic	Splenic artery aneurysm, iatrogenic (1)*, trauma, benign tumor (2), malignancy
Intrahepatic	Trauma, hepatic artery aneurysm (3), cirrhosis (4), iatrogenic (5), benign tumor, malignancy
2. Portal vein obliteration	
Extrahepatic	Malignancy, inflammation—pancreas (6), omphalitis, cirrhosis (7), iatrogenic-splenectomy (8, 9), idiopathic (10), congenital portal vein malformation
Intrahepatic (presinusoidal)	Schistosomiasis, sarcoidosis, amyloidosis, idiopatic (10), Hodgkin's disease, chronic myelogenous leukemia
3. Hepatic vein obliteration	
Intrahepatic (posthepatic)	Cirrhosis (11), veno-occlusive disease (VOD)
Extrahepatic	Budd–Chiari syndrome (primary, secondary), constrictive pericarditis, congestive heart disease

* Numbers in parentheses denote the case numbers in the text.

Classification of portal hypertension

The causes of portal hypertension may be classified into (1) arterio-portal shunting in which arterial blood flows into the portal vein, (2) stenotic or obliterative processes in the portal vein system, and (3) stenotic or obliterative processes in the hepatic vein system. The location of increased resistance may be divided into 'extrahepatic' and 'intrahepatic', and the latter 'presinusoidal', 'sinusoidal', and 'postsinusoidal'. The former is divided into 'prehepatic' and 'posthepatic'.

1. Arterio-portal shunt
(a) Extrahepatic: a shunt may form through a splenic artery aneurysm, as a result of ligation of vessels at the time of resection of an abdominal organ (Case 1), in association with a hemangiomatous change in the pancreas (Case 2), etc.
(b) Intrahepatic: a shunt may develop as a result of trauma to the liver, through an hepatic artery aneurysm (Takayasu *et al.* 1985*a*) (Case 3), due to cirrhosis (Case 4), needle biopsy, PTCD, PTC, etc. (Case 5) (Okuda *et al.* 1978), and a rare shunt may form in association with a benign neoplasm such as hemangioma, and a malignant neoplasm such as HCC and angiosarcoma.

2. Obliteration of the portal vein
(a) Extrahepatic: this frequently occurs in adults as a result of direct malignant invasion from the pancreas and stomach, and inflammation of the pancreas. Stomach cancer may cause a hepatopetal intraportal tumor invasion, though it is very rare (cf. Case 16 of intravascular HCC invasion). It may be due to thrombosis in a major (right first-order) portal branch in cirrhosis (Okuda *et al.* 1985*b*) (Case 7), thrombosis extending from the hilum into intrahepatic portal branches that follows splenectomy (Broe *et al.* 1981) (Cases 8 and 9), occlusion of the portal trunk without demonstrable cause, etc. Some children visit the hospital because of hematemesis, a chief complaint; they have portal vein trunk occlusion and subsequent formation of cavernous transformation that followed infection, such as omphalitis and appendicitis.
(b) Intrahepatic: this is called prehepatic or presinusoidal, and is caused by narrowing of the portal venules as a result of inflammation and fibrosis of the portal tract and portal venous wall. Typical examples are schistosomiasis (japonica, mansoni), sarcoidosis, amyloidosis (Suzuki *et al.* 1976), and idiopathic portal hypertension (IPH) (Okuda *et al.* 1984*a*) (Case 10). For the differential diagnosis of these disorders, needle biopsy is required. Hemodynamically, wedged hepatic venous pressure is significantly lower than portal venous presure.

3. Obliteration of the hepatic vein
(a) Intrahepatic: this is caused by hepatic vein obstruction or narrowing (postsinusoidal), typically seen in alcoholic cirrhosis

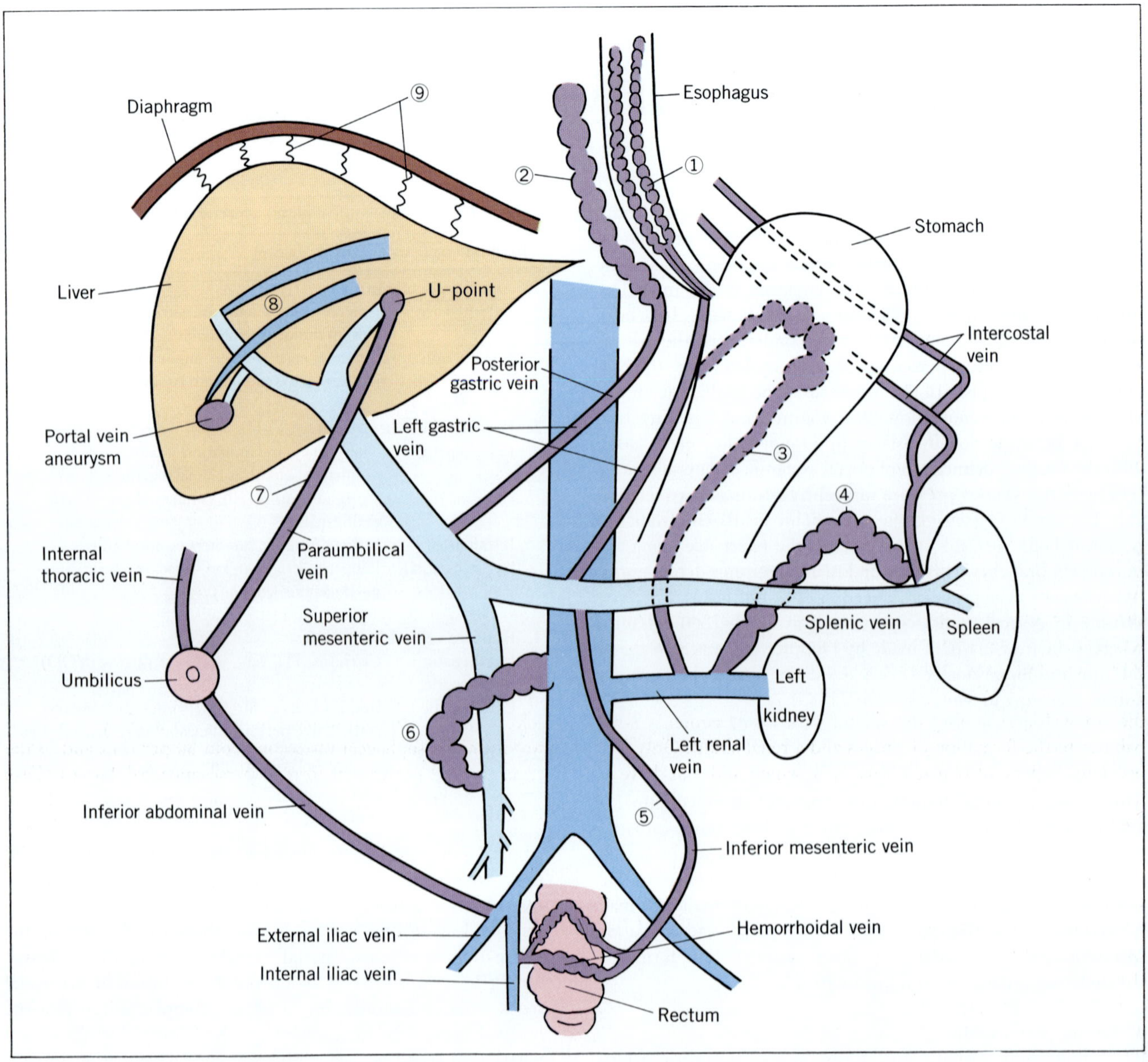

Fig. 11.1 Schematic representation of various extrahepatic and intrahepatic portal-system shunting routes: (1) left gastric-esophageal varices; (2) left gastric-paraesophageal and esophageal varices; (3) posterior gastric-renal vein; (4) splenic-renal vein; (5) inferior mesenteric-hemorrhoidal-internal iliac vein; (6) superior mesenteric vein-inferior vena cava (meso-caval); (7) paraumbilical-inferior abdominal wall vein or internal thoracic vein; (8) intrahepatic portal-hepatic vein; (9) Sappey's veins.

in which fibrosis around the central vein (perivenular fibrosis) and perisinudoidal fibrosis are the prominent histological features. Compression by regenerative nodules upon sublobular veins that lack protective fibrous sheaths and are vulnerable to external pressure increases resistance in these veins (Case 11). As the cirrhotic process progresses, arteries and portal veins gradually undergo morphologic alterations. Long-term use of Jamaican bush tea (which contains pyrrolizidine alkaloids) produces centrilobular necrosis, inflammation, and endophlebitits of the central vein (veno-occlusive disease, VOD). Hepatomegaly and ascites ensue. This is extremely rare in Japan. In cirrhosis and VOD, wedged hepatic vein pressure and portal vein pressure are close to each other, unlike presinusoidal portal hypertension.

(b) Extrahepatic: a typical case is obstruction of the inferior vena cava (IVC), the so called membranous obstruction of the IVC, in its hepatic portion. As will be discussed in the next chapter, this is endemic in certain global regions, and the cause is unclear. Classical Budd–Chiari syndrome in the western countries in which large intrahepatic hepatic veins are thrombosed, may be regarded intrahepatic as well as extrahepatic as far as the location is concerned. Secondary Budd–Chiari syndrome may be caused by a neoplasm arising in the liver and the kidney, compressing upon the IVC. The patient presents with ascites, hepatomegaly and abdominal pain. Constrictive pericarditis and right-side heart failure produce similar clinical features as will be discussed subsequently.

Spontaneous reversal of portal venous flow

Retrograde flow within the intrahepatic portal veins (hepatofugal portal outflow) is a common occurrence following portacaval shunt. However, whether spontaneous retrograde flow would occur within the major portal vein had long been disputed until we demonstrated several such cases by direct portography in patients with advanced cirrhosis (Okuda *et al.* 1973*b*; Moreno *et al.* 1975; Takayasu *et al.* 1982*b*). The frequency of spontaneous retrograde portal flow studied by PTP was 1 per cent among cirrhotics in our hands.

Portal systemic shunting route

As portal venous pressure increases, a variety of portal systemic shunting routes develop (Fig. 11.1), some contributing to the formation of esophageal varices. We studied these collaterals by PTP and demonstrated that not only the left gastric and short gastric veins, but a distinct vein draining the posterior wall of the stomach and joining the splenic vein also frequently contributes to the formation of varices and a renal shunt. Only few previous papers recognized this vein which did not have a name; we called this the 'posterior gastric vein' (Kimura *et al.* 1990). Of the 414 cases studied, 181 (42 per cent) had a distinct posterior gastric vein, and the frequency of this vein forming esophageal varices was 81 per cent and a left renal shunt 23 per cent. The so-called coronary vein depicted in old anatomy textbooks was never recognized. Clearly, the right and the left gastric veins do not form a loop along the lesser curvature of the stomach.

Other large shunting routes include the paraumbilical vein, left renal shunts arising along the splenic vein, inferior mesenteric hemorrhoidal vein, etc. Most of them bypass the liver. However, hemodynamic studies clearly show the presence of intrahepatic shunting (Ueda *et al.* 1967; Okuda *et al.* 1977*g*), but imaging seldom delineates intrahepatic shunting, except for opacification of the hepatic vein during portal venography.

There are a number of disorders that cause portal hypertension, but the collateral routes are random, unrelated to the cause of portal hypertension. The calibers of collateral routes increase up to a certain point with rising portal venous pressure, but thereafter portal venous pressure seems to decline somewhat because of the dilatation of the collaterals and reduced resistance (Ohnishi *et al.* 1985*a*). Sustained portal hypertension despite enlarging collaterals is explained by increased blood flow within the abdomen (hyperdynamic circulation) with increased cardiac output. In our study, shown in Table 11.2, each patient had at least one major shunting route, and conversely the majority of patients having a major collateral route had portal venous pressure greater than 200 mmH_2O. Therefore, if a hepatofugal collateral vein is demonstrable by one of the imaging modalities, the diagnosis of portal hypertension can be made indirectly without pressure measurement.

Table 11.2 Frequencies of major portosystemic shunts studied by PTP in 460 patients with portal hypertension

Type of shunt	Frequency (%)
Left gastric vein → esophageal and paraesophageal varices	76
renal shunt	12
Posterior gastric vein → esophageal varices	81*
renal shunt	23*
Short gastric vein → esophageal varices	84*
renal shunt	18*
Paraumbilical vein → internal thoracic, lower abdominal wall vein	24
Splenic → renal shunt	35
Others (inferior mesenteric vein → hemorrhoidal vein, etc)	4

* They add up to more than 100 per cent, because both coexist.

Left gastric vein

As shown in Table 11.2, this is an important collateral because it frequently feeds esophageal varices (Case 13). When this vein was selectively catheterized in patients with portal hypertension, it was forming esophageal varices in about 80 per cent and in the remaining 20 per cent it formed paraesophageal varices (Case 14) which do not rupture, or a renal shunt (Case 15). Some collateral goes into the pulmonary vein (Sano *et al.* 1982). Of the 414 cases in whom the cephalad extension of the esophageal and paraesophageal varices was opacified, contrast medium was drained into the azygos vein in 228 (55 per cent) and into the subclavian brachiocephalic vein in 166 (40 per cent). Histoanatomically, the left gastric vein commonly crosses the esophagogastric junction in a bundle of thin veins. On the venogram, they are seen running in parallel (parallel pattern) (Takashi *et al.* 1985*b*), and this area is called the palisade zone (Vianna *et al.* 1987). They are distinguished from paraesophageal collaterals. These veins in the lamina propria coalesce in the submucosa after crossing the muscularis mucosae in the lower esophagus to form large winding varices. This area is frequently the site of rupture and is called the critical zone (Arakawa and Kage 1987). In some others, one or two large varicose veins cross the esophagogastric junction, and Hashizume et al (1988) called it a bar type against the former type which they called the palisade type. Paraesophageal varices (Case 14) often form a large varix in the mediastinum or around the heart (Takayasu *et al.* 1982*a*), sometimes requiring differential diagnosis from malignant lymph node metastasis by a CT study. The left gastric vein can be identified by CT, and in the hands of skilled ultrasonographers, the flow direction and velocity may be determined by Doppler US. For the opacification of the gastric varices, selective left gastric arteriography (Ariyama *et al.* 1978) (Case 16) and enhanced CT (Balthazar *et al.* 1987) may prove useful.

Posterior gastric vein
This vein drains the posterior aspect of the stomach and enters the splenic vein between the left gastric and the short gastric (Kimura *et al.* 1990). Normally, this vein is indistinct and had no name previously, but in portal hypertension it is somehow frequently enlarged and participates in the formation of esophageal and gastric varices, and of a renal shunt (Table 11.2). Because it is located closer to the kidney than is the left gastric, it more often forms a shunt with the left renal vein than do other veins.

Paraumbilical vein
This vein originates in the umbilical portion of the left portal vein, traverses through the medial aspect of the left lobe (S^{IV}) and the falciform ligament where the umbilical vein existed during fetal life, toward the umbilicus. After reaching the umbilicus, it runs immediately beneath the peritoneum either cephalad into the internal thoracic vein or caudad into the veins in the lower abdominal wall, eventually draining into the vena cava (Case 18). Dilated veins radiating from the umbilicus called *caput medusae*, a term derived from Greek mythology, were considered as a classical sign of portal hypertension. However, this clinical feature is very uncommon and more often one large vein is seen emerging to the surface near the umbilicus. One often auscultates a venous hum or feels a vibration (Cruveilhier-Baumgarten syndrome) (Ohkubo *et al.* 1978). Although the original description of this syndrome was an anomalous umbilical vein circulation due to failed closure of the umbilical vein at the time of birth, the vast majority of *caput medusae* cases are due to portal hypertension and an enlarged paraumbilical vein. Once closed the umbilical vein never reopens, and the collateral running along the closed umbilical vein is the paraumbilical. A large paraumbilical vein may be mistaken for an hepatic malignancy on scintigraphy (Takayasu *et al.* 1983) (Case 19) or dynamic CT (Case 20). It can be studied well by US (Case 21) and Doppler US; the course is not always straight and is sometimes winding within the liver. It should not be mistaken for a small hepatic lesion (cf. Fig. 17.1, p.451).

Spleno-gastro-renal shunt
This collateral route mainly involves the short gastric, posterior gastric, and left gastric veins, and may be called gastro-renal shunt. However, the exact origin is rarely identified on imaging and for practical purposes, it has been called spleno-renal shunt because winding veins are seen near the splenic hilum readily identified by US (Takayasu *et al.* 1984*c*). It often reaches a large caliber and causes hepatofugal flow of a large volume of blood coming from the superior mesenteric vein otherwising going into the portal vein. It may contribute to a lowering of the portal venous pressure (Ohnishi *et al.* 1984*a*; Okuda et al 1984*a*), as does Warren's distal splenorenal shunt. We have seen cases in whom esophageal varices disappeared after formation of a large renal shunt. It also contributes to the development of portal systemic encephalopathy. When we compared 7 cases with repeated encephalopathy and 12 non-encephalopathic cases of portal hypertension, the average size of the shunt was 17.6 ± 5.0 mm in the former and 5.5 ± 3.5 mm in the latter (Takashi *et al.* 1985). In the presence of a large renal shunt, the left gastric vein seldom forms esophageal varices as shown in Table 11.3; only one of the 7 encephalopathic with a large renal shunt had esophageal varices, which were mild.

Other collaterals
Other collateral routes which are less common include one from the superior mesenteric vein to the IVC (meso-caval) through the Retzius veins with (Case 23) or without varix formation, from the portal trunk to the IVC (Case 24), from the superior mesenteric to the hemiazygos (very rare) (Case 25), from the inferior iliac through hemorrhoidal veins to the IVC (Case 26), etc. Hemorrhoids and colonic varices are rather common in portal hypertension (Saitoh *et al.* 1989) because of the last mentioned route.

Intrahepatic shunts develop as a result of extensive structural disorganization of the lobules in cirrhosis. Radiocolloid particles instilled within the portal vein at the hilum are transported through such shunts to be trapped in the lung (Okuda *et al.* 1977*g*), and on portography the hepatic vein is opacified in an early phase (Ohnishi *et al.* 1985*b*) (Case 18). It is not uncommon to see an opacified hepatic vein in the late phase of portography, however. Intrahepatic portal veins may communicate with the hepatic vein through a portal vein aneurysm (Takayasu *et al.* 1984*d*) (Case 27).

In cirrhosis, intrahepatic portal vein branches become smaller, hardened, and more linear, and branching is reduced as seen on the portogram (Case 29), clearly contrasted by the normal portogram (Case 28). As the right lobe increasingly shrinks, the spatial relationship between the right anterior and posterior segments is altered, and they tend to separate, the former shift-

Table 11.3 Clinical characteristics of seven cases of portal hypertension with encephalopathy

Age/sex	Disease	Varices	GI-bleed	Encephalopathy	NH_3 (μg/dl)
52/M	Cirrhosis	Cardiac	—	+, 4 years	200
47/M	Cirrhosis	Esophageal, minimal	—	+, 1 year	278
46/F	Cirrhosis	Cardiac	—	+, 2 years	240
59/M	Cirrhosis	No	—	+, 2 years	170
59/M	IPH*	Cardiac	—	+, 1 year	205
50/M	IPH	No	—	+, 20 years	209
46/M	Budd–Chiari	No	—	+, 2 years	149

* Idiopathic Portal Hypertension.

ing cranially and latter caudally, with little overlapping in the anterior view. The left lateral area and the caudate lobe undergo hypertrophy in compensation.

MR imaging in portal hypertension

Various collateral vessels that have developed in portal hypertension can be demonstrated as signal free structures owing to flow void (Bradley and Waluch 1985). If the blood flow is very slow, however, a paradoxical enhancement with increased signal is demonstrated. Both slow blood flow and tumor or bland thrombus appear as increased signal intensity in the vessel. These can be differentiated by means of the dual-echo technique; the signal intensity due to slow blood flow increases on the second echo (Waluch and Bradley 1984), and the signal intensity due to a thrombus decreases (Bradley and Waluch 1985). Gradient echo pulse sequence is another option to define the differences; slow blood flow is hyperintense and thrombus is hypointense.

MR angiography with the time-of-flight technique is a non-invasive diagnostic tool which depicts the venous and portal system in the abdomen (Edelman *et al.* 1989). The new MR angiography using fast spoiled GRASS (gradient recalled steady state) images is available to shorten the examination time (Murakami *et al.* 1994). Portal systemic collaterals can be imaged without contrast medium.

Therapy

The most serious complication of portal hypertension is bleeding, more frequently from esophageal varices than from gastric varices. Bleeding from the gastric mucosa is also frequent due to portal hypertensive gastropathy, accounting for nearly one-half of all upper GI bleedings (Baxter and Dobbs 1988). For the prevention of variceal bleeding, various surgical procedures are employed such as selective shunt operations [distal splenorenal (Warren *et al.* 1967), left gastric-vena caval (Inokuchi *et al.* 1984), meso caval, etc.], and non-shunting operations (transthoracic and transabdominal eshophageal transection (Sugiura and Futagawa 1984), Hassab operation, etc.). More recently, non-surgical techniques have been developed such as percutaneous transhepatic obliteration using the PTP technique (PTO) (Lundquist and Vang 1974; Okuda *et al.* 1982*b*) (Case 30), endoscopic sclerotherapy (Terblanche et al 1979; Westaby *et al.* 1989) (Case 31), and ligation (Van Stiegmann *et al.* 1986) (banding), transjugular intrahepatic portal venous shunt (TIPS) (Colapinto *et al.* 1982; Lossle *et al.* 1992), etc.

Earlier expectations of PTO turned to disappointment because of frequent recurrence and rebleeding of varices, and a risk of embolisim of the lung and brain. The exact indications for TIPS have not been established, although if successfully carried out, varices and ascites disappear immediately. The venous-portal anastomosis may be thrombosed or occluded requiring reshunting. Sclerotherapy involves injection of a sclerosing agent into varices which sometimes passes into the portal vein and the superior mesenteric vein to cause complications (Seidman *et al.* 1984; Deboever *et al.* 1989). The ligation method, which has no such complication, is gaining in popularity.

In patients with HCC and esophageal varices, surgical treatment of varices is not commonly done in Japan, and more often endoscopic sclerotherapy is carried out prior to resection. For HCC patients with hypersplanism due to splenomegaly, a two-step approach is usually made in Japan, namely splenectomy combined with Hassab operation followed by hepatic resection.

Portal hypertension—Case 1: Extrahepatic arterio-portal shunt developing after total gastrectomy. This patient underwent total gastrectomy for gastric cancer 2 years earlier, and came to the hospital complaining of postprandial precordial distress.

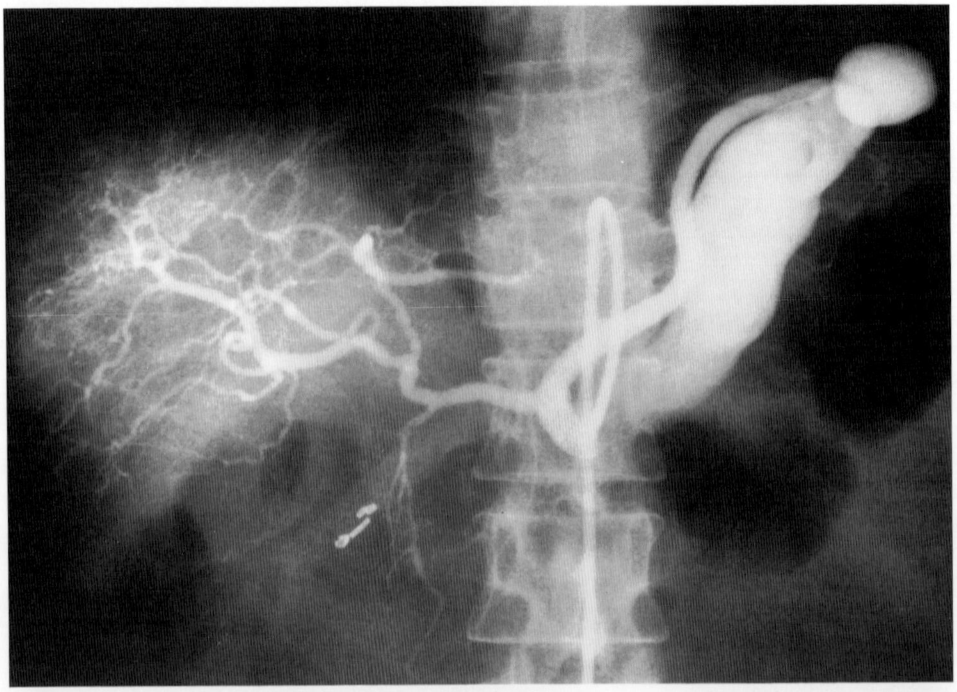

(a) Celiac arteriogram (early phase): an aneurysmal dilation of the vessel at the end of the splenic artery and a markedly dilated splenic vein are seen.

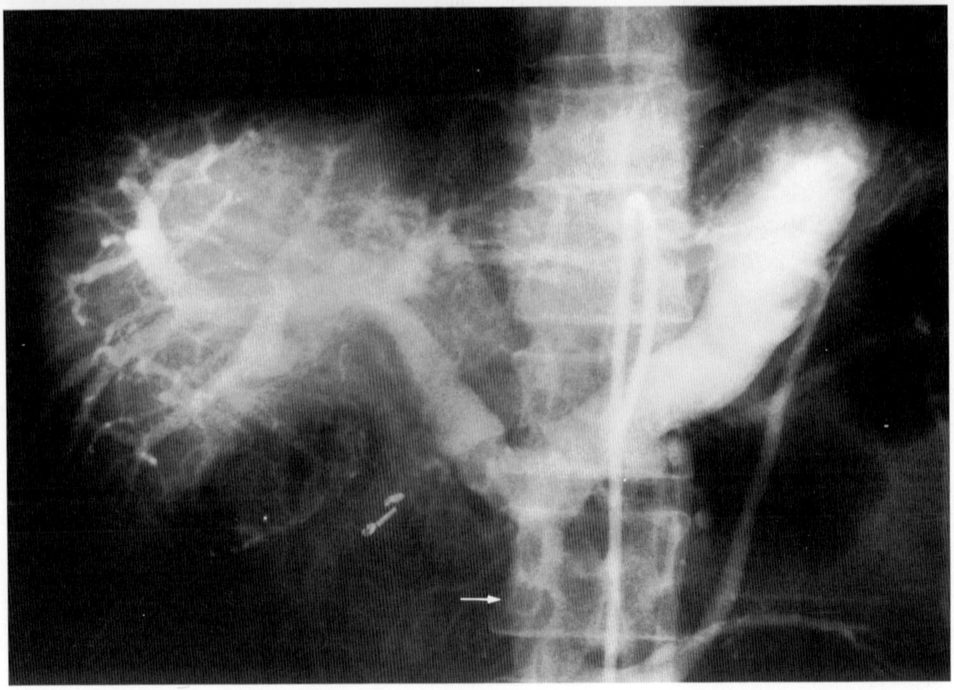

(b) Celiac arteriogram (late phase): the splenic vein is flowing hepatopetally in the portal vein as well as hepatofugally into the superior mesenteric vein (→).

Portal hypertension—Case 2: Extrahepatic arterio-portal shunt (congenital) in the body of the pancreas. This patient came to the hospital because of cirrhosis and esophageal varices.

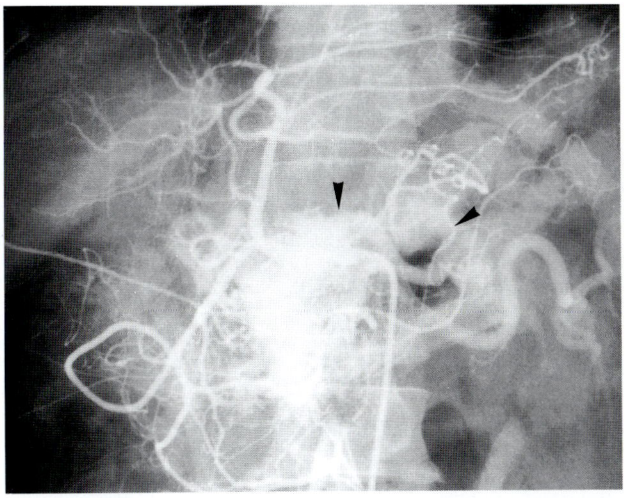

a

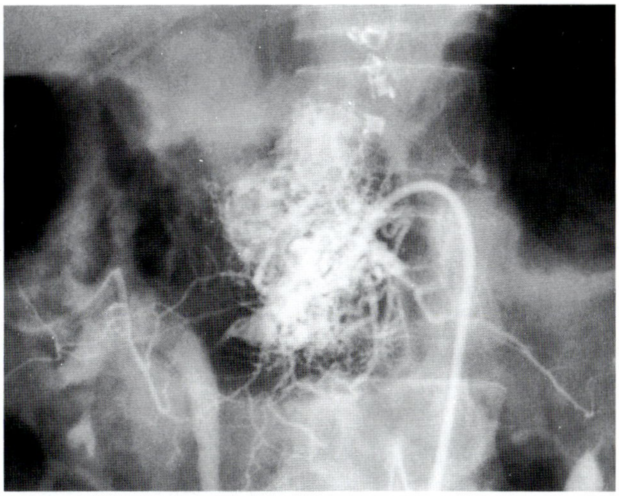

b

(a) Celiac arteriogram (early phase): An irregularly shaped pooling of contrast medium was first seen in the body of the pancreas. It was followed by opacification of the superior mesenteric vein and then the splenic vein (▶).

(b) Selective dorsal pancreatic arteriography: numerous dilated arteries and their anastomoses are seen in the body of the pancreas and its vicinity.

(c) PTP (catheter tip in the portal trunk): retrograde flow of the splenic vein (→) and a huge gastro-renal shunt are obvious.

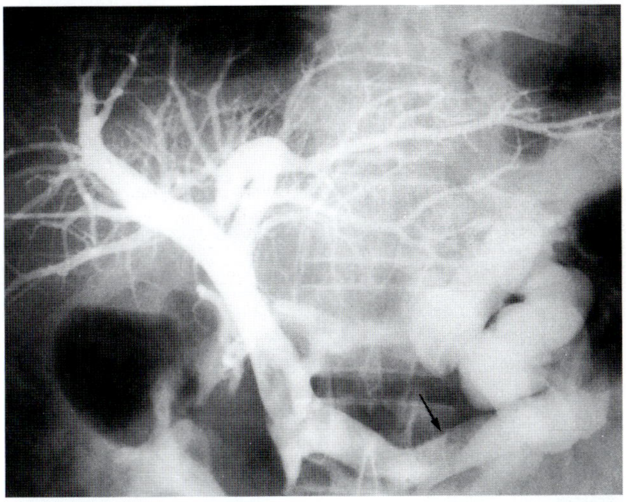

c

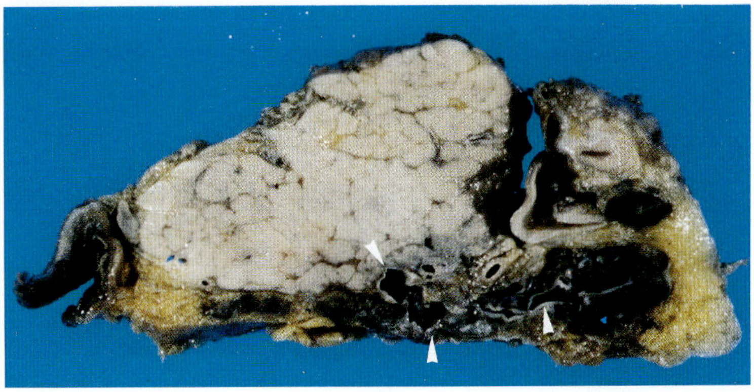

(d) Section of the pancreas at autopsy: esophageal transection combined with splenectomy was carried out for varices, but the patient eventually died of hepatic failure. Autopsy revealed multiple dilated vascular lumina (▶) in the dorsal aspect of the head and body of the pancreas.

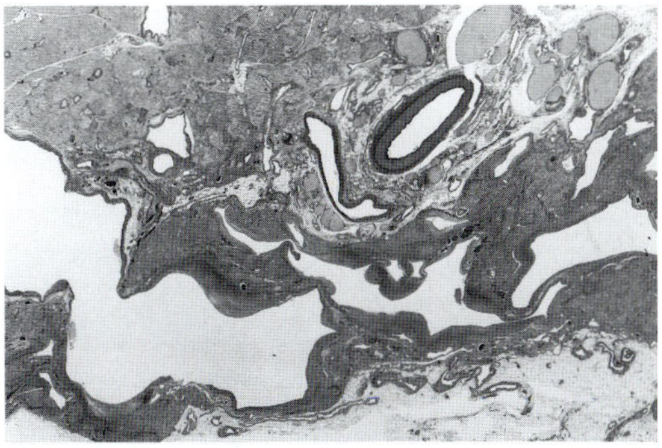

(e) Histology: the vascular lumina consisted of dilated blood vessels lined by thickened endothelium. It was assumed that these vessels caused communications between the pancreatic artery and vein, and blood therefrom flowed into the portal vein. The liver was cirrhotic.

Portal hypertension—Case 3: Intrahepatic arterio-portal shunt through an aneurysm of the hepatic artery. This patient with advanced cirrhosis underwent endoscopic sclerotherapy and splenectomy several years earlier for variceal bleeding. No history of trauma.

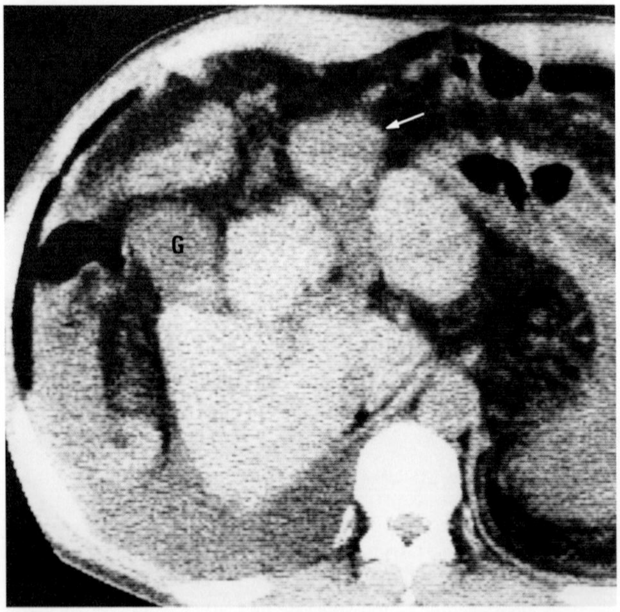

(a) Plain CT: the liver is markedly shrunk. A tumor-like lesion (→) is seen in the area corresponding to the falciform ligament. G, gallbladder.

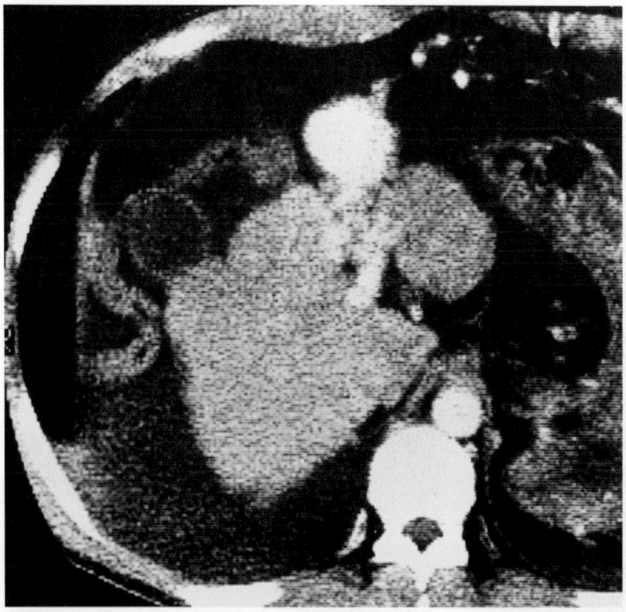

(b) Dynamic CT (early phase): the tumorus lesion and the main portal vein of the left lobe were opacified.

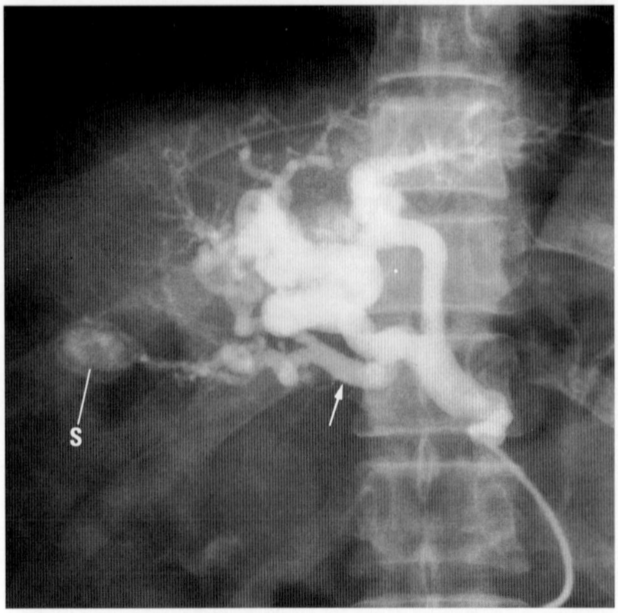

(c) Hepatic arteriogram (early phase): dilated middle and left hepatic arteries were opacified. S, gallstone: →, right hepatic artery

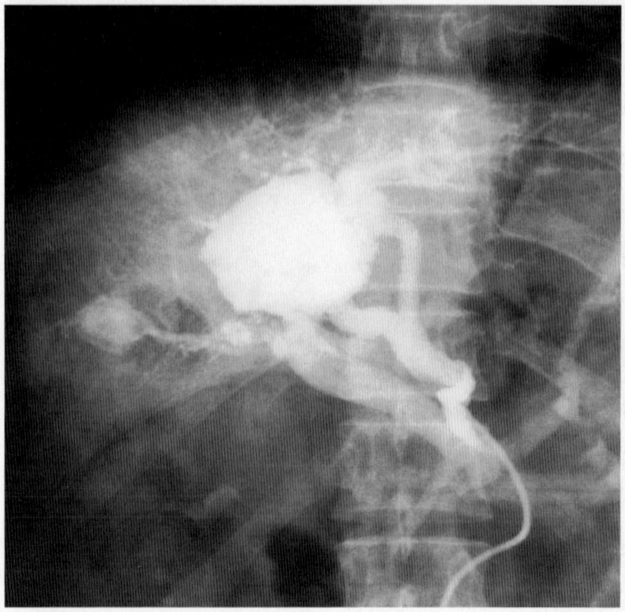

(d) Hepatic arteriogram [1.5 s after (c)]: contrast medium flowed retrogradely into the portal vein through a dilated vessel (aneurysm).

Portal hypertension—Case 4: Intrahepatic arterio-portal shunt associated with cirrhosis. This patient underwent cholecystectomy for gallbladder carcinoma, and during the follow-up, she developed ascites and an abnormal lesion in S^{VIII}. She entered hospital for suspected hepatic metastasis of gallbladder carcinoma.

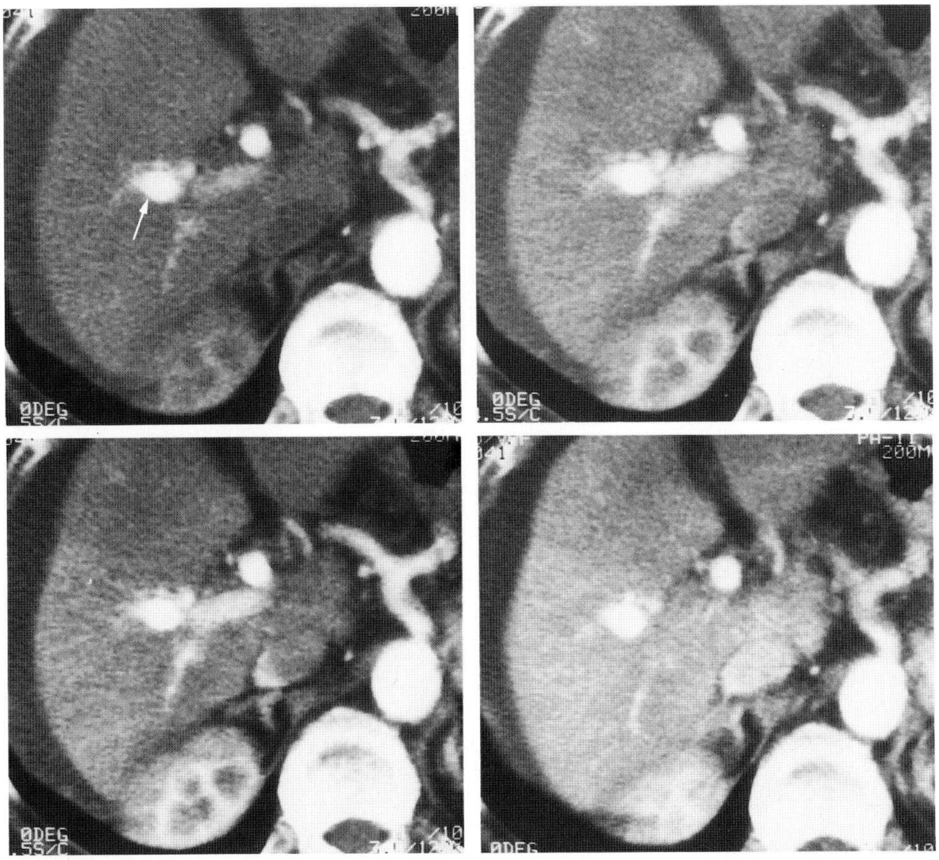

(a) Dynamic CT (same slice level): a dilated portal vein branch (→) was opacified in an early phase (1, 2) followed by slow enhancement of the right lobe (3, 4).

1	2
3	4

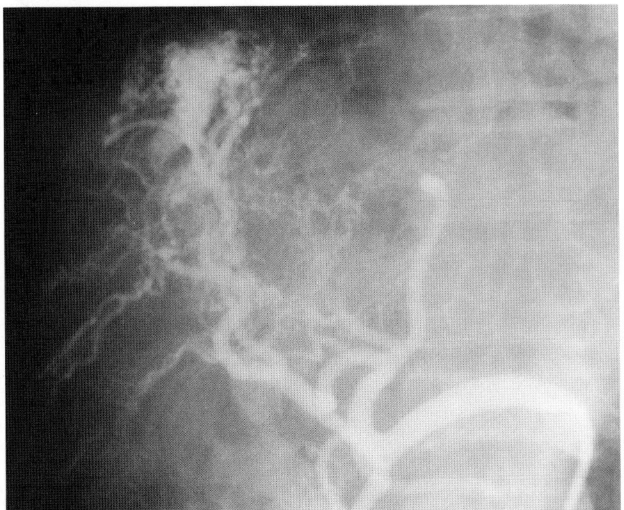

(b) Common hepatic arteriogram (early phase): arterio-portal communications were found in the anterior superior area of the right lobe (S^{VIII}).

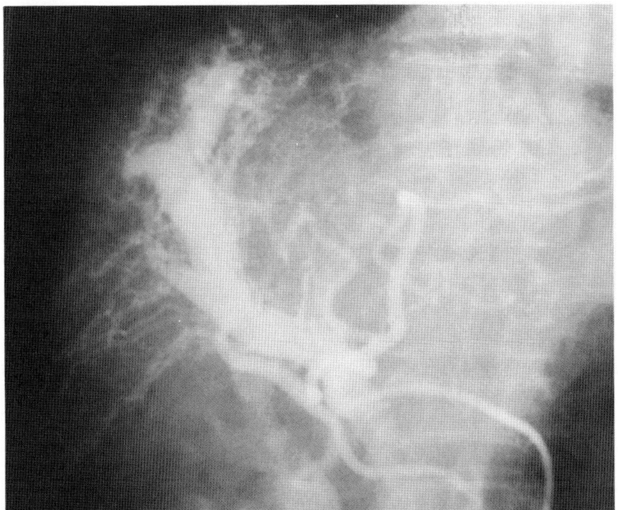

(c) Common hepatic arteriogram (1 s later): contrast medium regurgitated into a dilated anterior superior portal vein branch and further into the portal trunk. It was assumed that advanced cirrhotic changes produced these communications. The abnormal lesion in S^{VIII} suspected to be a metastasis was due to a dilated portal branch.

Portal hypertension—Case 5: Intrahepatic arterio-portal shunt caused by needle puncture.

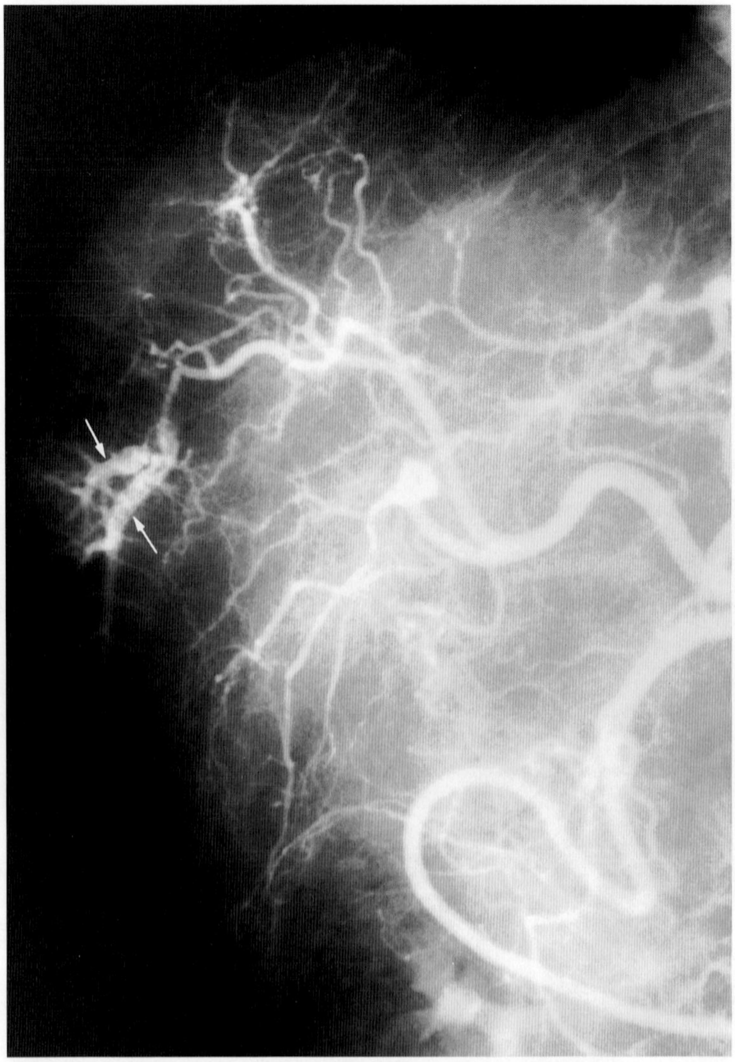

This is a communication between a peripheral arterial branch and small portal branches (→) caused by PTP. Most small-sized communications like this one will spontaneously disappear. However, if it is large, it will not close by itself, and may cause portal hypertension. We have seen a case which developed splenomegaly and bled from varices. According to Okuda *et al.* (1978), an arterio-portal fistula occurred in 5.4 per cent after needle biopsy, in 3.8 per cent after PTC, and 26.2 per cent after portal vein catheterization. In other words, the thicker the needle the more frequent the fistula formation.

Portal hypertension—Case 6: Extrahepatic portal vein obstruction associated with recurrent pancreatitis. This man with a 20-year history of excessive drinking came to the hospital because of severe abdominal colic.

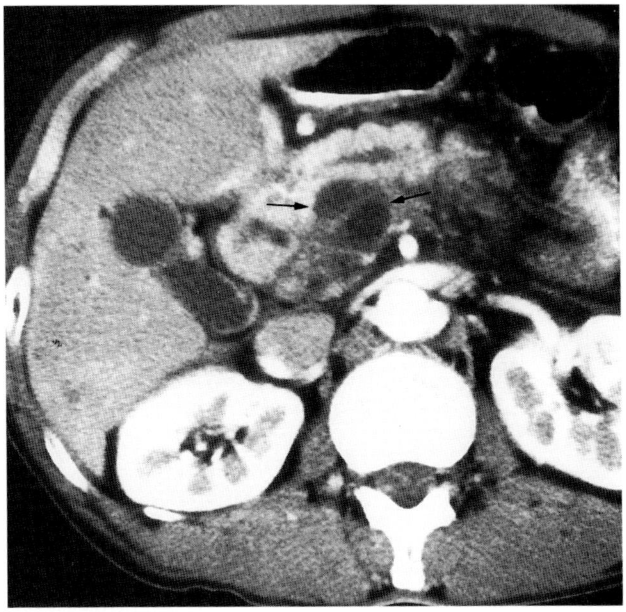

(a) Dynamic CT (early phase): a dilated pancreatic duct and a 2.5 cm low-density mass (→) are recognized. As it shows continuity to the superior mesenteric vein on further caudal CTs, portal vein thrombosis was suspected.

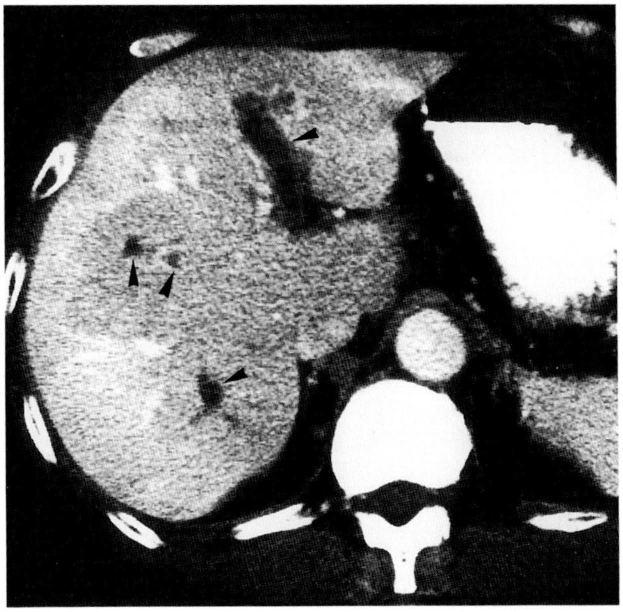

(b) Dynamic CT [section at the hilum level, made shortly after (a)]: a leaf-shaped low-density area extending from the hilum toward the periphery and high-density areas containing hepatic veins in the periphery (perihilar attenuation difference) are seen. Intrahepatic portal veins were not enhanced and remained low in density due to thrombosis.

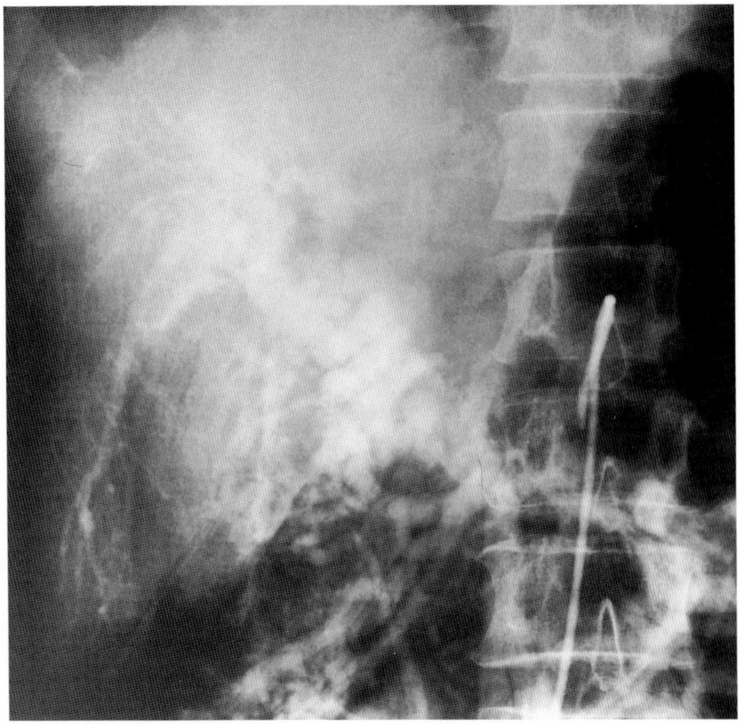

(c) Superior mesenteric arterial portogram: the portal vein is occluded from its origin and replaced by winding hepatopetal veins forming cavernous transformation.

Portal hypertension—Case 7: Obstruction of the right main portal vein associated with advanced cirrhosis.

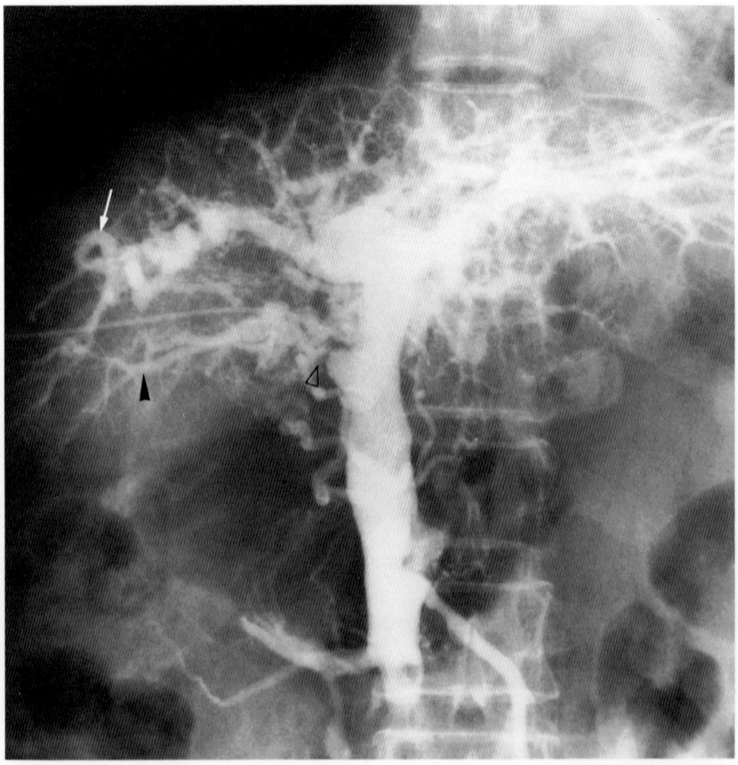

(a) PTP: the portal vein system was opacified from the catheter placed in the transverse portion of the left portal vein. The right portal vein is occluded at its origin (▶). The periphery of the right portal vein is opacified in part from the hepatopetal collaterals around the occlusion. The portal trunk runs vertical in this patient because of marked atrophy of the right lobe, perhaps as a result of occlusion of the right portal vein. The winding portal branches in the medial aspects of the left lobe (→) are frequently collaterals subsequent to occlusion of peripheral portal branches.

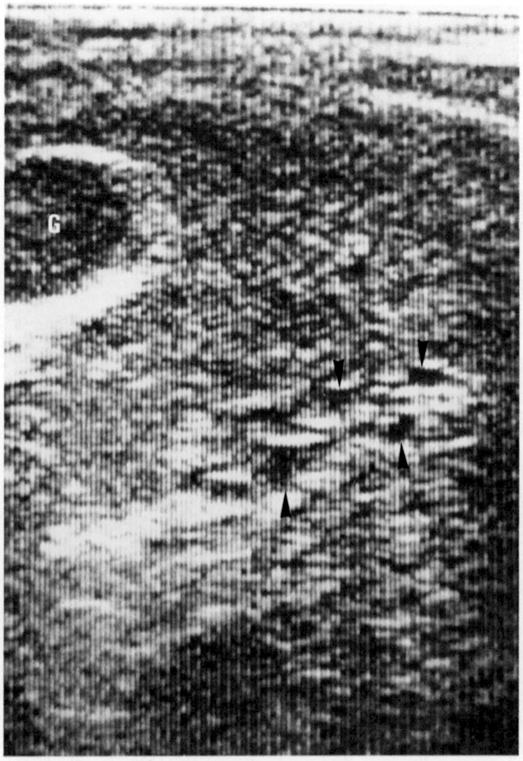

(b) US (right intercostal scan): the normal portal vein structure is not recognized. Sections of winding and bending portal branches (▶) are seen. G. gallbladder.

Portal hypertension—Case 8: Occlusion of the portal vein at the hepatic hilum following splenectomy. In this patient, splenectomy and Hassab operation were carried out following varical bleeding. He entered the hospital because of rebleeding.

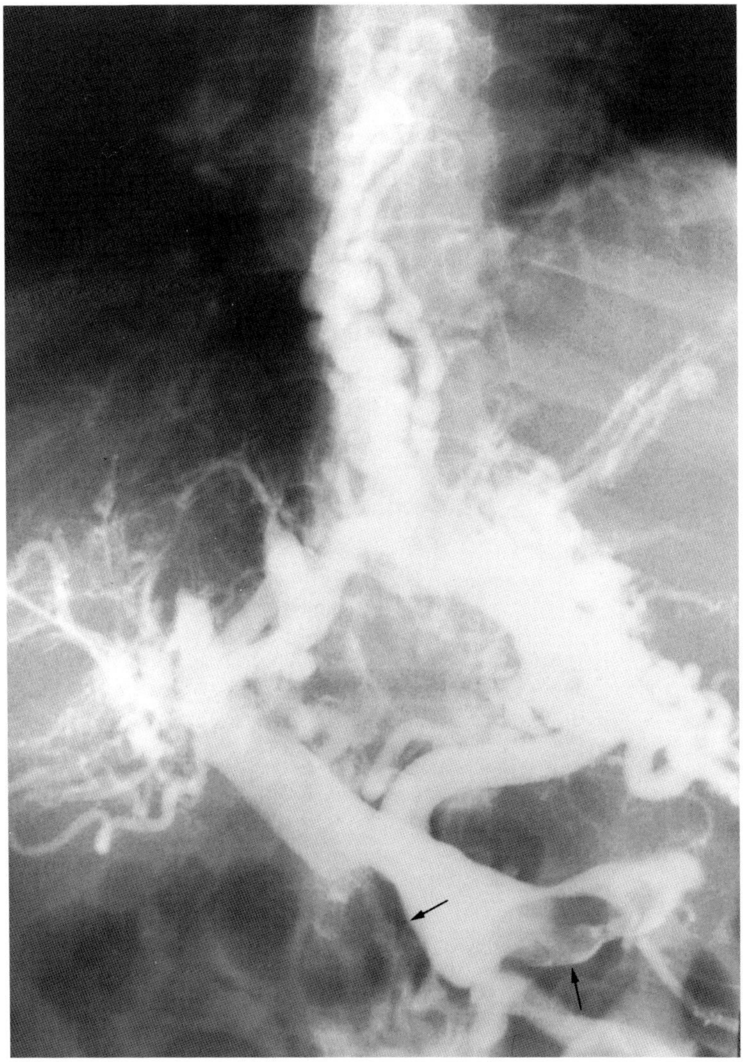

PTP: two large filling defects (→) are seen in the splenic vein and portal trunk. Except for the beginning of the left portal vein, no intraheptic portal vasculature is recognized. Thrombosis was a postsplenectomy event caused by sudden increase in platelet count. The hilar occlusion of the portal vein could have been a result of an embolizing blood clot that formed within the splenic vein. Development of extensive esophageal varices fed by the dilated left gastric vein is obvious.

Portal hypertension—Case 9: Postsplenectomy thrombosis of the portal vein at the hilum and intrahepatic portal branches. In this patient, splenectomy was carried out for marked hypersplenism preliminary to resection for HCC. Subsequent CT study demonstrated multiple thrombi in the intrahepatic and extrahepatic portal veins.

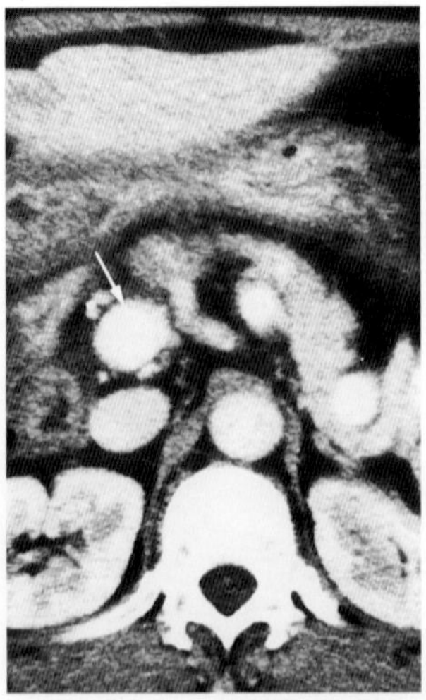

(a) Dynamic CT (preoperative): this was made before splenectomy. The portal trunk is patent (→).

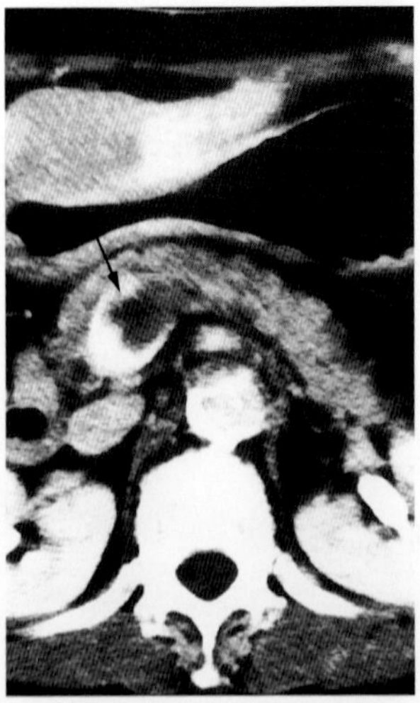

(b) Portal-CT (2 weeks postoperative): superior mesenteric arterial portal-CT demonstrated a filling defect in the splenic vein that extended into the portal vein (→).

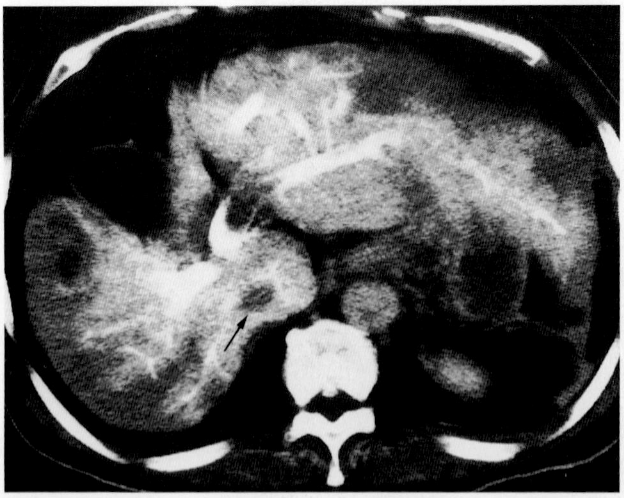

(c) Portal-CT [a slice further cranial from (b)]: the umbilical portion up to the beginning of P^{II} of the left portal vein shows filling defects. There are many wedge-shaped areas of non-enhancement in the peripheral portion of both lobes, suggestive of portal occlusion. The portal vein appeared normal on the superior mesenteric arterial portogram, and these thrombi were demonstrated only by portal-CT. The frequency of thrombosis following splenectomy is about 13 per cent (Yamashita *et al.* 1988). The suspected causes include, beside thrombocythemia, splenic vein congestion, damage to the vascular wall, and subsequent inflammation. →, inferior vena cava.

Portal hypertension—Case 10: Changes in the intrahepatic portal veins in idiopathic portal hypertension. A 72-year-old woman was admitted because of variceal bleeding

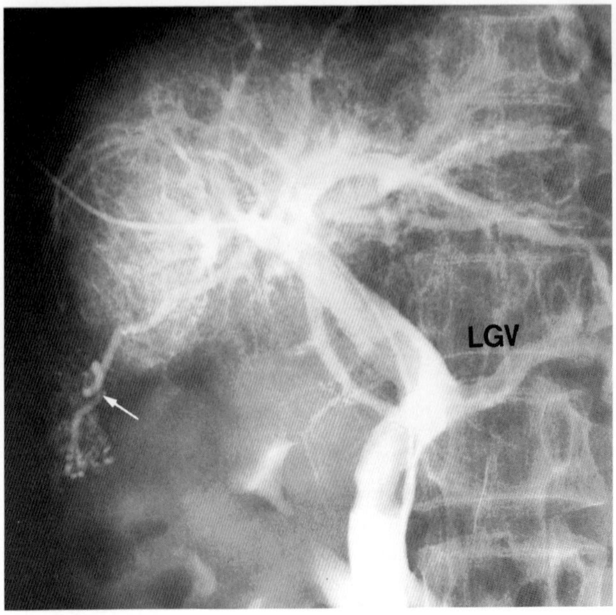

PTP: intrahepatic portal branches are difficult to identify except for P^{II} and P^{III}. The U- and P-points are obscure. The patent branches are accompanied by thin brush-like vessels. In the periphery of the presumable P^{VI}, a peculiar winding branch (→) is recognized. These changes are thought to be secondary to occlusive changes of the peripheral portal branches, representing recanalization and/or collaterals. LGV, left gastric vein. For details of portal changes see Futagawa *et al.* (1980).

Portal hypertension—Case 11: Hepatic vein changes in advanced cirrhosis.

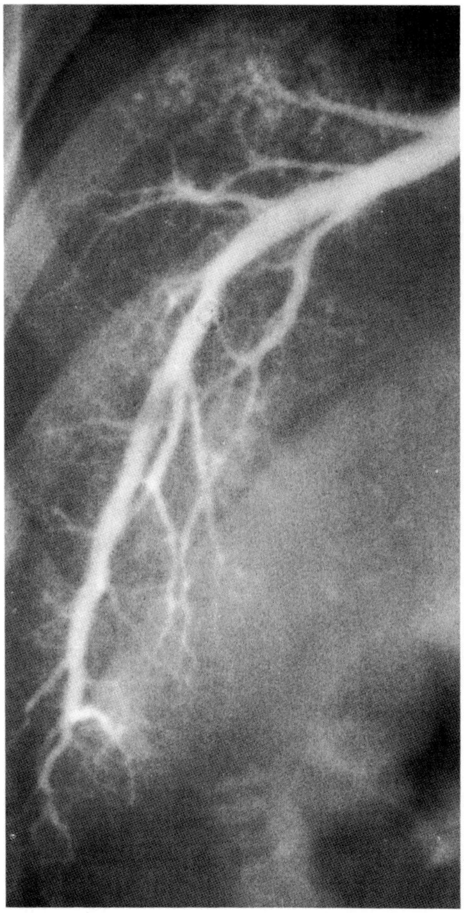

a

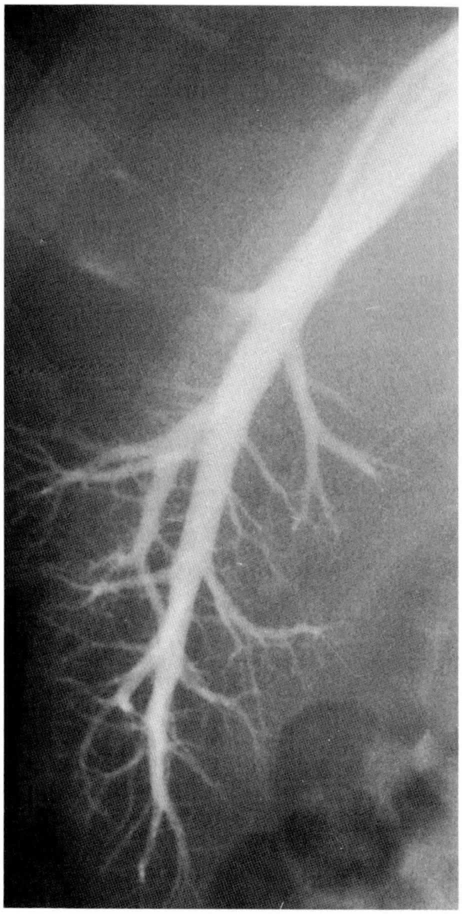

c

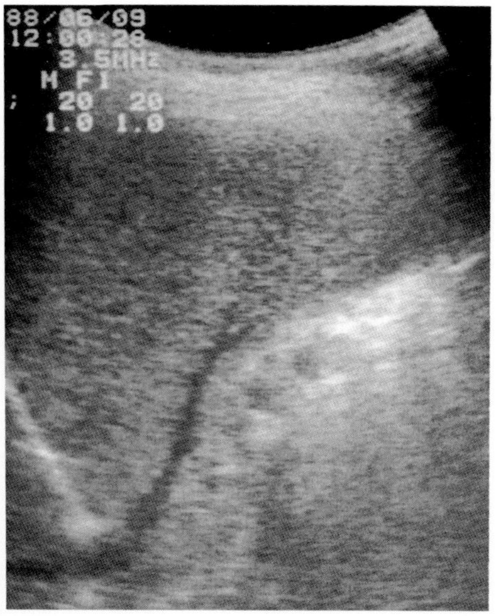

b

(a) Selective right hepatic venogram of a liver with advanced cirrhosis: the venous wall is hardened, the calibers diminished, and the number of branchings smaller compared with that in a normal venogram (c).

(b) US: in a liver with advanced cirrhosis, the right hepatic vein is narrow and the wall irregular as in the venogram.

(c) Selective right hepatic venogram of a normal liver: the venous wall is smooth, calibers are large, and the branching angles are sharp.

Portal hypertension—Case 12: Spontaneous reversal of portal blood flow in a liver with advanced cirrhosis.

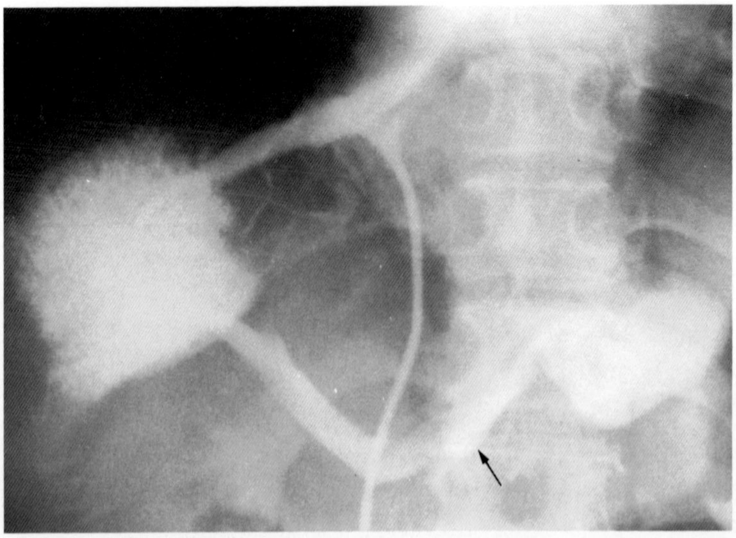

(a) Retrograde portography: retrograde portography was carried out from a catheter wedged into the right hepatic vein. Following opacification of the liver parenchyma, the portal vein trunk and a large hepatofugal collateral as an extension of the left gastric vein (→) was recognized.

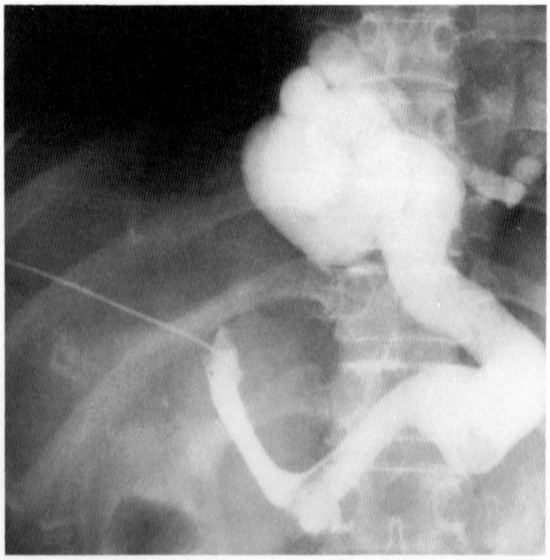

(b) PTP: contrast injection was done with the catheter tip near the hilum. Contrast medium did not enter the liver, and all flowed retrogradely into the left gastric vein that was forming large varices, and flowed further toward the azygos vein system.

Portal hypertension—Case 13: Left gastric venography and delineation of the parallel pattern at the esophagogastric junction.

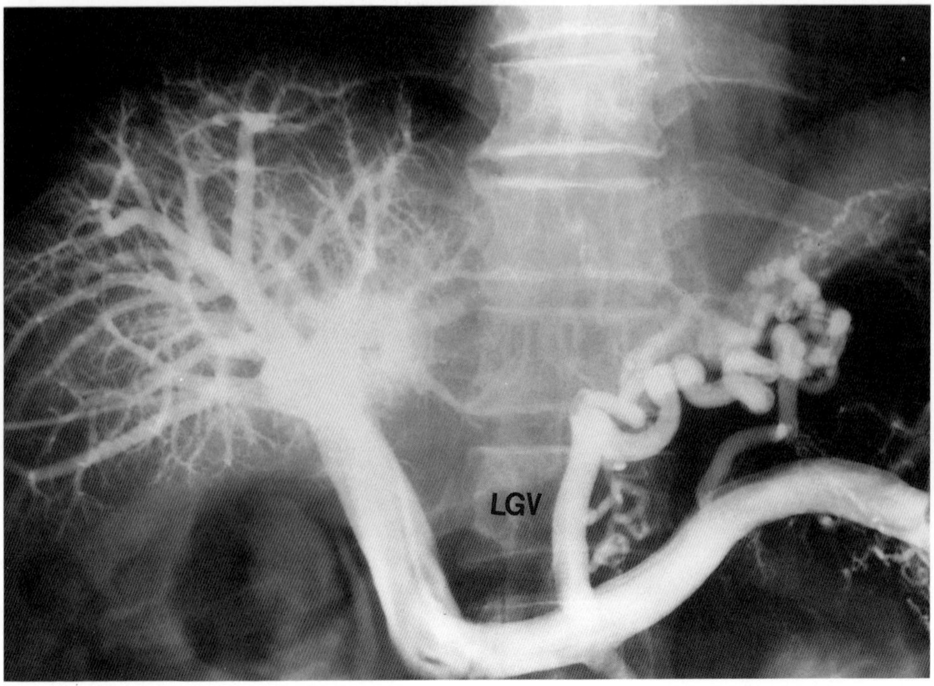

(a) PTP: two collateral veins, the left gastric (LGV) and posterior gastric, are recognized.

Case 13 (contd.)

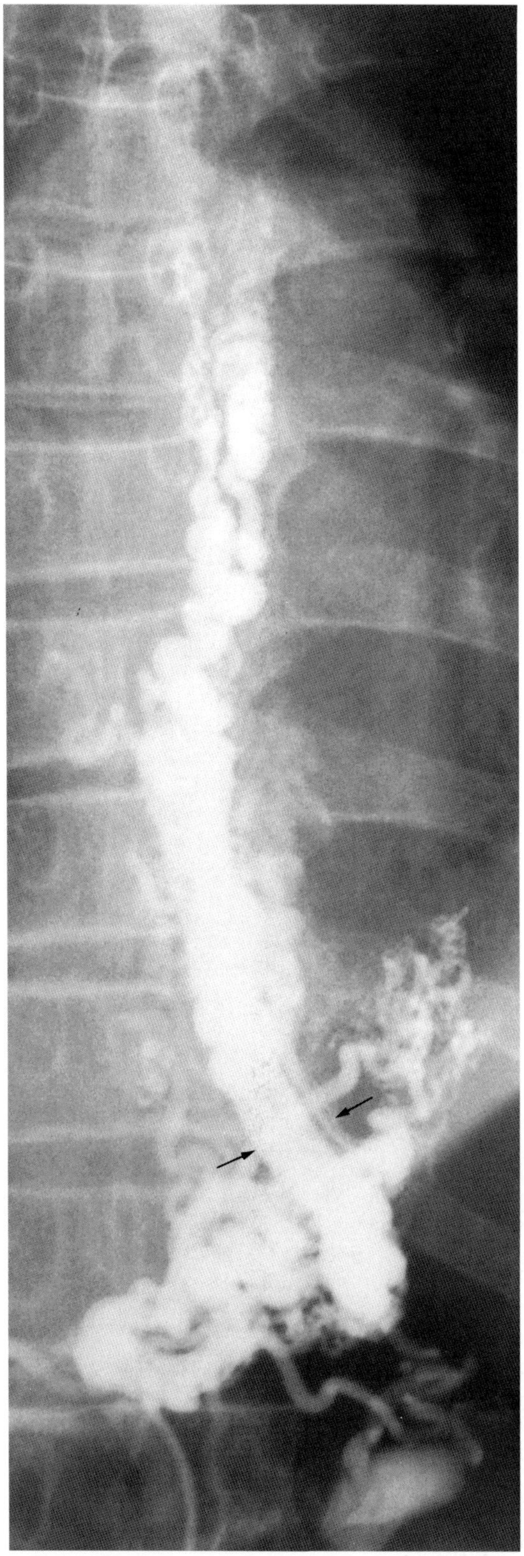

(b) Selective left gastric venogram: many thin straight veins (→) are seen running parallel (parallel pattern) at the esophagogastric junction.

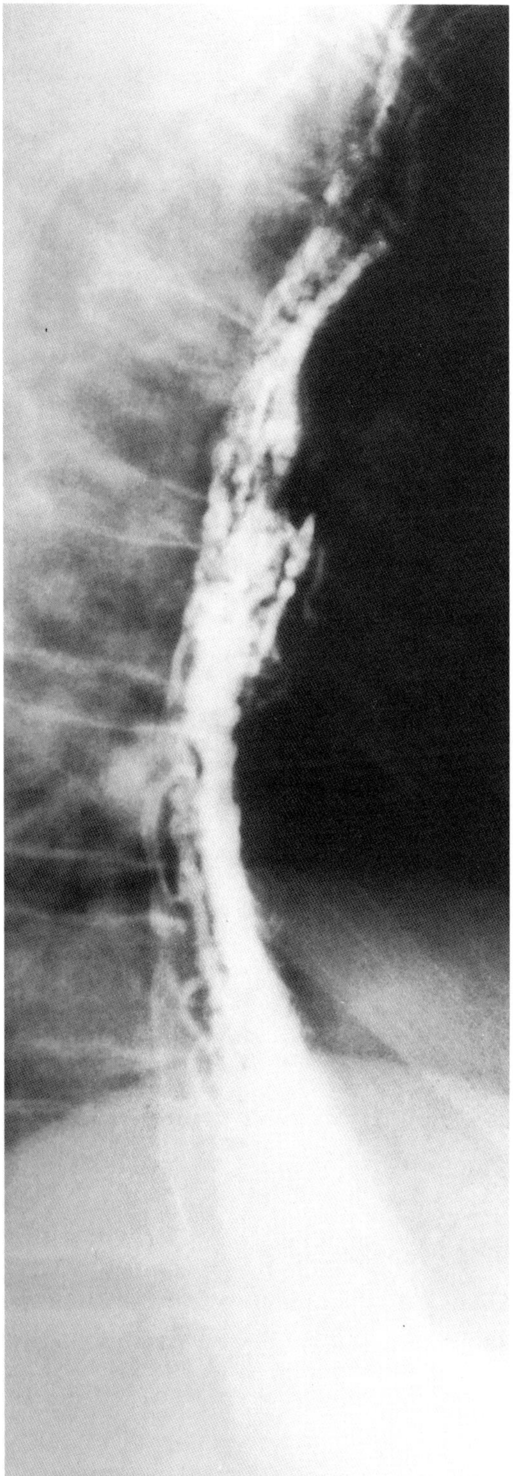

(c) Selective left gastric venogram [lateral view of (a)]: varicose veins run cephalad in front of the vertebral column up to the left brachio-

Portal hypertension—Case 14: The left gastric vein flowing into paraesophageal varices.

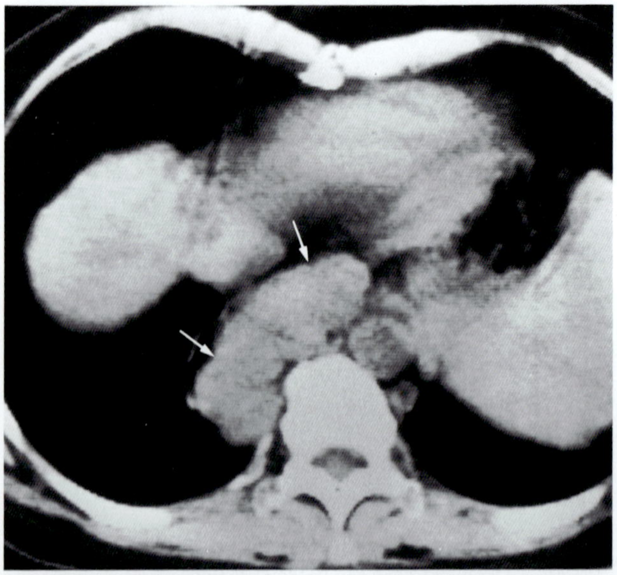

(a) Plain CT: there is a mass in the mediastinum (→ which is suggestive of lymph node metastases.

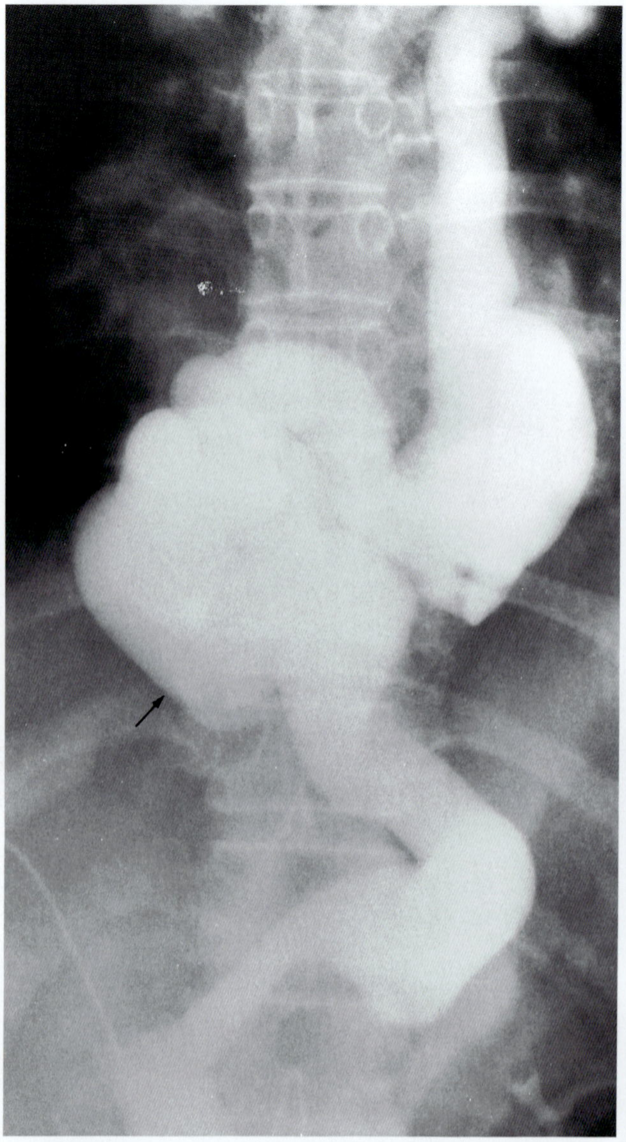

(b) PTP: blood in the superior mesenteric vein does not go to the liver. It flows into large paraesophageal varices (→), thenceforth to the hemiazygos and to the azygos vein. Since this collateral does not cross the esophagogastric junction, no parallel pattern is seen (same as Case 12, p.370).

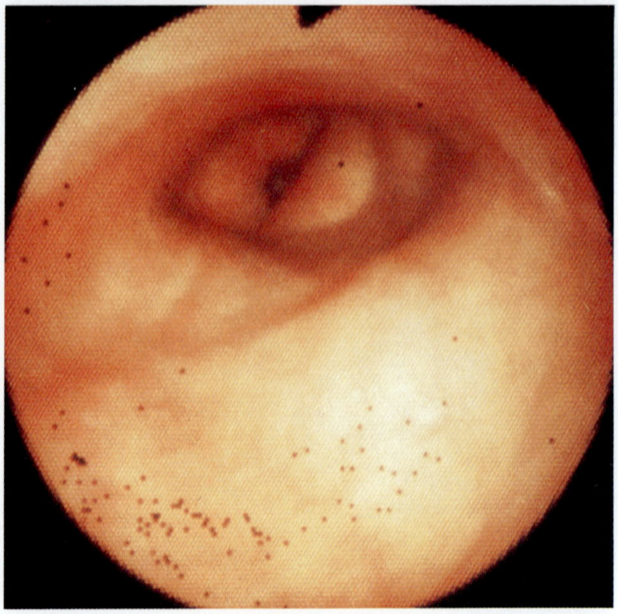

(c) Endoscopy of the esophagus: there are no obvious varices. Serpentine crisscrossing elevations in the submucosa perhaps represent compression from outside the esophagus as suggested by PTP.

Portal hypertension—Case 15: Gastro-renal shunt frequently found in patients with gastric varices.

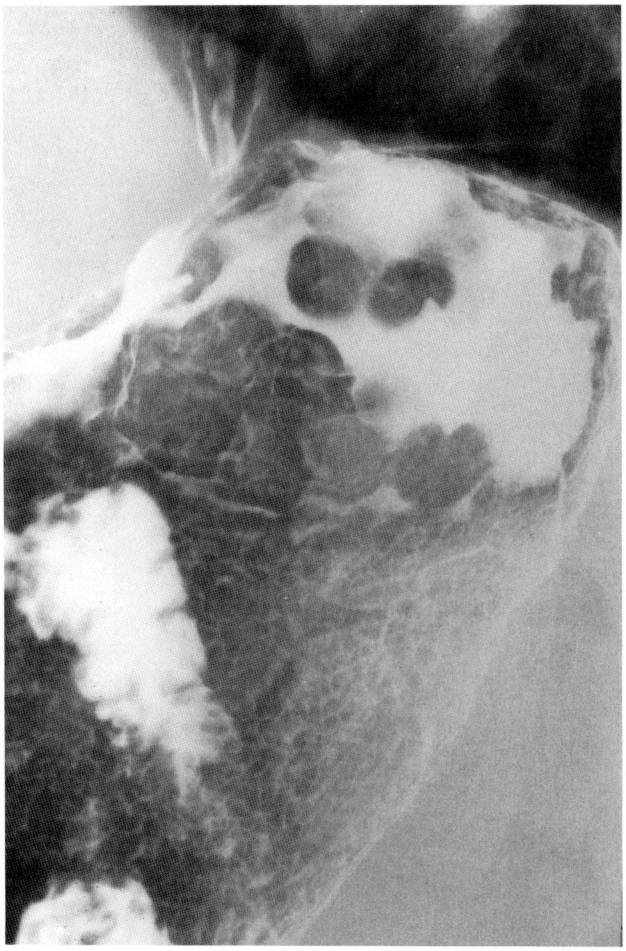

(a) Double-contrast barium study of the stomach: a number of nodular elevations are seen in the formix. Since there is continuity between these nodules, a diagnosis of gastric varices is possible. Most patients with gastric varices have a large gastro-renal shunt, and esophageal varices are absent or minimal.

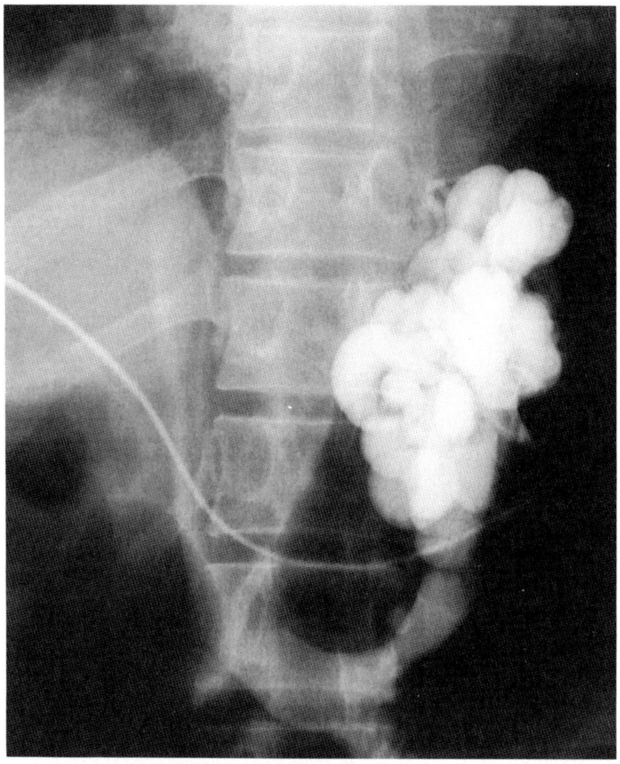

(b) Selective left gastric venography: winding varices were demonstrated in the posterior aspect of the fornix of the stomach, and a left renal-inferior vena cava communication was recognized.

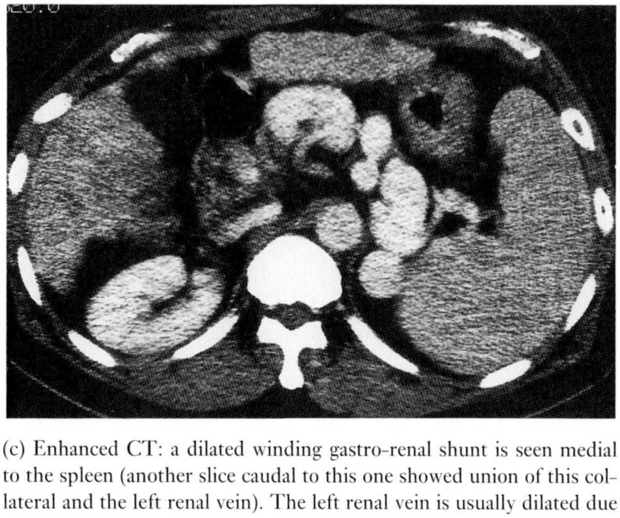

(c) Enhanced CT: a dilated winding gastro-renal shunt is seen medial to the spleen (another slice caudal to this one showed union of this collateral and the left renal vein). The left renal vein is usually dilated due to increased blood flow.

Portal hypertension—Case 16: Opacification of esophageal varices by selective left gastric arteriography.

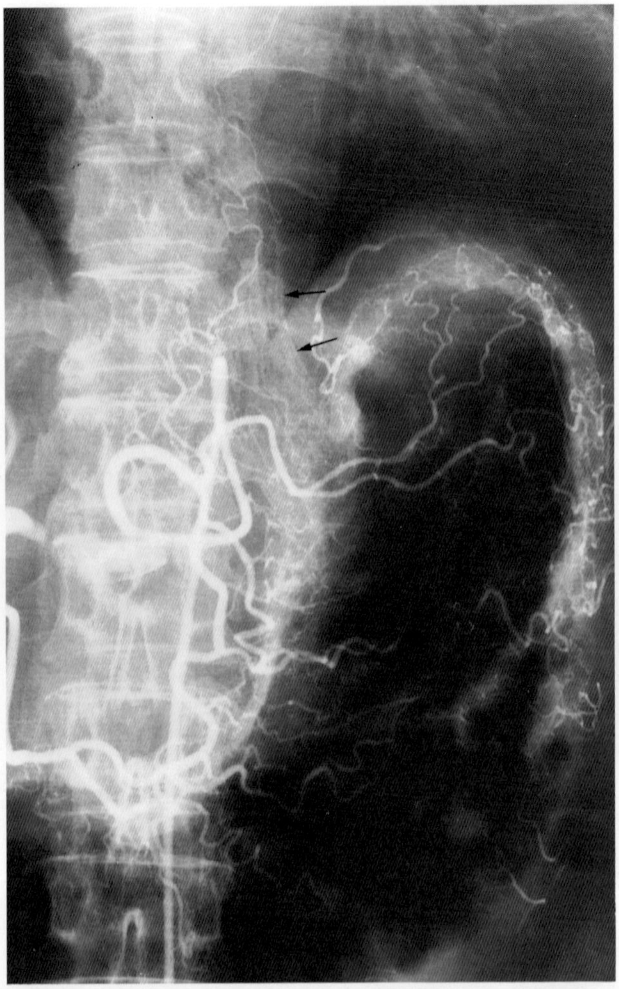

(a) Selective left gastric arteriography (arterial phase): following injection of one ampoule of papaverine hydrochloride, 30 ml of contrast medium was injected (6 ml/s). →, a fine arterial plexus supplying the lower esophagus.

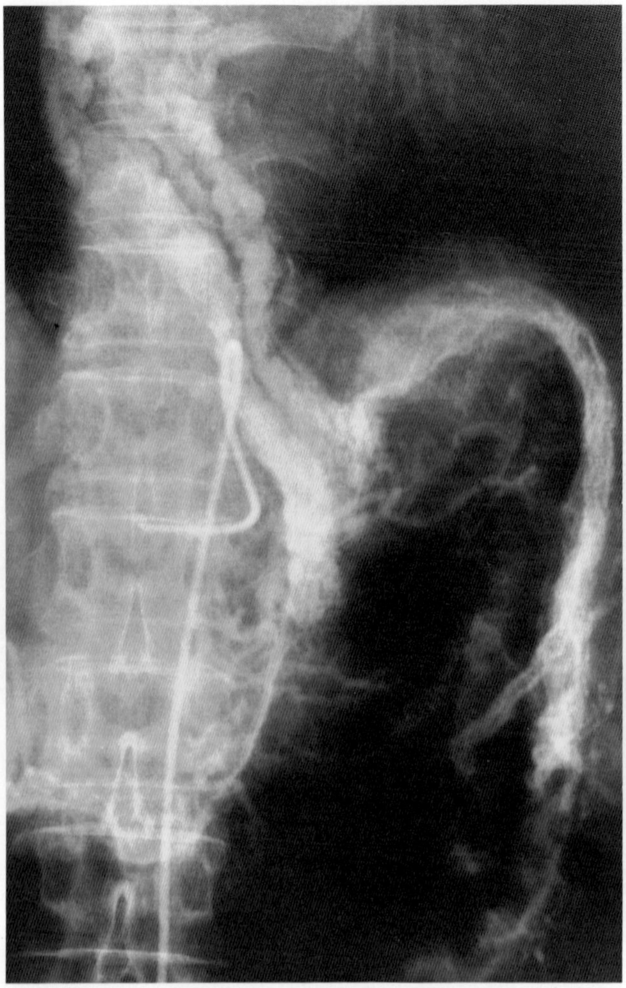

(b) Selective left gastric arteriography (venous phase): esophageal varices are clearly opacified.

Portal hypertension—Case 17: Delineation of esophageal varices by enhanced CT.

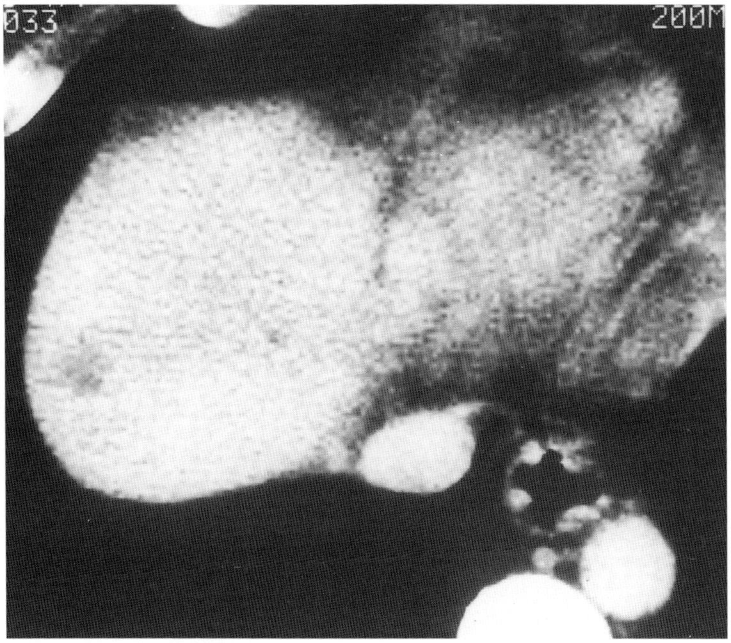

(a) Enhanced CT: four dilated veins are seen protruding in the esophageal lumen.

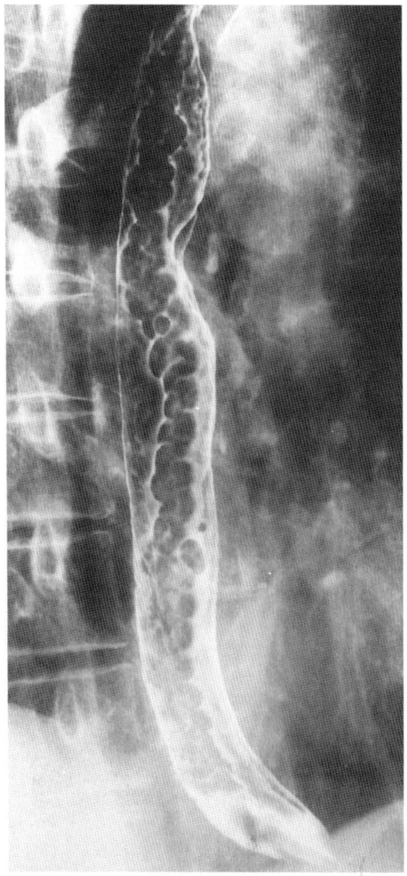

(b) Double-contrast barium study of the esophagus: marked varices are seen in the esophagus.

Portal hypertension—Case 18: A collateral route of the paraumbilical-external iliac-inferior vena cava.

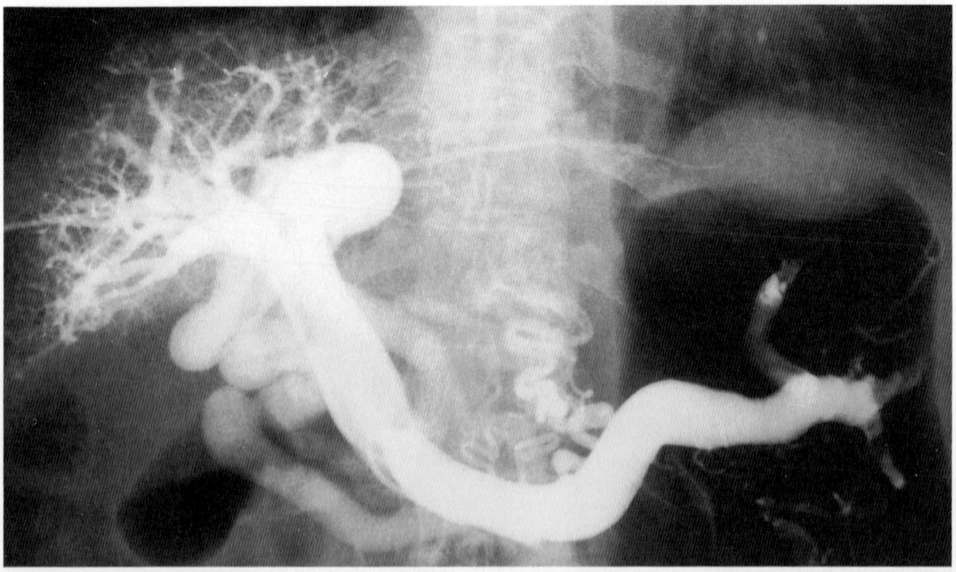

(a) PTP (early phase): the left portal vein is markedly dilated at its origin, and several dilated paraumbilical veins are seen coursing caudally.

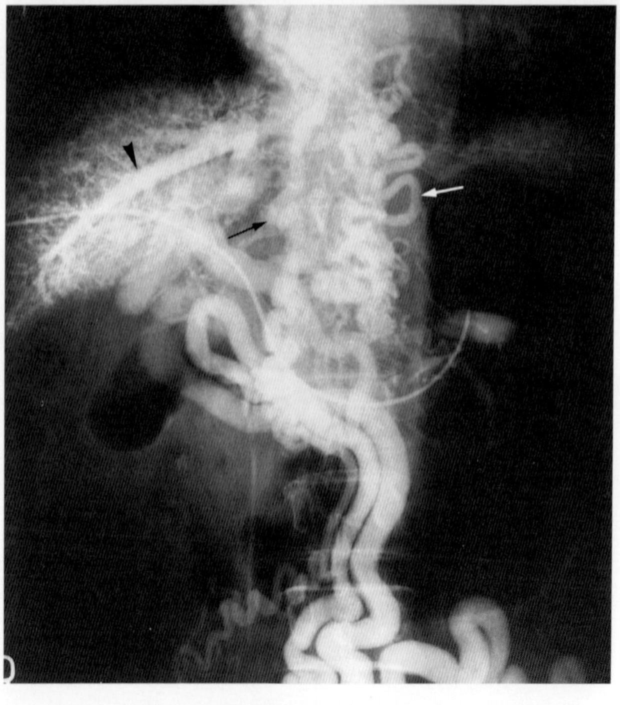

(b) PTP (late phase, 16 s): the paraumbilical veins are flowing into dilated veins of the lower abdominal wall. The internal thoracic veins (→) are also recognized. Reflecting extensive intrahepatic shunts, the right hepatic vein (▶) was opacified in a relatively early phase of portography.

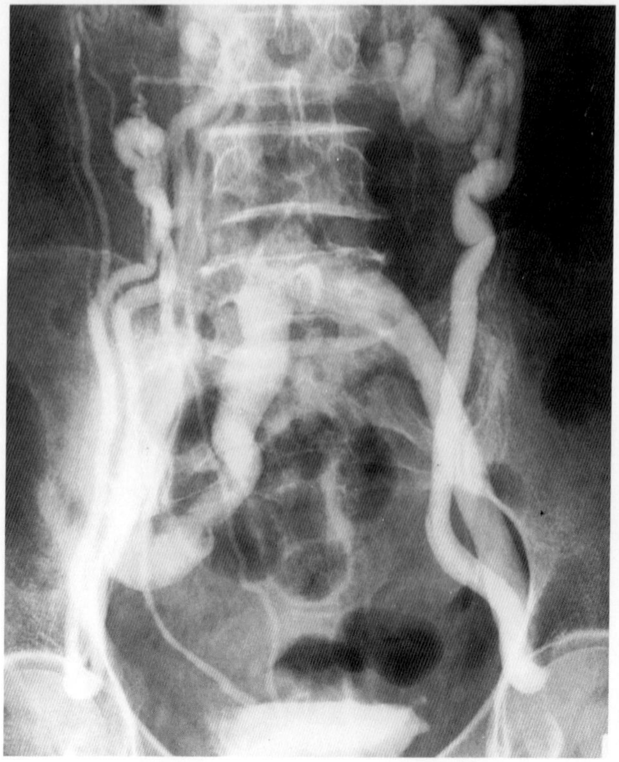

(c) PTP (late phase, 20 s): the caudal extension of the paraumbilical veins through the lower abdominal wall veins opacified the external iliac vein bilaterally, and the contrast medium flowed into the inferior vena cava.

Portal hypertension—Case 19: A dilated paraumbilical vein mistaken for hilar carcinoma on the scintigram.

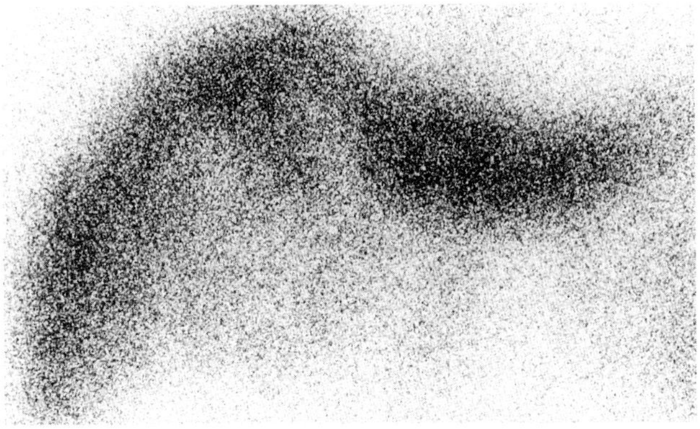

(a) Hepatic scintigram (^{99m} Tc-phytate): two cold areas simulating double peaks are recognized in the hilum on this scan. Hilar carcinoma was suspected.

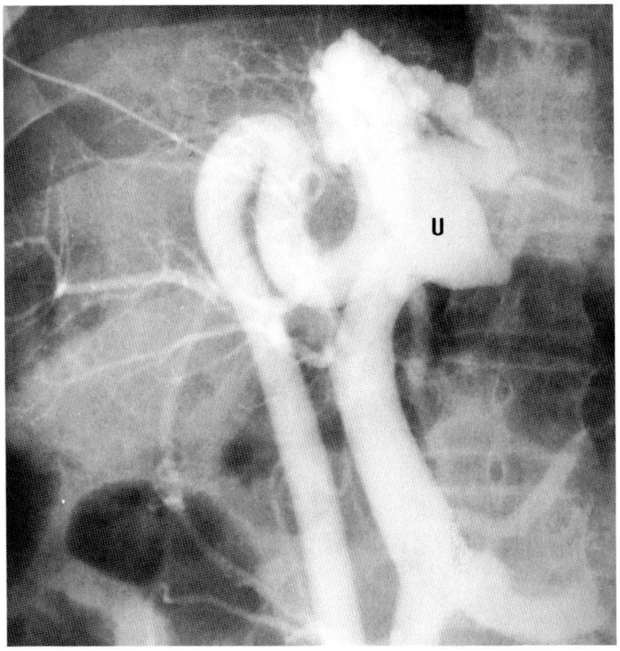

(b) PTP: a large winding paraumbilical vein arises from the umbilical portion of the left portal vein (U). The winding paraumbilical vein and the dilated umbilical portion correspond to the two peak-shaped cold areas on the scintigram. The paraumbilical vein is stealing a considerable portion of portal venous flow, and very little contrast medium is going into the liver; this accounts for the atrophy of the liver.

Portal hypertension—Case 20: A collateral paraumbilical vein simulating HCC.

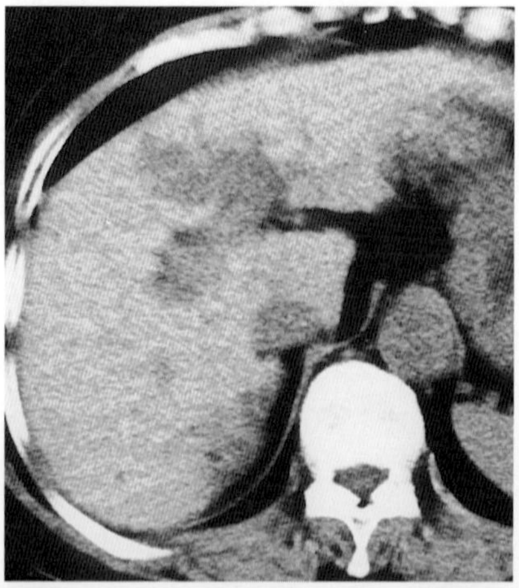

a

(a) Plain CT: a low-density area is seen lateral to the umbilical portion of the left portal vein.

(b) Dynamic CT made by the table incremental method (1–6): the lesion in question was enhanced like a tumor (1). However, as the slice moved caudally, it became clear that it was a dilated paraumbilical vein (2–5). The most caudal slice (6) shows several subcutanous veins as its continuation running cephalad. Grossly, the subcutanous veins resembled *caput medusae*. The collateral paraumbilical vein usually arises from the umbilical portion of the left portal vein, passes part of S^{IV}, and leaves the liver.

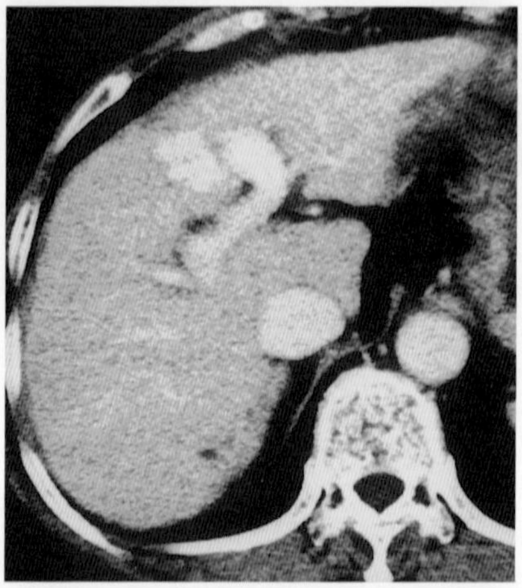

b–1

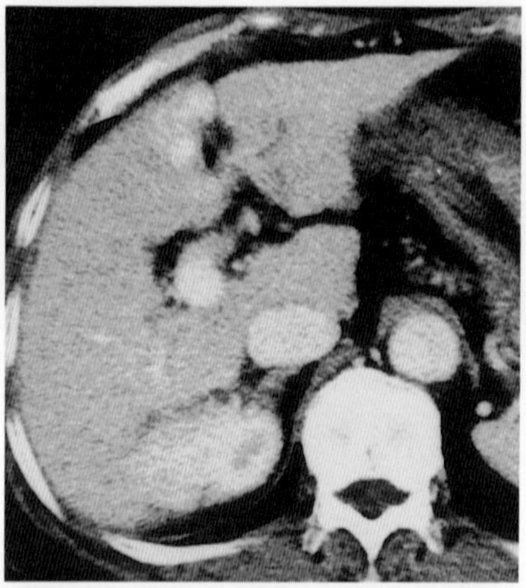

b–2

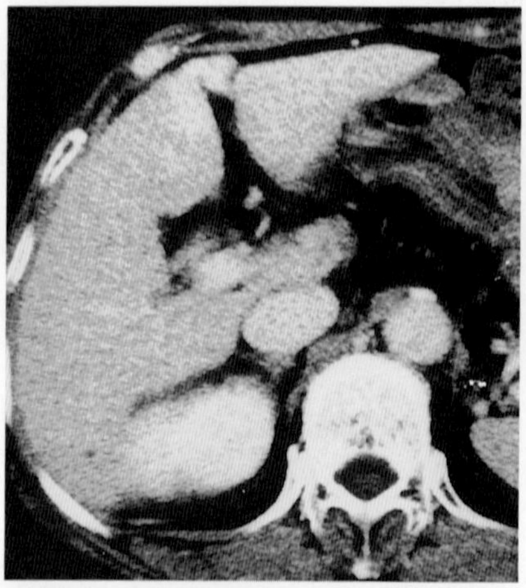

b–3

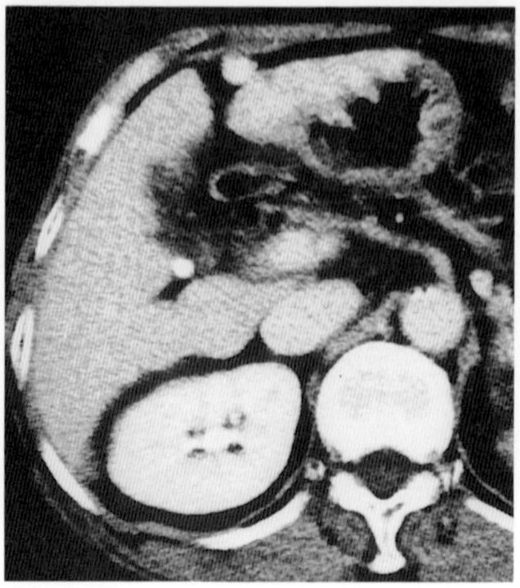

b–4

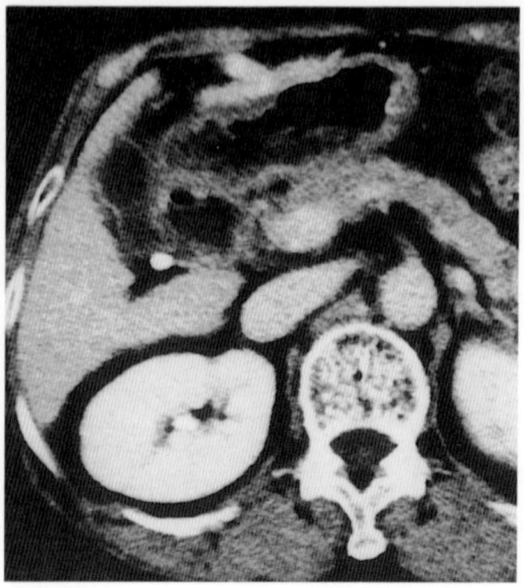

b–5

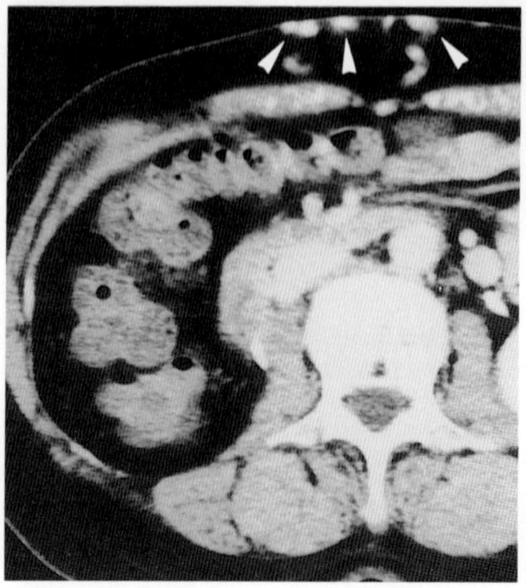

b–6

Portal hypertension—Case 21: Delineation of the paraumbilical vein by US.

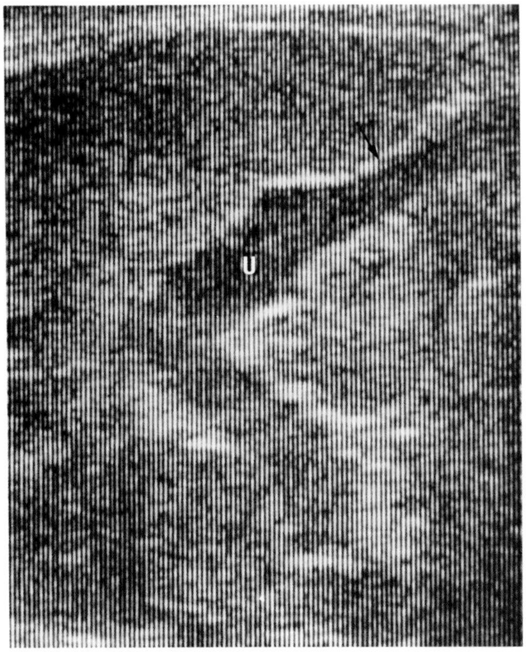

US (sagittal scan of the left lobe): a paraumbilical vein (→) which is somewhat smaller than the transverse-umbilical portion (U) of the left portal vein is seen as its continuation.

Portal hypertension—Case 22: A huge spleno-renal shunt as a cause of frequent attacks of portal systemic encephalopathy.

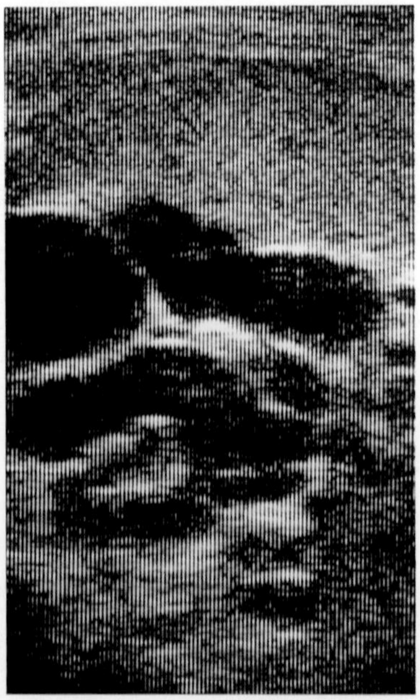

(a) US (left intercostal scan): varices consisting of winding dilated veins are seen near the splenic hilum. That these are not cysts is readily demonstrated if Doppler US is done.

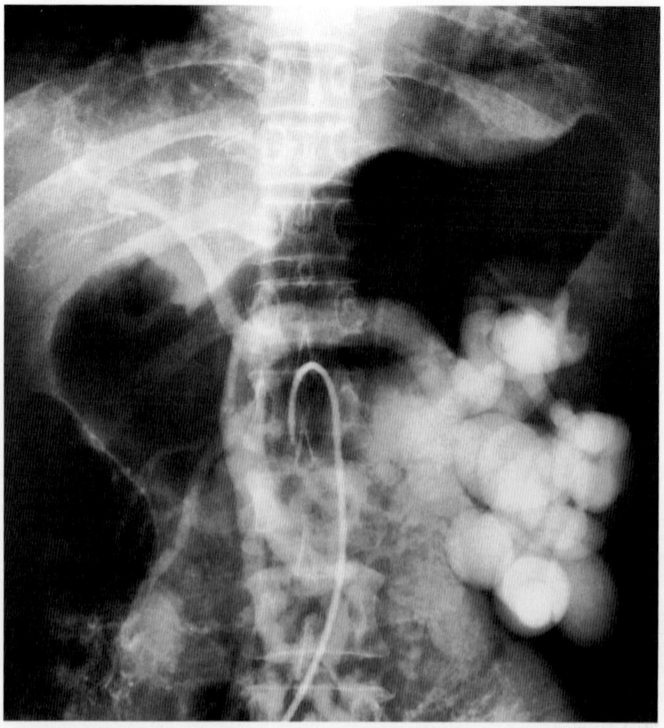

(b) Superior mesenteric arterial portogram: a large varicose spleno-renal shunt is apparent. The bulk of the superior mesenteric venous flow is diverted into the splenic vein hepatofugally; the portal vein is small with little hepatopetal flow. Development of a large renal shunt decreases portal venous pressure preventing the development of esophageal varices, but it causes portal systemic encephalopathy.

Portal hypertension—Case 23: A large meso-caval shunt.

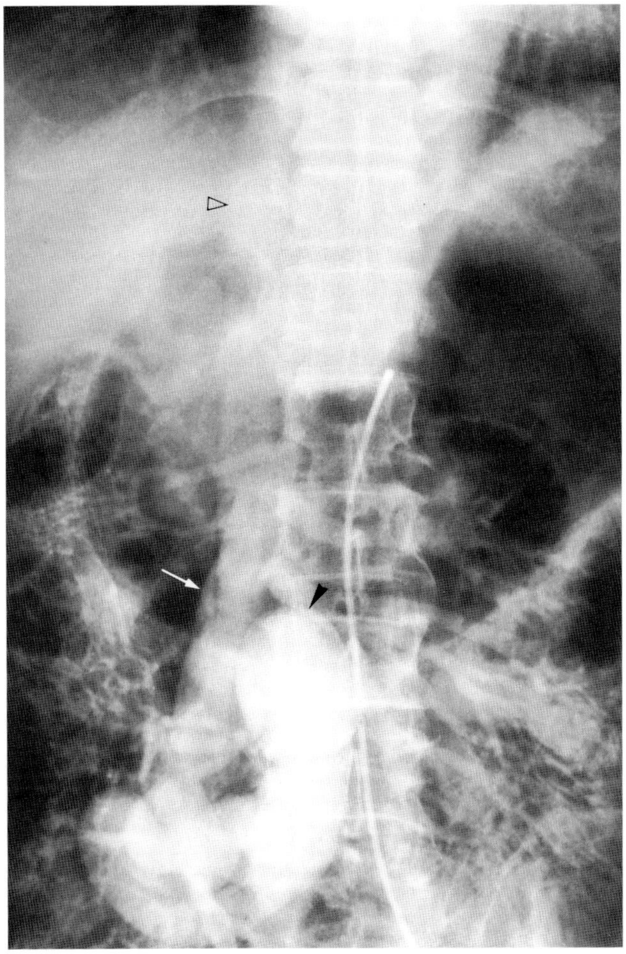

(a) Superior mesenteric arterial portogram: contrast medium flowed downward in a dilated superior mesenteric vein (→), turned around and ran cranially to enter the inferior vena cava (▷) after forming varices (▶). In our experience, there is no hepatopetal flow in the portal vein in the presence of a large meso-caval shunt.

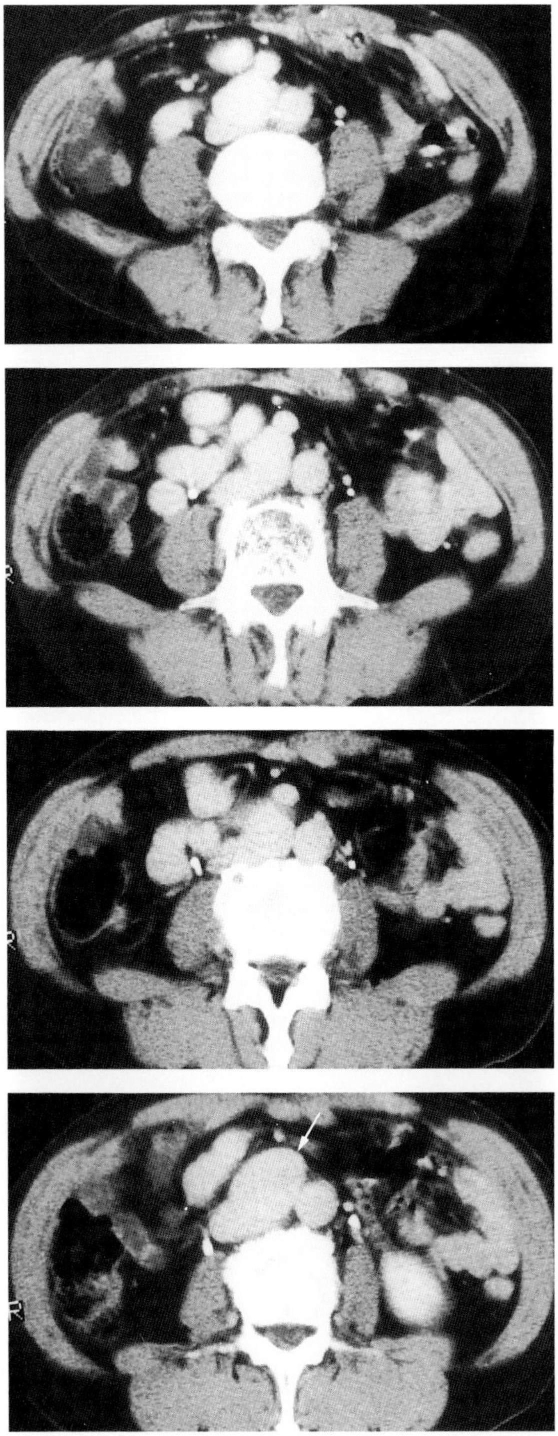

1

2

3

4

(b) Dynamic CT (1–4, table was moved cephalad from down): many dilated veins are seen behind the aorta and inferior vena cava (1–3). In slice #4, transition of contrast medium from a varix (→) to the vena cava is seen posterior to it.

Portal hypertension—Case 24: The superior mesenteric vein flowing directly into the inferior vena cava.

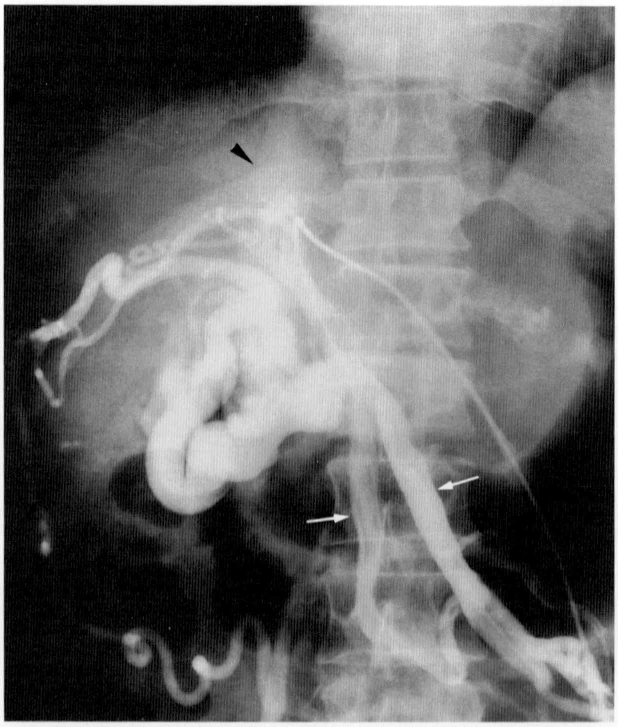

PTP: most of the contrast medium in the superior mesenteric vein (→) flows into the inferior vena cava (▶) through winding collaterals near the portal vein trunk.

Portal hypertension—Case 25: A collateral connecting the superior mesenteric and the azygos vein.

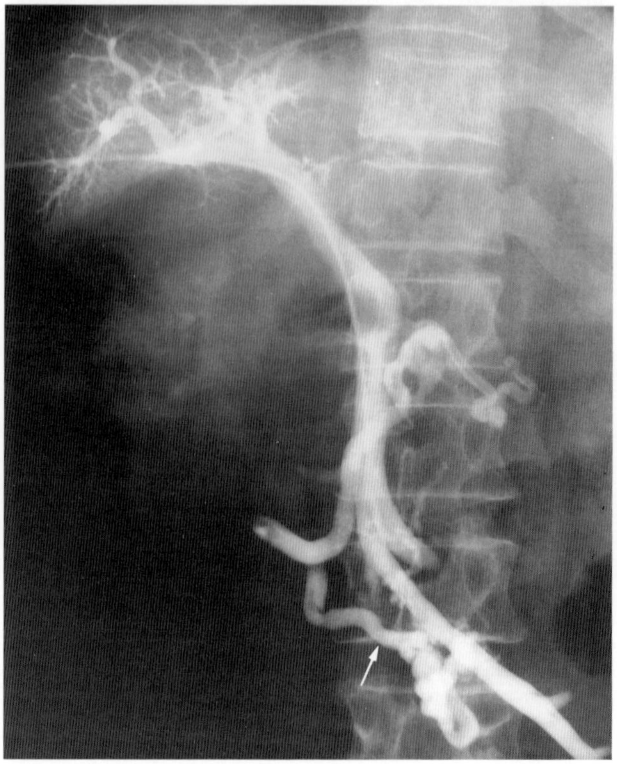

(a) PTP (early phase): a branch of the superior mesenteric vein is forming a collateral (→).

Case 25 (contd.)

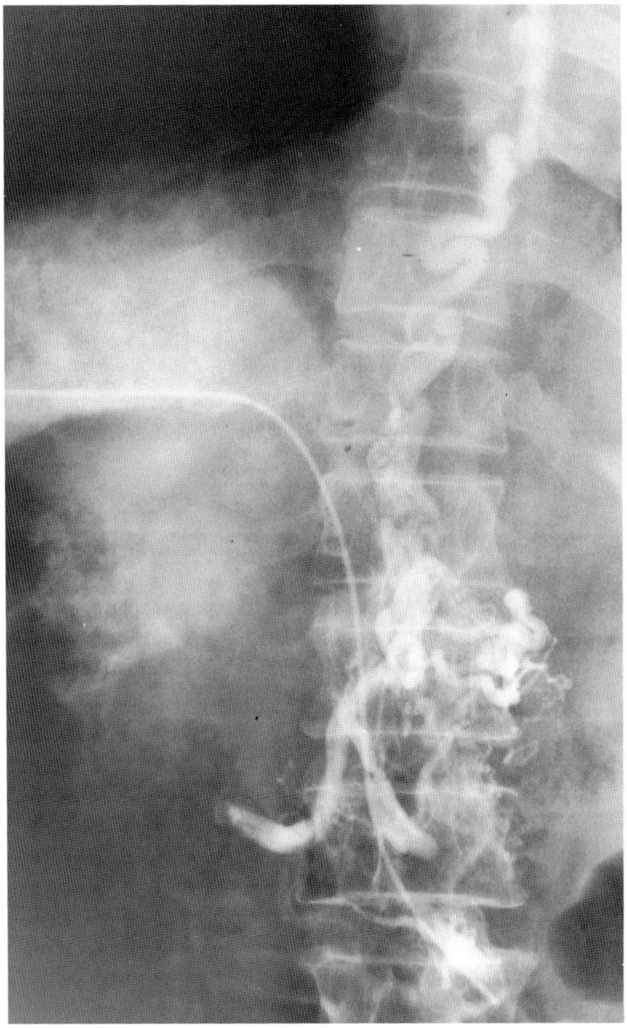

(b) PTP (late phase): this collateral vein opacified the azygos vein anterior to the vertebral column, and then the hemiazygos.

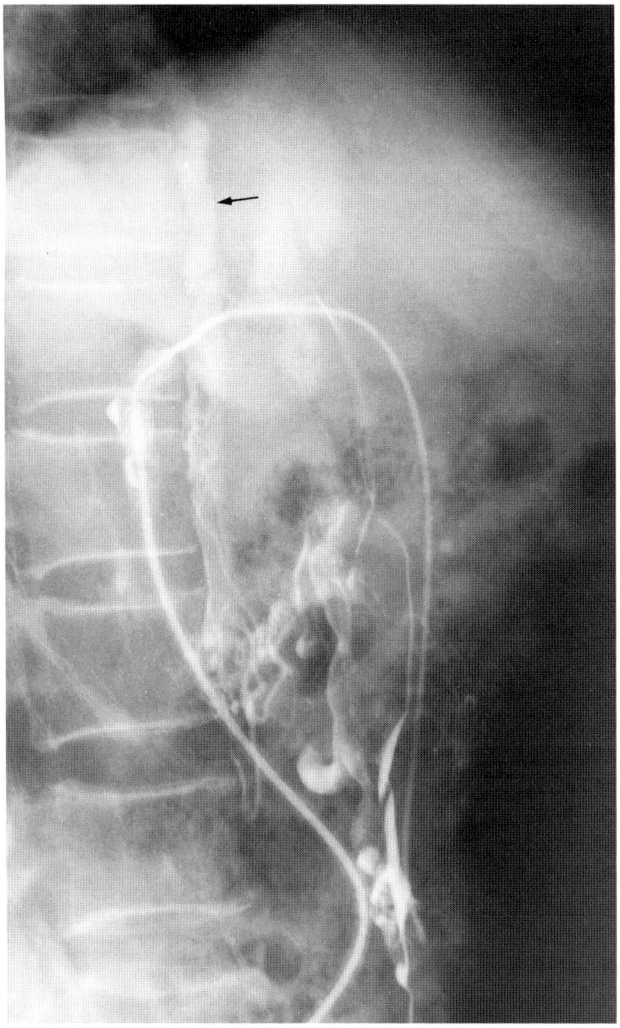

(c) Lateral view: the azygos vein (→) is seen running cephalad in front of the vertebral column.

Portal hypertension—Case 26: Hemodynamics of the hemorrhoidal veins.

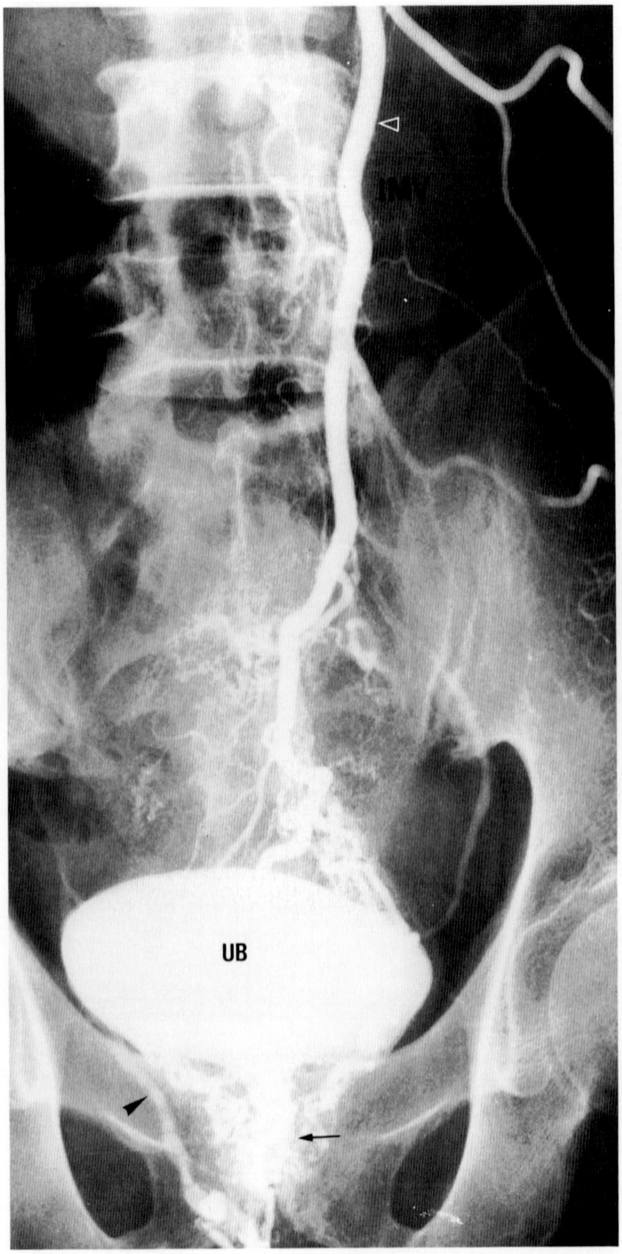

Selective inferior mesenteric venography (at the time of PTP): a hepatofugal inferior mesenteric venous flow (▷), hemorrhoidal veins as its continuation (→), and a collateral going to the right internal iliac vein (▶) are recognized. The patient had suffered from hemorrhoids associated with cirrhosis for years. UB, contrast medium in the urinary bladder.

Portal hypertension—Case 27: Portal-hepatic vein shunt through an intrahepatic venous aneurysm. A 75-year-old man with cirrhosis came to the hospital because of a suspected liver tumor.

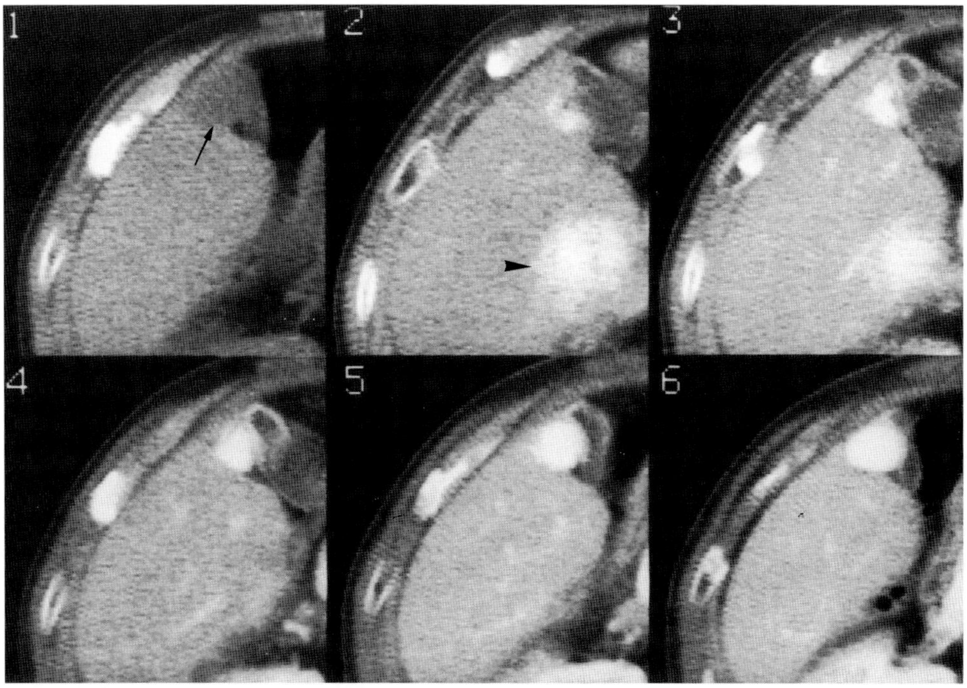

(a) Plain CT (1) and dynamic CT (2–6): in #1, a low-density area (→) was seen lateral to the gall-bladder. Slices were cut with the table incremental method starting from the level 3 cm cranial to it (2–6). An abnormal vessel was recognized arising near the gall-bladder and running caudally. ▶, HCC in the posterior segment. It had no relation to this vasculature.

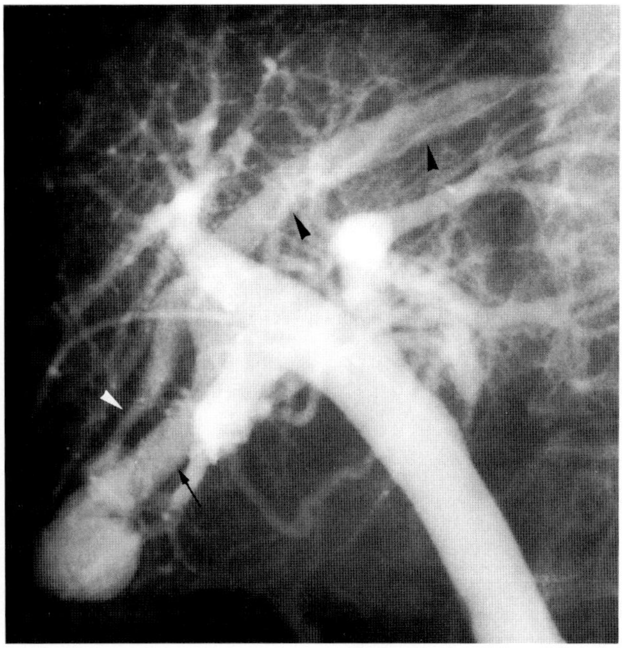

(b) PTP (anterior view): as superior mesenteric arterial portography showed a faintly opacified aneurysm-like structure, PTP was carried out. It demonstrated a 2 cm portal aneurysm continuous from a dilated portal branch, P^{V} (→). A communication between the portal vein and the middle hepatic vein (▶) through this aneurysm was recognized.

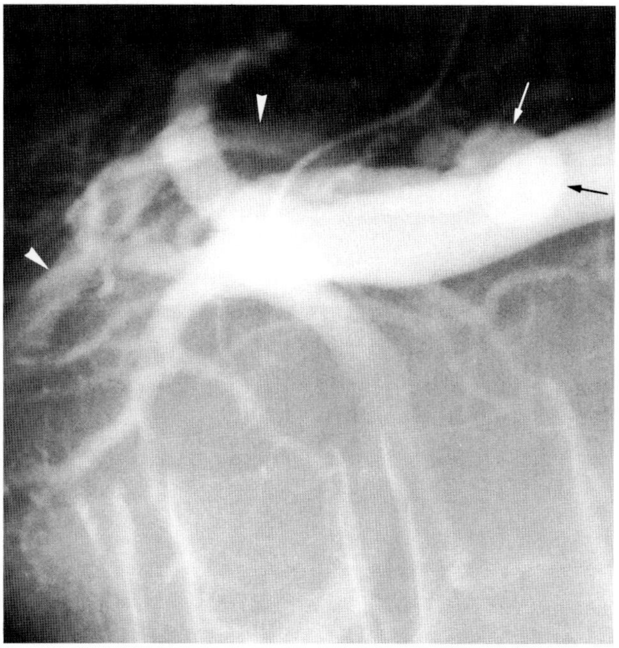

(c) PTP (right lateral view): portal aneurysm (→) and the middle hepatic vein (▶) are more easily identified.

Portal hypertension—Case 28: Opacification of normal intrahepatic portal vein system.

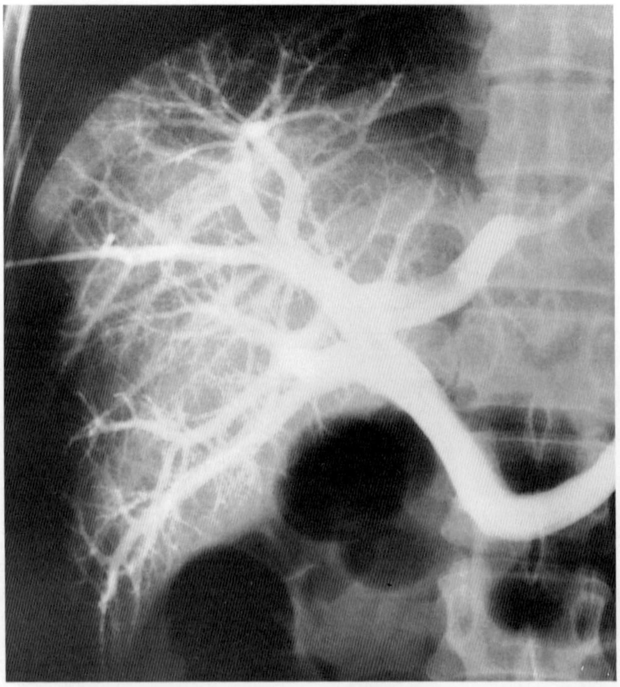

(a) PTP (early phase): intrahepatic portal vein branches are clearly opacified and identifiable.

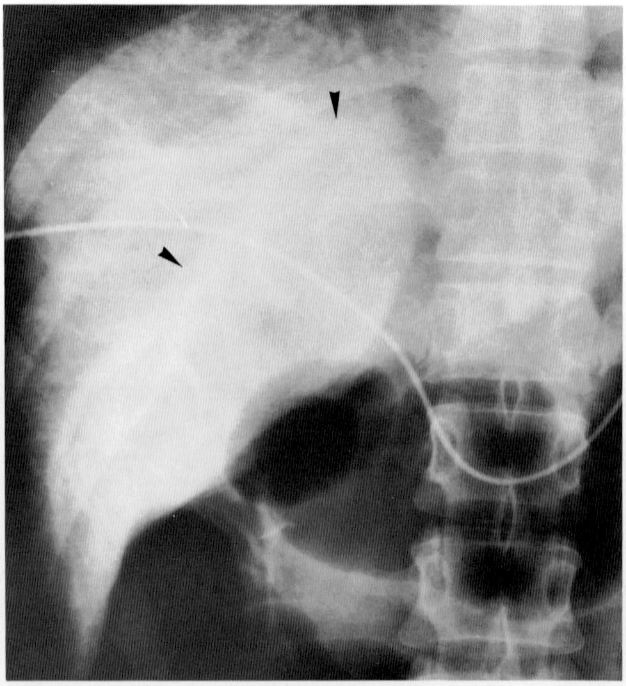

(b) PTP (late phase): after the liver parenchyma has been homogeneously stained, the right hepatic vein (▶) is faintly seen.

In this case, the posterior portal branch occurs independently from the portal trunk (independent type). The intrahepatic branches are smoothly extending and the vessel walls are also smooth. It may be conceived from these vessels that the posterior and anterior segments of the right lobe have some overlapping in the frontal view, while the former occupies the inferior part and the latter the superior part. The right hepatic vein runs in between.

Portal hypertension—Case 29: Portal vein changes in advanced cirrhosis.

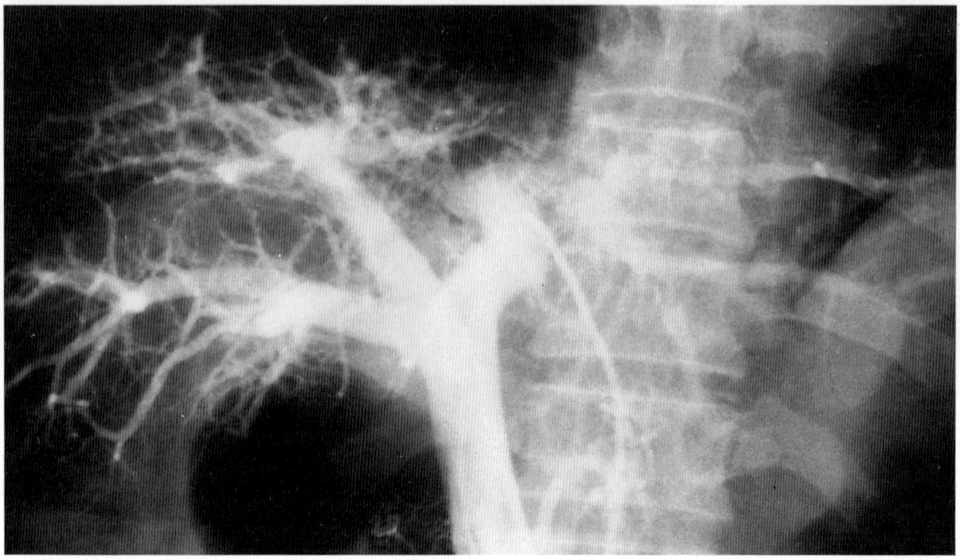

PTP: due to advanced cirrhoses, portal branches are narrowed and straightened, and the number of peripheral branches reduced. As the right lobe atrophies (common in Japan), the anterior and posterior portal branches are separated by being shifted cranially and caudally, respectively.

Portal hypertension—Case 30: Percutaneous transhepatic obliteration (PTO) of collateral veins for the treatment of esophageal varices.

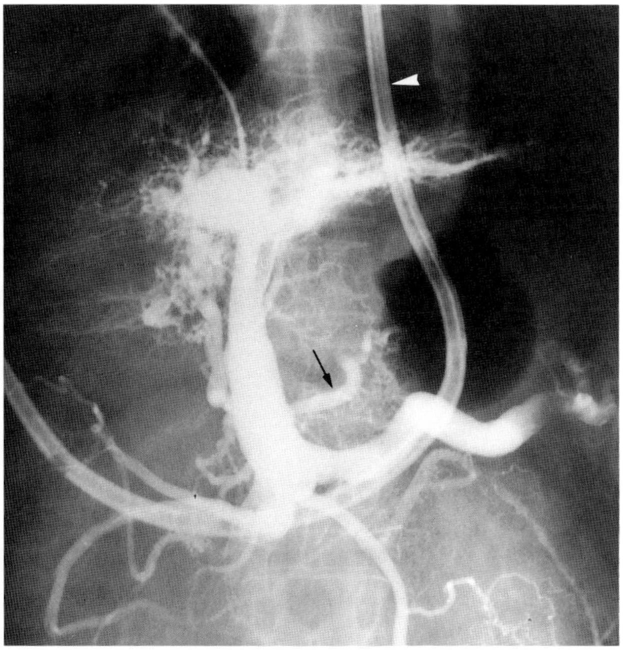

(a) PTP: the catheter was inserted toward the splenic vein through the umbilical portion of the left portal vein. The liver is markedly atrophied. The left gastric vein (→) is dilated, but varices are not opacified because the S-B tube (▶) is inflated.

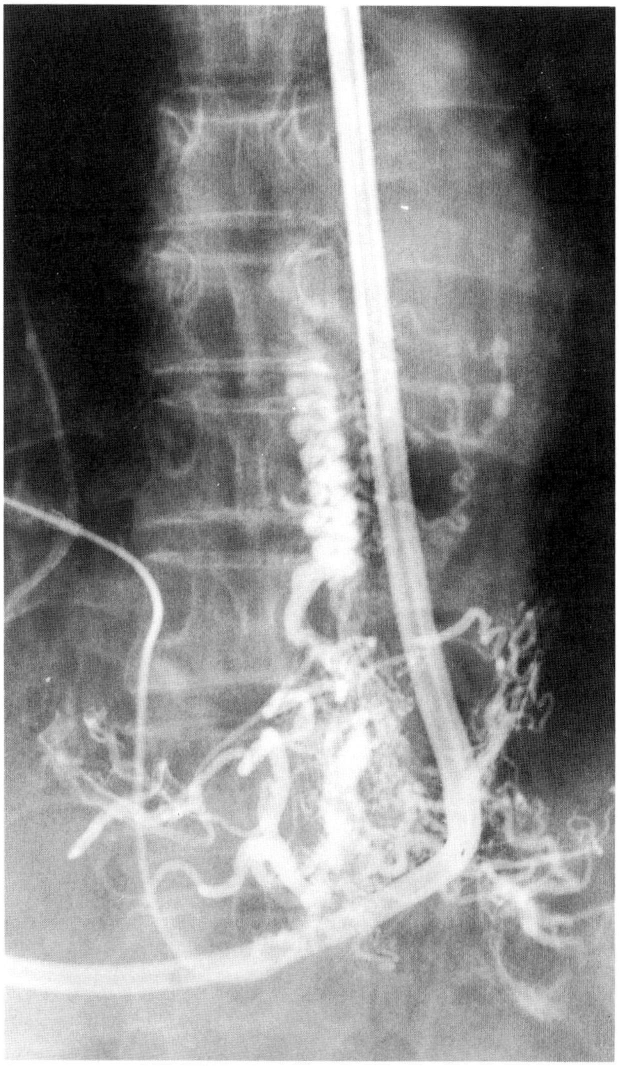

(b) Selective left gastric venography: the catheter was inserted into the left gastric vein, and contrast medium injected while the S-B tube was deflated. The esophageal varices were opacified, and 50 per cent glucose was injected followed by injection of Gelfoam sponge particles mixed with thrombin powder. Acute bleeding was successfully controlled. There was, however, recurrent bleeding 1 month later.

Portal hypertension—Case 31: Sclerotherapy for esophageal varices. This patient with HCC and cirrhosis was rushed to the hospital because of acute bleeding. Variceal bleeding was seen by endoscopy.

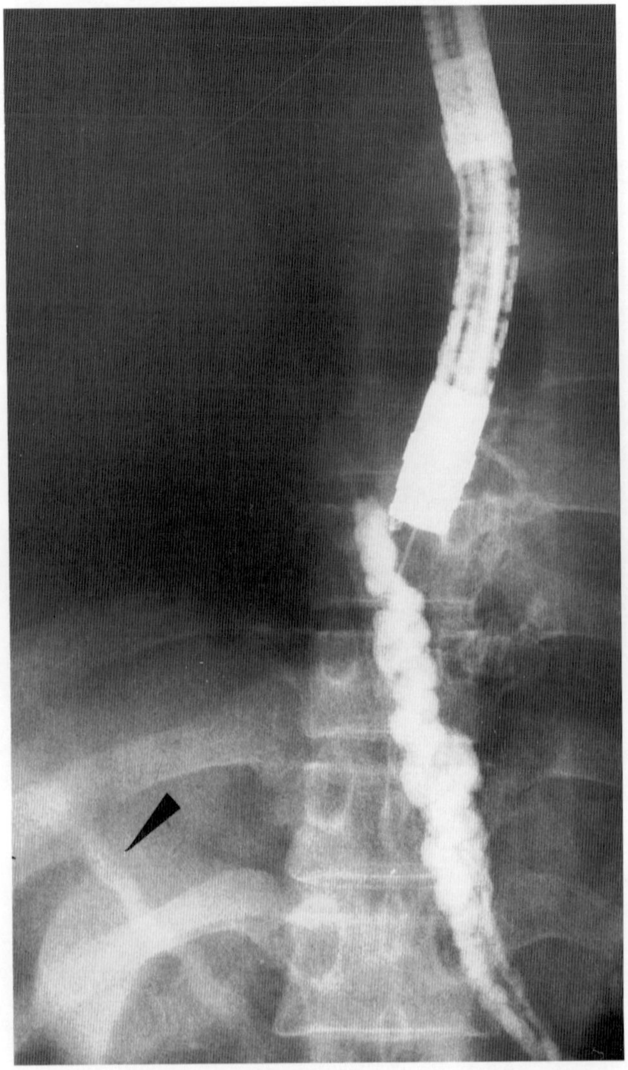

Endoscopic opacification of esophageal varies: under endoscopic vision, a needle was inserted into the varices, the needle position was confirmed by injecting contrast medium, and ethanolamine oleate was injected for hemostasis. Some of the intravariceally injected contrast medium flowed into the portal vein trunk (▶) which was faintly opacified.

12

Budd–Chiari syndrome

Budd–Chiari syndrome is defined as occlusion of the hepatic veins and their tributaries (Leevy *et al.* 1994). Another definition would be an outflow block to hepatic venous system at any site including the inferior vena cava (IVC). Outflow block can be caused not only by the hepatic vein occlusion, but also obstruction of the IVC above the opening of the hepatic veins. In the western countries where this syndrome was first documented, hepatic vein thrombosis is the most common cause (Mitchell *et al.* 1982), frequently associated with a hypercoagulable state such as myeloproliferative disease, coagulation factor deficiency, systemic lupus erythematosus (SLE) (Terabayashi *et al.* 1986), etc.; it may be called classical Budd–Chiari syndrome. In other regions of the world, IVC obstruction within the hepatic portion of the IVC without a known cause is much more common; it may be called 'idiopathic'. In Japan, 90 per cent of the cases are idiopathic (Okuda H. *et al.* 1995). Clinically, this syndrome is characterized by abdominal pain, ascites, hepatomegaly, and ankle edema, and in chronic cases by dilatation of the veins in the abdominal wall and splenomegaly. Hepatic vein outflow block may also develop secondarily to neoplasms of the liver, adrenal, kidney, etc., and to vasculitis caused by SLE and Beçhet disease. Idiopathic Budd–Chiari syndrome seems to be decreasing in Japan, but with modern imaging techniques, intra- and extrahepatic collateral veins are being found in asymptomatic cases (Makuuchi *et al.* 1984; Takayasu *et al.* 1994*b*).

Primary Budd–Chiari syndrome

The classical Budd–Chiari syndrome may be diagnosed by US (Case 1) from thrombosed large hepatic veins and an enlarged liver, and from the clinical symptoms. It is a severe disease with a high mortality for which liver transplantation is indicated. The idiopathic type Budd–Chiari syndrome is less severe at the onset, and tends to run a chronic course. The IVC occlusion may be preceded by mural thrombosis with incomplete obstrution. Prominent abdominal wall veins with cephalad blood flow are visible. For some ill defined mechanism, thrombosis occurs in the hepatic portion of the IVC, and when it organizes, it turns into fibrous obstruction (Kage *et al.* 1992). As it ages, it may be calcified. The term 'membranous IVC obstruction' is commonly used, but it is a misnomer, because more often the obstruction is much thicker than a membrane. The congenital malformation theory (Hirooka and Kimura 1970; Simson 1982) for the genesis of the obstruction fails to explain late onset of the disease (Okuda 1982). The caudate lobe is often markedly enlarged as a compensation for other lobes that are not functioning well due to congestion. On colloid scintigraphy, more activities are seen in the center and left of the liver in the anterior view (Case 3), because perfusion through the short and inferior right hepatic veins is compensatorily increased as a result of the occlusion of the major hepatic veins, causing accumulation of the colloid in the middle portion of the liver (Tavill *et al.* 1975).

The imaging features of the IVC obstruction studied by US (Makuuchi *et al.* 1984) and CT (Takayasu *et al.* 1994*b*) are:

1. Remarkable intrahepatic venous anastomoses and enlargement of the inferior right hepatic vein.
2. Occlusion of the orifices of major hepatic veins and/or IVC at the level of the diaphragm. Calcification may be present in the occluding lesion.
3. On CT, dilatation of the azygos/hemiazygos vein along the vertebral column and the anterior longitudinal vertebral veins of the vertebral venous plexus is recognized, along with IVC thrombosis.
4. Compensatory hypertrophy of the caudate lobe.
5. Transient dilatation of the IVC normally seen by US on the Valsalva maneuver is not recognized.

The final diagnosis is made by inferior cavography (Fig. 12.1). To determine the size and extent of the occluding lesion, and the therapeutic strategy, simultaneous opacification of the superior and inferior vena cava is required. When the IVC is completely occluded, winding venous anastomoses are seen within the liver, and the bulk of the blood that has entered the liver flows out into the IVC through the inferior right hepatic vein, thenceforth to the cavo caval shunts (Case 4). In the absence of sufficient outflow through the hepatic veins, the portal vein necessarily flows retrogradely. IVC obstruction may be incomplete (partial Budd–Chiari syndrome (Maguire *et al.* 1977)). If the obstruction is thin (membrane), its perforation with a catheter and balloon dilatation using the pressure-resistant Gruntzig balloon catheter (percutaneous transluminal angioplastly, PTA) (Yamada *et al.* 1983*b*) is the therapy of choice. If the occlusion is too thick and firm, a laser may be employed (Furui *et al.* 1988). Otherwise, a shunt may be surgically produced between the IVC and the right atrium or the subclavian vein. MR imaging is very useful in the assessment of the therapeutic effect on the IVC (Stark *et al.* 1986) (Case 1).

Histopathologically, centrilobular congestion and necrosis are the early changes which subsequently turn to fibrosis. Perhaps the compensatory liver cell regeneration that follows necrosis is the cause of frequent complication by HCC. In South African blacks, nearly one-half of the patients with IVC obstruction develop HCC (Simson 1982). When Nakamura *et al.* (1968) collected case reports in Japan, association with HCC was found in 41 per cent of them. However, this figure is

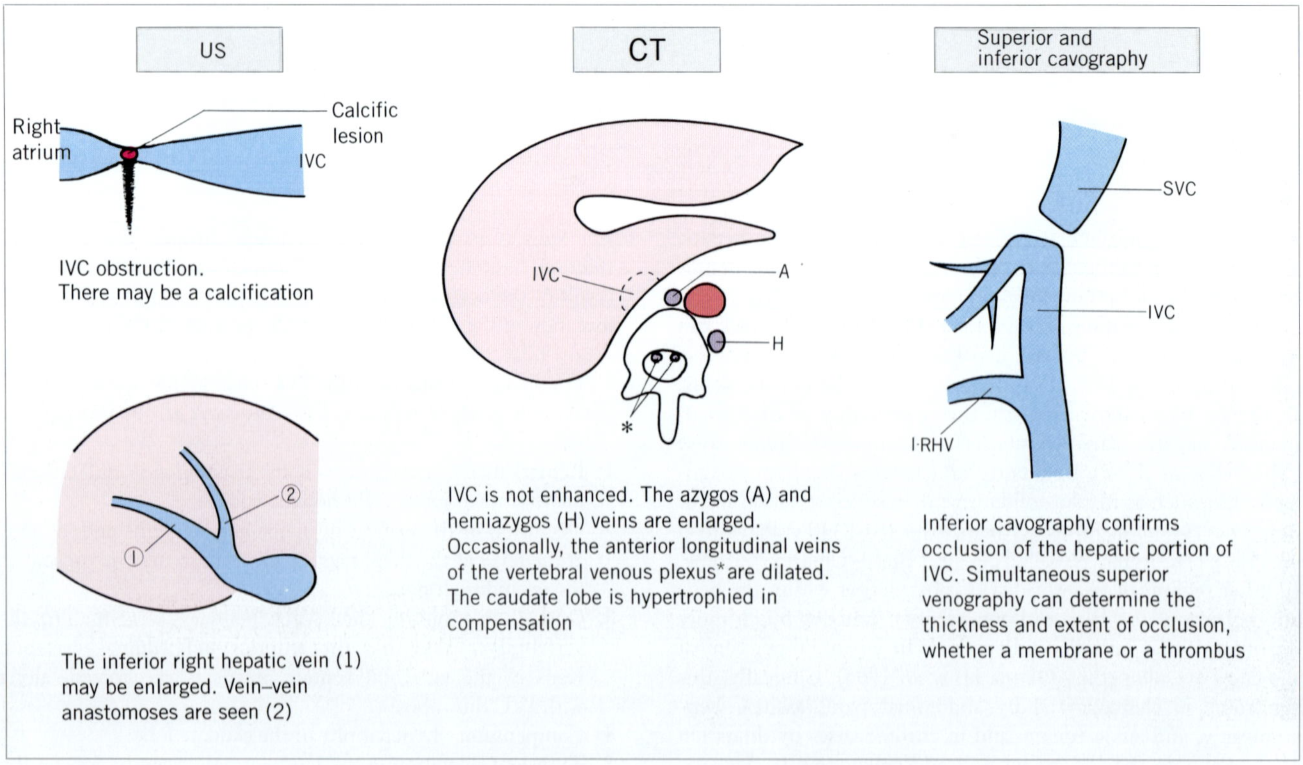

Fig. 12.1 Imaging characteristics of Budd–Chiari syndrome.

grossly biased, and a recent national study in Japan demonstrated an incidence of 6.4 per cent out of 157 authentic cases in 15 years (Okuda H *et al.* 1995). At the National Cancer Center Hospital, Tokyo, three of four cases had multicentric HCC (Case 1).

Secondary Budd–Chiari syndrome

The pathophysiology of secondary obstruction of the IVC is the same as the primary. When the hepatic portion of the IVC is occluded by a mass developing in the liver, and if the inferior right hepatic vein is patent, intrahepatic venous anastomoses will expedite blood flow into the right atrium through patent major hepatic veins (Takayasu *et al.* 1985*c*) (Case 5). Accurate vascular diagnosis is mandatory for surgical intervention. In a mass growing from below such as renal carcinoma, the inferior right hepatic vein is usually involved, and no such flow would occur. Thrombosis of the IVC can now be adequately studied by CT (Case 6). Complete obstruction of the IVC, whether by a thrombus or a tumor, is diagnosed when the IVC is not opacified and remains a low-density area on enhanced CT. If it is due to a tumor, the caliber of the IVC is enlarged, whereas thrombosis does not alter the venous caliber, and there is no continuity with the primary cancer lesion. The presence and absence of blood flow within the occluding lesion can be determined by Doppler US. In an early phase of dynamic CT, the IVC may be opacified in such a way that it simulates thrombosis (pseudo IVC thrombosis) (Case 7). One has to be familiar with this phenomenon which is explained by a time difference for contrast medium in entering the IVC between the blood perfusing through the lower limbs and that perfusing abdominal organs.

Congenital anomalies of the inferior vena cava

Various congenital abnormalities in the formation of the IVC and its course are known (Royal and Callen 1979). Left sided IVC (Case 8) and bilateral IVCs may be incidentally discovered during an imaging study. They do not have any clinical relevance, but occasionally it may be mistaken for lymph adenopathy, and for a collateral vein during the operation. In patients with left sided IVC who undergo an operation on the liver or kidney, the opening of the draining vein into the IVC has to be determined by imaging.

Budd–Chiari syndrome—Case 1: Diagnosis and therapy of Budd–Chiari syndrome complicated by HCC. A 24-year-old man came to the hospital for epigastric pain. US detected two mass lesions and IVC obstruction.

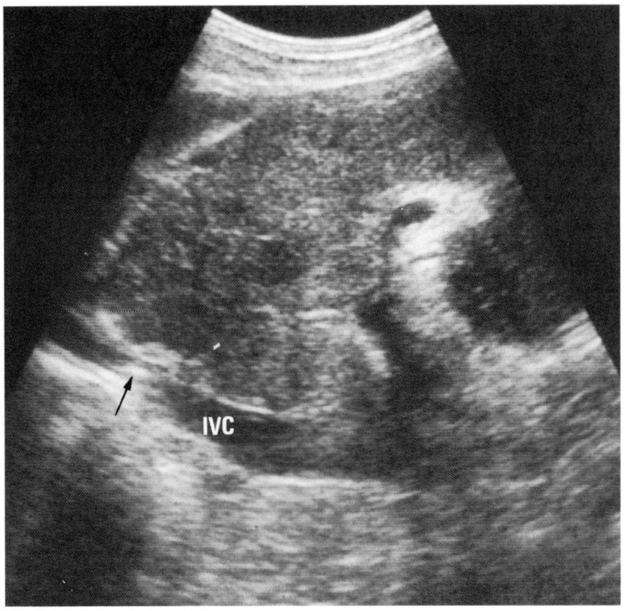

(a) US (epigastric sagittal scan): obstruction (→) of the hepatic portion of the IVC (IVC) is recognized. No dilatation of the IVC caliber occurred on the Valsalva maneuver.

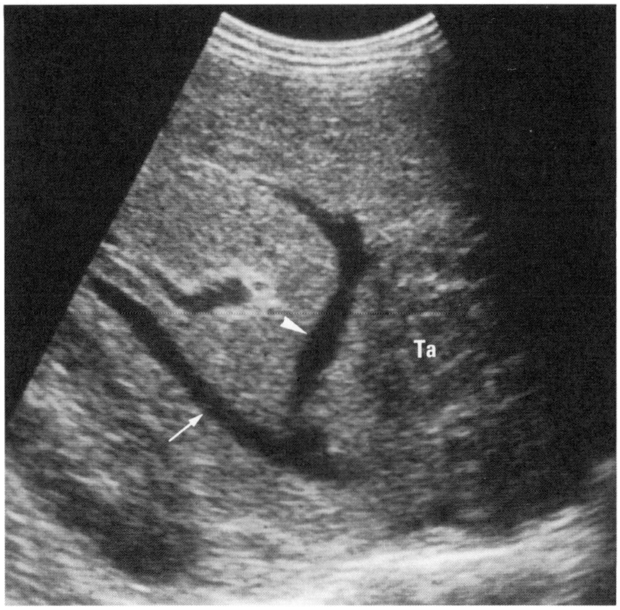

(b) US (right subcostal scan): the inferior right hepatic vein is dilated (→), and a communication (▶) with the middle hepatic vein is also evident. These kinds of vein-to-vein anastomoses are commonly seen in IVC obstruction. The central portion of the middle hepatic is occluded by tumor compression.

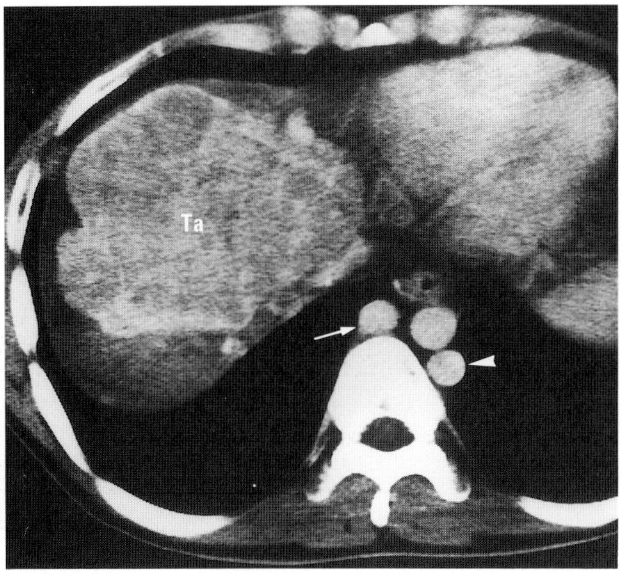

(c) Dynamic CT: dilated azygos (→) and hemiazygos veins (▶) are seen on both sides of the aorta. A confluent multinodular HCC (Ta) is seen occupying the right anterior superior subsegment (S^{VIII}).

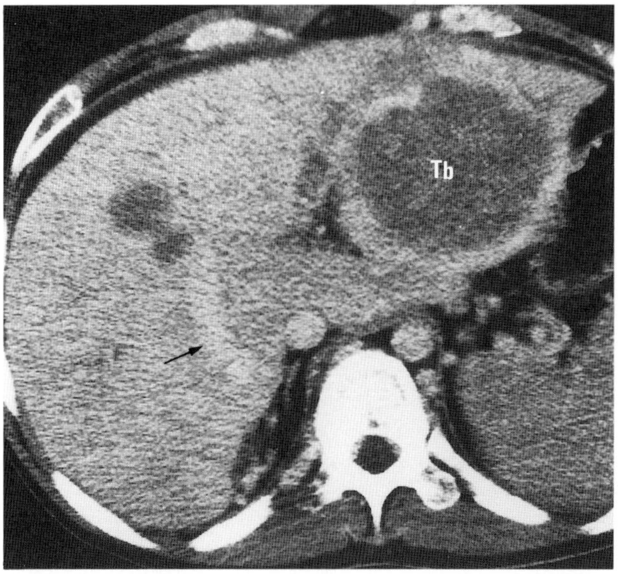

(d) Dynamic CT (hilar level): an anastomosing channel (→) between the middle and inferior right hepatic veins is recognized. Another nodular HCC (Tb) is seen in the left lobe laterally.

Case 1 (contd.)

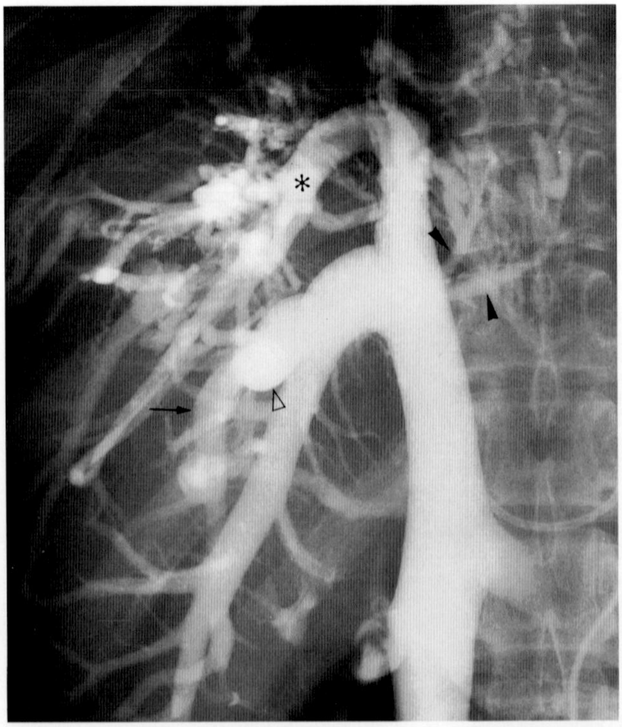

(e) Inferior vena cavography: the IVC is completely occluded immediately above the orifice of the right hepatic vein (*) at the diaphragmatic level. The middle hepatic vein (→) occluded by the tumor (Ta) flows into dilated IVC through an anastomosing vein (▷). The blood flows further down into the bilateral renal veins thenceforth into the azygos vein system. The two short hepatic veins that drain the caudate lobe are recognized (▶).

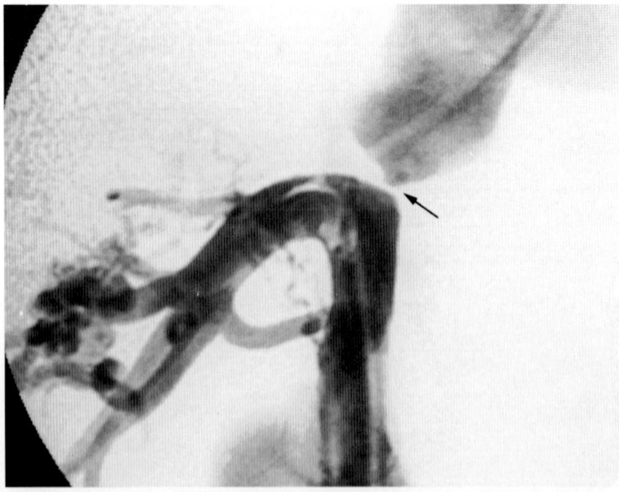

(f) Simultaneous superior and inferior cavography: a membrane several milimeters thick (→) is recognized. The IVC exists above the membrane for a length of 2 cm up to the right atrium as shown by the catheter inserted into the superior vena cava up to the membrane. It provides information important for the subsequent therapy.

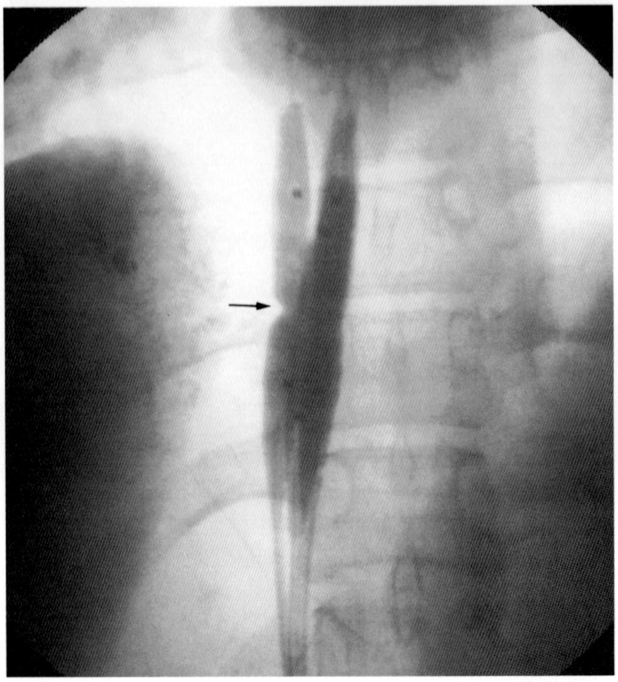

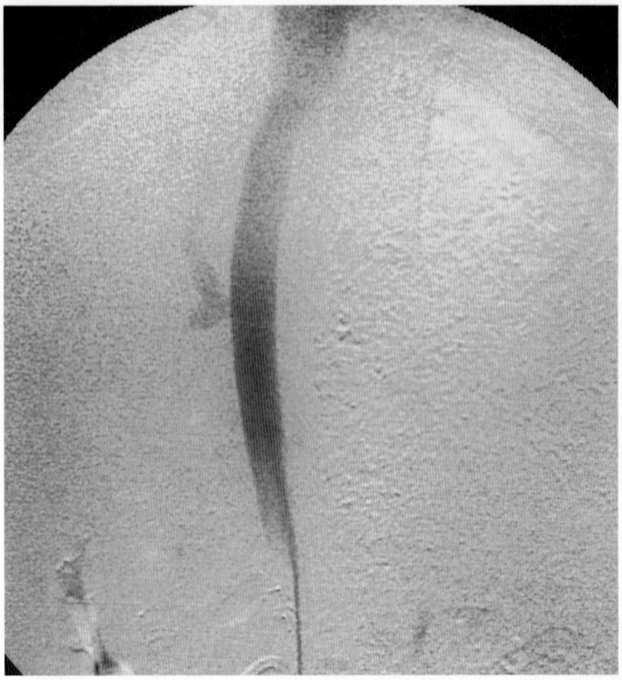

(g) (left) Inflated therapeutic balloons (during treatment): the membrane was perforated by a firm guide-wire in the IVC, followed by insertion of three to four Grunzig balloon catheters of increasing sizes for enlargement of the perforation. Since the membrane was firm, it caused an indentation of the balloon (→).

(h) Inferior cavography (post-treatment): after perforation and dilatation of the opening, contrast medium was injected. It showed satisfactory enlargement of the opening and flow of contrast into the right atrium.

Case 1 (contd.)

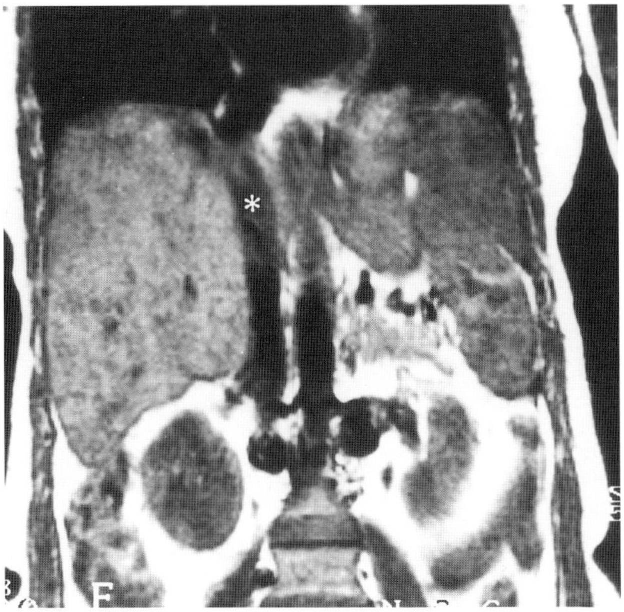

(i) MR imaging (pretreatment; T1-weighted, 600/15): blood is stagnant below the obstruction with IVC and is seen as hyperintense (flow void phenomenon)

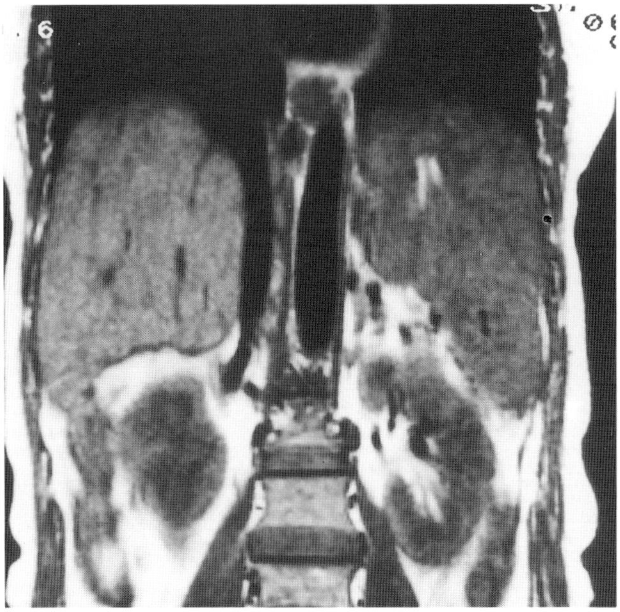

(j) MR imaging (post-treatment; T1-weighted, 600/15): MR image made 5 days after percutaneous transluminal angioplasty (PTA) displays opening of the IVC which now is of low intensity.

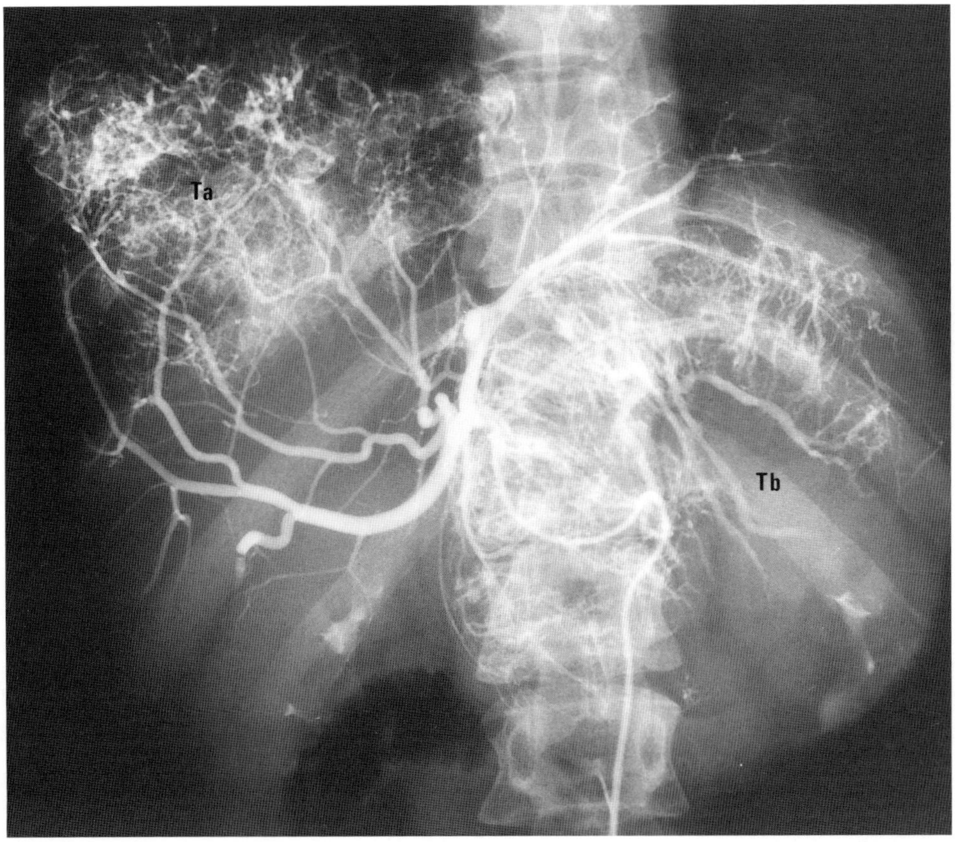

(k) Hepatic arteriogram: a hypervascular tumor is seen in each lobe (Ta, Tb). In general, HCC complicating Budd–Chiari syndrome demonstrates morphologic differences in individual tumors, suggesting multicentric emergence.

Budd–Chiari syndrome—Case 2: Budd–Chiari syndrome with a thrombus within the IVC and an enlarged inferior right hepatic vein.

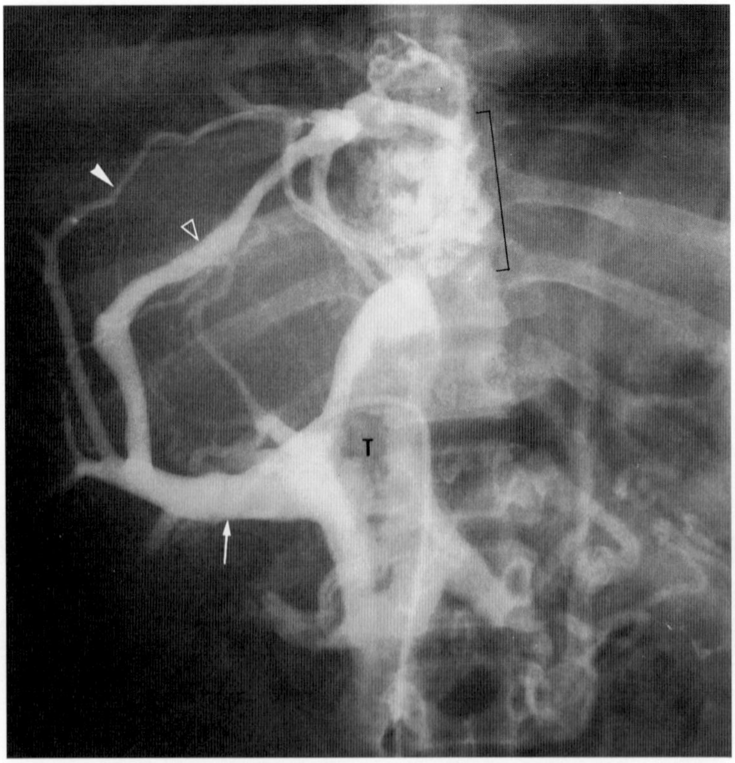

(a) Inferior cavogram: the hepatic portion of the IVC is occluded for several centimeters (⊔). The caudal portion from the occlusion is dilated and contains a secondary thrombus (T). The middle hepatic (▷) and right hepatic (▶) veins communicate with the IVC at a cranial level, but the bulk of blood flow in the hepatic veins enters a dilated inferior right hepatic vein (→).

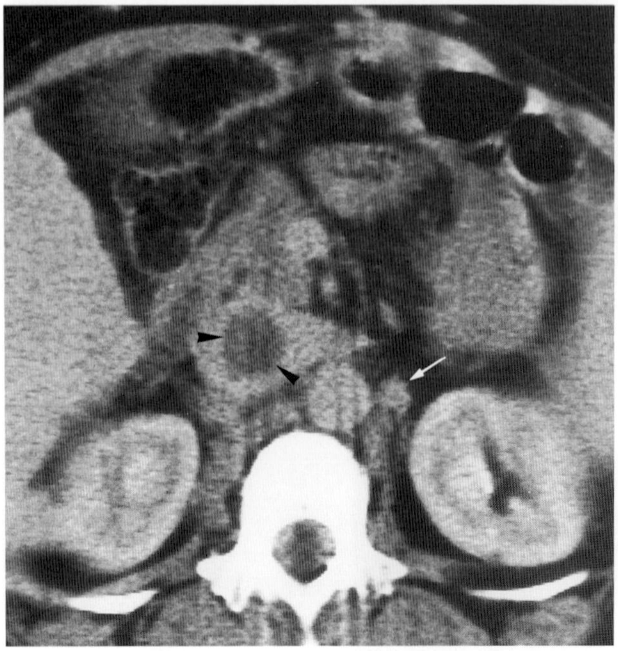

(b) Enhanced CT: this is the level of the opening of the left renal vein into the IVC. Dilated IVC and a cylindrical thrombus (▶) seen as a low-density area are recognized. The hemiazygos vein (→) is dilated.

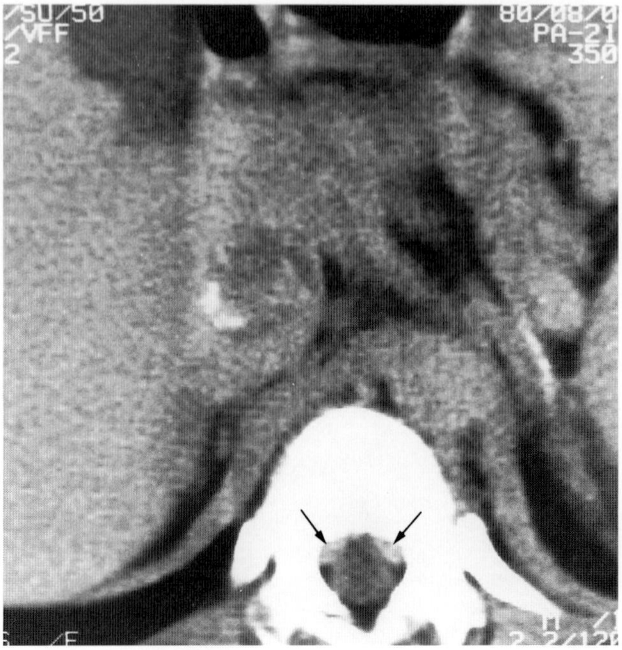

(c) Enhanced CT [cranial from (b)]: as one of the collaterals, bilateral anterior longitudinal vertebral veins of the vertebral venous plexus (→) are identified. Partial calcification of the thrombus within the IVC is also recognized.

Budd–Chiari syndrome—Case 3: Compensatory hypertrophy of the caudate lobe in Budd–Chiari syndrome.

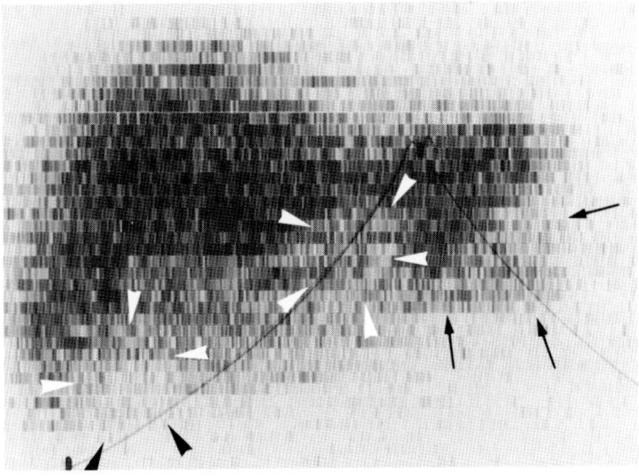

(a) Hepatic scintigram (^{99cm}Tc-phytate): an enlarged caudate lobe (→) is seen to the left laterocaudally. Two cold areas (▶) are due to complicating HCC.

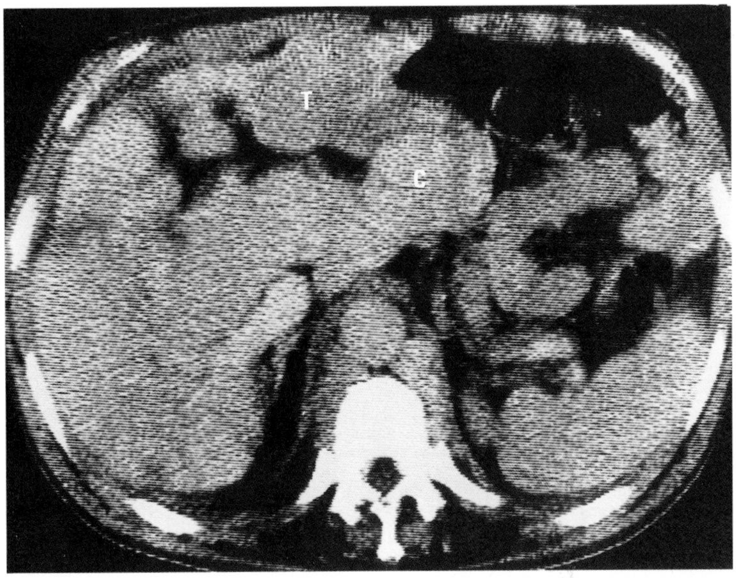

(b) Enhanced CT: a markedly enlarged caudate lobe (C) is seen near the hilum. An enlarged inferior right hepatic vein flowing into the IVC is a common finding in Budd–Chiari syndrome. T, HCC.

Budd–Chiari syndrome—Case 4: Budd–Chiari syndrome with a possibly (?) malformed hepatic portion of the IVC. During the follow-up of a patient by US after resection for a colon cancer, a solitary metastasis and multiple vascular structures were found in the liver.

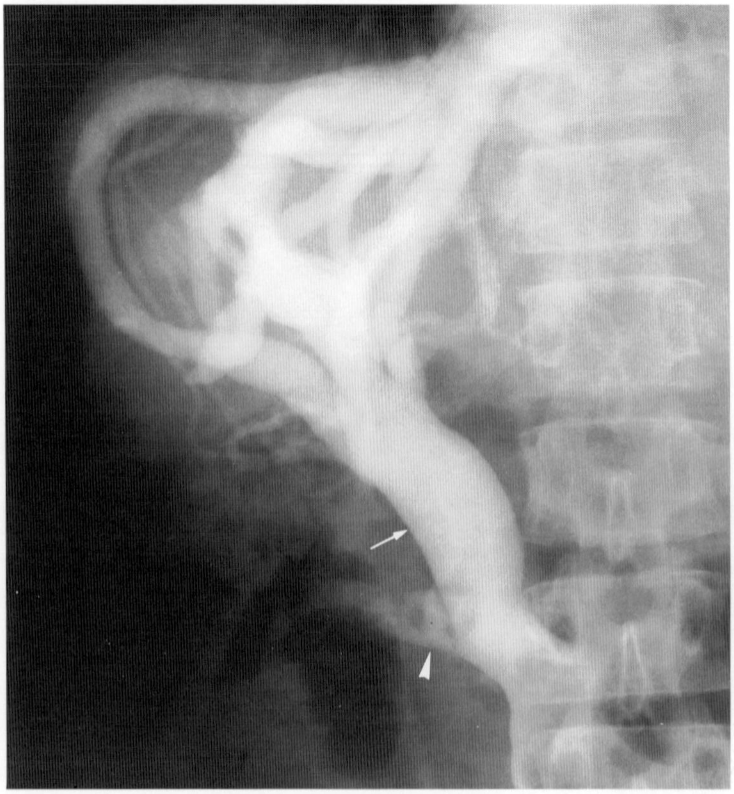

(a) Inferior cavogram: the IVC is not recognized above the opening of the right renal vein (▶). Instead, the IVC flows into the right atrium through numerous markedly dilated hepatic veins as a continuation of a large collatoral vein (→) within the liver.

(b) (opposite) Cavo-CT: while contrast medium was injected through the IVC with the table incremental method, moving 8→1 CT images were made. From these images, one can recognize the many large hepatic veins flowing into the right atrium while communicating with each other. The middle hepatic vein (→) can be identified from the position of the gallbladder. The IVC can be followed cranially, but its caliber is very small (▶). Although it could not be determined whether this is a congential hypoplasia of the IVC, or secondary narrowing following inflammation or mural thrombosis, the latter seems more likely.

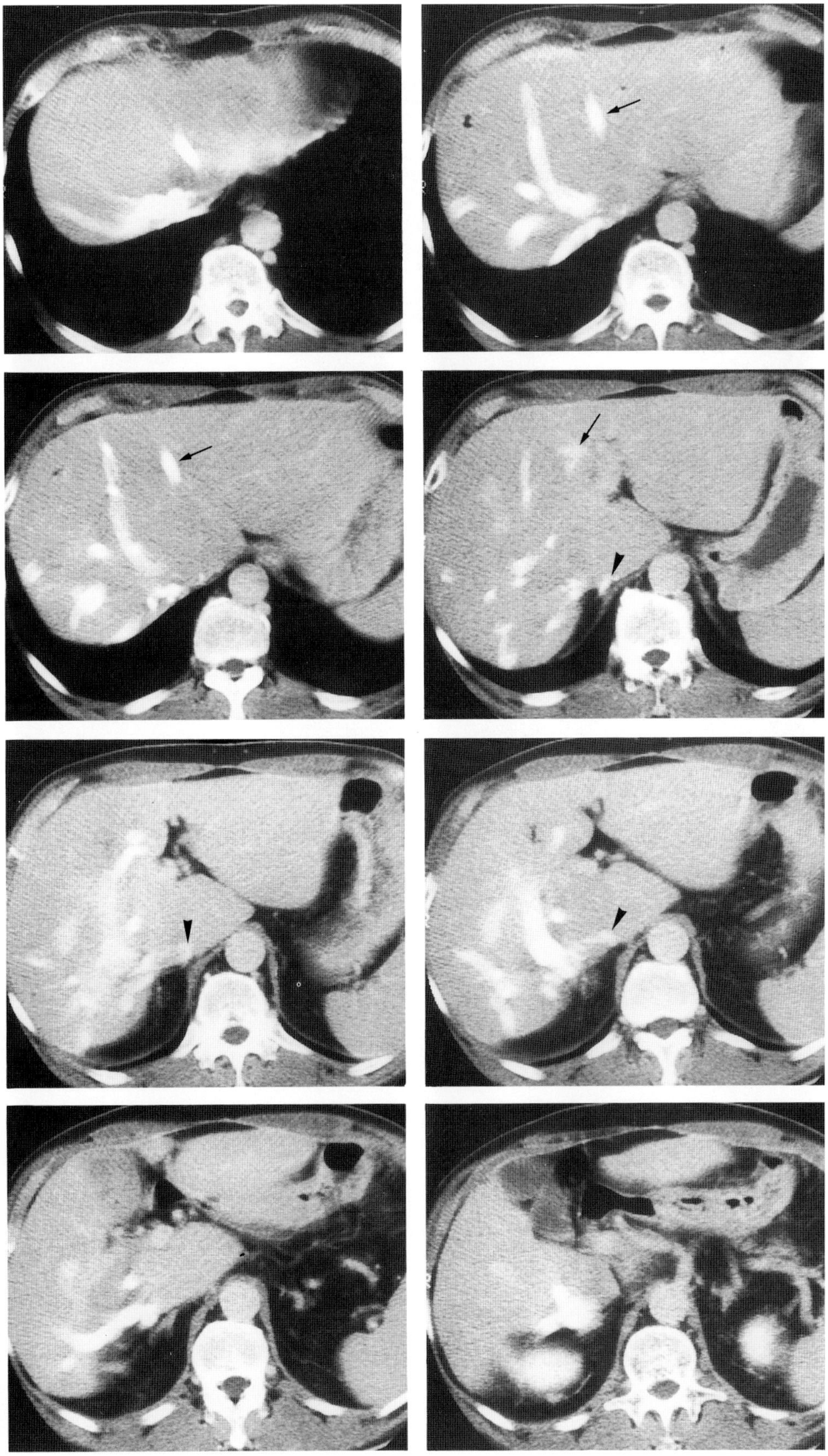

1	2
3	4
5	6
7	8

Budd–Chiari syndrome—Case 5: Secondary Budd-Chiari syndrome due to a huge lipoma of the right hepatic lobe.

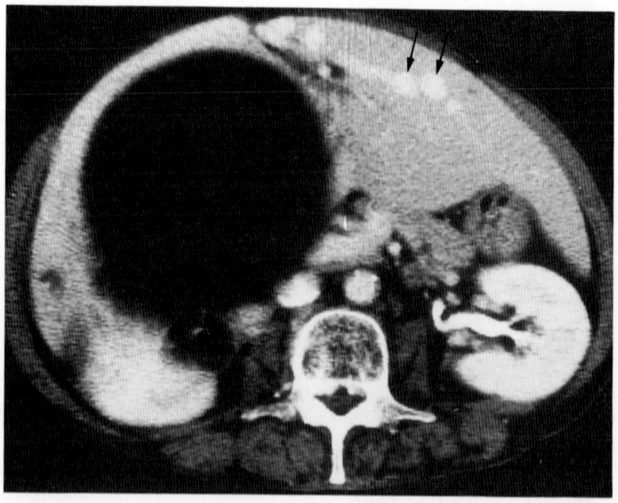

(a) Enhanced CT: a huge lipoma in the right lobe, its compression onto the IVC (seen in cranial slices) and enlarged hepatic veins in the left lobe (→) are apparent (same as Case 1).

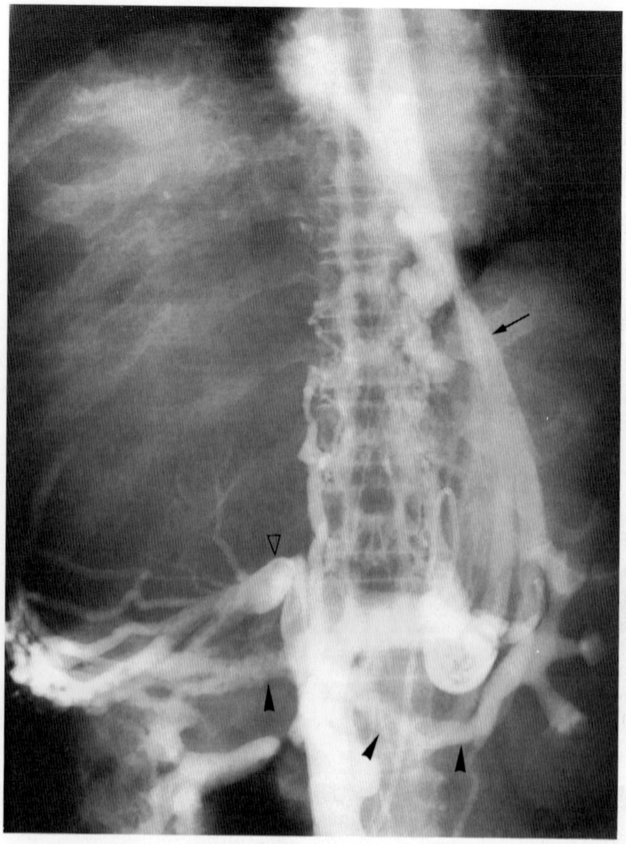

(b) Inferior cavogram: the IVC is completely occluded above the inferior right hepatic vein (▷). Several collaterals (▶) are flowing into the left hepatic vein (→) through the inferior right hepatic. The dilated left hepatic veins seen on the CT are clearly opacified. After resection of this lipoma, the compression was relieved and IVC started flowing.

Budd–Chiari syndrome—Case 6: Secondary Budd–Chiari syndrome due to thrombosis involving the IVC and bilateral iliac veins. A middle-aged woman presented with edema of the lower extremities and abdominal distension.

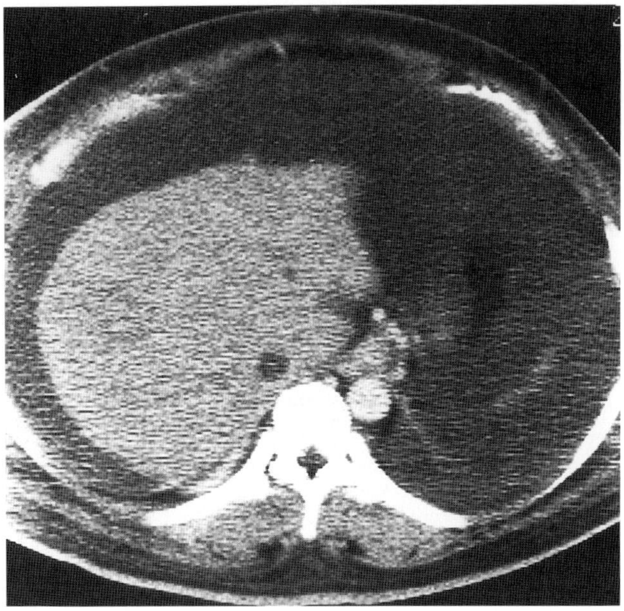

(a) Enhanced CT: the IVC was not enhanced, and was seen as a low-density area in all the cranial and caudal slices. A diagnosis of IVC thrombosis was made. Massive ascites was also evident.

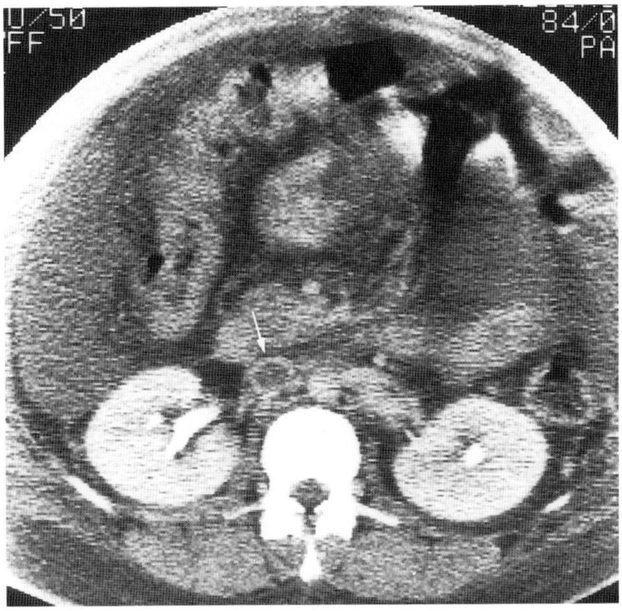

(b) Enhanced CT (level of the renal hilum): as in (a), only the wall of the IVC (→) not its lumen was enhanced.

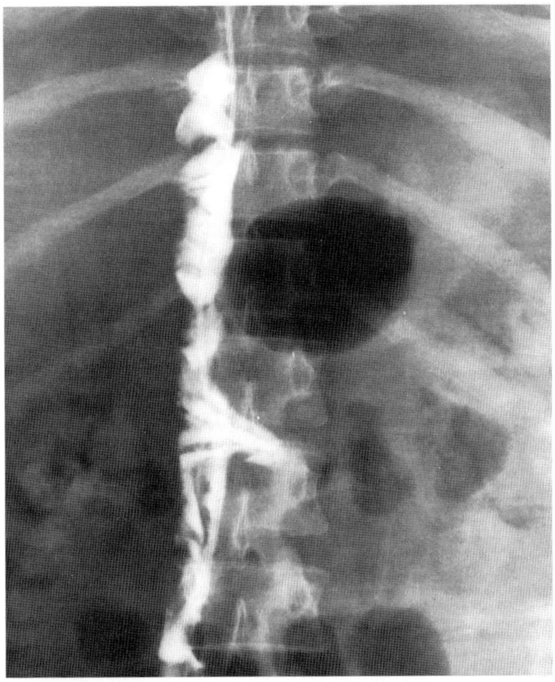

c

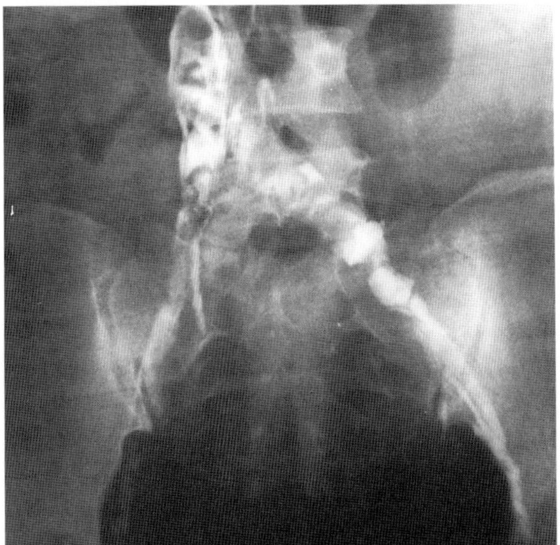

d

(c) Inferior cavogram: the catheter was inserted from the external jugular vein, and the hepatic portion of the IVC was found to be completely occluded.

(d) Inferior cavogram (further caudal): the catheter could be pushed down further, and contrast medium injected slowly. It opacified up to the external iliac vein bilaterally, revealing extensive thrombosis in the IVC; the left renal vein was also involved. The cause of thrombosis remained undetermined.

Budd–Chiari syndrome—Case 7: Pseudothrombosis of the IVC seen in an early phase of dynamic CT.

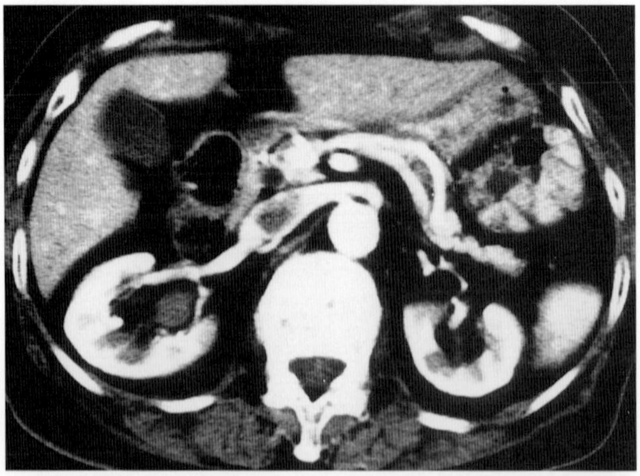

(a) Dynamic CT (early phase): a low-density area is seen in the IVC in the hilum of the right kidney. This may be mistaken for an IVC thrombus.

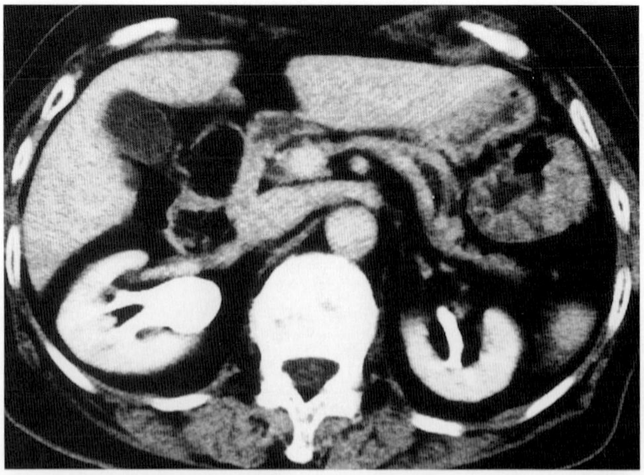

(b) Dynamic CT (late phase): the IVC is now homogeneously enhanced. This phenomenon is explained by the difference in the concentration of contrast medium between the renal venous flow and the flow coming from the limbs. The former is higher than the latter in density, and laminal flow is produced.

Budd–Chiari syndrome—Case 8: Left-sided IVC and its spatial relation to the hepatic vein.

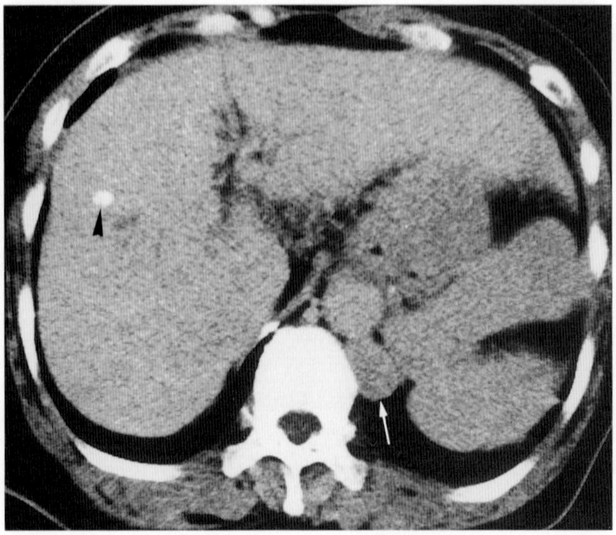

(a) Enhanced CT (late phase): a nodular lesion (→) is seen to the left of the aorta posteriorly. This has continuity with the same lesion in other slices. Since no IVC is seen in the right side, the diagnosis of left-sided IVC is possible. There is a Lipiodol deposit in an HCC (▶).

Case 8 (contd.)

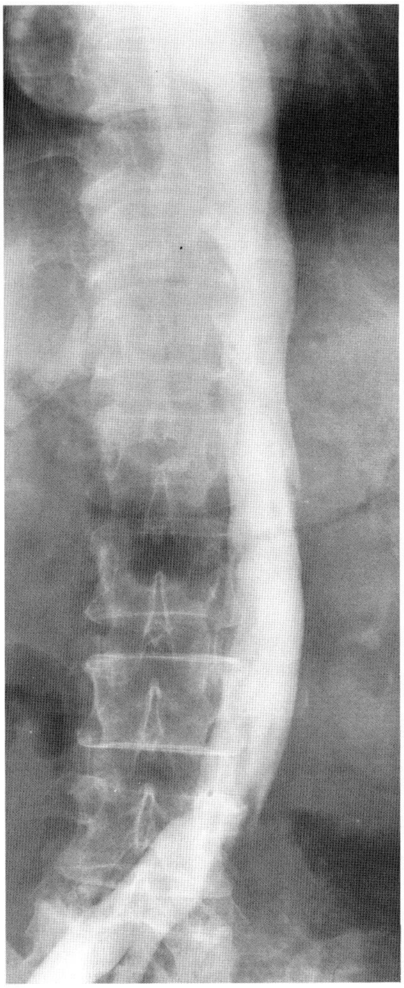

(b) Inferior cavogram: the IVC runs to the left of the vertebral column.

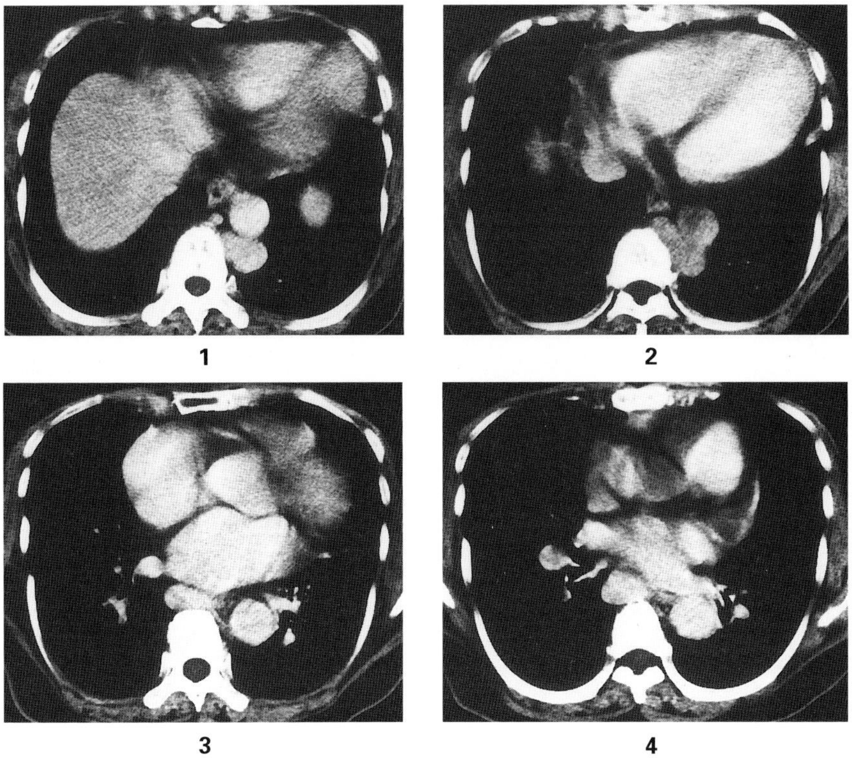

(c) Dynamic CT: the dynamic CT images from the caudal to the cranial levels (1–4) were analyzed. When it was followed cranially, it ran between the aorta and the vertebral column and entered the azygos (2) and thereon into the superior vena cava.

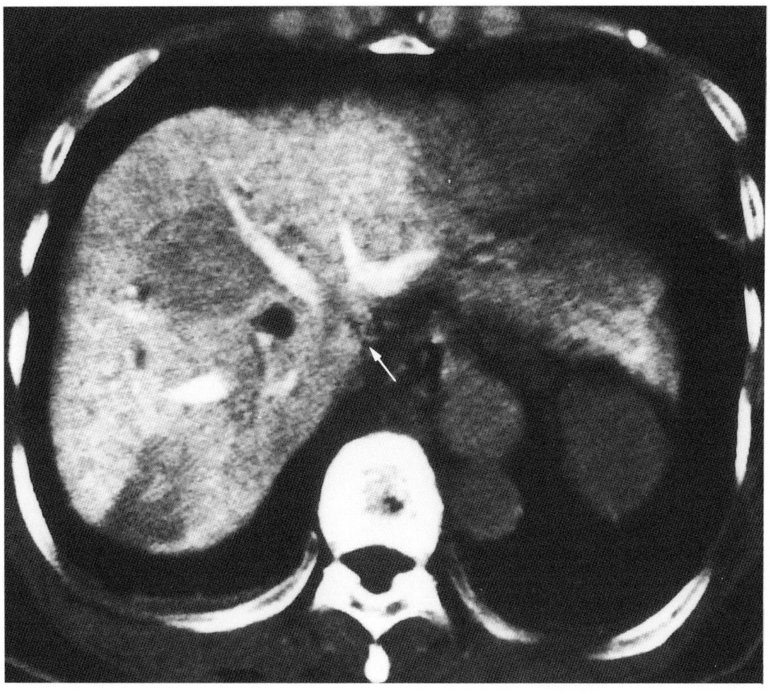

(d) Portal-CT (late phase): in left sided IVC, the opening of the hepatic veins has to be determined if an operation is contemplated. In the late phase image of portal-CT, the hepatic veins were flowing into the right atrium through a small remnant IVC (→).

II. Examination

13

Computed tomography

13.1 Introduction

Progress in computed tomography (CT)

CT is an indispensable diagnostic modality in the study of parenchymal organs that has developed to the current status after its first report by Hounsfield before the British Radiological Society meeting in 1972. The advantages of CT are its excellent spatial and density resolutions. In conventional roentgenography, differences greater than 10 per cent in X-ray absorption are required for recognition whereas in CT only a 0.5–1 per cent difference is necessary. With a spatial resolution of 0.35–0.5 mm, a recent machine requires only 30 ms to make one slice section.

The principle of CT is as follows: a very thin slit like X-ray beam is passed through the body and the rate of penetration is detected by a detector system (sodium iodide crystal or xenon gas ionization chamber) opposite to the X-ray tube. The X-ray beam rotates around the body by 180° to 360°, the CT values (attenuation coefficient) for individual pixels within the transverse section of the body are calculated by the computer, and digitalized values are converted to black/white densities.

The third-generation machine [Fig. 13.1(a)] is a rotation scanner with a movable X-ray tube and detector system. A broad fan of X-rays covering the entire object angularly faces a detector field consisting of 200–600 detectors which is moved around the body. The scanning time is between 1 and 4 s. The fourth-generation scanner [Fig. 13.1(b)] is a rotation system for the X-ray tube with stationary detectors. A fan shaped beam of X-rays covering the entire object angularly moves in a circle within the stationary detector array of 300–1000 detectors. The briefest scanning time amounts to 3–8 s. A further improvement from the fourth-generation scanner is the nutate/rotate system such as TCT 900S (Fig. 13.2). In this machine, the X-ray tube is located outside the detector system; the detector ring (2304 cadmium tungstate scintillators) moves in and out (nutates) in such a way that the detectors in front of the X-ray tube move away avoiding X-rays and the detectors on the opposite side from the X-ray tube receive the X-rays. Since the X-ray tube is always outside the detector, the distance between the X-ray focus and the detectors is large, permitting use of a high heat capacity X-ray tube with a large focus that can generate a larger X-ray beam. It thus enables continuous scanning for 30 s at a high speed. Since the detector system is inside the X-ray tube, it uses many small-diameter detectors tightly arrayed in a smaller ring arrangement. With this system the spatial resolution is improved to 0.35 mm, much better than the third- and fourth-generation scanners. In this system, the rotating part and the stationary part are in a slipping contact with multiple electrically conductive brushes that permit exchange of electricity and signals (slip ring system); the electrical cables supplying power to the X-ray tube are no longer necessary and the X-ray tube rotates continuously in one direction, much improving the time resolution.

A more recent development for faster CT scanning is the helical (spiral) CT system (Kalender *et al.* 1990; Vock *et al.* 1990) in which the X-ray tube is rotated continuously while the patient table is moved through the gantry. Therefore, the path of the X-ray shows a helix or a spiral on the surface of the patient (Fig. 13.3). Consecutive volumetric data of the entire liver are acquired within about 20 s, and the incidence of missing to slices due to respiratory misregistration has been reduced considerably (Kalender *et al.* 1990; Remy Jardin *et al.* 1993). With helical CT, arterial- and portal-CT have become more useful in detecting small hepatic lesions with three-dimensional reconstruction (Soyer *et al.* 1991). Three-dimensional reconstruction of portal-CT data is also helpful in simultating the surgical operation (Bluemke and Fishman 1993).

In the ultrafast electron beam scanner, Imatron, primarily developed for the study of the beating heart, an electron beam is used without moving the table (Fig. 13.4). It has the capability of imaging a single section in 50–100 ms with a moving focus of X-rays while sweeping an electron beam along a tungsten target arranged in a ring surrounding the patient. This may also be used in the diagnosis of diseases of the abdominal organs in the future.

Pixels and the partial averaging phenomenon

The CT image consists of small areas (pixels, usually 1×1 mm; pixel × thickness is called voxel) given on an analog gray scale of 16–32 grades for digitalized absorption rates. Therefore, theoretically a spatial resolution smaller than the pixel is impossible. If the study object is small, 5 mm or so, it is necessary for a better diagnosis to reduce the slice thickness to 5 mm, or do overlapping scan in which part of one slice is superimposed on part of the next slice. The lesion on the CT image, hence the CT value, may not be accurately displayed, because it depends on the slice thickness (Figs. 13.5, 13.6).

If the lesion is higher in density than the surrounding parenchyma (such as a tumor retaining Lipiodol, and a tumor enhanced on arterial-CT) it is more readily detected than is a low-density lesion (such as a cyst, a lesion that turns low-density on portal-CT) in a slice of the same thickness. For a small low-density lesion, it is necessary to reduce the thickness to 5 mm (Fig. 13.7).

The relative value of average X-ray absorption by pixels is called the CT value (Hounsfield unit, HU) which is set at 0 for water, −1000 for air, and +1000 for twice the water absorption. However, these absolute values vary with the condition of the

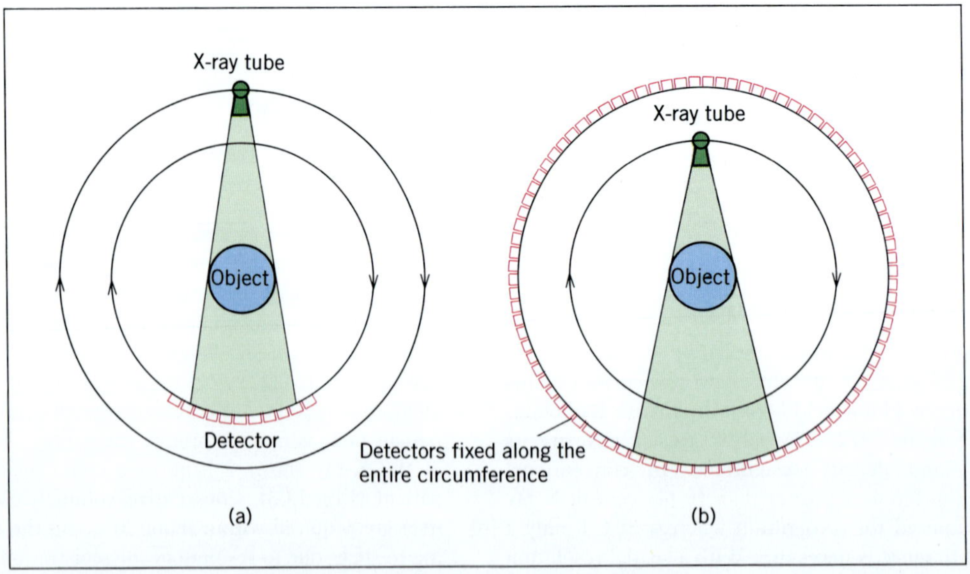

Fig. 13.1 The third and fourth generation CT scanners.
(a) The third-generation scanner (rotate/rotate system): the X-ray tube and detectors rotate together in the same direction. The former is outside to the latter.
(b) The fourth-generation scanner (rotate/stationary system): the detectors are fixed outside to the X-ray tube, and only the latter rotates in the inner circle.

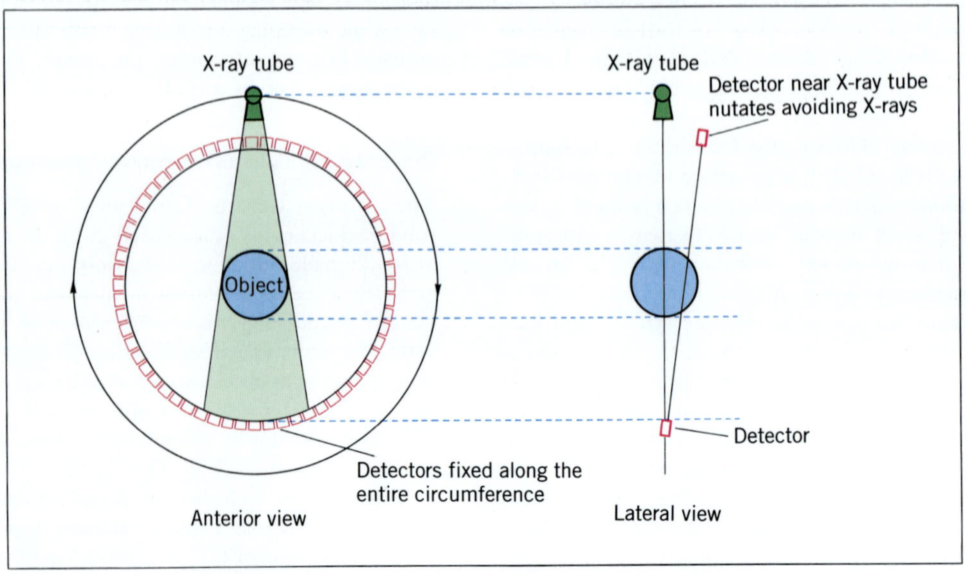

Fig. 13.2 New CT scanner based on the nutate/rotate system. The X-ray tube outside to the fixed detectors rotates continuously. The detectors right in front of the X-ray tube nutate to avoid the X-ray beam while the detectors opposite to the tube receive X-rays.

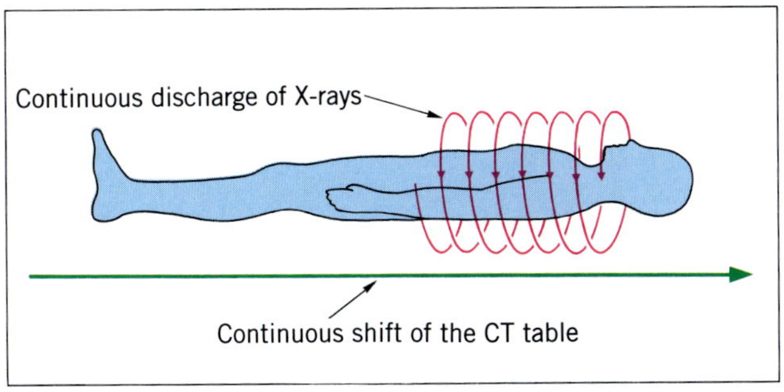

Fig. 13.3 Helical (spiral) CT. While the X-ray tube continuously rotates, the CT table is continuously moved. A special software program is required. One can choose various slice thicknesses (2, 5, 7 and 10 mm), and speed of table movement (2, 5, 7 and 10 mm/s). With a slice thickness of 5 mm and a speed of table movement of 5 mm/s, it takes only 30 s to cut the entire liver.

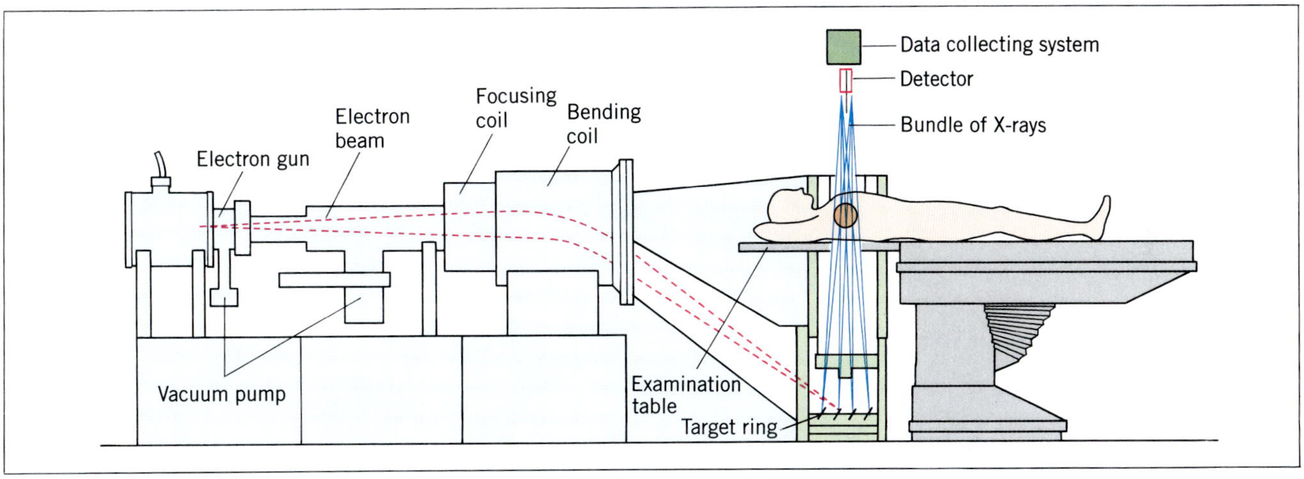

Fig. 13.4 Lateral view of the ultrafast CT scanner, Imatron (stationary detector/rotating electron beam). Electron beams shot from the electron gun are bent by the magnetic field (coil) and focused on four target rings. The X-rays generated from the rings are rotated by the coil for ultrafast scanning. The four target rings each receiving two electron beams produce eight slices from a tissue 8 cm thick in 0.25 s.

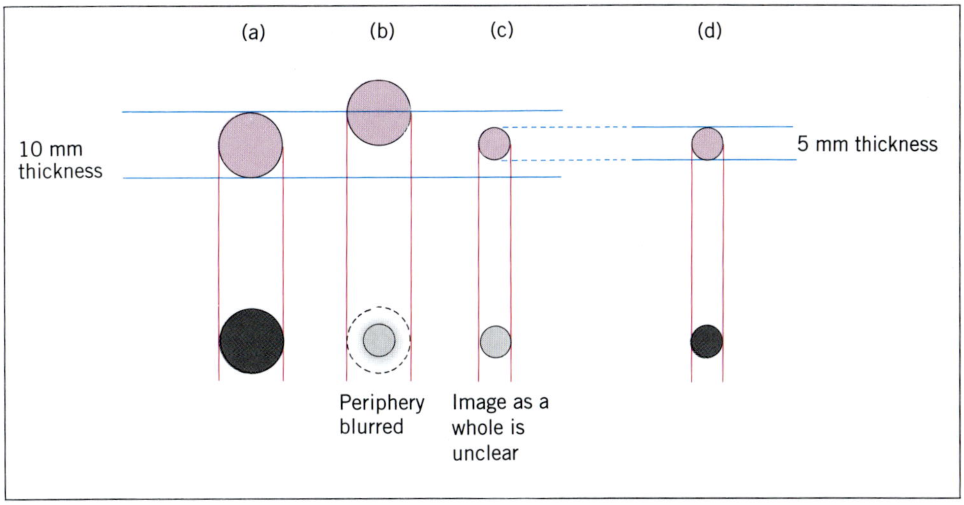

Fig. 13.5 Partial volume phenomenon. When a tumor 1 cm in diameter is scanned in a 1 cm slice, it will be clearly visualized if the tumor is in the center of the slice (a); it will be blurred with a poor contrast if only part of the tumor is in the slice (b). If the tumor is small, 5 mm in diameter, it is not clearly seen in a 1 cm thick slice (c), but will be discretely recognized if it is placed in the center of a 5 mm slice (d).

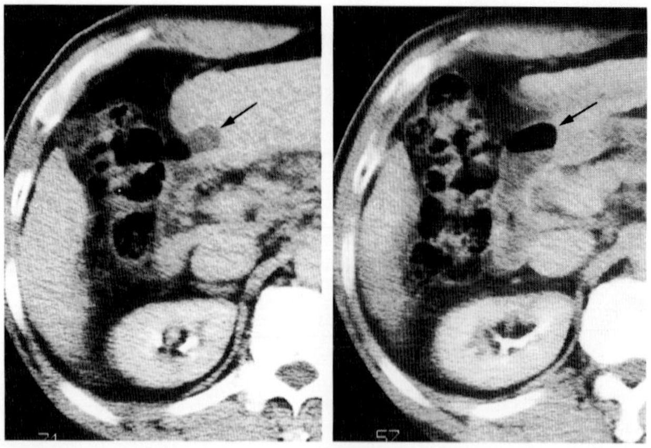

a b

Fig. 13.6 Pseudotumor lesion due to partial volume averaging. (a) Enhanced CT: in the caudal part of the left lobe a tumor-like lesion of a water density is seen (→). (b) Slice 1 cm caudal to (a): no liver tissue is seen in the same region; it was gas (→) in the duodenum.

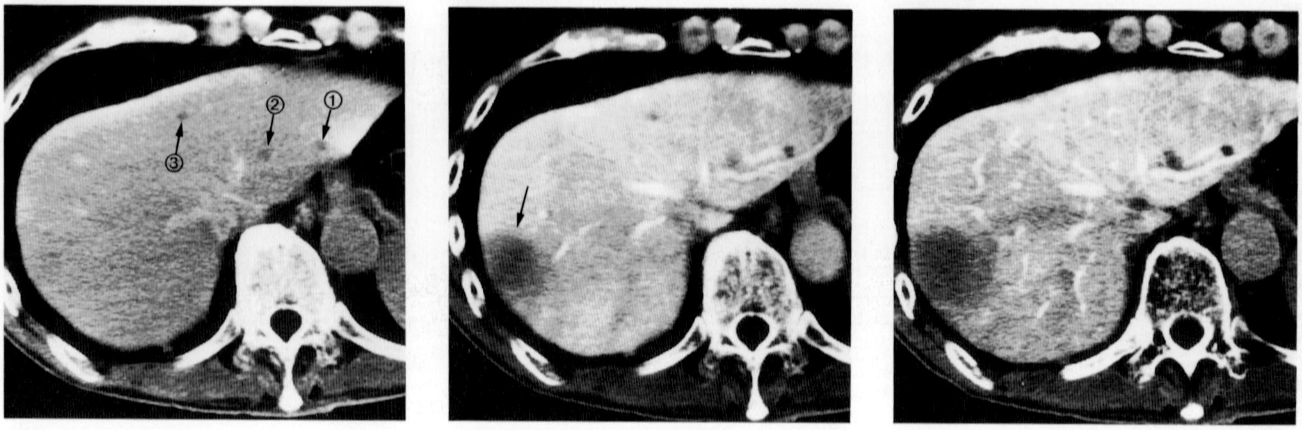

a b c

Fig. 13.7 Thin slicing proved diagnostic in differentiating a small cyst and a small metastasis from colon cancer.

(a) Enhanced CT (late phase, 10 mm slice): three 5 mm low-density masses (1), (2), (3) are seen in the left lobe. With this image, it was difficult to determine whether these were cysts or metastases.

(b) Portal-CT (10 mm slice): lesion (1) was diagnosed as a cyst from its low density, but the other two could not be diagnosed. →, an obvious metastasis.

(c) Portal-CT (5 mm slice): (1) and (2) are clearly cysts. Lesion (2) now looks like a snowman. Lesion (3) was also diagnosed as a cyst in the slice cranial to this image. The metastatic lesion (→ in (b)) was resected successfully.

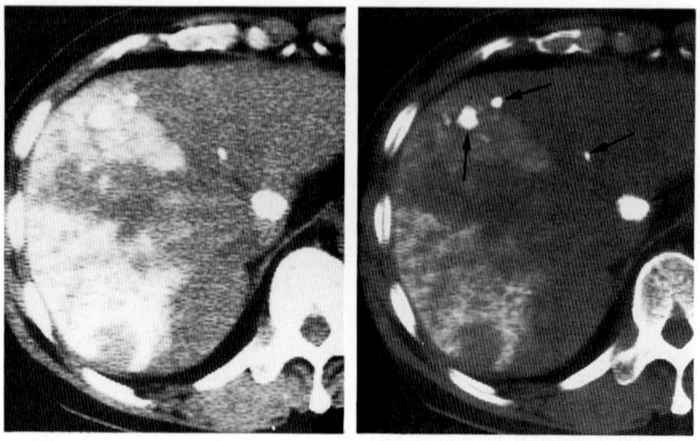

a WL 40, WW 264 **b WL 200, WW 800**

Fig. 13.8 Changes in the display condition have made diagnosis easier in a CT made after arterial injection of Lipiodol: (a) WL 40, WW 264; (b) WL 200, WW 800. With the window level (WL) set at 40 HU and window width (WW) at 264 (a), the mass was buried in non-specific deposition of Lipiodol in this monitoring image. However, when the display conditions were changed to those for bone study, the lesions (→) came to be clearly delineated (b).

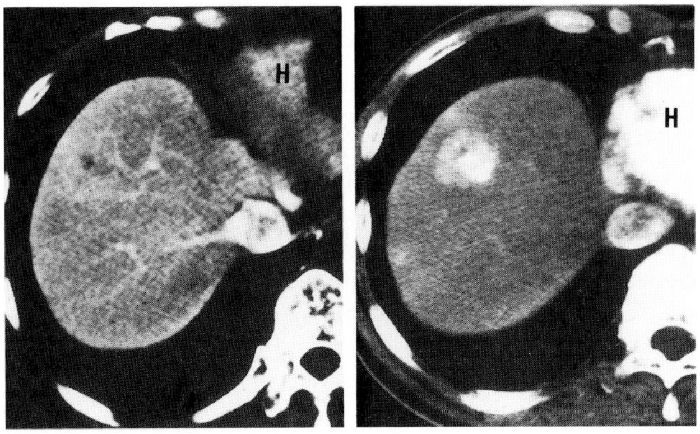

a b

Fig. 13.9 Differences in slice level due to different respiration phase, and obscurity of the lesion as a result of different scanning times: (a) inspiration phase, venous phase; (b) expiration phase, arterial phase. At a glance, the two slices appear to be of the same level: (a) was made at another hospital during the inhaling phase, and (b) was made at our hospital during the exhaling phase. Therefore, in (a) the heart (H) and the vertebra are more caudal than in (b). Contrast medium was injected under the same conditions (100 ml/3 ml/s) for both (a) and (b), and the lesion in S^{VIII} was not clearly opacified in (a) as in (b). In other words, for a hypervascular lesion scanning ought to be begun while the arteries are predominantly opacified as in (b). In a phase when hepatic veins are opacified, hypervascular lesions may become isodense as in (a).

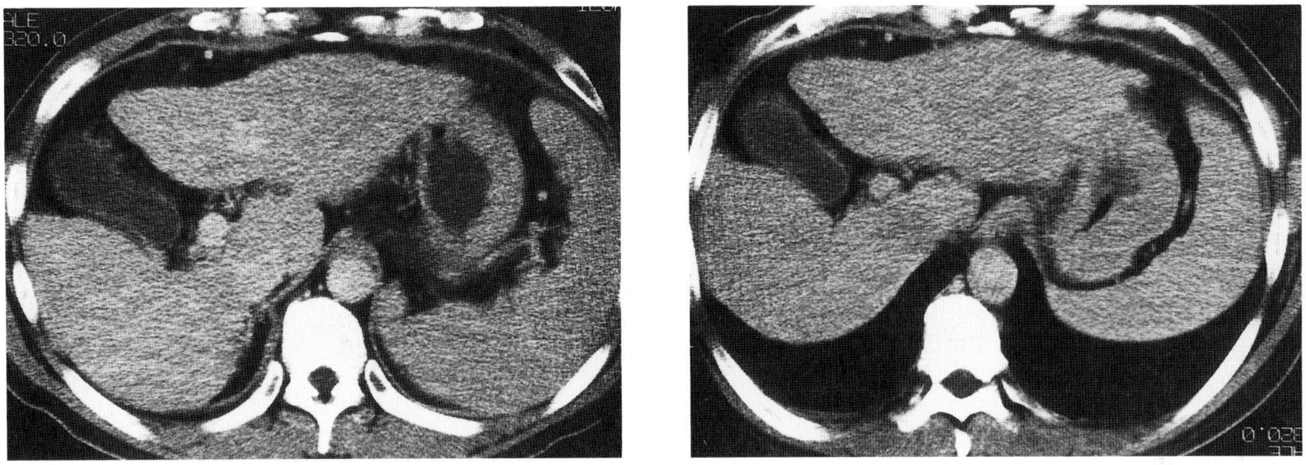

a b

Fig 13.10 Displacement of the liver due to posture changes: (a) supine position; (b) prone position. If the scan is made in a prone position (b), the liver and spleen move anteriorly due to their weights, and also caudally as a result of compression from the abdominal wall. Therefore, if the CT images made with two different positions are compared in a same level (the left lobe is in its largest section in this case), the CT slice made in the prone position (b) is more cranial to one made in the supine position (a).

object, the method of scanning, and with partial volume averaging, and they are used only as a relative reference in diagnosis. The CT value is useful particularly in distinguishing a tumor that has a fat element, hence a minus CT value from internal necrosis and old blood clot (Case 1, p.100; Case 2, p.101).

Window level and window width

While monitoring the CT image, one ought to bring the middle of the gray scale to the CT value of the image to be studied (to adjust the window level), and then determine the window width for best quality images. For the liver, the window level is set at 40–60 HU for plain CT and 80–100 HU for enhanced CT, and the window width is tightened to 100–150 for plain CT and 200–250 for enhanced CT. For the study of Lipiodol retention after its arterial injection, the window level is increased and width widened for better imaging (Fig. 13.8). The greater the window level, the smaller the size of mass as it is seen, and conversely the lower the window level the larger the tumor diameter. Therefore, for comparison of lesion sizes, the scanning conditions should be made equal.

Displacement of the liver by respiratory movements and posture changes

We usually do the scanning with the patient in a state after expiration (breathing out). If breathing is not fully stopped, or while the patient is breathing in, the cranial border of the liver may be distorted due to contraction of the diaphragm, or the liver is rotated dorsally and the slices may not be made exactly in parallel. For these reasons, CT slices made at another hospital may not be the same and an obvious lesion may not be in the same slice; the scanning conditions are to be considered in interpreting the images (Fig. 13.9).

If the scanning is done in a prone position, the liver as a whole shifts caudally (Fig. 13.10). The lateral decubitus position may have an advantage for moving a gallstone for better visualization, for recognizing adhesion and infiltration, and for assessing the amount of fluid collection.

13.2 Conventional CT (via a peripheral vein)

Conventional CT consists of (1) plain CT and (2) enhanced CT in which contrast medium is injected into a peripheral vein. For the first CT examination, plain CT of the abdomen is important because it may reveal intrahepatic stones, calcifications within a tumor, bleeding (Fig. 13.11), and sometimes Lipiodol retention due to TAE. For enhanced CT, rapid (bolus) injection of contrast medium (2–3 ml/s) and continuous scanning are important (dynamic CT). Drip infusion CT is to be avoided in the diagnosis of tumor, because it may turn the mass and parenchyma isodense, preventing existence diagnosis for a tumor (Fig. 13.12). The antecubital vein is usually punctured for injection, but when this vein is not suitable, the dorsalis pedis vein may be used. However, if undiluted contrast medium is injected into this vein, it may produce a streak artefact due to concentrated contrast medium in the IVC, interfering with liver study (Fig. 13.13). Therefore, this vein is used only for demonstrating IVC occlusion, and tumor growth into the IVC from adrenal and renal malignancies.

Existence diagnosis for a tumor

To determine the number of tumors, sequential scanning is made while moving the table, starting 35-45 s after rapid intravenous injection of contrast medium (2–3 ml/s) (table incremental method) (Fig. 13.14). One has to be careful not to be too late in starting the scan (Fig. 13.9). With TCT900S, one slicing takes 1 s, and in the table incremental technique 2 s, and therefore only six to seven slices may be made during one breathhold. An ordinary liver needs 12–15 slices of 1 cm to cut the entire organ. Therefore, two sessions of slicing and one to two additional slices will be required for this purpose. The usual timing for this method is schematically given in Fig. 13.15. Even such a high-speed scan with TCT900S has several problems. The early scanning from the diaphragm to the liver hilum is made during the arterial phase, and the images are suitable for diagnosis of a hypervascular tumor. However, the subsequent scans from the hilum to the caudal end of the liver have to wait about 20 s, during which time the patient is allowed to breathe, and no scan is made. Thus, the arterial phase ends before the caudal half of the liver is scanned, and these slices are made during the portal phase. A hypervascular tumor may be seen as a low-density or isodensity mass. For this reason, a hypervascular mass is recognized either as a high-density or low-density lesion depending on its location. To minimize this difficulty, as many slices as possible are made while the patients is inhaling oxygen. However, even with oxygenation, the whole liver is not scanned during one breathhold. To prevent oversights, we do additional slicing after 5 min as late enhanced CT.

In the presence of a mass in S^{VI} and daughter lesions nearby, a reversed order of scans may be made (from caudal to cranial) to avoid overlooking the daughters. As a routine, three series are carried out on a new patient, plain CT, early phase enhanced CT, and late phase enhanced CT. However, if only limited time is available, we prefer early and late phase enhanced CT because late phase enhanced CT provides such findings as fill-in in hemangioma and peripheral low density in adenocarcinoma, which are necessary to make quality diagnosis and minimize tumor oversight. In patients in whom a metastatic

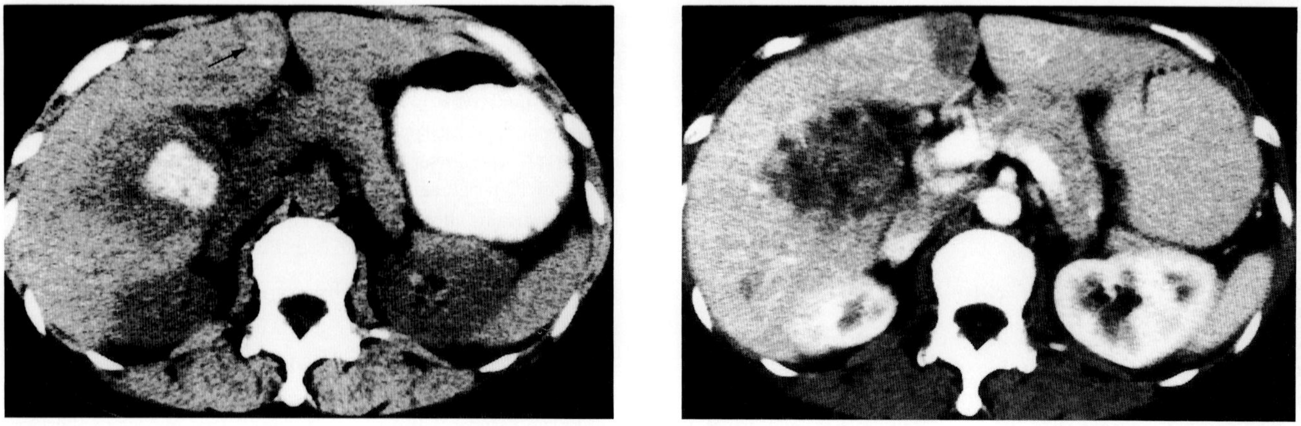

a b

Fig. 13.11 Hepatic metastasis from colon carcinoma in which plain CT demonstrated bleeding and calcifications. Plain CT (a) (WL 35, WW 172) shows a 5 cm low-density lesion with a high-density area (bleeding) in the center. Another metastatic lesion with a fine calcification (→) is seen in S^{IV}. Enhanced CT (b) (WL 94, WW 200) displays both lesions as low-density masses, and bleeding and calcification are not recognized.

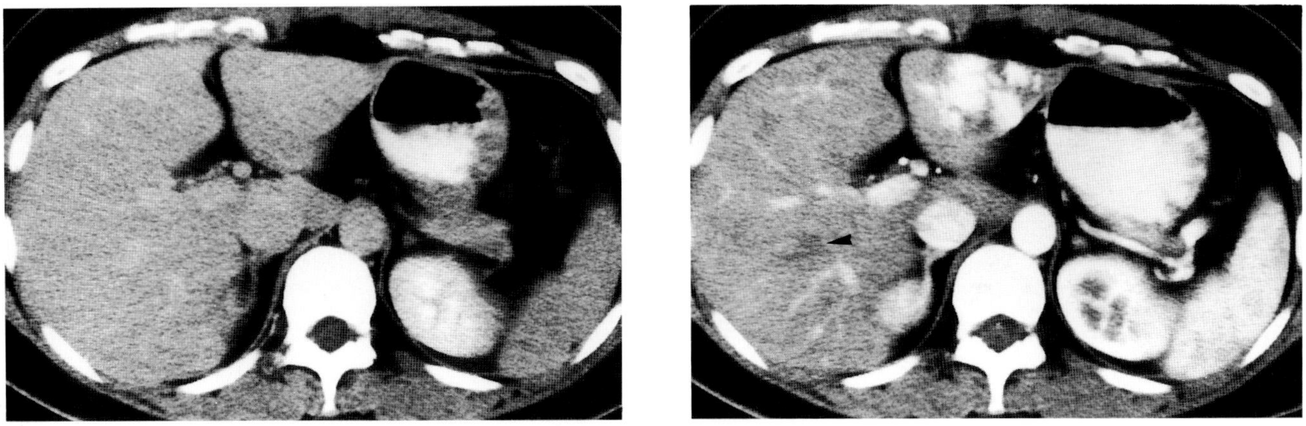

a b

Fig. 13.12 Drawback of drip infusion CT.
Enhanced CT by drip infusion (a) shows intrahepatic vasculature only faintly, and recognition of the tumor is not possible. By contrast, dynamic CT (b) clearly demonstrates hemangiomas in the left lobe; it also permits distinction between portal veins and hepatic veins (▶).

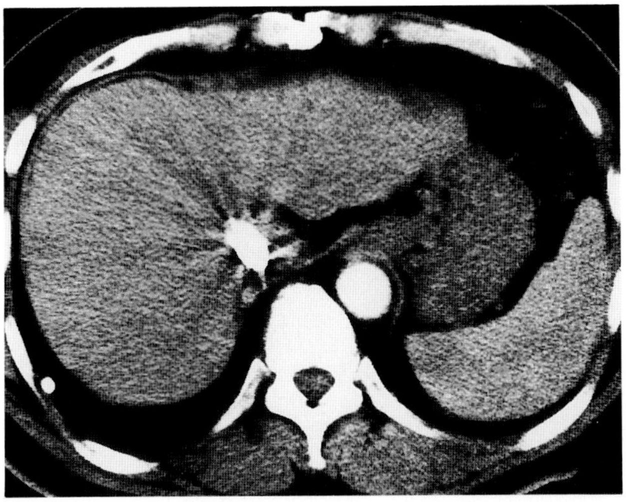

Fig. 13.13 Artefact arising from the inferior vena cava. In this patient, the antecubital vein was collapsed and contrast medium was injected into the dorsalis pedis vein. Contrast medium reached the IVC in high concentrations producing a streak artefact that interfered with interpretation. To study the patency of the IVC, slow injection at 0.5 ml/s or so and a somewhat delayed scanning are desirable.

liver tumor is suspected by other diagnostic procedures and tumor markers, and in whom the number of tumors is important, such lesions are expected to be seen as low-density masses, and therefore the start of scanning may be delayed by about 10 s near the portal phase (Fig. 13.16). In occasional cases, the heart may be seen by partial volume averaging in the area where the left lobe is normally seen, or the adipose tissue near the caudal end of the left and right lobes causes partial volume averaging and interferes with quality diagnosis. One can place a sensor in the area in question, and compare it with contiguous cranial and caudal slices for differential diagnosis. If even these manipulations have failed in differential diagnosis, the thickness of the slice is reduced to 5 mm, and the incremental scan is made with 3 mm slices for better diagnosis. Sometimes, reconstruction of sagittal and/or frontal slices may further assist in diagnosis. In this study of multiple small lesions in the liver, an arbitrary x- and y-axes may be drawn on the film for comparison of neighboring slices to avoid missing small lesions (Fig. 13.17).

Quality diagnosis for a tumor

Quality diagnosis follows existence diagnosis. To this end, dynamic CT is done in the slice which contains the mass. Contrast medium, 60 ml, is injected from a peripheral vein at a speed of 2–3 ml/s and scanning started at 25–30 s. The temporal changes in the internal structure and density changes are interpreted (Fig. 13.18). Also the timing of injection and scanning varies with the CT scanner.

If the internal structure and intratumor vasculature (centripetal in HCC and other neoplasms; centrifugal in FNH) are important for differential diagnosis, more information can be gained by dynamic CT done in the same slice. For quality diagnosis of a small lesion, say about 1 cm, dynamic CT done in the same slice may not reveal the same lesion. In that case, a multi-dynamic study may be made in which two to three slices are made repeatedly around the lesion in question while moving the table (Fig. 13.19).

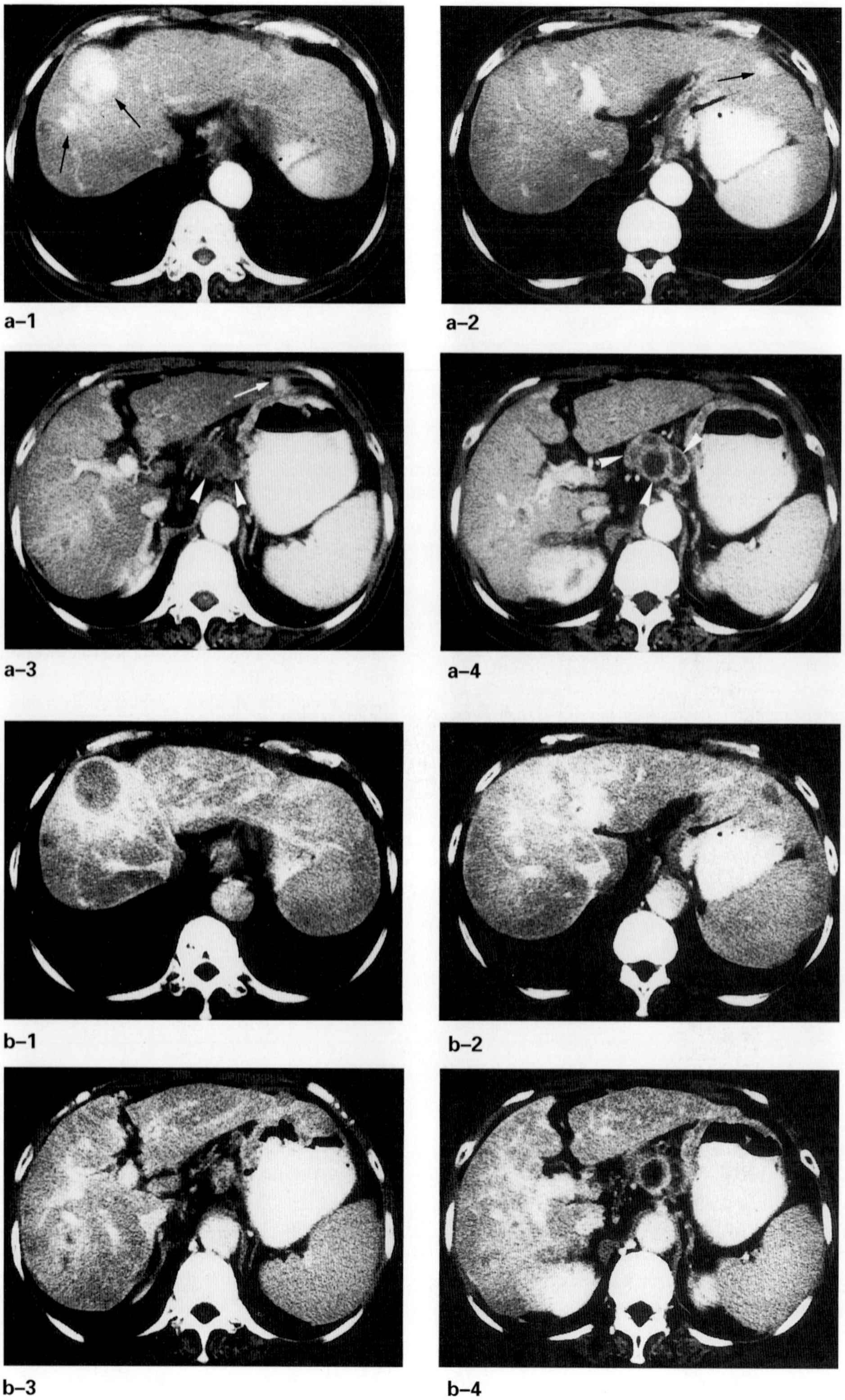

Fig. 13.14 Dynamic CT by the table incremental technique. With a moving table, sequential dynamic CT scanning was made for arterial (a) and venous (b) phases. In the arterial phase (a), multiple HCCs are seen as high-density lesions (→) and in the venous phase (b) made 8 min later the same lesions are seen as low-density ones. Both existence and quality diagnoses were possible in one scanning procedure. Lymph node metastases were also found along the lesser curvature of the stomach (▶).

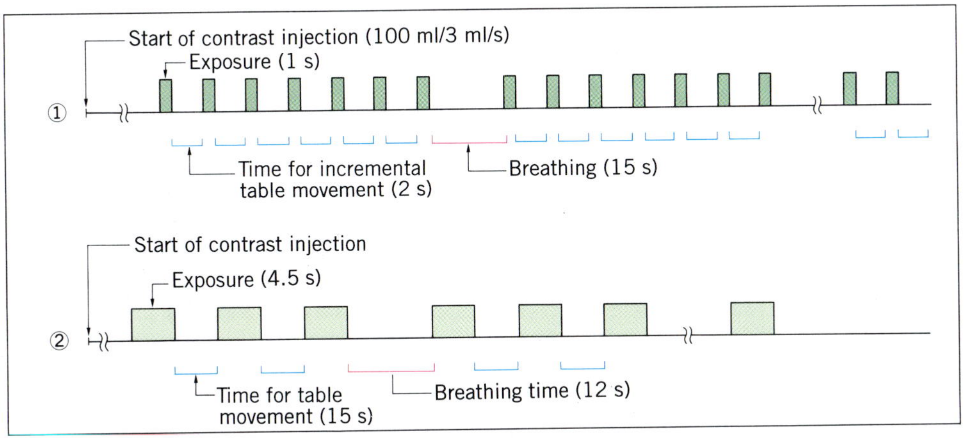

Fig. 13.15a Timing for dynamic CT scan with contrast medium injected from a peripheral vein. The scan begins 30–40 s after the start of contrast injection. (1) Program for high-speed CT (such as TCT900S). Seven slices are made, then the patient breathes, and another seven slices are made. (2) Program for moderate or slow speed CT (such as TCT 60). Slices are made in sequence, three at a time.

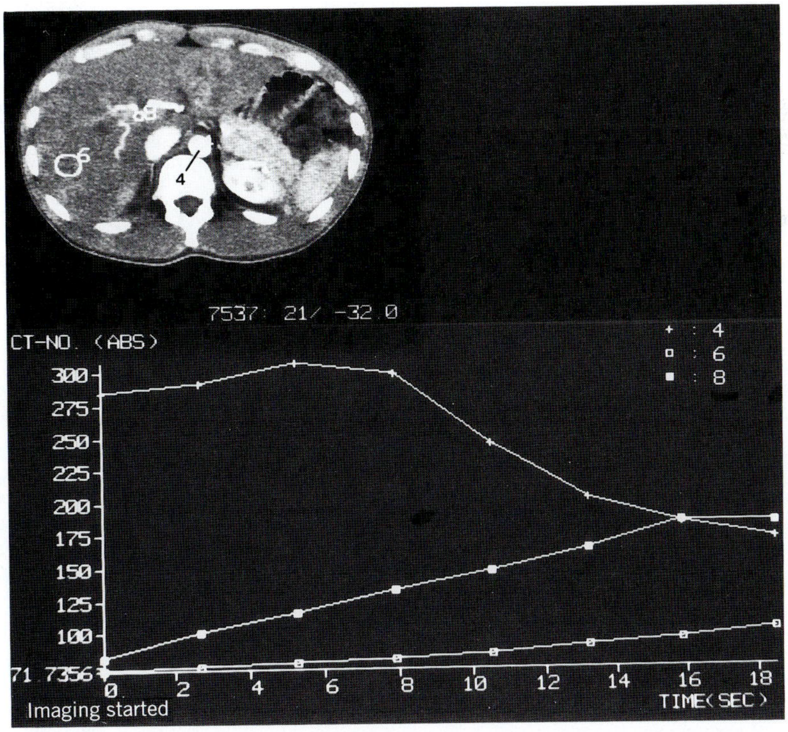

Fig. 13.15b Time-density curve in high-speed dynamic CT with contrast injected from a peripheral vein. Eight sequential slices were made beginning 30 s after the start of contrast injection, 90 ml/3 ml/s. The density of the aorta (+ : 4) reached the peak of 300 HU at 4.5 s, and dropped sharply thereafter. The density of the portal vein at the hilum (■ : 8) rose linearly, followed by that of the parenchyma (□ : 6) with a slower inclination. From this chart, it is clear that before 16 s the ar-teries are opacified earlier than the portal veins, and after 16 s tumors, even hypervascular ones, may become low-density areas because contrast in portal blood overwhelms the arterial contrast making quality diagnosis difficult.

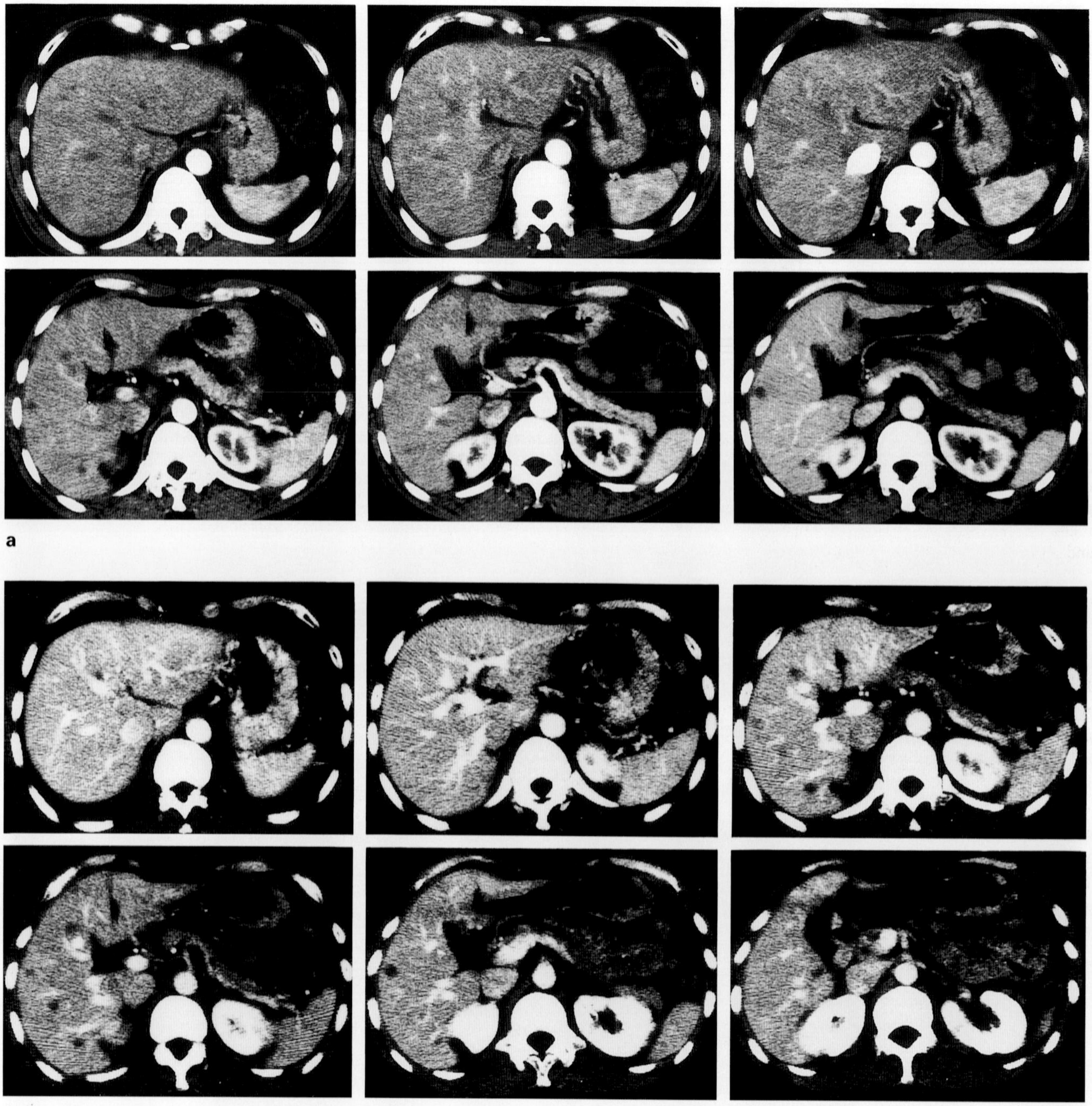

Fig. 13.16 For metastatic liver cancer, the start of contrast medium injection should be slightly delayed in dynamic CT: (a) 35 s from start of contrast injection (100 ml/2 ml/s); (b) 50 s from start of contrast injection. In (a) enhancement of the parenchyma is weak, hepatic veins are not well visualized, and differential diagnosis of hepatic veins and metastatic tumors is not easy. For the diagnosis of the latter (adenocarcinoma) (b) is better than (a).

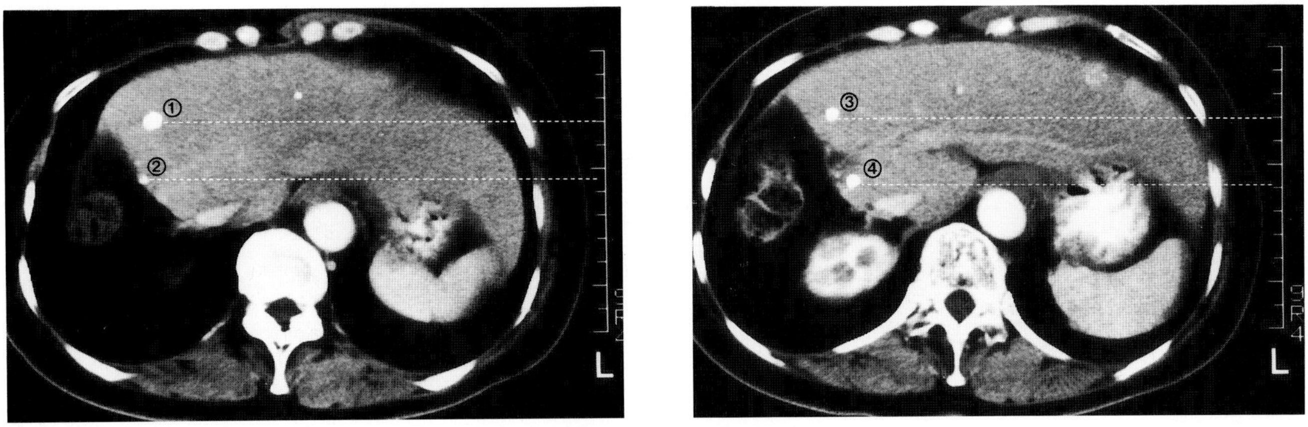

a b

Fig. 13.17 Existence diagnosis of small intrahepatic lesions based on graphic axes: (b) is a slice 1 cm caudal to (a). CT images cannot be placed on top of one another for the study of multiple small lesions in the liver, because many images are made on one large film, unlike angiograms which can be placed on top of one another for more accurate interpretation. Therefore drawing axes on the film may prove helpful. In this illustrative situation to determine whether or not the two lesions (1) and (2) on CT (a) are the same as (3) and (4) on CT (b), the locations of these lesions are plotted against the *X*- and *Y*-axes—the scale to the right is used as the *Y*-axis. Thus, lesion (1) is at 3 cm on the *Y*-axis and 20 cm on the *X*-axis (3, 20), and lesion (3) is also at (3, 20), suggesting (1) and (3) to be identical; they show partial volume averaging. When (2) and (4) were similarly analyzed (2) was (5.5, 20.5) and (4) was (5.7, 19) indicating that the two are different lesions.

Treatment of the patient prior to study

Eating is avoided before enhanced CT. When differential diagnosis from lymph node metastasis is required, the patient is encouraged to drink as much diluted Gastrografin (2 cups (9 ml) of 76 per cent Gastrografin diluted with 300 ml water yielding a 2.3 per cent solution) as possible. Anticholinergic drugs which were used in the past are no longer necessary because artefacts derived from bowel movement have become very rare with rapid CT scanning, except in special situations. Barium in the GI tract frequently produces streak artefacts (Fig. 13.20) and therefore it is better to schedule CT before barium examination.

13.3 Angio-CT

Angio-CT is a combination of angiography and CT. Using the angiographic technique, the catheter is inserted into the hepatic artery (arterial-CT) (Prando *et al.* 1979; Moriyama 1980; Moss *et al.* 1982; Freeny and Marks 1983) or superior mesenteric artery (portal-CT) (Moriyama 1980; Hisa *et al.* 1980; Matsui *et al.* 1983), and scan is made while contrast medium is being injected. This modality is indispensable in patients scheduled for surgery. In either technique, hepatic angiograms are done before angio-CT.

Hepatic arterial-CT

This was done in the past for the detection of small lesions (mainly secondaries of HCC). However, the best timing for arterial-CT is difficult to determine, and distinction between HCC and regenerative nodules is usually not feasible by this technique alone. For this reason, portal-CT and Lipiodol-CT are now more often used for the same purpose. Angio-CT is indicated in patients in whom conventinonal CT and angiography have failed to make quality diagnosis [HCC not enhanced (Case 14, p.123)] and borderline lesions including early HCC, FNH (Case 1, p.84), and hepatocellular adenoma (Case 1, p.78)). This modality permits study of temporal changes in the internal structure and in the tumor size, hence more accurate diagnosis. Dynamic CT was previously made at the level of the slice that had the largest diameter of the mass, but more recently hepatic arterial-CT is frequently done of the whole liver for quality diagnosis of multiple borderline lesions. About half of patients have anatomical variations in the origin and course of the hepatic artery, and repeated catheterization is required for the study of both lobes in such patients, reducing the diagnostic usefulness of this modality.

Technique

In subjects having a normal vascular anatomy, the tip of the catheter is placed in the common hepatic artery, and in those who have a variant artery, it is placed in the artery supplying the targeted area of the liver. For a CT scanner that has a good density resolution (such as TCT900S) the contrast medium is diluted 1:3. For dynamic CT in a same slice, scanning is begun with the start of injection of contrast medium (10–20 ml) at a rate of 1 ml/s. If the table is moved incrementally for scanning, the amount of contrast medium is adjusted with the capability of the CT machine (number of sequential slices that can be made). Formerly, contrast medium was injected for each slice, but with more recent machines, six to eight slices are made in one sequence (Fig. 13.21).

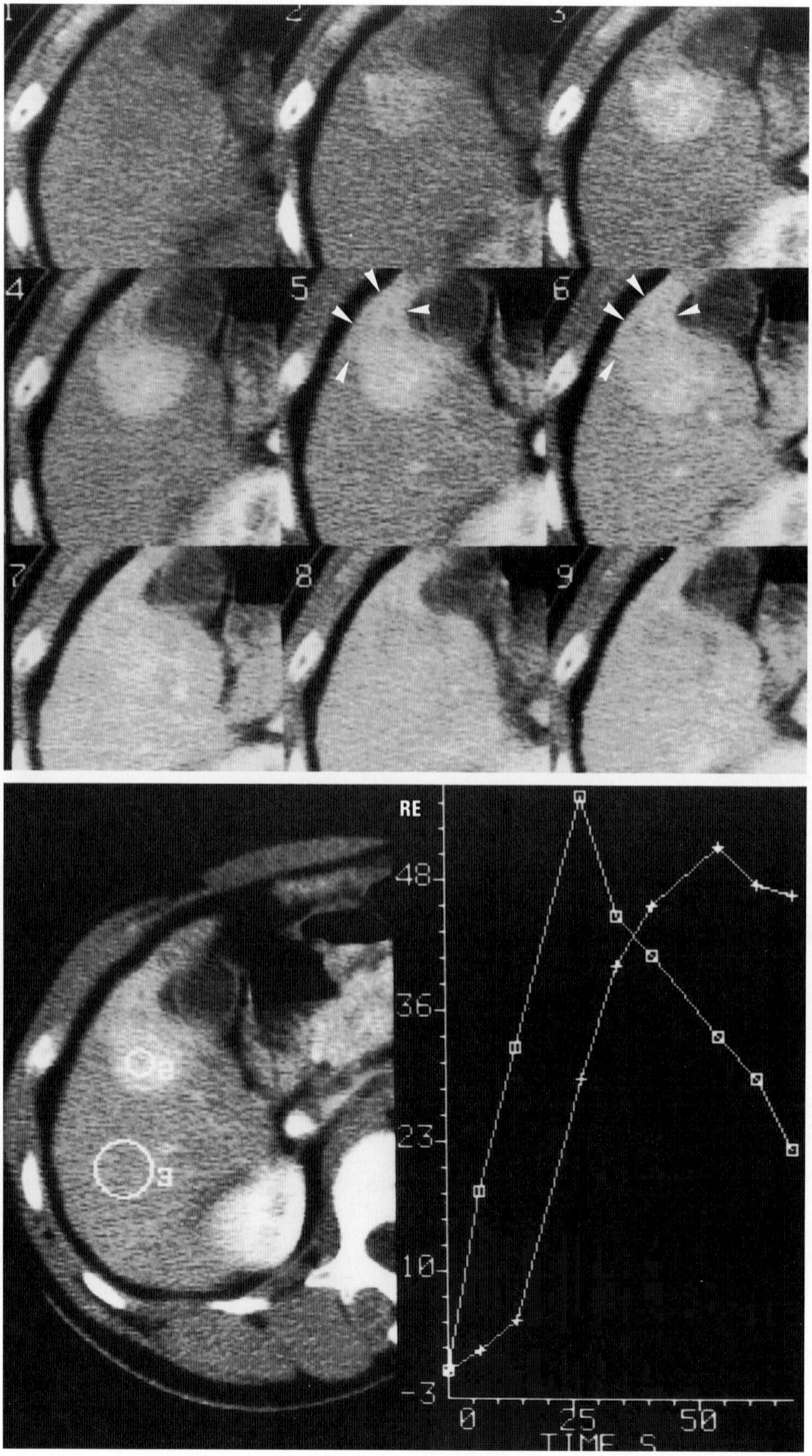

Fig. 13.18 Quality diagnosis based on temporal enhancement pattern in dynamic CT study. (a) Plain CT (1) shows a low-density area in S^{V}. This lesion is markedly enhanced in the arterial phase (2–4) and a slightly delayed phase (5, 6). In the parenchymal phase (7), it has turned isodense and then hypodense. This pattern of enhancement is typical of HCC. The enhanced region (▶) to the periphery of the tumor is due to an arterio-portal shunt. (b) Time–density curves over the tumor (□ : 2) and non-tumor parenchyma (+ : 3) demonstrate early enhancement over the tumor followed by parenchymal enhancement. RE (*Y*-axis) is the CT value after contrast injection subtracted by preenhancement CT value. The *X*-axis starts 35 s after the beginning of contrast injection.

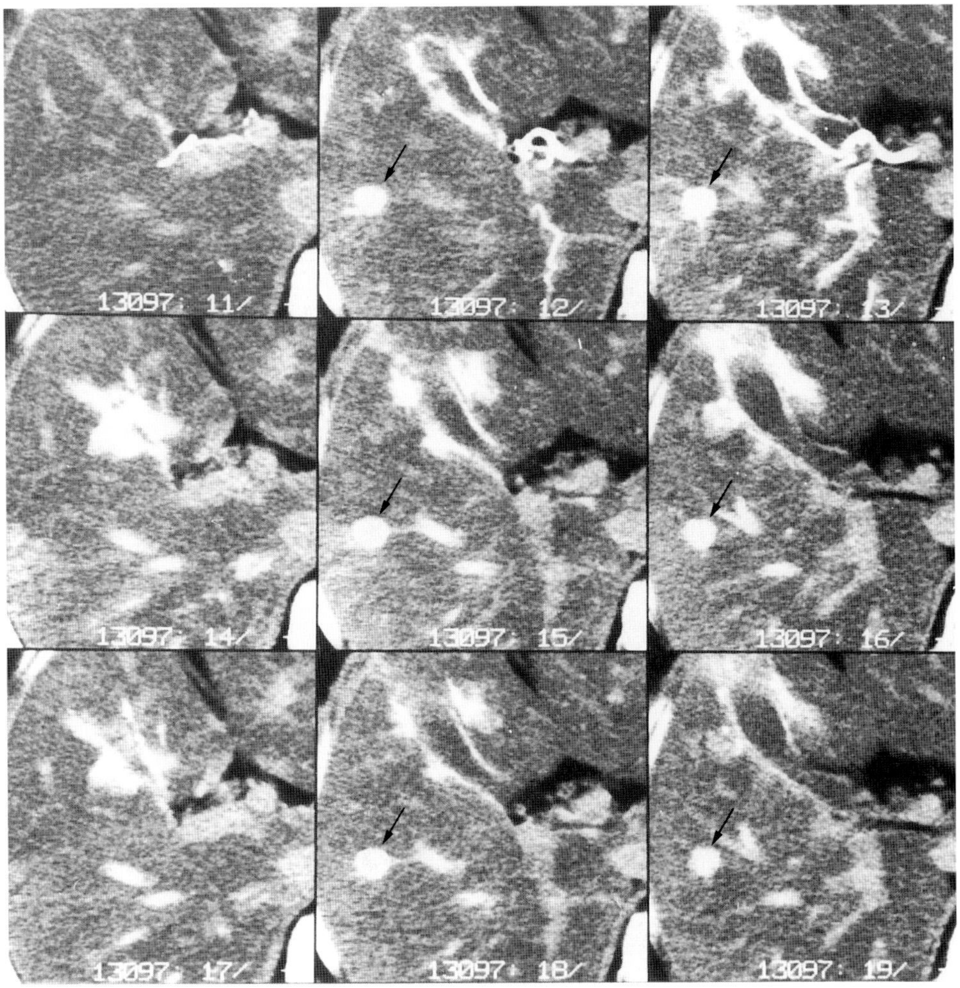

Fig. 13.19 Multidynamic CT for a small lesion. For quality diagnosis of a 1.2 cm tumor (→), arterial-CT with 5 mm slices was made by moving the table (5 mm each time, multidynamic CT). The three slices in the top row were made by the table incremental method, the table returned to the original level and another three slices (middle row) made in exactly the same way. It was repeated again (lower two). The lesion was markedly enhanced and remained so in the late phase, and the diagnosis was hemangioma. This kind of repeated slicing by the incremental method prevents missing a small lesion in the slice.

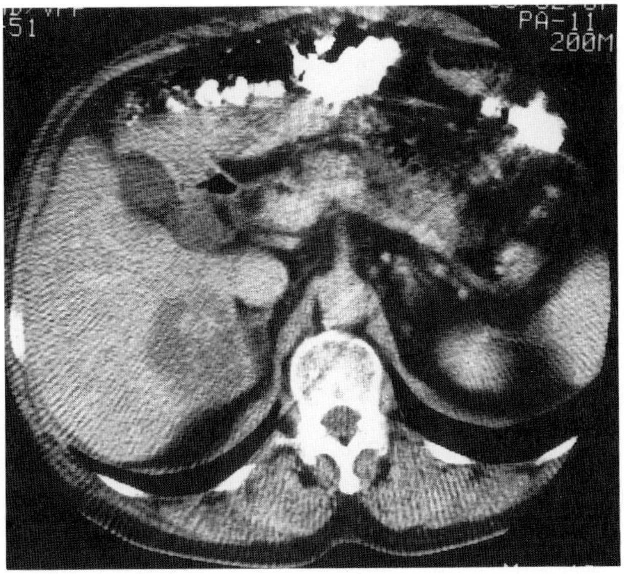

Fig. 13.20 Artefact due to barium. A barium study was done 3 days earlier. Barium in the colon is producing a strong streak artefact. Administration of a cathartic 1 day before the CT study may not expel all the barium. It is better to schedule CT before the barium study.

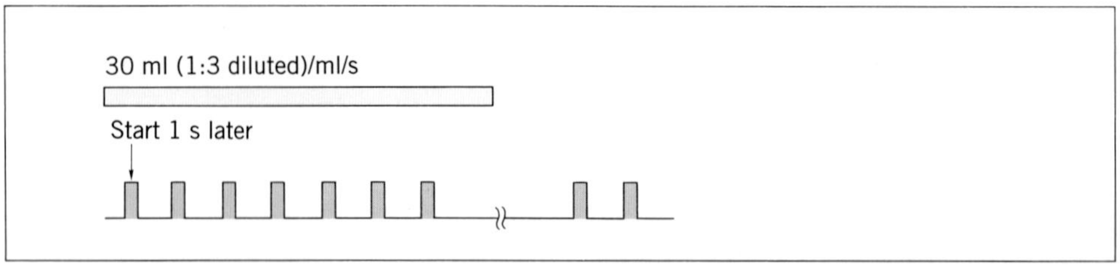

Fig. 13.21a Hepatic arterial-CT. The conditions for rapid CT scan with incremental table movement. A total of 30 ml of 1:3 diluted contrast medium is injected from the common hepatic or proper hepatic artery at a speed of 1 ml/s. Seven sequential scans are made beginning 1 s from the start of injection. If necessary, the same procedure is repeated. To cover the entire liver, it has to be done at least twice.

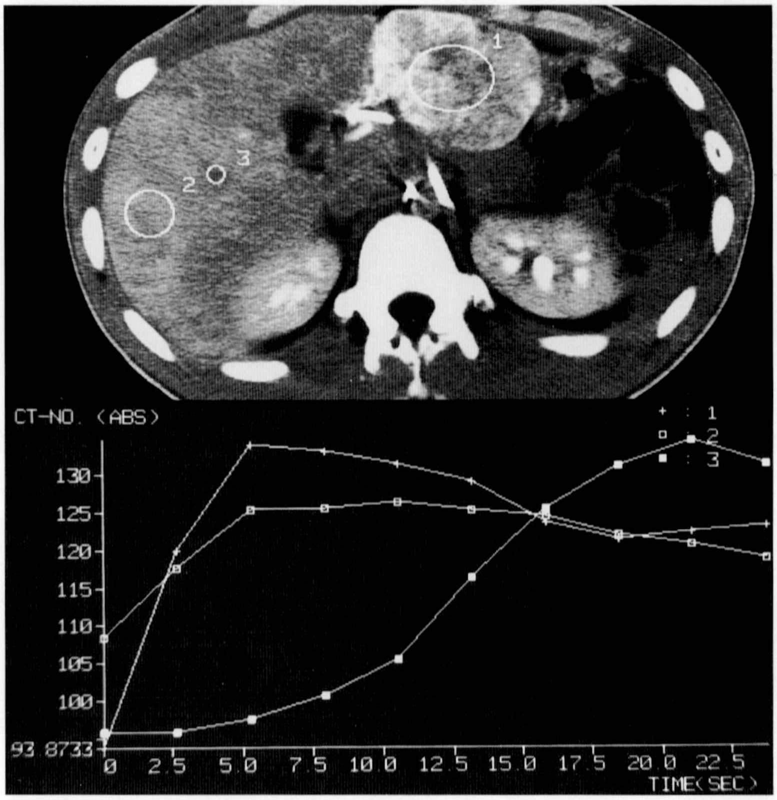

Fig. 13.21b Time–density curve during arterial-CT. Ten slices were made in the left lobe laterally in the same slice. In an HCC (+ : 1), a rapid increase in CT value is seen, and a less rapid increase in the parenchyma (□ : 2). The peak value is greater in HCC, but after 15 s the CT values become similar, and HCC is isodense, making its diagnosis difficult. The CT value of the hepatic vein (■ : 3) after 15 s surpasses that of the parenchyma. In other words, the hepatic vein is most clearly delineated in this phase.

The reason for placing the catheter in the common hepatic artery and not in the proper hepatic is to avoid wedging the catheter in the artery (it occurs in the proper hepatic artery) which blocks the natural blood flow, hence inhomogeneous enhancement. Using a recently developed thin catheter (thinner than 5F), such wedging can be prevented, and arterial-CT is now possible carried out from the proper hepatic artery—image quality is improved because of more arterial blood flow. With the catheter in the common hepatic, contrast medium enters the portal vein through the gastroduodenal artery after 10 s, and subsequent slices may become portal-CT. Therefore, it is desirable to complete the study in 12–15 s. If the table incremental method is used for dynamic CT, the amount of contrast medium should be so increased as to obtain predominantly arterial contrast CT images up to the last slice.

Portal-CT

This modality is very useful for existence diagnosis and important as a preoperative study, particularly in patients with HCC and metastatic carcinoma (Fig. 13.22). All tumors not supplied by the portal vein are seen as low-density masses. It clearly opacifies the intrahepatic vasculature and expedites segment diagnosis, necessary for the selection of the operative procedure.

Fig. 13.22 Portal-CT excels other modalities in detecting small lesions in the liver. In the hepatic arteriogram (a), at least five mildly stained mass lesions are recognized. In portal-CT (b), five lesions are clearly seen in the four slices made at the level designated (└──┘) in (a). Lesions superimposed in the anterior view cannot be separated on the angiogram. Portal-CT excels in delineating the vasculature, particularly the hepatic veins, enabling segment diagnosis. →, middle hepatic vein; ▶, right hepatic vein.

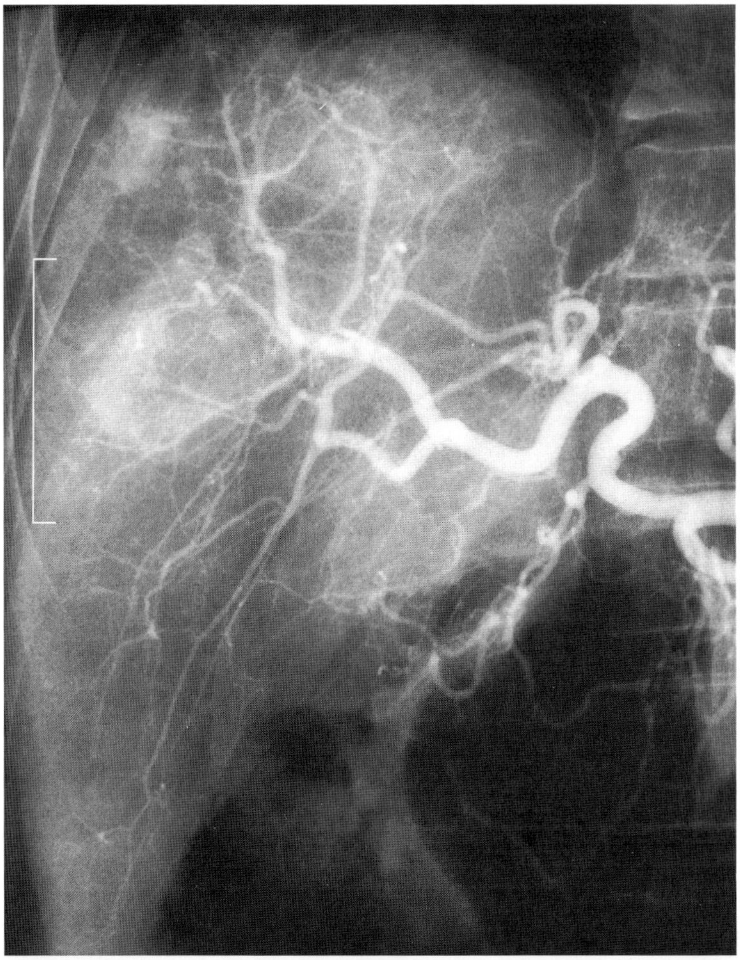

a

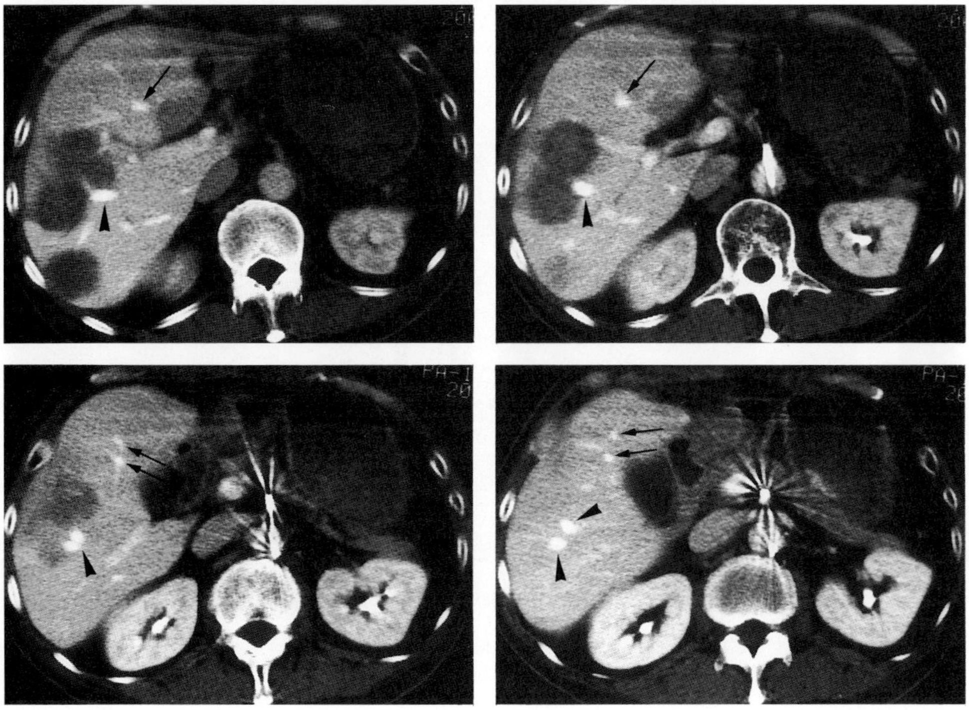

b

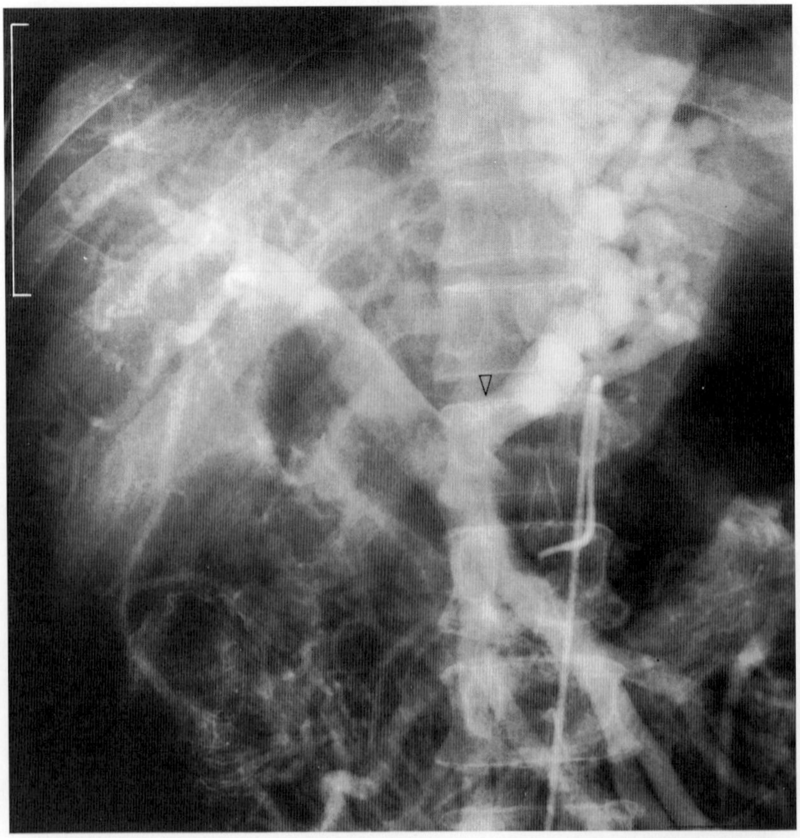

a

Fig. 13.23 Portal-CT produces poor images in the presence of large extrahepatic collaterals. The superior mesenteric arterial portogram (a) shows a dilated hepatofugal left gastric vein (▷) due to cirrhosis, and decreased portal venous flow into the liver. Portal-CT (b) demonstrates many non-specific low-density areas which are not readily distinguished from real tumors (→). These six slices were made in the area designated (└─┘) in (a). ▶, right hepatic vein. Esophageal and para-esophageal varices are recognized in these images.

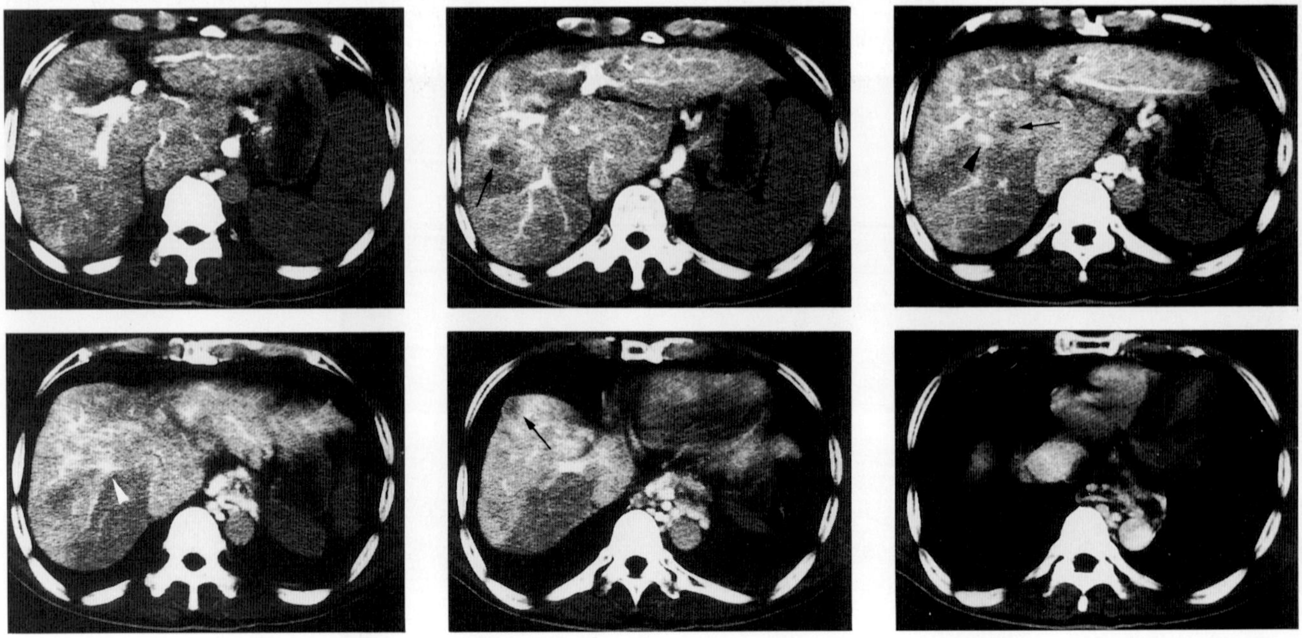

b

However, quality diagnosis is not possible with portal-CT and it has to be preceded by other imaging studies for that purpose. As we emphasize late phase enhanced CT images, our recommendation is that late enhanced CT of the whole liver be made following angiography. It will disclose a peripheral low-density area (Muramatsu *et al.* 1986) if exists, and facilitate quality diagnosis of the lesion that portal-CT will reveal. If a tumor thrombus or clot is in a segment portal branch or its central portion, or in the presence of hepatofugal portal flow as a result of arterio-portal shunt, contrast medium does not enter the peripheral portal branches, leaving a large area without enhancement (low density); it hampers detection of tumors in that area. In patients with portal hypertension in whom the bulk of the superior mesenteric venous flow goes through collaterals into the systemic circulation, portal-CT is not indicated (Fig. 13.23) (Oliver *et al.* 1995). One has to grasp extrahepatic portal hemodynamics when portal-CT is contemplated.

Hemangioma is already isodense or slightly high in density at the time when portal-CT is done, because of preceding angiography, and contrast between the mass and parenchyma may be too small to be diagnostic. With portal-CT, such false positive findings are uncommon, but they do occur. Besides the partial volume averaging seen in the perphery of the liver as in conventional CT, a localized low-density area may be created if the liver has accessory portal branches not derived from the portal trunk (Fig. 13.24 see also Fig. 1.19, p.15) (Takayasu *et al.* 1990*a*; Fernandez and Bernardino 1991; Nelson *et al.* 1992; Soyer *et al.* 1993; Matsui *et al.* 1994). A similar false positive phenomenon may be seen if the cystic vein blood flows into the portal vein throught the liver bed (Case 10, p.339) (Matsui *et al.* 1987*b*). A collective interpretation based on other imaging findings is necessary.

Technique

The catheter tip is placed in the superior mesenteric artery (it is important to go beyond the pancreatic arcade), 60–70 ml, depending on the number of slices, of 1:3 diluted contrast medium is injected, and CT scan started 25 s later (Fig. 13.25). If the superior mesenteric artery is occluded or stenosed, the splenic artery is used for portal-CT, but contrast medium stays in the spleen too long to make good images, particularly in patients with splenomegaly due to cirrhosis. The anatomical factors that influence the prognosis of HCC patients include the portal vein in the hilum and openings of major hepatic veins into the IVC, and accurate anatomical information is required. For more vascular information, we start the table incremental scan starting from the hilum proceeding cranially, followed by scanning from the hilum to the caudal direction. In this way, scanning follows natural blood flow (portal vein → parenchyma → hepatic vein), making vascular identification, hence segment diagnosis, easy. By dividing the liver at the level of the hilum and scanning twice in sequence, the time to start the scan can be determined from the experience with the first scanning. If it was not appropriate, a correction can be made for the second

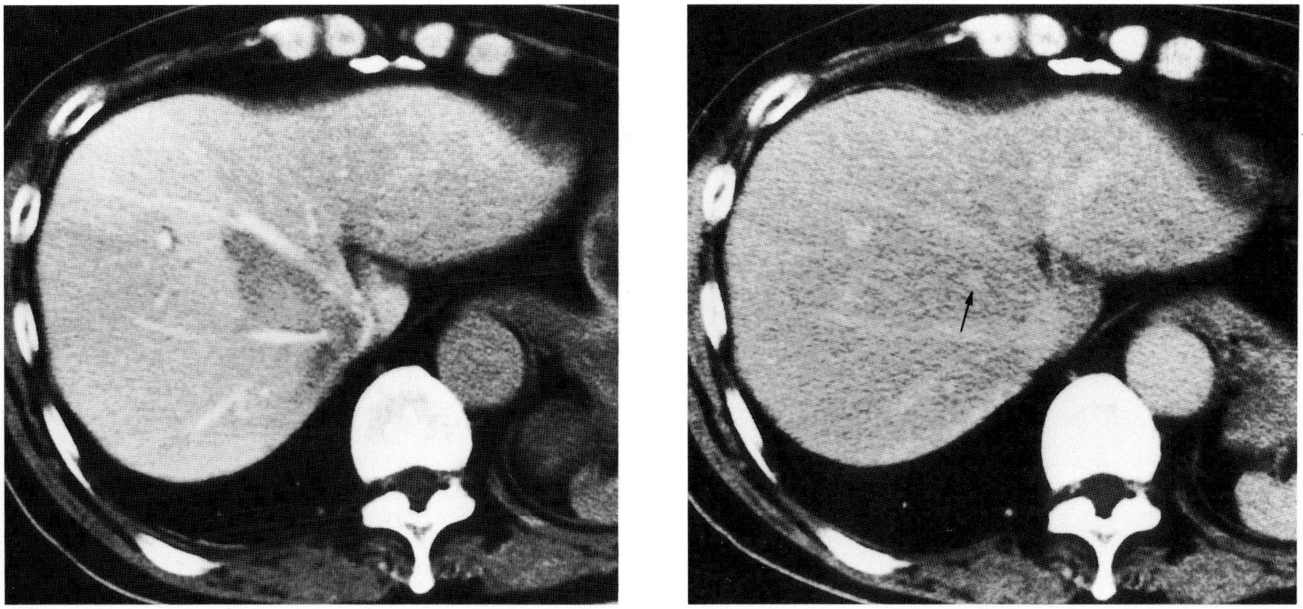

a **b**

Fig 13.24 False positive results in portal-CT. A 4 cmHCC was found in S^{III} and portal-CT (a) was made as a preoperative study. It showed a triangular area of low density between the right and middle hepatic veins. Conventional enhanced CT (b) did not demonstrate the same, nor was abnormality found in the same region during the operation. When (a) and (b) were compared, $P^{VIII}{}_{d}$ (→) seen in (b) was not recognized in (a), and it was assumed that for some reason the portal flow in $P^{VIII}{}_{d}$ was reduced, or this area had its own accessory portal branches. Angiography failed to demonstrate arterio-portal shunting in $S^{VIII}{}_{d}$.

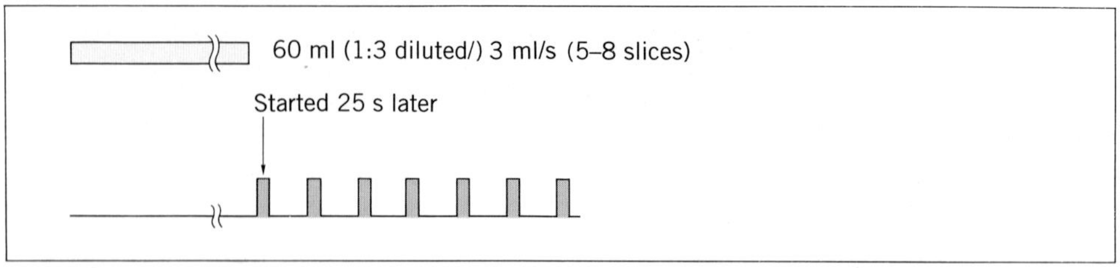

Fig. 13.25a Scan timing for portal-CT with rapid table incremental dynamic CT. Seven sequential CT slices are made with 60 ml of 1:3 diluted contrast medium. Scanning is begun 25 s after the start of contrast injection into the superior mesenteric artery. Following the natural blood flow, scanning is started from the hilum proceeding cranially up to the diaphragm, and then from the hilum proceeding caudally.

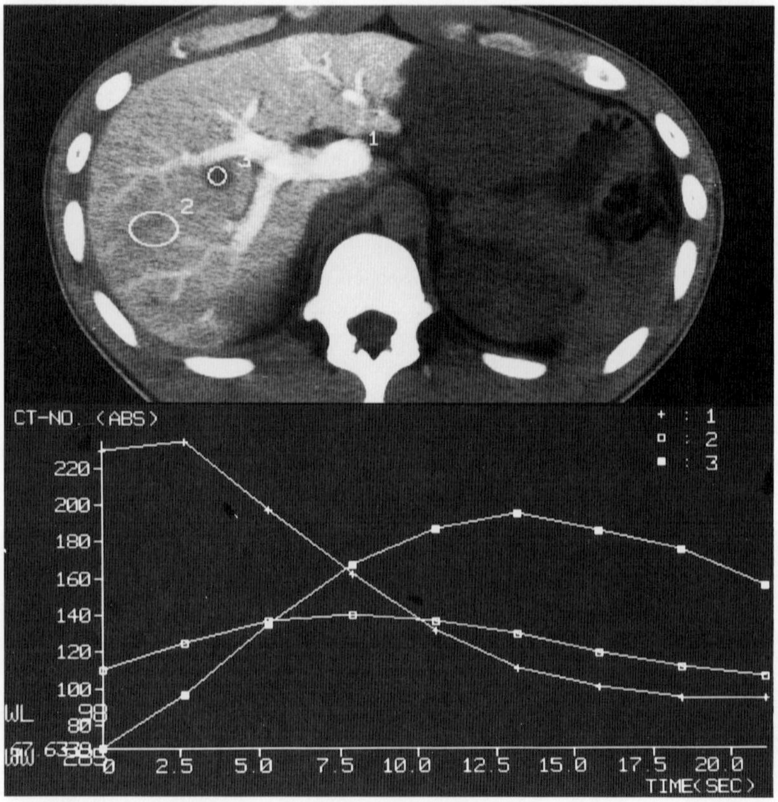

Fig. 13.25b Time-density curves for various hepatic regions during portal-CT. Nine dynamic CT images are made in the same level after injection of 60 ml of 1:3 diluted contrast medium at 3 ml/s. The CT value of the portal vein (+ : 1) reaches a peak in 2.5 s and declines rapidly thereafter. Liver parenchyma (□ : 2) maintains a relatively constant value of 100–140 HU, suggesting its constant capability of delineating abnormalities. The hepatic vein (■ : 3) slowly gains density, and after 13 s or so it has the highest value, corroborating the fact that late CT images show hepatic veins clearly.

sequential scan to avoid a failure. An important merit of this method is simplicity of the procedure and acquisition of information on the entire liver irrespective of arterial variations.

In portal-CT, all tumors are seen as low-density areas (similar to cold areas on the scintigram) and when compared with Lipiodol-CT (similar to hot areas on the scintigram); it is subject to partial volume averaging to a greater extent and less able to delineate small lesions. If the catheter is wedged in a peripheral branch of the superior mesenteric artery, and portal-CT is made, the liver may be enhanced inhomogeneously due to laminar flow (the specific gravity of contast medium is greater than that of blood, and the former tends to flow in a layer in the lower aspect within the blood vessel). The left lobe is influenced by the laminar flow to a greater extent (Fig. 13.26) and the angiographer has to take a special caution to avoid wedging of the catheter.

13.4 PTP-CT

This is a combination of percutaneous transhepatic portography (PTP) and dynamic CT, developed by one of the authors in 1980 (Takayasu *et al.* 1981) for the purpose of existence diagnosis of HCC, assessment of the extent of tumor invasion, and

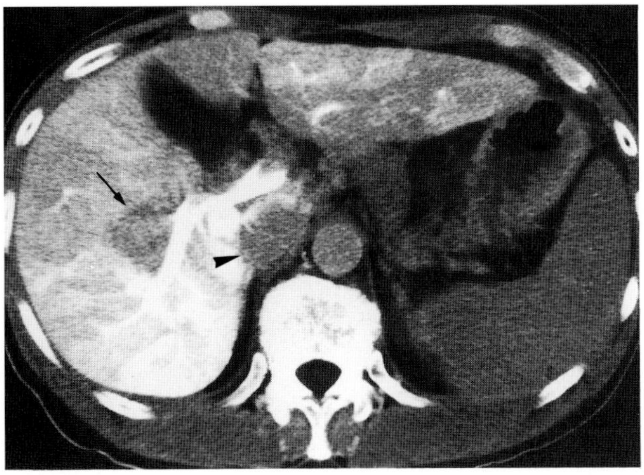

a

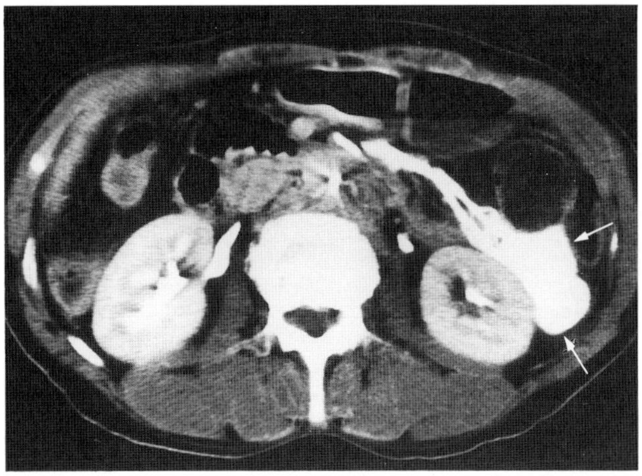

b

Fig. 13.26 Laminar flow in portal-CT:
(a) laminar flow in portal-CT; (b) localized opacification of the small bowel due to catheter wedging in a branch of the superior mesenteric artery. During the transport of this patient from the angiography room to the CT room, the tip of the catheter was wedged in a branch of the superior mesenteric artery, and during the portal-CT procedure, contrast medium entered mainly into the posterior aspect of the liver as a result of laminar flow due to gravity. Other areas of the liver did not receive sufficient contrast medium, making the diagnosis of a tumor (→) less definitive than otherwise (▶, IVC).

If a CT image like (a) was obtained in portal-CT, scanning of areas supplied by the superior mesenteric artery would demonstrate localized opacification of the small bowel, clarifying the cause. Re-portal-CT may be made after slightly withdrawing the catheter for a better diagnosis.

diagnosis of intrahepatic collaterals in portal hypertension. This technique is useful in the evaluation of portal hemodynamics, but is too invasive for cancer diagnosis; portal-CT has replaced this technique. However, it has been revived more recently because PTPE is increasingly done in the management of HCC in Japan, and PTP-CT assists in confirming the selective catheterization of the intended portal branch.

13.5 Lipiodol-CT

This technique was first developed by a group at Kumamoto University for the purpose of targeted chemotherapy of HCC (Konno *et al.* 1984), and then for the detection of very small HCC (Yumoto *et al.* 1985; Ohishi *et al.* 1985). The behavior of Lipiodol after intraarterial injection is discussed in Chapter 19. Plain CT made 7–10 days after Lipiodol injection into the hepatic artery will disclose very small HCCs, particularly intrahepatic secondaries of HCC (Fig. 13.27). Lipiodol will be distributed throughout the liver immediately after its injection (Fig. 13.28), but it disappears slowly from the non-cancerous tissue. A hypervascular cancer, particularly HCC, retains it and shows up as a discrete Lipiodol-retaining area on CT. The exact mechanism of Lipiodol disposal by normal tissue is not well understood, but the absence of Kupffer cells and normal lymphatics may explain Lipiodol retention in cancer tissue.

If Lipiodol alone is injected without an anticancer agent or Gelfoam embolization, it may be cleared from the tumor faster, sometimes as soon as 3 days. With added Gelfoam embolization, Lipiodol remains longer, facilitating detection of small lesions. Lipiodol retention is influenced by vascularity. In other words, it is retained by HCC and hypervascular metastatic cancer, but does not remain in or only minimal amounts are retained by a hypovascular well differentiated HCC, cholangiocarcinoma, and metastatic cancer. Early HCC and borderline lesions that are not well vascularized do not retain Lipiodol, and such characteristics are being utilized in differential diagnosis. Hemangioma also takes up Lipiodol, and may retain it for a long period of time, interfering with subsequent studies. When quality diagnosis has not been established for a mass lesion, unnecessary Lipiodol injection ought to be avoided.

False positive findings may occur when Lipiodol is retained in a fan shaped peripheral area (Fig. 13.29), around the gallbladder (Fig. 13.29, 13.30) and immediately beneath the liver capsule Fig. 13.29). Follow-up CT will assist in distinction from a real tumor (Fig. 13.29) in most cases.

Technique

If Adriamycin (20 mg) or a water-soluble anticancer agent is used, it is dissolved in 2.5 ml of 60 per cent Urografin, mixed with Lipiodol (5 ml) and vigorously stirred. This procedure is sometimes called 'lipiodolization' (Kanematsu *et al.* 1989) in which an angiography agent with a specific gravity similar to that of Lipiodol is used to facilitate thorough mixing of water and fat. Lipiodolization produces small (50–300 μm) droplets of Urografin (Fig. 13.31). The amount of Lipiodol is adjusted with the dose of Adriamycin. Injection is done very slowly avoiding back flow, through a catheter passed as peripheral as possible into the tumor-feeding artery.

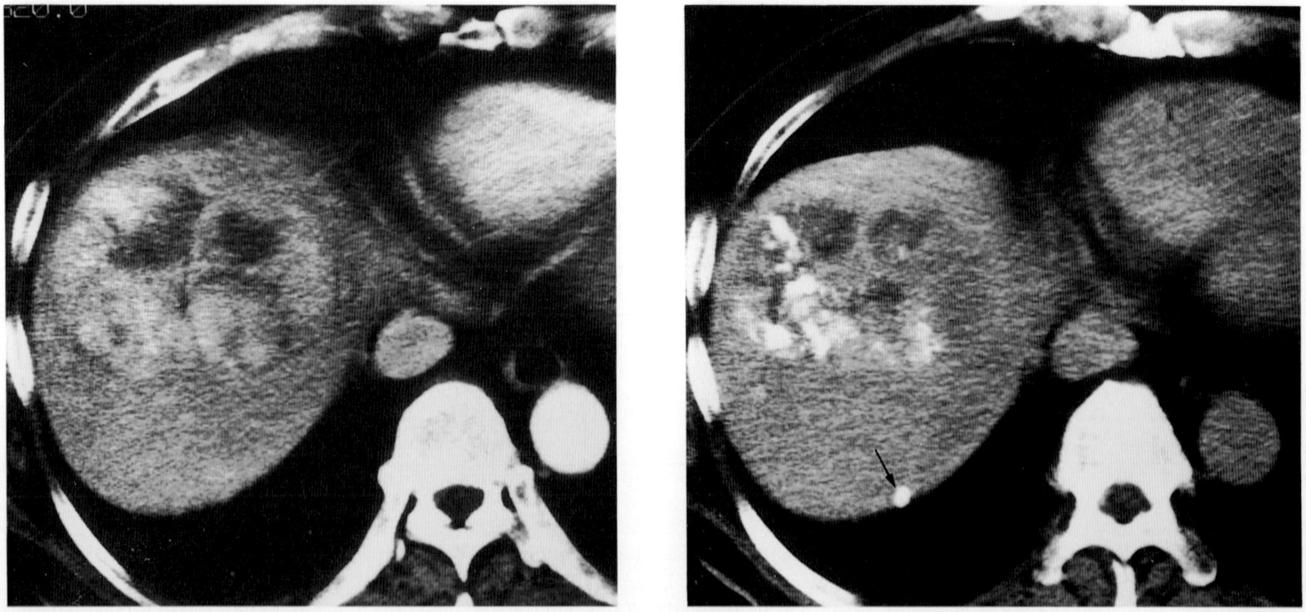

a b

Fig. 13.27 A small lesion (intrahepatic metastasis) found by Lipiodol-CT. The main mass is opacified as a typical HCC in the early phase (a) of dynamic CT. Lipiodol-CT (b) made after Lipiodol-TAE demonstrates a 4 mm Lipiodol-retaining intrahepatic secondary (→), posterior to the main mass. Re-examination of the earlier CT image (a) identified this lesion as a very faint stain hardly recognizable without the information from (b). This lesion evaded detection by US and angiography.

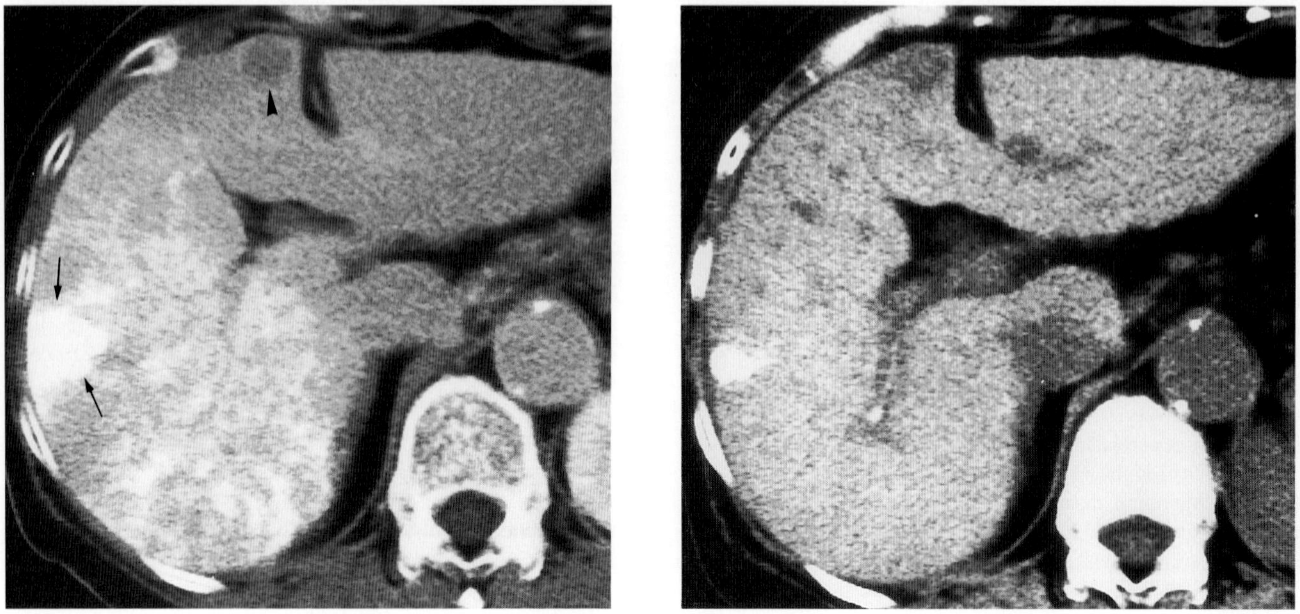

a b

Fig. 13.28 Non-specific Lipiodol retention by non-tumor parenchyma following arterial injection of Lipiodol. Lipiodol-TAE was carried out from the right hepatic artery. Plain CT (a) made immediately after injection shows a wedge-shaped strong retention (→) in S^{V} (due to arterio-portal shunt), and inhomogeneous Lipiodol retention in the right lobe. In the plain CT (b) made 40 days later, the non-specific Lipiodol retention has disappeared, leaving only the HCC that has retained Lipiodol. The lesion (▶) in S^{IV} is a cyst.

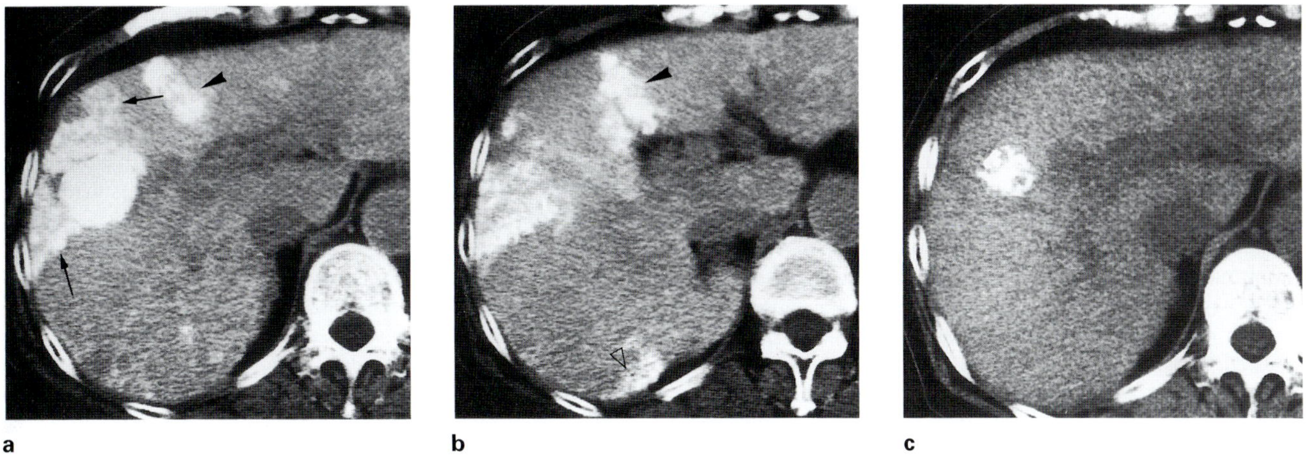

Fig. 13.29 False positive finding in Lipiodol-CT (HCC). Plain CT (a) made immediately after arterial injection of Lipiodol (5 ml) + Adriamycin (20 mg) shows a tumor in S^{V} and a fan-shaped Lipiodol retention in its periphery (→). In the slice (b) 1 cm caudal to (a), heavy deposition of Lipiodol is seen near the gallbladder along the Cantlie line (▶). Another area of non-specific Lipiodol retention is seen subcapsularly (▷). Follow-up CT (c) made 44 days later demonstrates Lipiodol retention only in HCC, and the non-specific retention has disappeared. A 2.5 cm HCC was resected along with the gallbladder. The gallbladder was normal except for the Rokitansky–Aschoff sinuses.

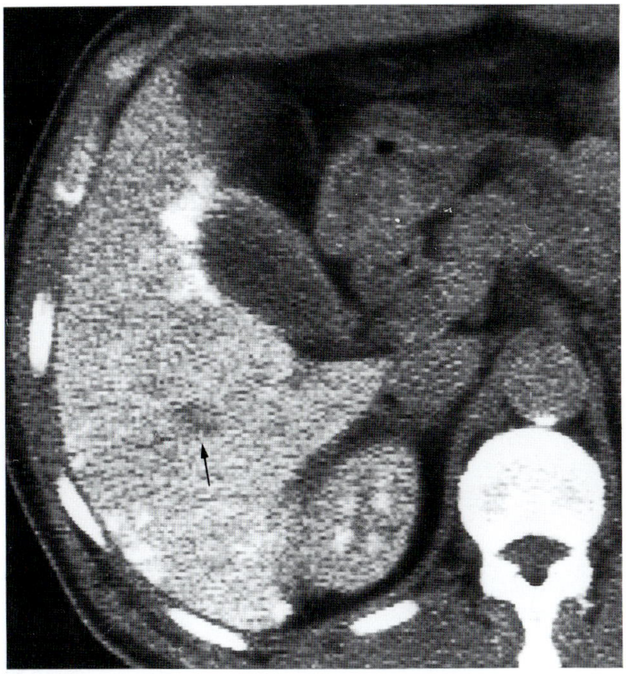

Fig. 13.30 False positive finding (hepatic metastasis from rectum carcinoma). Lipiodol was injected into the hepatic artery in this patient with rectum carcinoma metastatic to the liver. This plain CT made immediately after injection shows Lipiodol retention in the liver parenchyma adjacent to the gallbladder fundus. At the time of operation, no pathologic finding was seen in this region or in the gallbladder. →, metastasis.

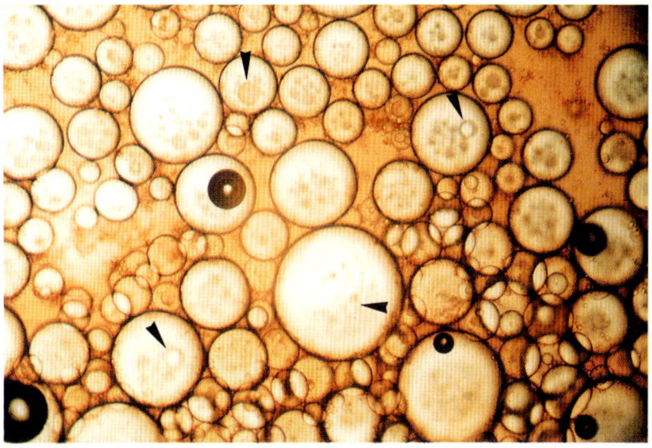

Fig. 13.31 Microscopic view of the mixture of Urografin containing Adriamycin and Lipiodol. Within large Lipiodol droplets are seen small light yellow Urografin droplets (▶) that contain Adriamycin.

13.6 Cholangio-CT

This modality, in which CT is made during cholangiography, has the advantages of clearly delineating the lumen of the bile duct, which conventional CT cannot do, and of providing extraductal information (Stockberger *et al.* 1994). Direct cholangiography, either PTC or ERC, gives information on the ductal lumen, but is incapable of evaluating pathology in the extraductal tissue (tumor extension outside the bile duct and lymph node metastasis). Some intrahepatic ducts are superimposed over others, obscuring the details. Cholangio-CT is possible using conventional intravenous cholangiography, but cholangiography carried out through a PTCD tube gives much superior images of bile ducts providing information on occluding lesions and ductal communications, and the drainage effect can be evaluated (Fig. 13.32). In addition, it will delineate an occluding extraductal lesion and mural infiltration, and assist in differential diagnosis between bile duct carcinoma and inflammation.

If dynamic CT is combined with cholangiography, information on the portal veins and arteries near the bile duct occlusion necessary in patients scheduled for surgery may be gained. Cholangio-CT may also assist in the differential diagnosis of an elevated mucosal lesion of the gallbladder, deformity due to adenomyomatosis (Case 6, p.335), displaced gallbladder (Fig. 13.33), etc.

Technique
In the absence of occlusion along the extrahepatic biliary system, drip infusion cholangiography [DIC, 100 ml of Biliscopin (50 mg of iodine/ml)] is carried out, and CT scan is made after 20 min for the study of the running course of the ductal system, and after 40 min for the gallbladder examination. If the hepatic bile duct is occluded, opacification of the biliary system is inadequate by DIC, and therefore cholangiography through the PTCD tube is desirable. Contrast medium of 2 per cent in concentration (1 ml of 60 per cent Angiografin in a test ampoule is diluted with 30 ml saline to which 1g/A of Gentamicin is added) is injected through the drainage tube to a total amount of 15–20 ml while monitoring patient discomfort, and CT scan started immediately. If the area between the hepatic hilum and the head of the pancreas is the target, only the necessary length of the bile duct is scanned; namely, the table incremental method is used with a 5 mm table shift for 5 mm slices. Information necessary for surgery is thus gained, such as the running course, mural thickness and periductal infiltration. When possible, oral contrast medium (Gastrografin) is used for the delineation of the duodenum and better interpretation.

Fig. 13.32 Cholangio-CT:
(a) Cholangiography through the PTCD tube, (b) Cholangio-CT, (c) Cholangio-CT [slice 5 mm caudal to (b)].

Cholangio-CT (b, c) were made during cholangiography through the PTCD tube. The intrahepatic biliary tree is clearly delineated (→), bile duct in the caudate lobe). This technique permits study of extra-ductal changes and evaluation of drainage effects.

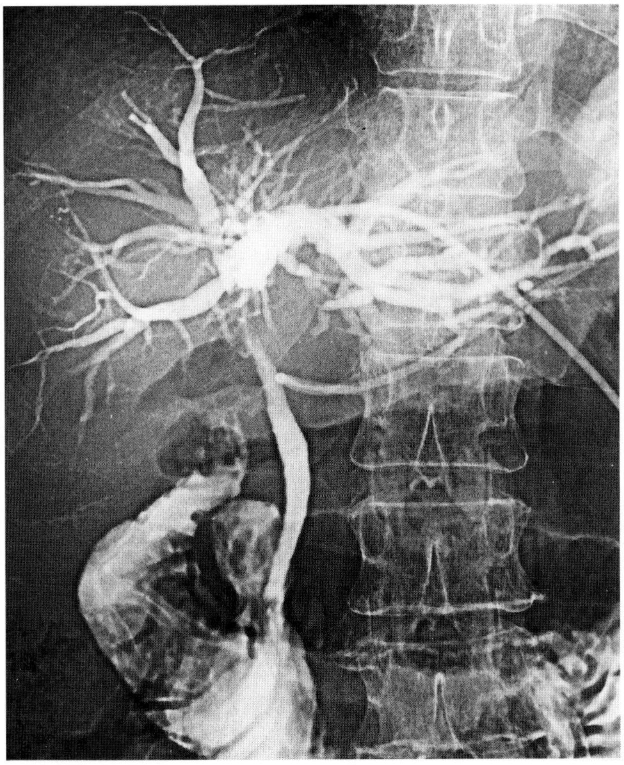

a

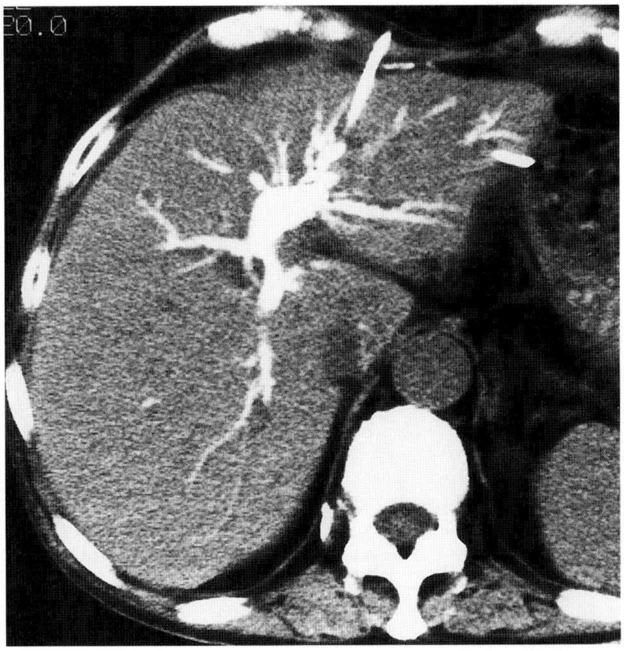

b

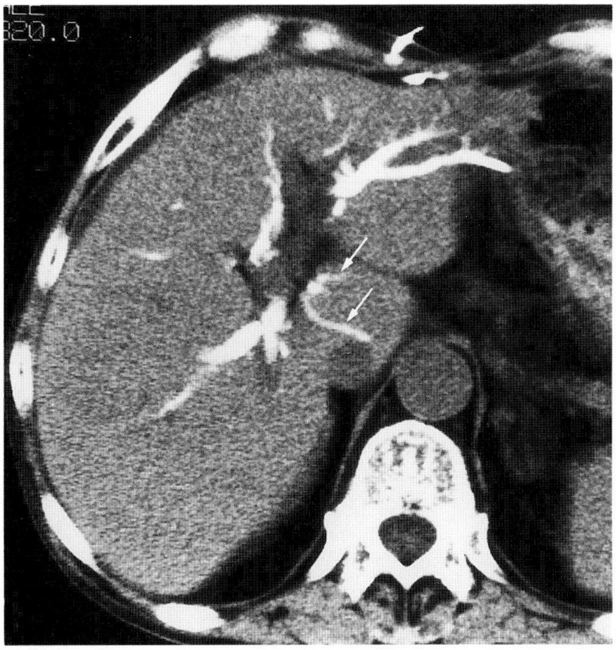

c

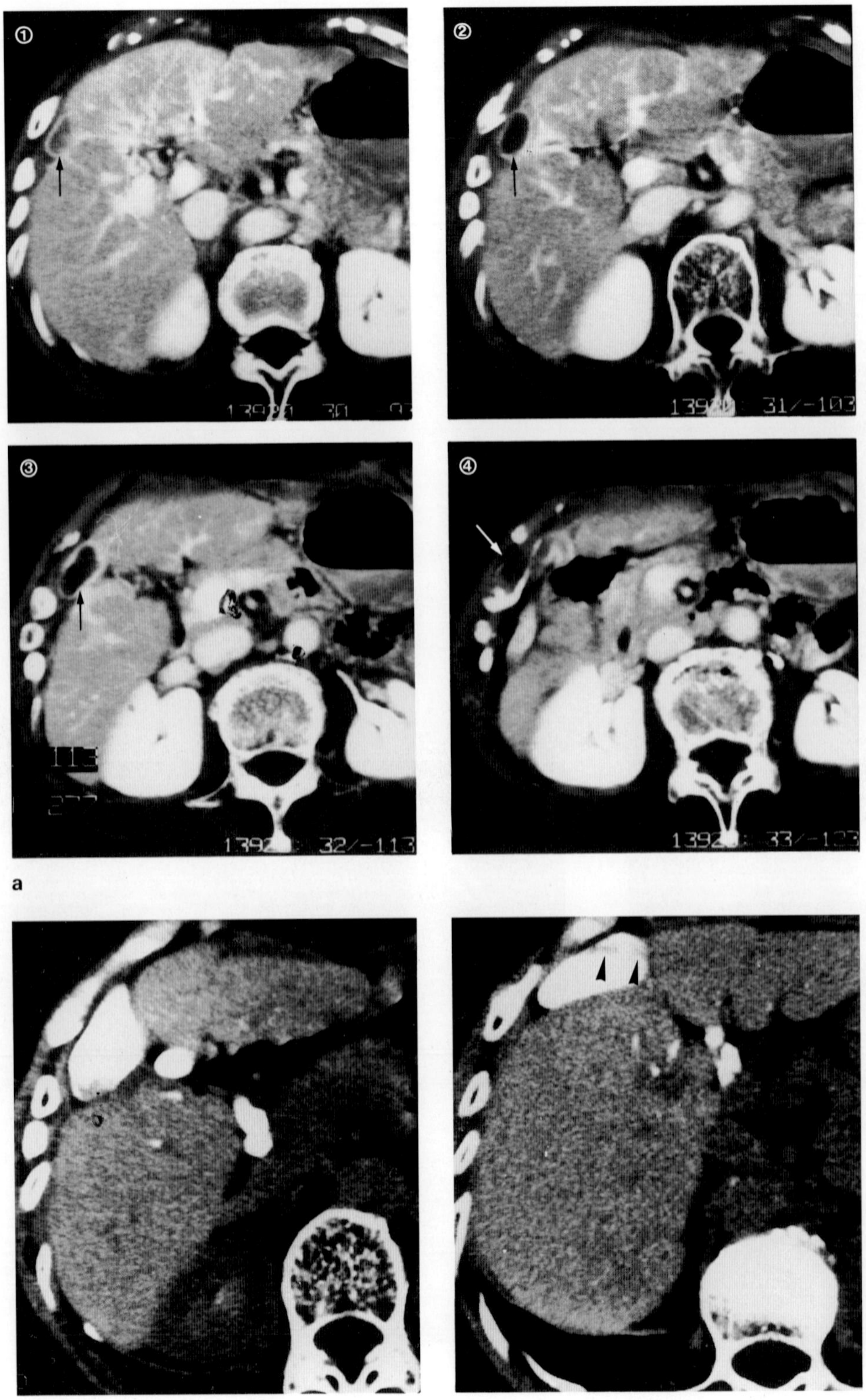

a b c

Fig. 13.33 Marked displacement of the gallbladder for which cholangio-CT was useful. A 63-year-old woman came to the hospital because of fever and abdominal pain. Enhanced CT (a) was made while moving the table incrementally. It demonstrated an oval-shaped lesion of water density in the liver surface (→). It was partially calcified (4), and differential diagnosis between inflammation (abscess) and a displaced gallbladder was required. CT scan was repeated 40 min after the start of DIC (Biliscopin). The lesion in question was filled with the contrast medium, and the diagnosis became obvious. On the CT (c) made in the prone position, a shift of filling defect was recognized (▶), suggesting stones.

14

Angiography

The significance and role of angiography in diagnosis change with time, and it seems to have become more important than before. In the past, angiography was done mainly for tumor diagnosis, but with the advent of CT and US, quality diagnosis has become easier, and it is now needed for more thorough examination such as angio-CT and Lipiodol-CT, and for embolization therapy. For greater efficacy of embolization treatment, catheterization of a peripheral feeding artery is desirable; considerable progress has recently been made in the technique of catheterization and in the quality of equipment, such as the catheter, guide-wire, catheter sheath, and non-ionized low-osmotic pressure contrast agent, digital subtraction angiography (DSA), etc.

A new catheter has been developed in which the wall has an embedded metal mesh (Torquon catheter) for better torque maneuver, and a lumen enlarged for a high flow as the new wall material resists a higher pressure. A tapered catheter (Fig. 14.1) in which the outer diameter of the tip is smaller than before, is now available. The coaxial parent-baby catheter in which a 3F baby catheter passes the parent catheter has been so improved that it can be passed into further peripheral arteries (Hosoki *et al.* 1989; Takayasu *et al.* 1990*b*).

A new type of guide-wire has also become available. An ultra elastic alloy core covered by hydrophilic polymer (Radifocus, Thermo) (Fig. 14.2) is changing the whole angiographic procedure. In the past, the guide-wire was used only up to the common or proper hepatic artery, but with this new guide-wire which can be sent into a more peripheral artery, the whole catheterization technique has become guide-wire dependent (Fig. 14.3) (Takayasu *et al.* 1988*b*). The core of Radifocus guide

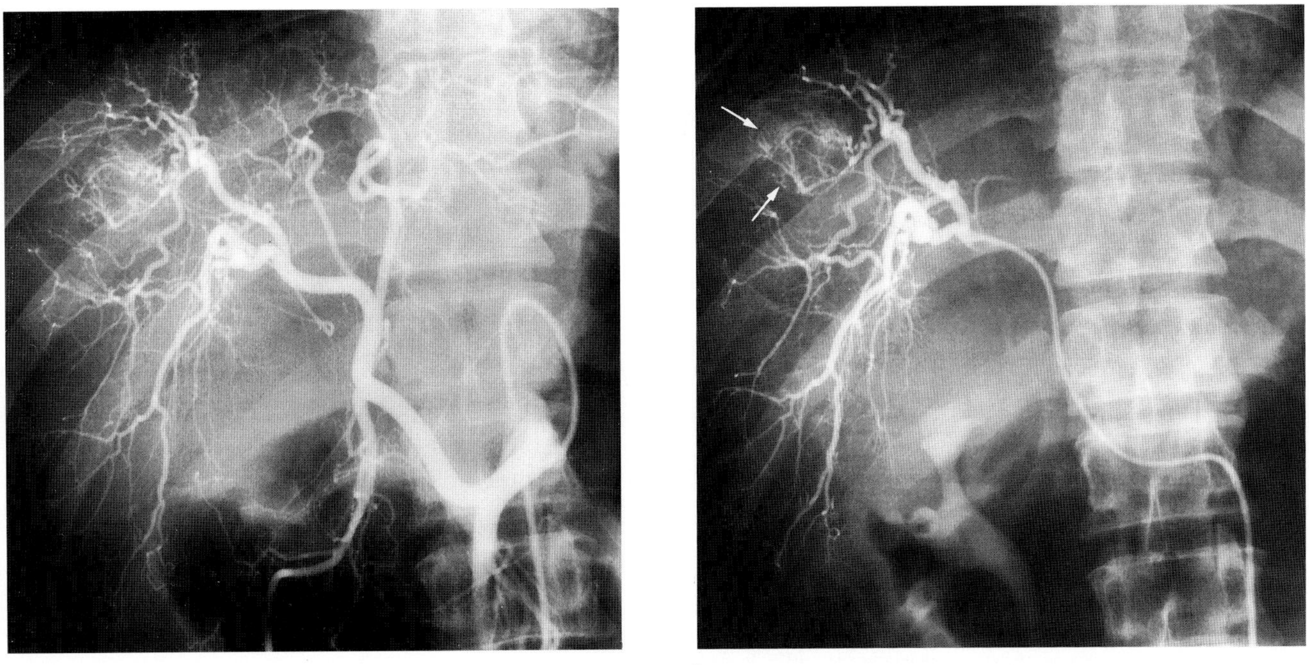

a **b**

Fig. 14.1 Hepatic arteriograms:
(a) made with a conventional catheter,
(b) made with a tapered catheter. Selective catheterization of the hepatic artery arising from the superior mesenteric artery was difficult in the past, particularly in a patient as shown here, in whom the common hepatic and superior mesenteric arteries share a common trunk. The catheter could not be passed beyond the gastroduodenal artery (a). However, with the advent of the radifocus type of guide-wire, it can now be passed into a peripheral artery. The catheter used first is withdrawn and is replaced by a tapered catheter (thickness of the tip for the length of 12–15 cm is made smaller), the procedure being called 'catheter exchange' (b). →, HCC in S^{VIII}.

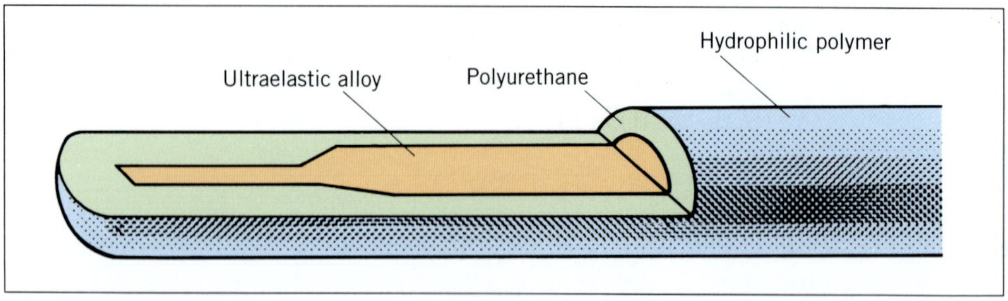

Fig. 14.2 Section diagram of a Radifocus type guide-wire. This has a ultraelastic alloy core in the center (the tip is thin for a length of 3 cm) which is embedded in polyurethane, and the surface is covered by a hydrophilic polymer. There are two types, one having a straight tip and the other with a tip bent in a J shape.

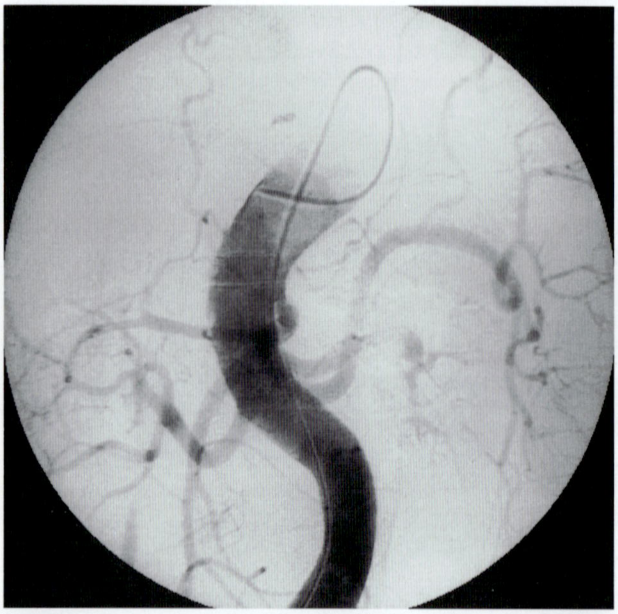

a

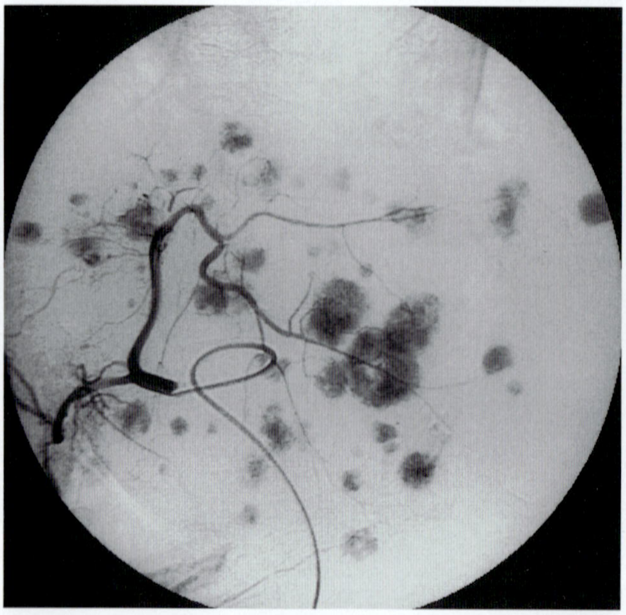

b

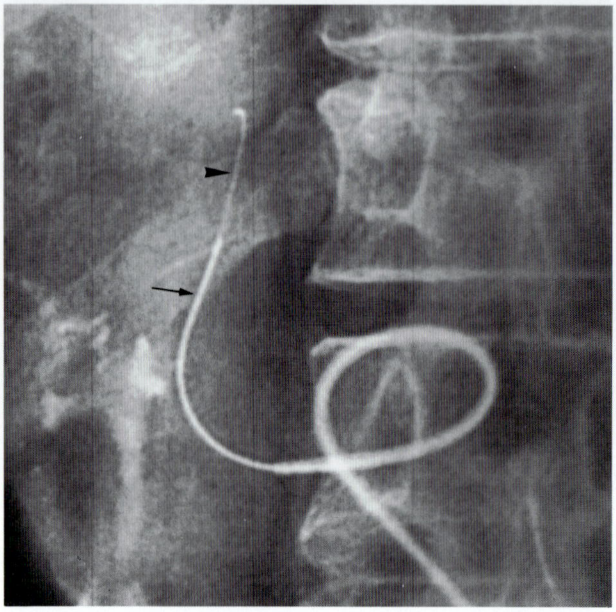

c

Fig. 14.3 Opacification of the proper hepatic artery using a new guide-wire that leads the catheter:
(a) aortography by IADSA;
(b) common hepatic arteriography by IADSA;
(c) the proper hepatic artery reached with a supercatheter. The aortogram made by IADSA (a) shows a marked winding of the aorta; the celiac artery arises from its left side forming a celiaco-mesenteric trunk. The catheter was passed into the common hepatic artery (b) but it was too long to permit catheterization of the proper hepatic artery. The proper hepatic artery could be reached by the use of a supercatheter through the parent catheter (c). TAE using Lipiodol + Adriamycin and Gelfoam sponge particles became possible. →, supercatheter; ▶, removable core within the supercatheter.

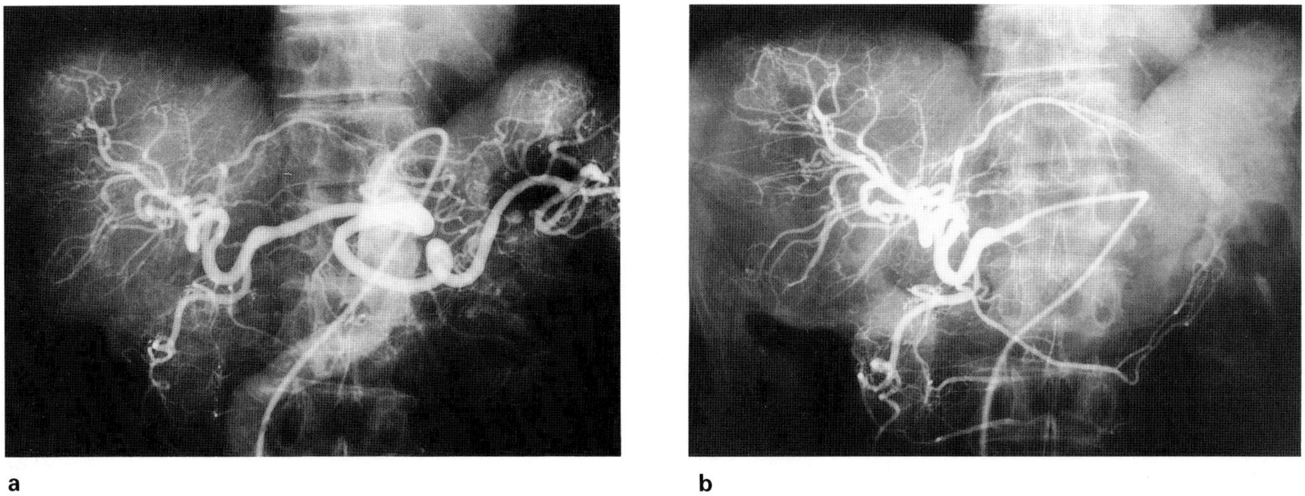

Fig. 14.4 Hepatic arteriography using a long sheath. Before the advent of the long sheath (a), the catheter could not be passed selectively into the hepatic artery if the aorta was markedly winding or bent. Contrast medium was injected with the catheter tip in the celiac artery partially opacifying the aorta. Six months later when the long sheath (25 cm, 7.5F) became available (b), the proper hepatic artery was reached with it, and proper hepatic arteriography and Lipiodol-TAE were successfully carried out.

wire can now be pulled out and a 3F hydrophilic polymer catheter that can do both opacification and embolization can be passed through it.

The development of a long 25 cm sheath now permits selective hepatic arteriography in patients who have a markedly winding iliac artery or aorta (Fig. 14.4). In the past, selective hepatic arteriography was not possible in such patients. Aneurysm is no longer a contraindication for hepatic arteriography (Fig. 14.5).

There are two types of low osmotic pressure contrast media, non-ionized (Iopamidol, Iohexol, Metrizamide) and ionized (Ioxaglate). The osmotic pressures of these newer contrast media are lower than the previous ones (Diatrizoate Meglumine, Angiografin) minimizing the pain and burning sensation that might be experienced during contrast injection. The frequency of nausea and vomiting has decreased from the previous figure of 13 per cent to 3 per cent (Katayama *et al.* 1990). The viscosity has also been reduced, permitting the use of a thin catheter (2.5–3.0F) for contrast injection. If one combines DSA with it, a clear angiogram can be made with a small amount of diluted contrast medium.

The disadvantages of low osmotic pressure contrast media include possible blood clot formation within the catheter. The catheter has to be flushed with a heparin saline before use. Allergic shock with the previous ionized contrast media usually occurs within 5 min or so, but the reaction to low-osmotic-pressure agents is a delayed allergic one, such as drug eruptions that appear several hours to several days after angiography (Mikkonen *et al.* 1995). The patient has to be watched carefully for some time after the procedure. Another disadvantage is its high cost. The new contrast media cost seven times that of Angiografin.

There are two techniques for DSA, namely intravenous DSA (IVDSA) and intraarterial DSA (IADSA). In our hospital, the latter is mainly used, and therefore that will be described here.

Advantages of IADSA

1. Intrahepatic arteries are fully opacified with a small amount of contrast medium (one-third of the amount previously used).
2. It will delineate small lesions, particularly in the area superimposed on the vertebral column (lateral area of the left lobe) (Fig. 14.6).
3. If a patient has Lipiodol in the liver due to previous lipiodolization, it can be erased for the evaluation of tumor stain which is indicative of cancer cell viability.
4. The angiograms are monitored as real-time images, and the operator can proceed with the diagnostic and therapeutic procedures while observing the fluoroscopic monitor.

Disadvantages of IADSA

This method uses a computer to digitize information on the contrast concentrations within blood vessels, and reconstitute such information into images. For this reason it has the following disadvantages.

1. Certain artefacts are produced due to respiratory movements and peristalsis of the bowel during imaging (Fig. 14.7).
2. Diagnosis of small lesions and encasement may be difficult because the images have been reconstructed.
3. The area of DSA imaging is too small to cover the entire abdomen as does the conventional angiogram.

We combine conventional angiography and DSA in our practice considering the advantages and disadvantages of DSA.

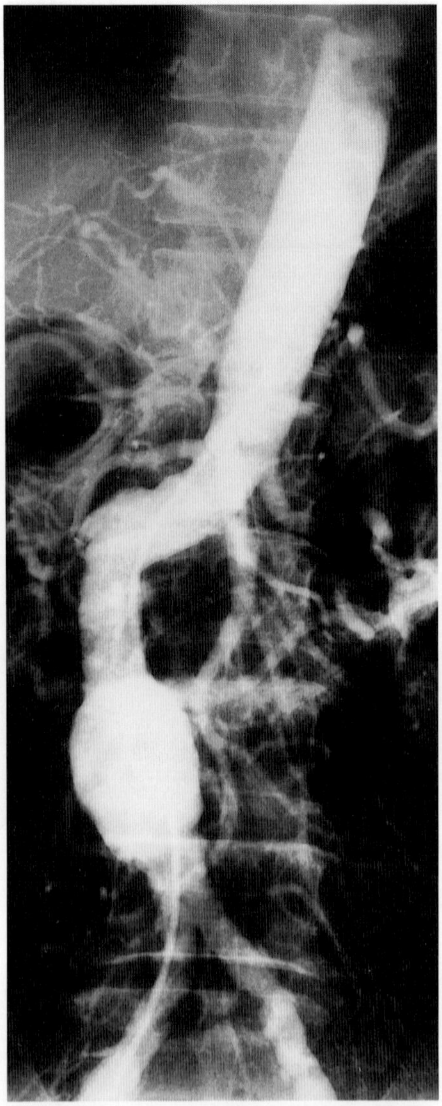

Fig. 14.5 Hepatic arteriography made possible by the use of a long sheath in a patient with an aneurysm of the abdominal aorta. In this patient, the abdominal aorta was bent, winding, and had an aneurysm. With the previous technique, it was not possible to catheterize the hepatic artery. By the use of a long sheath, exchange of the guide-wire and the catheter has become easier and safer.

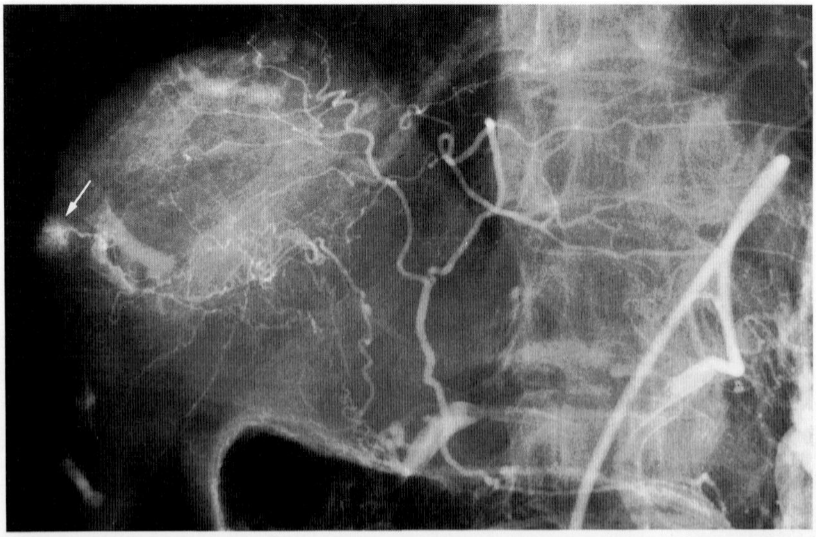

a

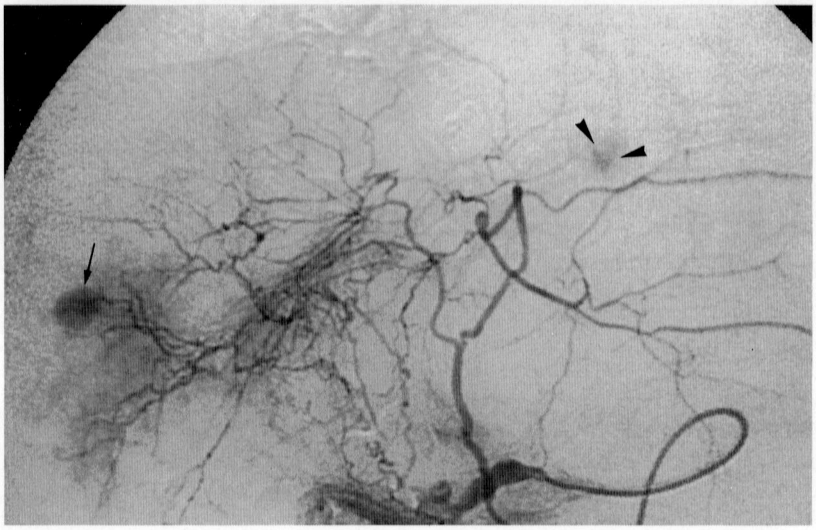

b

Fig. 14.6 Delineation by IADSA of a small lesion superimposed on the vertebral column. Conventional angiography (a) detected only one hypervascular lesion of 1 cm (→) in the right lobe. IADSA (b) demonstrated yet another small lesion (▶) in the left lobe that was superimposed on the vertebral column.

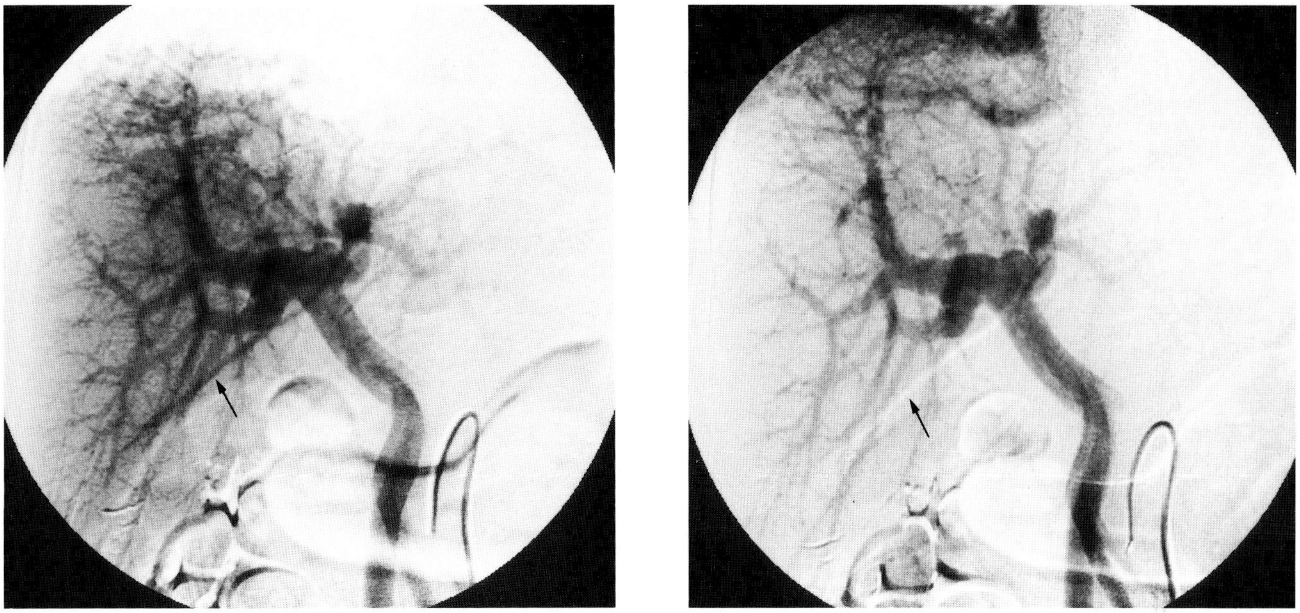

a b

Fig. 14.7 Artefact due to respiratory movements in IADSA. In this late phase film of superior mesenteric arterial portography (a), a linear structure (→) is seen arising from the U-point simulating a blood vessel. In its early phase (b), however, the same blood vessel-like structure was white and unenhanced (→), suggesting that this was a pseudo image due to a slight respiratory movement of the liver.

Hepatic arteriography

The Seldinger method through the femoral artery is the usual approach except in patients who have an occlusion of the abdominal aorta (Fig. 14.8) or in whom a long-term indwelling catheter is scheduled. The sequence of procedures is as follows: first celiac arteriography, then superior mesenteric arterial portography, and after the study of the celiac arteriogram, selective catheterization is carried out for proper hepatic arteriography or left/right hepatic arteriography.

The celiac arteriogram provides information on the vasculature within the upper abdomen that includes possible variant origin, course of the hepatic artery, presence of arterio-portal or anterio-pulmonary venous communications (Fig. 14.9), portal hypertension, feeding artery, occlusion of an artery due to a previous embolization procedure, etc.

The superior mesenteric arterial portogram demonstrates the patency of the portal vein or the site of occlusion, which is important information required for embolization therapy.

Some angiographers attempt proper hepatic arteriography immediately, but this should be avoided because passage of the catheter to the periphery may cause a spasm or subintimal damage to the artery which prevents subsequent angiography; even the intended embolization treatment may not be realized.

Without air in the stomach, as introduced by administration of a gas-producing agent, a so-called vanishing tumor that simulates a tumor vessel may be seen in the stomach fundus. During angiography, therefore, the stomach ought to be fully distended. To facilitate exchange of catheters, we use a long sheath (5F, 25 cm) together with loop-the-loop catheters (Waltman type) (Fig. 14.10). While having the patient breathe deeply, the guide-wire is passed as peripheral as possible, and the catheter is advanced over it (guide-wire first technique); catheter exchange with an indwelling guide wire is commonly done for superselective angiography (Reuter and Redman 1977). It is important not to wedge a thick catheter in a peripheral artery (Fig. 14.11). The recently developed parent-baby catheter (coaxial catheter system) and its improvement now enable catheterization of peripheral arteries with the baby catheter; the whole angiographic methodology is undergoing change.

To obtain a good quality portogram via the superior mesenteric artery, it is important to pass the catheter beyond the origin of the inferior pancreatic artery (pancreatic arcade). As a vasodilator, prostaglandin E_1 (20 μg/A) dissolved in 10 ml saline is injected immediately before contrast injection. This agent increases blood flow within 30 s, and there is no further increase in flow with a larger dose; it only increases the duration of increased flow (Cho *et al.* 1975). About 90 per cent of the prostaglandin is inactivated by one passage through the lung.

In portography, the left portal vein is sometimes opacified poorly. Contrast medium has a greater specific gravity than blood and tends to flow along the posterior aspect of a large blood vessel. The right posterior portal vein tends to be opacified better than other branches whereas the left portal vein which is located most anteriorly gets less contrast medium due to the gravity difference (Fig. 14.12). For the same reason, if P^{III}I and P^{IV} are well opacified and P^{II}, which is more posterior to them, is not opacified, a pathological change should be sus-

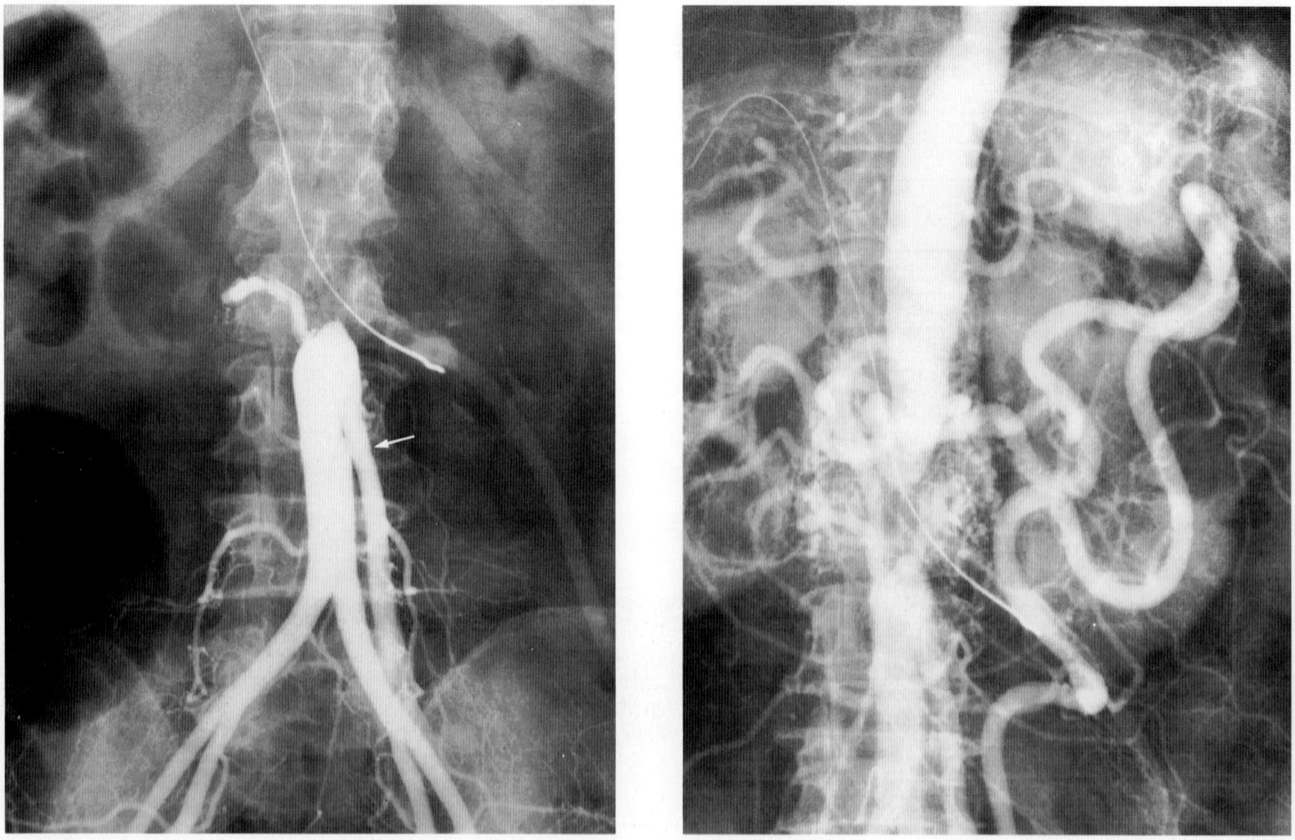

a b

Fig. 14.8 Hepatic arteriography in a patient with an occluded abdominal aorta. Angiography from the right femoral artery (a) showed a complete occlusion of the abdominal aorta at the level immediately above the origin of the inferior mesenteric artery (→), and the targeted hepatic artery could not be opacified. The left axillary artery was then entered (b) by passing the catheter toward the occlusion and contrast medium injected. It revealed a stenosis of the aorta immediately below the bilateral renal arteries, and complete occlusion below the stenosis. The aorta below the occlusion was opacified through dilated superior mesenteric and inferior mesenteric arteries (Leriche syndrome). In the past, translumbar aortography (Dossantos method) was done, but currently this is seldom carried out.

pected in P^{II}, and the cause should be determined using other imaging procedures. The most common complication of angiography is subcutaneous hematoma at the site of catheter entry. We have seen a patient in whom a pseudoaneurysm at the puncture site suddenly ruptured 1 week later requiring a prosthesis for the femoral artery, and in another the puncture site was too caudal and a pseudoaneurysm slowly enlarged and had to be resected (Fig. 14.13). The main cause in these cases was repeated punctures by an inexperienced angiographer. In several cases, it took more than two hours for hemostasis. The reason was the use of a large sheath (7.5F) in elderly patients with arteriosclerosis, in patients with thrombocytopenia, and in patients in whom the earlier puncture site was repunctured. For the management of all these problems, we use the hands, sometimes alternating with a helper, for compression hemostasis; this is always successful. We still believe that 'compression hemostasis is better than any other hemostatic procedure'. The tip of the sheath should not be irregular, and a good one with a minimal resistance in piercing the tissue ought to be selected. The hepatic artery may be damaged by the catheterization procedure and manipulation of the guid wire, and the damage may be indirectly associated with an aberrant course of the vessel, such as intimal injury, aneurysm formation (Case 6, p.491), and extravasation. Aneurysm usually develops following intimal damage. Repeated angiography in such patient usually demonstrates healing of the aneurysm that follows thrombus formation. In about half of the patients the artery with the subintimal injury remains occluded (Soo *et al.* 1982), and therefore the catheterization procedure should be carried out with the utmost caution.

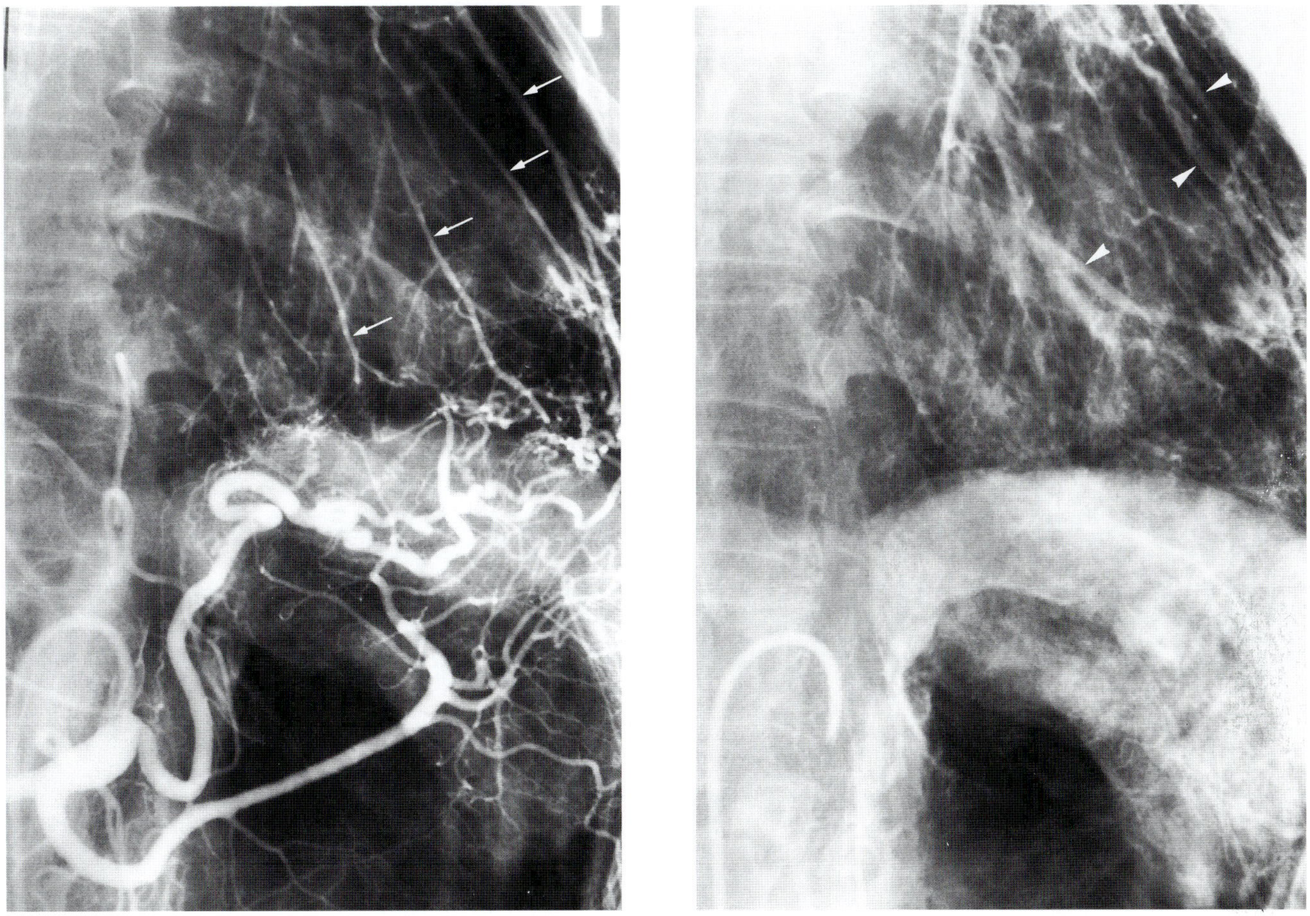

a b

Fig. 14.9 Communication between the hepatic artery and pulmonary veins. Celiac arteriography (arterial phase) (a) displayed a dilated left inferior phrenic artery and many communicating pulmonary arteries (→). In the venous phase (b), the blood coming from the celiac artery entered numerous pulmonary veins (▶) running from the diaphragm toward the pulmonary hilum. In this kind of patient precautions are necessary in the TAE procedure.

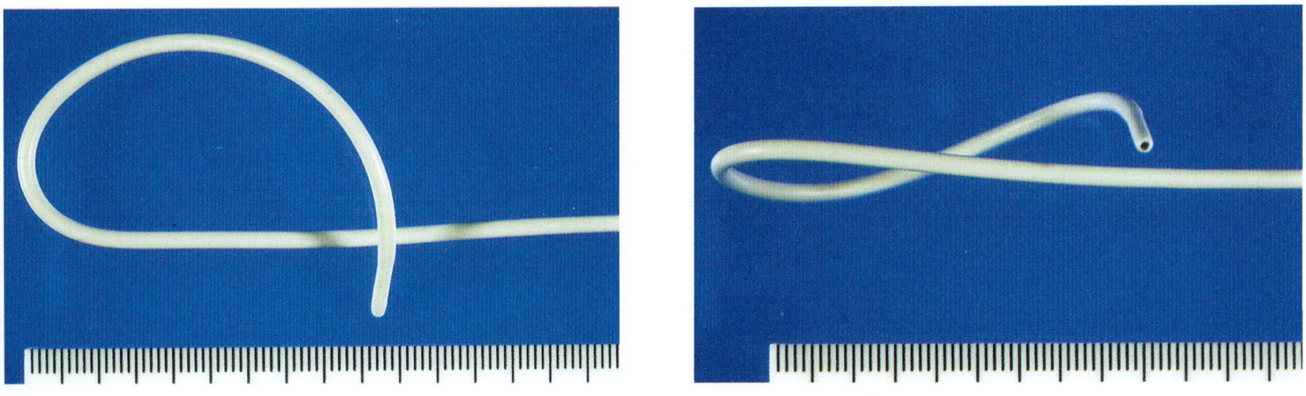

a b

Fig. 14.10 Loop-the-loop (Waltman) type catheter: (a) frontal view; (b) lateral view. The catheter tip has a three-dimensional bending that facilitates entry into the hepatic artery. After entry into the aorta, the tip assumes this shape in the aortic arch.

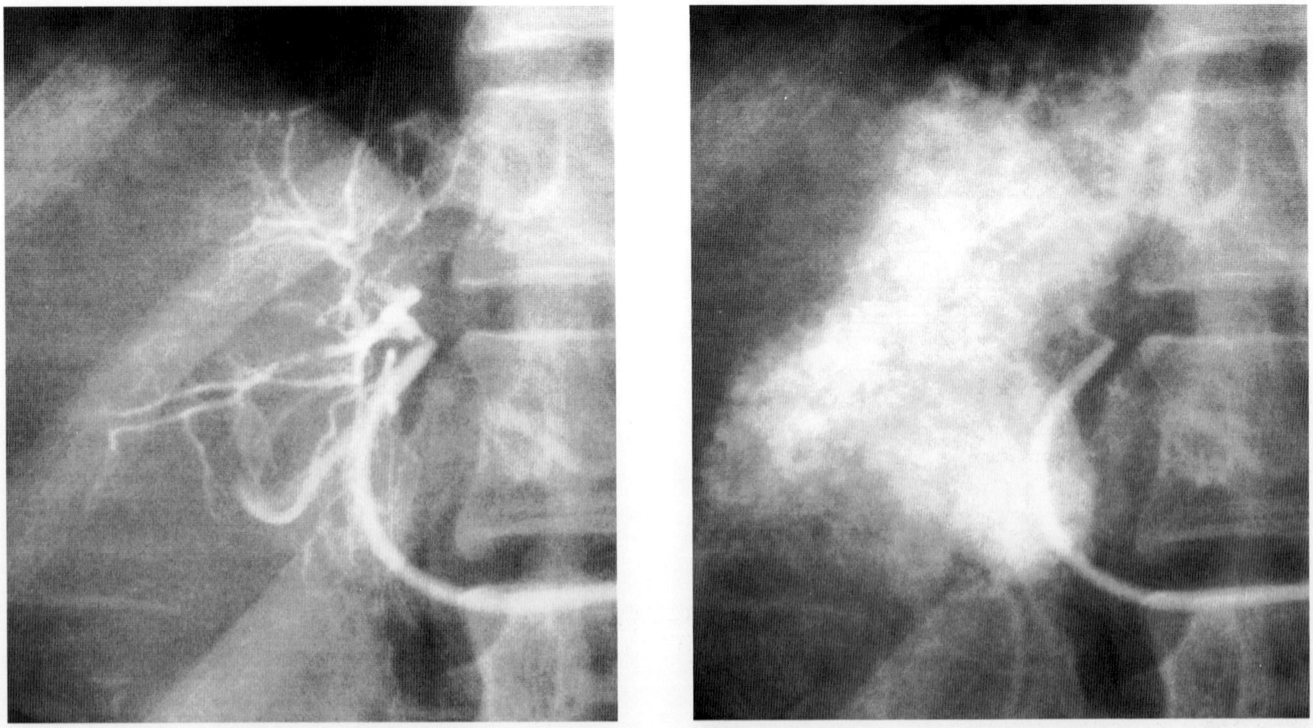

a b

Fig. 14.11 Wedging of a thick catheter. If a large caliber catheter is used, it gets wedged in a peripheral artery, and an irregular contrast passage results (a). In the venous phase (b), contrast medium does not flow out, making distinction of tumor and parenchyma difficult. Such wedging should be avoided.

Hepatic venography

As in hepatic arteriography, Seldinger's method is usually employed with a catheter inserted by femoral vein puncture. This technique can be used not only for venography, but also for the measurement of wedged hepatic vein pressure (WHVP) after wedging the catheter tip into the peripheral hepatic vein, and for retrograde portography in which contrast medium is injected through the catheter in a wedged position (Fig. 14.14). A round tipped long catheter is frequently used for this purpose. A catheter with a balloon may also be used for selective hepatic venograpyy (Fig. 14.15) and panhepatography, in which all hepatic veins are opacified (Mutou 1980) (Fig. 14.16). The need for hepatic venography has been reduced after the advent of CT and MR imaging, and it is now required mainly for the diagnosis and treatment of Budd–Chiari syndrome. For the diagnosis of Budd–Chiari syndrome due to IVC obstruction, sandwich opacification of the hepatic portion of the IVC with combined superior and inferior cavography is carried out. The hepatic vein may be visualized in the late phase of arteriography and portography, providing important information for surgery.

Portography

Portography is important in the diagnosis of portal hypertension and for the study of portal hemodynamics. Previously, splenoportography was the only non-surgical technique with which portal venous pressure could be measured and the portal vein opacified. In this method, the spleen is punctured with a thick needle, pulp pressure measured, and contrast medium injected. The drawbacks are possible massive bleeding in patients with portal hypertension and splenomegaly, and non-opacification of the portal vein in the presence of a large splenorenal shunt (it used to be mistaken for portal vein occlusion). To overcome these problems, several other techniques were developed such as umbilico-portography (transumbilical portography) (Chiandussi *et al.* 1967; Wiechel 1979) and operative portography (Moore and Bridenbauch 1950). In the former, the occluded umbilical vein in the ligamentum teres is reopened, and the catheter pushed into the left portal vein through the reopened umbilical vein for contrast injection. In the latter, during an operation a catheter is inserted into the portal vein through one of the mesenteric veins. Some surgeons make a small incision in the abdominal wall and insert catheters into the gastroepiploic veins (trans gastroepiploic portography) (Okuda and Iio 1976), or the omental vein is catheterized after peritoneoscopy (Yamamoto and Reynolds 1964).

These techniques are invasive and some are not repeatable. Currently, percutaneous transhepatic portography (PTP) carried out under US guidance using a long stylet (Kimura *et al.* 1981) is the most useful and practical. It permits direct measurement of portal venous pressure and direct opacification of the portal vein and intrahepatic portal branches (Okuda *et al.*

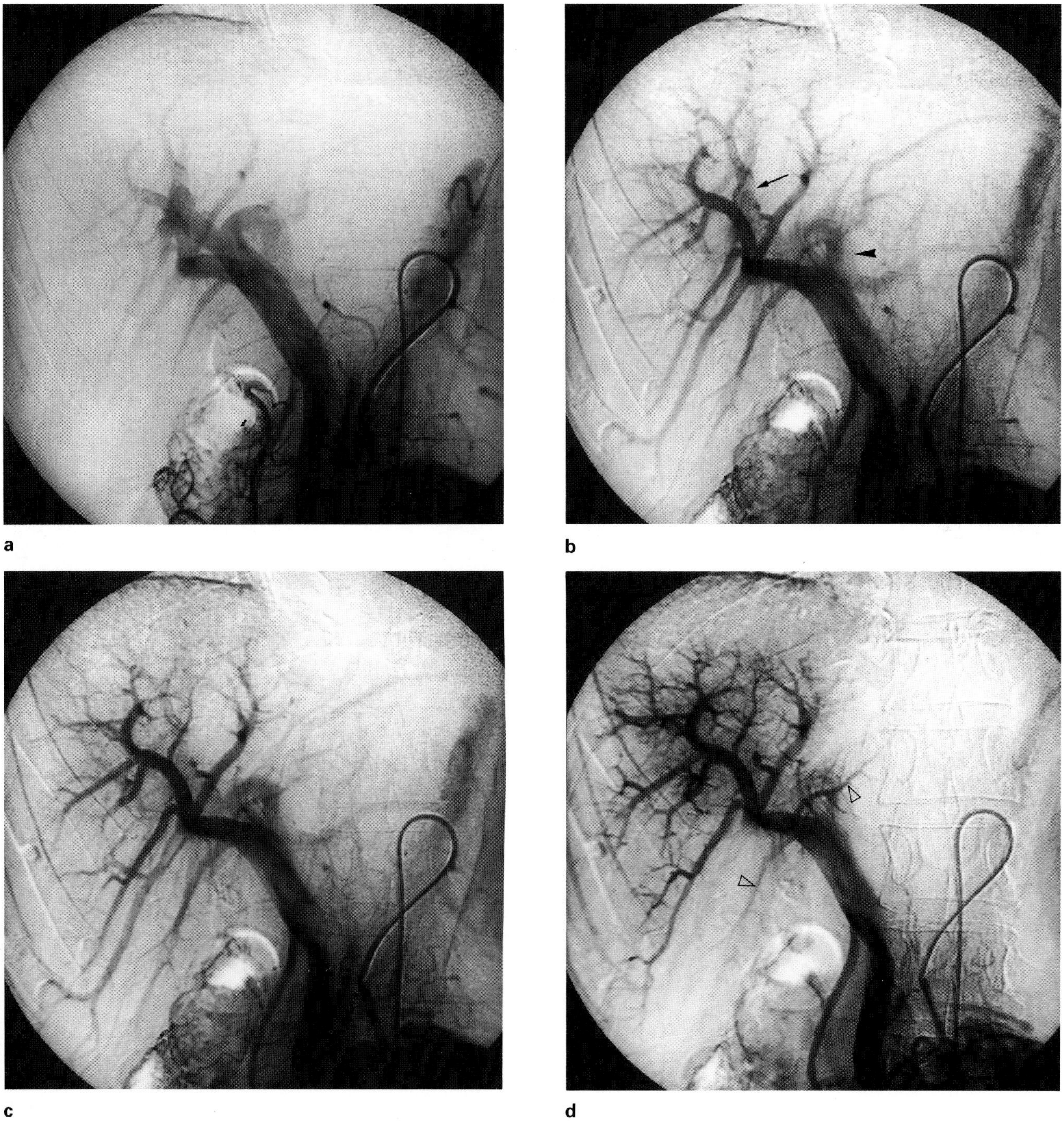

Fig. 14.12 Laminar flow in superior mesenteric arterial portography. These (a–d) are superior mesenteric arterial portograms in sequence. Since the catheter tip is wedged in a branch of the superior mesenteric artery, contrast medium is flowing slowly in the portal vein in which heavier contrast medium runs along the posterior aspect of the lumen. Because of this laminar flow, the right posterior portal vein is more clearly opacified (b, c, d), and the right anterior portal vein (b, →) and the left portal vein (b, ▶) are only faintly opacified. For the same reason, the caudate lobe branch deriving from the posterior aspect of the bifurcation of the right and left portal veins and running toward the left medially (d, ▷) is often clearly opacified.

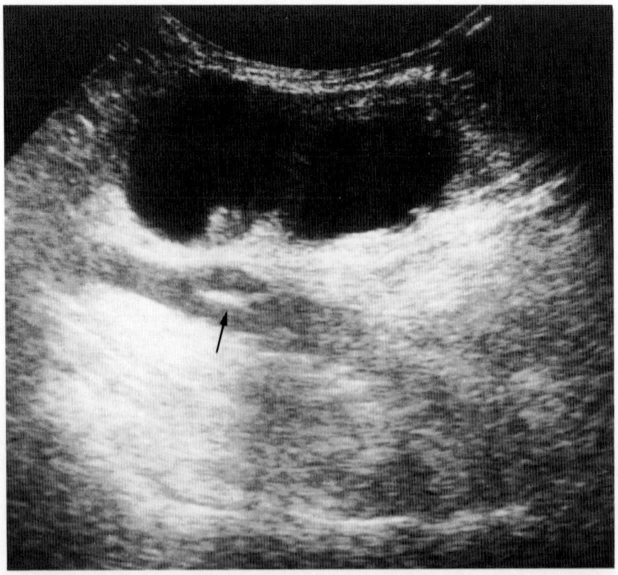

a

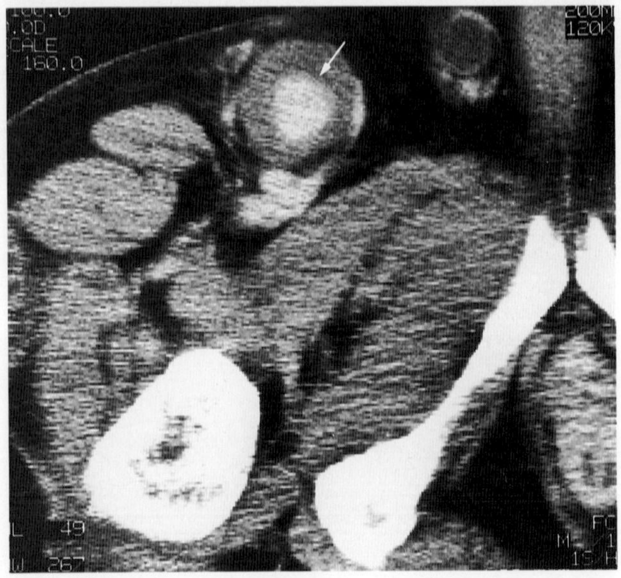

b

Fig. 14.13 Complication of angiography (pseudoaneurysm). As the puncture site was far down from the level of the head of the femur, compression hemostasis was difficult. Several days later, the puncture site slowly bulged, and US (a) demonstrated a cystic lesion (pseudoaneurysm), 6 cm on the longitudinal axis, anterior to the bifurcation (→) of the femoral and deep femoral arteries. The lesion contained a high-echo structure. Enhanced CT (b) clearly opacified the lumen (→) of the pseudoaneurysm, suggesting its communication with the femoral artery; it was resected.

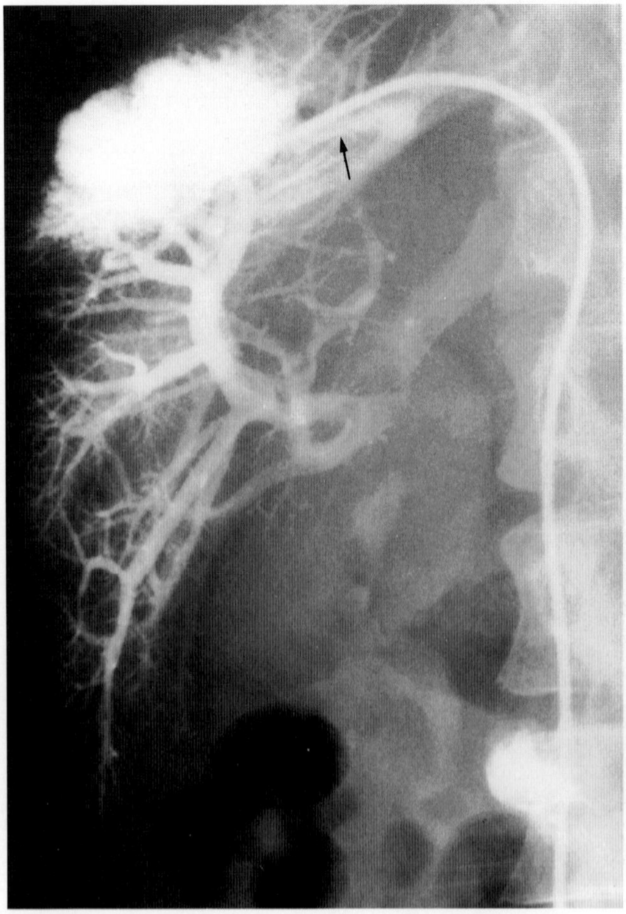

Fig. 14.14 Retrograde portography. The catheter tip is wedged in the right hepatic vein (→), and contrast medium injected under pressure. Contrast medium enters the portal vein (P^{VIII}, P^{V}) through the sinusoids, producing a retrograde portogram. This technique was used in the past mainly in patients with obstruction in the portal trunk or in the first-order portal vein (right and left), in whom arterial portography did not opacify the peripheral portal branches. Diagnosis of portal vein occlusion can now be made with ease using US and CT.

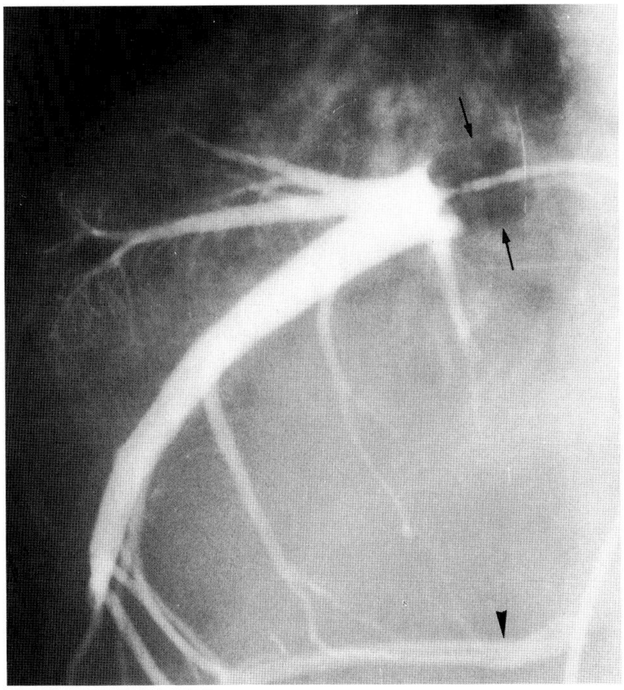

Fig. 14.15 Selective hepatic venography. With a balloon inflated (→) at the opening of the right hepatic vein into the IVC, creating a situation similar to wedging, contrast medium is injected slowly. It enters other veins (inferior right hepatic, ▶) through vein–vein anastomoses. In idiopathic portal hypertension and Budd–Chiari syndrome (IVC obstruction) such communications are extensive.

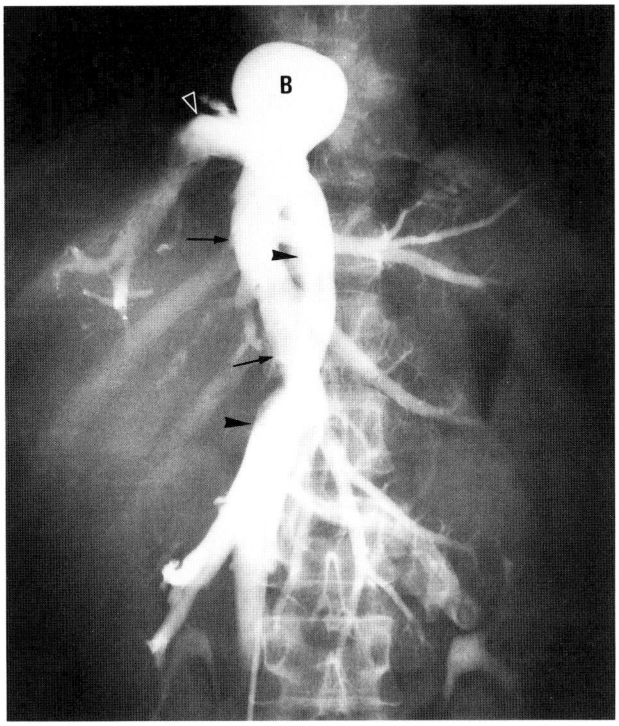

Fig. 14.16 Panhepatography using a balloon catheter. In this technique, the IVC is occluded by inflating the balloon (B) at the tip of the catheter, and contrast medium injected through a side hole below the balloon, opacifying all hepatic veins simultaneously. In this patient, a huge HCC in the right lobe is displacing the IVC (▶) to the left. The middle hepatic vein (▷) is also compressed and stenosed, and only the left hepatic vein (→) is opacified.

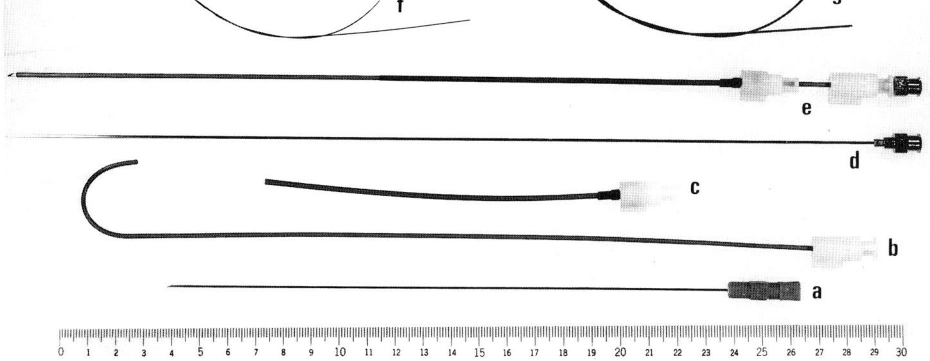

Fig. 14.17 Equipment for percutaneous transhepatic portography: (a) PTC needle (21G, 20 cm); (b) PTP catheter (J-tipped, 5F, 30 cm); (c) sheath (5F, 13 cm); (d) PTP needle (19G, 30 cm); (e) PTP puncture set (c+b+d); (f) long stylet (0.4 mm, 50 cm); (g) guidewire (0.035″, 50 cm).

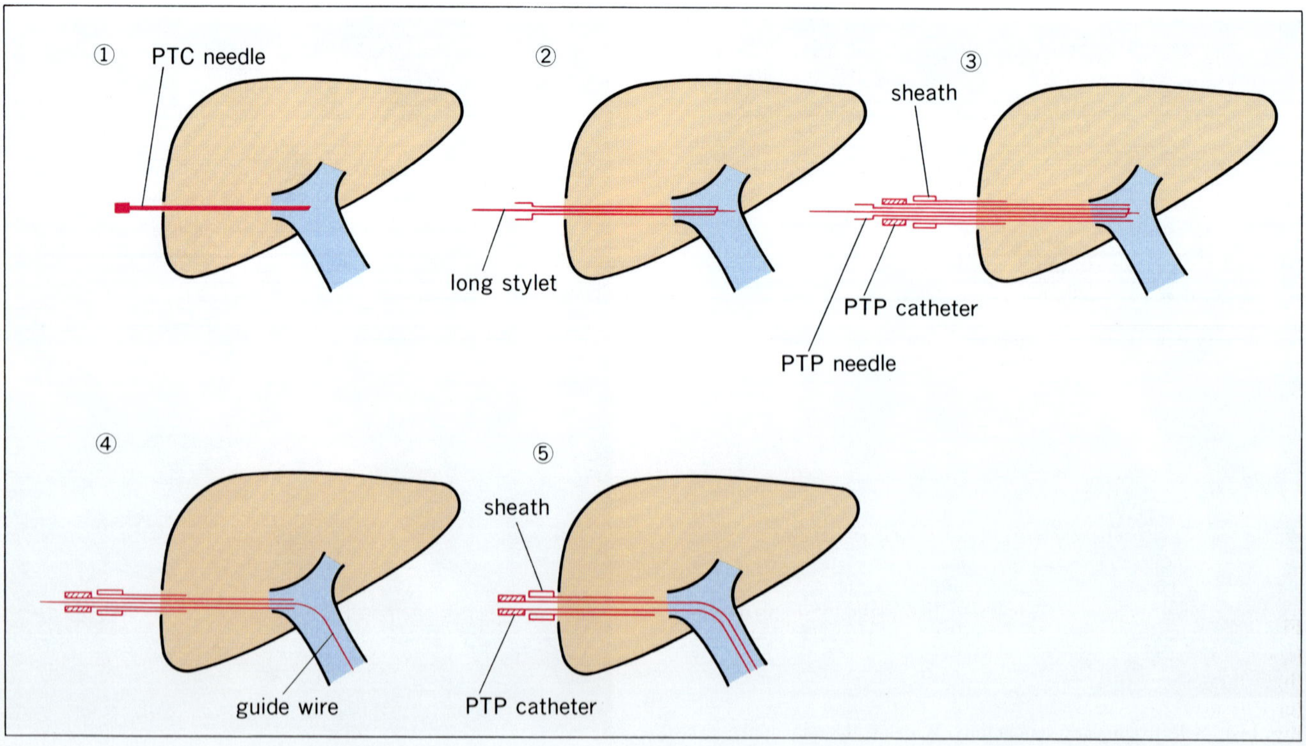

Fig. 14.18 The technique for percutaneous transhepatic portography.

(1) A portal vein branch is punctured with a PTC needle under US guidance. When entering the right lobe one aims at the anterior portal vein, and when entering from the left lobe one aims at the umbilical portion of the left portal vein. Hemostasis is easier if entry is made from the right anterior portal vein.

(2) The inner needle (stylet) is removed, blood withdrawn, and then contrast medium injected to confirm the portal vein. The long stylet is inserted through the PTC needle to secure that portal vein. The needle moves at the time of withdrawal, during contrast injection, and with the patient's respiration, and therefore a pediatric extension tube (50 cm) is connected to the needle to cushion its movements. More recently, a stylet with a J-shaped guide-wire attached to its tip has been developed; it facilitates passage of the stylet more centrally making the procedure easier.

(3) The PTC outer needle is withdrawn (leaving the stylet) and the PTP puncture set (the sheath over a straight PTP catheter, which in turn is over the PTP needle) is pushed in over the stylet up to its tip. In this procedure, it is important to monitor under fluoroscopic control that the stylet is not bent between the abdominal wall and the liver. When the puncture set is pushed forward, it may push the stylet further due to friction, and therefore one should hold back the stylet at that time.

(4) The long stylet and the PTP needle are pulled out together, blood withdrawn through the catheter, contrast medium injected to confirm the portal vein, and the guide-wire (0.035″, 50 cm) pushed into it. If a large portal vein has been entered, entry of the guide-wire is easy, but in a small portal branch it is not and careful manipulation is required. It is important that the patient does not breathe deeply in order to prevent shift in the position of the catheter tip.

(5) After confirming that the guide-wire has gone further centrally beyond the portal trunk, the catheter is advanced and the sheath pushed further all the way up to its base.

1977*g*). It will also opacify portal-systemic collateral veins. Embolization of the left gastric vein and intrahepatic portal branches is also possible with this technique (Lunderquist and Vang 1974). It has been used to localize a hormone-producing tumor in the pancreas by collecting blood from different sites of the pancreas (Burcharth 1979). Indirect portography includes transarterial portography and retrograde portography.

Technique for PTP and embolization

The equipment used for PTP is shown in Fig. 14.17, and the procedure is diagramatically depicted in Fig. 14.18: (1) a thin PTC needle (21G, 20 cm) (Okuda *et al.* 1974) is inserted into a portal vein branch in the liver under US guidance; (2) the inner needle is removed, a 50 cm long stylet is sent in through the outer needle up to the portal branch to secure its position, (3) while the long stylet is kept still, the PTC outer needle is removed and a PTP set (19G 30 cm PTP needle within a 5F 30 cm PTP catheter, which in turn is covered by a 5F 13 cm sheath) is inserted sliding over it under X-ray fluoroscopy; (4) after the PTP needle has reached the tip of the long stylet (after penetration of the portal vein wall) the PTP needle and stylet are withdrawn; blood is withdrawn to be certain that the catheter is in the portal branch, then the guide wire is passed toward the central direction; and (5) the catheter and the sheath are pushed further to conclude the procedure.

For the embolization of the left gastric and short gastric veins (percutaneous transhepatic obliteration, PTO) and an intrahepatic portal vein branch (PTPE), a catheter with a specially

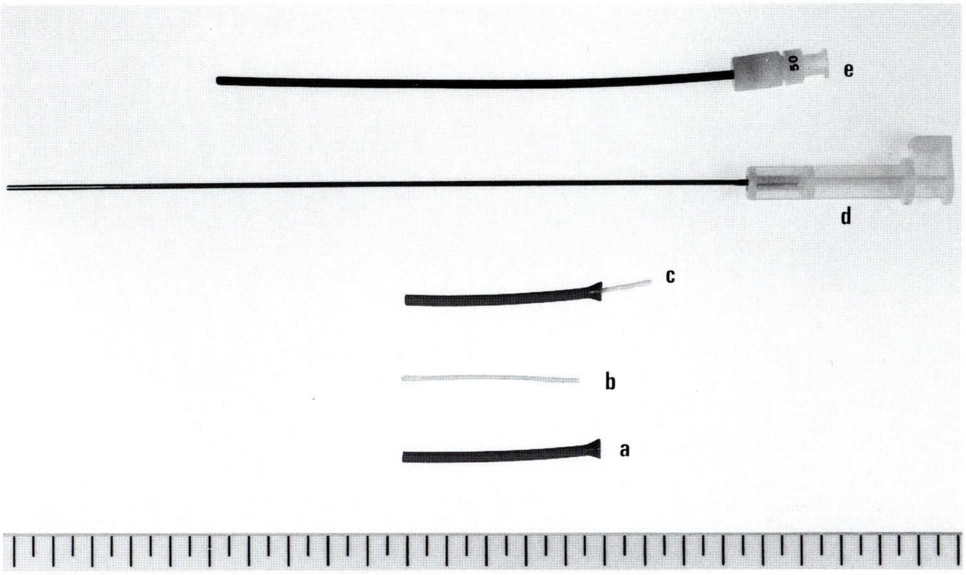

Fig. 14.19 Equipment used for hemostasis at termination of the PTP procedure:
(a) Cartridge, 8F, 5 cm;
(b) Gelfoam sponge twist (a little shorter than the cartridge to faciliate pushing it out);
(c) This shows how the Gelfoam twist goes into the cartridge at the time of use. The Gelfoam should be sticking out from the cartridge by 1–2 mm; this makes fitting it into the sheath easier.
(d) Push bar (1.5 mm, 19 cm). More recently, the same size catheter with a closed tip has been used to ease the patient's breath-hold.
(e) Sheath used in PTP (5F, 13 cm).

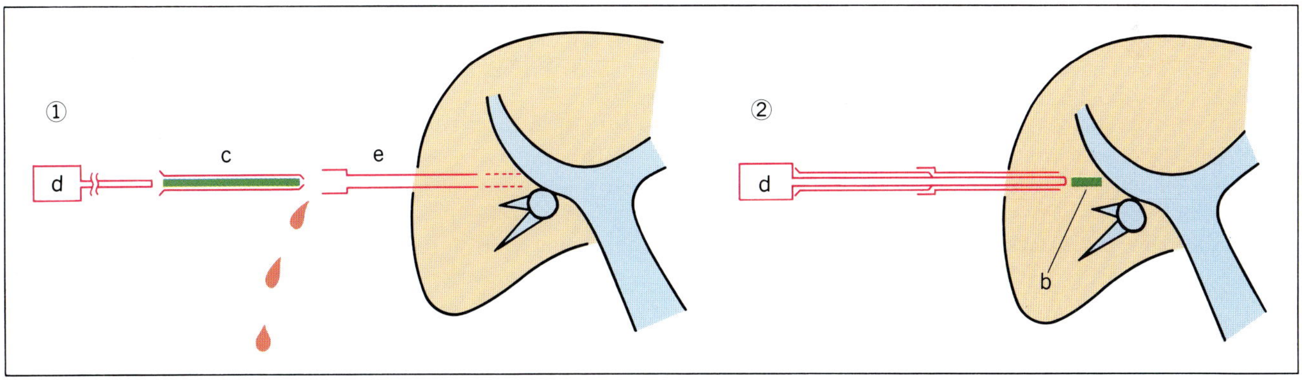

Fig. 14.20 Diagrammatic depiction of the hemostatic procedure at the end of PTP.

(1) The catheter is removed leaving the sheath (e), and the sheath withdrawn a little back into the liver parenchyma. While the push bar (d) is slightly in the cartridge (c), the cartridge tip is placed in the entrance of the sheath.

(2) Under fluoroscopic control, the push bar is advanced and the Gelfoam (b) is pushed out of the cartridge, plugging the puncture hole. If necessary, the same procedure is repeated one or two more times while pulling out the sheath further to conclude hemostasis. If contrast medium is added to the Gelfoam, one can confirm hemostasis (see Fig. 14.21).

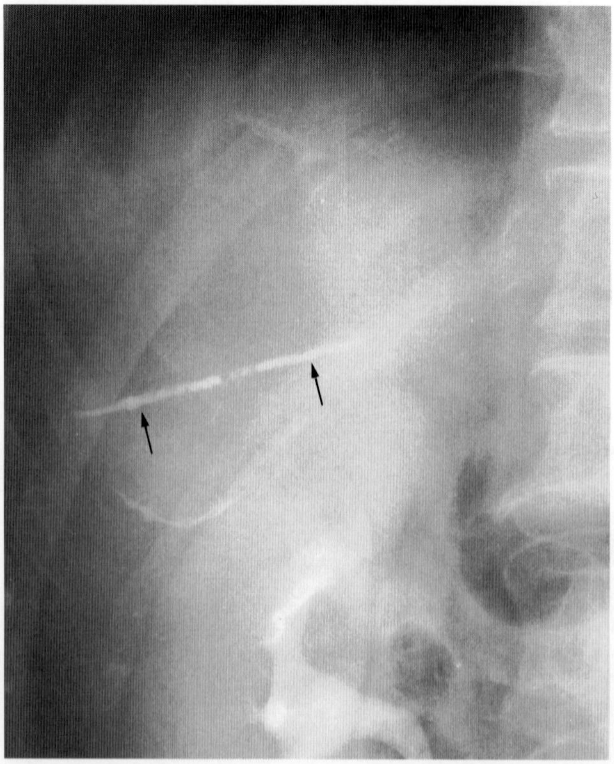

Fig. 14.21 Hemostasis at the end of PTP. After withdrawal of the catheter, a Gelfoam sponge twist containing contrast medium (→) is pushed into the puncture track through the sheath that has been left.

Table 14.1 Various materials used for embolization

Solid	Gelfoam	T
	Ivalon	P
	Steel coils	P
	Detachable balloons	P
	Blood clot	T
	Oxycel	T
	Avitene	S/P
	Blood vessel intima	S/P
	Silk streamers	P
	Nylon brushes	P
	Barium-impregnated silicone spheres (BISS)	P
	Lead shot and steel balls	P
	Plastic spheres and glass beads	P
	Tantalum powder and barium particles	P
Liquid	50% dextrose	P
	Absolute ethyl alcohol	P
	Bucrylate (IBCA)	P
	Ethibloc	P
	Sotradecol	P
	Varicocid	P
	Silicone rubber	P
	Hot contrast medium	P
	Thrombin	S/P
	Hypertonic saline	S/P
	Lipiodol	S/P
Other	Balloon occlusion catheter	T
	Electrocoagulation	P
	Thermocoagulation	P

T, temporary; S/P, semipermanent; P, permanent [after Gregson (1988)].

shaped tip may be passed to the targeted vein following portography, and absolute ethanol and Gelfoam sponge are used for PTO, and Gelfoam powder for PTPE. For hemostasis after the procedure, we use Gelfoam sponge (Fig. 14.19) cut to a size of 1.5 [×] 1.5 [×] 45 mm which is then twisted into a stick to be passed into the sheath to plug the hole (Fig. 14.20). By this plugging technique, the frequency of post procedure bleeding into the abdominal cavity, hence complications, has been dramatically reduced (Takayasu *et al.* 1988*d*) (Fig. 14.21).

Materials for arterial and portal embolization

A number of different materials are available and used for different purposes and at different sites (Table 14.1) (Gregson 1988). In Japan, small particles of Gelfoam sponge cut into a size of 0.5–1.0 mm (Fig. 14.22(a)) which are subsequently absorbed into tissue, are usually used for arterial embolization. Gelfoam powder (40–60 μm) (Fig. 14.22(b)) is too small in size and is no longer used because it frequently causes complications such as bile duct necrosis (Case 2, p.487) and hepatic infarct. However, when a very thin catheter (smaller than 3F) is used, sponge particles are too large to pass through, and Gelfoam powder is required in its place. In the USA unabsorbable Ivalon is commonly used. This has an advantage of being made in various sizes, but is expensive; it has no further advantage over Gelfoam.

A steel coil (Fig. 14.23) is suitable for occluding a large artery in its central site, but it may soon reopen because its periphery is patent, and collaterals form rather quickly. Thus, the net effect of steel coil embolization is similar to that of arterial ligation. Therefore, it is more suited for the treatment of large arterio-portal and arterio-venous shunts, and of bleeding from the GI tract [advanced stomach cancer (Fig. 14.24), bleeding from an anastomosis site, and hemobilia] rather than in the treatment of liver cancer.

It is said that to recognize extravasation by angiography, bleeding exceeding 0.5 ml/min is necesary (Nusbaum and Baum 1963). To accurately lodge the steel coil at the target site, one should carefully explore the path by passing the guide-wire fluoroscopically before placing the coil in the catheter. To embolize an intrahepatic portal branch, we use Gelfoam powder in order to send in as much embolizing material as possible. The use of Gelfoam powder prevents recanalization of the occluded portal branch and formation of collateral veins that occur after portal vein ligation (Case 12, p.573).

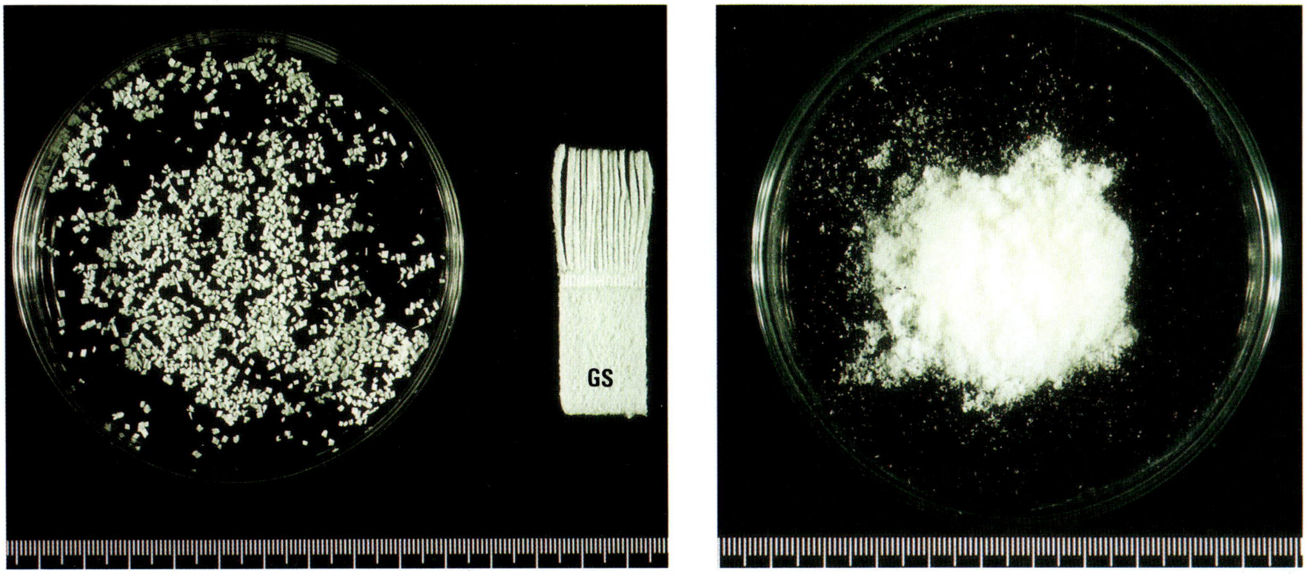

a b

Fig. 14.22 Materials used for embolization. (a) Gelfoam sponge: a plate of Gelfoam sponge (GS) (5.5 × 2 cm) is compressed and made thin using the hands. It is cut by scissors into 0.5 mm wide strips which are then cut across in 0.5 mm widths to yield small 0.5 × 0.5 mm particles. Manipulation of these particles is easier if they are placed in saline in a Petri dish. (b) Gelfoam powder: since the particle size is very small, it is used mainly for PTPE.

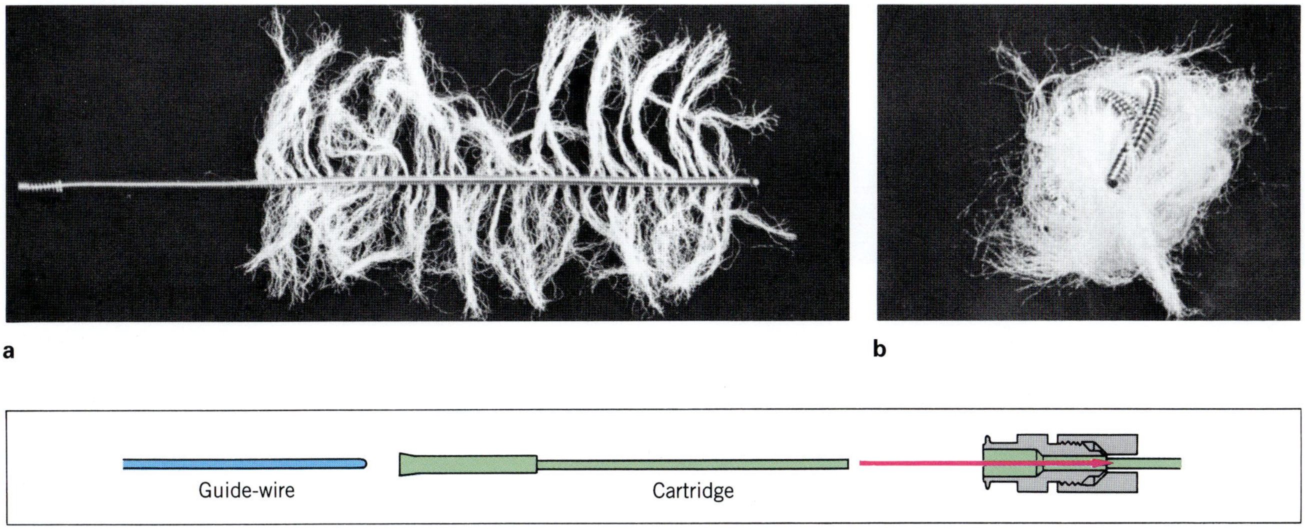

Fig. 14.23 Stainless steel coil. The front part of the coil (guide-wire without a core) has many pieces of cotton wool sewed in (a), and it is normally placed inside the cartridge (c). When pushed out of the cartridge, it rolls up to turn into a woollen ball (b). Using a straight soft guide-wire of a caliber that fits the cartridge, the steel coil in the cartridge is pushed into the catheter, and placed in the targeted vessel at the aimed site.

Fig. 14.24 Hemostasis of GI bleeding with a steel coil. Celiac arteriography (a) demonstrated extravasation of contrast medium (→) near the splenic artery. To identify the exact vessel that was bleeding, common hepatic arteriography was done (b). It showed bleeding from the right gastric artery (▶), but the caliber of this artery was too narrow to be catheterized. Therefore, the arteries around the right gastric, namely the right hepatic and common hepatic arteries, were embolized with three steel coils (▷). Extravasation was no longer seen on repeat celiac arteriography (c).

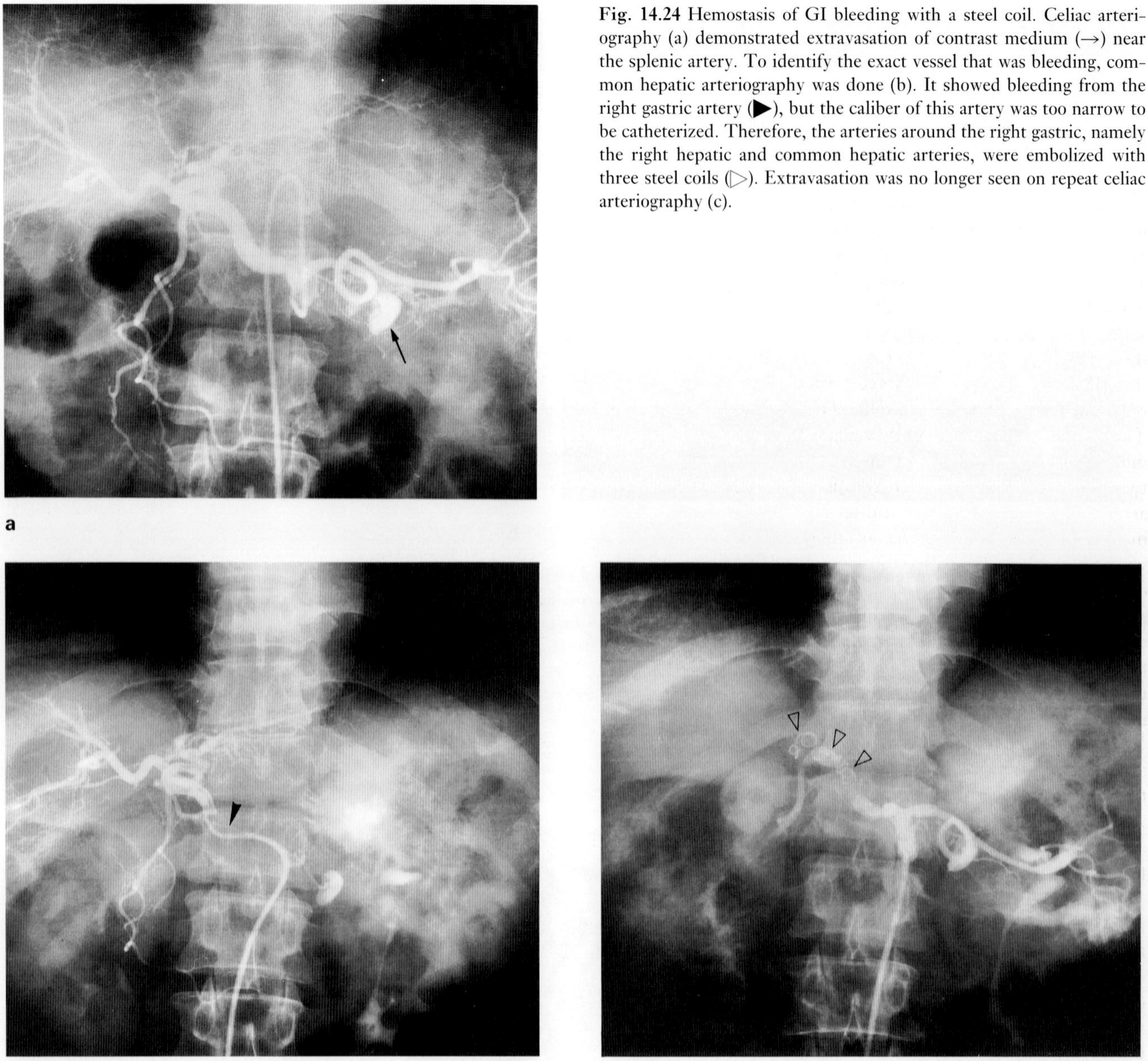

a

b

c

15

Ultrasonography

The origin of medical ultrasonography (US) is traced back to underwater US devices for military purposes. Attempts were made in the early 1950s to utilize reflecting ultrasound to detect gross abnormalities in the body. When a pulse of high frequency sound waves is transmitted into the body, reflections of sound occur at tissue interfaces as the wave front advances, and the returning echoes can be recorded by the same transducer that generated the sonic wave. The reflected echoes are recorded on a cathode-ray oscilloscope (A-mode) for analysis. The A-mode was subsequently replaced by the B (brightness)-mode by the introduction of intensity modulation linked to a two-dimensional display with the use of mechanical scanning arm. Using a potentiometer and an X–Y axis position-sensing mechanism, the point source of the echo can be displayed within several millimeters on a plane. As the transducer moves over the skin surface, a B-scan image forms (contact compound scan). This was used mainly in obstetrics and cardiology. Gray scale signal processing was introduced around 1974. The display was on a bistable scope in black and white; the gray scale display provides information about tissue texture because of the many shades of gray in the image (Goldberg 1977; Taylor 1978). The transducer was also improved thereafter. The sector scan in which an arch-like movement of the probe gives a real-time effect, was followed by the development of the linear array transducer in which the probe contains 12–240 small oscillators arranged linearly in parallel; they are activated electronically through an electronic switch which activates a group of successive oscillators at a time while activation continuously shifts to produce a linear ultrasound beam. It is combined with other mechanisms to produce electronic focusing and small-angle deflection for the improvement of the image and resolution (Weill 1978). The most important feature of this system is a real-time effect of the image, because a frame rate of 30 frames per second provides a continuous dynamic image on the screen (Ferrucci 1979). By changing the direction of one beam, tubular structures, such as bile ducts and blood vessels, are readily identified and followed in either direction. A large area of the body or organ can be quickly screened by changing the touch angle of the linear probe, or sliding it on the skin. The operator can construct a three-dimensional visual impression (Okuda 1981).

Various types of transducer are now available, but the convex probe is most useful. It permits study of most of the immediate subphrenic area of the right lobe which was called earlier the dead-angle, reducing the frequency of false negative results. As with CT, US has axial and lateral resolutions. The former is the capability of recognizing two points separately along the beam axis, and the latter two points separately along the axis perpendicular to the beam. The axial resolution has been improved with electronic focusing along the long axis and with an acoustic (silicone) lens along the short axis. The lateral resolution can be improved by increasing the beam frequency and shortening the wavelength. However, this will weaken the ultrasonic beam, and is only applicable to organs on or near the surface (thyroid, breast), and intraoperative US (8–10 MHz). The currently used transducers have an axial resolution of about 1 mm and a lateral resolution of about 2 mm.

Thickness of US images

In the US image, as with CT, the two-dimensional image contains three-dimensional information, because it has a certain thickness (slice thickness). This slice thickness is not uniform, but varys with the effect of the acoustic lens attached to the surface of the probe. Namely, when the beam width is narrowed, the lateral resolution is sacrificed, and two different structures may be superimposed and appear to be in the same slice. Because of this phenomenon, the duodenum may mimic a tumor in the gallbladder, and the needle tip inserted under US guidance may appear as if it were in a blood vessel. A similar phenomenon also occurs with other slice imaging techniques such as CT and MR imaging.

Phenomena characteristically associated with US

Ultrasound has a property similar to light within a certain range of wavelength, and is reflected by an object like the diaphgram that strongly reflects the US beam, producing a miror phenomenon (Fig. 15.1). If the beam hits an object perpendicularly, the beam traverses back and forth between the probe surface and the object, and produces the multiple-reflection phenomenon. A typical case is an artefact layer within the gallbladder (Fig. 15.2). The comet sign or comet tail artefact, in which an intramural stone and adenomyomatosis produce an echogenic tail, is a diagnostically useful artefact (Fig. 15.3)

The ultrasound beam has a directivity that is determined by its strength and wavelength. If the directivity is measured in front of the transducer, it shows besides the main lobe perpendicular to the transducer surface, two small side lobes at angles to the main axis. If a strong beam reflector exists in the direction of a side lobe, it produces an artefactual image seen in the same slice, called the 'side lobe' (Fig. 15.4).

An ultrasound beam cannot penetrate air, gas (bowel), stone, or calcification (in tumor), and produces an anechoic zone behind. This phenomenon is called 'acoustic shadow or shadowing' (Fig. 15.5). Although this interferes with the study of structures within the shadow, it is a useful diagnostic sign that assists in differentiating between a polyp and a stone. The beam enters the sides of a round structure such as liver cancer at an oblique angle, and an anechoic line or band is produced behind it (lateral shadow) (Fig. 15.6). This phenomenon is particularly distinct in the presence of a fibrous capsule because of the large difference in the speed of penetration of the beam in tissue. In contrast to an acoustic shadow, the beam is not much attenuated when penetrating a cyst or a tumor with a liquefied interior, and the echoes in the area behind it are enhanced and exaggerated (posterior echo enhancement). This phenomenon may prove diagnostic in the differential diagnosis of a small cyst and a small hypoechoic solid mass (Fig. 15.7).

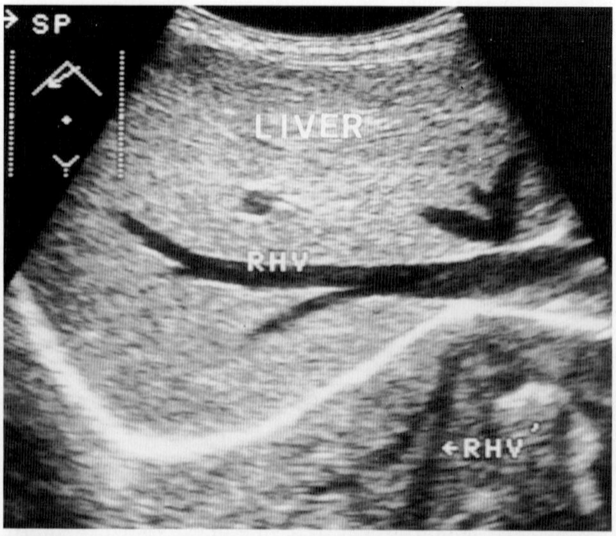

Fig. 15.1 Artefact due to the mirror phenomenon. The diaphragm is acting as a mirror, and a pseudo image (RHV') of the right hepatic vein (RHV) is seen behind the diaphragm in a symmetrical position.

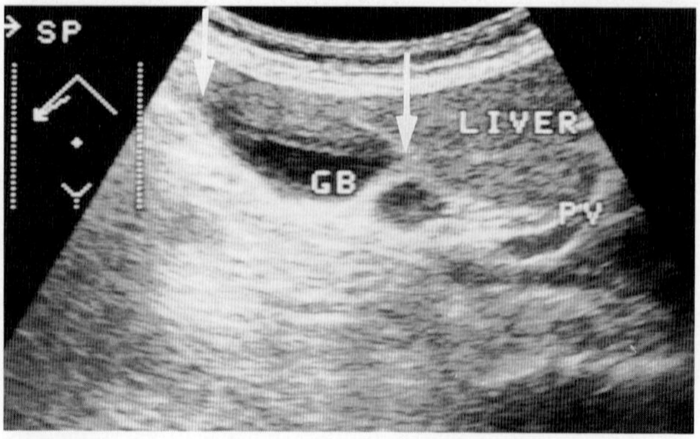

Fig. 15.2 Artefact due to multiple reflections occurring between the transducer and reflecting object. The ultrasonic beam generated from the transducer in contact with the body surface hits the liver surface perpendicularly, and is reflected back to the transducer repeatedly. This phenomenon produces a linear pseudo image (between → and →) at a site in a distance between the transducer and object, multiplied by an integer. The pseudo image will disappear with a posture change and respiratory movement. GB, gallbladder.

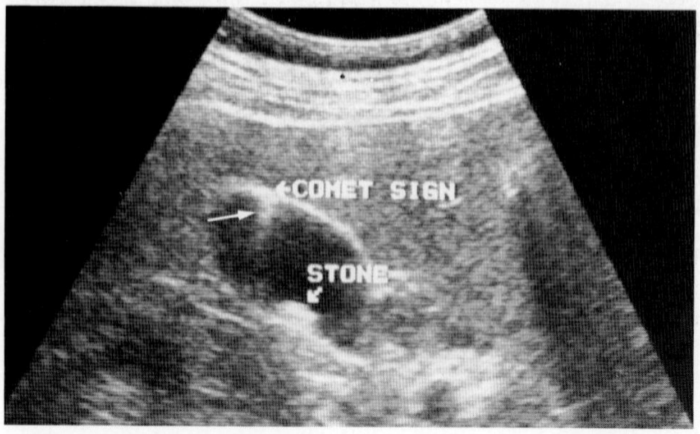

Fig. 15.3 The comet sign produced by a stone within the gallbladder wall. This stone in the gallbladder wall produced a so-called comet sign or comet tail echo (→), which is thought to be a type of artefact related to multiple reflections.

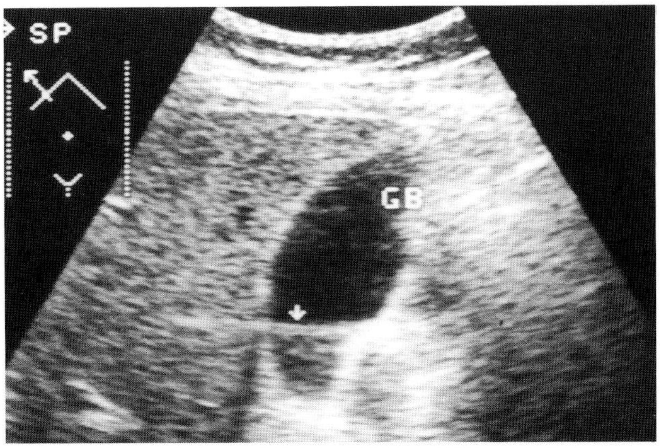

Fig. 15.4 Artefact due to a side lobe. Due to a side lobe produced by the transducer, a horizontal line (→) that does not exist is seen crossing the gallbladder and liver parenchyma as an artefact.

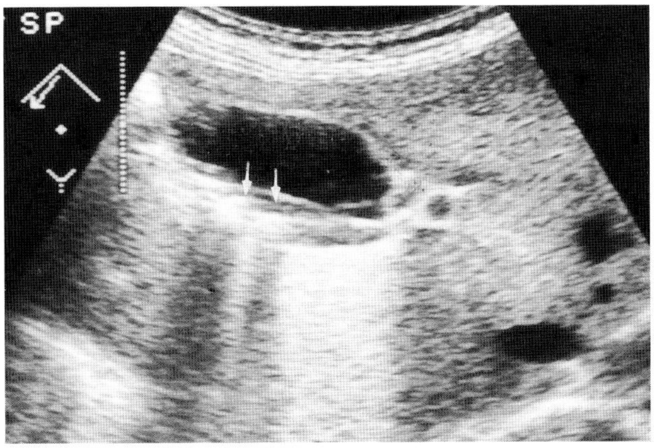

Fig. 15.5 Acoustic shadow resulting from gallbladder stones. Two stones (→) in the gallbladder produce two bands of acoustic shadow behind. This is an important feature that assists in differentiation from polyp.

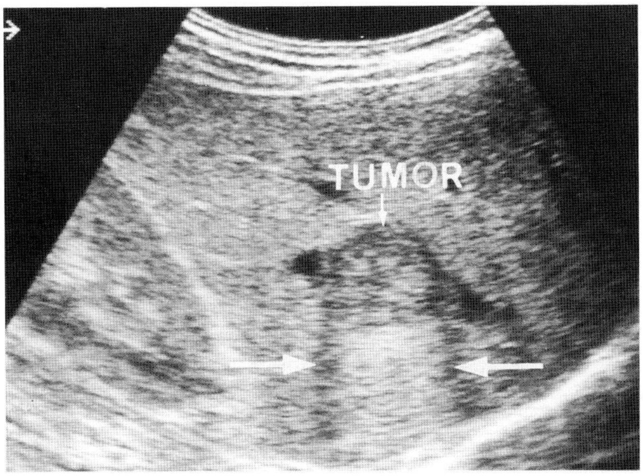

Fig. 15.6 Lateral shadows produced at the sides of a global object. A linear acoustic shadow (→) is seen running posteriorly in both sides of this HCC with a fibrous capsule.

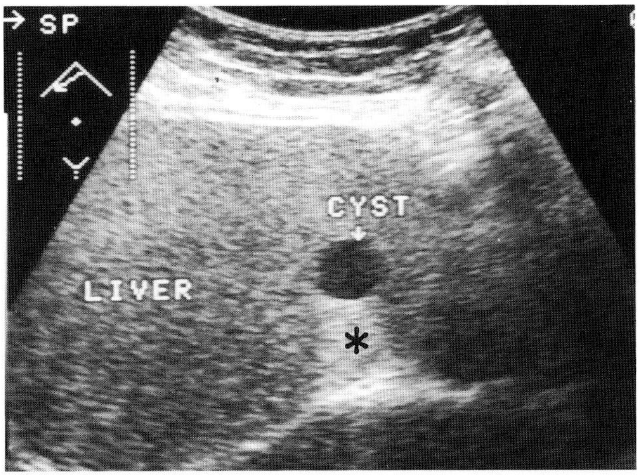

Fig. 15.7 Posterior echo enhancement produced by a simple cyst. A band-shaped hyperechoic zone is seen posterior to this cyst (*, posterior echo enhancement). This finding is important in the differential diagnosis of a small cyst and a small solid mass.

16

Magnetic resonance imaging (MRI)

16.1 Historical background and principle

In 1946 Block and Purcell independently reported their observations on nuclear magnetic resonance (NMR) for which they received the Nobel Prize. The potential of NMR to obtain images of the human body was suggested from an NMR image of a water-filled capillary in the early 1970s, and the first image of a human finger was reported in 1976. Certain atomic nuclei that have unpaired protons or neutrons possess an intrinsic spin, generating a small magnetic field, analogous to a microscopic bar magnet. The most abundant of the naturally occurring spinning nuclei in the body is the hydrogen nucleus or proton. Other nuclei that possess spin but are much less abundant include ^{23}Na, ^{31}P, and ^{13}C. If such randomly oriented spinning nuclei are placed within a static magnetic field, they align with the lines of force of the field. The spinning protons, for instance, wobble (precess) about the axis of the main magnetic field at a rate given by the Larmor frequency. These two motions of the proton are analogous to the movement of a child's spinning top. The precessional motion is slow relative to the faster spinning motion. Some of the protons line up parallel (in keeping with a lower energy level) and other antiparallel (higher energy level) to the magnetic field. There is only a small excess of protons in the lower energy state to produce a net magnetization in line with the field; it is upon this small excess that the potential NMR signal depends.

When a radiofrequency (RF) field is applied at the same frequency as the precessing nuclei and at right angles to the main magnetic field, it excites or 'flips' the small excess of protons in the lower energy level into a higher energy state. Energy is absorbed during this transition as the protons in the lower energy level move into a higher energy state. The energy absorbed during this transition is subsequently released as electromagnetic waves to the environment as the protons relax back to their lower energy state and equilibrium (resonance phenomenon). This release of energy can be recorded as an electrical signal. The relaxation of the protons back to equilibrium and the lower energy state is termed spin-lattice relaxation or longitudial relaxation. It is an exponential decay process and has a time constant referred to as 'T1'. Immediately after the RF pulse is applied the excited protons precess together, in synchronism or in phase with each other, at the resonant frequency. During relaxation, however, they quickly get out of phase due to small variations in local magnetic fields. This loss of phase is termed spin-spin relaxation or transverse relaxation. It is also an exponential and possesses the time constant 'T2'.

Magnetic resonance systems for clinical use include the magnet, radiofrequency (RF) coils, gradient coils, computer, display unit, and digital storage facilities. There are currently three main types of magnet used in MR imaging: permanent magnet, resistive magnet, and superconducting magnet. Each has its merits and demerits, but the details shall not be discussed here. While the first two types of magnet can generate a maximum magnetic field of 1.0 to 0.3 Tesla (T)—T equals 10 kilogauss—the superconducting magnet produces a much higher field strength of 1.5 to 2 T, perhaps the upper limit for body imaging. Such homogeneous high field strength permits the production of high quality images and has enabled MR spectroscopy. Although the magnet field is stable with the superconducting magnet, it requires liquid helium and nitrogen to keep the electric resistance to near zero (4° K).

There are two broad categories of RF coils used in imaging which may be likened to radio antennas. The volume coil, which is most commonly used, completely surrounds the part of the body being imaged, and receives the same amount of signal from deep and superficial tissues. For abdominal scanning, a 50 cm body coil is usually used. A second type is a surface coil. It is used to obtain high-resolution images of relatively superficial body structures. The gradient system is used to generate small magnetic fields that are added to the main field to select slices and to encode position in the images. It consists of a set of three gradient coils, one for each dimension or axis, that are resistive electromagnets capable of being switched on and off and varied rapidly and precisely. It thus permits slices of tissue in transverse, coronal, or sagittal planes.

As the transmitted RF pulse and the MR signal take place at different times, the coil can act as both transmitter and receiver. The strength of radio wave or degree of whiteness or blackness (signal intensity) depends on four tissue factors, namely proton density, flow, T1 and T2 relaxation values as well as on pulse repetition time (TR), echo delay time (TE) and inversion time (TI) which are imaging parameters and are controlled by the operator. Proton density is the number of resonating hydrogen nuclei present in a particular volume of tissue following application of an RF pulse. In tissue, the concentration of such protons is related primarily to water content and secondarily to lipid content. Since signal intensity is directly proportional to proton density, gas and cortical bone demonstrate extremely low signal intensity (appearing black).

Flow is a function of the speed at which hydrogen nuclei move through the region being imaged, and the percentage of protons in the region that are moving. Flowing blood can appear black, white or any shade of gray depending on various factors. The relationship of these four factors to signal intensity may be simply described as:

Signal intensity	Proton density	T1	T2	Blood flow
High (white)	High	Short	Long	Stationary, slow
Low (black)	Low	Long	Short	Turbulent, fast

16.2 Pulse sequences and fast imaging techniques

The conventional RF pulse sequences used in imaging are total or partial saturation recovery (SR), inversion recovery (IR), and spin echo (SE). These sequences give different weighting in the received signal to proton density, T1, and T2; SR gives a similar weight to these three parameters, while IR emphasizes T1. These sequences have their own advantages and disadvantages with regard to scanning time, information on tissue (water and lipid), chemical shift effects, etc. Because of the limited space in this book, and the rapidly progressing instrumentation and techniques, these aspects cannot fully be covered, and readers are referred to recent textbooks on MR imaging.

For some time after the advent of MR imaging a major drawback of this modality was the long scanning time required, but with subsequent progress, various fast imaging techniques have become available, particularly after the introduction of the shielded gradient coil and digitization of RF. Of particular note is the development of the fast low-angle shot (FLASH) technique by Haase *et al.* in 1986 in which gradient echo is combined with a low flip angle. A scanning time of the order of a few seconds now permits use of contrast medium for dynamic studies, as with dynamic CT. The conventional SE depends on a rather slow pulse repetition time and echo delay time, but the new fast scanning techniques use different physical conditions. Various modifications of FLASH have since been developed, such as spoiled FLASH, refocused FLASH, fast imaging with steady-state free precession (FISH), the contrast enhanced Fourier-acquired steady-state technique (CE FAST), and turbo FLASH. Other new fast scanning techniques include fast SE, echo planar imaging (EPI), magnetization prepared rapid gradient echo (MP RAGE), etc.

In the past, the vasculature of the liver and other organs could only be delineated by angiography, but with the improvement of MR imaging, vasculature can now be studied non-invasively and without contrast medium by MR imaging. It is very useful for the study of portal-systemic shunts in portal hypertension. For MR angiography (MRA), several techniques are available, such as the time-of-flight (TOF) method that utilizes the inflow effect (Sevic *et al.* 1991; Miki *et al.* 1991) and the phase contrast (PC) method (Dumoulin and Hart 1986). Both can be either two dimensional (2D) or three dimensional (3D). 2D TOF is suited for the delineation of slow flow and 3D TOF for high flow, and for the portal systemic collateral study, the former is most suitable. NMR can also be applied to the measurement of flow speed, such as portal venous flow speed. For that purpose, the direct bolus tracking method is used in which a plane perpendicular to the blood vessel is excited with the gradient magnetic field Gz. The subsequent Gz generates a gradient echo after an interval of TE. The flow speed is calculated from the distance of fluid displacement (Shimizu *et al.* 1986), and this technique, called direct bolus imaging (DBI), has been utilized for the measurement of portal venous flow velocity (Tamada *et al.* 1989). The other technique, called the presaturation method, is primarily for measuring rapid blood flow, but it may be used to delineate the two venous systems in the liver, portal, and hepatic veins in one image. Very slow flows such as spinal fluid can now be turned into images, and so can bile flow. MR cholangiography has been developed by Wallner *et al.* (1992) and Morimoto et al (1991) using 2D and 3D fast imaging with a flow sensitive gradient-echo pulse sequence CE-FAST. This method is totally non-invasive, not requiring contrast medium, and in the future may become the first imaging choice in patients with suspected obstructive jaundice.

16.3 Contrast medium for MR imaging

Unlike the contrast medium in conventional radiography in which the contrast is produced by differences in X-ray absorption, contrast medium in MR imaging exerts its effect by shortening the relaxation time for protons that surround the molecule of the contrast agent. Only paramagnetic substances (magnetized parallel to the field when placed in a magnetic field) have such a property. The agents that shorten T1 relaxation time are called negative contrast agents. As a positive contrast agent, gadolinium (Gd) in various chemical forms is most commonly used, and for negative contrast, ferric iron (Fe 3+) which is superparamagnetic, is frequently used. Depending on its chemical form and purpose, some are used intravenously and others orally. Colloid preparations given intravenously, such as ferric iron colloid (Ferrite), are taken up by the Kupffer cells, turning liver parenchyma to lower intensity, and mass lesions will have increased contrast.

The currently available contrast media for hepatic MR imaging include Gd-diethylenetriamine pentaacetate, a chelate of Gd (Gd-DTPA), iron oxide Fe_3O_4 (SPIO, Ferrite), manganese (II) *N*, *N'*-dipyridoxylethylene diamine-*N*, *N'*-diacetate 5, 5'-bis (phosphanate) (Mn-DPDP), etc. Some are not yet widely available at the time of writing. Each agent has its own characteristics in the way of tissue uptake, distribution, and speed of excretion. The degree of ionization of the compound is also related to the degree of toxicity.

Gd-DTPA is non-specifically distributed in the interstitial space of cancerous and non-cancerous tissues (Carr *et al.* 1984; Weinmann *et al.* 1984; Ohtomo *et al.* 1987). Imaging of the liver is based on exploitation of differences in blood flow between the two tissues, namely hepatocellular carcinoma is usually more hypervascular than non-cancerous portion in the arterial dominant phase of dynamic MR imaging. Therefore, bolus injection of contrast medium and dynamic imaging are indispensable. The hemodynamics of Gd-DTPA after the administration into the blood vessel is very similar to that of the ionic contrast medium used in dynamic CT.

SPIO (Saini *et al.* 1987; Ferrucci and Stark 1990) is cleared from circulation by the reticulendothelial system, especially Kupffer cells in the non-tumorous hepatic parenchyma, which appears as an area of low signal intensity (negative enhancement). In contrast, malignant liver tumors do not have Kupffer cells, and therefore the tumor is demonstrated as a mass of relatively high signal intensity. Sixty minutes after the injection of SPIO, MR imaging is made, and T2-weighted images are found to be superior to unenhanced T2-weighted images in the detection of focal hepatic lesions (Winter *et al.* 1993). Chondroitin sulfate iron colloid is also used for the same purpose as SPIO, but in a limited number of cases (Kato *et al.* 1993), because of a high rate of adverse reactions; this agent has not yet been put to wide clinical use.

Mn-DPDP is a paramagnetic agent primarily taken up by hepatocytes and eliminated with the bile (Elizondo *et al.* 1991), and is composed of a chelate of pyridoxal-5′-phosphate, the active coenzyme form of vitamin B_6. It is assumed that the transport of Mn-DPDP into hepatocytes occurs through the following four steps: receptor, sinusoid, hepatocyte, and cytoplasmic transport (Chilton and Brown 1990). Shortening of T1 relaxation is its predominant paramagnetic effect, and therefore liver parenchyma appears significantly increased in signal intensity on T1-weighted images (positive enhancement). The number of non-enhanced malignant liver lesions was reported to increase in T1-weighted Mn-DPDP enhanced SE images more than in T2-weighted images. There was no uptake of this agent by metastases, cyst, or hemangioma. In contrast, the uptake of Mn-DPDP by normal hepatocytes explains the increase of signal intensity in focal nodular hyperplasia and regenerative nodules as well as HCC cells that are functionally similar to hepatocytes (Hamm *et al.* 1992).

Other paramagnetic contrast agents recently introduced for MR imaging include Gd (4s)-4-(4-ethoxybenzyl)-3,6,9-tris (carboxylatomethy) 3,6,9-triazaundecandioic acid disodium salt (Gd-EOB-DTPA) introduced as Gd-DTPA convalently linked to the lipophilic ethoxybenzyl moiety that exhibits high hepatobiliary specificity combined with high T1 relaxivity (Schumann-Giampieri *et al.* 1992). Liver metastases in a rodent model were demonstrated as lesions of relatively low signal intensity in the signal increased liver parenchyma (positive enhancement) by the spin echo technique (Muhler *et al.* 1992). This agent shows dual elimination, 75 per cent being excreted through the liver and bile and 25 per cent through the kidney.

17

Needle biopsy

In the past, needle biopsy was done blindly or under X-ray control. Recently, it has become possible to biopsy or puncture a mass or an area of interest under the control of US (Ohto *et al.* 1980; Holm and Kristensen 1985) and CT. Although needle biopsy is very diagnostic, it is not without problems. The tissue obtained by biopsy may not contain cancer cells in patients with neoplasms, but cancer cannot be ruled out because it could have been missed (risk of false negative). The same problem applies to hemangioma when a thin needle is used; if only blood is suctioned, a definitive diagnosis cannot be made (Fig. 17.1). A thick needle is more diagnostic (Fig. 17.2), but it entails the risk of bleeding in hemangioma (Takayasu and Uesaka 1987*d*).

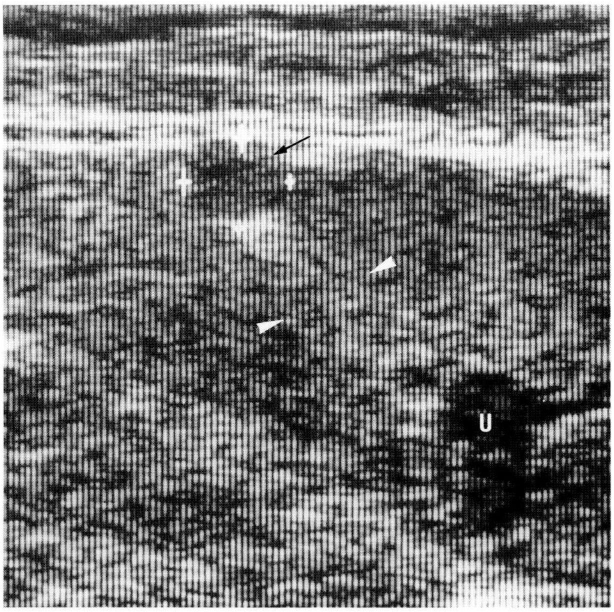

Fig. 17.1 Only blood was withdrawn by suction biopsy using a 21G needle. During the follow-up of this patient with cirrhosis, a 1.3 cm hypoechoic lesion (→) was found immediately beneath the capsule caudal to the umbilical portion (U) of the left portal vein. An HCC was strongly suspected. Enhanced CT failed to provide diagnostic information, and suction biopsy with a 21G needle was carried out under US guidance through non-tumoros parenchyma. Only blood was withdrawn. After return to the ward, her blood pressure slowly came down, and emergency laparotomy was carried out with a suspicion of abdominal hemorrhage. Bleeding was from an enlarged paraumbilical vein on the liver surface, and hemostasis was achieved by ligation of this vein. In retrospect, there was a high-echo band (▶) connecting the mass in question and the umbilical portion. No communication between the umbilical portion and the paraumbilical vein was recognized (Takayasu and Uesaka 1987*d*).

Another problem is complications associated with the procedure. Needle tract seeding is a serious one, although this is an uncommon event (Sakurai *et al.* 1983; Cedrone *et al.* 1992; Goletti *et al.* 1992). The incidence is somewhat correlated with the caliber of the needle. Bleeding into the free abdominal cavity and formation of an arterio portal shunt (Okuda *et al.* 1978) are other problems.

Tissue diagnosis is most important in patients who have a diffuse liver disease, but for those with a localized lesion such as a suspected neoplasm, the diagnostic strategy may differ. At the National Cancer Center Hospital, Tokyo, we have adopted the following guidelines. Needle biopsy is not required in a patient who is scheduled for an operation and in whom imaging study has been adequate. More effort should be made to make the diagnosis as accurate as possible by collective imaging diagnosis that includes arterial- and portal-CT. In patients with an advanced and inoperable cancer, biopsy may become necessary before giving chemotherapy.

In recent years, intraoperative needle biopsy has come to be done frequently because intraoperative US is more sensitive than preoperative imaging for small lesions (cf. Table 4.6, p.107), and nodular borderline lesions (benign regenerative nodule, dysplastic nodule, and early HCC) that require differential diagnosis are frequently found during an operation. Even intraoperative US cannot differentiate them. Intraoperative biopsy and quick diagnosis based on frozen sections are necessary to decide whether a newly found lesion should be or need not be resected. If the diagnosis was 'malignant', that nodule

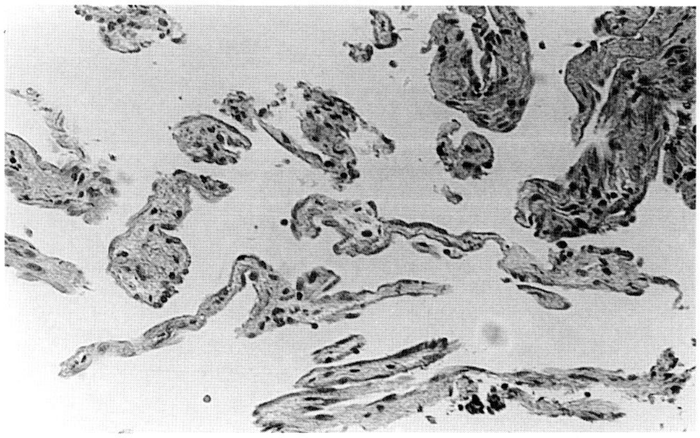

Fig. 17.2 Hemangioma diagnosed by biopsy using a 19G Tru Cut needle. Suction biopsy was done using a 22G needle for a mass that was not stained by angiography, and only blood came out. Therefore, biopsy was repeated with a 19G Tru Cut needle. The biopsy specimen was that of hemangioma demonstrating vascular endothelium, and the operation was called off.

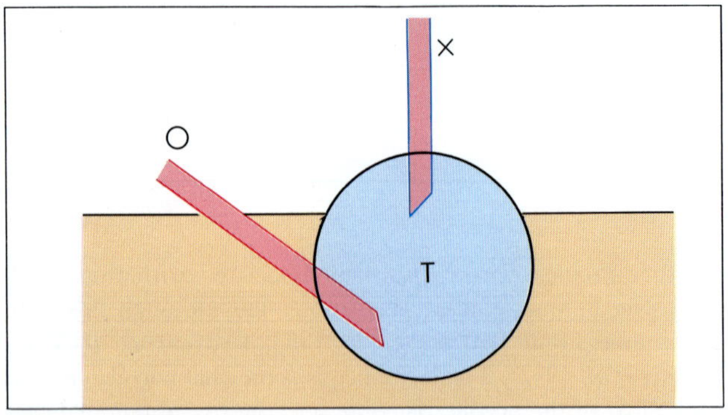

Fig. 17.3 Needle biopsy for a mass protruding from the liver surface. If the mass is punctured directly from the tumor surface (X), it may bleed and spread cancer cells over the peritoneum. It is safer to puncture it at an angle through non-tumoros parenchyma (O). T, tumor.

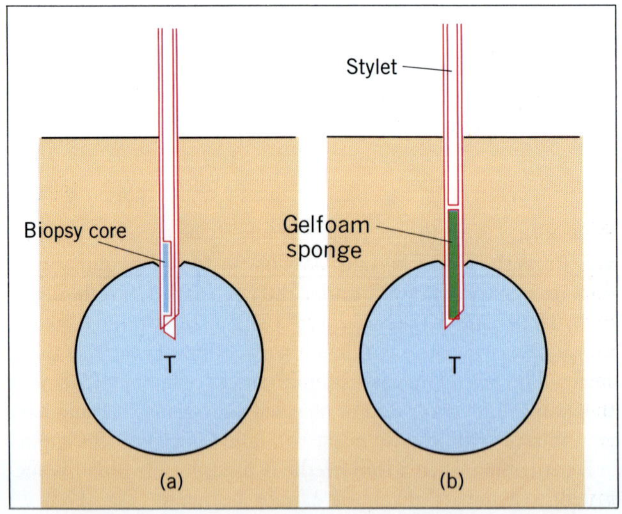

Fig. 17.4 Hemostasis after biopsy with a Tru Cut needle. After a tissue core (T) has been cut with a 19G Tru Cut needle, the inner needle alone is withdrawn for confirmation of the success of the procedure (a), and then a Gelfoam twist is pushed into the outer needle using a stylet as done for hemostasis after PTP (b).

including the needle tract is resected. For intraoperative biopsy, our surgeons use a thick (14G) Tru Cut needle.

Technique

In Japan, where US is very widely used by gastroenterologists/hepatologists, US is used for guiding the needle. In the USA, CT is more commonly used for aiming. CT has an advantage over US in a very fat patient, and for an adrenal tumor. Relatively thin 21–23G needles are usually used.

Local anesthesia and the puncture technique are the same as for PTP and PTC. If the mass to be aimed at is deep seated, more than 2 cm from the liver surface, it is possible to puncture it perpendicularly from the liver surface, but if the tumor is protruding from the surface, it should be punctured at an angle so that the needle goes through non-tumorous parenchyma before reaching the target (Fig. 17.3). In this situation, the respiratory movements bend the needle, and a flexible thin needle is safer. The amount of tissue obtained by a flexible needle may not be sufficient, and therefore we sometimes use a thicker 19G Tru Cut needle. When a thick needle is used, it is safe to do the hemostatic procedure after tissue acquisition using a Gelfoam sponge as done after PTP (Fig. 17.4).

18

Reappraisal of imaging diagnosis using resected specimens

Postoperative reappraisal of preoperative imaging diagnosis is very important. Not only can one compare the preoperative US findings and US images obtained with the specimen immersed in water (Fig. 18.1), but one can also analyze the preoperative imaging features for clarification of some of the questions and ambiguities with reference to the resected specimen. One can thus improve the interpretation of images, and apply the newly gained knowledge and experience to future practice.

One of the commonly used methods for appraisal is soft X-ray of a specimen containing Lipiodol. With soft X-ray, very small (2–3 mm) lesions retaining Lipiodol are often discovered (cf. Case 11, p.475). It can also be used for identification of calcification (Case 13, p.195). Microangiography is another method in which barium is injected into a blood vessel in the specimen (cf. Case 2, p.57; Case 19, p.284).

It has to be realized that the resected liver specimen does not have a blood flow, and one may encounter some unphysiological phenomena. Air enters the vessel systems of the specimen, and when placed in water and studied by US and CT, the image mimics pneumobilia, and the examination is often hampered by the air. On CT examination of an immersed specimen (Fig. 18.2), the necrotic area within the mass is recognizable, but the viable region may not be seen clearly because of the lack of blood flow. By contrast, US of an immersed specimen permits recognition of a nodule-in-nodule, halo, and lateral shadow, and facilitates comparison of preoperative imaging diagnosis and pathology. For the purpose of microangiography, blood vessels at the dissection edge of the specimen ought to have a long excess suture so that subsequent cannulation may be facilitated. A hepatic artery tends to be buried within the liver like a rubber cord after dissection. A 120 per cent (v/w) barium solution mixed with gelatin, with a dye (carmine for red; Berlin blue for blue) if necessary, is injected. A radiograph is made in a direction that corresponds to the preoperative angiogram. Subsequently, the specimen is cut into slices in the same plane as the preoperative CT plane. The slices are re-studied by soft X-ray in comparison with the preoperative angio-CT.

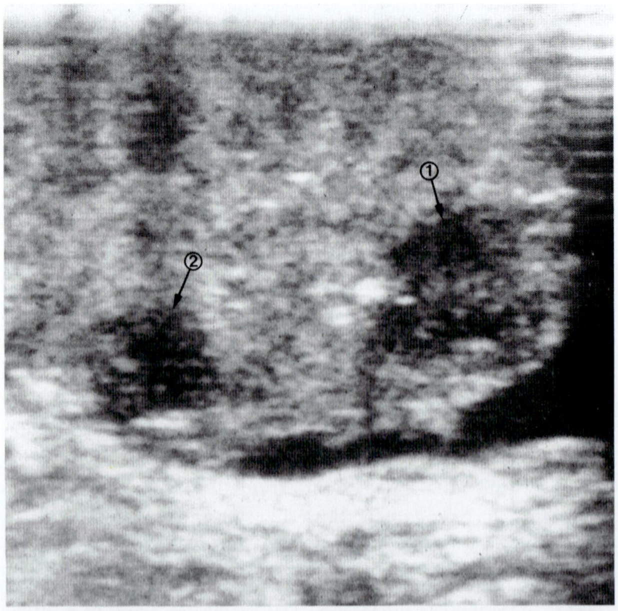

a

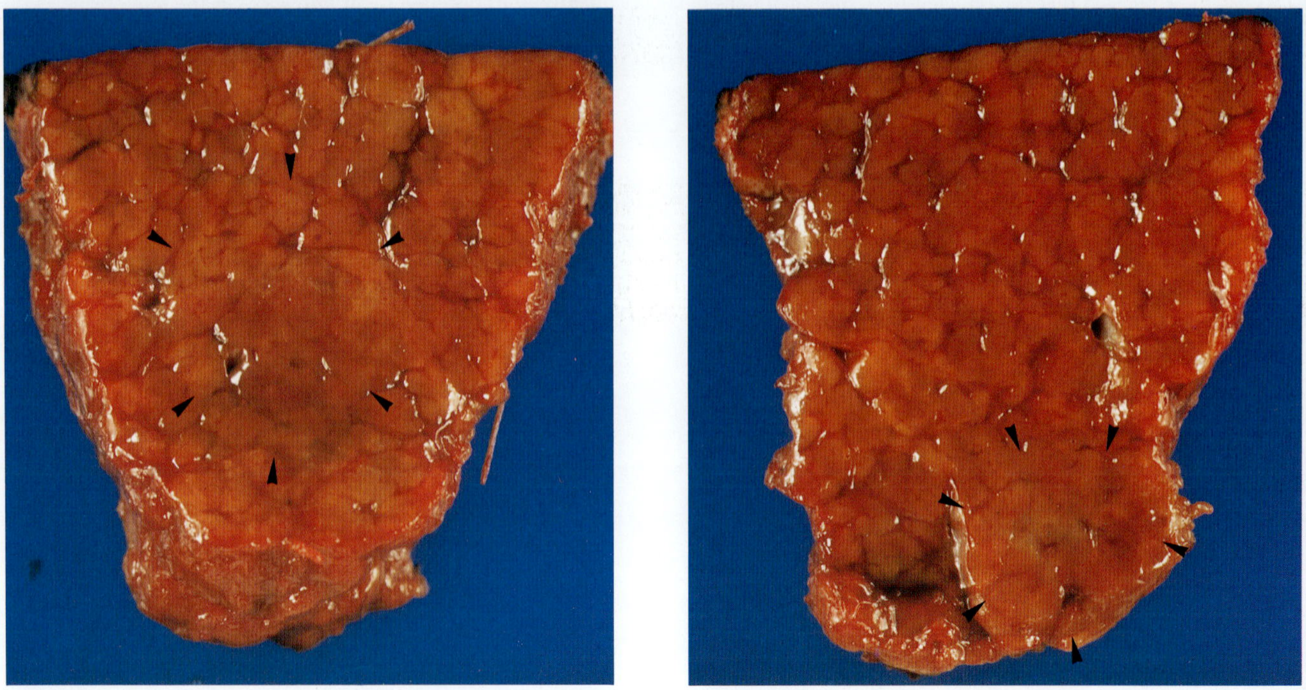

b

c

Fig. 18.1 US image of the resected specimen in water. US of a resected specimen immersed in water (a) demonstrates two low-echo lesions, (1) and (2). On the cut surface of the specimen (b, c), it is difficult to grossly identify these lesions. However, with the knowledge of immersion US, one may be able to identify lesions (1) in (b) (▶, 1.5 cm), and lesion (2) in (c) (▶, 0.7 cm). Histologically, (1) displayed an increased cellularity but no malignant feature, and was diagnosed as atypical adenomatous hyperplasia. The other lesion, (2), was adenomatous hyperplasia.

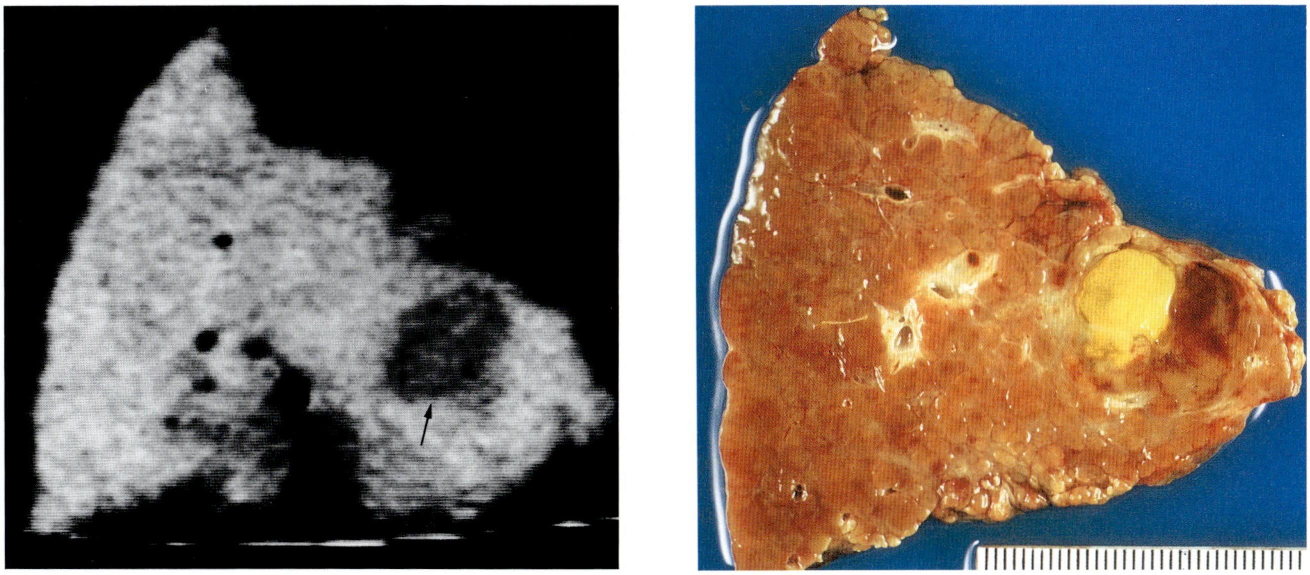

a b

Fig. 18.2 CT image of the resected specimen immersed in water. CT made of the resected specimen immersed in water (a) demonstrates a 1 cm low-density lesion near the dissection margin (→). Vessels in the specimen are seen as air densities. The mass actually measured 2.2 cm, and only the necrotic yellow portion was recognized by CT, leaving the remaining viable region unrecognizable.

III. Therapy

19

Transcatheter arterial embolization (TAE) therapy

19.1 TAE THERAPY

TAE is a technique in which an intraabdominal artery is occluded for the management of GI bleeding (Goldstein *et al.* 1975; Chuang and Wallace 1981) and treatment of malignancies of the kidney and liver (Wallace 1976). It was started based on animal studies (Cho *et al.* 1976) in the USA. Subsequently, it began to be employed for the treatment of inoperable HCC in Japan (Yamada *et al.* 1983*a*) and the results were found to be much better than those obtained with systemic chemotherapy (Okamura *et al.* 1982; Nakamura *et al.* 1984; Takayasu *et al.* 1984*b*; Ohnishi *et al.* 1984*c*; Furui *et al.* 1984). With additional use of Lipiodol (Konno *et al.* 1983; Yumoto *et al.* 1985; Takayasu *et al.* 1987*c*; Nakamura *et al.* 1988), anticancer effects have been enhanced further. It also has some therapeutic benefit on tumor thrombus and intrahepatic metastases. This method has had a considerable impact on the diagnosis and treatment of HCC, and is currently the leading modality among therapeutic techniques for HCC with a wide range of indications. Attempts have also been made to irradiate HCC with radioactive Lipiodol (Kobayashi *et al.* 1986; Park *et al.* 1986). Only about 20 per cent of HCC patients are resectable, and the remaining inoperable cases are currently treated non-surgically (Liver Cancer Study Group of Japan 1990), and TAE is the leading modality, carried out in increasing numbers at our cancer center hospital (Fig. 19.1). Preoperative TAE previously practised is no longer done except for special cases. TAE is also given to patients with recurrence.

Embolizing material, therapeutic efficacy and problems studied with resected specimens

There are currently three methods: (A) Lipiodol alone; (B) Lipiodol + cytotoxic agent (Adriamycin) suspension; (C) Lipiodol + cytotoxic agent and additional injection of Gelfoam (gelatine sponge). These embolizing materials had never been fully evaluated for antitumor effects based on resected specimens. We have compared these three materials for the frequency of complete necrosis (Table 19.1). The results clearly showed that Lipiodol + Adriamycin + Gelfoam had the best anticancer

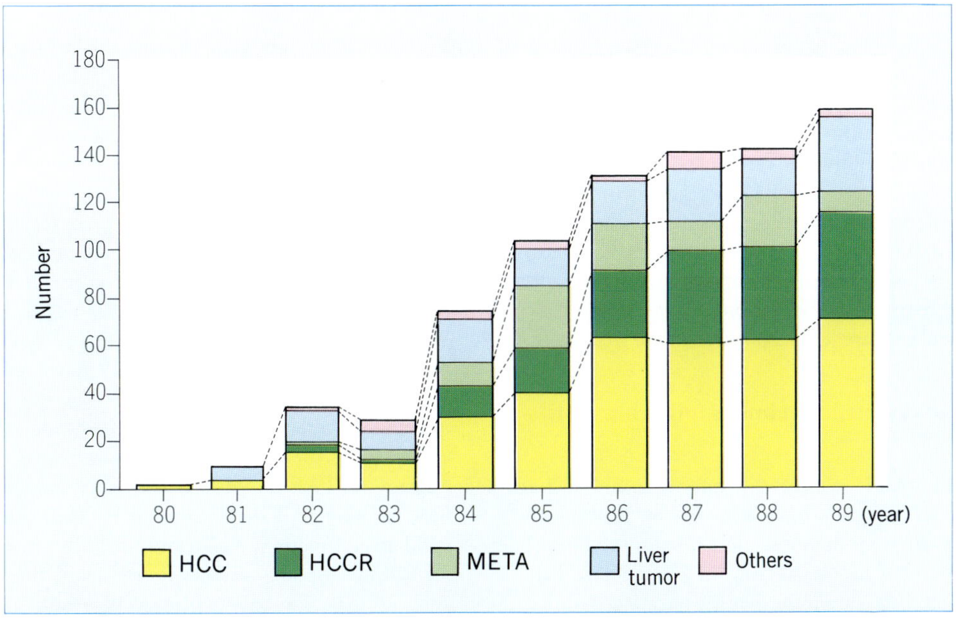

Fig. 19.1 Number of TAE procedures carried out at the National Cancer Center Hospital, Tokyo, in the past 10 years. In the past 10 years, 828 TAE procedures have been carried out; the number greatly increased in the latter 5 years during which 681 (82 per cent) pro-cedures were made. Of the total of 828, 684 were for HCC (yellow) [including 351 inoperable cases and 146 preoperative procedures, 187 for postoperative recurrence (HCCR) (dark green)], 103 for metastatic cancer (META) (light green), and others (liver tumor, blue; others, pink).

Table 19.1 Embolizing material and anticancer effect studied with resected specimens

Group	Embolizing material	Area of necrosis in (%) main mass	Frequency of complete necrosis (%)			Frequency (%) of lesions with more than 80% necrosis	
			Main mass	Daughter mass	Portal tumor thrombus	With fibrous capsule	Outside capsule
A (n = 6)	Lipiodol alone	5 ± 5	0 (0/6)	0 (0/10)	0 (0/1)	0 (0/3)	0 (0/2)
B (n = 15)	Lipiodol + Adriamycin	46 ± 10	13 (2/15)	6 (2/36)	0 (0/11)	0 (0/10)	0 (0/6)
C (n = 10)	Lipiodol + Adriamycin + Gelfoam	91 ± 9	83 (10/12)	53 (10/10)	17 (1/6)	67 (2/3)	0 (0/1)

A total of 33 lesions in 31 cases were analyzed. There was no difference in tumor size between the three groups.

effect (Takayasu *et al.* 1987*c*). Ohnishi et al (1984*c*) used Mitomycin C microcapsules of 225 μm in size, but the results were not compared with Gelfoam embolization.

None of the HCCs treated by Lipiodol alone (A) showed complete necrosis (Case 1), suggesting that its embolization effect is minimal. By contrast, the degree of necrosis varied from zero to 100 per cent with Lipiodol + Adriamycin suspension, only 13 per cent showing complete necrosis (Case 2). In the case of a large HCC, administration of 40 ml of Lipiodol failed to give an anticancer effect (Case 3). Injection of Lipiodol + Adriamycin followd by Gelfoam particles produced considerable necrosis for a large HCC (Case 4). A nearly 100 per cent necrosis was induced to a portal tumor thrombus (Case 5). These results suggest that Lipiodol + Adriamycin is more effective for small HCC, and addition of Gelfoam particles improves the efficacy regardless of tumor size (Fig. 19.2). However, in some patients who were very similar to Case 2, Lipiodol + Adriamycin did not produce necrosis at all, and in these patients a very low susceptibility of cancer cells to Adriamycin was suggested. There is a certain correlation between the gross type of tumor and the therapeutic effect. Namely, better results are usually obtained for a solitary encapsulated HCC whereas the results are much poorer for fused small nodules even with additional Gelfoam particle embolization (Kanai *et al.* 1987). Tumors of low vascularity are less responsive to the treatment.

Soft X-ray study of resected specimens following TAE treatment

In Case 7, a small nodule within the tumor on its section appears viable because it seems to be growing by pushing the capsule. Soft X-ray does not demonstrate Lipiodol retention in this nodule as contrasted by the necrotized areas where Lipiodol retention is seen. It was thought that the encapsulated nodule which did not respond to the treatment grew in an expanding fashion and protruded into the main mass during the period from TAE to resection.

The areas retaining Lipiodol are usually necrotized. Sometimes, Lipiodol is seen in small tumor vessels (Case 2), and as the mass shrinks Lipiodol is condensed. Necrosis occurs with the individual tumor nodule within an incompletely necrotized main mass (Case 8). Lipiodol does not enter a preexisting central necrosis (Case 9). A soft X-ray study sometimes demonstrates the pattern of tumor growth. An example is Case 10, in which the center of the resected mass retained Lipiodol, but the growth around it did not. When grossly studied in the cut section, it was assumed that the outer layer of the mass not retaining Lipiodol was clearly a new concentric expanding growth while the Lipiodol-containing interior did not change in size. When soft X-rayed a resected specimen sometimes reveals 1–2 mm daughter nodules that preoperative imaging and intraoperative US failed to find; histological investigation becomes necessary.

TAE for inoperable HCC patients

In a 10-year period from January 1980 to December 1989, TAE was carried out in 212 inoperable HCC cases and also in 88 cases of postoperative recurrence, totalling 684 procedures in 300 cases. The 1-, 3- and 5-year survival rates were 64.6 per cent, 28.7 per cent and 8.5 per cent, respectively (Fig. 19.3).

TAE in patients who were inoperable from the beginning

The 5-year survival rate in 212 inoperable cases for which TAE was carried out was 10.5 per cent (Fig. 19.4). The correlation between tumor size and survival (n = 69) is shown in Fig. 19.5. With increasing tumor size, the survival rate decreases, and all those with an HCC smaller than 2 cm lived for more than 5 years (Takayasu *et al.* 1989*f*). As the mass enlarges, the frequency of tumor infiltration past the fibrous capsule, intra- and extrahepatic metastases, and vascular invasion increases. The efficacy of TAE is reduced with such tumors, and the results become poor. All these cases of HCC smaller than 2 cm had good liver function, and came to the hospital for surgery, but for various reasons resection could not be done. The results suggest that not only will resection but TAE as well prove efficacious in such patients. Of the prognostic factors analyzed, tumor size was the most important. Complete cure is seldom expected with only one TAE session. In our practice, the majority of patients are followed by a CT study and AFP measurements, and TAE is repeated whenever a recurrence is suspected. Occasionally, tumor regression with a marked reduction of AFP level is experienced (Case 12). Portal tumor thrombosis is thought to be difficult to treat, but Lipiodol-TAE may

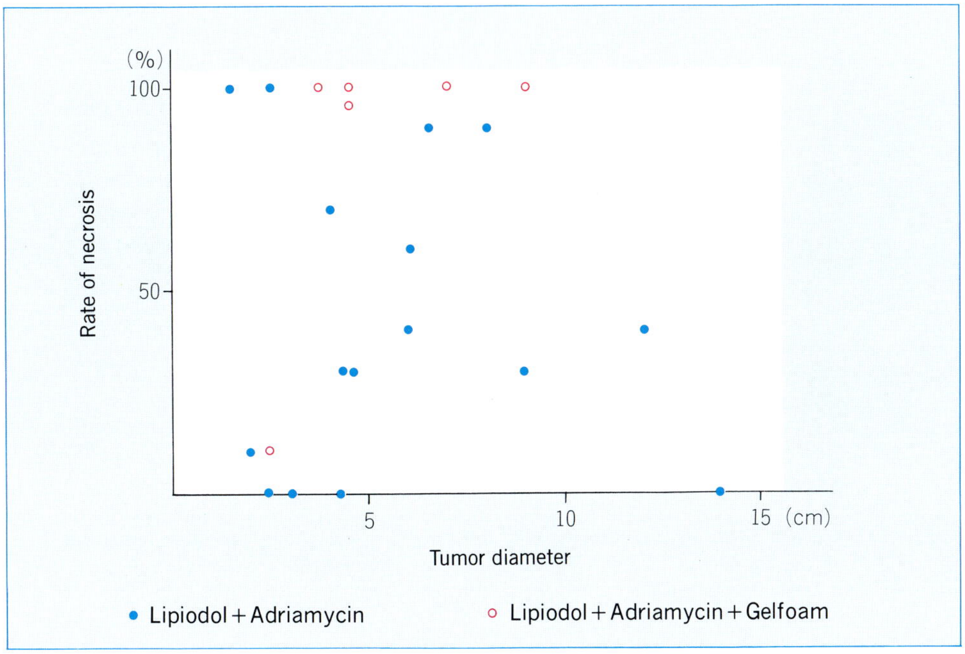

Fig. 19.2 Correlation between the size of the tumor and the rate of necrosis among different embolic materials. Rate of necrosis = area of necrosis in the largest tumor section/tumor area (%).

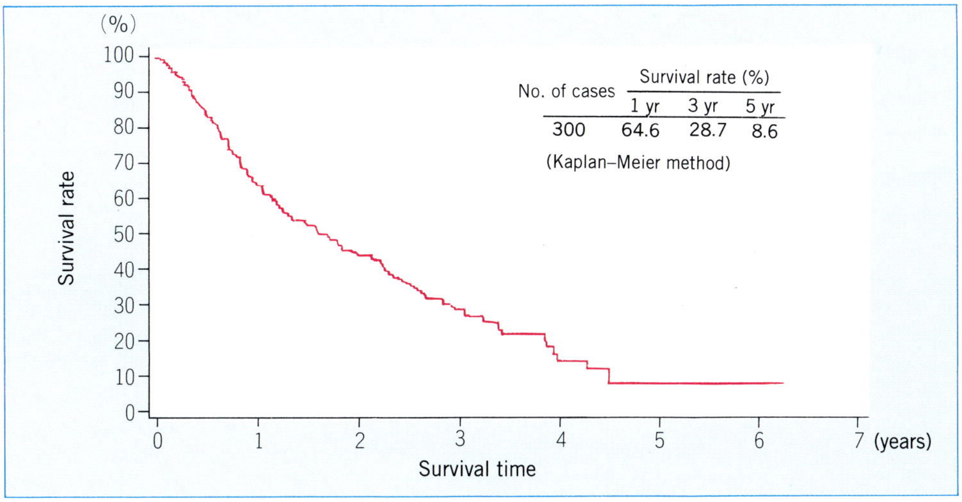

Fig. 19.3 Results of TAE in 300 inoperable cases of HCC (including 88 of postoperative recurrence).

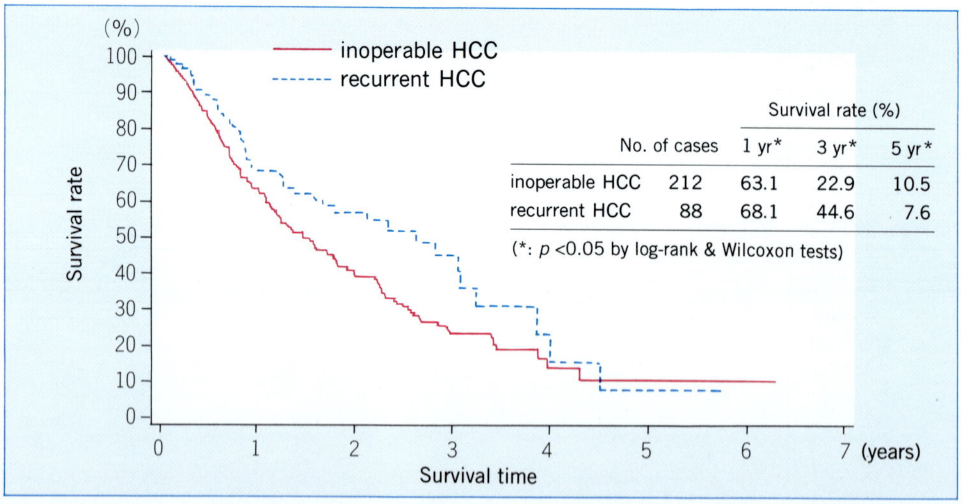

Fig. 19.4 Comparison of TAE effects between inoperable cases ($n = 212$) and postoperative recurrence cases ($n = 88$). With the log-rank and Wilcoxon tests, there were significant differences in 1-, 3-, and 5-year survival rates between the two groups.

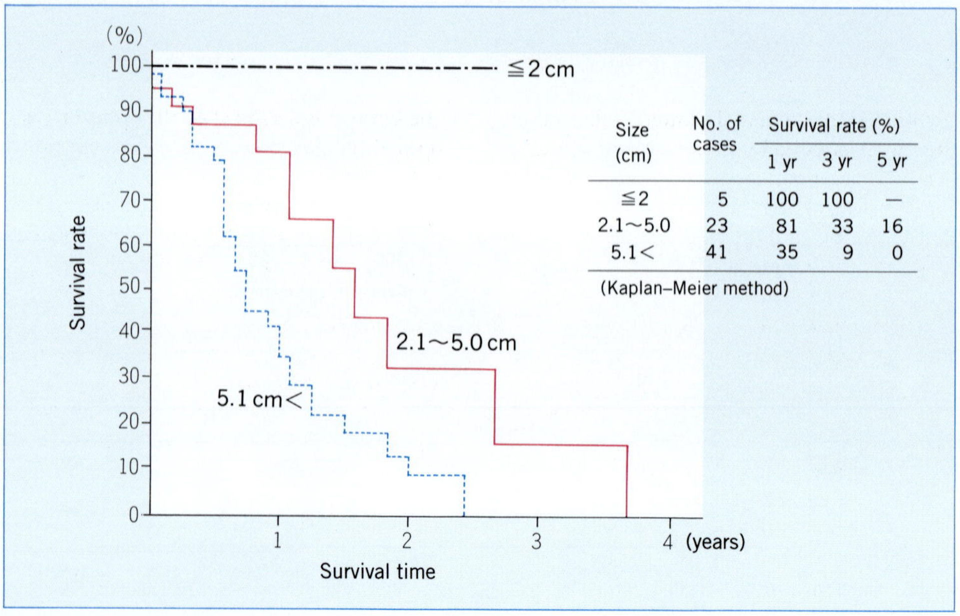

Fig. 19.5 Prognosis and tumor size in inoperable cases following TAE ($n = 69$).

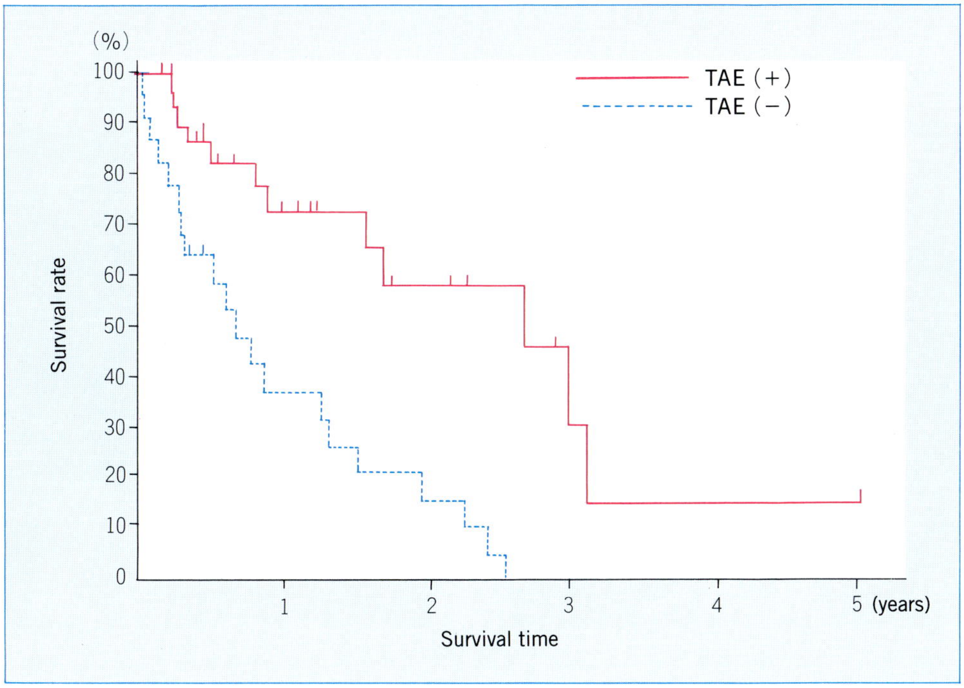

Fig. 19.6 Prognosis of patients with postoperative recurrence treated (n = 32) and not treated (n = 23) by TAE.

induce Lipiodol retention in the tumor thrombus, followed by remarkable improvement as assessed by angiography (Case 13).

Nakamura *et al.* (1988) observed the phenomenon in which Lipiodol injected into the artery entered the portal vein through arterio-portal communications, and developed the technique called segmental TAE in which simultaneous embolization of the feeding artery and the portal vein is carried out by segmental catheterization (Nakamura *et al.* 1990). Matsui *et al.* (1993) reported on subsegmental TAE with a 4-year survival rate of 67 per cent.

TAE for postoperative recurrence

However carefully the preoperative imaging diagnosis and intraoperative US have been carried out, tumor recurrence is almost inevitable after resection. At the National Cancer Center Hospital, Tokyo, 56 per cent of 123 patients who underwent resection for HCC had recurrence in the remnant liver after an average of 14.5 months (Takayasu *et al.* 1989*e*). The diagnosis of recurrence is best achieved with a combination of CT and AFP measurement. TAE proved effective when those treated and not treated by TAE were compared for prognosis (Fig. 19.6). TAE significantly prolonged survival, and the longest survivors were those treated by TAE repeatedly. The patients who underwent resection usually have a functional liver reserve that can tolerate repeated TAE, and therefore additional TAE should not be delayed when it is indicated.

In Case 15, recurrence was detected 1 year after two central segments had been resected. Three courses of TAE that consisted of Gelfoam+Adriamycin were given. The existing hepatic artery was occluded by the procedure, and collaterals developed through the superior mesenteric artery. Considering the risk of sending Gelfoam particles into the superior mesenteric artery, only Lipiodol and Adriamycin were injected for six sessions. The patient is still living 6.5 years after six such TAE sessions and a re-resection for recurrence. In Case 16, tumor thrombosis developed in the portal vein despite repeated TAE for recurrent HCC in the residual liver; it caused deterioration of liver function and made the prognosis very poor. All those who have developed tumor thrombosis in the portal vein (particularly in the right) usually have poor prognosis irrespective of treatment.

Preoperative TAE

Preoperative TAE was carried out in the past with the rationale of reducing tumor viability and minimizing the posibility of intraoperative spread for the prevention of postoperative recurrence. In a retrospective study, Nagasue *et al.* (1989) found no benefit in preoperative TAE. No prospective randomized study assessing the relationship between preoperative TAE and postoperative recurrence has been available. Considering the complications, to be described below, we are of the opinion that resection should be done as early as possible in operable patients. However, in patients with a very large cancer which has a risk of rupture or in which operation is deemed difficult because of size, and who will be on the waiting list for a couple of months, TAE may be indicated just to make the best use of available time.

TAE therapy—Case 1: Intrahepatic artery injection of Lipiodol alone (tumor remaining 100 per cent viable). A 36-year-old man. AFP (−) and CEA (−).

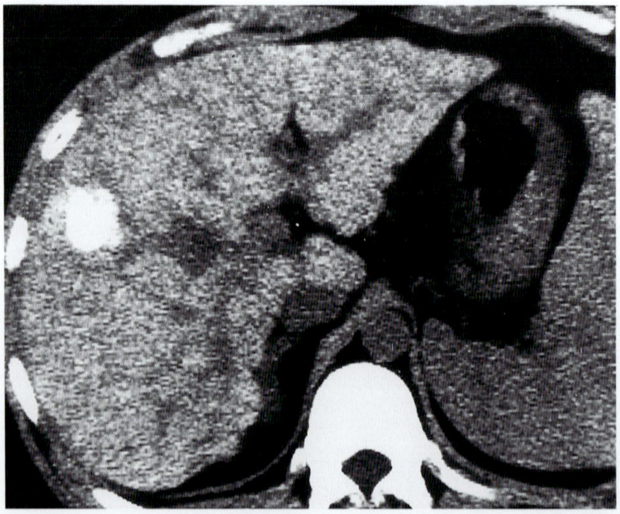

(a) Plain CT (10 days after arterial injection): this is a plain CT made 10 days after 6 ml of Lipiodol was injected into the hepatic artery. Lipiodol retention is seen in a mass in S^{VIII}.

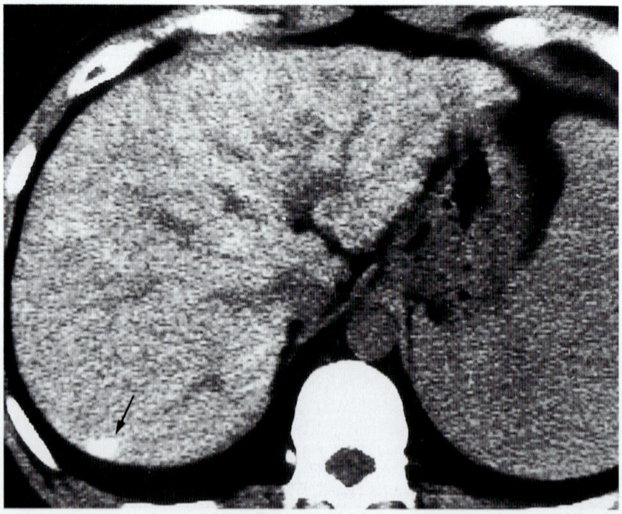

(b) Plain CT [1 cm cranial to slice (a)]: Lipiodol retention is seen in a mass in S^{VII}.

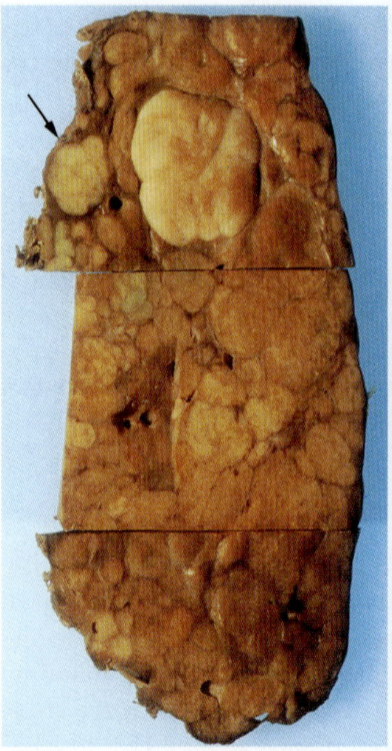

c

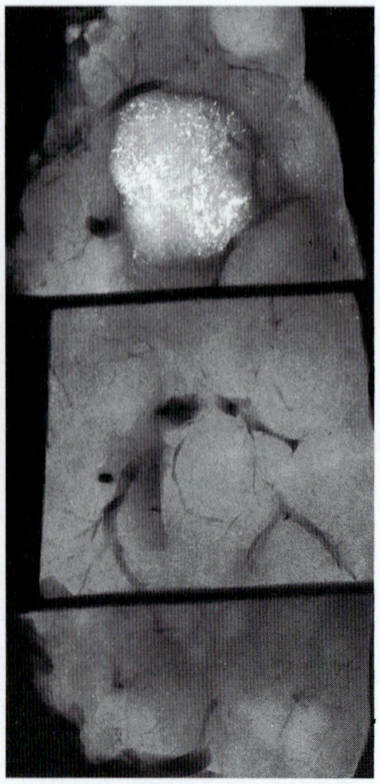

d

(c) Cut section of resected specimen (tumor in S^{VIII}): soft X-ray (d) shows good retention of Lipiodol in the mass. Histologically, this was Edmondson's grade I–II, with no necrosis. →, this looked like a daughter nodule, but had no Lipiodol, and histologically it was a regenerative nodule.

(d) Soft X-ray film of (c).

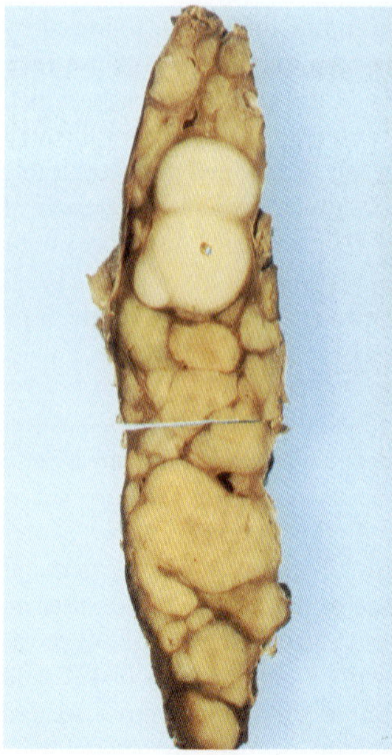

e

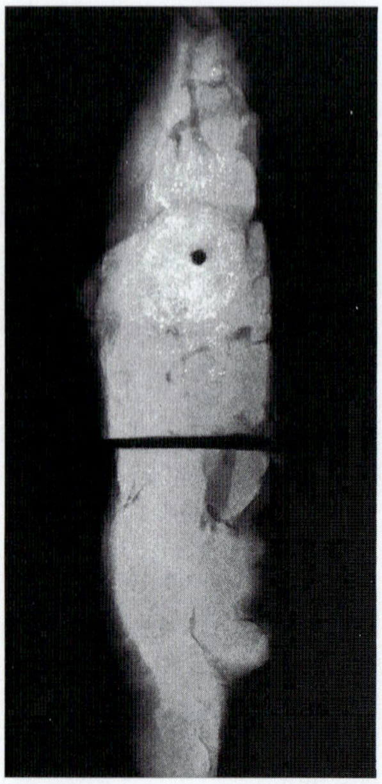

f

(e) Cut section of resected specimen (tumor in S^{VII}): there are two cancer nodules. Soft X-ray (f) showed Lipiodol retention, but there was no necrosis histologically (Edmondson's grade I).

(f) Soft X-ray film of (e).

TAE therapy—Case 2: Complete necrosis of a small HCC induced by intraarterial injection of Lipiodol + Adriamycin. A 64-year-old woman. AFP 5950 ng/ml.

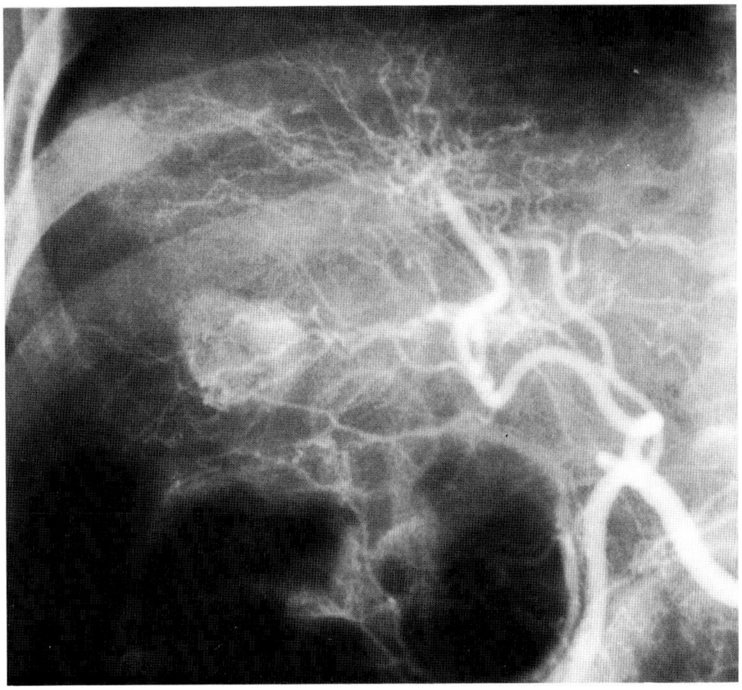

(a) Hepatic arteriogram: a mass is seen in S^{VI}. Lipiodol (5 ml) + Adriamycin (20 mg) was injected into the proper hepatic artery.

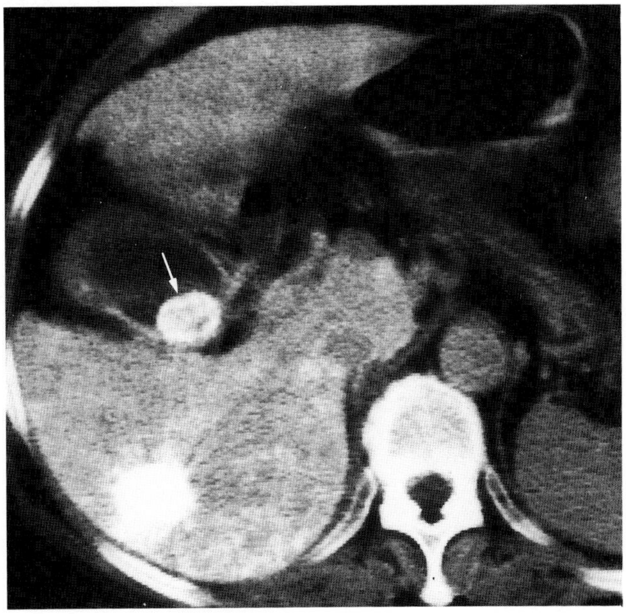

(b) Plain CT (immediately after arterial injection): adequate retention of Lipiodol is seen in the mass. →, stone in the gallbladder.

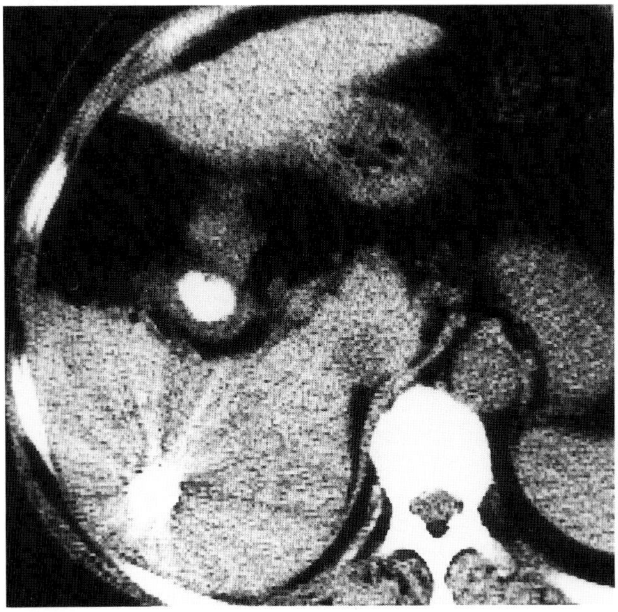

(c) Plain CT (78 days after arterial injection): the size of the mass has been reduced to 18 mm from 28 mm with condensation of Lipiodol producing a radiating artefact in the surrounding area. AFP decreased to 0 ng at 55 days postinjection.

Case 2 (contd.)

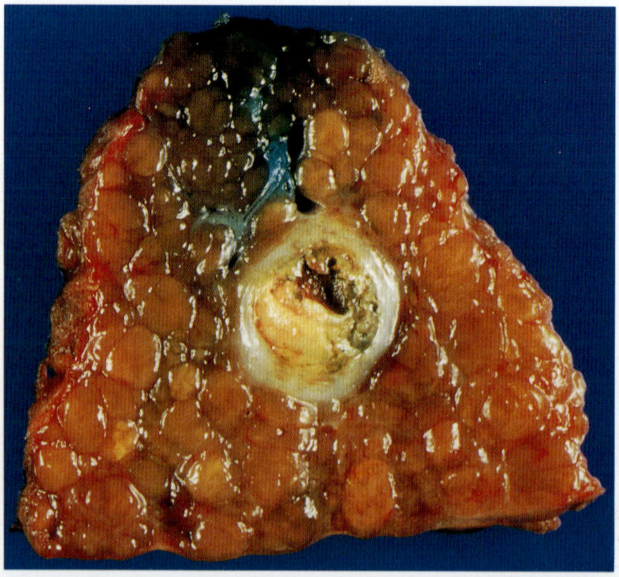

(d) Cut section of resected specimen: the mass was completely necrotized and surrounded by a thick fibrous capsule. The green color seen above the mass is indigocarmine dye injected during the operation to determine the area for resection.

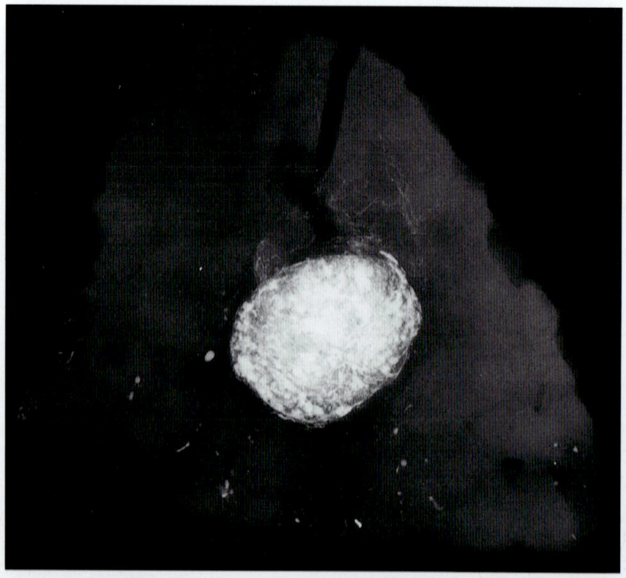

(e) Soft X-ray of (d): fine reticular and dotted retention of Lipiodol is seen in the mass.

TAE therapy—Case 3: Large HCC in which no necrosis was induced by arterial injection of Lipiodol + Adriamycin. A 65-year-old man with normal AFP and CEA.

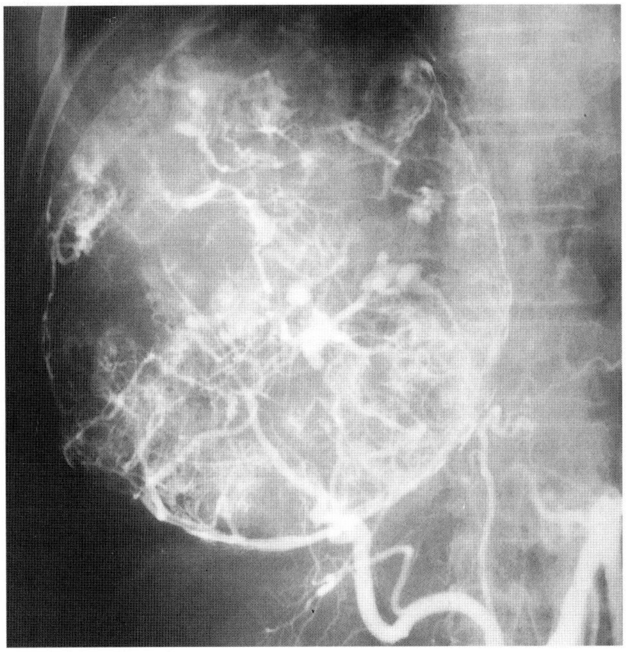

(a) Celiac artriogram (preoperative): a huge HCC (15 × 12.5 cm) is seen in $S^{VIII-IV}$. The cranial portion of the mass is not adequately opacified because of its supply from the inferior right phrenic artery.

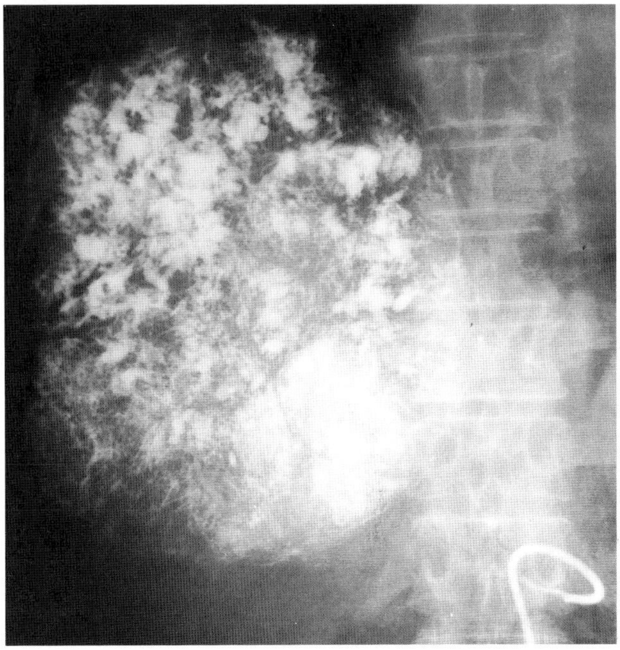

(b) Plain CT (immediately after treatment): Lipiodol (30 ml) + Adriamycin (40 mg) was injected into the right hepatic artery and inferior right phrenic artery. This plain abdominal film was made immediately after injection. It shows large amounts of Lipiodol retained in the mass.

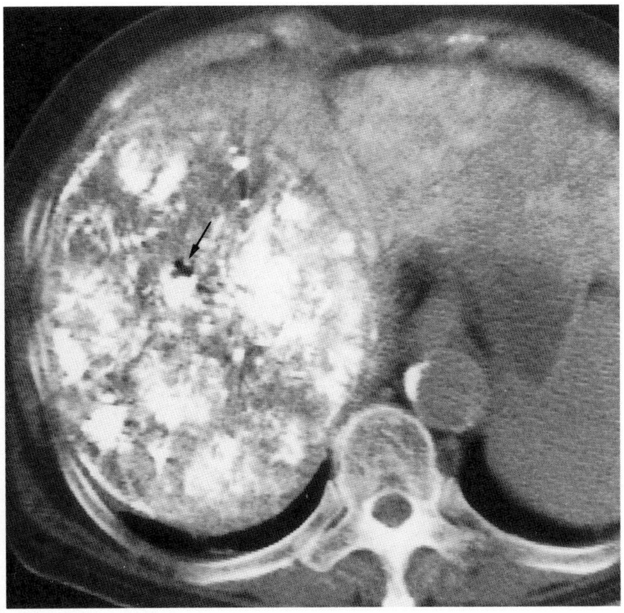

(c) Plain CT (immediately after treatment): each tumor nodule has Lipiodol retention. A spot-like low density (→) is air introduced into the tumor during the catheterization procedure.

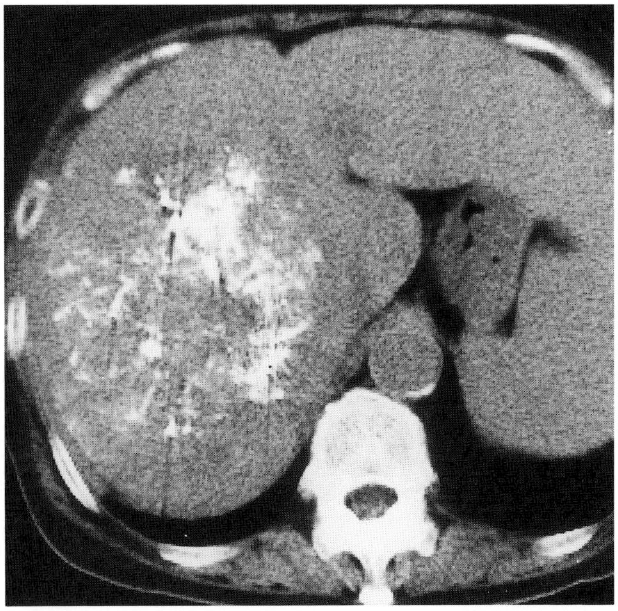

(d) Plain CT (58 days post-treatment): Lipiodol in the mass has been much reduced, some disappeared.

Case 3 (contd.)

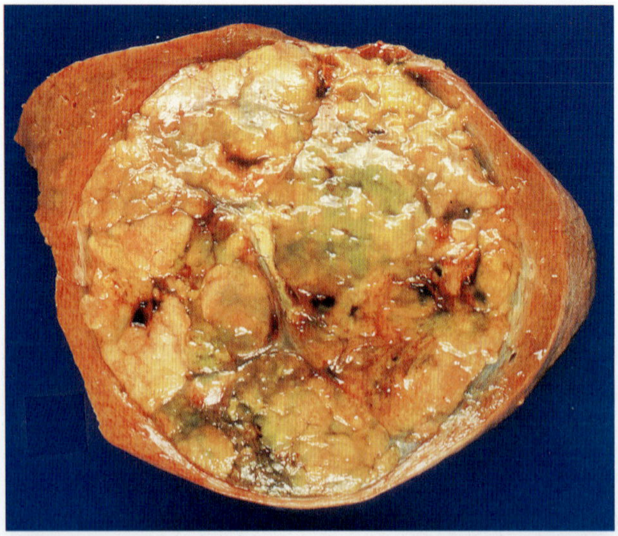

(e) Cut section of resected specimen: central bisegmentectomy was carried out. The interior of the mass was partitioned into many nodules by fibrous septa, some nodules being green because of bilirubin production. Histologically, no necrosis was seen at all. Formation of a fibrous capsule around the mass was recognized.

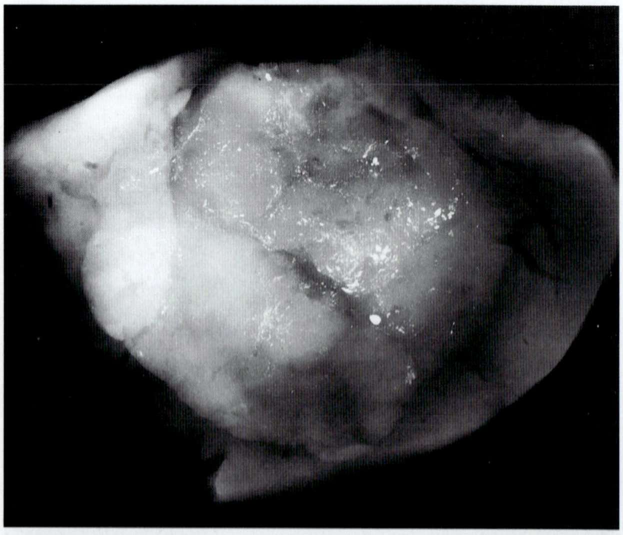

(f) Soft X-ray of (e): retention of Lipiodol has been further reduced from the follow-up CT (d).

TAE therapy—Case 4: Marked shrinkage of a large HCC caused by repeated TAE using Lipiodol + Adriamycin + Gelfoam particles. A 45-year-old man. AFP, 13 000 ng/ml.

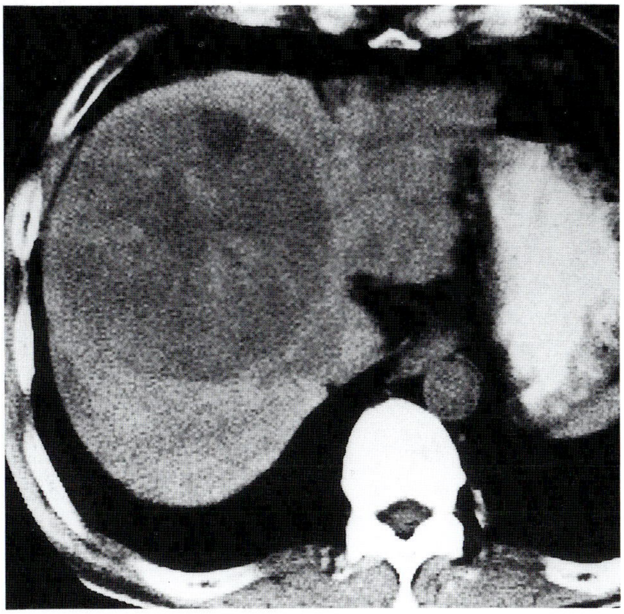

(a) Plain CT (preoperative): a 9 cm mass is seen in $S^{VIII-IV}$. Two session of Lipiodol-TAE and one session of Lipiodol-TAI (transarterial injection) were given in 1 year. AFP dropped to 0 ng/ml.

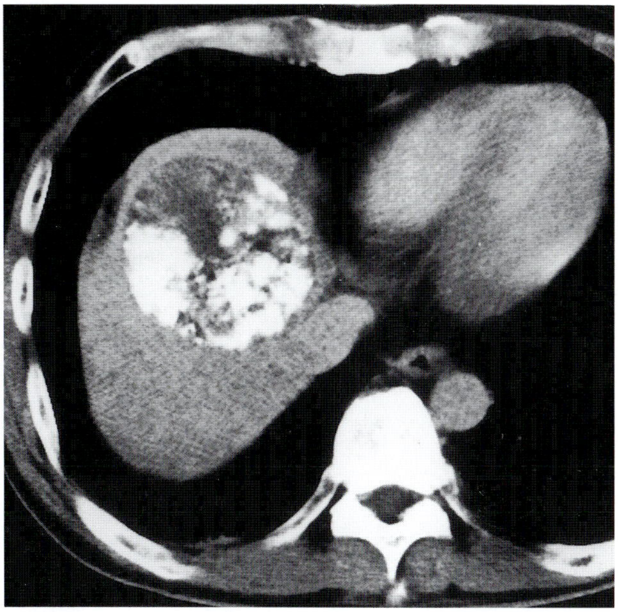

(b) Enhanced CT (10 months post-treatment): in a late phase of enhanced CT (8 min), the mass measures 6.5 cm, much reduced in size. One-quarter of the area of mass does not have Lipiodol. The viability of tumor cells in this area was the cause of concern.

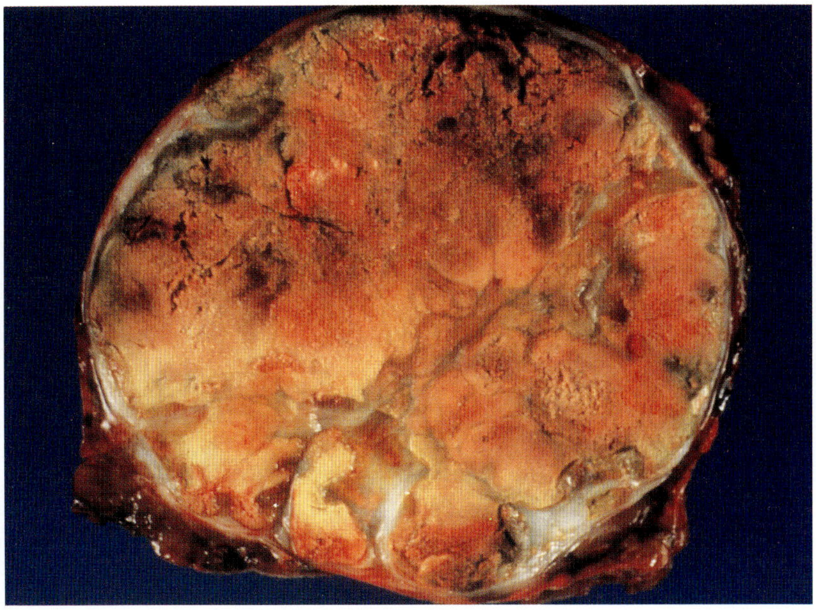

(c) Cut section of resected specimen: the whole tumor was completely necrotic with no viable cancer cells.

TAE therapy—Case 5: Marked necrosis of hepatic vein tumor thrombus induced by Lipiodol + Adriamycin + Gelfoam particles (Lipiodol-TAE). A 48-year-old man. AFP, 165 ng/ml.

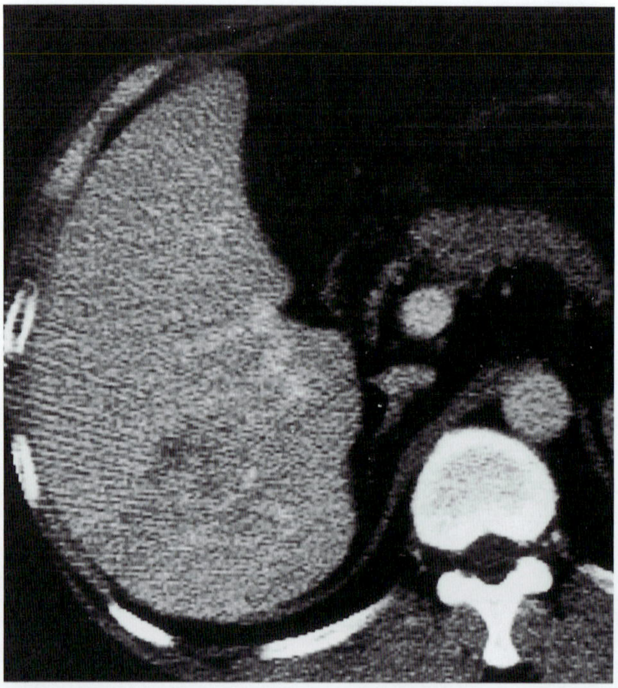

(a) Enhanced CT (pretreatment): a 3 cm low-density tumor is seen in S^{VI}. No tumor thrombus is recognized.

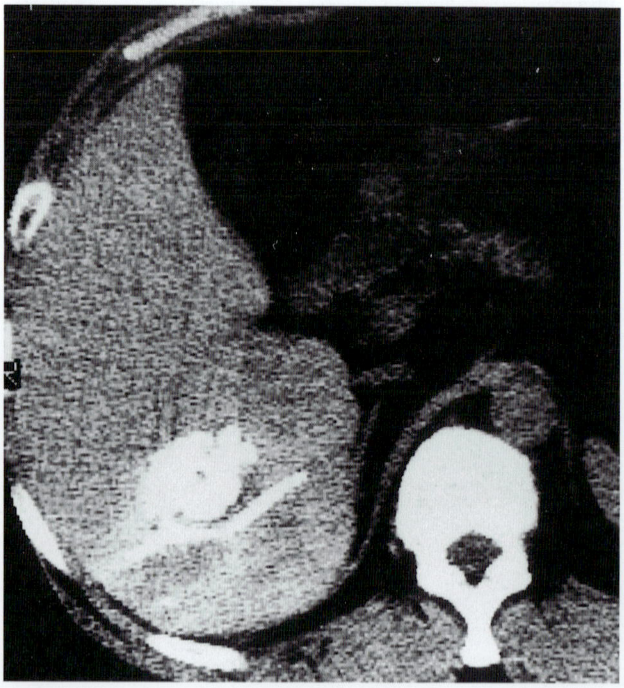

(b) Plain CT (4 days post-treatment): beside the mass, Lipiodol retention is seen in a tumor thrombus within the inferior hepatic vein as a cord-like density posterior to it.

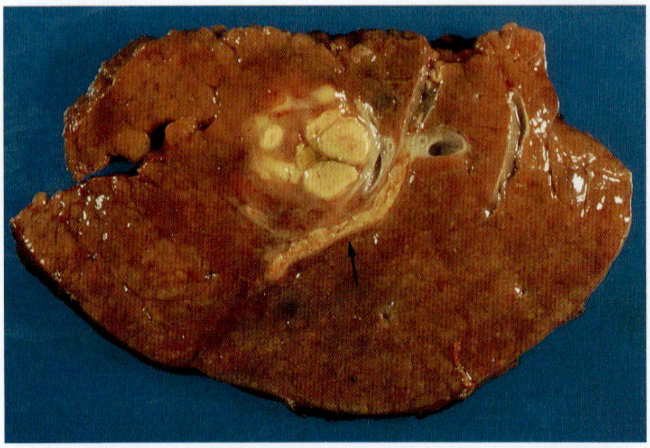

(c) Cut section of resected specimen: the main mass was totally necrotized. The tumor thrombus (→) within the inferior right hepatic vein was also necrotized, but histologically a small portion of the thrombus contained viable cancer cells.

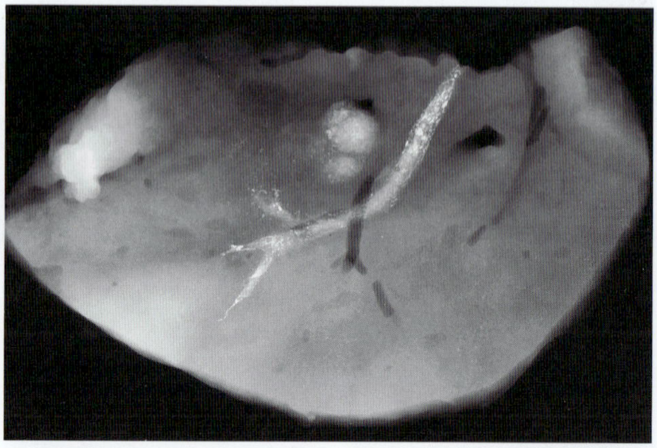

(d) Soft X-ray of (c): good Lipiodol retention is seen in the mass as well as in the tumor thrombus.

TAE therapy—Case 6: Confluent multinodular HCC not responding to Lipiodol-TAE.

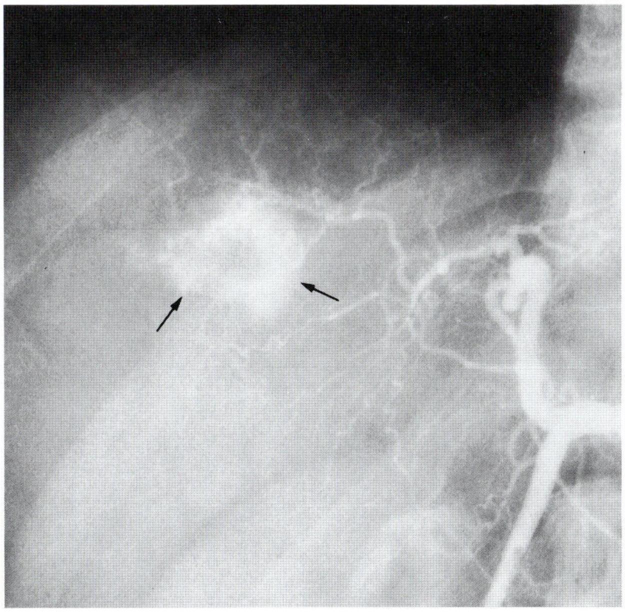

(a) Left hepatic arteriogram (pretreatment): an irregularly bordered tumor stain (→) with a non-stained center is seen in S^{IV}.

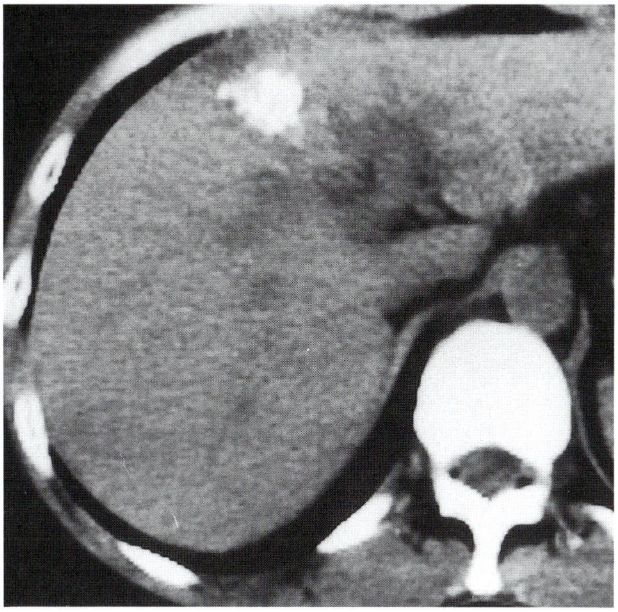

(b) Plain CT (13 days post-treatment): Lipiodol is retained as dots within the mass.

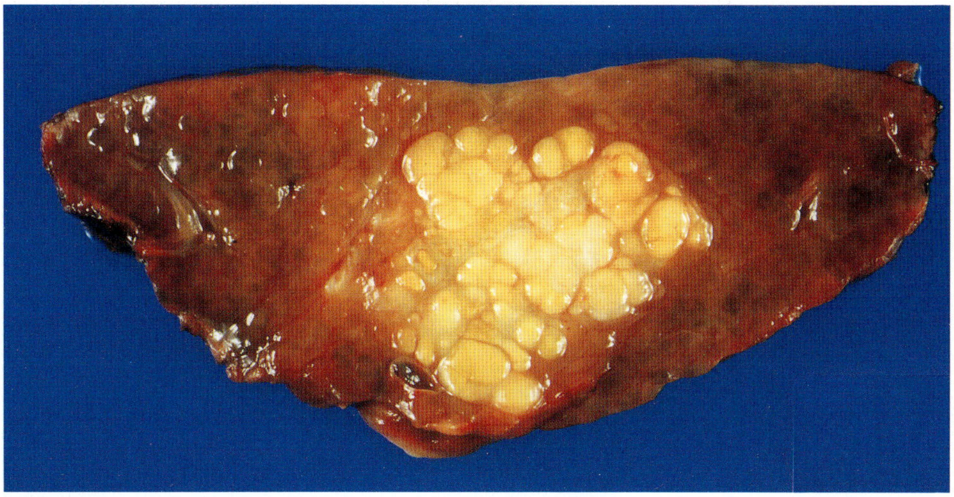

(c) Cut section of resected specimen: many small 2–5 mm nodules are confluent (multinodular fused type). Histopathologically, this was Edmondson's grade II > III with practically no necrosis, and not encapsulated.

TAE therapy—Case 7: Growth of tumor cells within a fibrous capsule, suggested by comparison of soft X-ray and resected specimen.

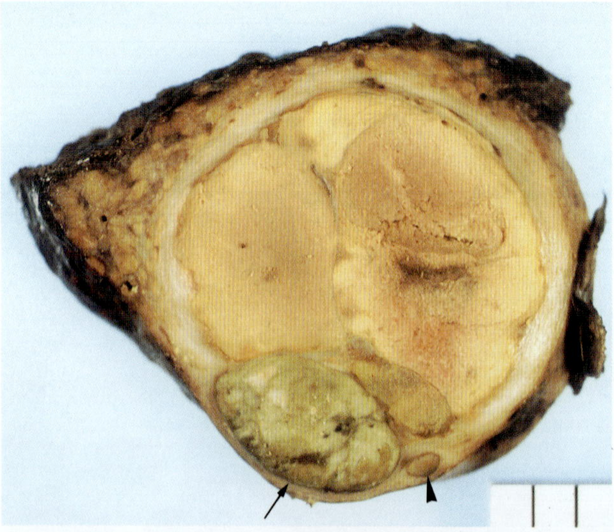

(a) Cut section of resected specimen: at a glance, this nodule appeared to be a viable one (→) within the main mass, but on a closer look it turned out to be growing within the fibrous capsule. Another small nodule is seen within this thick capsule (▶).

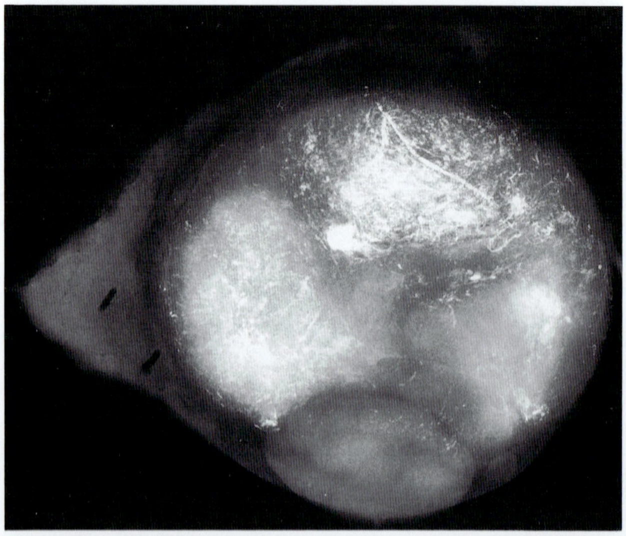

(b) Soft X-ray of (a): the growing nodule did not contain Lipiodol, and it was assumed that the main mass was necrotized by Lipiodol-TAE; a small tumor remaining in the capsule grew during the period from Lipiodol injection to operation. It looked as though a tumor nodule within the mass did not respond at the time of TAE.

TAE therapy—Case 8: Nodule-wise response of HCC to Lipiodol-TAE.

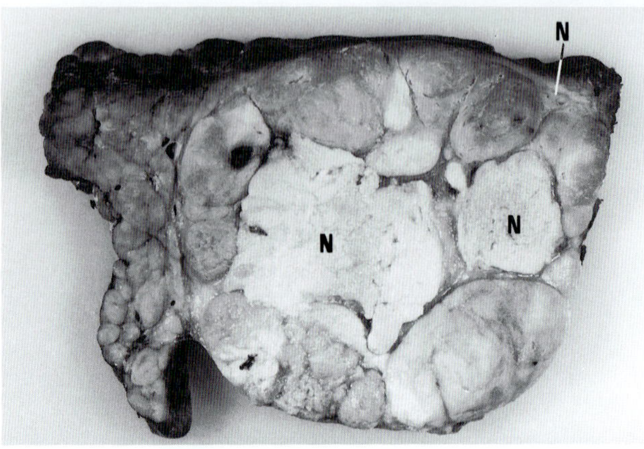

(a) Cut section of resected specimen: a number of tumor nodules are arranged in a mosaic pattern. Nodule-wise necrosis in which some nodules are necrotized (N) and others not, is recognized.

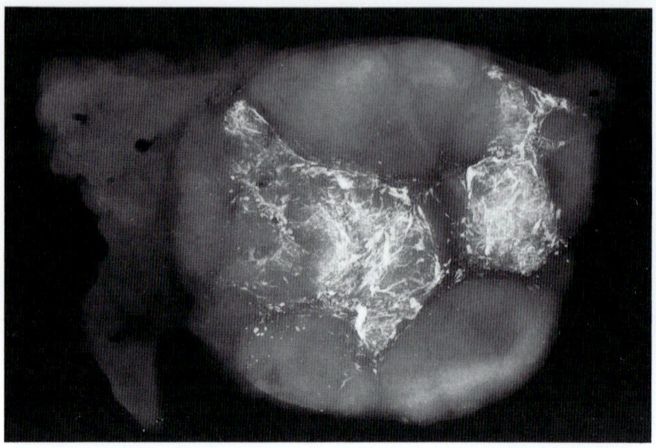

(b) Soft X-ray of (a): necrosis and Lipiodol retention correspond well.

TAE therapy—Case 9: No Lipiodol retention occurs in the area which is already necrotic.

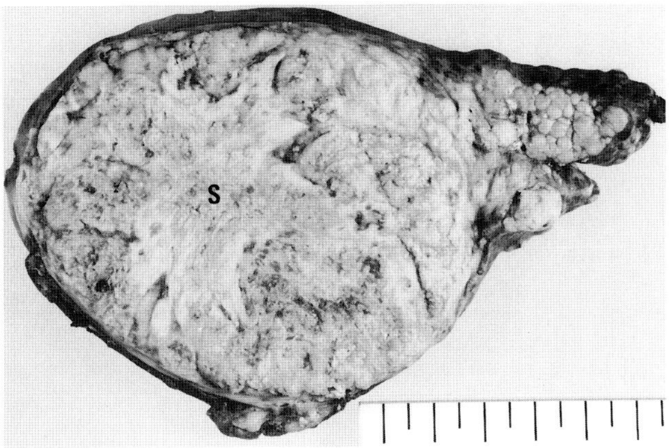

(a) Cut section of resected specimen: this is a large HCC nodule with a stellate fibrous scar (S) in the interior. The interior was not enhanced by dynamic CT.

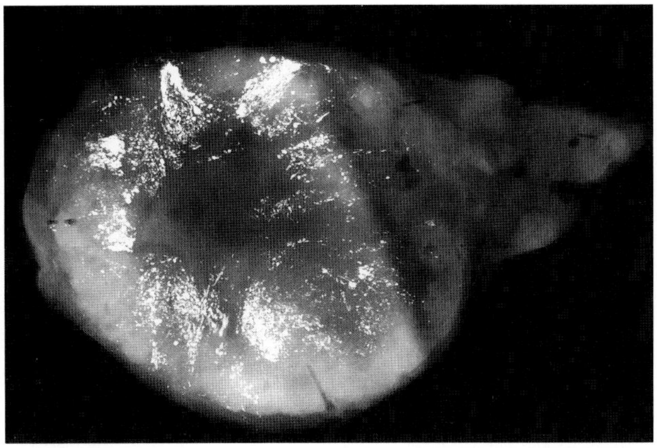

(b) Soft X-ray of (a): Lipiodol is retained in viable nodules in the periphery, but the center has no Lipiodol. In other words, Lipiodol does not flow into the tissues already necrotic at the time of TAE, and a soft X-ray does not show it.

TAE therapy—Case 10: HCC growth pattern assumed by comparison of soft X-ray film and resected specimen. A 63-year-old woman. AFP 142 ng/ml.

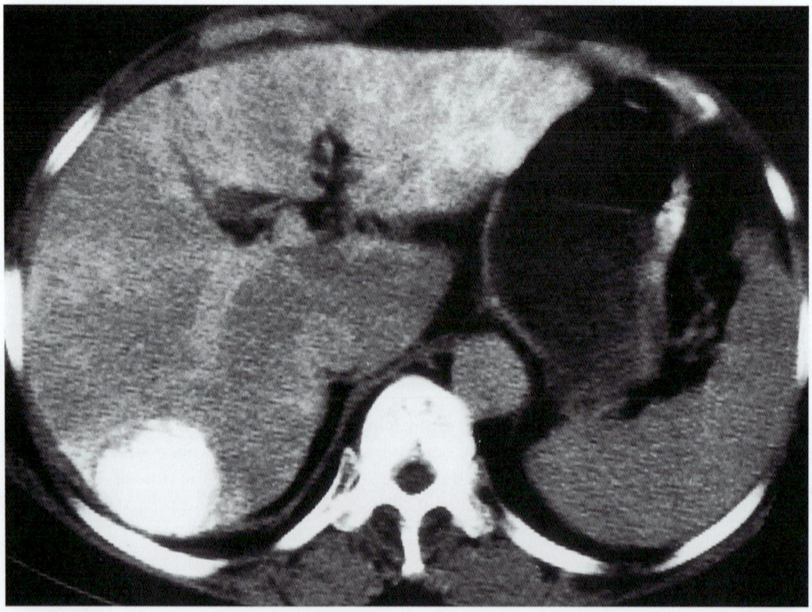

(a) Plain CT (immediately after treatment): this CT made immediately after arterial injection of Lipiodol–Adriamycin demonstrated good Lipiodol retention by a mass (3.5 cm) in S^{VI} and a good anticancer effect was anticipated.

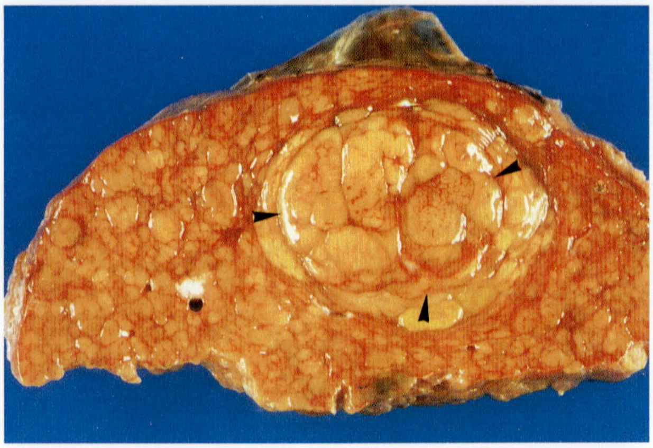

(b) Cut section of resected specimen: nevertheless, when studied grossly and histologically there was no necrosis in the specimen resected 29 days after arterial injection. Compared with the soft X-ray (c), Lipiodol retention was confined to an area of 3.5 cm in diameter. The tumor size was 4.5 cm, and it was found that only the concentric 3.5 cm nodule within the tumor boundary (▶) contained Lipiodol. The outer portion surrounding the Lipiodol-retaining mass did not have Lipiodol, suggesting that this portion grew concentrically outward after Lipiodol-TAE. It may represent one of the growth patterns of HCC.

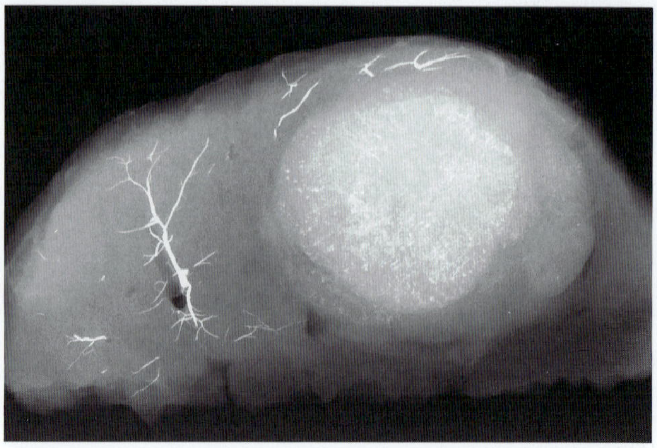

(c) Soft X-ray of (b): the diameter of the Lipiodol containing area was 3.5 cm.

TAE therapy—Case 11: A 2 mm intrahepatic metastasis detected by soft X-ray.

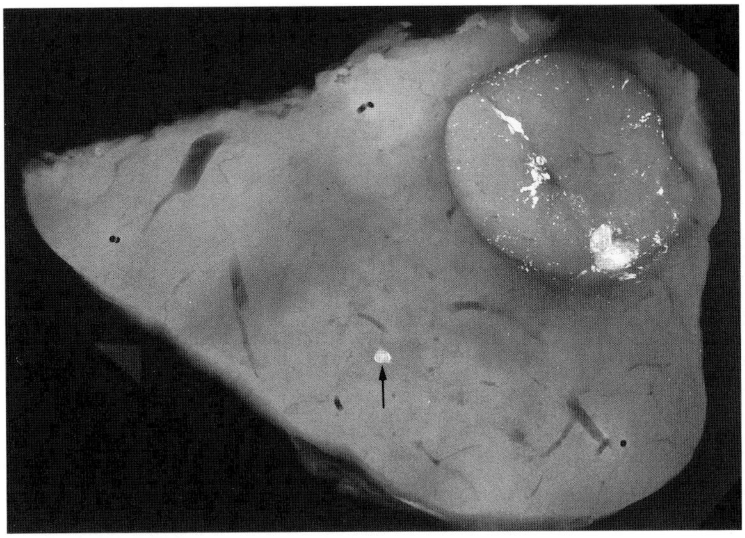

(a) Soft X-ray of resected specimen: this small 2 × 1 mm intrahepatic metastasis (→) was found by soft X-ray in addition to the main mass.

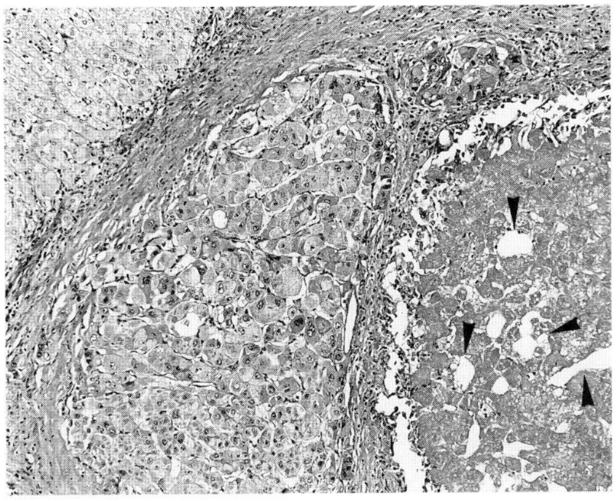

(b) Histopathology: this small lesion was HCC. The right area of this photomicrograph represents necrosis induced by Lipiodol-TAE that contained fat droplets (▶, Lipiodol), and the left side viable cancer cells. This lesion was thought to have grown from cancer cells implanted via the portal vein.

TAE therapy—Case 12: Marked reduction of AFP and shrinkage of HCC following Lipiodol-TAE (non-operated case). A 66-year-old woman. As her liver function was poor, Lipiodol-TAE was carried out. AFP 1335 ng/ml.

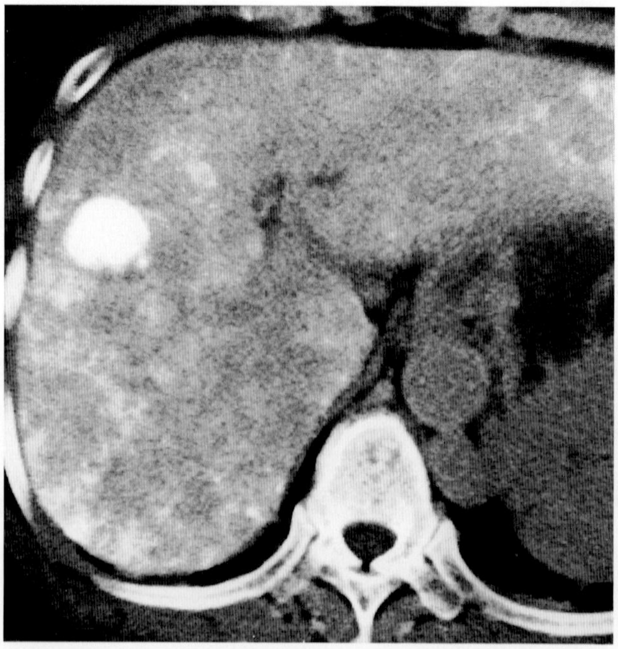

(a) Plain CT (immediately after treatment): TAE with Lipiodol (5 ml) + Adriamycin (20 mg) + Gelfoam particles was carried out through the proper hepatic artery. This plain CT made immediately after TAE demonstrates a 27 × 21 mm mass in S^{VIII} that has retained Lipiodol (same as Case 8, p. 400).

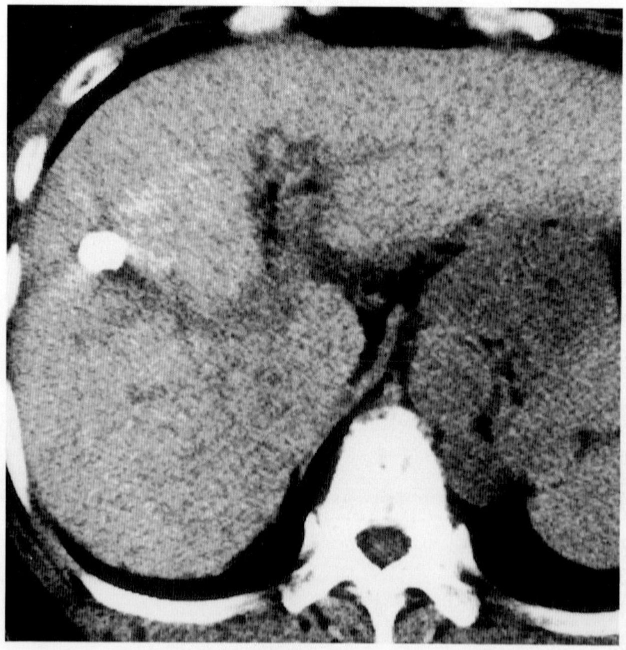

(b) Plain CT (5 months post-treatment): the mass has shrunk to 15 × 12 mm, and AFP decreased to 6 ng/ml.

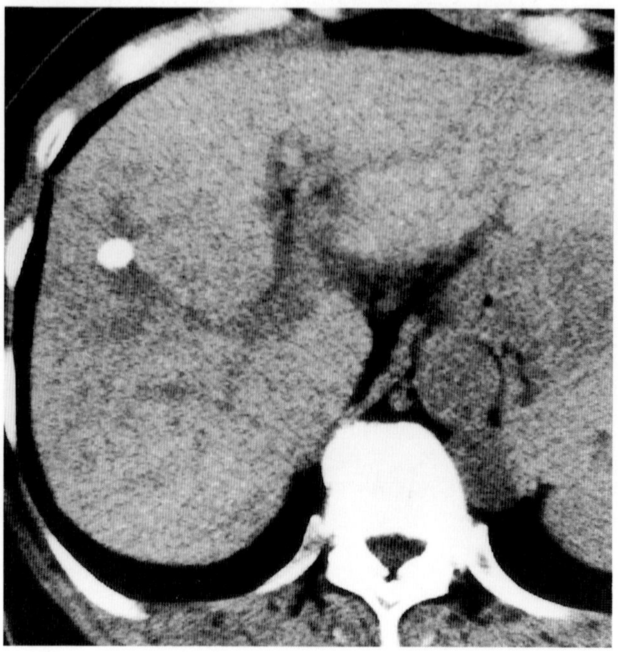

(c) Plain CT (13 months post-treatment): the mass has been reduced further to 9 × 6 mm in size.

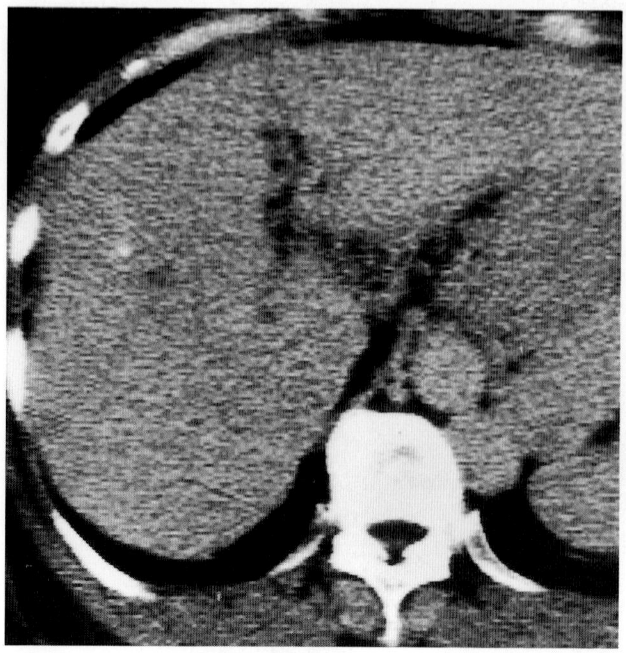

(d) Plain CT (2 years and 5 months post-treatment): the tumor is near extinction. It eventually disappeared.

TAE therapy—Case 13: Reduction in size of a portal vein tumor thrombus by Lipiodol-TAE.

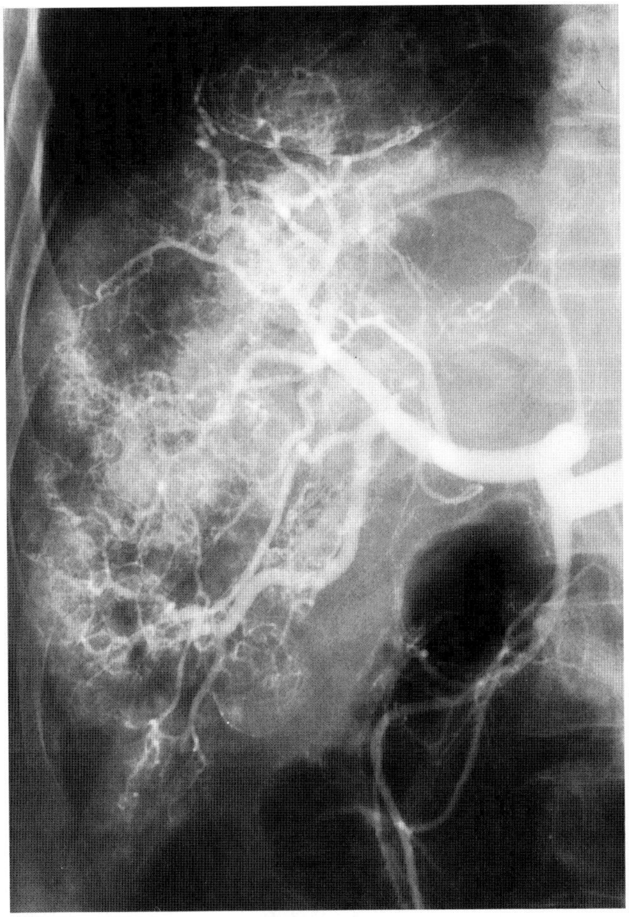

(a) Hepatic arteriogram (early phase, pretreatment): a large mass is occupying almost the entire right lobe.

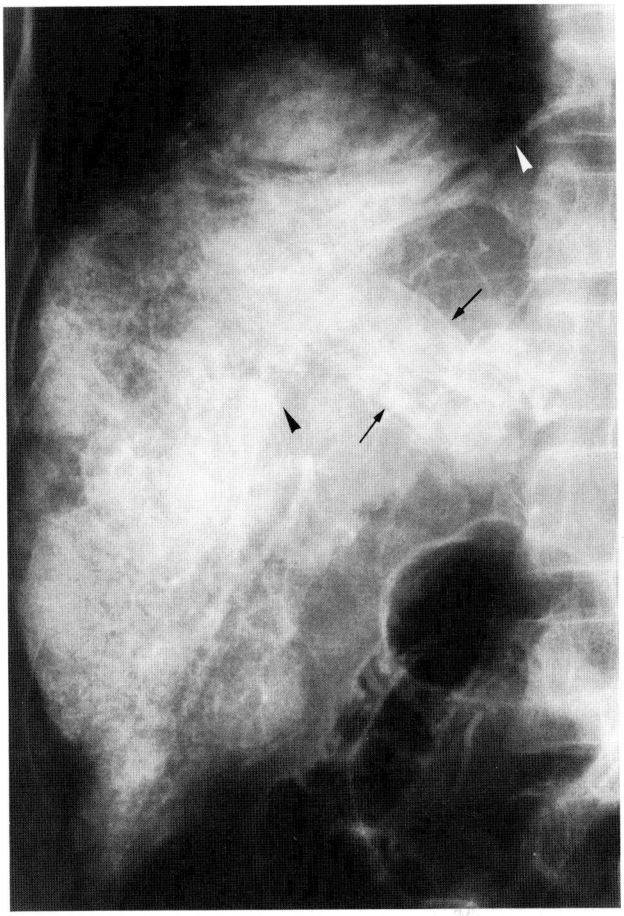

(b) Hepatic arteriogram (late phase, pretreatment): a dilated right portal vein contains a tumor thrombus (→). ▶, hepatic vein.

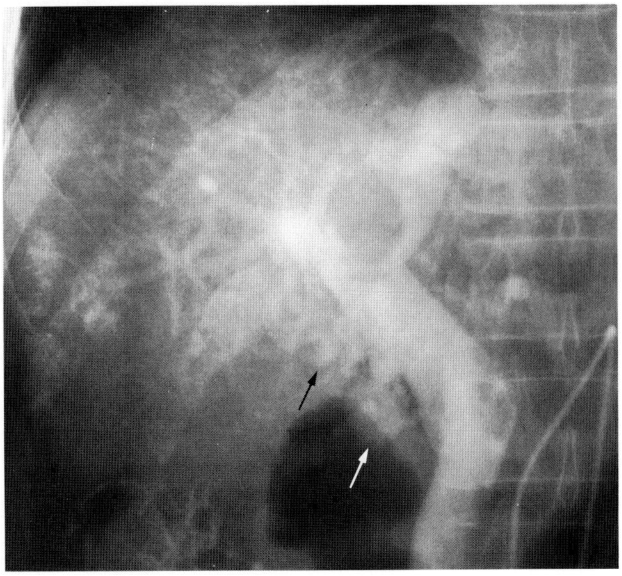

(c) Portogram (pretreatment): the right anterior portal vein is not opacified, and a filling defect due to a tumor thrombus growing from the transverse portion of the left portal vein toward the portal trunk is seen. The posterior portal vein is patent as it is independent of the others. Cavernous transformation is also recognized (→). Lipiodol-TAE was carried out from the proper hepatic artery.

Case 13 (contd.)

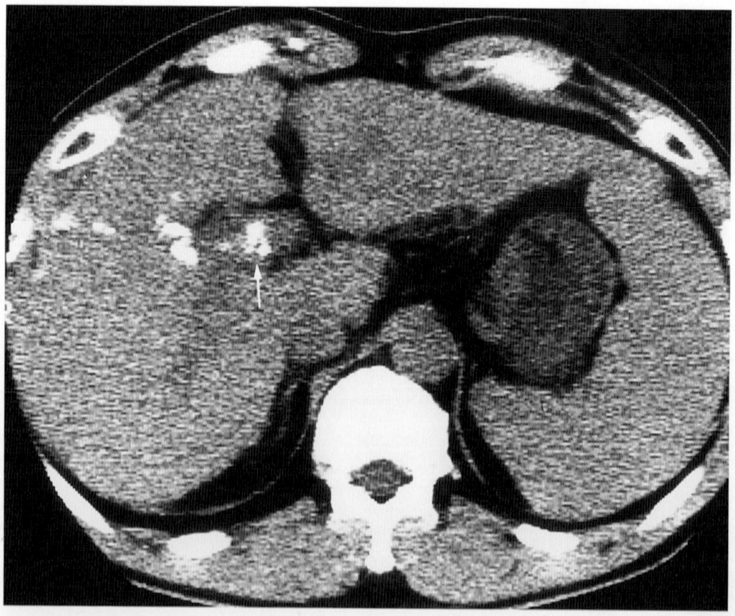

(d) Plain CT (immediately after treatment): Lipiodol retention is seen within the right portal vein (→).

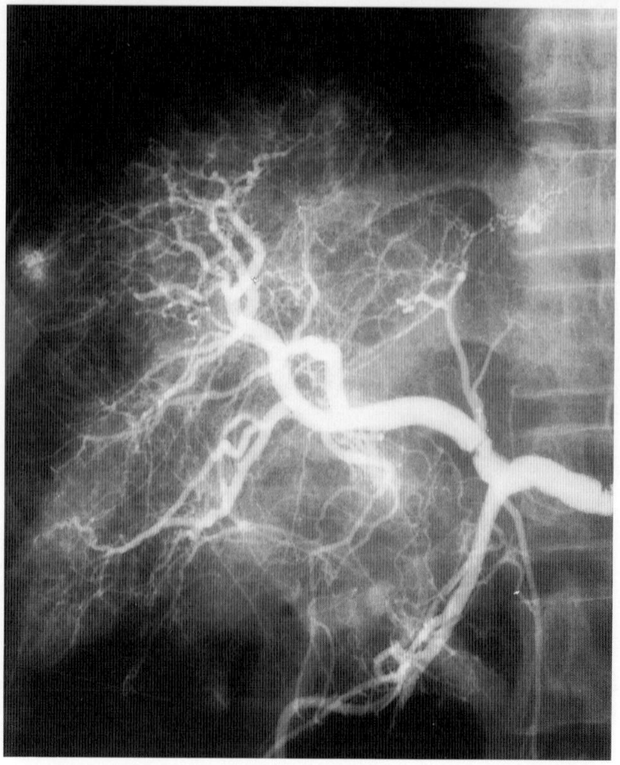

(e) Hepatic arteriogram (1 year and 2 months post-treatment): tumor vessels have been much reduced in number and caliber.

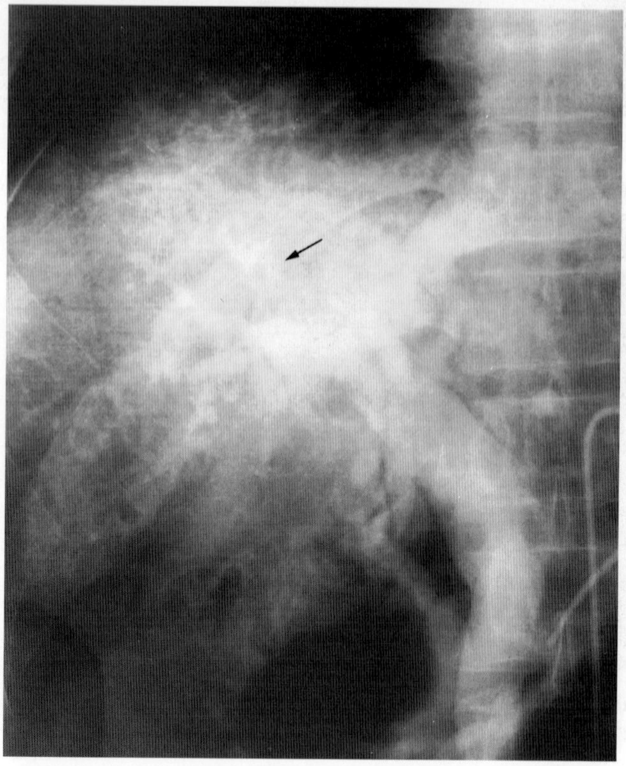

(f) Portography (1 year and 2 months post-treatment): although a small filling defect is still seen in the transverse portion of the left portal vein, the right anterior portal vein is now reopened (→). The cavernous transformation has also been reduced in size.

TAE therapy—Case 14: Successful treatment of postoperative recurrence by intraarterial injection of Lipiodol-Adriamycin. A 63-year-old man. AFP 3911 ng/ml.

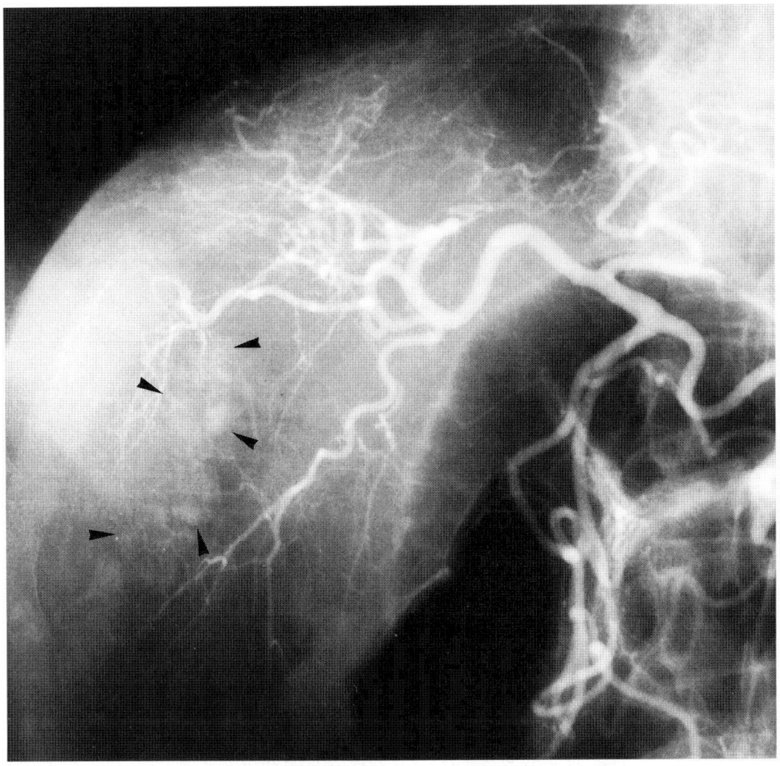

(a) Proper hepatic arteriogram: a recurrent lesion in S^{VI} was treated with Lipiodol (5 ml) + Adriamycin (20 mg) injected from the proper hepatic artery.

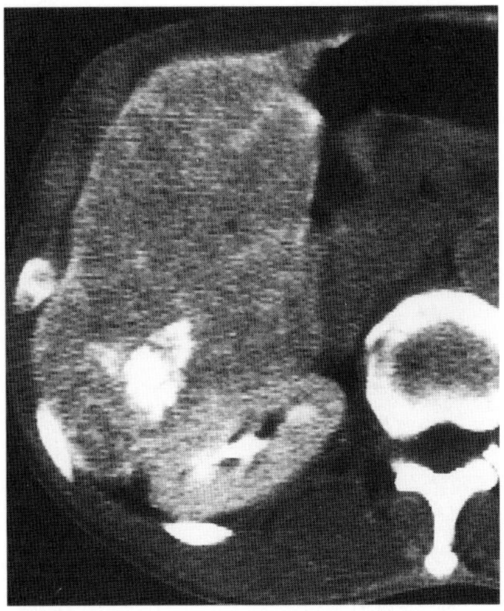

(b) Plain CT (immediately after treatment): good Lipiodol retention is seen in the tumor (30 × 20 mm).

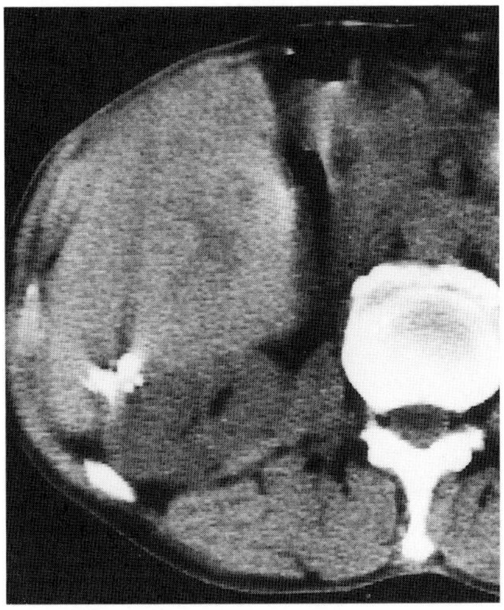

(c) Plain CT (40 days post-treatment): tumor size has been reduced to 15 × 9 mm with a normal AFP level.

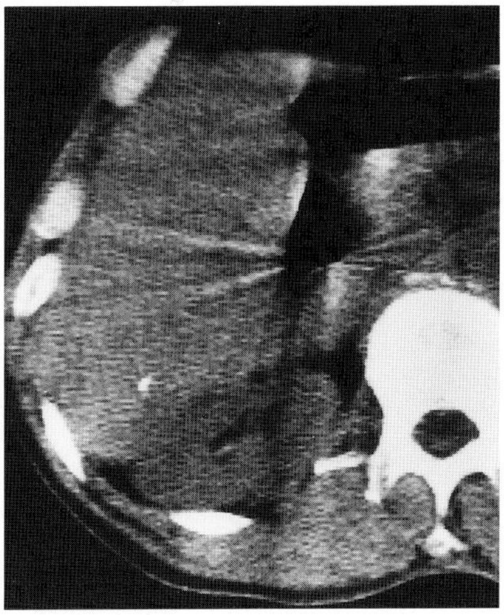

(d) Plain CT (2 years and 4 months post-treatment): The mass is now 6 × 3 mm. It subsequently disappeared on a follow-up CT. There has been no recurrence as of 6 years post-treatment.

TAE therapy—Case 15: Long survival gained by frequent arterial injections of Lipiodol + Adriamycin from the pancreatic arcade artery for a recurrence.

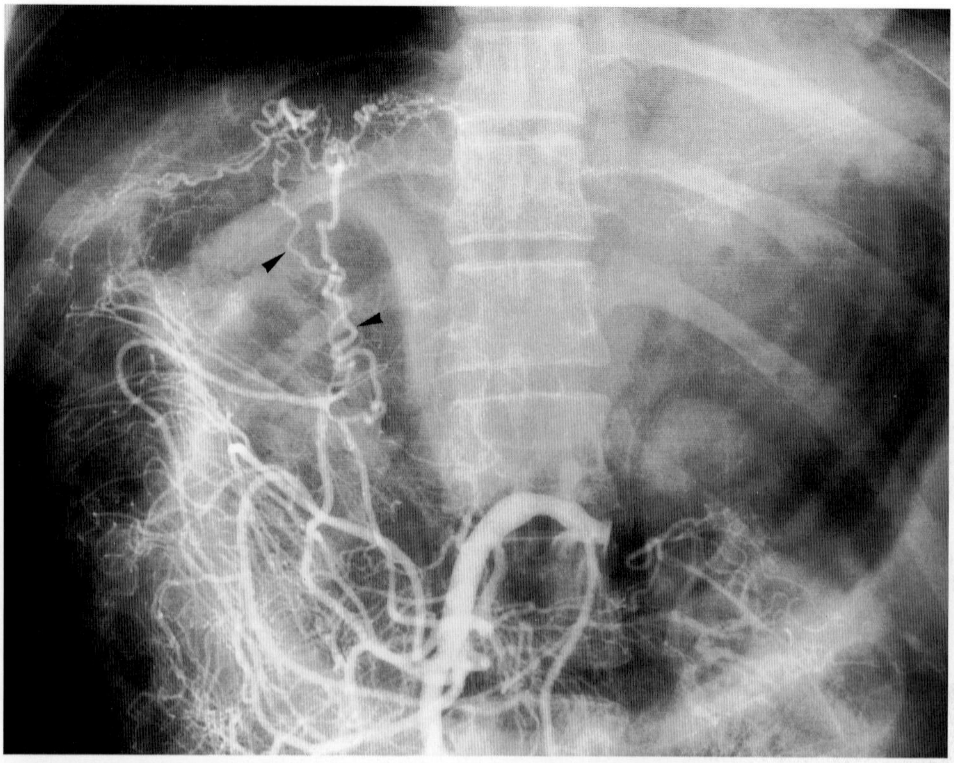

(a) Hepatic arteriogram: the hepatic artery was occluded by repeated TAE, and the mass was opacified by contrast medium injected from the pancreactic arcade artery, a branch of the superior mesenteric artery, through the epicholedochal plexus (▶) which was supplying the tumor.

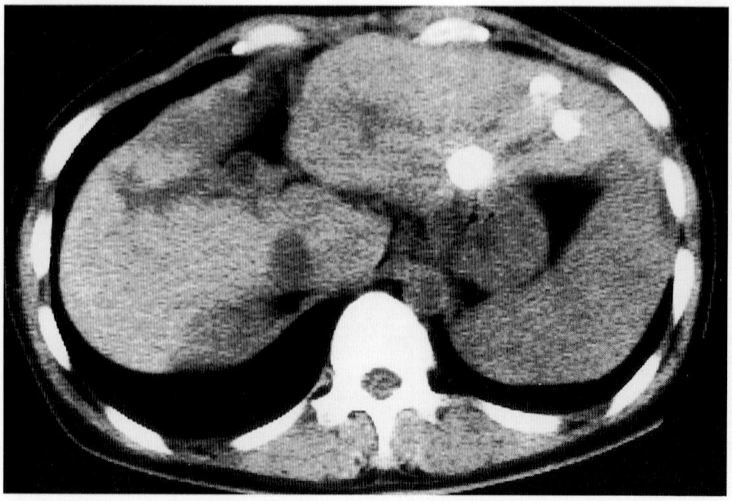

(b) Plain CT: in this plain CT made after arterial injection of Lipiodol-Adriamycin, a number of Lipiodol-containing recurrent lesions are recognized. Unlike Gelfoam particles, Lipiodol does not induce severe complications even though it enters the superior mesenteric artery. Lipiodol has made it possible to treat this kind of case with a complicated vascular anatomy. This patient, after six sessions of arterial injection of Lipiodol-Adriamycin, lived for 6.5 years after recurrence (same as Case 4).

TAE therapy—Case 16: Worsening of liver function due to repeated TAE for recurrence in the remnant liver. Extended right lobectomy was carried out for a large 11.5 cm HCC 10 months earlier, and follow-up CT found recurrent lesions in the residual liver.

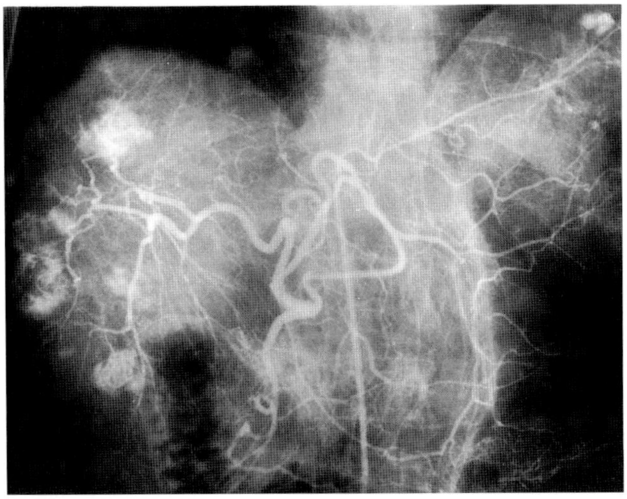

(a) Hepatic arteriogram (10 months postoperatively): this hepatic arteriogram displays multiple recurrent lesions of similar sizes in S^{VI}. The left lobe also has a small lesion. The first TAE with Gelfoam + Adriamycin was carried out.

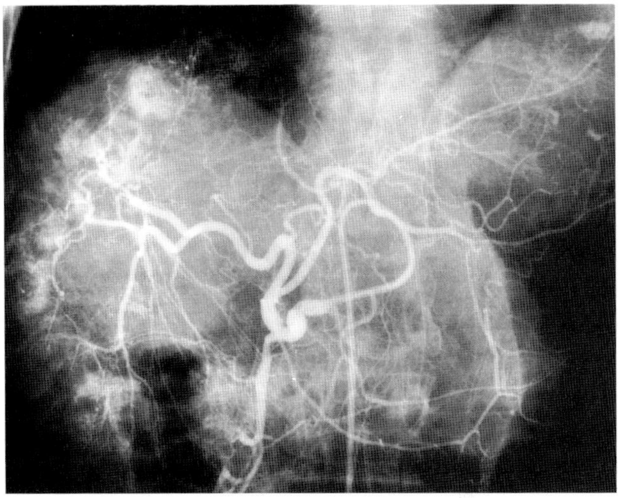

(b) Hepatic arteriogram (6 months after the first TAE): there are more recurrent lesions than in the previous angiogram. This time, TAE with Lipiodol + Adriamycin + Gelfoam was carried out.

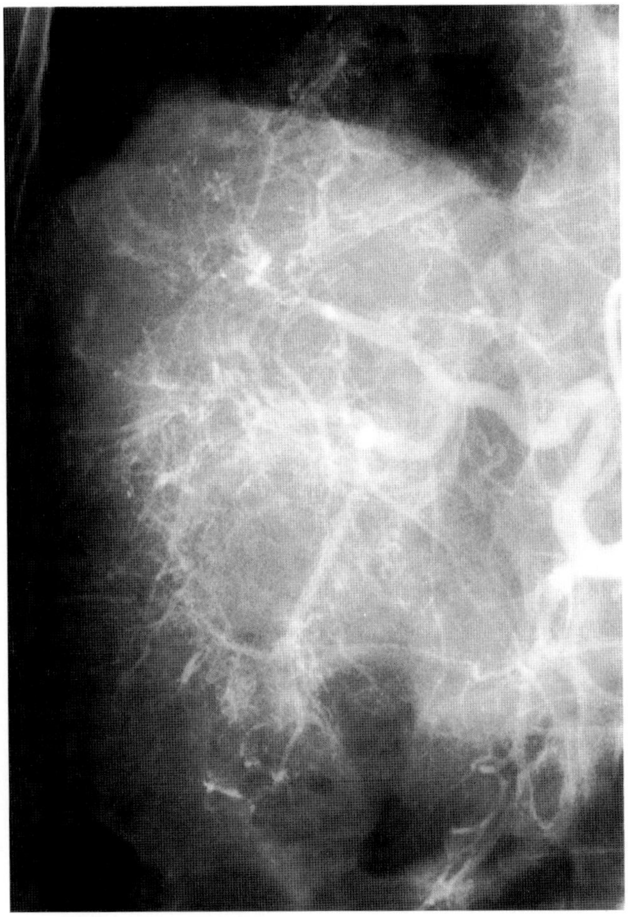

(c) Hepatic arteriogram (11 months after the second TAE): at this stage, the thread and streaks sign (tumor thrombus) is seen in P^{VI}. A third TAE session was done, but the patient rapidly went downhill, and died 1 year and 3 months after the first TAE for the recurrence.

19.2 Combination of TAE and PTPE

TAE alone may not be sufficiently effective for HCC, particularly for tumor cells residing within the capsule which has a dual blood supply. Attempts have been made to obtain better results by occluding the portal flow supplying the capsule and periphery of the tumor. Namely, the portal vein is embolized (PTPE) after TAE by percutaneous transhepatic portal vein catheterization (PTP) (Nakao *et al.* 1986). In our unit at the National Cancer Center Hospital, Tokyo, the first PTPE in the world was carried out in June 1982 in a patient with hilar carcinoma for the purpose of expanding surgical indications (Makuuchi *et al.* 1990). This patient (Case 1) had two 4 cm HCCs. As an additional preoperative therapy, we embolized the right portal vein and carried out TAE 3 days later. The tumors shrank slowly but progressively from 4 to 2 cm and 4.5 to 3 cm. The operation was deemed unnecessary and called off. Atrophy of the right lobe also occurred. However, histopathological investigation of resected specimens in such cases found that tumor necrosis was often incomplete; we have to determine further the best interval between TAE and PTPE, and study histological events that follow the procedure.

PTPE alone has a deleterious effect and will expedite tumor growth as arterial blood supply increases in compensation (Case 2). It has been suggested that it will also expedite metastasis to the lung as the portal vein acting as an outflow vessel for HCC is closed and the hepatic vein takes its place. Therefore, TAE should be done within a very short period prior to PTPE.

Combined therapy—Case 1: HCC for which combined Lipiodol-TAE and PTPE proved effective. Two HCCs were found, one in $S^{VIII-VII}$ and the other in S^{VI}. PTPE was carried out followed by Lipiodol-TAE as an additional preoperative therapy.

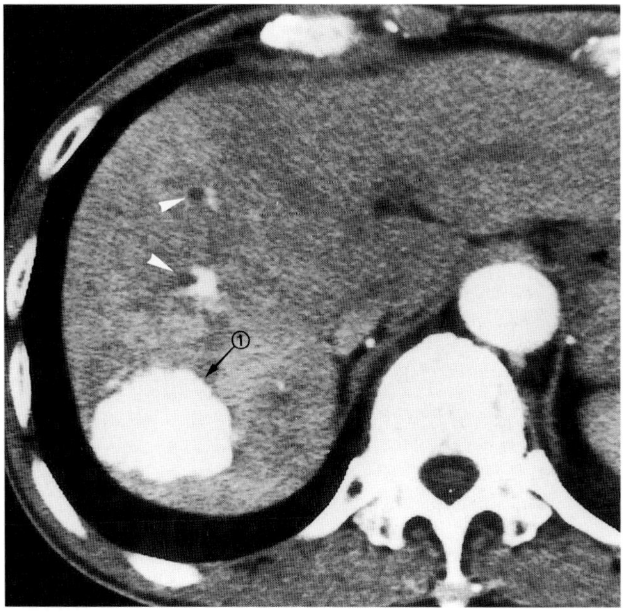

(a) Dynamic CT (tumor in $S^{VIII-VII}$ after PTPE and Lipiodol-TAE): a 4 cm mass retaining Lipiodol is seen in $S^{VIII-VII}$ (1). The portal vein has already been occluded by PTPE, and portal branches are seen as low-density areas (▶) accompanied by reopened arterial branches.

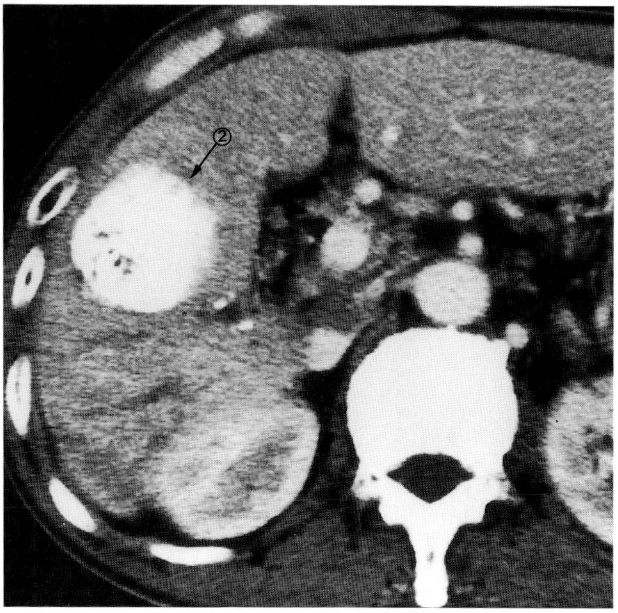

(b) Dynamic CT [tumor in S^{VI}, a slice caudal to (a)]: a 4.5 cm mass with good Lipiodol retention (2) is seen in S^{VI}.

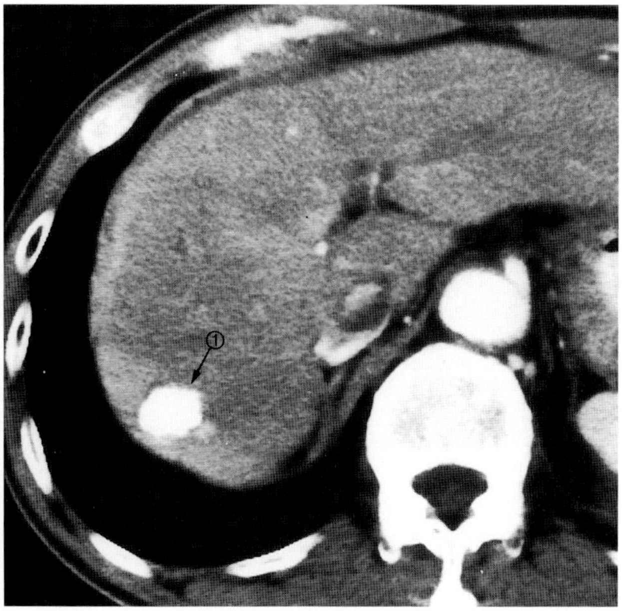

(c) Dynamic CT ($S^{VIII-VII}$, 9 months later): tumor (1) has shrunk to 2 cm.

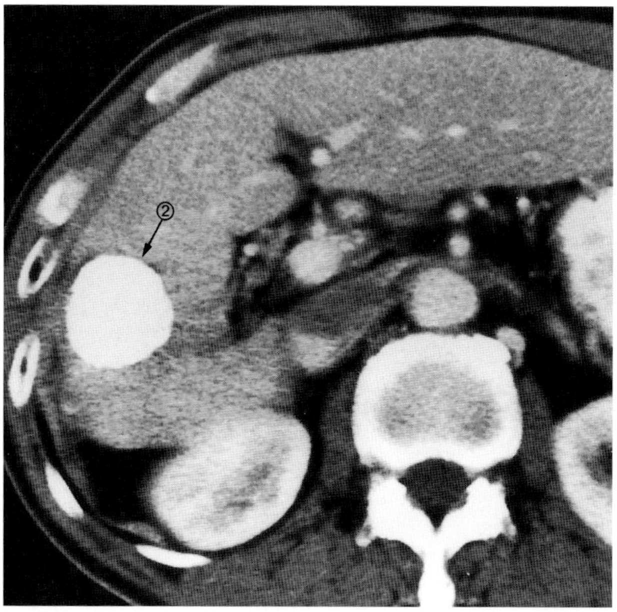

(d) Dynamic CT [S^{VI}, a slice caudal to (c)]: tumor (2) has also shrunk to 3 cm.

Combined therapy—Case 2: Early intrahepatic metastases as a result of PTPE without TAE. Liver metastasis from gastric cancer. Hepatic resection was scheduled for the multiple lesions in the right lobe, and PTPE of the right portal vein was carried out without TAE.

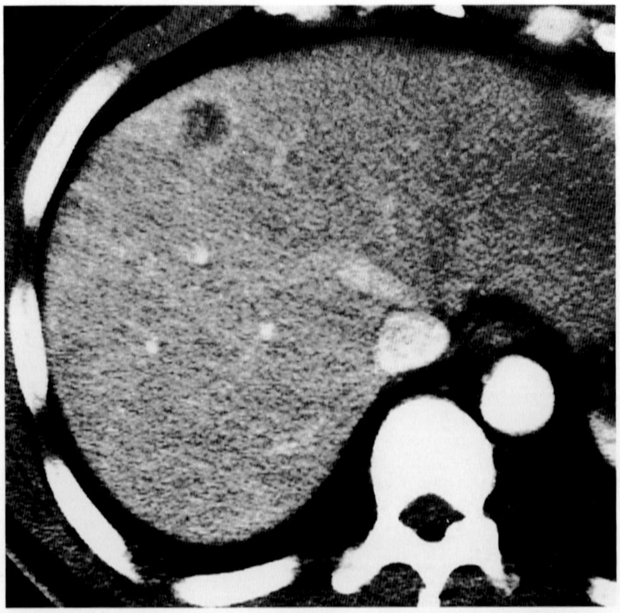

(a) Dynamic CT (before PTPE): one mass was seen on the Cantlie line before PTPE.

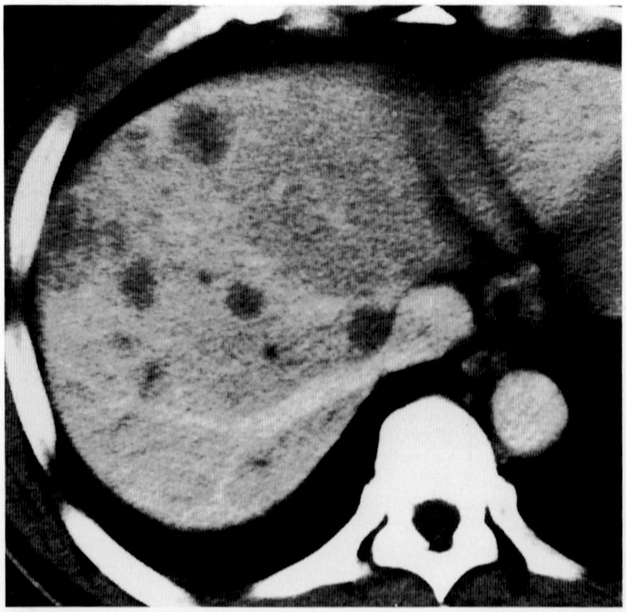

(b) Dynamic CT (15 days after PTPE): the same level slice as (a) now shows multiple new metastatic lesions as low-density areas beside embolized portal vein branches.

19.3 Complications of TAE

Complications of TAE include a transient embolization syndrome such as fever, right upper quadrant pain, nausea and vomiting due to arterial occlusion, and specific troubles as a result of mislodging of embolizing material outside the liver. Attempts have to be made to avoid and minimize these complications and to manage them properly.

Gallbladder infarction

Gallbladder infarction is the most common complication of TAE when Gelfoam particles are used, whether singly or in combination with Lipiodol, although the use of Lipiodol somewhat reduced its incidence (Kuroda *et al.* 1983; Takayasu *et al.* 1985*b*) (Case 1). Acute right upper quadrant pain follows TAE, and US may demonstrate swelling of the gallbladder, as in acute cholecystitis. Depending upon the time of study, the gallbladder may be seen much shrunk as a result of mural thickening and fibrosis; in the process of gallbladder shrinkage, a tumorous protrusion of the gallbladder wall secondary to the infarct may be recognized by US, and comparison with the pre-TAE image becomes necessary. Most cases recover with a rest and fasting, but perforation into the abdominal cavity has been reported (Sato *et al.* 1986).

Bile duct necrosis

Small-sized particulate material for embolization such as Gelfoam powder (250 μm) may embolize the peribiliary arterial plexus and cause localized necrosis of the bile duct (Makuuchi *et al.* 1985*b*). A similar event may follow arterial ethanol injection (Doppman and Girton 1984). The patient develops jaundice and elevation of serum alkaline phosphatase and gamma-GTP following TAE (Case 2). Bile leakage within the liver may result from bile duct necrosis (biloma), which may be mistaken for necrosis of the lesion induced by TAE.

Liver infarct

If small-sized embolizing materials such as Gelfoam powder and Lipiodol enter the portal vein system through very fine arterio portal shunts, it will result in embolization of peripheral arteries and portal branches, and a wedge shaped infarct may occur (Case 4). A similar liver infarct could be produced when TAE and PTPE are carried out with a short interval.

Damage to the hepatic artery

When an arterial branch in the liver is occluded, the peribiliary arterial plexus enlarges in compensation (Case 5). Damage to the intima of the right or left hepatic artery causes its occlusion, and a compensatory arterial supply may come from the epicholedochal plexus. A pseudoaneurysm may develop (Long *et al.* 1980) as a result of intimal and medial damage by the catheterization procedure (Soo *et al.* 1982). Inadvertent damage to the arterial wall produces arterial occlusion and may give the same result as TAE (Takayasu *et al.* 1986*b*) (Case 6).

Splenic infarct

Gelfoam injected into the hepatic artery may regurgitate back into the splenic artery as a result of sudden changes in the hemodynamics within the celiac artery following TAE (Case 7). When a pain develops in the left flank immediately after TAE, splenic infarct should be suspected; CT will demonstrate multiple wedge-shaped low-density areas in the spleen (Takayasu *et al.* 1984*a*). The diagnosis is not difficult.

Small bowel infarct

We have seen a patient in whom Gelfoam particles entered the superior mesenteric artery that was replacing the hepatic artery, and ileus ensued (Takayasu *et al.* 1988*a*).

Others

HCC necrosis induced by TAE may rupture into the adominal cavity (Nakao *et al.* 1988). HCC may undergo sarcomatous changes histologically following TAE and arterial chemotherapy (Kakizoe *et al.* 1987). The superior adrenal artery that branches off the right inferior phrenic artery may be embolized when embolization of the latter is carried out (Takayasu *et al.* 1988*a*) (Case 9). In one report, a transient paralysis of the lower extremities developed as a result of embolization of the vertebral artery coming off the intercostal artery (Uchino *et al.* 1987). Therefore, special precautions are required in TAE of the intercostal artery. The embolizing material may spill over into the aorta and embolize the kidney (Tegmeyer *et al.* 1977) and the inferior mesenteric artery. Irrespective of the embolizing material, some patients develop an ulcer in the stomach and duodenum due to stress. Embolizing material may also embolize a gastric artery and results in a deep ulcer resistant to treatment. Therefore, it is our practice to prescribe drugs for ulcers after TAE.

Complication of TAE—Case 1: Gallbladder infarct due to cystic artery embolization. A 65-year-old man.

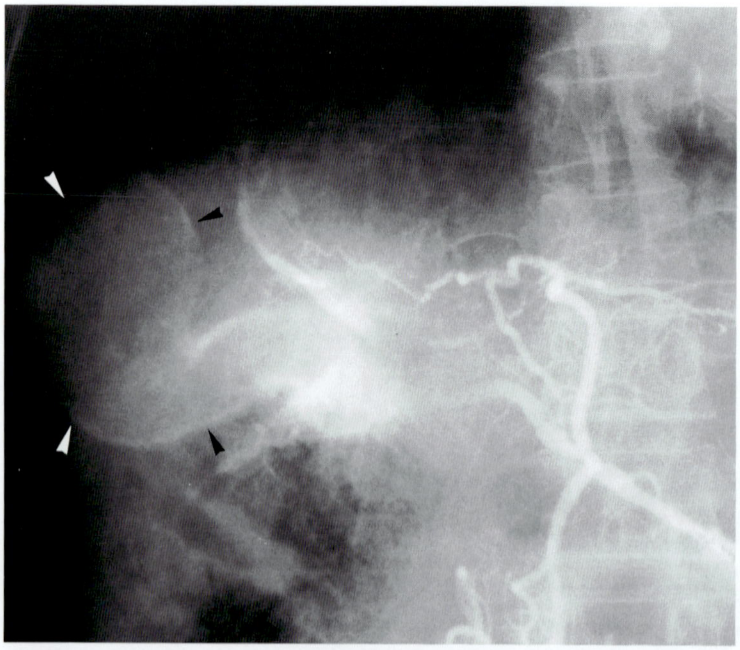

(a) Celiac arteriogram (immediately after TAE): Gelfoam sponge particles alone were injected into the right hepatic artery for an HCC in S^{VIII}. This celiac arteriogram made immediately after TAE shows complete occlusion of the right hepatic artery and the cystic artery. The gallbladder is silhouetted (▶) by the contrast medium remaining in the gallbladder wall.

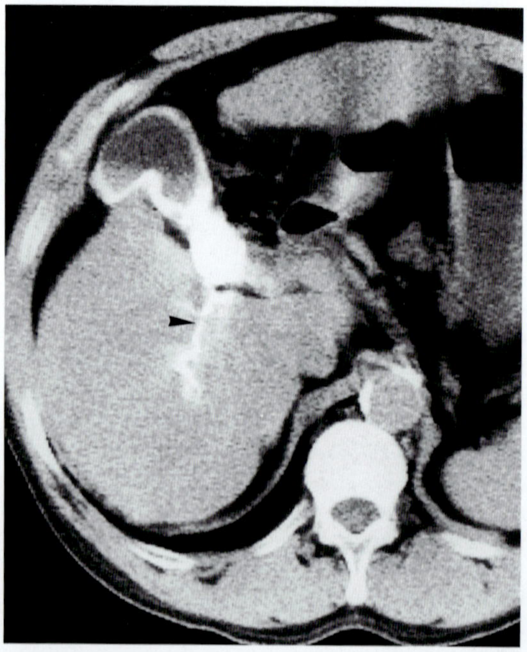

(b) Plain CT (immediately after TAE): the patient complained of right upper quadrant pain, and the gallbladder wall was clearly seen with retained contrast medium. ▶, completely occluded right posterior hepatic artery.

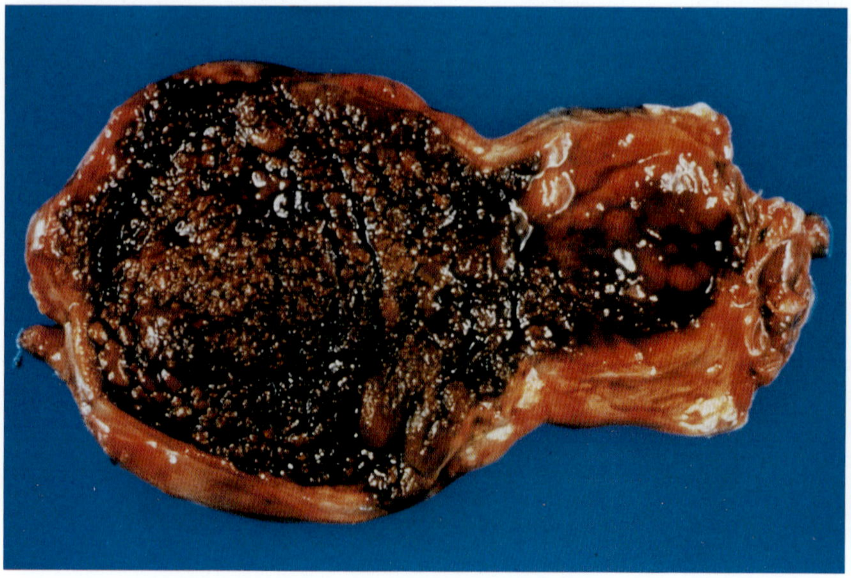

(c) Removed gallbladder, opened: the gallbladder wall was thickened, firm, and atrophied. The mucosa was dark red, and showed coagulation necrosis. Several black stones were found (not shown).

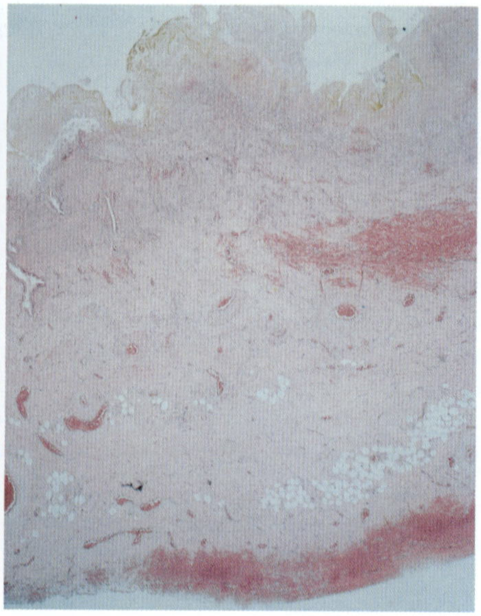

(d) Histopathology: the gallbladder was necrotic and replaced by fibrous tissue.

Complication of TAE—Case 2: Bile duct necrosis caused by Gelfoam powder. A 47-year-old man. TAE using Gelfoam powder was carried out from the proper hepatic artery for an HCC in S^{VIII}. Subsequently, serum alkaline phosphatase, gamma-GTP, and LAP were progressively elevated reaching peak levels three to four times normal in 1 month.

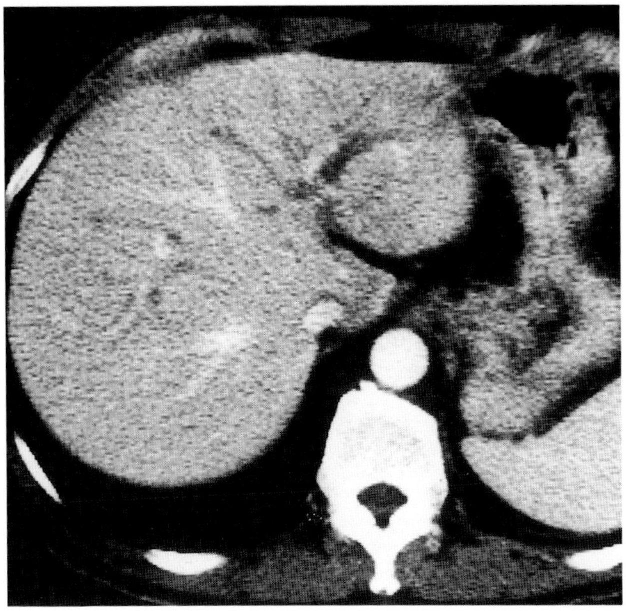

(a) Enhanced CT (1 week after TAE): bile duct dilatation not seen before TAE is now evident. A wedge-shaped infarct is also seen cranial to this slice (not shown).

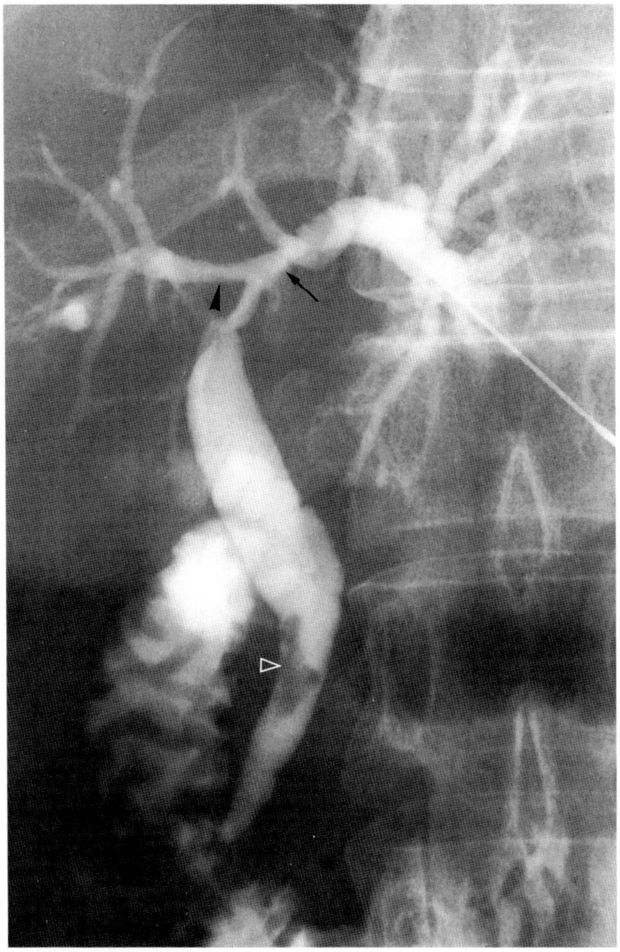

(b) PTC (1 week after TAE): stenosis (→) of the left hepatic duct and dilatation of its peripheral branches are seen. The right hepatic bile duct is also narrowed (▶). There is a filling defect in the common bile duct inferiorly (▷). On histological examination, it was a necrotic material associated with bile sediments.

Complication of TAE—Case 3: Intrahepatic bile duct necrosis mistaken for a new lesion during repeated TAEs. A 66-year-old man. TAE with Gelfoam powder was carried out for multiple HCCs in S^{IV}, three sessions in 3 months. He was referred to us because of re-elevation of serum AFP.

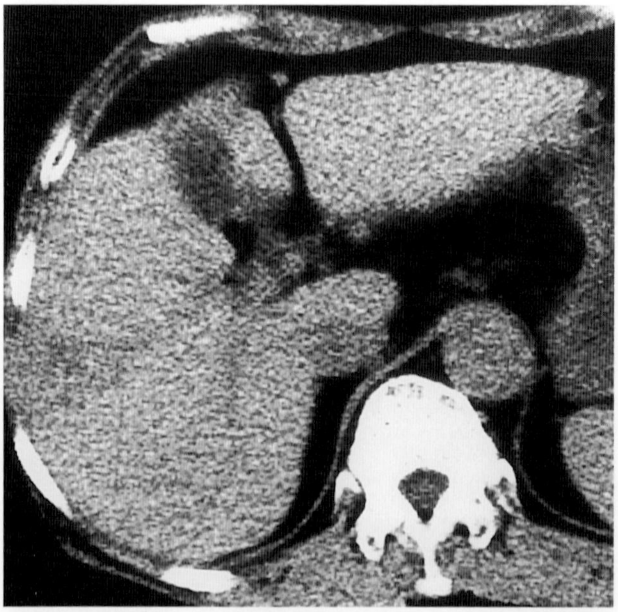

(a) Plain CT (76 days after the last TAE): beside the lesions in S^{IV}, a wedge-shaped low-density lesion is now seen in S^{V}.

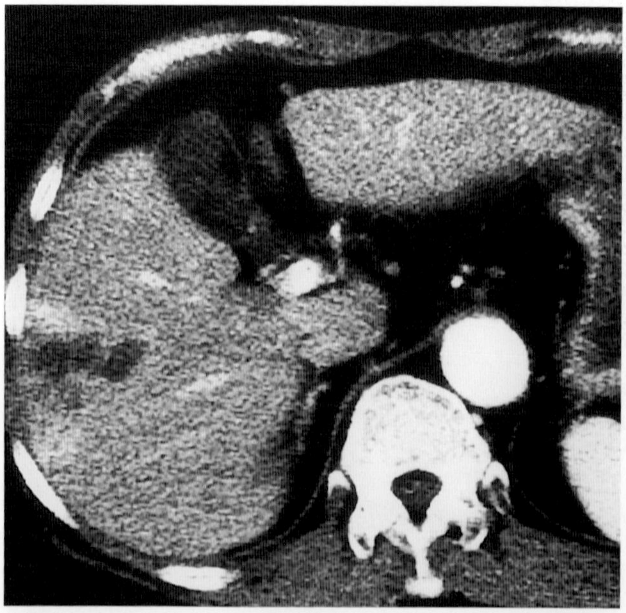

(b) Enhanced CT [early phase, same day as (a)]: the periphery of this lesion is enhanced.

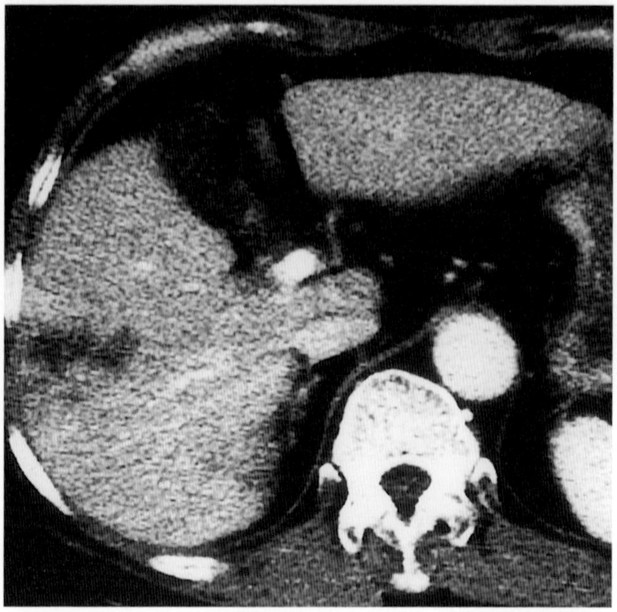

(c) Enhanced CT (mid-phase).

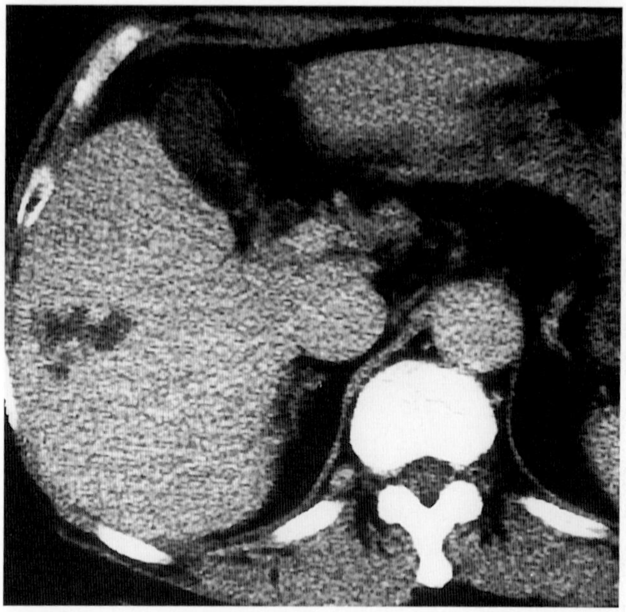

(d) Enhanced CT (late phase): a worm-shaped low-density lesion is now clearly discerned. It was assumed that this lesion not found earlier underwent necrosis responding to repeated TAE.

Case 3 (contd.)

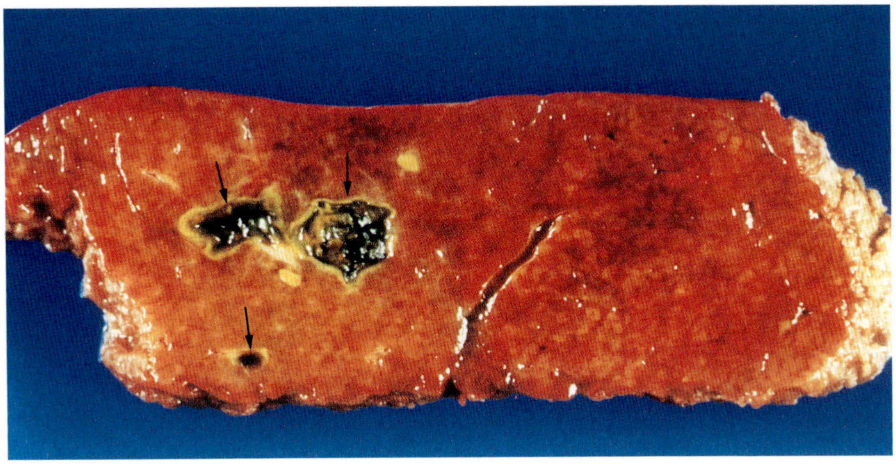

(e) Cut section of resected specimen: the S^{V} lesion thought to be a tumor turned out to be a biloma (→) due to bile leakage as a result of bile duct necrosis. The blood vessels, bile duct, and supporting tissue in the same portal tract were also necrotic. The diagnosis was bile duct necrosis induced by Gelfoam powder. The original lesions in S^{IV} were necrotized, but there were many minute metastases consisting of viable cancer cells (same as Case 14, p.515).

Complication of TAE—Case 4: Liver infarct caused by TAE with Gelfoam powder.

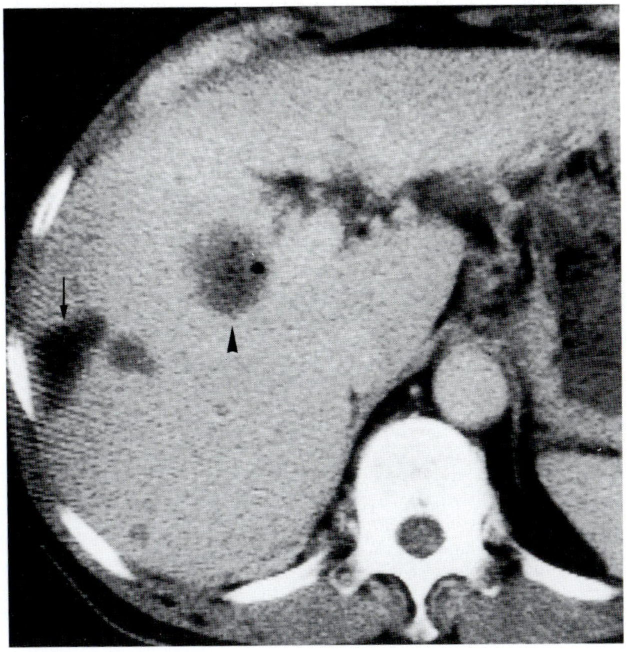

(a) Plain CT: adequate antitumor effect was obtained by TAE using Gelfoam powder (▶), but a characteristic wedge-shaped infarct (→) also resulted.

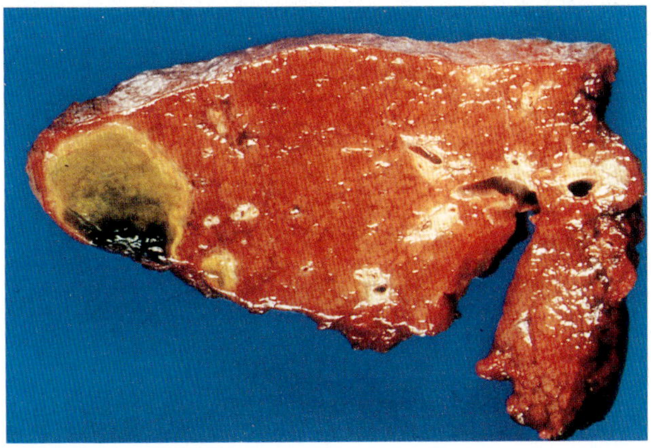

(b) Cut section of resected specimen: the infarcted area was yellow green with coagulation necrosis and the liver surface over it was depressed.

Complication of TAE—Case 5: Damage to the hepatic artery.

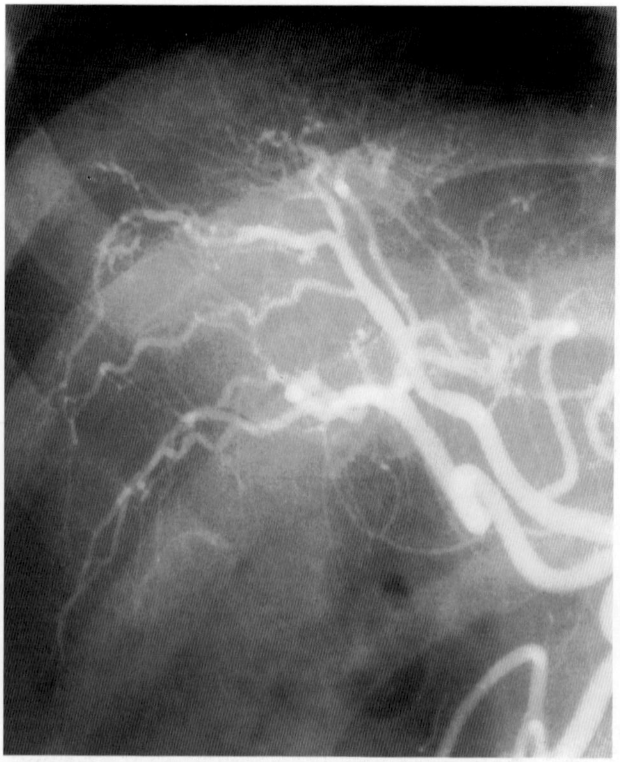

(a) Hepatic arteriogram (before TAE): due to underlying cirrhosis, arteries are winding and bending.

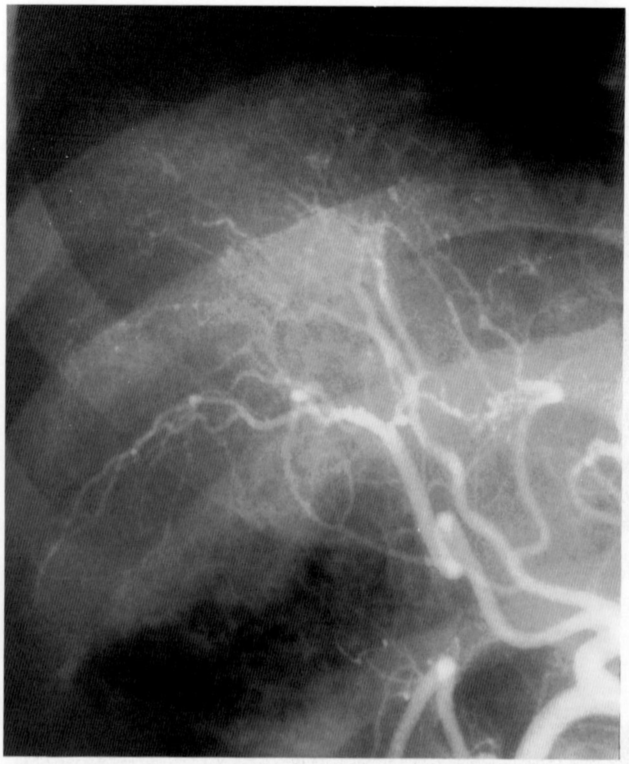

(b) Hepatic arteriogram (28 days after TAE): arteriography was repeated after TAE in which small particles of Gelfoam sponge were used. The A^{VIII} artery shows interruptions and stenoses. There are also many fine vessels connecting the interrupted arteries.

Complication of TAE—Case 6: Marked necrosis of HCC induced by iatrogenic damage to the hepatic artery.

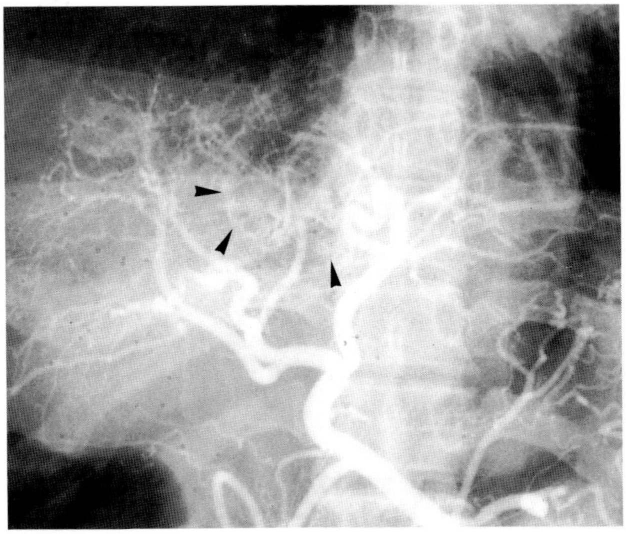

(a) Hepatic arteriogram: a hypervascular tumor is seen in S^{IV} (▶).

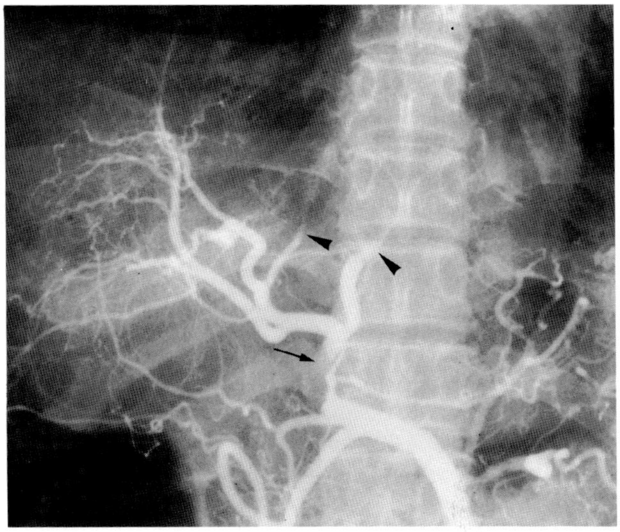

(b) Hepatic arteriogram (immediately after intimal damage): when the catheter was advanced towards the periphery for the purpose of TAE, it caused severe subintimal damage in the proper hepatic artery (→). An interruption is also seen in the left and middle hepatic arteries (▶).

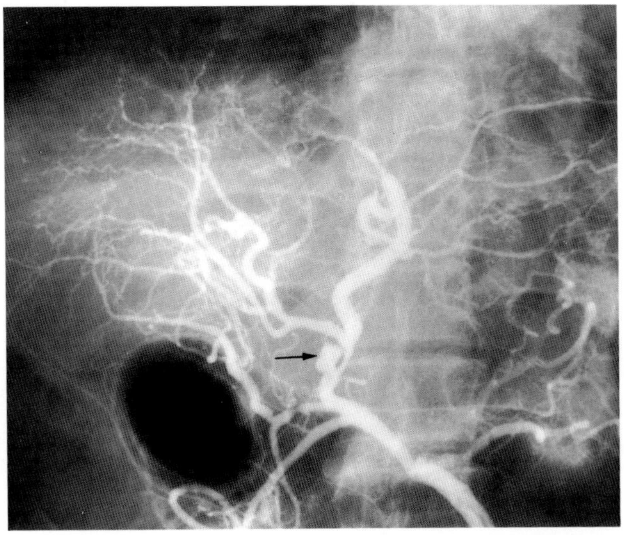

(c) Hepatic arteriogram [26 days after (b)]: reopening of the proper hepatic artery and an aneurysm (→) are recognized. No more tumor stain is seen in S^{IV}.

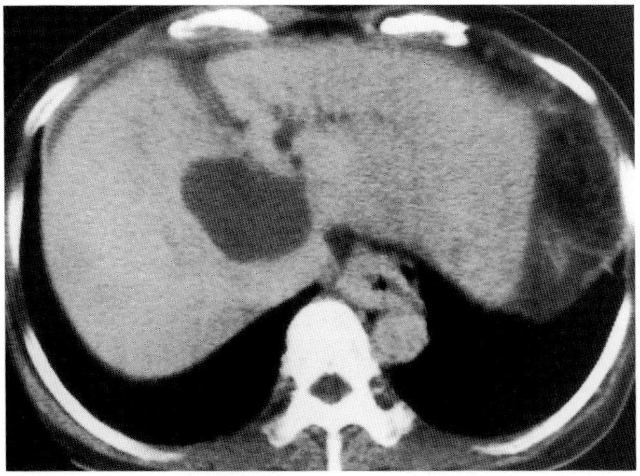

(d) Enhanced CT [same time as (c)]: a cystic unenhanced lesion is seen in $S^{IV-VIII}$, and dilated bile ducts in the left lobe are apparent. As no CT was made before the first arteriography (a), it could not be determined whether the cystic lesion was a pre-existing cyst or necrosis of HCC induced by hepatic artery damage. Needle biopsy yielded only necrotic tissue.

The patient died 2.5 years later due to hepatic failure. Autopsy disclosed the cystic lesion to consist of liquefied necrosis and coagulation necrosis, and histologically only very few viable HCC cells were seen outside the fibrous capsule.

Complication of TAE—Case 7: Splenic infarct. TAE was carried out for mutiple recurrent lesions in the remnant liver using Gelfoam sponge particles + Adriamycin. During the procedure under fluoroscopy, sponge particles were seen regurgitating into the splenic artery.

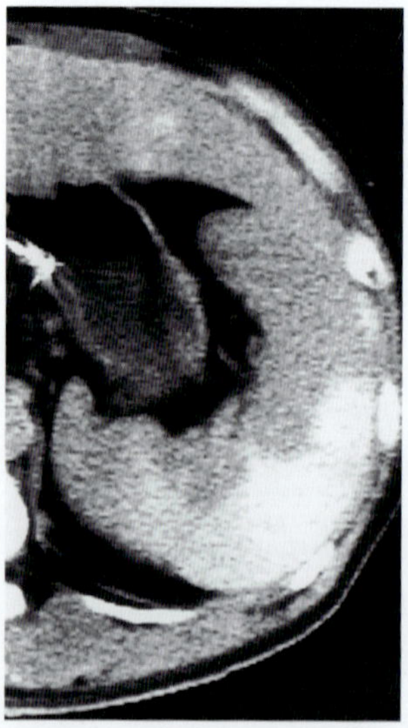

(a) Plain CT (immediately after TAE): a wedge-shaped high-density area is seen in the spleen.

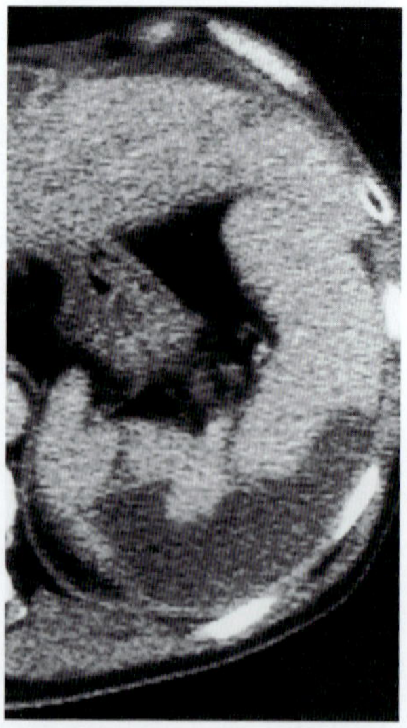

(b) Enhanced CT (7 days after TAE): a wedge-shaped low-density area is seen subcapsularly.

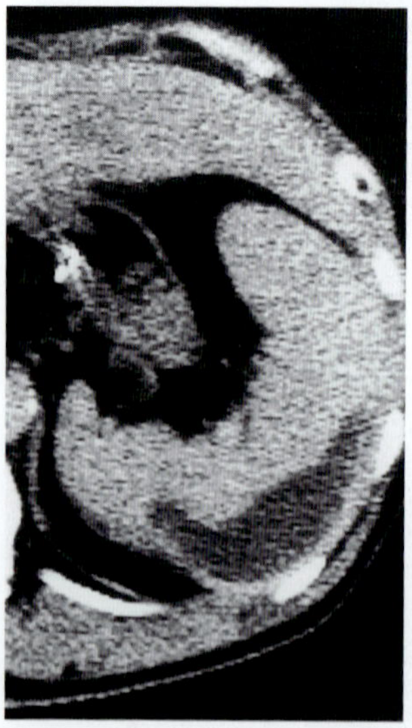

(c) Enhanced CT (34 days after TAE): the infarct is becoming smaller.

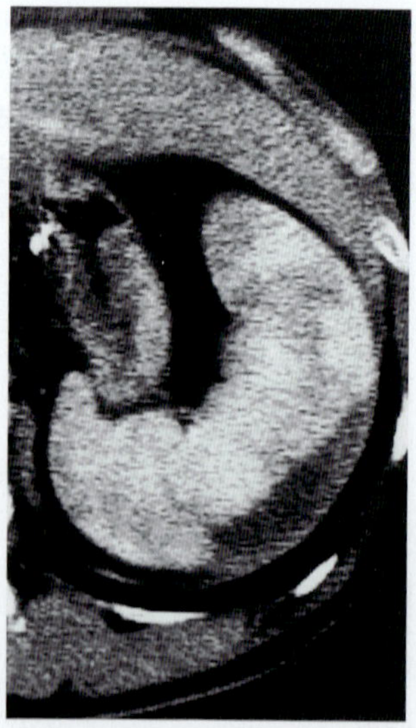

(d) Enhanced CT (3 months after TAE): the infarct has been reduced further in size.

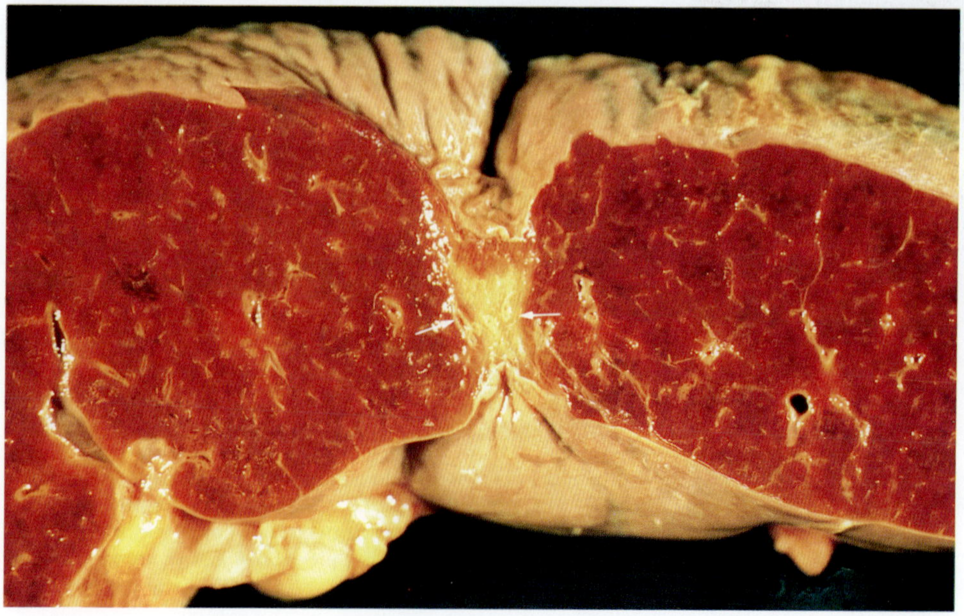

(e) The spleen at autopsy: the surface had an indentation, and the cut surface showed a firm scar (→).

Complication of TAE—Case 8: Small bowel infarct iatrogenically induced by TAE through the right hepatic artery replaced by a superior mesenteric arterial branch.

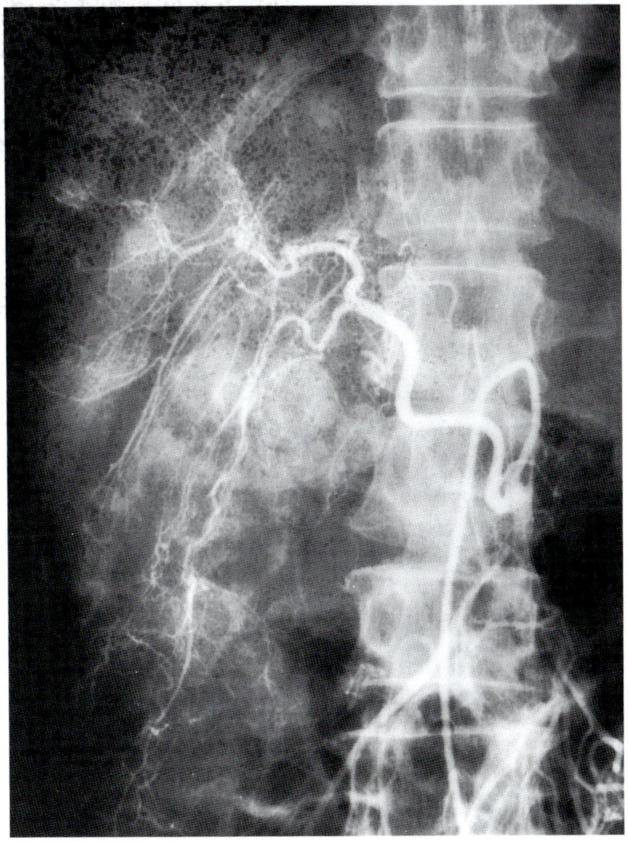

(a) Hepatic arteriogram: contrast medium was injected into the right hepatic artery coming from the superior mesenteric artery, disclosing multiple HCCs in the right lobe. Gelfoam sponge particles and Mitomycin C (10 mg) were injected for TAE. Some sponge particles were seen flowing into the superior mesenteric artery.

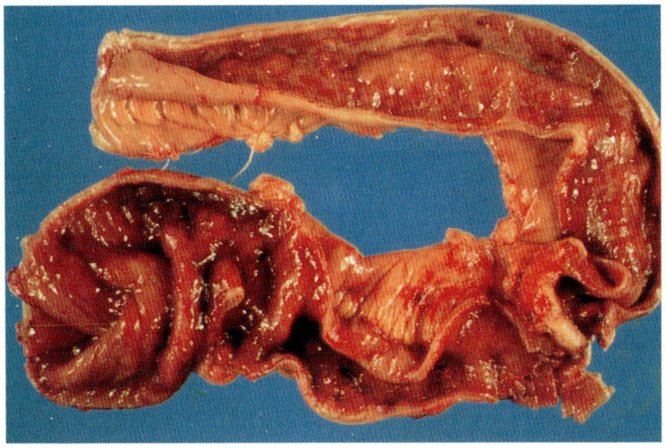

(b) Resected ileum: the patient complained of right lower abdominal pain after TAE, and the test for occult blood in the feces was positive for two days. Ileus then developed. The abdomen was opened and ileum near its end was resected for a length of 30 cm, and extended right hepatectomy was carried out. The patient lived for 2 years postoperatively.

Compication of TAE—Case 9: Adrenal infarct induced by TAE of the inferior phrenic artery.

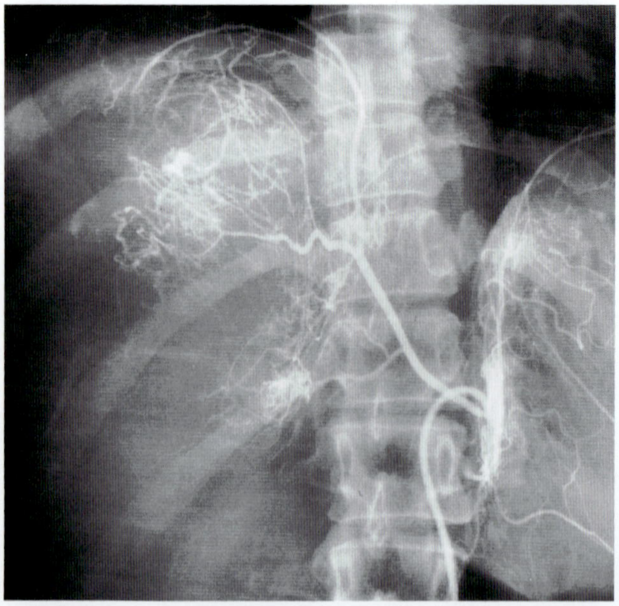

(a) Bilateral inferior phrenic arteriogram: the right inferior phrenic artery was one of the feeding arteries of large metastatic cancer occupying the right lobe. It was embolized with Gelfoam sponge particles and Adriamycin.

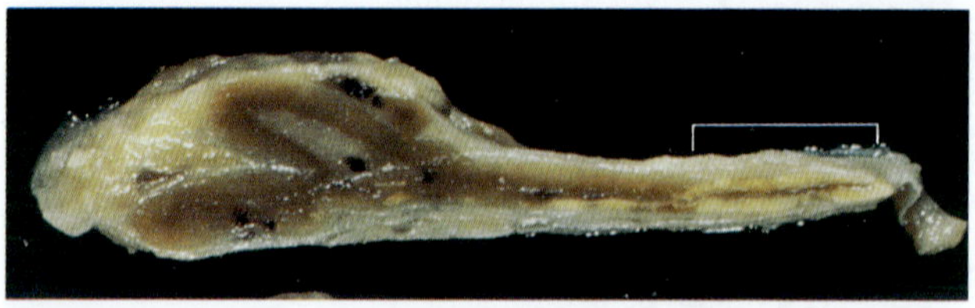

(b) The adrenal at autopsy (1.5 months after TAE): the patient died from hepatic failure, and was autopsied. A coagulation necrosis (└─┘) was found in the cranial one-third of the right adrenal.

19.4 Complications of PTPE

Complications of PTPE are uncommon. However, we had one patient in whom a thrombus formed in the portal trunk following PTPE.

Complication of PTPE—Case 1: Thrombus formation in the portal trunk following PTPE.

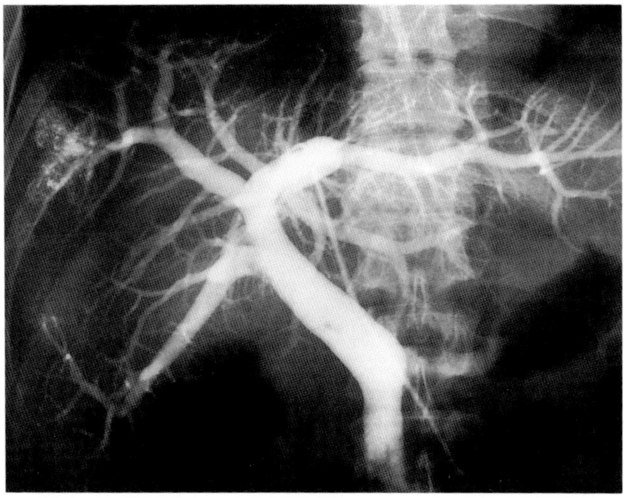

(a) PTP (before PTPE, anterior view).

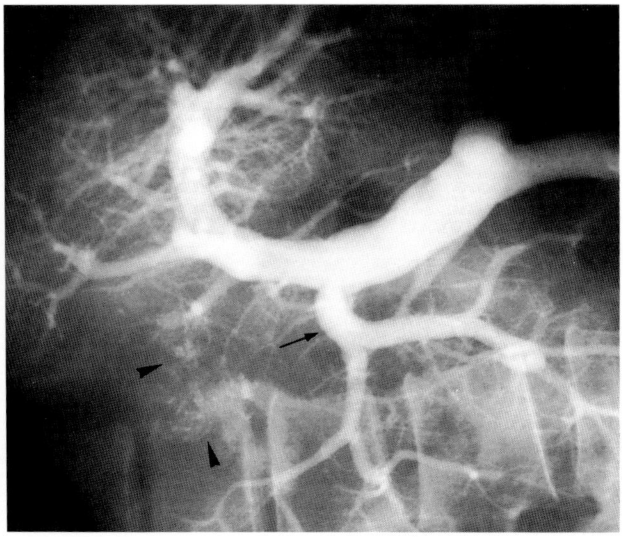

(b) PTP (before PTPE, right lateral view): as the Lipiodol-containing tumor (▶) was in the right posterior segment, only the posterior portal vein (→) was embolized.

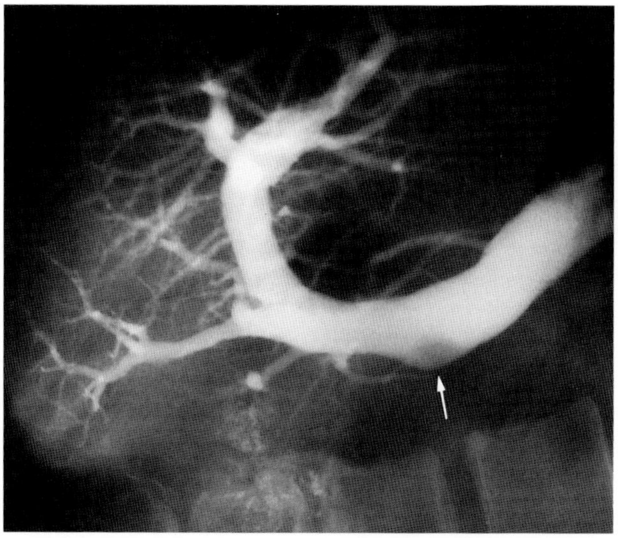

(c) PTP (PTP was repeated 1 week after PTPE, right lateral view): a filling defect is seen at the beginning of the right posterior portal vein protruding into the portal trunk (→, thrombus).

19.5 Complications due to an indwelling catheter in the hepatic artery

An indwelling catheter in the hepatic artery is increasingly used for repeated or continuous administration of anticancer drugs for inoperable HCC and metastatic liver cancer. Previously, the catheter was placed operatively, but more recently, it has been passed through the femoral or subclavian artery into the hepatic artery and the drugs are periodically injected through a reservoir (port) implanted subcutaneously. Complications due to the indwelling catheter and repeated injections of drugs are also increasing, such as collapse of the hepatic artery and subsequent mislodging of Gelfoam particles (splenic infarct) or transit of the drug into non-hepatic organs (such as the spleen) causing infarct and ulcers of the GI tract (Chuang *et al.* 1981). Anticancer drugs may also cause arteritis, hence bile duct necrosis (Case 1) and obstructive jaundice (Botet *et al.* 1985; Pien *et al.* 1985). Such jaundice has to be differentiated from parenchymal jaundice. We have recently seen several cases of portal vein obstruction (thrombosis) (Takayasu *et al.* 1990*d*). One has to be aware of these complications. Injection of ^{99m}Tc-macroaggregated albumin (MAA) through the catheter is a useful diagnostic procedure that will determine the patency of the hepatic artery and flow distribution within the liver. Angio-CT with a catheter is also helpful.

Complication due to an indwelling hepatic artery catheter—Case 1: Sclerosing cholangitis caused by arterial injection of anticancer drugs through an indwelling catheter. A 34-year-old man. A catheter was placed in the gastroduodenal artery by laparotomy for an advanced hepatic metastasis from sigmoid colon cancer, and 6 mg of MMC and 500 mg of 5FU were administered by a subcutaneously implanted infusion pump once a week. The patient developed jaundice at the time when 70 mg of MMC and 7750 mg of 5FU had been given.

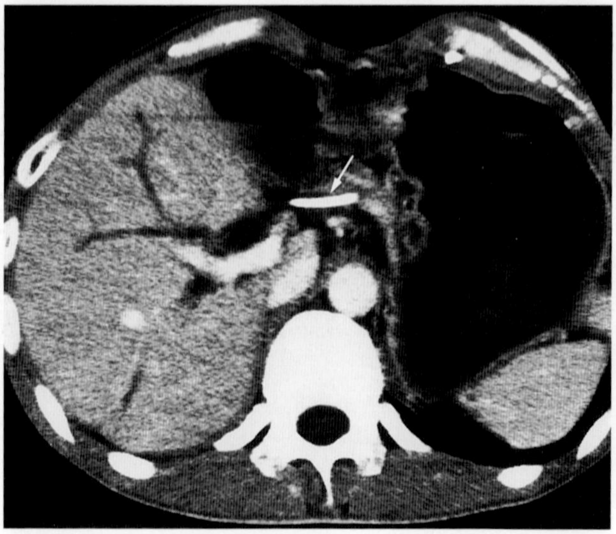

(a) Dynamic CT: moderate dilatation of intrahepatic bile ducts is seen. The metastatic lesion did not enlarge during the treatment. →, indwelling catheter.

Case 1 (contd.)

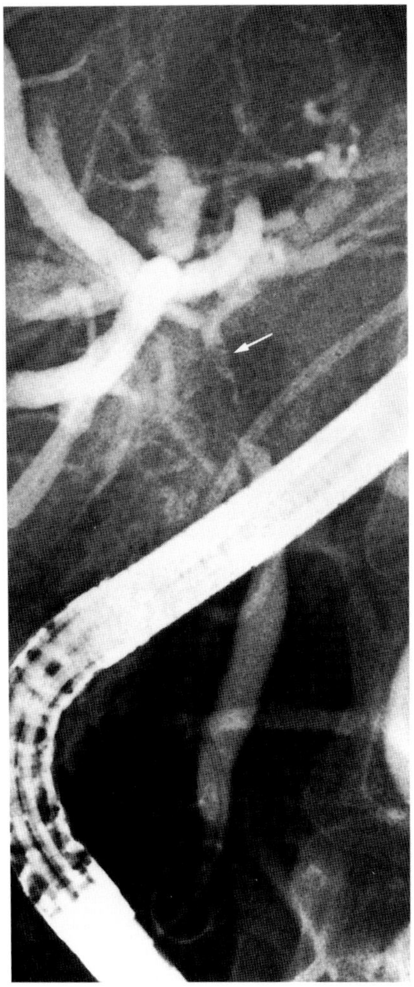

(b) ERC: stenosis is seen in the common hepatic duct (→), and the left and right hepatic ducts. The peripheral bile ducts are dilated.

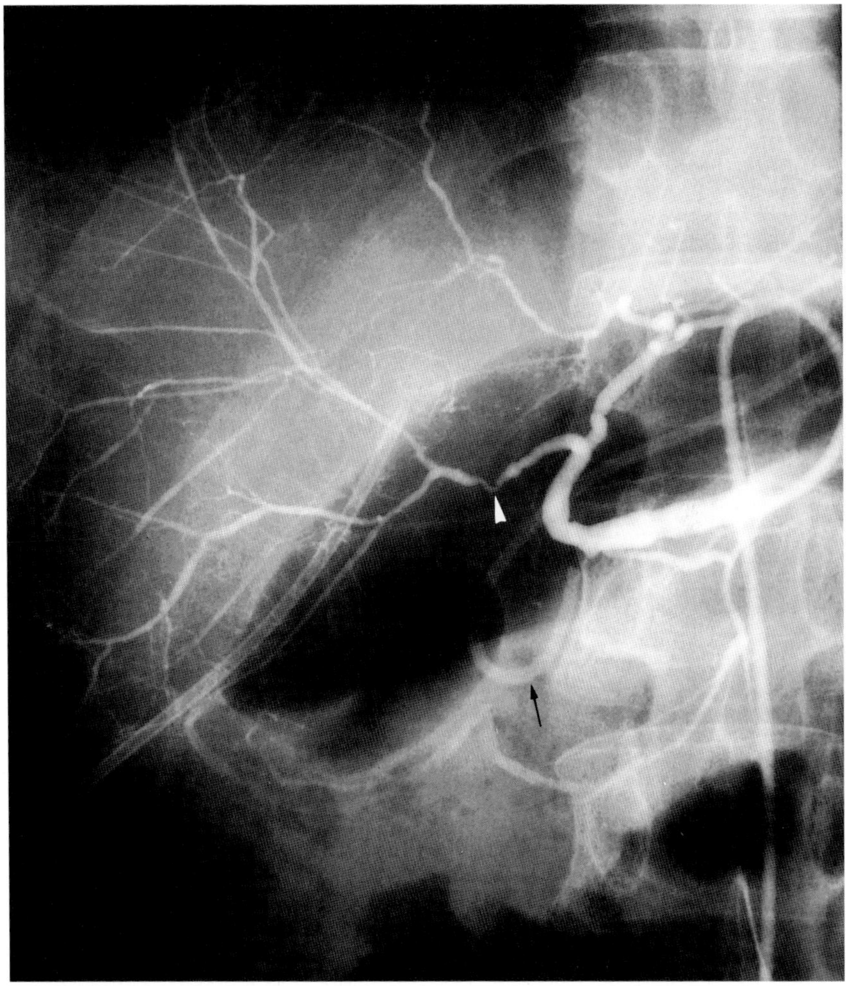

(c) Hepatic arteriogram: the right hepatic artery is narrowed and hardened (▶) from its origin toward the right anterior and posterior arteries. The diagnosis was arteritis due to the anticancer agents and subsequent sclerosing cholangitis. It improved after cessation of medication and administration of steroids. →, tip of the catheter placed in the gastroduodenal artery.

Complication due to an indwelling hepatic artery catheter—Case 2: Portal thrombosis due to arterial injection of anticancer drugs through an indwelling catheter. In this patient, hepatic metastasis from a transverse colon carcinoma was found. Resection of the transverse colon and hepatic artery catheterization were carried out. Arterial injection was discontinued because of anemia at 7 months when a total of 7550 mg of 5FU and 72 mg of MMC had been given.

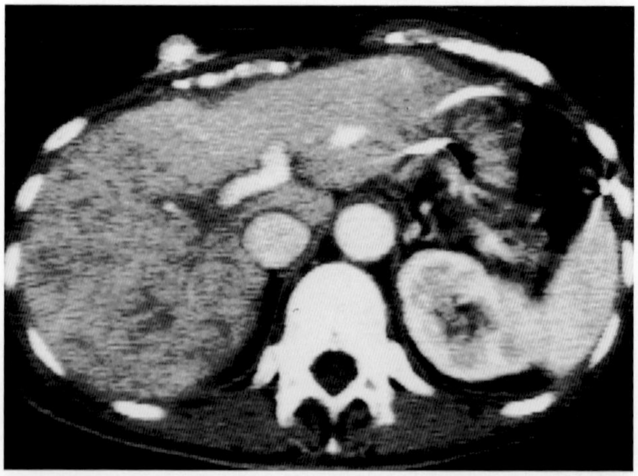

(a) Enhanced CT (7 months after treatment): the right lobe to the right of the Cantlie line is enhanced inhomogeneously, and the branches of the right portal vein seen in the pretreatment CT(b) are no longer opacified. Since there was no increase in arterial flow compensating for the reduced portal venous flow, damage to the right hepatic artery was suspected. Total bilirubin was elevated to 1.7 mg/dl, but alkaline phosphatase remained normal.

For the explanation of portal thrombosis, the possibility of transit of anticancer agents into the portal vein through small intrahepatic arteries and inflammation of the portal vein that ensued was entertained (cf. Fig. 1.36, p.25).

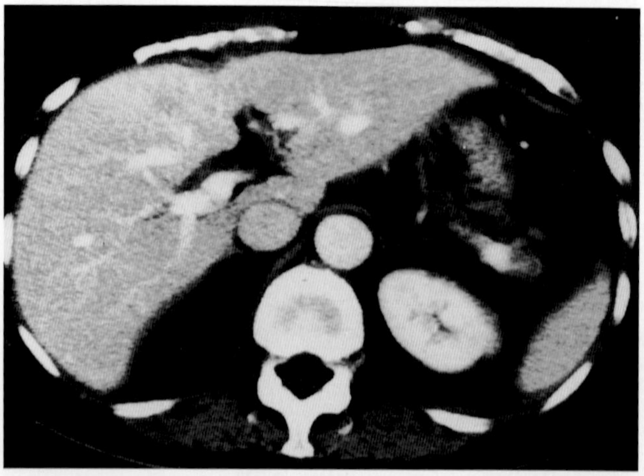

(b) Enhanced CT (pretreatment): both lobes are enhanced homogenously with patent right and left portal veins.

20

Surgical treatment

Among non-systemic treatments, surgery for HCC would be the most efficacious were it not for postoperative recurrence. Cirrhosis, a preneoplastic state, exists in more then 80 per cent of patients, and tumorigenesis is often multicentric, making the therapy very difficult. Currently, operation is deemed safe in patients of clinical stage I (no ascites, bilirubin < 2 mg/dl, albumin > 3.5 g, 15 min ICG retention < 15 per cent, and prothrombin > 80 per cent) and a cancer stage of 2 or less. In patients in a more advanced stage, the extent of resection is carefully estimated from the expected remnant liver function (Okamoto *et al.* 1984). The analysis of prognosis of 427 HCC cases excluding operative and hospital deaths who underwent resection at the National Cancer Center Hospital, Tokyo, after 1972 showed the 1-year, 3-year, 5-year and 10-year survivals to be 82.9 per cent, 57.0 per cent, 40.6 per cent and 22.7 per cent, respectively (Yamasaki *et al.* 1991). Purely surgical results are difficult to assess, and were perhaps lower than these figures because many of them underwent interventional treatments such as TAE, for recurrence (Sasaki *et al.* 1987; Takayasu *et al.* 1989*e*, 1992*d*).

The frequency of re resections for recurrence (Nagasue *et al.* 1986; Lange *et al.* 1989) may have been somewhat reduced because of the development of TAE and percutaneous ethanol injection (PEI) (see Chapter 21). Small lesions not seen by preoperative imaging may be found by intraoperative US (Makuuchi *et al.* 1987*a*; Makuuchi *et al.* 1991), and even intraoperative US may miss small lesions which MR imaging can pick up. Efforts are being made by surgeons not to miss such lesions during the operation.

A new but imminent problem is the identification and differentiation of early HCC and dysplactic nodules (still called adenomatous hyperplasia in Japan). Histological distinction of preneoplastic lesions already committed and those not yet committed to transform is extremely important, but has not yet been achieved. Some recent imaging studies aimed at such differential diagnosis with limited success (Takayasu *et al.* 1989*a*, 1995*a*; Matsui *et al.* 1989, 1990; Kudo *et al.* 1992*a*, *b*).

An absolute cure is possible only with liver transplantation for a small HCC carried out before extrahepatic metastasis has taken place (Iwatsuki *et al.* 1988). However, in countries where HCC is endemic, potential recipents far outnumber donors. The surgical results have been much improved in recent years in Japan with a remarkable reduction in operative deaths due mainly to more accurate diagnosis and estimation of remnant liver function (Okuda *et al.* 1980; Liver Cancer Study Group of Japan 1990). From the point of view of a radiologist and an internist, more frequent reduction surgery seems desirable in which a large mass is resected together with several small secondaries. There are no non-surgical approaches to a large cancer, a tumor thrombus around the first-order portal vein, and metastases to the adrenal and lymph nodes, and a more positive surgical strategy is needed.

Imaging diagnosis and operability

Staging of liver cancer is possible by preoperative imaging, utilizing various modalities. Determination of the T factor is possible (Takayasu *et al.* 1990*f*) in more than 90 per cent of the cases with conventional dynamic CT, US, and sometimes with additional portal-CT and Lipiodol-CT. Portal vein tumor thrombosis can be diagnosed with relative ease in the second- or higher-order central branches of the portal vein. For the assessment of the N factor, CT excels other modalities, and assessment of the M factor can be made with a combination of US, CT, MR imaging, bone scintigraphy, and chest radiograph.

Operability of HCC that has a tumor thrombus in the second-order portal branch

In the past, diagnosis of patency of the second-order portal branch depended on portal phase of angiography. In other words, tumor thrombosis was suspected when a second-order portal branch was not opacified clearly in the portogram. Based on past experience of having frequent postoperative recurrence, resection was not indicated in such patients at our cancer center hospital. However, with the advent of US and CT, we now can determine the nature of the changes along the portal vein up to the second-order branches, and surgical management of portal thrombosis has to be reassessed.

In Case 1, tumor thrombosis of the right posterior portal vein was diagnosed preoperatively, and during the operation a tumor thrombus was found in the right hepatic vein. Resection of the right lobe encompassing these tumor thrombi was carried out. The patient is still living five years postoperatively. We have another case in whom tumor thrombosis of the inferior right hepatic vein was found by intraoperative US, and a similar resection was carried out. He is still alive 10 years after the operation. These experiences suggest that intrahepatic vascular invasion does not always suggest a poor prognosis (Fujii *et al.* 1993).

Resectability of a mass in close proximity to a large blood vessel, and utility of the inferior right hepatic vein for extended hepatectomy

The spatial relationship betwen the carcinoma and the portal vein, hepatic vein and the inferior vena cava can be determined with US and CT. However, resectability varies with the nature

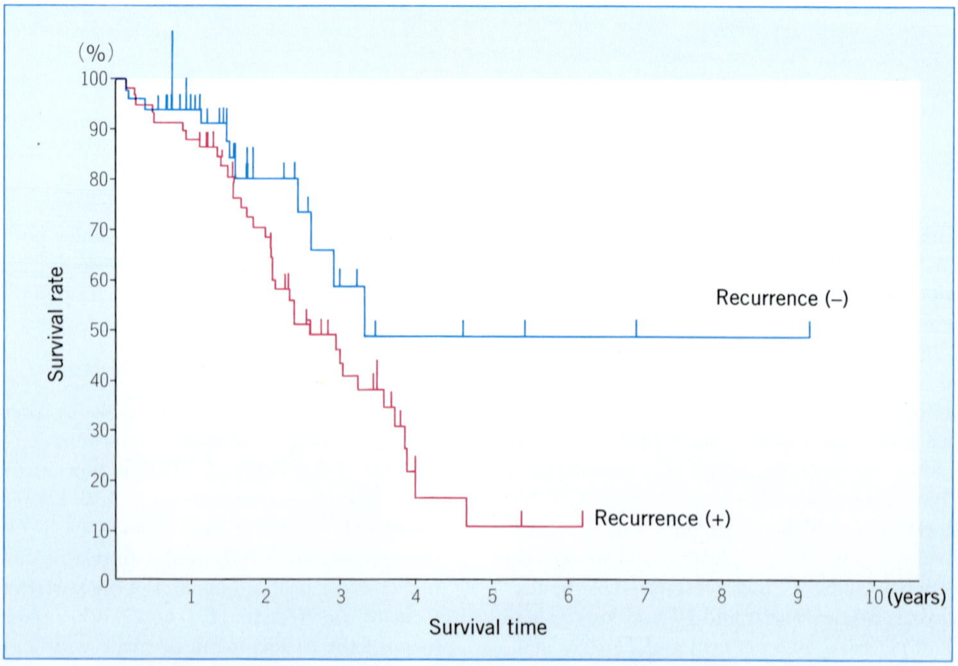

Fig. 20.1 Prognosis in patients with (n = 58) and without (n = 49) postoperative recurrence.

of tumor, such as HCC (Case 2) and adenocarcinoma (bile duct carcinoma and adenocarcinoma metastatic to the liver, Case 3), even though the mass is close to a large vessel. Therefore, quality diagnosis of the mass is important, because HCC grows in an expanding fashion and may readily be detached from the vessel during operation, whereas an adenocarcinoma tends to infiltrate into the vascular wall and is difficult to separate, making resection impossible in most instances. Most large carcinomas occupying $S^{VIII-VII-IV}$ invade the right hepatic vein, necessitating resection of this vein. Under such circumstances, the operative technique of Makuuchi *et al.* (1987*b*) in which the inferior right hepatic vein is kept as a drainage vein for the posterior segment is a good one based on anatomical considerations (Case 4).

Cases in which resection is difficult because of the anatomical location, despite small tumor size

There are cases in which the tumor is small but located at the origin of the portal vein or the hepatic vein; its removal requires extensive resection of non-cancerous parenchyma. For a liver with a low functional reserve, this is not possible (Case 5). If a small lesion is deep seated separate from the main mass which is close to the surface and resectable, the former may be treated by PEI intraoperatively (Case 6).

Postoperative recurrence in the remnant liver

Of the 123 patients in whom HCC smaller than 5 cm was resected between March 1977 and July 1985 at the National Cancer Center Hospital, Tokyo, 107, excluding operative deaths, those with a positive margin, double cancers and deaths due to unrelated causes, were followed. Within 14.5 months postoperatively, 54 per cent of them developed recurrence (Takayasu *et al.* 1989*e*), and the survival of those without recurrence was significantly ($p < 0.02$) better in the period of four to six years postoperatively (Fig. 20.1). Clearly, postoperative recurrence is an important prognostic factor. It has already been discussed in the chapter on TAE that among recurrent cases, treatment with TAE significantly improves survival rate (Takayasu *et al.* 1992*d*).

Our multivariate analysis of prognostic factors (Takayasu *et al.* 1987*a*) has demonstrated that recurrence was more frequent in patients in whom: (1) there was more than one lesion in different segments and (2) HBsAg was negative; among those with a single lesion recurrence was more frequent when, (3) the tumor size was greater than 3 cm and (4) fibrous encapsulation was not complete (absent or incomplete capsule). In other words, recurrence is expected preoperatively to be less likely when the patient has a single encapsulated HCC smaller than 3 cm. The HBsAg status was not an important prognostic factor, because hepatitis C virus infection is more frequently involved.

The expression 'recurrence' is not a good one. At the moment, it is difficult to clearly determine whether recurrence is due to intraoperative seeding of cancer cells or a *de novo* emergence of a second primary, but both would occur according to the study on integration of viral DNA into cancer cell DNA (Esumi *et al.* 1986; Tsuda *et al.* 1988; Hsu *et al.* 1991). Recurrence with multiple lesions of similar sizes within 3 months postoperatively (Case 7) may well be due to the former mechanism while a single recurrent lesion appearing after a lapse of more than 5 years (Case 8) is more likely due to the latter. If the histology of a new lesion is very well differentiated, it is more likely to be a *de novo* emergence. Frequently, the AFP value varies between the time of the first diagnosis and that of the recurrence. A technique to prevent spread of cancer cells during operation ought to be developed.

Reduction surgery

Surgeons in general are not enthusiastic about reduction surgery, which offers little possibility of cure. However, in view of the recent progress in non surgical management such as TAE and PEI for a small HCC, we feel that a tumor greater than 10 cm should be resected even though the other lobe has a small lesion or two. It may have a life-prolonging effect (Case 9). Reduction surgery resorting to multidisciplinary therapy is to be encouraged. To expand the indications for reduction surgery, a new technique has recently been developed in which the portal vein supplying the tumor-bearing lobe is embolized by PTPE to induce atrophy of that lobe and compensatory hypertrophy of the contralateral lobe (Makuuchi *et al.* 1990). In Case 10, the operation was thought not to be indicated, but PTPE changed the situation and led to successful resection. Preoprative supplemental therapy in which PTPE is used needs further evaluation.

Surgical management of metastases to lymph nodes and distant organs

If metastases are found in lymph nodes and other organs, the cancer stage is either III or IV, and surgery is contraindicated at the moment. However, recent progress in interventional therapy now permits resection of lymph node metastasis (Case 7, distant metastasis of HCC, p.207) and a metastasis to the adrenal (Case 11) for long survival as long as the intrahepatic primary is under good control (Terpstra *et al.* 1984; Takayasu *et al.* 1989*c*). In the absence of effective interventional treatment, surgery is the best management for metastatic lesions. Therefore, a positive approach with careful assessment is desirable in patients with metastasis.

Ligation of the hepatic artery and the portal vein under laparotomy

In occasional cases, resection is found to be impossible upon opening the abdomen. In the past, this was a very common situation, and ligation of the hepatic artery (Balasagaram 1972; Nagasue *et al.* 1976) and/or the portal vein (Honjo *et al.* 1975) was then carried out. Hepatic artery ligation is immediately followed by the development of feeding arteries derived from the contralateral lobe, the epicholedochal plexus and adjacent tissues (Cases 12, and 13) annuling the therapeutic effect of arterial ligation. It is not known whether hepatopetal collaterals immediately develop following portal vein ligation. However, in one of our patients (Case 12), in whom an intrahepatic portal vein was ligated, hepatopetal flow subsequently developed in some of the pre-existing veins. In another patient (Case 13) in whom the beginning of the portal trunk was ligated, a large hepatopetal collateral developed to communicate with the intrahepatic portal veins. In either case, no antitumor effect was obtained even though both the artery and the portal vein were ligated, nor did hepatic infarct occur. It was assumed that reperfusion occurred soon after ligation.

A consideration on systematic subsegmentectomy

Systematic subsegmentectomy was developed by Makuuchi and co-workers in 1985 (Makuuchi *et al.* 1985*a*). In this technique the tumor is resected together with the feeding portal vein, based on the rationale that intrahepatic spread occurs through that portal branch. However, careful study of the resected specimens disclosed that such a spread (Case 14) is not so frequent, and that instead intrahepatic spread not expected from the portal vein anatomy is more common.

In Case 15, the preoperative diagnosis was a single HCC lesion in S^{III}, but S^{II} also had to be resected because of an inadvertent injury to the bile duct. The resected specimen when studied showed multiple 3–5 mm secondaries in S^{II}, and the resection of S^{II} which had not been scheduled proved succesful. In order for cancer cells to metastasize from the main mass in S^{III} to S^{II}, blood in P^{III} has to regurgitate to the umbilical portion of the left portal vein, and cancer cells subsequently become implanted. During the operation, a dye was injected into a branch of P^{II} in order to delineate the boundary between S^{III} and S^{II} ; all the dye regurgitated into P^{II}. It was assumed that there was a small arterio-portal shunt (regurgitation) in a branch of P^{II}. In other words, the main lesion was in S^{III} but cancer cells from it regurgitated into P^{II} for the subsequent spread in S^{II}. In fact, S^{IV} was free of metastases. It is known in portal hypertension that the flow within the portal trunk sometimes becomes to-and-fro in advanced cirrhosis. In such a liver, dislodgement of cancer cells to a distant segment is not surprising. We have seen a number of similar cases. In one patient, when HCC in S^{VIII} was resected, a tumor thrombus was found in P^{IV}, and in another the main mass was in S^{VIII}, and S^{VII} had many secondaries. It may be more reasonable to resect the target tumor in a cone shape that includes part of the neighbouring segments.

Postoperative complications, anatomical changes of the liver, and displacement of other organs following operation

Early complications within 1 month of operation include liver abscess, pleural effusion, and ascites. The most common site of abscess formation is the surgical margin (Case 16) and below the diaphgram. It may also be around the hepatoduodenal ligament. It is usually accompanied by fever that lasts for some time, and CT and US display abnormal fluid retention. However, even dynamic CT may not disclose the typical feature of abscess (mild ring stain in the periphery of the lesion), and distinction between abscess and retention of serous fluid (Case 17) or postoperative hematoma (Case 18) is difficult. If the interior shows high echoes, the possibility of abscess (Case 16) is strong, and bacterial study of the aspirate and drainage may be required. Pleural effusion is common in the right side (Case 19), and it may or may not be accompanied by ascites. Occasional cases may have pleural effusion for more than a year. The mechanism of this so called hepatic hydrothorax (Morrow *et al.* 1958) is still poorly understood. If it is due to a small hole in the diaphragm (Lieberman *et al.* 1966), a ball-bearing mechanism is operative and ascites is suctioned into the thorax (Okuda and Iio 1976). Massive effusion causes dyspnea, but this will spontaneously disappear in due time.

Marked compensatory hypertrophy of the residual (leftover) lobe occurs in 3 to 6 months after resection (Chen *et al.* 1991; Yamanaka *et al.* 1993); hypertrophy of the left lobe following right hepatectomy is particularly prominent. Hypertrophy seems to be more pronounced in a liver with a good function (Case 20). A small resection such as the removal of the left lateral area does not cause visible hypertrophy, or a hypertrophy only confined to the caudate lobe. The effects of surgery on other organs are their displacement (Letourneau *et al.* 1988). The neighbouring organs move to fill up the dead space created by resection. In the case of right hepatectomy, the right kidney and small bowel shift cranially (Case 23), and the pancreas head is displaced posteriorly. Following central bisegmentectomy, the duodenum may shift cranially for a remarkable distance (Case 24).

Surgery—Case 1: Five-year suvival after resection for an HCC with portal and hepatic vein tumor thrombosis. In this patient, a 5 × 7 cm mass and a tumor thrombus in the right posterior portal vein were detected preoperatively, and an operation was carried out. Intraoperative US further detected a tumor thrombus in the superficial right hepatic vein near the surface, and therefore the right posterior segment including the tumor thrombus was resected.

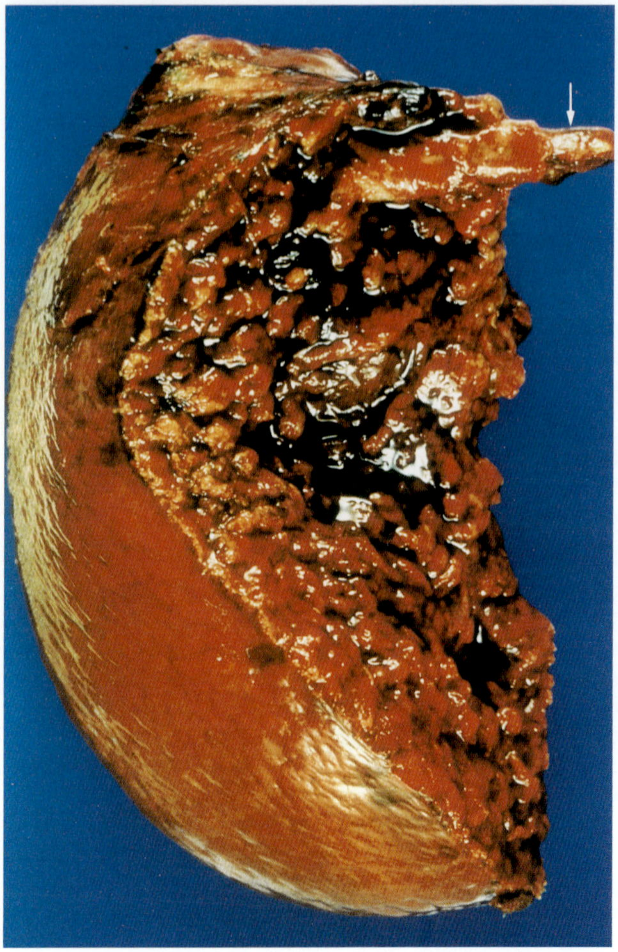

Resected specimen: a tumor thrombus in the superficial right hepatic vein protruding from the cut surface is recognized (→). The patient was well without lung metastasis up to 3.5 years postoperatively when a solitary recurrent lesion was found in S^{III} which was resected again. The AFP level of more than 200 000 ng/ml at the beginning turned negative when recurrence was found. The first tumor was Edmondson's grade III, poorly differentiated, but the recurrent lesion was moderately differentiated, grade II. Therefore, in this patient, multicentric tumorigenesis was suggested. He is still living, with normal social activities, 5 years after the first operation. Currently, there is no established surgical policy for tumor thrombosis, and expanded surgical indications seem desirable.

Surgery—Case 2: Resection of a huge HCC compressing and occluding the inferior vena cava.

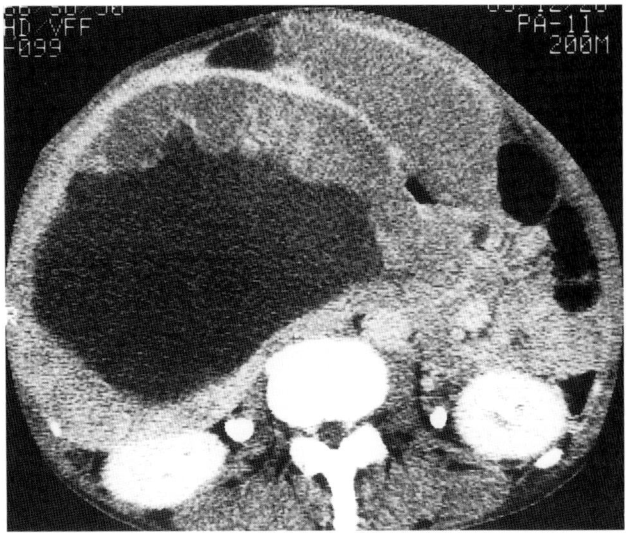

(a) Enhanced CT: the IVC is compressed and occluded by a huge HCC occupying the right lobe. The IVC cannot be identified by enhanced CT.

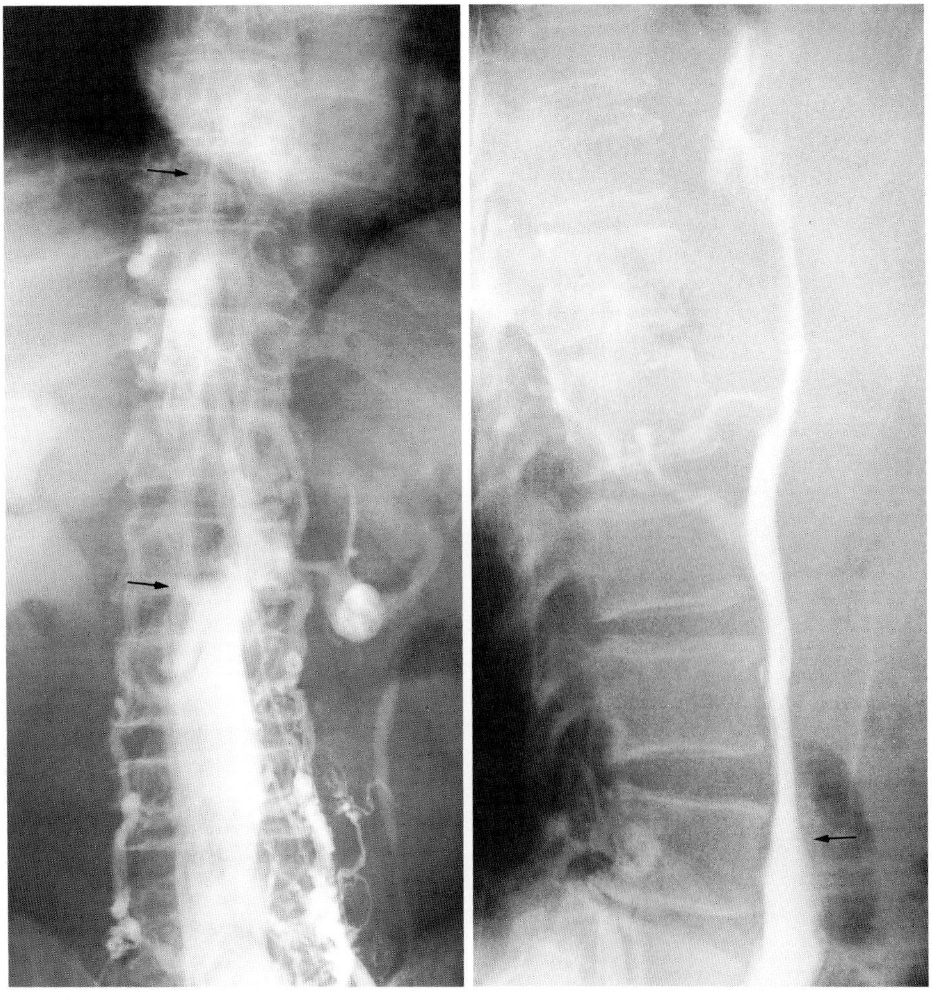

b c

(b) Inferior cavogram (anterior view): the hepatic portion of the IVC is not filled with contrast medium for a length of 17 cm (between → and →). Collateral ascending lumbar veins and an azygos system are seen along the vertebral column bilaterally.

(c) Inferior cavogram (right lateral view): the stenosis of the IVC further extends caudally in this film, starting near the origin of the IVC (→), and ending near the right atrium. The wall of the IVC is smooth. In this patient, the resected tissue containing the mass weighed 5500 g. The mass could be easily separated from the IVC, and the IVC fully opened postoperatively. Unlike adenocarcinoma, HCC in close proximity to the IVC is mostly separable from it (same as Case 3, p. 148).

Surgery—Case 3: Metastatic tumor diagnosed by CT as infiltrating onto the IVC, hence not resectable. In this patient, a 5 cm metastasis from cecum carcinoma was found by CT in $S^{VIII\text{–}IV}$ and in part in S^{I}.

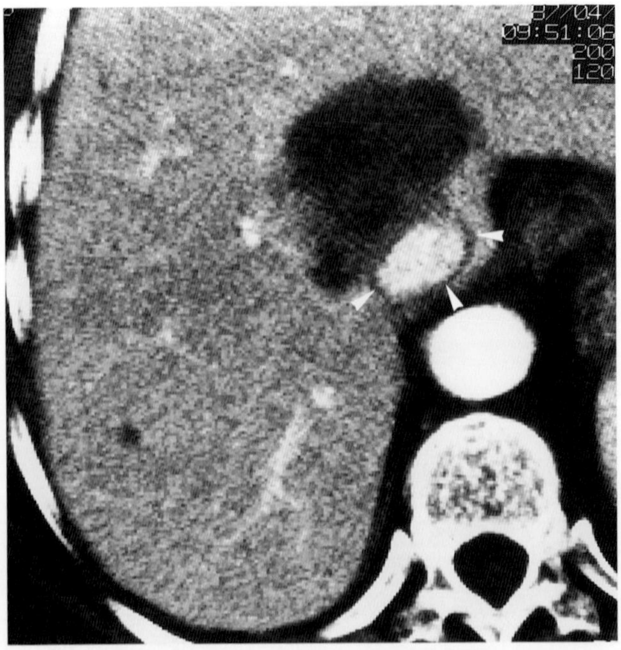

Dynamic CT (early phase): the IVC wall (▶) normally seen as a low-density ring in an early phase is obscured at the site in contact with the tumor due to cancer infiltration. The tumor–IVC contact spans nearly half the circumference, suggesting extensive infiltration, hence difficulty in resection.

Laparotomy was done, but the mass was firmly adherent to the IVC, not detachable, and resection was not carried out.

Surgery—Case 4: Extended central bisegmentectomy utilizing the inferior right hepatic vein as a drainage vein for conserved S^{VI}.

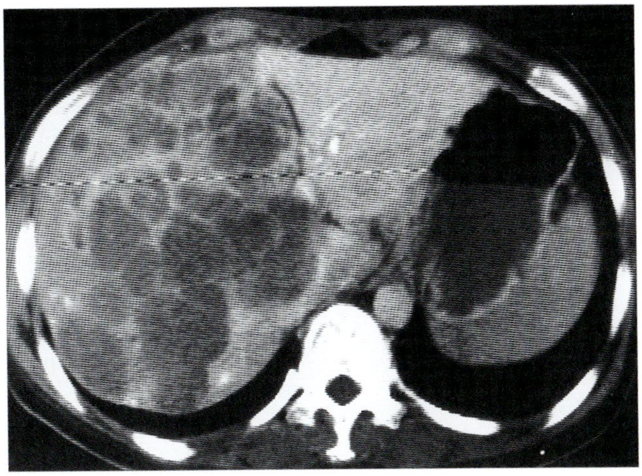

(a) Portal-CT: a huge HCC is seen occupying S^{IV}, S^{VIII}, and S^{VII}. Both the right and middle hepatic veins are buried in the mass and not recognized.

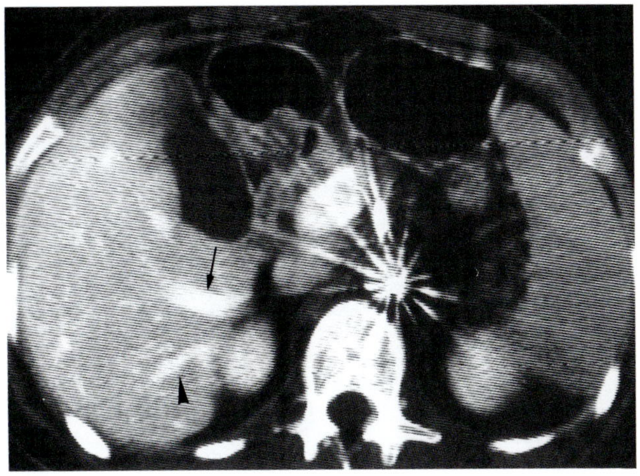

(b) Portal-CT [slice caudal to (a)]: the inferior right hepatic vein entering the IVC (→) and its branch (▶), both enlarged, are seen.

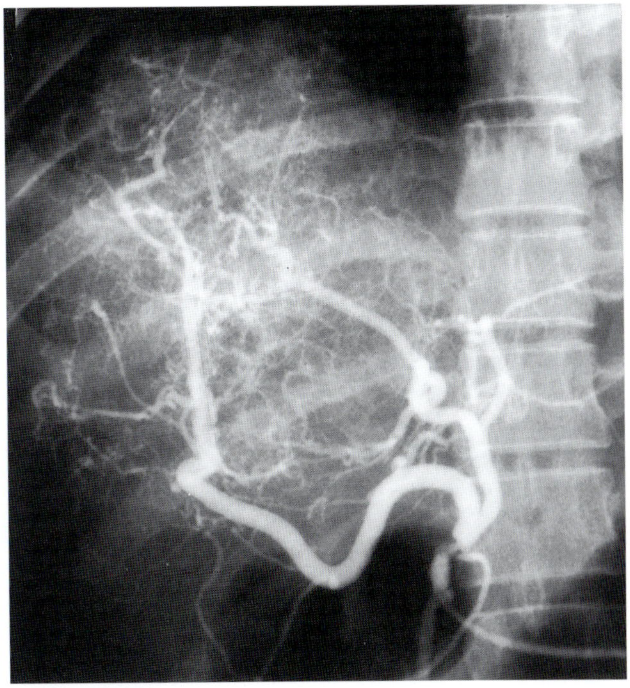

(c) Heptic arteriogram: a huge HCC is occupying the right lobe and S^{IV} except for S^{VI}.

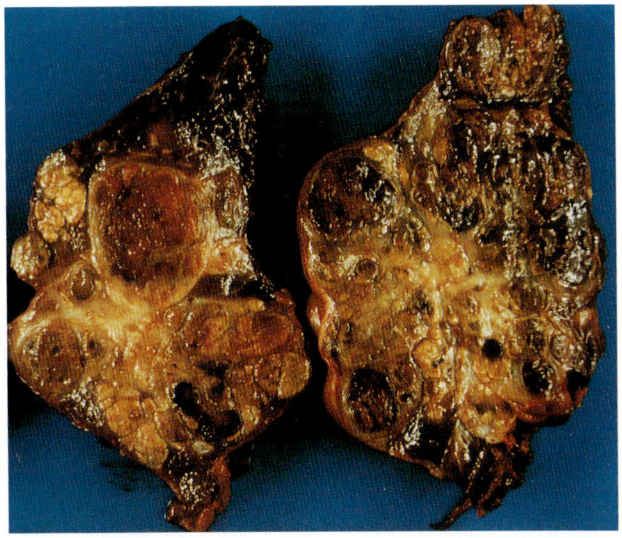

(d) Cut section of resected specimen: extended central bisegmentectomy including the right and middle hepatic veins was carried out. It was a confluent multinodular HCC (Edmondson's grade III > II). Postoperative recurrence occurred, but it was controlled by repeated Lipiodol-TAE, and the patient lived for quite a long time (same as Case 15, p. 480).

Surgery—Case 5: Small HCC not resectable because it was riding on the portal vein bifurcation in a liver with a poor function.

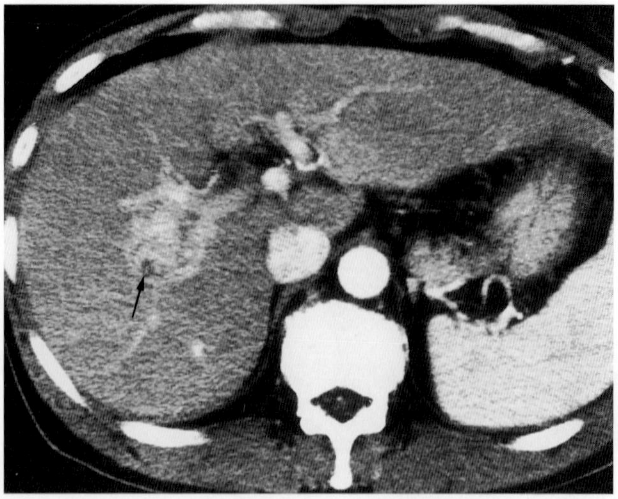

Enhanced CT: the mass is only 2.5 cm, but is located at the bifurcation of the anterior and posterior portal veins in the right lobe. The right hepatic vein (→) is buried in it. Since the liver function was poor, resection was called off and TAE was done instead.

Surgery—Case 6: Combination of resection and introperative ethanol injection.

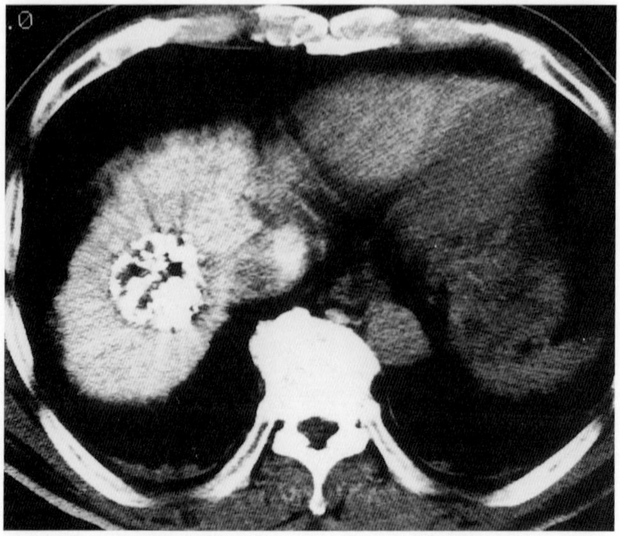

(a) Portal-CT: the main mass with Lipiodol retention is seen in S^{VIII}.

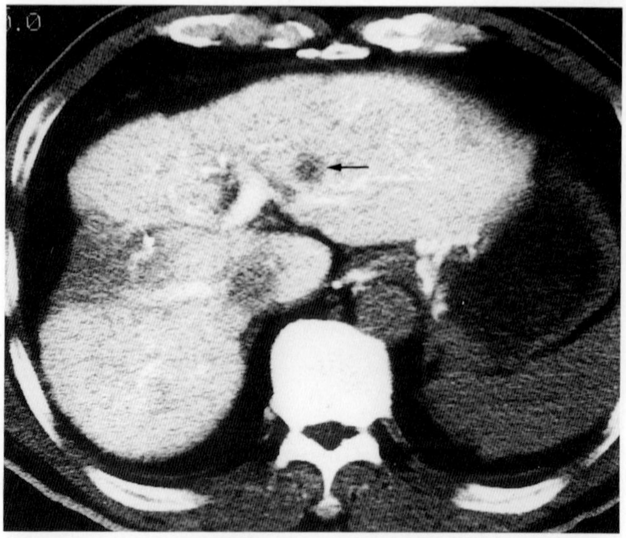

(b) Portal-CT [slice caudal to (a)]: a 1 cm mass (→) was found at the junction of P^{II} and P^{III}. Preoperative study showed a poor liver function (total bilirubin 1.5 mg/dl, ICG.R_{15} 39 per cent), and only partial resection of S^{VIII} was carried out. For the S^{II-III} lesion, ethanol (4.5 ml) was injected under US guidance intraoperatively. The latter lesion has since disappeared, and there has been no recurrence.

Surgery—Case 7: Early postoperative recurrence with multiple lesions that resembled plum blossom on angiogram. Lipiodol-TAE was carried out preoperatively, and a 5.5 cm HCC in S^{VIII} was resected. It was 100 per cent necrotized. However, at 1 month postoperatively, AFP started rising, and CT demonstrated multiple recurrent lesions in the remnant liver.

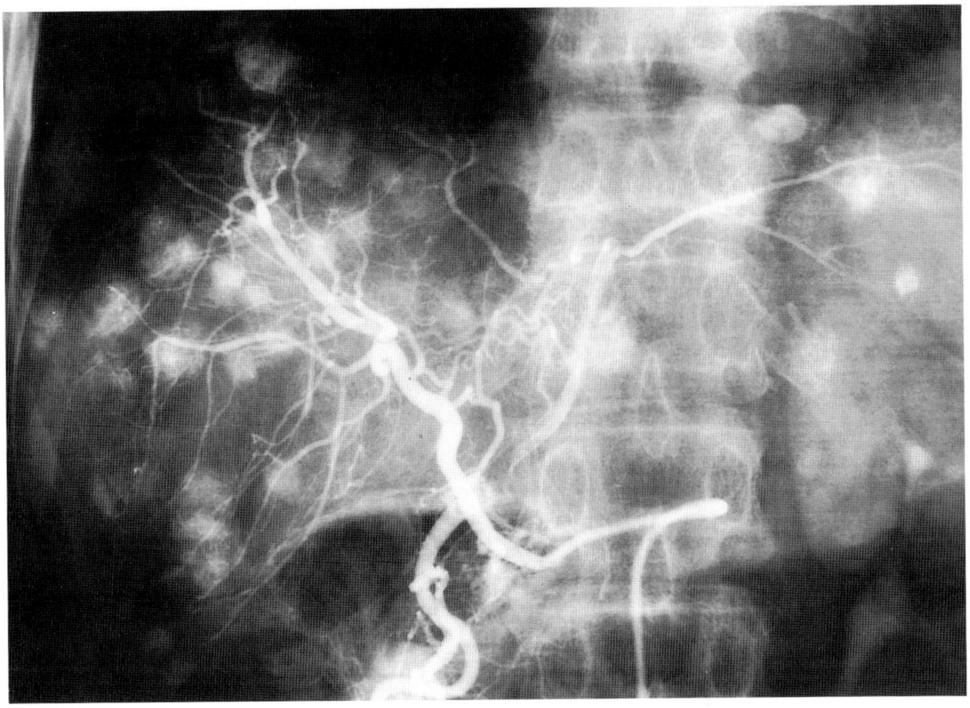

Hepatic arteriogram (4 months postoperative): multiple lesions of about 1 cm are seen looking like plum blossom. There was no arterio-portal shunt or tumor thrombus.

Surgery—Case 8: Recurrence 6 years after resection.

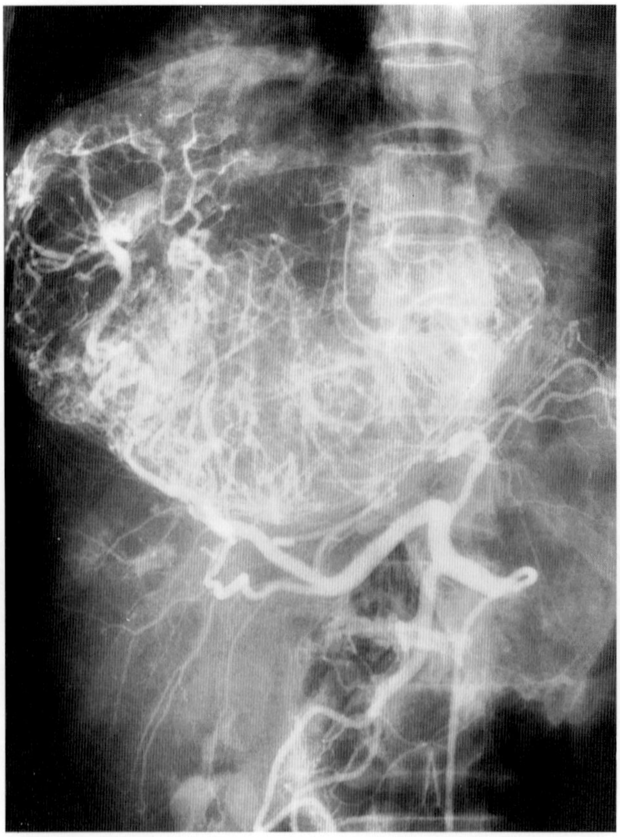

(a) Hepatic arteriogram (first time, preoperative): a 15 cm HCC is seen in $S^{VIII–IV}$. Central bisegmentectomy was carried out.

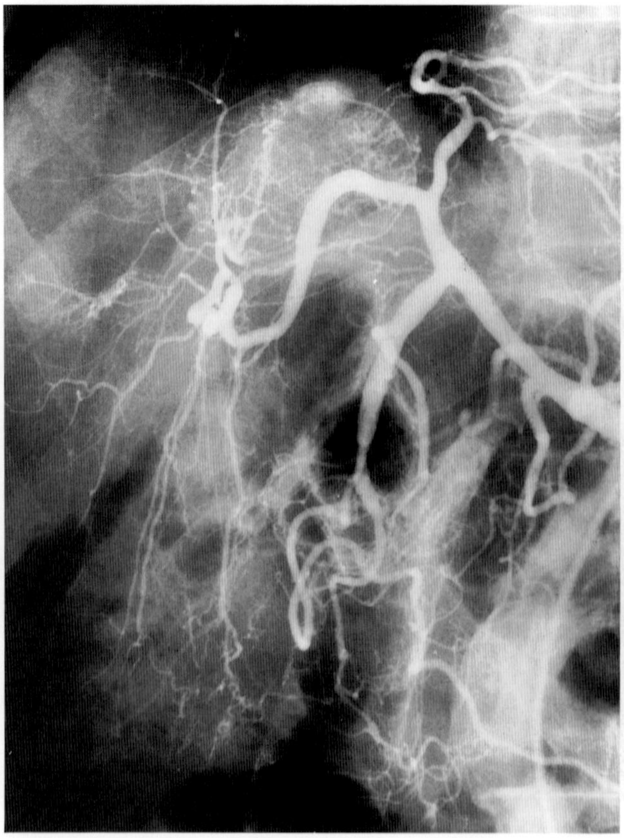

(b) Hepatic arteriogram (6 years postoperatively): serum AFP remained normal and the patient was living normally. Six years after the operation, dynamic CT found a recurrent lesion. Angiography showed a 5 cm solitary mass in S^{VII}, and it was resected. In the resected specimen, there were four secondaries, several millimeters in size, around the main mass.

Surgery—Case 9: Successful reduction surgery.

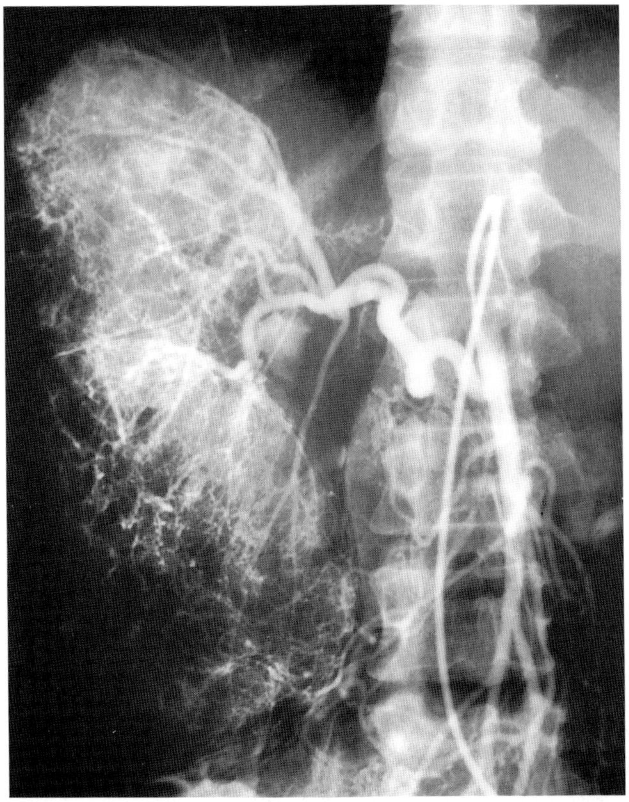

(a) Right hepatic arteriogram: two large masses are being supplied by the right hepatic artery derived from the superior mesenteric artery. Left hepatic arteriography found two small lesions in the left lobe laterally (not shown).

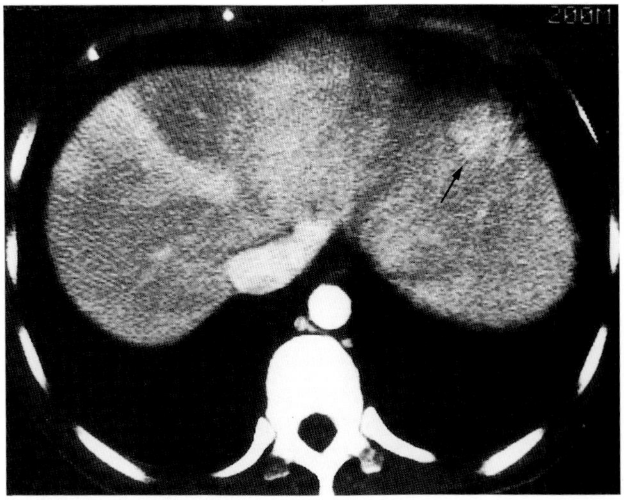

(b) Dynamic CT: beside the main mass, a 3 cm lesion (→) is seen in the left lobe laterally.

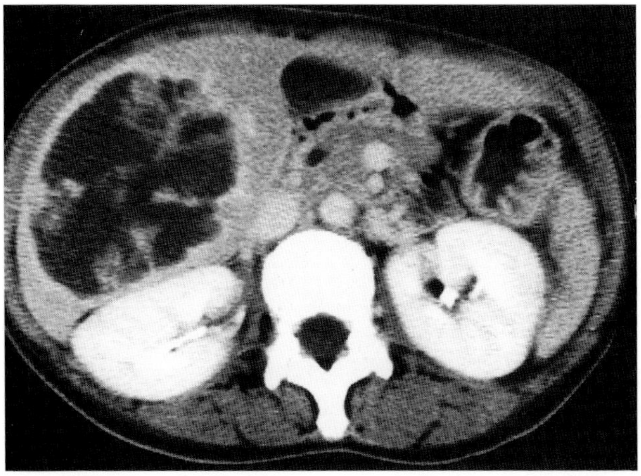

(c) Dynamic CT (after TAE): the bulk of the main mass has been necrotized, and right hepatectomy and a wedge resection of the left lateral area were carried out. Against expectations, there was no recurrence for some time. At 4.5 years postoperatively, a 1.5 cm recurrent lesion was found in the left lateral area which was resected. Both the primary and the recurrent lesions were of mixed type hepatocholangioma, suggesting that an intrahepatic secondary grew very slowly. The patient is doing well 3.5 years after the second operation.

Surgery—Case 10: A primarily inoperable HCC turning resectable with additional PTPE therapy.

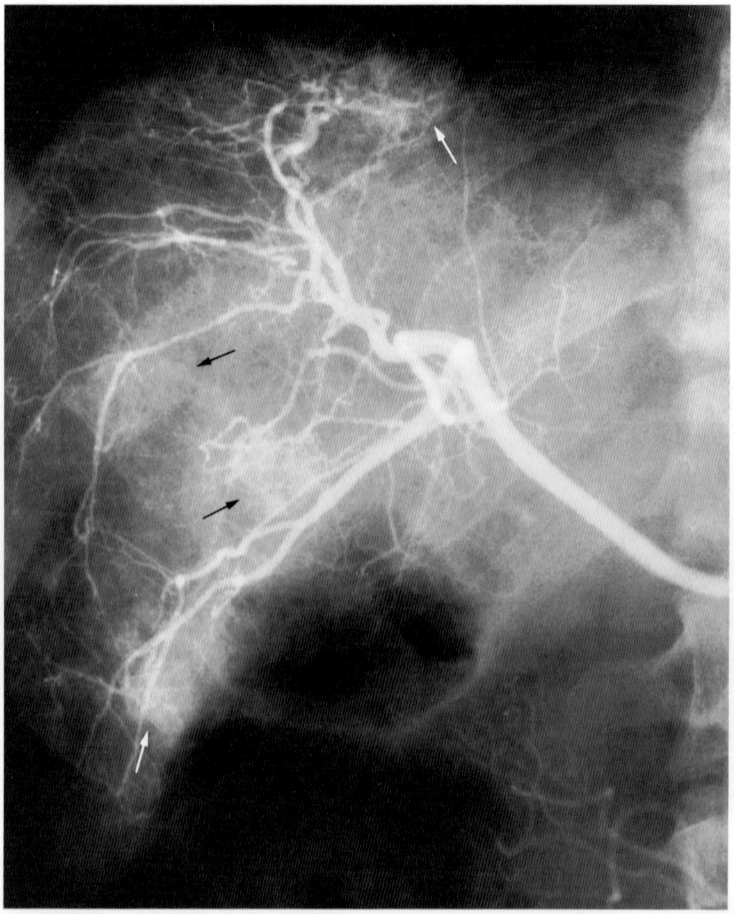

(a) Right hepatic arteriogram: four lesions are seen scattered in the right lobe (→). Lipiodol-TAE was carried out.

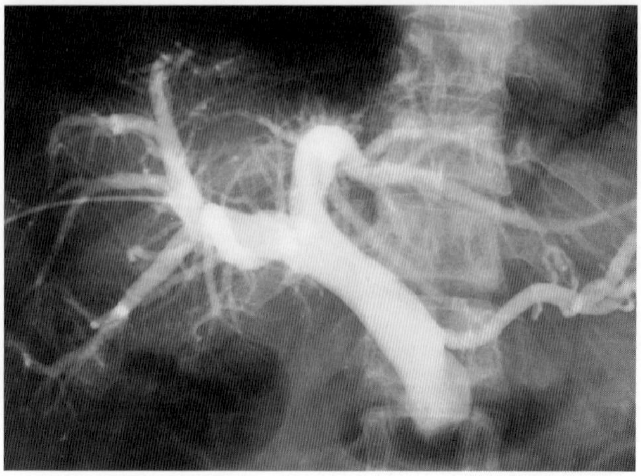

(b) PTP (before PTPE): the left lobe was too small for right hepatectomy. In order to expand surgical indication and turn this case operable, PTPE was carried out.

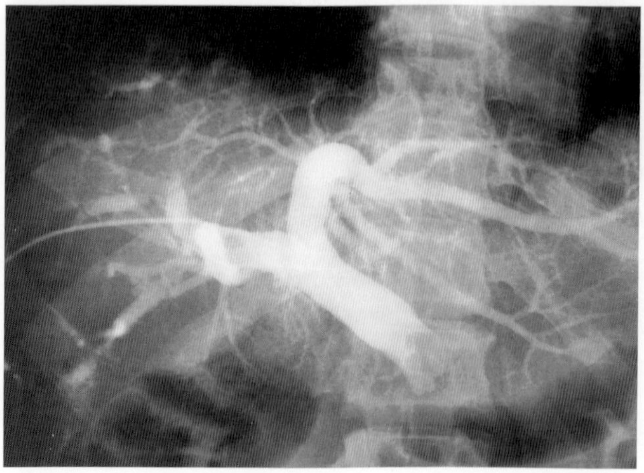

(c) PTP (after PTPE): the portal vein supplying the right lobe (to be resected) was embolized. Portal venous pressure rose by 80 mmH_2O after PTPE.

Case 10 (contd.)

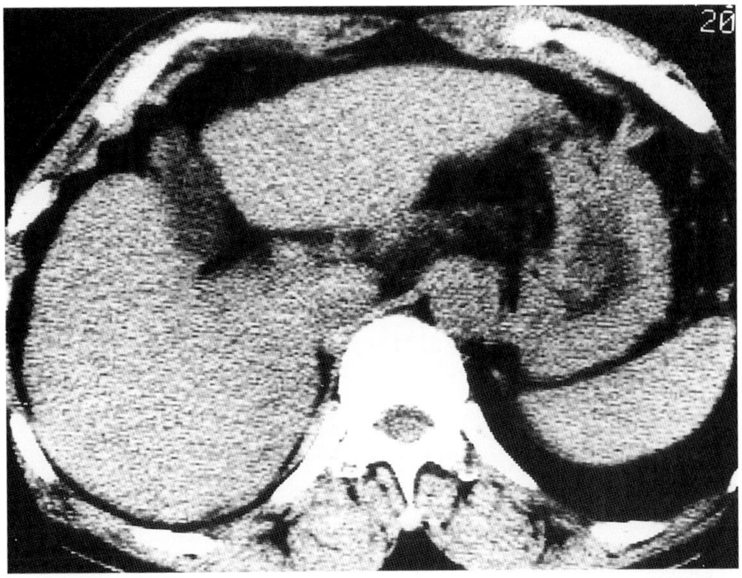

(d) Plain CT (before PTPE): the lateral surface of the right lobe is smooth and round.

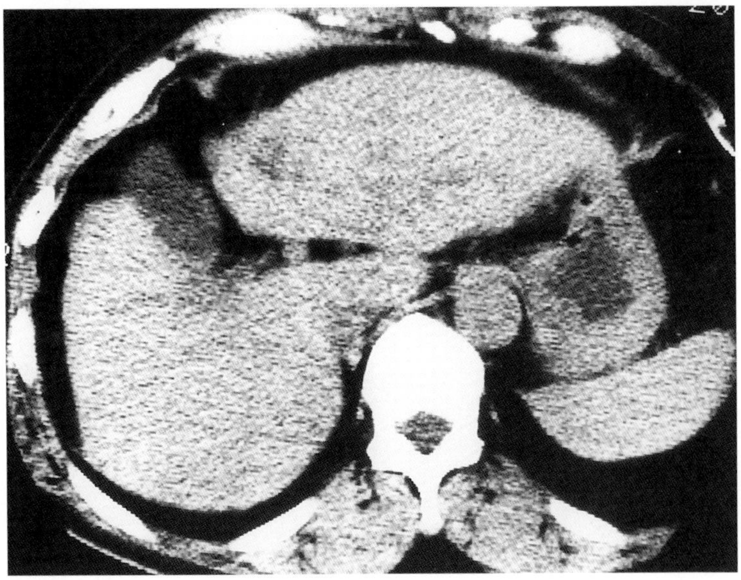

(e) Plain CT (4 months after PTPE): atrophy of the right lobe and compensatory left lobe hypertrophy (rounded) are recognized.

Surgery—Case 11: Successful management of recurrent hepatic lesions by Lipiodol-TAE, enabling resection of metastasis to the adrenal gland. A 2.7 cm solitary HCC in S^{V} was resected 1.5 years earlier. A metastasis to the right adrenal was found by CT.

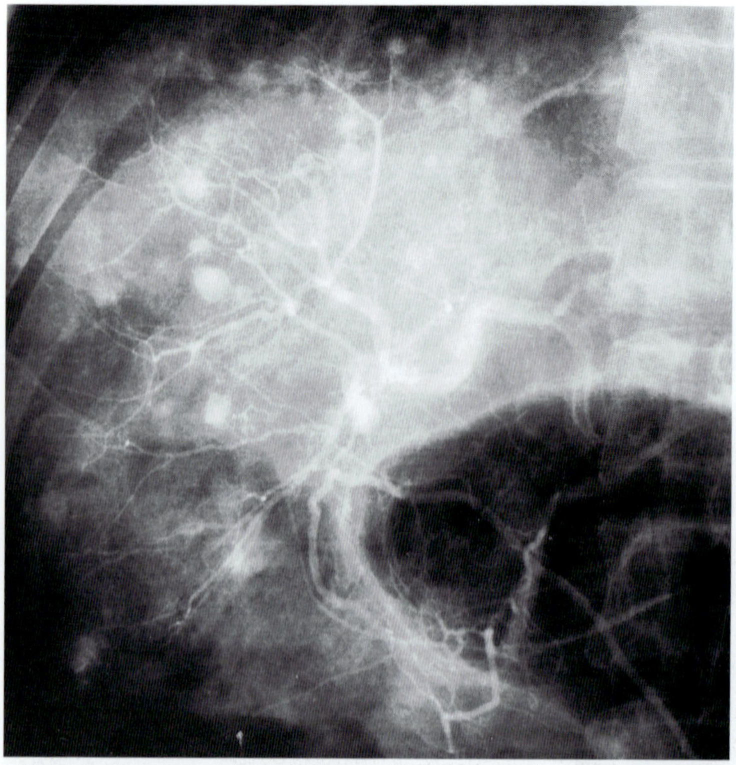

(a) Hepatic arteriogram: right adrenal arteriography demonstrated a metastatic lesion in the adrenal. Subsequent hepatic arteriography found small multiple lesions in the remnant liver. Lipiodol-TAE was carried out.

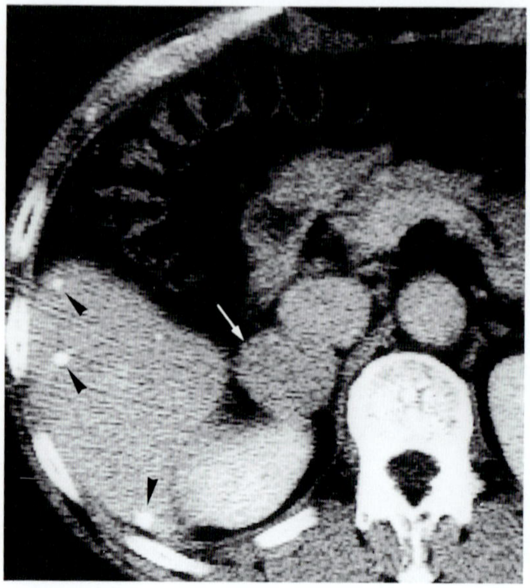

(b) Enhanced CT (after Lipiodol-TAE): the recurrent lesions are under control (▶). A round metastasis is seen in the right adrenal gland (→).

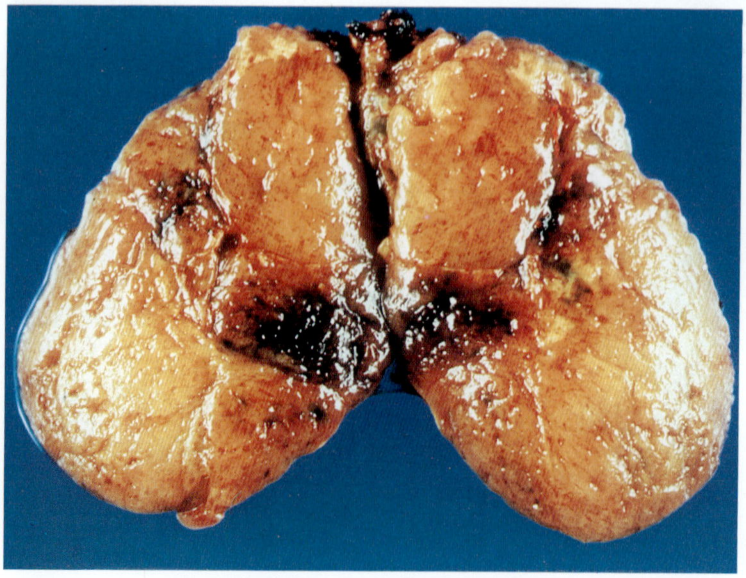

(c) Resected adrenal: the right adrenal gland with a metastasis was removed. The cut surface (5.5 × 4.0 cm) showed metastatic HCC with some bleeding. Histologically, it was Edmondson's grade II.

Surgery—Case 12: Reperfusion of an intrahepatic artery and a portal vein following their simultaneous division. A 48-year-old man. There was a 12 cm HCC in the right lobe, and the right hepatic artery and the right portal vein was ligated and divided simultaneously for the purpose of right hepatectomy. However, during the operation, when the right lobe was about to be freed, it was found to be tightly adherent to the IVC (not due to infiltration), and not separable. No resection could be done. Angiography was repeated 6 months later.

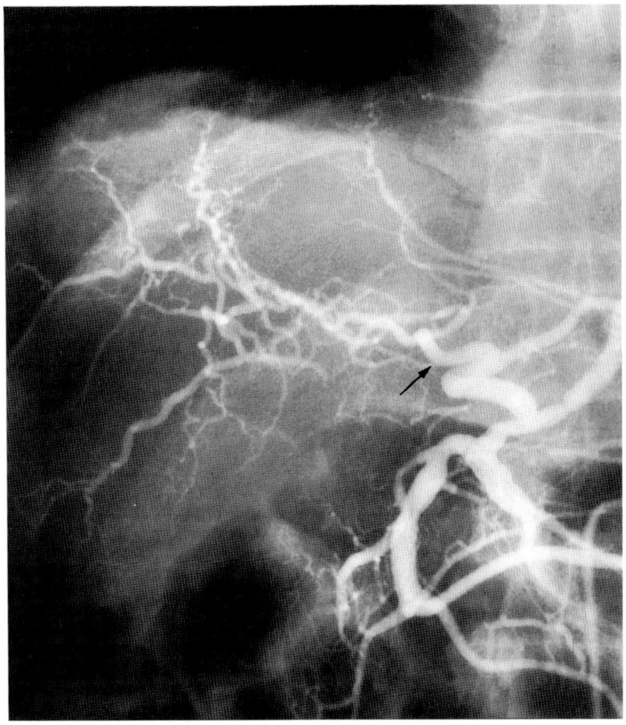

(a) Hepatic arteriogram (early phase): the right hepatic artery has been divided at →, but the anterior and the posterior branches were opacified through the middle hepatic artery.

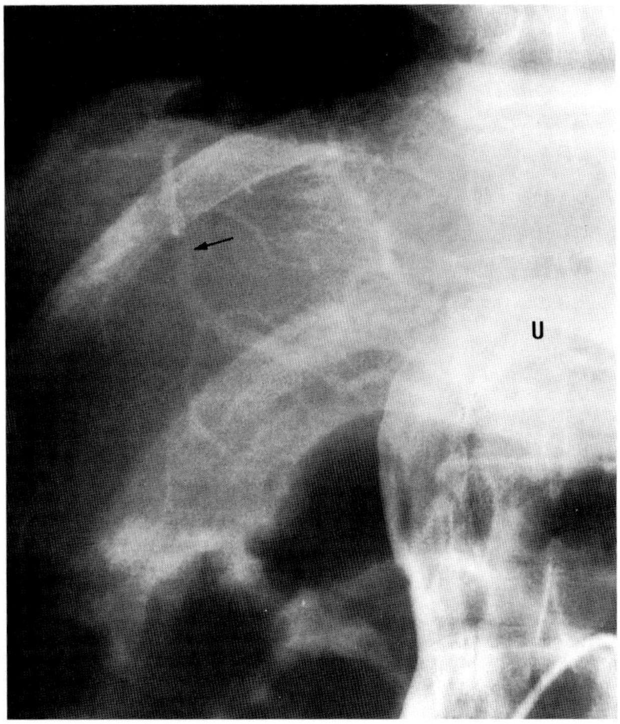

(b) Superior mesenteric arterial portogram: the divided right anterior portal vein P^{IV}, is opacified through intrahepatic venous anastomoses (→). The caliber of this vein is smaller than normal. U, the umbilical portion.

Surgery—Case 13: Restoration of arterial and portal perfusion in the liver after simultaneous ligation and division of the hepatic artery and portal vein extahepatically. A 65-year-old man was operated on for rectum carcinoma 2 years earlier. Four metastatic lesions were recently found in both lobes, and intraarterial infusion chemotherapy (13 000 mg of 5FU and 12 mg of MMC) was carried out. He suddenly vomited blood, and emergency laparotomy found a perforated duodenal ulcer and abscess formation in the hepatic hilum. During the operation, profuse bleeding occurred in the hilar region necessitating simultaneous ligation and division of the common hepatic artery and the origin of the portal vein. Gastrectomy followed.

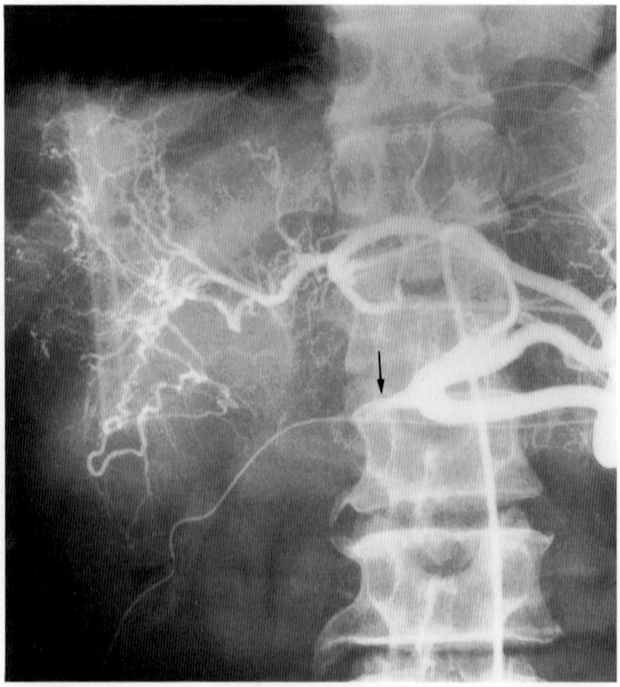

(a) Celiac arteriogram (22 days postoperatively: the common hepatic artery had been divided and only a small portion was opacified (→). The left hepatic artery was opacified through the left gastric artery, and contrast medium entered thereon into the right hepatic arterial branches.

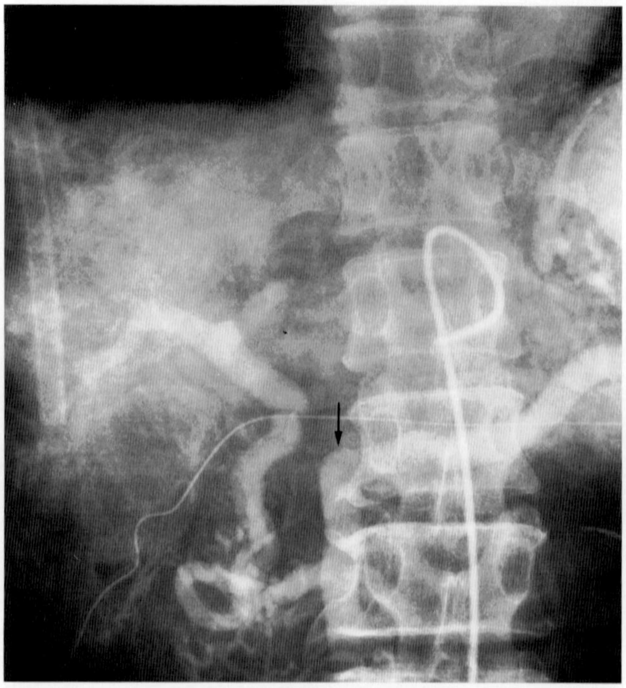

(b) Superior mesenteric arterial portogram (22 days postoperatively): the beginning of the portal vein is completely occluded (→). Contrast medium flowed retrogradely into the pancreatic arcade vein, and further into the intrahepatic portal branches. Hepatic failure due to dual ligation did not develop. There was a mild elevation of serum enzymes derived from the liver. The patient died 9 months later from hepatic failure as a result of growing metastatic cancer.

Surgery—Case 14: Systematic subsegmentectomy that permitted successful resection of the main mass as well as multiple small secondaries.

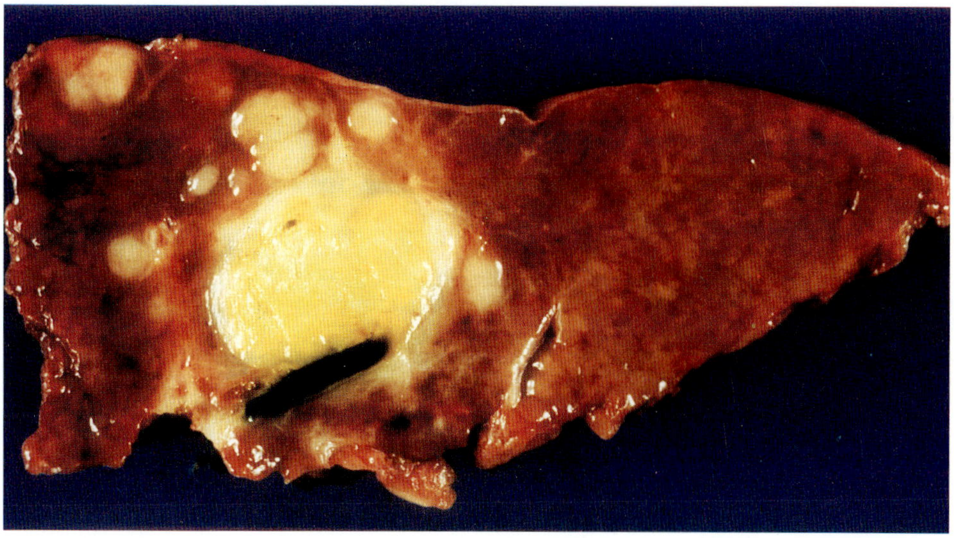

Cut section of resected specimen: systematic subsegmentectomy mimicking partial resection of S^{V} was carried out. The main mass had been necrotized by repeated TAE, but there were many secondaries (10 in this cut surface alone). If an enucleation procedure had been done, the secondaries would have been left over.

Surgery—Case 15: Systematic subsegmentectomy that could have left small secondaries unresected.

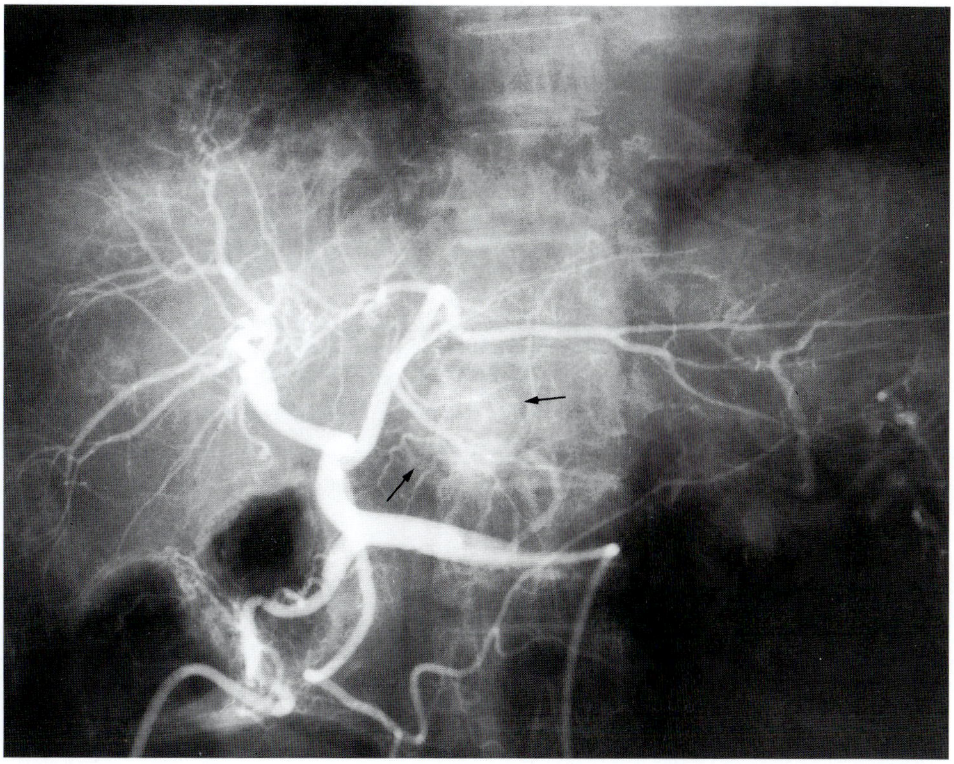

(a) Hepatic arteriogram: a 2.5 cm mass (→) is seen in S^{III}.

Case 15 (contd.)

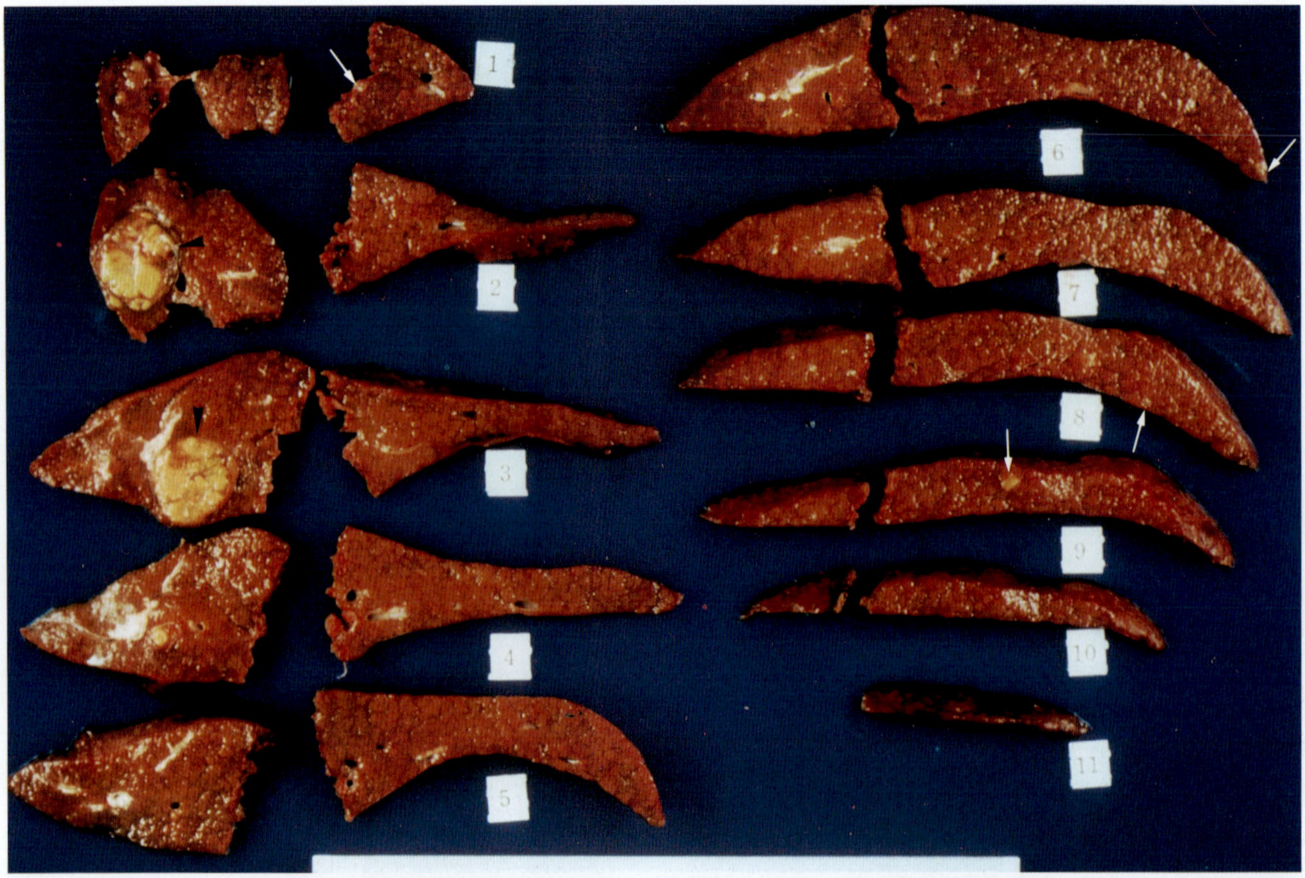

(b) Cut sections of resected specimen: S^{III} subsegmentectomy was the primary intention (S^{III} to the left), but an intraoperative technical error caused damage to the bile duct, and S^{II} (to the right) had to be additionally resected. Beside the main mass in S^{III}, S^{II} contained several small secondaries (→).

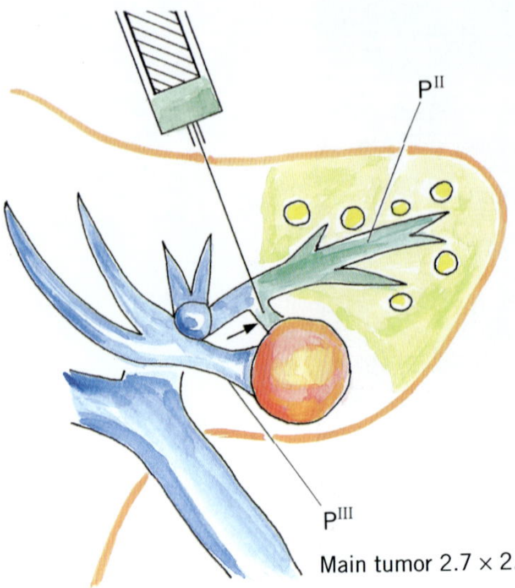

(c) Suggested mechanism for the metastases from the main mass in S^{III} to S^{II}: the main mass (red) is in S^{III} and for secondaries (yellow) to occur in S^{II}, it is generally assumed that cancer cells regurgitated into the umbilical portion of the left portal vein, and therefrom entered P^{II}. In this patient, intraoperative US found involvement of the first branch of P^{II} and P^{III}, and to delineate the separating line indigocarmine (5 ml) was injected into the first branch of P^{II}. All the dye regurgitated into S^{II} through arterio-portal shunts, suggesting that cancer cells were most likely transported through the same route.

Similar hemodynamic events are expected to be occurring in patients, namely, cancer cells are transported not only by the portal vein in the tumor-bearing subsegment, but also by other portal veins in the vicinity.

Surgery (complication)—Case 16: Liver abscess at the surgical margin. For an HCC in $S^{VI-VIII}$, enucleation combined with microwave heat coagulation was carried out. Ten days later, the patient started running a low-grade fever.

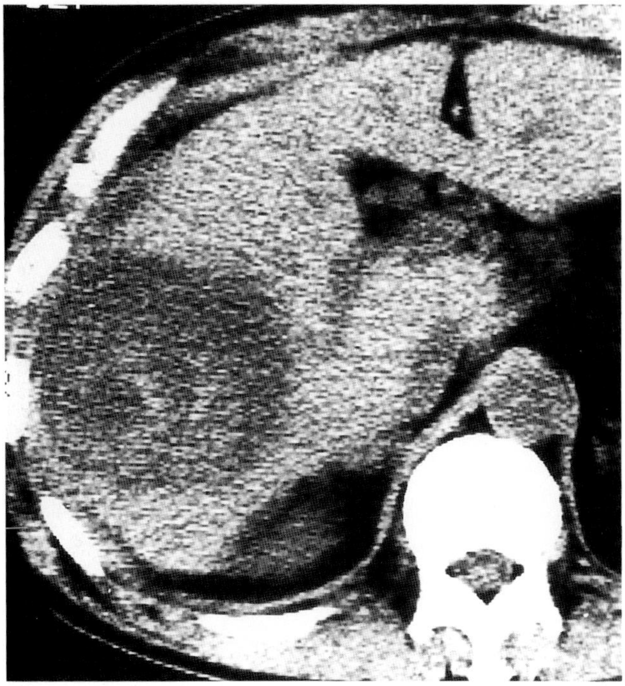

(a) Plain CT (10 days postoperatively): An 8 cm low-density lesion is seen in S^{VI} that has a high-density structure internally. A hematoma or an abscess was suspected.

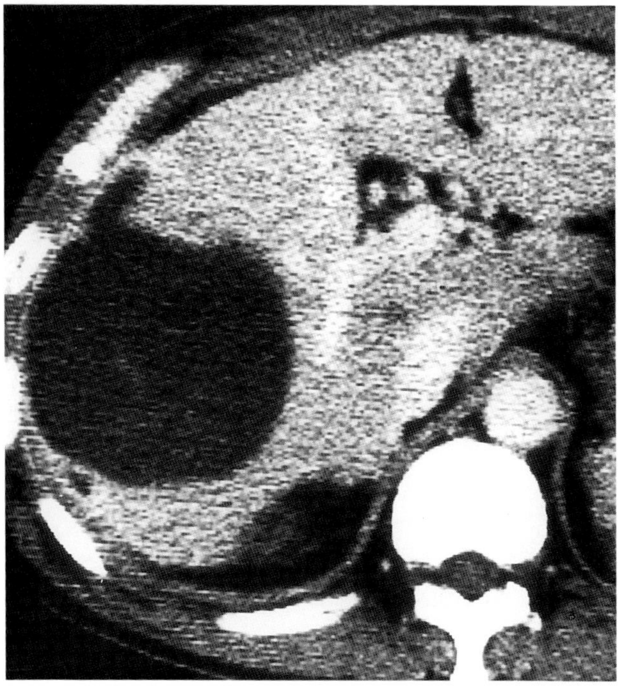

(b) Enhanced CT (10 days postoperatively): the lesion was not enhanced, nor did the periphery show ring enhancement. The late phase scan showed the same.

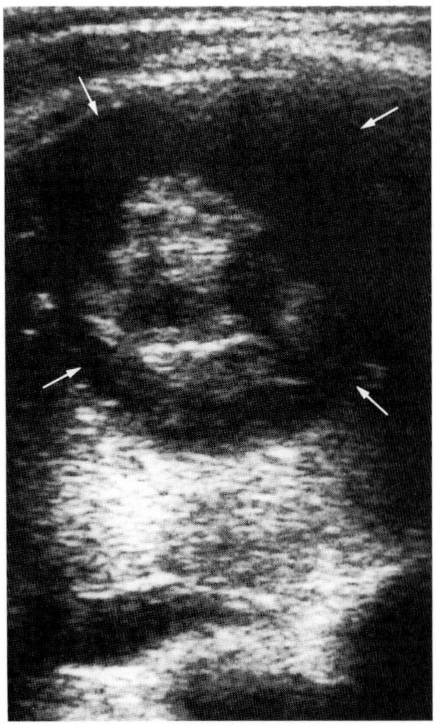

(c) US (10 days postoperatively): the mass (→) is hypoechoic and a high-echo interior is recognized. With a suspicion of abscess, puncture was carried out, yielding a chocolate colored fluid. The lesion was drained, and with the administration of antibiotics, the patient recovered.

Surgery (complication)—Case 17: Serous exudate accumulating at the surgical margin. Partial resection was done for an HCC in $S^{VIII-VI}$ in the right lobe.

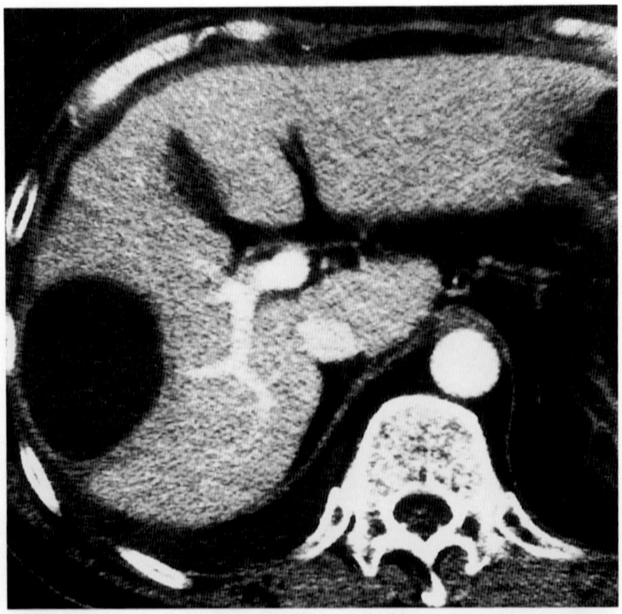

(a) Enhanced CT (1 month postoperatively): an oval-shaped area of fluid retention is seen in the surgical margin. There is no ring enhancement. At the time of this CT study, there was no fever or symptom suggestive of abscess.

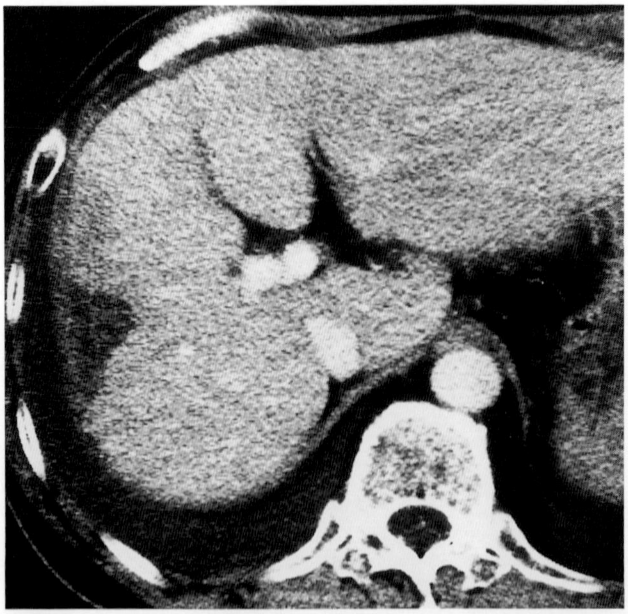

(b) Enhanced CT (5 months postoperatively): the fluid has been reduced and the tissue defect is being filled by an increasing hepatic mass. There is also some pleural effusion.

Surgery (complication)—Case 18: Subphrenic hematoma following hepatic resection. For two HCC lesions in S^{V} and S^{I}, partial resection and PEI were done along with splenectomy. Postoperatively, fever of 38°C continued, and a CT study was done.

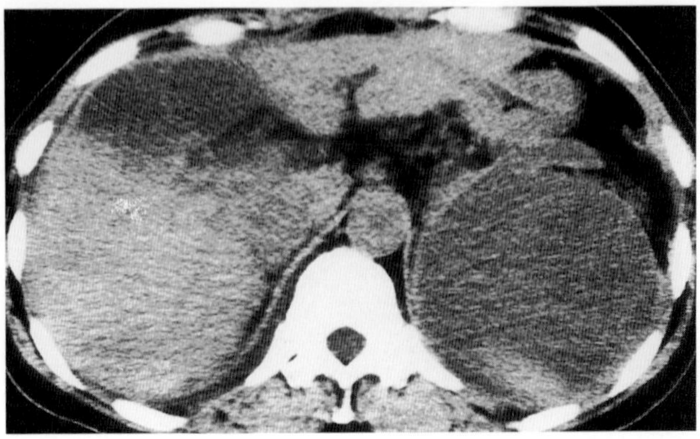

(a) Plain CT (21 days postoperatively): a 9 cm low-density lesion is seen behind the stomach which contained a high-density structure posteriorly.

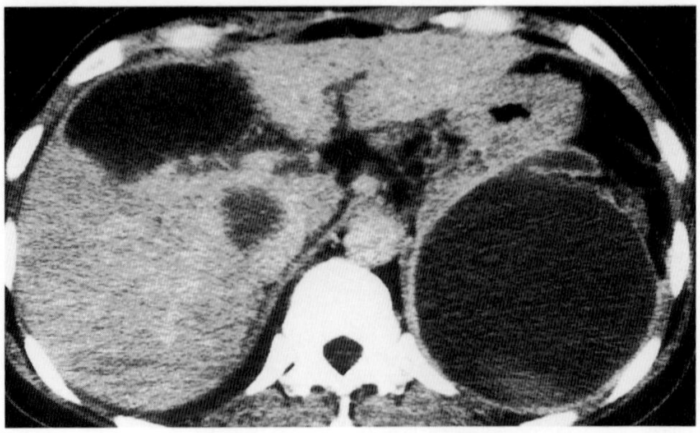

(b) Enhanced CT (21 days postoperatively): the interior of the lesion was not enhanced at all, and an abscess was suggested. Aspiration changed the diagnosis to hematoma. A small collection of fluid was seen in S^{V} that ensued resection, and aspiration yielded a serous fluid.

Surgery (complication)—Case 19: Right-sided pleural effusion following hepatic resection.

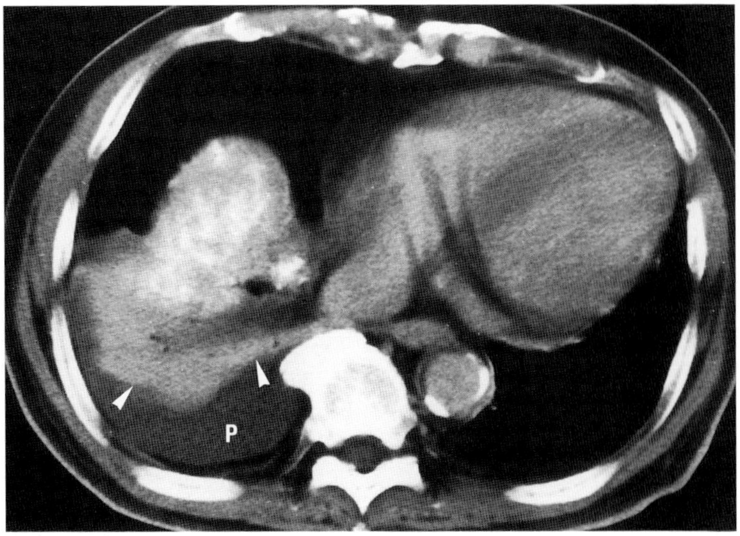

Lipiodol-CT: the posterior segment of the right lobe was resected. CT made immediately after the operation demonstrated pleural effusion in the right thorax, and atelectasis of the lower lobe of the lung. This state lasted for a year, and the fluid decreased thereafter. Lipiodol retention produced by the treatment for recurrent lesions is also seen.

Surgery (deformity)—Case 20: Hypertrophy of the remnant liver that appeared as normal liver. Right hepatectomy was done for a hepatic metastasis from colon cancer.

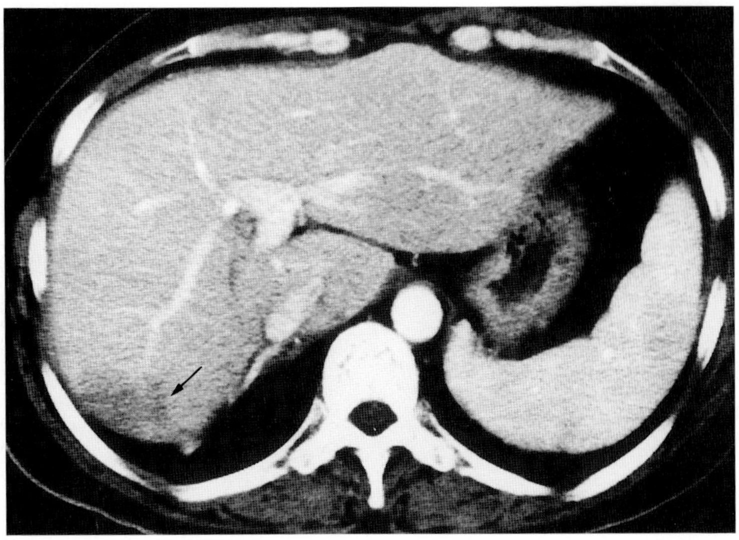

Enhanced CT (1 year postoperatively): the left lobe is hypertrophied in compensation, making the general contour of the liver appear normal. However, the dilated portion of the portal vein is the umbilical portion of the left portal vein, and the branch supplying the seemingly right lobe is not P^{V}, but is an enlarged P^{IV}. The low-density area (→) at the surgical margin represents parenchymal changes that follow resection.

Surgery (deformity)—Case 21: Hypertrophied liver which has a portal vein system appearing normal. A 15-year-old girl. Right lobectomy was done for hepatoblastoma.

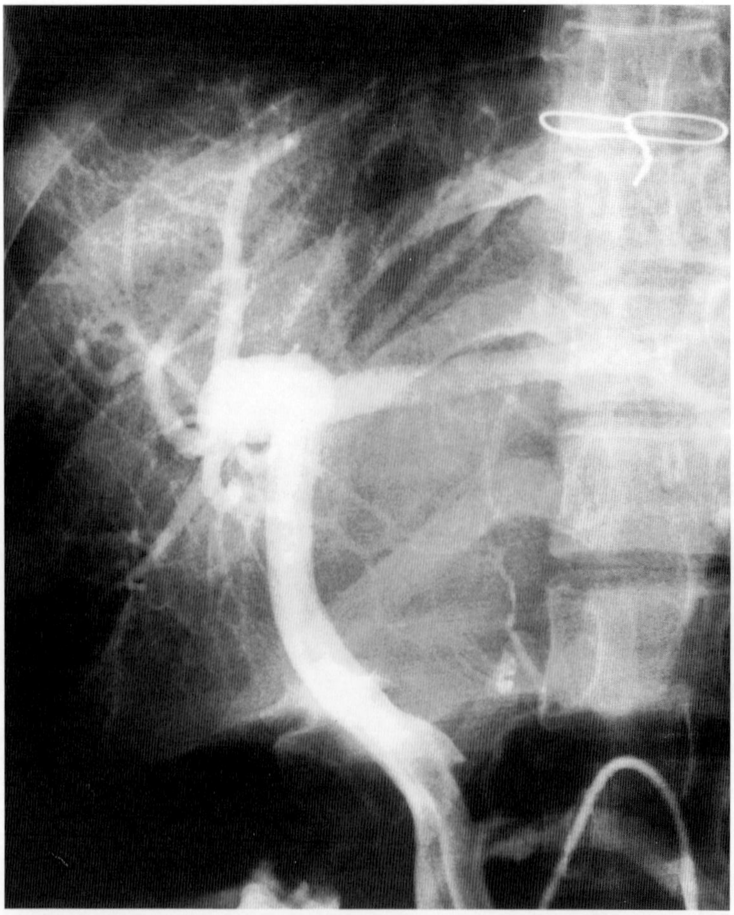

(a) Angiogram (portogram, 13 months postoperatively): the vessels seem stretched. The right anterior and right posterior portal veins seem to exist, but actually they are the left medial (P^{IV}) and left lateral inferior (P^{III}) branches.

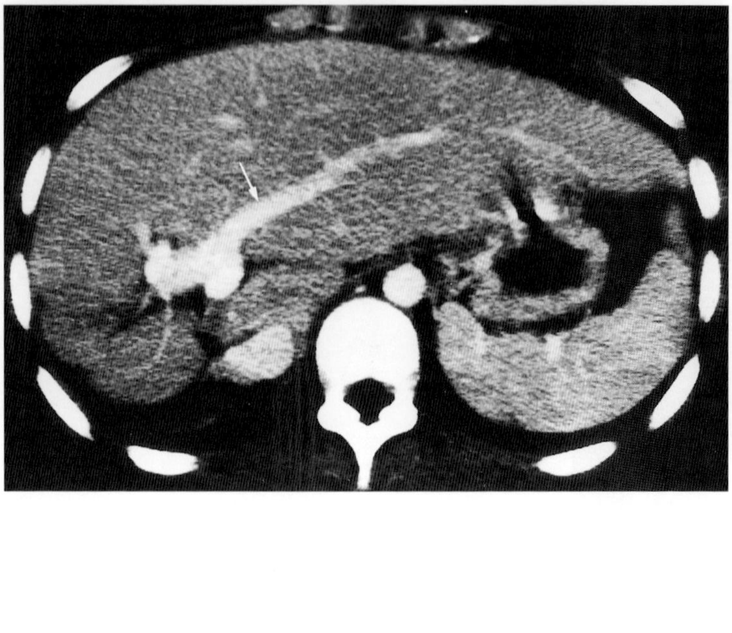

(b) Enhanced CT (13 months postoperatively): the remnant left lobe has extended, filling the entire abdominal cavity anteriorly. The umbilical portion is slanted toward the right, and P^{II} is much enlarged (same as Case 1, p. 237).

Surgery (deformity)—Case 22: Compensatory hypertrophy of the caudate lobe following left lateral resection.

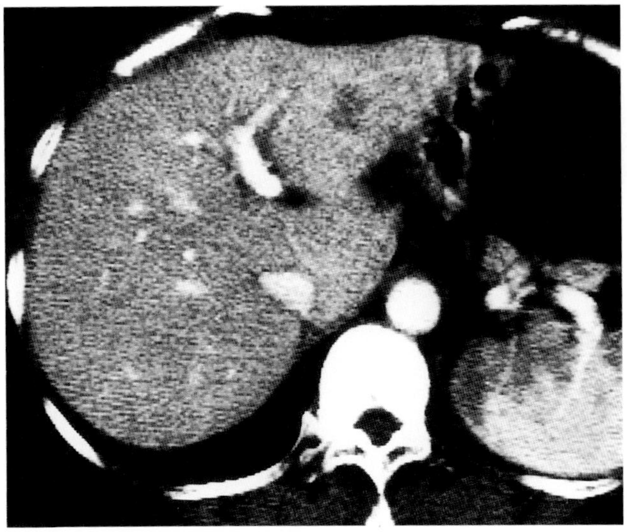

(a) Enhanced CT (preoperative): a 2 cm lesion was found in the left lobe laterally, and left lateral resection was carried out.

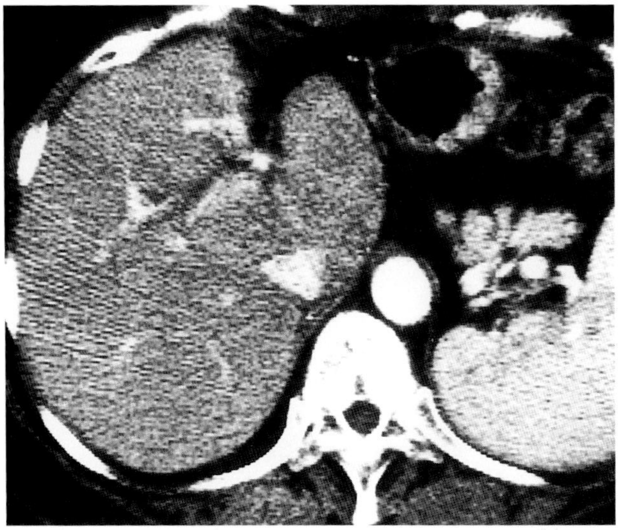

(b) Enhanced CT (8 months postoperatively): the left caudate lobe which was somewhat larger than normal preoperatively is now enlarged, protruding anteriorly.

Surgery (induced displacement)—Case 23: Cranial displacement of the right kidney following right lobectomy. Right lobectomy was carried out for HCC.

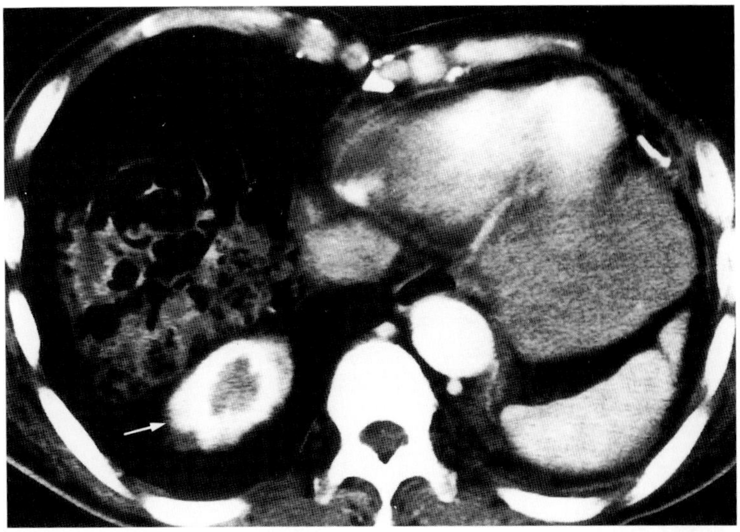

Enhanced CT (2 years 8 months postoperatively): the right kidney (→) is markedly displaced cranially, and so is the small bowel seen anterior to it.

Surgery (induced displacement)—Case 24: Elevation of the gastric antrum following central bisegmentectomy. Central bisegmentectomy was carried out.

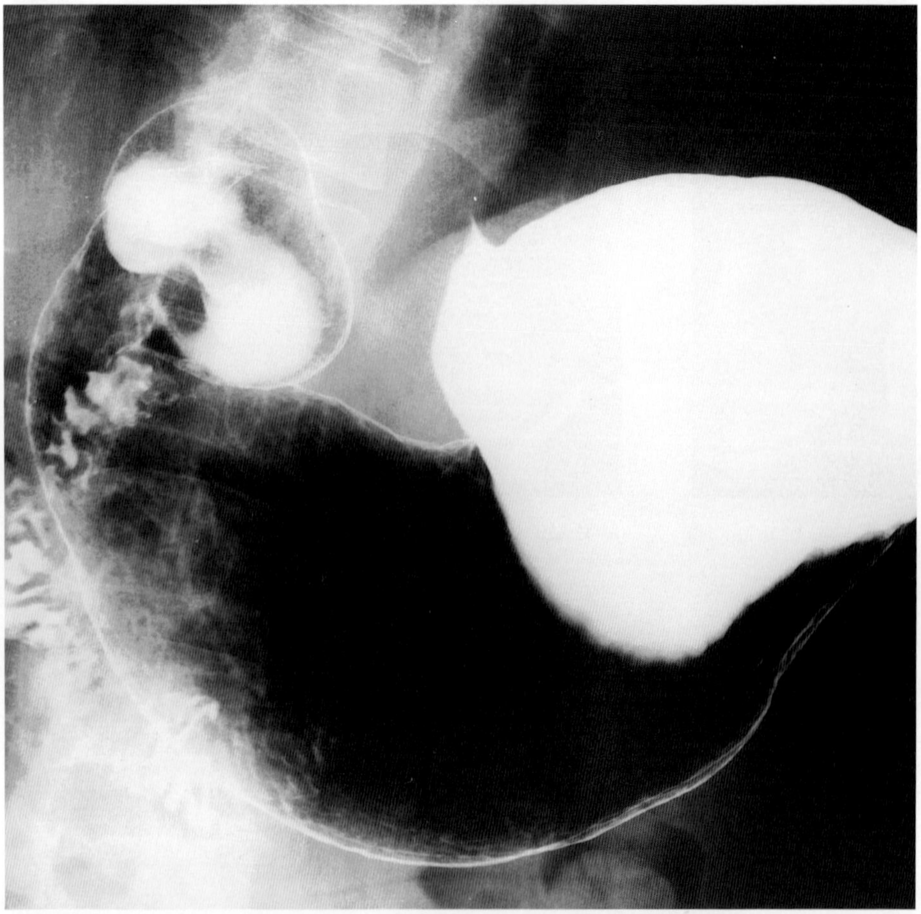

(a) Upper GI barium study (5 years postoperatively): the antrum of the stomach and the duodenum are displaced cranially (elevated) making the fornix appear somewhat caudally shifted relative to the antrum.

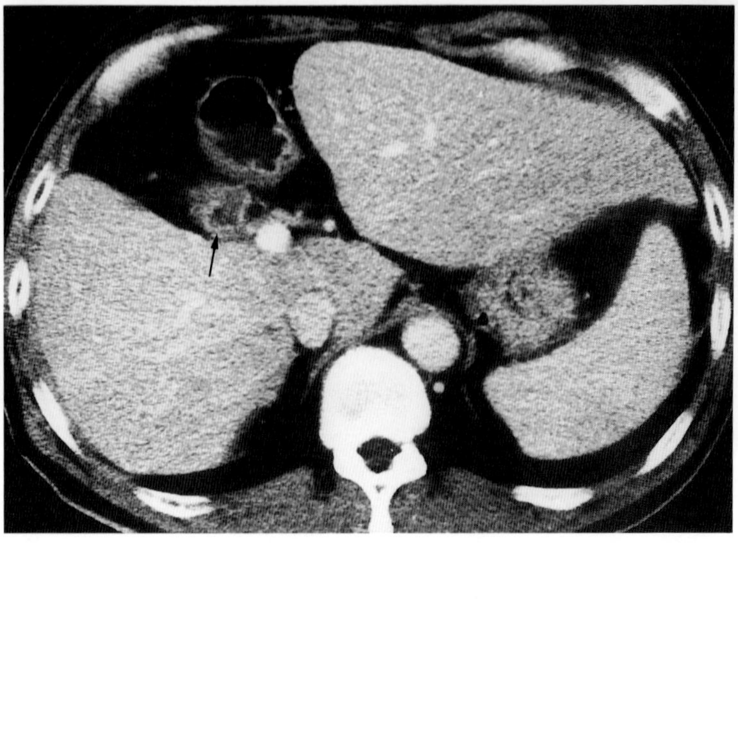

(b) Enhanced CT (5 years postoperatively): the resected void area now contains the gastric antrum and the descending part of the duodenum (→) close to the portal vein.

21

Percutaneous ethanol injection (PEI) therapy

This therapy in which absolute ethanol is injected into a small HCC under US guidance was first developed by one of the authors and his group at the Department of Medicine, Chiba University, in 1983 (Sugiura *et al.* 1983); it was quickly adopted by a number of radiologists and hepatologists (Livraghi *et al.* 1986; Shiina *et al.* 1987). It is currently used throughout the world (Sheu *et al.* 1987; Vilana *et al.* 1992). The original study aimed at killing HCCs less than 3 cm in size and fewer than three in number (Ebara *et al.* 1990). The results have been estimated to be equivalent to those of surgery in comparable cases (Okuda 1993). This therapy is particularly useful in patients with advanced cirrhosis in whom a small HCC has evolved, a situation frequently experienced in the screening program for patients with hepatitis C virus induced cirrhosis in Japan and Italy. It may be combined with other treatments as part of multidisciplinary therapy (Tanikawa 1992).

The instrument for PEI consists of a 22 gauge Chiba needle (Okuda *et al.* 1974), a short extension tube, and a 5 ml syringe. Under local anesthesia, a 22 gauge needle is introduced into a tumor or its marginal area through a puncture probe under US guidance. Absolute ethanol is slowly injected from the syringe while it is being withdrawn little by little to produce as much necrosis as possible inside and around the mass. The amount of ethanol injected each time is 2–6 ml. The injection is repeated twice a week for up to 10 sessions or more, depending on the tumor size. This procedure is repeated until the original US pattern is completely replaced by another pattern that persists for some time in the tumor. A PEI-induced necrotic area is seen hypoattenuating at both early and late phases of enhanced CT (Ebara *et al.* 1995).

This therapy may be used in patients in whom repeated TAE destroyed the tumor feeding artery, who have a hypovascular HCC which would not retain much Lipiodol, and in whom sufficient resection could not be made because of poor liver function (Case 6, p.506). However, PEI cannot be done for a lesion not well visualized by US, or for multiple lesions. Complications include portal vein thrombosis which may require differential diagnosis from tumor thrombosis (Case 1). Other complications include liver abscess (Isobe *et al.* 1990) and bile duct occlusion due to ethanol entry causing jaundice.

Some radiologists and hepatologists have expanded the indication to the treatment of portal tumor thrombus (Livraghi *et al.* 1990) and tumors up to 5 cm in size (Livraghi *et al.* 1992) and even larger tumors (Shiina *et al.* 1990), but the results have not yet been fully evaluated. Tanaka *et al.* (1991) used PEI and TAE in combination for the treatment of large encapsulated HCC in patients who are poor surgical risks. Beside ethanol, any substance that would cause death of cancer cells may be used. Attempts have been made with concentrated acetic acid (Ohnishi *et al.* 1994) similarly injected into the tumor. Seki *et al.* (1994) used a microwave coagulator inserted percutaneously to destroy cancer growing within a large bile duct.

PEI—Case 1: Portal vein thrombosis following intratumor ethanol injection.

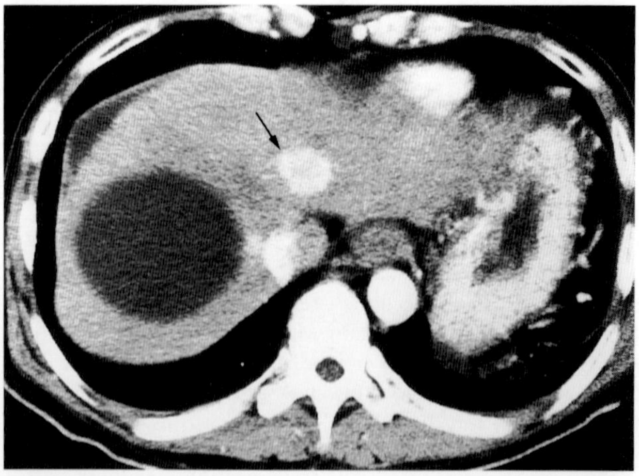

(a) Enhanced CT: during the follow-up of this patient after resection, a recurrent lesion (→) was found by CT, and PEI was carried out.

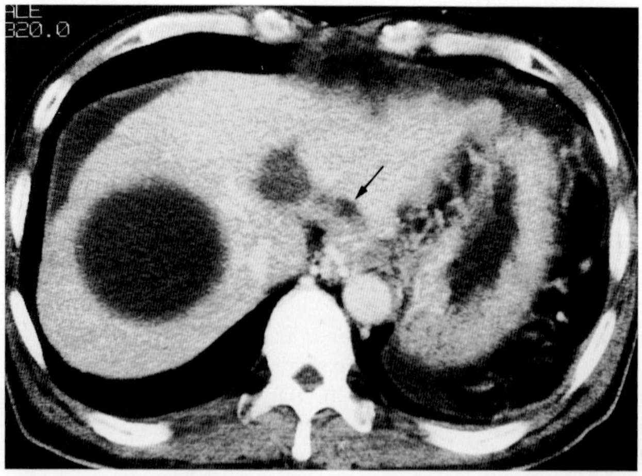

(b) Enhanced CT (1.5 months post-PEI): the recurrent lesion was not enhanced, suggesting successful treatment, but a cord-like unstained structure was recognized (→).

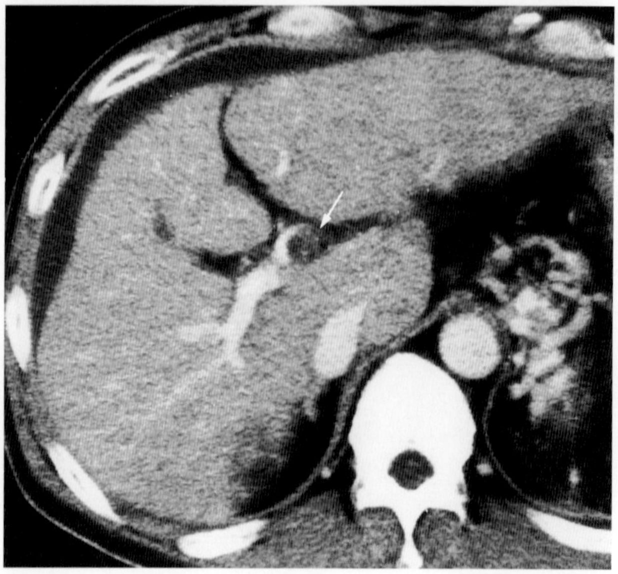

(c) Enhanced CT [slice caudal to (b)]: a filling defect was seen in the left portal vein (→) which did not exist in the pretreatment CT. The likely diagnosis was thrombosis induced by ethanol that entered the portal vein during the PEI procedure.

22

Radiation therapy

Radiation therapy for liver cancer had nearly been abandoned until recently. It was revived in the 1980s at Chiba University (Ohto *et al.* 1987), and at the National Cancer Center Hospital (Aoki *et al.* 1994). We are also giving radiation therapy (total dose, 50–60 Gy, 200 rad/dose) to patients in whom TAE has not been very successful. Case 1 described on p.183 had an HCC primary to the left caudate lobe, and early in the course developed tumor thrombosis in the left portal vein and multiple intrahepatic secondaries. The primary lesion and portal tumor thrombosis were irradiated with a total dose of 50 Gy, and Lipiodol-TAE repeated for the secondaries; the patient lived for 2.5 years. However, liver atrophy may follow radiation (Case 1) with ascites formation and deterioration of liver function. Therefore, this therapy should be given only to patients who have a good liver function (Child A, and some Child B patients).

Case 2 had advanced HCC complicating alcoholic cirrhosis. Intrahepatic secondaries became smaller by three sessions of TAE, but the main mass did not respond, and radiation therapy (50 Gy) was given. Subsequently, the main mass slowly shrank, and there has been no recurrence for 3.5 years. In this patient, liver function quickly improved after he stopped drinking, and the improved liver function could well be one of the reasons for long survival. It has been our practice to wait 1 month or so after Lipiodol TAE before radiation, because of our early experience in which a patient in whom radiation was begun immediately after TAE developed unexpected hepatic failure. Some patients develop ascites and deterioration of liver function associated with marked liver strophy following irradiation given to a large area of the liver.

Recently, heavy particle radiation using the proton beam has been developed (Chuvilo *et al.* 1984; Tsujii *et al.* 1992). It has a Bragg peak which limits the distribution of beams, resulting in both a marked reduction in the amount of radiation that reaches non-targeted areas and an increase in the amount of radiation hitting the target. Matsuzaki *et al.* (1994) used low-energy protons generated by a booster synchrotron in inoperable HCC cases (50–87 Gy) singly or in combination with TAE. Size reduction was obtained in 92 per cent with irradiation alone and in 100 per cent with the combination. There was no serious parenchymal damage because these protons had a Bragg peak. Particles heavier than proton (such as carbon) can be used, and phase I/II study is in progress. However, the cost for such facilities is prohibitive.

There was a time when ^{192}Ir was used through the PTC tube for extrahepatic bile duct carcinoma, but the determination of the extent of the tumor was inadequate, and the management of PTCD difficult. Since the results were poorer than expected, this method is seldom used.

Radiation therapy—Case 1: Combined hepatocholangioma of the mixed type responding to irradiation which entailed atrophy of the right lobe.

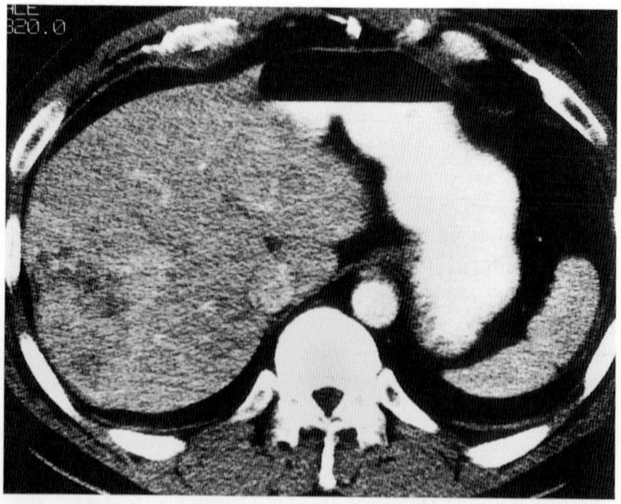

(a) Enhanced CT (pretreatment): a 7 cm wedge-shaped lesion in the right lobe was enhanced. The patient developed cerebral infarct as a result of atrial fibrillation developing during angiography, and the intended TAE and operation were called off. Parallel opposing irradiation (60 Gy) was carried out.

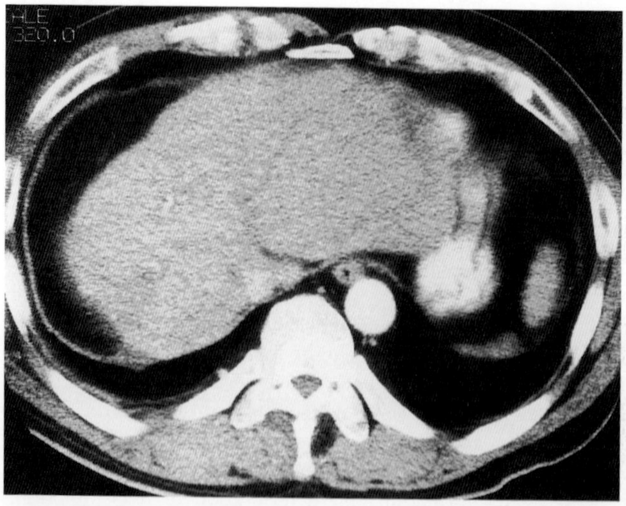

(b) Enhanced CT (6 months post-treatment): the right lobe is markedly atrophied with compensatory hypertrophy of the left lobe. Serum AFP dropped from the pretreatment value of 308 ng/ml to 20 ng/ml post-treatment.

Radiation therapy—Case 2: Advanced HCC that responded to irradiation combined with TAE. Multiple tumors were found in the liver.

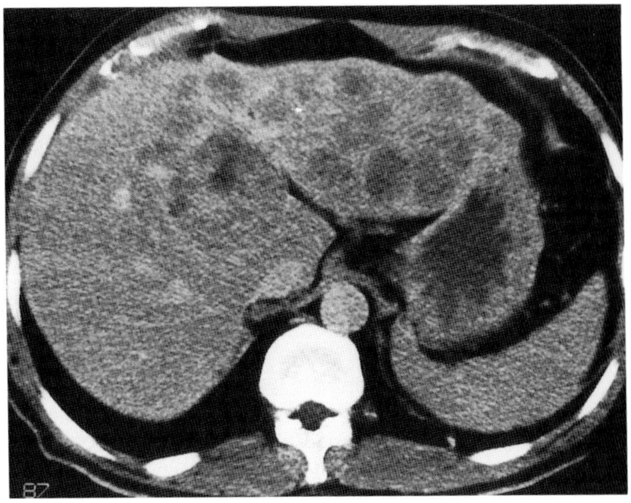

(a) Enhanced CT (pretreatment): in this late phase image, a 5 cm main mass is seen in S^{IV} and multiple lesions in the left lobe. The diagnosis was HCC, and angiography also disclosed six secondaries in the right lobe. Lipiodol-TAE was carried out.

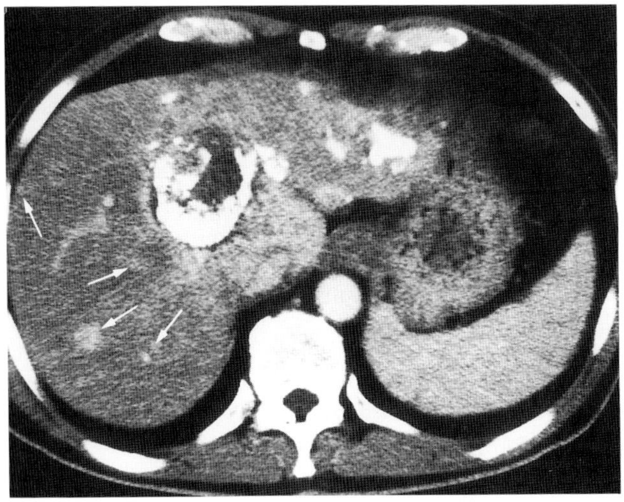

(b) Enhanced CT (after the first TAE): despite the first TAE, new lesions appeared (→). TAE was repeated followed by irradiation (50 Gy) against the main mass.

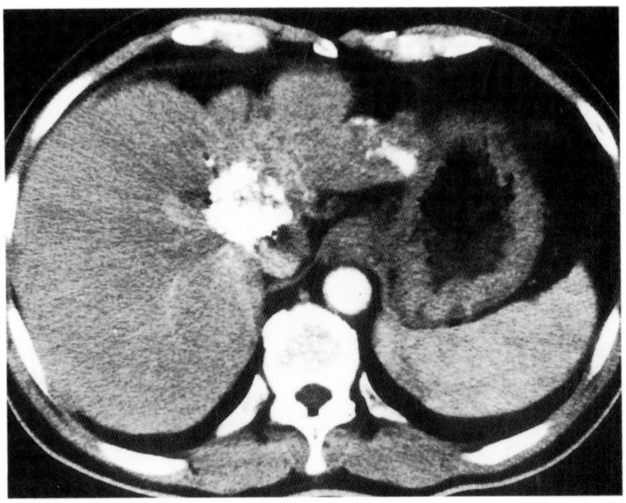

(c) Enhanced CT (3 years after the first treatment): the main mass has shrunk and the left lobe has been markedly atrophied. No new lesion has since developed, and the patient is doing well.

23

Systemic chemotherapy

Systemic chemotherapy is generally regarded as unrewarding in HCC (Okazaki 1976; Falkson and Coetzer 1987; Okada *et al.* 1992). At the National Cancer Center Hospital, Tokyo, phase II studies were carried out with doxorubicin (Adriamycin), Tegaful, UFT, Etoposide, Mitoxantrone, Cisplatin, and gamma-interferon in 141 patients with HCC, but partial response was obtained in only 10 (7.0 per cent). Drug-wise, the number of responders was one each for doxorubicin, Tegafur, UFT, and Etoposide, two for Mitoxantrone, zero for gamma-interferon, and four for Cisplatin. Cisplatin had a response rate of 15 per cent and was the best (Okazaki *et al.* 1992). The prognosis of the 86 who did not respond to chemotherapy was analyzed with respect to additional TAE whether it was given (n=20) or not (n=66). As shown in Fig. 23.1, the survival curve was significantly better with additional TAE (Okazaki *et al.* 1988). Based on these results, we feel that TAE should be given preference as an additional therapy in patients who have HCC only in the liver and who did not respond to systemic chemotherapy. The results in these six responders were equivalent to those obtained with TAE. A reliable test should be developed for determining the sensitivity of cancer cells to various chemotherapeutic agents.

There was a time in Japan when intraarterial single dose (one-shot) chemotherapy was advocated over systemic chemotherapy with a rationale that higher concentrations of anticancer agents would reach the cancer (Kubo and Shimokawa 1976), but subsequent studies have failed to corroborate its superiority to systemic chemotherapy.

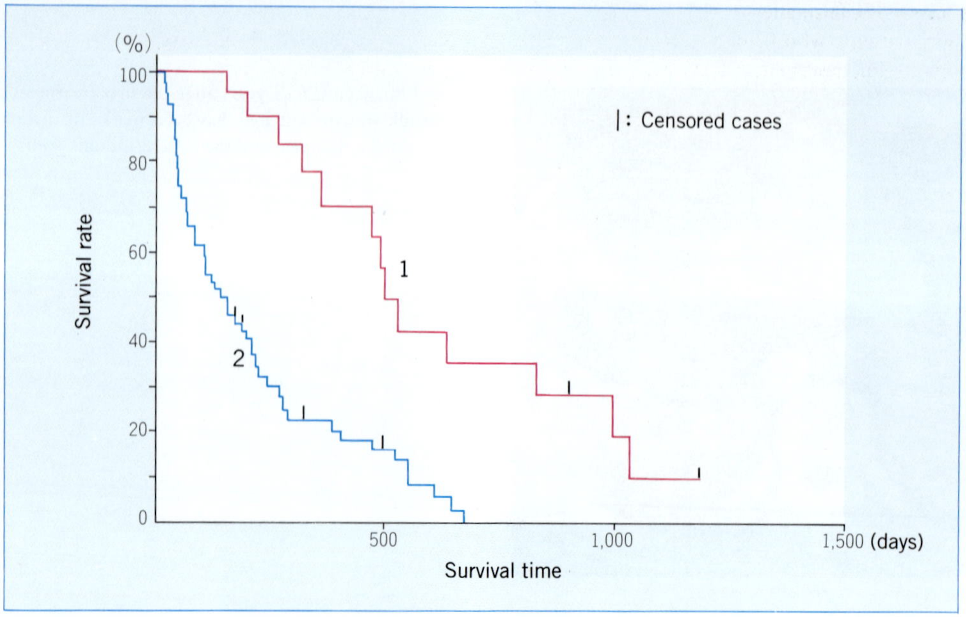

24

Selection of the best treatment modality for HCC

As already discussed, various therapeutic modalities are available for HCC, such as TAE, surgery, PEI, radiation, systemic chemotherapy, etc. The first four aim at a localized target in the liver (local therapy) and the last one is to be applied to patients with distant metastases. The policy at our cancer hospital in the selection of modality for the first treatment is to prefer surgery to other approaches when the liver function is good (serum bilirubin less than 2.0 mg/dl, no ascites) with no extrahepatic metastasis, even though the lesions are multiple and located in both lobes. The reason is that despite frequent postoperative recurrences, a long survival can be expected in those who do not develop recurrence. For the patients with moderately reduced liver function (mainly Child B) who have multiple lesions but no tumor thrombosis in the portal trunk, TAE is preferentially considered.

Indication for PEI has been extended at many centers to patients who have several HCC smaller than 3 cm, but in reality there are not so many patients who fulfil such criteria for PEI. The major determinants for treatment selection are the degree of liver dysfunction and of tumor growth (Okuda *et al.* 1985*b*; Ohnishi *et al.* 1987). We have been irradiating patients who have portal tumor thrombosis occupying up to the beginning of the second-order portal branch and who did not respond to TAE, but the results varied; some developed acute hepatic failure, and others fared well. As already discussed, a proton beam that has a Bragg peak permits greater doses of radiation to hit the targeted lesion with very little radiation damage to the untargeted areas (Tsujii *et al.* 1992; Matsuzaki *et al.* 1995); it may have a bright future.

For recurrence in the residual liver, reoperation is generally difficult, and TAE or PEI is frequently used. Some carry out both TAE and PEI in combination for the first treatment and for recurrence (Tanaka *et al.* 1991), or TAE combined with radiation (Pechoux *et al.* 1994), the so called multidisciplinary therapy. A prospective randomized trial comparing TAE and PEI is required in patients with HCC, but in reality it is difficult. Therefore, we are about to embark on such a trial in patients with recurrence.

25

Evaluation of therapeutic effects

Before the advent of modern imaging techniques, the evaluation of therapeutic effects was based on the Karnofsky score which grades the general physical status of the patient. Later, palpation, radioisotope study, and more objective means were used for measuring the size of tumor for evaluation of treatment efficacy. For the assessment of therapeutic effects of systemic and arterial chemotherapy, we used the 'Criteria for Direct Evalustion of Therapeutic Effects on Solid Tumors', the guidelines proposed by the Japanese Society for Cancer Therapy (1986). However, these guidelines are not always applicable to newer therapeutic modalities, as will be discussed below. We perhaps need simpler and more widely applicable guidelines that can be used in developing countries.

TAE therapy

For the evaluation of TAE effects, we usually depend on tumor staining. Enhanced CT and AFP measurement are easily done, and are most reliable. The evaluation based on CT images and that based on AFP changes generally correspond well. However, there will be a discrepancy between these two in the presence of an extrahepatic metastasis and when viable lesions smaller than 1 cm (which CT cannot detect) remain in the liver.

In patients who were treated by TAE in which only Gelfoam and an anticancer drug were used, necrotic and viable areas in the tumor were clearly distinguished from the degree of stain on enhanced CT, and the assessment agreed well with the histological study of the resected specimens (Takayasu *et al.* 1984*b*) (Case 1). Enhanced CT also permits diagnosis of post-TAE regrowth within the tumor (Case 2). After the introduction of Lipiodol to TAE, evaluation of effects by CT alone become difficult. If Lipiodol once retained in the tumor disappears, enhanced CT is still of value in assessing the effect (Case 3), but in the presence of retained Lipiodol, this is not the case. In some with ample Lipiodol retention, no antitumor effect is demonstrable (cf. Case 1, p.464) whereas in others with a similar retention there is a satisfactory effect. At the moment, the CT features suggestive of good antitumor effects with TAE are: (1) good Lipiodol retention, (2) the area not enhanced by contrast CT if it does not retain Lipiodol, (3) shrinking of the tumor size, and (4) increase in Lipiodol density in the mass (Case 2, p.465). With heavy Lipiodol retention, an artefact radiating from the tumor is often seen in the CT image.

Following TAE with Gelfoam and an anticancer agent, gas forms in the tumor within two to three days. It is assumed that sudden interruption of blood flow in the feeding artery produces carbon dioxide generated by anaerobic breakdown of reticulocytes, and free molecular oxygen derived from oxidized hemoglobin-bound oxygen (Rankin 1979). Gas formation is more pronounced when the TAE effect was good (Case 4). US readily recognizes intratumor gas as high echoes, but they may interfere with US evaluation of the internal structural changes.

Surgical treatment

Enhanced CT is very useful in the diagnosis of marginal recurrence, and recurrence in the residual liver (Case 5). Within 1 month of the operation, the surgical margin in the remnant liver may be enhanced in some patients as a result of the tissue repair process (Case 6). It has to be differentiated from marginal recurrence. In the former, the enhancement disappears with time whereas in the latter it increases in size.

Intratumor ethanol injection therapy

A necrotic area induced by PEI in the tumor is not enhanced whereas the viable region is stained on enhanced CT (Case 7), and the evaluation is virtually the same as in TAE therapy (Joseph *et al.* 1993; Ebara *et al.* 1995). However, during the repair process after PEI, proliferating capillaries may be mildly enhanced and distinction from a viable area becomes necessary. Since ethanol is injected beyond the tumor boundary, the size of the mass seen by imaging is frequently larger than the actual size, making it difficult to base the evaluation on tumor size. There has been an attempt to implant steel coils in the tumor as a landmark (Sheu *et al.* 1987). The tumor may undergo a change in shape (Case 8) and a linear unenhanced area may be produced by ethanol that leaked along the needle track.

Radiation therapy

Therapeutic evaluation is made from the change in size of the tumor. Some tumors responding to irradiation may show mild enhancement in the tumor periphery or interior (Case 9). It is assumed that tissue repair with capillary proliferation increases the uptake of contrast medium.

Arterial and systemic chemotherapy

Response to arterial one-shot administration of an anticancer agent and systemic chemotherapy is indicated by changes in tumor diameter. The tumor is reduced in size when responding to the therapy (Case 10). The degree of tumor shrinkage may be quantified according to the WHO Guidelines for the Clinical Evaluation of Antineoplastic Drugs (1979). Following chemotherapy calcification may develop within the tumor, but the incidence is rather low.

Evaluation based on MR imaging

As MR imaging does not pick up the signal of Lipiodol, it was thought to be useful in the evaluation of the effectiveness of TAE. However, this is not necessarily so when compared with Lipiodol-CT (Case 11). The changes that occur following TAE include, beside coagulation necrosis and fresh bleeding, liquefaction, exudation of plasma and changes of paramagnetic hemoglobin molecules with time, making the correlation of MR images and tissue changes difficult. Assessment of necrosis in a large mass retaining Lipiodol may be possible by MR imaging with contrast enhancement using Gd-DTPA (Murakami *et al.* 1993), but evaluation of small areas by MR imaging may be difficult. The effect of PEI can also be assessed by MR imaging (Kubota *et al.* 1989; Sironi *et al.* 1993). At the moment, evaluation by MR imaging has limitations, and further investigations comparing histopathology and imaging features are required.

Evaluation of therapeutic effects—Case 1: Evaluation of antitumor effect comparing CT images and cut section of resected specimen after TAE without Lipiodol.

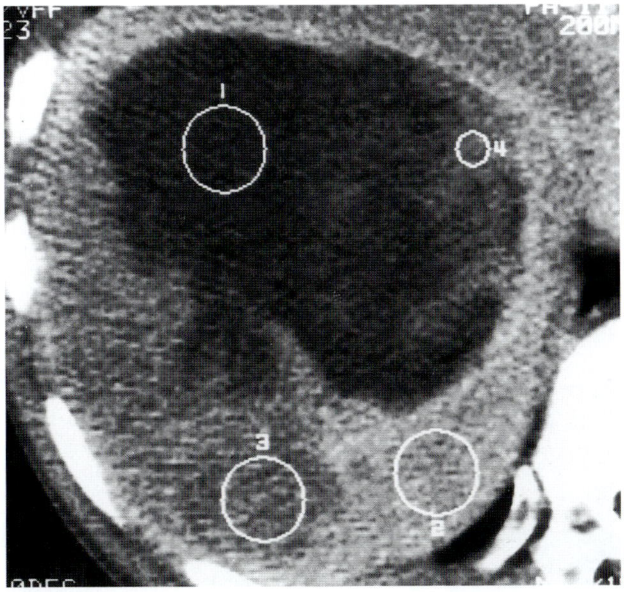

(a) Enhanced CT (54 days post-TAE): this was made 54 days after TAE in which Gelfoam + Adriamycin were used. The upper half of this 12 cm mass (1) is of low density (24 HU) with no enhancement. The right posterior (3) and medial (4) areas were slightly enhanced (75 HU).

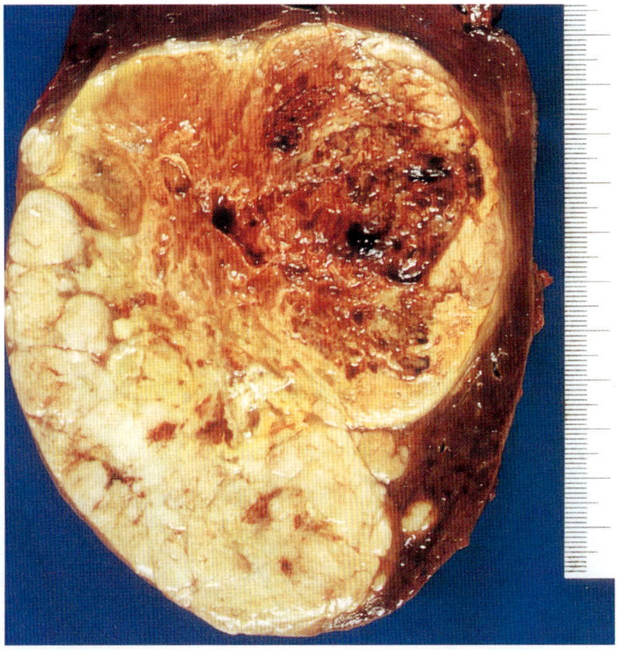

(b) Cut section of resected specimen (71 days post-TAE): the unstained area in the enhanced CT image was necrotic as contrasted by the enhanced area which consisted of viable cancer cells, closely corresponding to the CT image.

Evaluation of therapeutic effects—Case 2: Diagnosis by enhanced CT of regrowth within the mass after TAE.

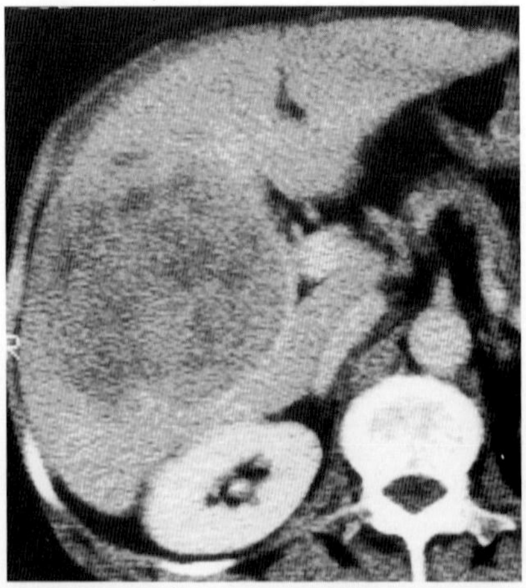

(a) Enhanced CT (before TAE): a 9 cm mass is seen in the right lobe. TAE with Gelfoam particles + Adriamycin was carried out.

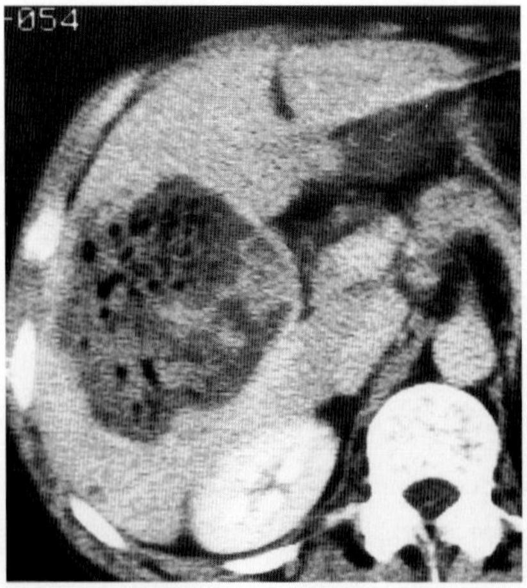

(b) Enhanced CT (4 days post-TAE): a large part of the mass has changed to a low-density area with multiple spots of gas. The left side of the tumor is stained and remaining viable cancer cells are suggested.

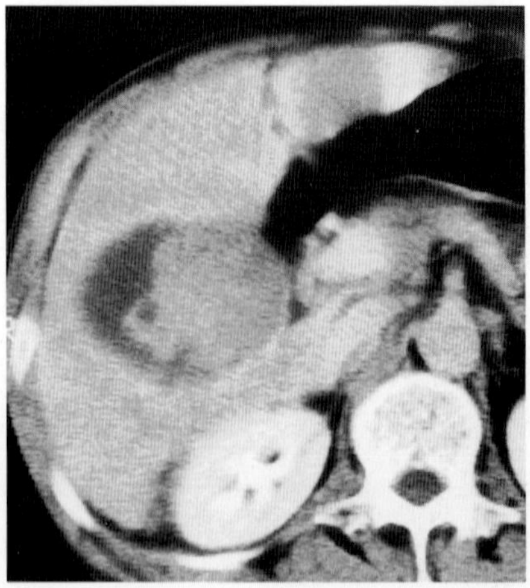

(c) Enhanced CT (1.5 months post-TAE): the area diagnosed as viable grew within the mass, but the size of the entire mass has shrunk from the pre-TAE size of 9 cm to 7 cm.

Evaluation of therapeutic effects—Case 3: Evaluation of antitumor effect by enhanced CT made after Lipiodol-TAE.

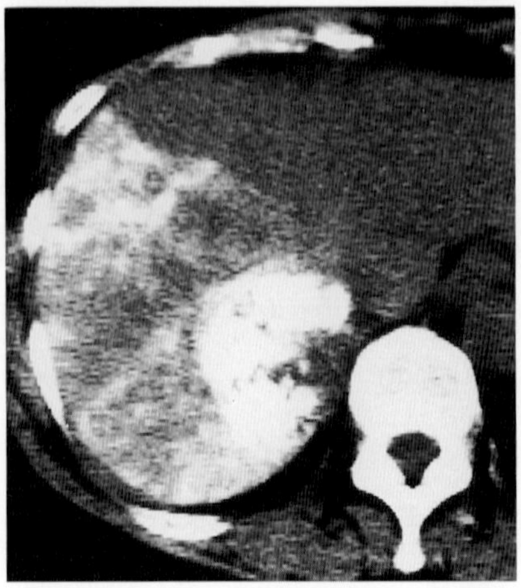

a

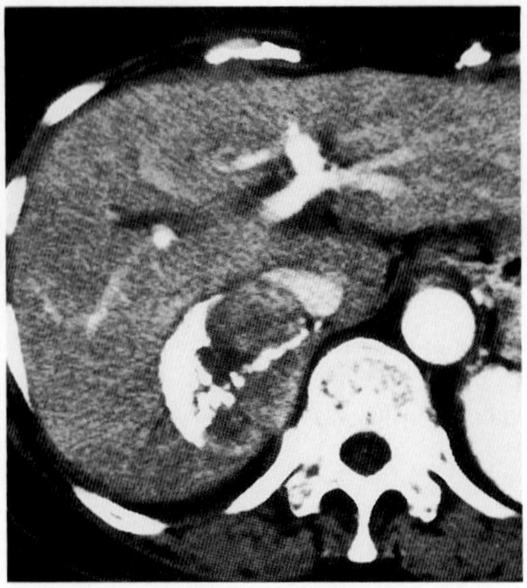

b

(a) Plain CT (immediately after Lipiodol-TAE): Lipiodol-TAE was done through the right hepatic artery, and this CT was made immediately thereafter. Lipiodol entered the mass except for a small medial area

.

(b) Enhanced CT (2 months after Lipiodol-TAE): enhancement is seen in one-third of the area to the right of the tumor, and in the remaining two-thirds Lipiodol has disappeared. This latter area was enhanced by contrast medium, suggesting its viability. Lipiodol retention does not necessarily indicate necrosis, and therefore evaluation of therapeutic effects is not always feasible with enhanced CT.

Evaluation of therapeutic effects—Case 4: Inaccuracy of US evaluation of TAE effects when compared with CT.

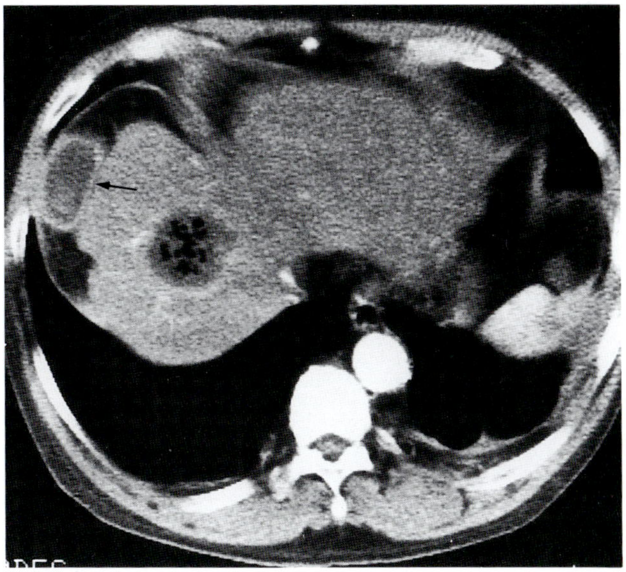

(a) Enhanced CT (2 weeks after TAE): although the tumor periphery is mildly enhanced, the interior has multiple gas holes with no enhancement, and necrosis was suggested. →, marked displacement of the gallbladder due to cirrhosis.

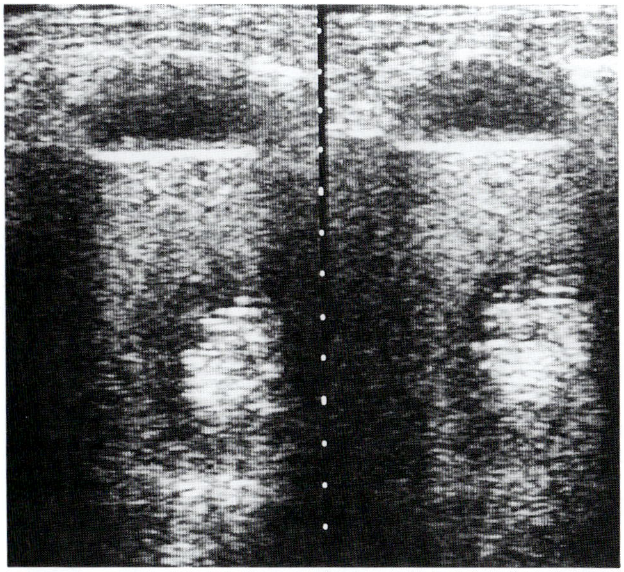

(b) US (right intercostal scan after TAE): the tumor periphery is hypoechoic, and the interior is homogeneously hyperechoic, hampering evaluation of the internal structure. Compared with CT, evaluation of antitumor effects with US is generally difficult.

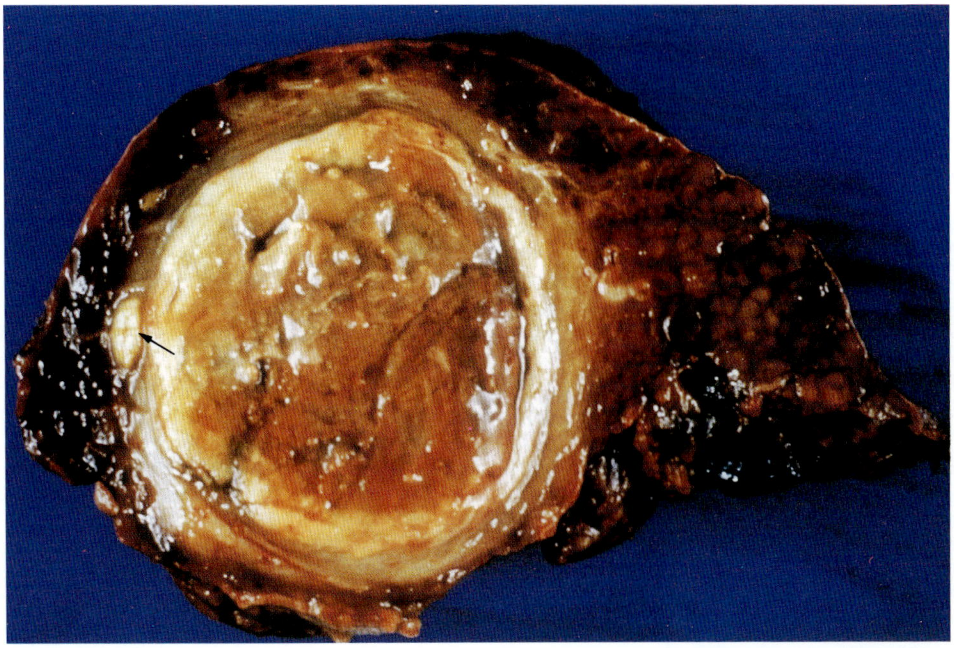

(c) Cut section of resected specimen: except for a small lesion (→) within the thick fibrous capsule, the entire mass has undergone coagulative necrosis.

Evaluation of therapeutic effects—Case 5: Marginal recurrence after resection. A 56-year-old man. The left lobe was resected in an emergency operation for tumor rupture. Tumor thrombosis was grossly recognized in the portal vein as well as in the hepatic vein, and the resection was not a curative one.

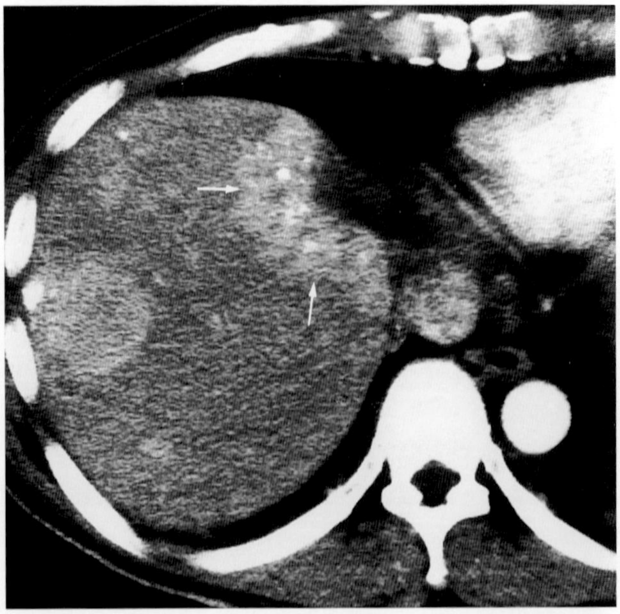

Enhanced CT (2 months postoperatively): a band-shaped irregular area (→) along the margin was enhanced. S^{VIII} also has a recurrent lesion. This kind of marginal recurrence is very uncommon.

Evaluation of therapeutic effects—Case 6: Non-specific enhancement along the margin seen by enhanced CT shortly after resection. A 51-year-old man. Partial resection was done for an HCC in S^{VII}. A recurrent lesion was suspected in the right lobe, and arterial-CT was done 1 week postoperatively.

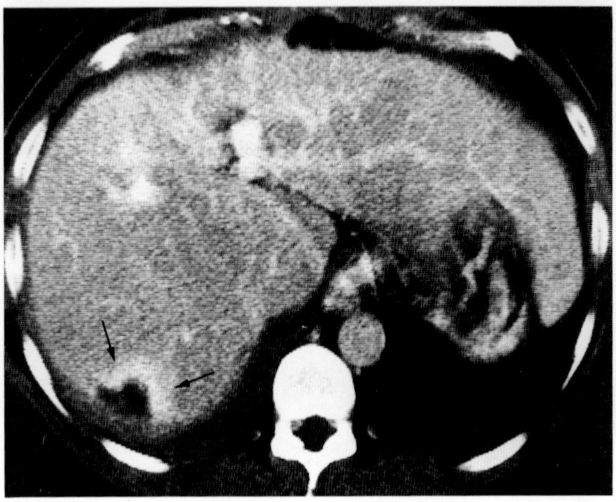

Arterial-CT (1 week postoperatively): the margin is enhanced (→). The enhancement decreases toward the diaphragm. This was interpreted as a change in the margin in reaction to the surgical intervention (same as Case 1, p. 111).

Evaluation of therapeutic effects—Case 7: Evaluation of PEI effect by enhanced CT. A 65-year-old woman. Because of poor liver function, PEI (6 ml) was given to HCC under laparotomy.

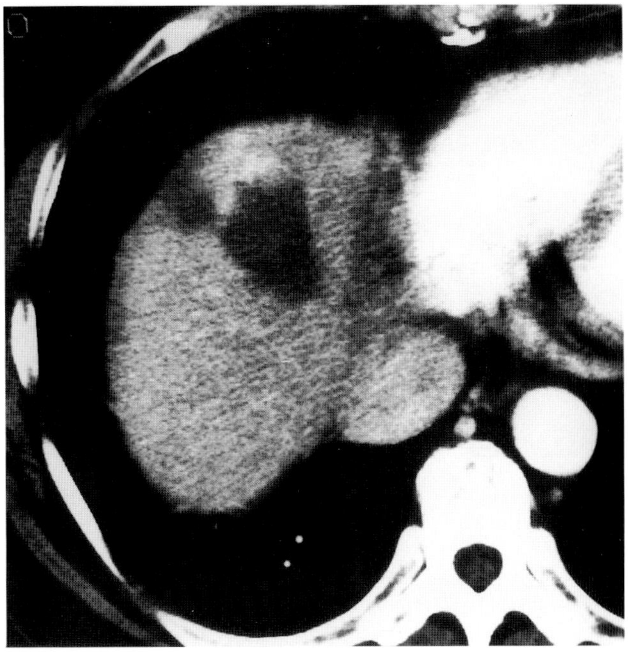

Enhanced CT (3 months after PEI): in this follow-up enhanced CT, the bulk of the mass was not enhanced, but a small anterior area was stained (viable). Before the therapy, the tumor was round, but its shape changed to a geometric one due to ethanol injected into the surrounding area.

Evaluation of therapeutic effects—Case 8: Change in shape of necrosis due to PEI. Four sessions of PEI were given to a recurrent HCC lesion in the left lobe.

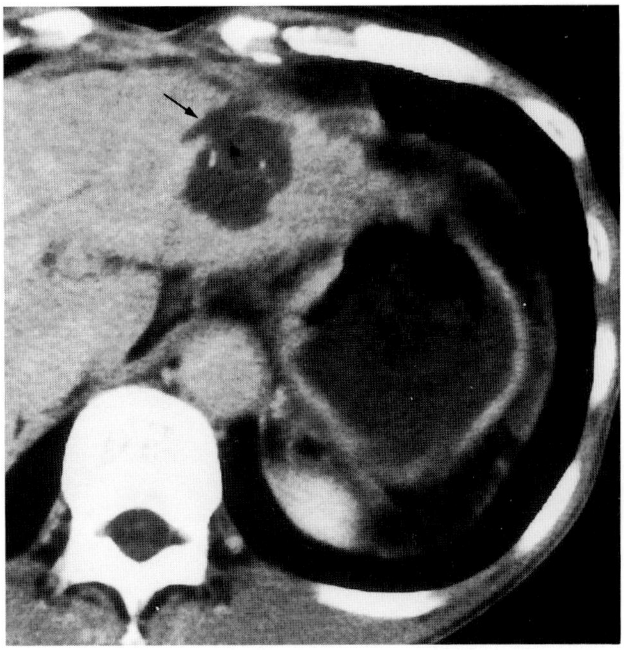

Enhanced CT (after PEI): the round lesion changed to rectangular, and a linear low-density area (→) of necrosis is now seen along the needle puncture track.

Evaluation of therapeutic effects—Case 9: Evaluation of radiation effects by CT. A 60-year-old man. Radiation therapy (64.8 Gy) was given to multiple HCC lesions and tumor thrombosis in the peripheral portal veins.

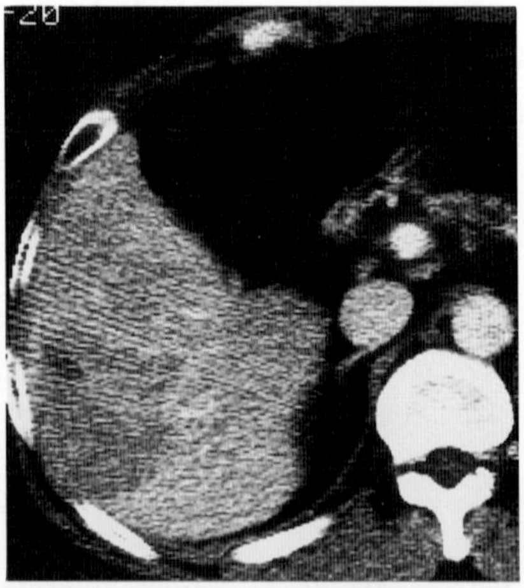

(a) Enhanced CT (before irradiation): a 5 × 5 cm irregularly bordered low-density lesion is seen in S^{VI}.

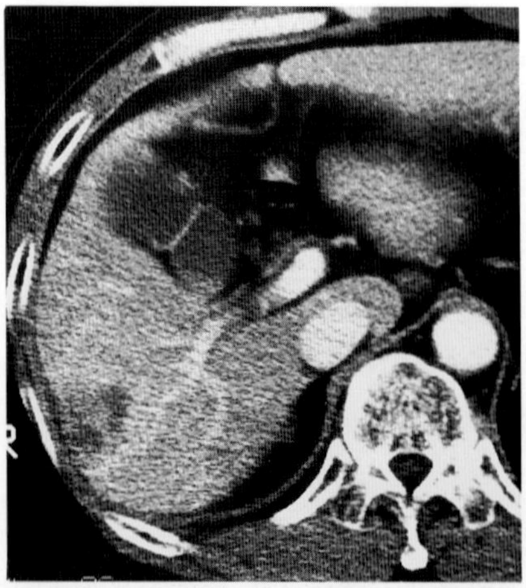

(b) Enhanced CT (2 months postirradiation): the mass in S^{VI} has been shrunk to a size of 3.6 × 3 cm. The periphery of the tumor is stained slightly.

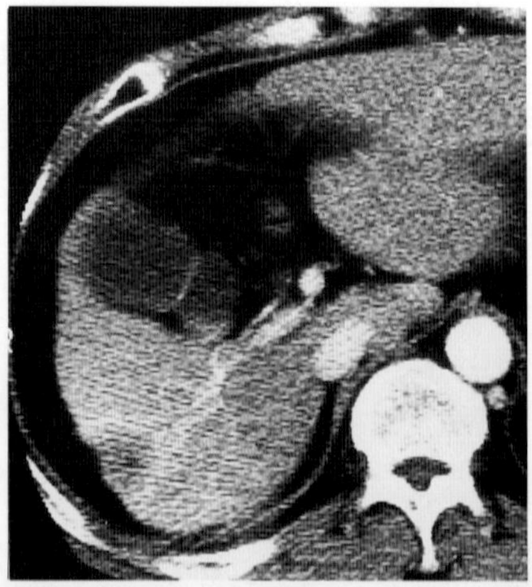

(c) Enhanced CT (9 months postirradiation): the mass in S^{VI} has been shrunk further to 2.8 × 2.5 cm with peripheral enhancement. After 1 year and 2 months local tumor growth was recognized to which repeat radiotherapy was given, but the patient died from hepatic failure 2 years 7 months later. Autopsy disclosed atrophy of the right lobe, scarring of the tumor, and many viable small lesions.

Evaluation of therapeutic effects—Case 10: Evaluation of therapeutic effects of systemic chemotherapy by enhanced CT. Etoposide, Adriamycin, and CDDP (EAP therapy) were given to multiple hepatic metastases from advanced gastric cancer (Borrmann type II).

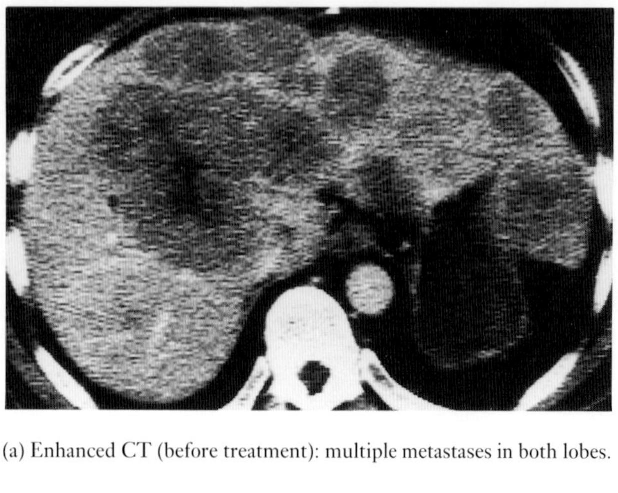

(a) Enhanced CT (before treatment): multiple metastases in both lobes.

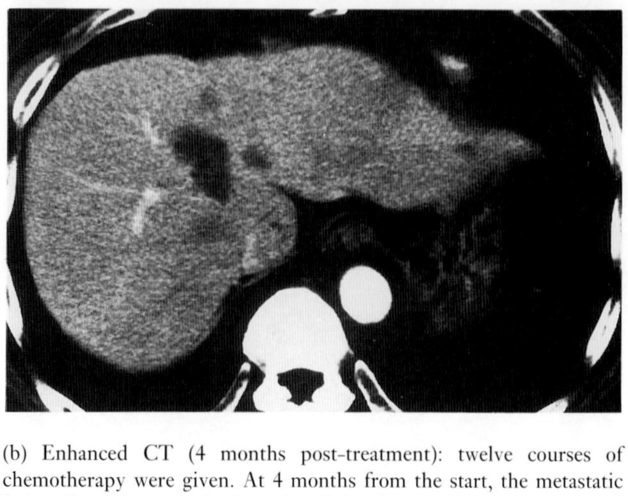

(b) Enhanced CT (4 months post-treatment): twelve courses of chemotherapy were given. At 4 months from the start, the metastatic lesions have been markedly reduced in size, leaving only one small lesion. The primary in the stomach has also disappeared.

Evaluation of therapeutic effects—Case 11: Evaluation of antitumor effects by MR imaging. TAE with Lipiodol + Adriamycin (40 mg) + Gelfoam was given to an HCC in S^{VIII}.

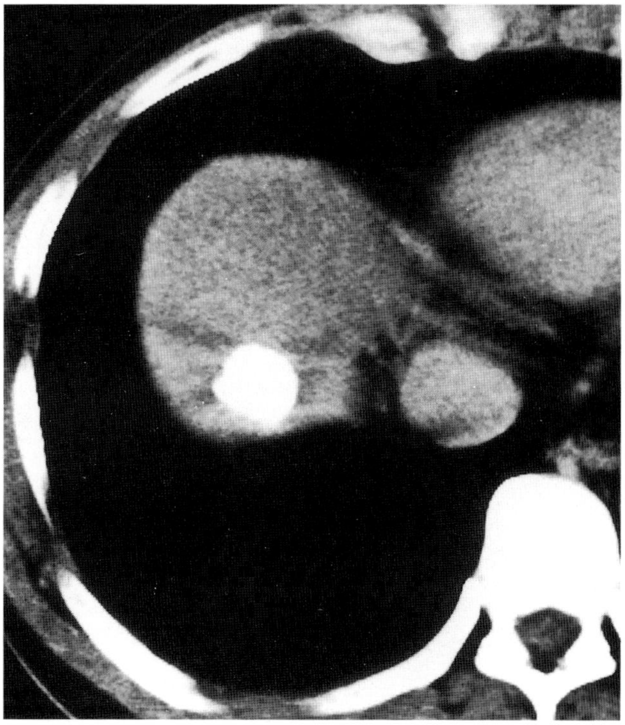

(a) Enhanced CT (1 month after treatment): the whole mass is occupied by Lipiodol. Since there is no enhanced area, a complete necrosis of the tumor was expected.

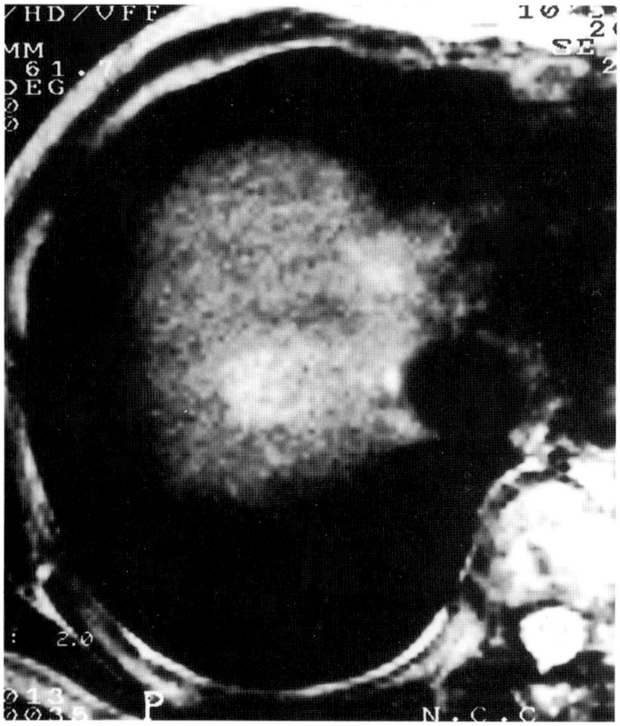

(b) MR imaging (T2-weighted): MR imaging by the spin-echo method was done 1 day after (a). On the T1-weighted image, the mass was of isointensity (not shown). On the T2-weighted image, it was of high intensity. These MR findings suggested that the mass was mostly viable. Resection was done 2 months later to disclose an encapsulated HCC which was completely necrotized. There was no bleeding or liquefying necrosis.

References

Akine, Y., Ogino, T., Kajiura, Y. *et al.* (1988). Ir-192 brachytherapy by an afterloading technique: initial experience at the National Cancer Center Hospital, Tokyo. *Radiation Med.*, **6**, 40–45.

Alberti-Flor. J.J., O'Hara M.F., Weaver F., *et al.* (1985). Malignant fibrous histiocytoma of the liver. *Gastroenterology*, **89**, 890–3.

Allen. R.A. and Lisa. J.R. (1949). Combined liver cell and bile duct carcinoma. *Am. J. Pathol.*, **25**, 647–55.

Amendola, M.A., Blane, C.E., Amendola, B.S., *et al.* (1984). CT findings in hepatoblastoma. *J. Comput. Assist. Tomogr.*, **8**, 1105–9.

Andreola, S., Lonbardi, L., Audisio, R.A., *et al.* (1990). A clinicopathologic study of primary hepatic carcinoid tumors. *Cancer*, **65**, 1211–18.

Anson, B.H., (1963). *An Atlas of Human Anatomy*. Saunders, Philadelphia.

Anthony, P.P., Telesinghe, P.U. (1986). Inflammatory pseudotumour of the liver. *J. Clin. Pathol.* **29**, 761–8.

Aoki, K., Takayasu, K., Kawano, T., *et al.* (1993). Combined hepatocellular carcinoma and cholangiocarcinoma: clinical features and computed tomographic findings. *Hepatology*, **18**, 1090–95.

Aoki, K., Okazaki, N., Okada, S., *et al.* (1994). Radiotherapy for hepatocellular carcinoma: clinicopathological study of seven autopsy cases. *Hepato-Gastroenterology*, **41**, 427–31.

Arai, K., Matsui, O., Takashima, T., *et al.* (1988). Focal spared areas in fatty liver caused by regional decreased portal flow. *A.J.R.*, **151**, 300–2.

Arakawa, M., Kage, M., Sugihara, S., *et al.* (1986*a*). Emergence of malignant lesions within an adenomatous hyperplastic nodule in a cirrhotic liver. Observations in five cases. *Gastroenterology*, **91**, 198–208.

Arakawa, M., Kage, M., Matsumoto, S., *et al.* (1986*b*). Frequency and significance of tumor thrombi in esophageal varices in hepatocellular carcinoma associated with cirrhosis. *Hepatology*, **6**, 419–22.

Arakawa, M., Kage, M. (1987). The anatomy and pathomorphology of esophageal varices. In *Portal hypertension. Clinical and physiological aspects* (ed. K. Okuda and J.-P. Benhamou), pp.415–28. Springer, Tokyo.

Araki, T., Itai, Y., Furui, S., Tasaka, A. (1980), Dynamic CT densitometry of hepatic tumors. *A.J.R.*, **135**, 1037–43.

Araki, T., Karikomi, M., *et al.* (1988). Hepatocellular carcinoma: metastatic abdominal lymph nodes identified by computed tomography. *Gastrointest. Radiol.*, **13**, 247–52.

Araki, T., Suda, K., Sekikawa, T., *et al.* (1990). Portal venous tumor thrombosis associated with gastric adenocarcinoma. *Radiology*, **174**, 811.

Ariyama, J., Shirakabe, H., Ikenobe, H., and Roberts, G.M. (1978). Comparison of barium swallow and left gastric angiography in the diagnosis of esophageal varices, with special reference to the management of variceal bleeding. *Gastrointes. Radiol.*, **3**, 1–6.

Arrivé, L., Fléjou, J.F., Vilgrain, V., *et al.* (1994). Hepatic adenoma: MR findings in 51 pathologically proved lesions. *Radiology*, **193**, 507–12.

Balasagarum M. (1972). Complete hepatic dearterialization for primary carcinoma of the liver: report of twenty-four patients. *Am. J. Surg.* 124, 340–5.

Balthazar, E.J., Naidich, D.P., Megibow, A.J., and Lefleur, R.S. (1987). CT evaluation of esophageal varices. *A.J.R.*, **148**, 131–5.

Baron, R.L., Campbell, W.L., Dodd, G.D. III. (1994). Peribiliary cysts associated with severe liver disease: imaging pathologic correlation. *A.J.R.*, **162**, 631–36.

Baxter, J.N., and Dobbs, B.R. (1988). Portal hypertensive gastropathy. *J. Gastroenterol. Hepatol.*, **3**, 635–44.

Bechtold, R.E., Karstaedt, N., Wolfman, N.T., and Glass, T.A., (1985). Prolonged hepatic enhancement on computed tomography in a case of hepatic lymphoma. *J. Comput. Assist. Tomogr.*, **9**, 186–9.

Becker, C.D., Hassler, H., and Tarrier, F. (1984). Preoperative diagnosis of the Mirizzi syndrome: limitations of sonography and computed tomography. *A.J.R.*, **143**, 591–6.

Belton, D.L., and Van Zandt, T.F., (1983). Congenital absence of the left lobe of the liver: a radiologic diagnosis. *Radiology*, **147**, 184.

Bengmark, S., and Hafstrom, L. (1969). The natural history of primary and secondary tumors of the liver. I. The prognosis for patients with hepatic metastases from colonic and rectal carcinoma by laparotomy. *Cancer*, **23**, 198–202.

Bernardino, M.E. (1979). Computed tomography of calcified liver metastases. *J. Comput. Assist. Tomogr.*, **3**, 32–5.

Bluemke, D.A. and Fishman, E.K. (1993). Spiral CT arterial portography of the liver. *Radiology*, **186**, 576–9.

Boijsen, E. and Abrams, H.L. (1965). Roentgenologic diagnosis of primary carcinoma of the liver. *Acta Radiol. (Diag.)*, **3**, 257–77.

Bookstein, J.J., Cho, K.J., Davis, G.B., and Dail, D. (1982). Arterioportal communications: observations and hypotheses concerning transsinusoidal and transvasal types. *Radiology*, **142**, 581–90.

Borow, M., Conston, A., Livornese, L., *et al.* (1973). Mesothelioma following exposure to asbestos: a review of 72 cases. *Chest*, **64**, 641–6.

Botet, J.F., Watson, R.C., Kemeny, N.K., *et al.* (1985). Cholangitis complicating intraarterial chemotherapy in liver metastasis. *Radiology*, **156**, 335–7.

Boulstein, P.A. (1978). Hepatic leiomyosarcoma. *Hum. Pathol.*, **9**, 713–15.

Bradley, W.G. Jr and Waluch, V. (1985). Blood flow: magnetic resonance imaging. *Radiology*, 154, 443–50.

Brady, J., Liberatore, F., Harper, P., *et al.* (1977). Angiosarcoma of the liver: an epidemiologic survey. *J. Natl. Cancer Inst.*, **59**, 1383–5.

Brandt, D.J., Johnson, C.D., Stephens, D.H., and Weiland, L.H. (1988). Imaging of fibrolamellar hepatocellular carcinoma. *A.J.R.*, **151**, 295–9.

Brasch, R.C., Wesbey, G.E., Gooding, C.A., and Koerper, M.A. (1984). Magnetic resonance imaging of transfusional hemosiderosis complicating thalassemia major. *Radiology*, **50**, 767–71.

Broe, P.J., Conley, C.L., and Cameron, J.L. (1981). Thrombosis of the portal vein following splenectomy for myeloid metaplasia. *Surg. Gynecol. Obstet.*, **151**, 488–92.

Buetow, P.C., Buck, J.L., Ros, P.R., and Goodman, Z.D. (1994). Malignant vascular tumors of the liver: radiologic-pathologic correlation. *Radiographics*, **14**, 153–66.

Burcharth, F. (1979). Percutaneous transhepatic portography. I. Technique and application. *A.J.R.*, **132**, 177–82.

Cantlie, M.A. (1898). On a new arrangement of the right and left lobes of the liver. *Proc. Anatomical Soc. Great Britain and Ireland 1898*, **32**, 4–9.

Carr, D.H., Brown, J., Bydder, G.M., *et al.* (1984). Gadolinium-DTPA as a contrat agent in MRI: initial clinical experience in 20 patients. *A.J.R.*, **143**, 215–24.

Cedrone, A., Rapaccini, G.L., Pompili, M., *et al.* (1992). Neoplastic seeding complicating percutaneous ethanol injection for treatment of hepatocellular carcinoma. *Radiology*, **183**, 787–8.

Charnsangavej, C., Chuang, V., Wallace, S., *et al.* (1982). Angiographic appearance of recurrent malignant melanoma before and after intra-arterial chemotherapy. *Radiology*, **142**, 347–9.

Chen D.S., Shue, J.C., Sung, J.L. *et al.* (1982). Small hepatocellular carcinoma—a clinicopathological study in thirteen patients. *Gastroenterology*, **83**, 1109–19.

Chen, M.F., Hwang, T.L., and Hung, C.F. (1991). Human liver regeneration after major hepatectomy: a study of liver volume by computed tomography. *Ann. Surg.*, **213**, 227–9.

Chiandussi, L., Juliani, G., Crecco, F., *et al.* (1967). Hepatic portography by direct catheterization of the portal vein through the round ligament of the liver (ligamentum teres). *A. J. Roentgenol*, **99**, 625–8.

Chilton, H.M., Brown, M.L. (1990). Radiopharmaceuticals for abdominal and gastrointestinal imaging: reticuloendothelial, hepatobiliary, and intestinal. In *Pharmaceuticals in medical imaging* (ed. D.P. Swanson *et al.*). pp.462–500. Macmillan, New York.

Cho, K.J. and Lunderquist, A. (1983). The peribiliary vascular plexus: the microvascular architecture of the bile duct in the rabbit and in clinical cases. *Radiology*, **147**, 357–64.

Cho, K.J., Chuang, V.P., and Reuter, S.R. (1975). Prostaglandin E_1 as pharmacoangiographic agent for arterial portography. *Radiology*, **116**, 207–9.

Cho, K.J., Reuter, S.R., and Schmidt, R. (1976). Effects of experimental hepatic artery embolization on hepatic function. *A.J.R.*, **127**, 563–7.

Choi, B.I., Park, J.H., Kim, Y.I., *et al.* (1988). Peripheral cholangiocarcinoma and clonorchiasis : CT findings. *Radiology*, **169**, 149–53.

Choi, B.I., Han, M.C., Park, J.H., *et al.* (1989). Giant cavernous hemangioma of the liver: CT and MR imaging in 10 cases. *A.J.R.*, **152**, 1221–6.

Choi, B.I., Han, M.C., Kim, C.W. (1990*a*). Small hepatocellular carcinoma versus small cavernous hemangioma: differentiation with MR imaging at 2.0 T. *Radiology*, **176**, 103–6.

Choi, B.I., Lee, G.K., Kim, S.T., and Han, M.C. (1990*b*). Mosaic pattern of encapsulated hepatocellular carcinoma: correlation of magnetic resonance imaging and pathology. *Gastrointest. Radiol.*, **15**, 238–40.

Choi, B.I., Takayasu, K., and Han, M.C. (1993). Small hepatocellular carcinomas and associated nodular lesions of the liver: pathology, pathogenesis, and imaging findings. Review article. *Am. J. Roentgenol.*, **160**, 1177–87.

Chuang, V.P., and Wallace, S. (1981). Hepatic artery embolization in the treatment of hepatic neoplasms. *Radiology*, **140**, 51–58.

Chuang, V.P., Wallace, S., Stroehlein, J., *et al.* (1981). Hepatic artery infusion chemotherapy: gastroduodenal complications. *A.J.R.*, **137**, 347–50.

Chuvilo, I.V., Goldin, L.L., Khoroshkov, V.S., *et al.* (1984). ITEP synchrotron proton beam in radiotherapy. *Int. J. Radiat. Oncol. Biol. Phys.*, **10**, 185–95.

Clain, J.E., Stephens, D.S., Charboneau, J.W. (1984). Ultrasonography and computed tomography in focal fatty liver: report of two cases with special emphasis on changing appearances over time. *Gastroenterology.*, **87**, 948–52.

Colapinto, R.F., Stronell, R.D., Birch, S.J., *et al.* (1982). Creation of an intrahepatic portosystemic shunt with a Grutzig balloon catheter. *Can. Med. Assoc. J.*, **126**, 267–8.

Collan, Y., Hakkiluoto, A., and Hastbacka, J. (1978). Ectopic liver. *Ann. Chir. Gynaecol.*, **67**, 27–9.

Collins, V.P., Loeffler, P.K., and Tivey, H. (1956). Observations on growth rates of human tumors. *A.J.R.*, **76**, 988–1000.

Conran, R.M., and Stocker, J.T. (1985). Malignant fibrous histiocytoma of the liver. *Am. J. Gastroenterol.*, **80**, 813–15.

Cook, G.B. (1966). A comparison of single and multiple primary cancers. *Cancer*, **19**, 959–66.

Couinaud, C. (1954). Lobes et segments hepatiques. Notes sur L'architecture anatomique et chirurgicale du foie. *Presse Med.*, **62**, 709–2.

Couinaud, C. (1957). *Le Foie. Etudes anatomiques et chirurgicales*, pp.187–208. Masson et Cie, Paris.

Craig, J.R., Peters, R.L., Edmondson, H.A., and Omata, M. (1980). Fibrolamellar carcinoma of the liver: a tumor of adolescents and young adults with distinctive clinicopathologic features. *Cancer*, **46**, 372–9.

Craig, J.R., Peters, R.L., and Edmondson, H.A. (1989). *Tumors of the liver and intrahepatic bile ducts.* Armed Forces Institute of Pathology, Washington DC.

Cremin, B.J., and Nuss, D. (1974). Calcified hepatoblastoma in a newborn. *Pediat. Surg.*, **9**, 913–15.

Cutillo, D.P., Swayne, L.C., Fasciano, M.G., and Schwartz, J.R. (1989). Absence of fatty replacement in radiation damaged liver. CT demonstration. *J. Comput. Assist. Tomogr.*, **13**, 259–261.

Dachman, A.H., Lichtenstein, J.E., Friedman, A.C., and Harttman, D.S. (1983). Infantile hemangioendothelioma of the liver: a radiologic-pathologic-clinical correlation. *A.J.R.*, **140**, 1091–6.

Dail, D.H., and Liebow, A.A. (1975). Intravascular Bronchioloalveolar tumor (abstr.). *Am. J. Pathol.*, **78**, 6a.

Dail, D.H., Liebow, A.A., Gmelich, J.T., *et al.* (1983). Intravascular, bronchiolar and alveolar tumor of the lung: An analysis of twenty cases of a peculiar sclerosing endothelial tumor. *Cancer*, **51**, 452–64.

Davis, G.L., Kissane, J.M., and Ishak, K.G. (1969). Embryonal rhabdomyosarcoma (sarcoma botryoides). of the biliary tree. *Cancer*, **24**, 333–42.

Deboever, G., Elegeert, I., and Defloor, E. (1989). Portal and mesenteric venous thrombosis after endoscopic injection sclerotherapy. *Am. J. Gastroenterol.*, **84**, 1336–7.

Dehner, L.P. (1978). Hepatic tumors in the pediatric age group. *Perspect. Pediatr. Pathol.*, **4**, 217–68.

Demaerel, P., Marchal, G., Van Steenbergen, W., *et al.* (1989). CT demonstration of right hepatic lobe atrophy. *J. Comput. Assist. Tomogr.*, **13**, 351–3.

DeMent, S.H., Mann, R.B., Staal, S.P., *et al.* (1987). Primary lymphomas of the liver. *Am. J. Clin. Pathol.*, **88**, 255–63.

Didier, D., Weiler, S., Rohmer, P., *et al.* (1985). Hepatic alveolar echinococcosis: correlative US and CT study. *Radiology*, **154**, 179–86.

Doppman, J.L., and Girton, M.E. (1984). Bile duct scarring following ethanol embolization of the hepatic artery: an experimental study in monkeys. *Radiology*, **152**, 621–6.

Düber, D., Storkel, S., Wagner, P-K., and Muller, J. (1984). Xanthogranulatous cholecystitis mimicking carcinoma of the gallbladder: CT findings. *J. Comput. Assist. Tomogr.*, **8**, 1195–8.

Ducommun, J.C., Goldberg, H.I., Korobkin, M., *et al.* (1979). The relation of liver fat to computed tomography numbers: a preliminary experimental study in rabbits. *Radiology*, **180**, 311.

Dumoulin, C.L., and Hart, H., Jr (1986). Magnetic resonance angiography. *Radiology*, **161**, 717–20.

Ebara, M., Ohto, M., Shinagawa, T., *et al.* (1986*a*). Natural history of minute hepatocellular carcinoma smaller than three centimeters complicating cirrhosis. A study of 22 patients. *Gastroenterology*, **90**, 289–98.

Ebara, M., Ohto, M., Watanabe, Y., *et al.* (1986*b*). Diagnosis of small hepatocellular carcinoma: correlation of MR imaging and tumor histology studies. *Radiology*, **159**, 371–7.

Ebara, M., Ohto, M., Sugiura, N., *et al.* (1990). Percutaneous ethanol injection for the treatment of small hepatocellular carcinoma. Study of 95 patients. *J. Gastroenterol. Hepatol.*, **5**, 616–26.

Ebara, M., Watanabe, S., Kita, K., *et al.* (1991). MR imaging of small hepatocellular carcinoma: effect of intratumoral copper content on signal intensity. *Radiology*, **180**, 617–21.

Ebara, M., Kita, K., Sugiura, N., *et al.* (1995). Therapeutic effect of percutaneous ethanol injection on small hepatocellular carcinoma; evaluation with CT. *Radiology*, **195**, 371–7.

Edelman, R.R., Wentz, K.U., Mattle, H., *et al.* (1989). Projection arteriography and venography. Initial clinical results with MR. *Radiology*, **172**, 351–7.

Edmondson, H.A. (1956). Differential diagnosis of tumors and tumor-like lesions of the liver in infancy and childhood. *Am. J. Dis Child*, **91**, 168–86.

Edmondson, H.A. (1958). Tumors of the liver and intrahepatic bile ducts. *Atlas of Tumor Pathology*, section, 7, fascicle, 25, pp.105–109. Armed Forces Institute of Pathology, Washington, D.C.

Edmondson, H.A. (1976). Benign epithelial tumors and tumorlike lesions of the liver. In *Hepatocellular carcinoma* (ed. K. Okuda and R. L. Peters), pp.309–30. Wiley, New York.

Edmondson, H.A., and Steiner, P.E. (1954). Primary carcinoma of the liver. A study of 100 cases among 48,900 necropsies. *Cancer*, **7**, 462–503.

Edmondson, H.A., Henderson, B., and Benton, B. (1976). Liver-cell adenomas associated with use of oral contraceptives. *New Engl. J. Med.* 294, 470–2.

Eggel, H. (1901). Ueber das primäre Carcinoma der Leber. *Beitr. Pathol. Anat.*, **30**, 506–604.

Elizondo, G., Gretz, C.J., Stark, D.D., *et al.* (1991). Preclinical evaluation of Mn-DPDP: new paramagnetic hepatobiliary contrast agent for MR imaging. *Radiology*, **178**, 73–8.

Ellis, G.L. and Kratichvil, F.J. (1986). Epithelioid hemangioendothelioma of the head and neck: a clinicopathologic report of twelve cases. *Oral Surg. Oral Med. Oral Pathol.*, **61**, 61–8.

Esumi, M., Aritaka, T., Arii, M., *et al.* (1986). Clonal origin of human hepatoma determined by integration of hepatitis B virus DNA. *Cancer Res.*, **46**, 5767–71.

Falk, H., Creech, J.L. Jr, Heath, C.W. Jr, *et al.* (1974). Hepatic disease among workers at a vinyl chloride polymerization plant. *J.A.M.A.* **230**, 59–63.

Falk, H., Herbert, J.T., Edmonds, L., *et al.* (1981). Review of four cases of childhood hepatic angiosarcoma—elevated environmental arsenic exposure in one case. *Cancer*, **47**, 382–91.

Falkson, G., and Coetzer, B. (1987). Chemotherapy of primary liver tumors. *Neoplasms of the Liver* (ed. K. Okuda and K.G. Ishak). pp.321–6, Springer, Tokyo.

Fang, Z.M., Yamashita, Y., Harada, M., *et al.* (1993). Intrahepatic cholangiocarcinoma: spin-echo and contrast-enhanced dynamic MR imaging. *A.J.R.*, **161**, 313–7.

Fechner, R.E., Roehm, J.O.F. Jr (1977). Angiographic and pathologic correlation of hepatis focal nodular hyperplasia. *Am. J. Surg. Pathol.*, **1**, 217–24.

Feng, W., Takayasu, K., Konda, C., *et al.* (1991). CT of nodular hyperplasia of the liver in non-Hodgkin lymphoma. *J. Comput. Assist. Tomogr.*, **15**, 1031–4.

Fernandez, M.P., and Bernardino, M.E. (1991). Hepatic pseudolesion: appearance of focal low attenuation in the medial segment of the left lobe at CT arterial portography. *Radiology*, **181**, 809–12.

Ferrell, L., Wright, T., Lake, J., *et al.* (1992). Incidence and diagnostic features of macroregenerative nodules vs small hepatocellular carcinoma in cirrhotic livers. *Hepatology*, **16**, 1372–81.

Ferrucci J.T. Jr. (1979). Body ultrasonography. *Engl. J. Med.*, **300**, 538–42.

Ferrucci, J.T., Stark, D.D. (1990). Iron oxide-enhanced MR imaging of the liver and spleen: review of the first 5 years. *A.J.R.*, **155**, 943–50.

Fong, J.A. and Ruebner, B.H. (1974). Primary leiomyosarcoma of the liver. *Hum. Pathol.*, **5**, 115–9.

Freeny, P.C. and Marks, W. (1983). Computed tomographic arteriography of the liver. *Radiology*, **148**, 193–7.

Freeny, P.C., Vimont, T.R. and Barnett, D.C. (1979). Cavernous hemangioma of the liver: ultrasonography, arteriography and computed tomography. *Radiology*, **132**, 143–8.

Friedman, A.C., Lichtenstein, J.E., Goodman, Z., *et al.* (1985). Fibrolamellar hepatocellular carcinoma. *Radiology*, **157**, 583–7.

Fujii, T., Takayasu, K., Muramatsu, Y., *et al.* (1993). Hepatocellular carcinoma with portal tumor thrombus: analysis of factors determining prognosis. *Japan. J. Clin. Oncol.*, **23**, 105–9.

Furui, S., Ohtomo, K., Itai, Y., and Iio, M. (1984). Hepatocellular carcinoma treated by transcatheter arterial embolization: progress evaluated by computed tomography. *Radiology*, **150**, 773–8.

Furui, S., Yamauchi, T., Ohtomo, K., *et al.* (1988). Hepatic inferior vena cava obstruction: Clinical results of treatment with percutaneous transluminal laser-assisted angioplasty. *Radiology*, **166**, 673–7.

Furui, S., Itai, Y., Ohtomo, K., *et al.* (1989). Hepatic epithelioid hemangioendothelioma: report of five cases. *Radiology*, **171**, 63–8.

Futagawa, S., Fukazawa, M., Musha, H., *et al.* (1980). Portographic liver changes in idiopathic portal hypertension. *Am. J. Roentgenol*, **134**, 917–23.

Futagawa, S., Fukazawa, M., Musha, H., *et al.* (1981). Hepatic venography in noncirrhotic portal hypertension. Comparison with cirrhosis of the liver. *Radiology*, **141**, 303–9.

Gabata, T., Matsui, O., Kadoya, M., *et al.* (1990). MR imaging of hepatic adenoma. *A.J.R.*, **155**, 1009–11.

Gaffey, M.J., Joyce, J.P., Carlson, G.S. and Esteban, J.M. (1990). Spontaneous regression of hepatocellular carcinoma. *Cancer*, **65**, 2779–83.

Gall, E. (1960). Primary and metastatic carcinoma of the liver. Relationship to hepatic cirrhosis. *Arch. Pathol.*, **70**, 753–9.

Gaulard, P., Zafrani, E.S., Mavier, P., *et al.* (1986). Peripheral T-cell lymphoma presenting as predominant liver disease. *Hepatology*, **6**, 864–8.

Gazelle, G.S., Lee, M.J., Hahn, P.F., *et al.* (1994). US., CT., and MRI of primary and secondary liver lymphoma. *J. Comput. Assist. Tomogr.*, **18**, 412–5.

Gazzangia, G.M., Faggioni, A., Bagarolo, C., *et al.* (1989). Percutaneous fibercholangioscopies. *Hepato-Gastroenterology*, **36**, 367–75.

Gen, E., Kusuyama, Y., Saito, K., *et al.* (1983). Primary fibrosarcoma of the liver with hypoglycemia. *Acta. Pathol. Japan*, **33**, 177–82.

Gibney, R.G., Hendin, A.P. and Cooperberg, P.L. (1987). Sonographically detected hepatic hemangiomas: absence of change over time. *A.J.R.*, **149**, 953–7.

Gibson, L.B., Sobin, L.H. (1978). *Histological typing of the tumors of the liver, biliary tract and pancreas*, (International histological classification of tumors. No. 20). WHO., Geneva.

Godwin, J.D. (1975). Carcinoid tumors: an analysis of 2837 tumors. *Cancer*, **36**, 560–9.

Goldberg, B.B. (1977). *Abdominal gray scale ultrasonography*. Wiley, New York.

Goldberg, H.I. (1980). CT scanning of diffuse parenchymal liver disease. In *Computed tomography, ultrasound, and x-ray* (ed. A.A. Moss and H.I. Golberg). pp.177–87. University of California Press, San Francisco.

Goldstein, H.M., Medellin, H., Ben-Menachem, Y., and Wallace, S. (1975). Transcatheter arterial embolization in the management of bleeding in cancer patients. *Radiology*, **115**, 603–8.

Goletti, O., De Negri, F., Pucciarelli, M., *et al.* (1992). Subcutaneous seeding after percutaneous ethanol injection of liver metastases. *Radiology*, **183**, 785–6.

Goodman, Z.D., Ishak, K.G., Langloss, J.M., *et al.* (1985). Combined hepatocellular-cholangiocarcinoma. A histologic and immunohistochemical study. *Cancer*, **55**, 124–35.

Goodman, Z.D. (1987). Benign tumors of the liver. In *Neoplasms of the liver* (ed. K. Okuda and K.G. Ishak). pp.105–25. Springer, Tokyo.

Gottfried, E.B., Steller, R., Paronetto, F. and Lieber, C.S. (1982). Spontaneous regression of hepatocellular carcinoma. *Gastroenterology*, **82**, 770–4.

Gregson, R. (1988). Embolic materials—a review. *J. Intervent. Radiol.*, **3**, 141–6.

Haase, A., Matthaer, D., Hanicke, W., *et al.* (1986). Dynamic digital subtraction imaging using fast low-angle shot MR movie sequence. *Radiology*, **160**, 537–41.

Halvorsen, R.A., Korobkin, M., Ram, P.C., *et al.* (1982). CT appearance of focal fatty infiltration of the liver *A.J.R.*, **139**, 277–81.

Hamada, M., Ohta, M., Yasuda, Y., *et al.* (1982). Hepatic calcification in schistosomiasis japonica. *J. Comput. Assist. Tomogr.*, **6**, 76–8.

Hamm, B., Vogl, T.J., Branding, G., *et al.* (1992). Focal liver lesions: MR imaging with Mn-DPDP: initial clinical results in 40 patients. *Radiology*, **182**, 167–74.

Hamrick-Turner, J., Abbit, P.L. and Ros, P.R. (1992). Intrahepatic cholangiocarcinoma: MR appearance. *A.J.R.*, **158**, 77–9.

Hamrick-Turner, J.E., Shipkey, F.H. and Cranston, P.E. (1994). Fibrolamellar hepatocellular carcinoma: MR appearance mimicking focal nodular hyperplasia. *J. Comput. Assist. Tomogr.*, **18**, 301–4.

Harbin, W.P., Robert, N.J. and Ferrucci, J.T., Jr (1980). Diagnosis of cirrhosis based on regional changes in hepatic morphology. *Radiology*, **135**, 273–83.

Hashizume, M., Kitano, S., Sugimachi, K. and Sueishi, K. (1988). Three-dimensional view of the vascular structure of the lower esophagus in clinical portal hypertension. *Hepatology*, **8**, 1482–7.

Healey, J.E. Jr and Schroy, P.C. (1953). Anatomy of the biliary ducts within the human liver. Analysis of the prevailing pattern of branchings and the major variations of the biliary ducts. *Arch. Surg.*, **66**, 599–616.

Hermanek, P. and Sobin, L.H. (ed.)(1987). *TNM classification of malignant tumors*, 4th revision. International Union Against Cancer, Geneva, Springer, Berlin.

Herzberg, A.J., MacDonald, J.A., Tucker, J.A., *et al.* (1990). Primary leiomyoma of the liver. *Am. J. Gastroenterol*, **85**, 1642–5.

Hirokawa, M., Ryu, M., Watanabe, K., *et al.* (1993). A case of fibrolamellar carcinoma of the liver. *Acta Hepatol Japan*, **35**, 29–35.

Hirooka. M. and Kimura, C. (1970). Membranous obstruction of the hepatic portion of vena cava. Surgical correction and etiologic study. *Arch. Surg.*, **100**, 655–63.

Hisa, N., Hiramatsu, K., Narimatsu, Y., *et al.* (1980). Detection of hepatic neoplasms by computed tomography in portal hepatogram phase. *Japan. J. Clin. Radiol.*, **25**, 529–34 (in Japanese).

Holm, H.H. and Kristensen, I.K. (ed.). (1985). *Interventional ultrasound.* Munksgaard, Copenhagen.

Honjo, I., Suzuki, T., Ozawa, K., *et al.* (1975). Ligation of a branch of the portal vein for carcinoma of the liver. *Am. J. Surg.* **130**, 296–302.

Horie, Y., Katoh, S., Yoshida, H., *et al.* (1983). Pedunculated hepatocellular carcinoma: report of three cases and review of literature. *Cancer*, **51**, 746–51.

Horiuchi, N., Kitamura, T., Tateishi, *et al.* (1973). Hepatoma originated in the retroperitoneal space. *Oncology*, **27**, 235–43.

Horowitz, M.E., Etcoubanase, E., Webber, B.L., *et al.* (1987). Hepatic undifferentiated (embryonal). sarcoma and rhabdomyosarcoma in children. *Cancer*, **59**, 396–402.

Hosoki, T., Hashimoto T., Masuike, M., *et al.* (1989). Slippery coaxial catheter system. *Radiology*, **171**, 858–59.

Hou, P.C. (1956). Relationship between primary carcinoma of the liver and infestation with *Clonorchis sinensis. J. Pathol. Bacteriol.*, **72**, 239–46.

Hsu, H.C., Chiou, T.J., Chen, J.Y., *et al.* (1991). Clonality and clonal evolution of hepatocellular carcinoma multiple nodules. *Hepatology*, **13**, 923–8.

Iha, H. (1994). Clinicopathological study on scirrhous hepatocellular carcinoma—A study of 12 resected cases. *Acta Hepatol. Japan*, **29**, 855–63.

Iio, M., Iuchi, M., Kitani, K., *et al.* (1971). Scintigraphic evaluation of the liver with schistosomiasis japonica. *J. Nucl. Med.*, **12**, 655–9.

Imaeda, T., Yamawaki, Y., Hirota, K., *et al.* (1989). Tumor thrombus in the branches of the distal portal vein: CT demonstration. *J. Comput. Assist. Tomogr.*, **13**, 262–8.

Imamura, M., Miyashita, T., Tani, T., *et al.* (1984). Cholangiocellular carcinoma associated with multiple liver cysts. *Am. J. Gastroenterol*, **79**, 790–5.

Imazato, M., Isobe, Y., Ueno and E., Yamada, A. (1990). Inflammatory pseudotumor of the liver, (Letter). *A.J.R.*, **154**, 201.

Inamoto, K., Sugiki, K., Yamasaki, H., *et al.* (1981). CT of hepatoma: effects of portal vein obstruction. *A.J.R.*, **136**, 349–53.

Ingold, J.A., Reed, G.B., Henry, S., et al.. (1965). Radiation hepatitis. *A.J.R.*, **93**, 200–8.

Inokuchi, K., Beppu, K., Koyanagi, N., *et al.* (1984). Fifteen years' experience with left gastric venous caval shunt for esophageal varices. *World J. Surg.*, **8**, 716–721.

International Union Against Cancer (1987). *TNM classification of malignant tumors*, 4th fully revised edition. Springer, Geneva.

Ishak, K.G. (1976). Mesenchymal tumors of the liver. In *Hepatocellular carcinoma* (ed. K. Okuda and R.L. Peters), pp.247–308. Wiley, New York.

Ishak, K.G. and Rabin, L. (1975). Benign tumors of the liver. *Med. Clin. N. Am.*, **59**, 995–1013.

Ishak, K.G., Willis, G.W., Cummins, S.D., *et al.* (1977). Biliary cystadenoma and cystadenocarcinoma. Report of 14 cases and review of the literature. *Cancer*, **38**, 322–38.

Ishak, K.G., Mesterhenn, I.A., Goodman, Z.D., *et al.* (1984). Epithelioid hemangioendothelioma of the liver: a clinicopathologic and follow-up study of 32 cases. *Hum. Pathol.*, **15**, 839–52.

Ishak, K.G., Anthony, P.P. and Sobin, L.H. (1994). *Histological typing of tumors of the liver.* Springer, Berlin.

Ishikawa, N., Nakagawa, S., Hirata, K., *et al.* (1989). Long-term follow-up of hepatitis using computed tomography. *J. Comput. Assist. Tomogr.*, **13**, 645–9.

Isobe, H., Fukai, T., Iwamoto, T., *et al.* (1990). Liver abscess complicating intratumoral ethanol injection therapy for HCC. *Am. J. Gastroenterol.*, **85**, 1646–8.

Itai, Y., Araki, T., Yoshikawa, K., *et al.* (1980*a*). Computed tomography of gallbladder carcinoma. *Radiology*, **137**, 713–18.

Itai, Y., Furui, S., Araki, T., *et al.* (1980*b*). Computed tomography of cavernous hemangioma of the liver. *Radiology*, **137**, 149–155.

Itai, Y., Moss, A.A., and Goldberg, H.I. (1982). Transient hepatic attenuation difference of lobar or segmental distribution detected by dynamic computed tomography. *Radiology*, **144**, 835–9.

Itai, Y., Ohtomo, K., Furui S., *et al.* (1985). Noninvasive diagnosis of small carvenous hemangioma of the liver: advantage of MRI. *A.J.R.*, **145**, 1195–9.

Itai, Y., Ohnishi, S., Ohtomo, K., *et al.* (1987*a*). Regenerating nodules of liver cirrhosis: MR imaging. *Radiology*, **165**, 419–23.

Itai, Y., Ohtomo, K., Kokubo, T., *et al.* (1987*b*). CT demonstration of fluid-fluid levels in nonenhancing hemangiomas of the liver. *J. Comput. Assist. Tomogr.*, **11**, 253–7.

Itai, Y., Ohtomo, K., Kokubo, T., *et al.* (1988). CT and MR imaging of postnecrotic liver scars. *J. Comput. Assist. Tomogr.*, **12**, 971–5.

Itai, Y., and Teraoka, T. (1989). Angiosarcoma of the liver mimicking cavernous hemangioma on dynamic CT. *J. Comput. Assist. Tomogr.*, **13**, 910–12.

Itai, Y., Ebihara, R., Tohno, E., *et al.* (1994). Hepatic peribiliary cysts: multiple tiny cysts within the large portal tract, hepatic hilum, or both. *Radiology*, **191**, 107–10.

Ito, Y., Kojiro, M., Nakashima, T. and Mori, T. (1988). Pathomorphologic characteristics of 102 cases of Thorotrast-related hepatocellular carcinoma, cholangiocarcinoma, and hepatic angiosarcoma. *Cancer*, **62**, 1153–62.

Itoh, K., Nishimura, K., Togashi, K., *et al.* (1987). Hepatocellular carcinoma: MR imaging. *Radiology*, **164**, 21–5.

Itsuji, T., Funatsu, K., Ishii, M., *et al.* (1987). Disappearance of lung metastases following arterial embolization for primary liver cancer. A case report. *Acta Hepatol. Japan*, **28**, 374–9 (in Japanese)

Iwatsuki, S., Starzl, TE., Todo, S., *et al.* (1988). Experience in 1,000 liver transplants under cyclosporin-steroid: a survival report. *Transplantation Proc.*, 20, Suppl, 1, 498–504.

Japanese Society of Biliary Surgery (1993). *General rules for surgical and pathological studies on cancer of biliary tract*, 3rd edn. Kanehara Press, Tokyo.

Japanese Society for Cancer Therapy (1986). Guidelines for the clinical evaluation of antineoplastic drugs. *J. Japan. Soc. Cancer Ther.*, **12**, 929–42.

Johnson, D.H., Vinson, A.M., Wirth, F.H., *et al.* (1984). Management of hepatic hemangioendotheliomas of infacy by transarterial embolization: a report of two cases. *Pediatrics*, **73**, 546–9.

Johnson, P.M., Grossman, F.M. and Atkins, H.L. (1967). Radiation induced hepatic injury. *A.J.R.*, **99**, 453–62.

Joseph, F.B., Bumgartem, D.A. and Bermardomp E. (1993). Hepatocellular carcinoma: CT appearance after percutaneous ethanol ablation therapy. *Radiology*, 186,553–6.

Kadoya, M., Matsui, O., and Nakanuma, Y., *et al.* (1990). Ciliated hepatic foregut cyst: radiologic features. *Radiology*, **175**, 475–7.

Kadoya, M., Matsui, O., Takashima, T., Nonomura, A. (1992). Hepatocellular carcinoma: correlation of MR imaging and histopathologic findings. *Radiology*, **183**, 819–25.

Kage, M., Arakawa, M., Kojiro, M. and Okuda, K. (1992). Histopathology of membranous obstruction of the inferior vena cava in the Budd-Chiari syndrome. *Gastroenterology*, **102**, 2081–90.

Kakizoe, S., Kojiro, M. and Nakashima, T. (1987). Hepatocellular carcinoma with sarcomatous change. Clinicopathologic and immunohistological studies of 14 autopsy cases. *Cancer*, **59**, 310–16.

Kalender, W.A., Seissler, W., Klotz, and Vock, P. (1990). Spiral volumetric CT with single-breath-hold tehnique, continuous transport, and continuous scanner rotation. *Radiology*, **176**, 181–3.

Kalovidouris, A., Pissiotis, C., Pontifex, G., *et al.* (1986). CT characterization of multivesicular hydatid cysts. *J. Comput. Assist. Tomogr.*, **10**, 428–31.

Kamiya, J., Nimura, Y. and Kondo, S. (1992). Precise diagnosis of bile duct carcinoma by percutaneous transhepatic cholangioscopy (PTCS). *Endosc. Digest.*, **4**, 317–21.

Kanai, T., Hirohashi, S., Upton, MP., *et al.* (1987). Pathology of small hepatocellular carcinoma. A proposal for a new gross classification. *Cancer*, **60**, 810–19.

Kasai, M. and Watanabe, I. (1970). Histological classification of liver cell carcinoma in infancy and childhood and its clinical evaluation. *Cancer*, **25**, 551–63.

Kasbach, H.H. and Merritt, K.K. (1940). Capillary hemangioma with extensive purpura. Report of a case. *Am. J. Dis. Child.*, **59**, 1063–70.

Katayama, H., Yamaguchi, K., Kozuka, T., *et al.* (1990). Adverse reaction to ionic and nonionic contrast media. A report from the Japanese committee on the safety of contrast media. *Radiology*, **175**, 621–28.

Kato, T., Sudo, Y. and Matsuo T. (1993). Chondroitin sulfate iron colloid as an MR contrast agent for the hepatic reticuloendotherial system. *J. Comput. Assist. Tomogr.*, **17**, 603–8.

Kawarada, Y. and Mizumoto, R. (1983). Angiomyolipoma of the liver. *Am. J. Gastroenterol.*, **78**, 434–9.

Kawashima, A., Suehiro, S., Murayama, S., *et al.* (1986). Focal fatty infiltration of the liver mimicking a tumor: sonographic and CT features. *J. Comput. Assist. Tomogr.*, **10**, 329–31.

Kelleher, M.B., Iwatsuki, S., Sheahan, D.G. (1989). Epithelioid hemangioendothelioma of liver. Clinicopathological correlation of 10 cases treated by orthotopic liver transplantation. *Am. J. Surg. Pathol.*, **13**, 999–1008.

Kerlin, P., Davis, G.L., McGill, D.B., *et al.* (1983). Hepatic adenoma and focal nodular hyperplasia: clinical, pathologic, and adiologic features. *Gastroenterology*, **84**, 994–1000.

Keslar, P.J., Buck, J.L. and Selby, D.M. (1993). Infantile hemangioendothelioma of the liver revisited. *Radiographics*, **13**, 657–70.

Kida, E., Uchimura, M. and Okamoto, K. (1987). Intrahepatic architecture of the bile duct and portal vein. *Tan-to-Sui*, **8**, 1–7.

Kikuchi, M., Makuuchi, M., Yamazaki, S., *et al.* (1987). Intraoperative ultrasonic detection of tumor thrombus in patients with metastatic liver tumor. *Acta Hepatol. Japan*, **28**, 92–7 (in Japanese).

Kimura, A., Makuuchi, M., Takayasu, K., *et al.* (1990). Ciliated hepatic foregut cyst with solid tumor appearance on CT. *J. Comput. Assist. Tomogr.*, **14**, 1016–18.

Kimura, K., Tsuchiya, Y., Ohto, M., *et al.* (1981). Single-puncture method for percutaneous transhepatic portography using a thin needle. *Radiology*, **139**, 748–9.

Kimura, K., Ohto, M., Saisho, H., *et al.* (1985). Association of gallbladder carcinoma and anomalous pancreaticobiliary ductal junction. *Gastroenterology*, **89**, 1258–65.

Kimura, K., Ohto, M., Matsutani, S., *et al.* (1990). Relative frequencies of portosystemic pathways and renal shunt formation through the 'posterior' gastric vein: portographic study in 460 patients. *Gastroenterology*, **12**, 725–8.

Kishikawa, T., Numaguchi, Y., Tokunaga, M. and Matsuura, K. (1977). Hemangiosarcoma of the spleen with liver metastases: angiographic manifestations. *Radiology*, **123**, 31–5.

Klatskin, G. (1965). Adenocarcinoma of the hepatic duct at its bifurcation with the porta hepatis. *Am. J. Med*, **28**, 241–56.

Knowles, D.M. II. and Wolff. M. (1976). Focal nodular hyperplasia of the liver. A clinicopathologic study and review of the literature. *Hum. Pathol*, **7**, 533–45.

Kobayashi, H., Hidaka, H., Kajiya, Y., *et al.* (1986). Treatment of hepatocellular carcinoma by transarterial injection of anticancer agents in iodized oil suspension or of radioactive iodized oil solution. *Acta Radiol. (Diagn.)*, **27**, 139–47.

Kobayashi, K., Sugimoto, T., Makino, H., *et al.* (1985). Screening methods for early detection of hepatocellular carcinoma. *Hepatology*, **5**, 1100–5.

Koga, A., Watanabe, K., Fukuyama, T., *et al.* (1988). Diagnosis and operative indications for polypoid lesions of the gallbladder. *Arch. Surg.* 123, 26–9.

Kojiro, M. and Nakashima, T. (1987). Pathology of hepatocellular carcinoma. In *Neoplasms of the liver* (ed. K. Okuda and K.G. Ishak), pp.81–104. Springer, Tokyo.

Kojiro, M., Kawabata, K., Kawano, Y., *et al.* (1982). Hepatocellular carcinoma presenting as intra-bile duct tumor growth. A clinicopathologic study of 24 cases. *Cancer*, **49**, 2144–7.

Kolbenstvedt, A., Kjølseth, I., Klepp, O., and Kolmannskog, F. (1980). Postirradiation changes of the liver demonstrated by computed tomograph. *Radiology*, **135**, 391.

Kondo, F., Wada, K., Nagato, Y., *et al.* (1989). Biopsy diagnosis of well-differentiated hepatocellular carcinoma based on new morphologic criteria. *Hepatology*, **9**, 751–5.

Konno, T., Maeda, H., Iwai, K., *et al.* (1983). Effect of arterial administration of high-molecular weight anticancer agent SMANCS with lipid lymphographic agent on hepatoma. *Europ. J. Cancer Oncol*, **19**, 1053–65.

Korobkin M., Kirks, D.R., Sullivan, D.C., *et al.* (1981). Computed tomography of primary liver tumors in children. *Radiology*, **139**, 431–5.

Korobkin, M., Stephens, D.H., Lee, J.K., *et al.* (1989). Biliary cystadenoma and cystadenocarcinoma: CT and sonographic findings. *A.J.R.*, **153**, 507–11.

Kosuge, T., Makuuchi, M., Ozaki, H., *et al.* (1991). Primary lymphoma of the common bile duct. *Hepato-Gastroenterol.*, **38**, 235–8.

Kubo, Y. and Shimokawa, Y. (1976). Arterial injection chemotherapy. In *Hepatocellular carcinoma* (ed. K. Okuda and R.L. Peters), pp.477–90. Wiley, New York.

Kubo, Y., Okuda, K., Musha, H. and Nakashima, T. (1978). Detection of hepatocellular carcinoma during a clinical follow-up of chronic liver disease. Observations in 31 patients. *Gastroenterology*, **74**, 578–82.

Kubota, Y., Nakano, T., Seki T., *et al.* (1989). Validity of MR imaging for monitoring effects of percutaneous ethanol injection for HCC. *Hepato-Gastroenterology*, **36**, 262–5.

Kudo, M., Tomita, S., Tochio, H., *et al.* (1991). Hepatic focal nodular hyperplasia: specific findings at dynamic contrast-enhanced US with carbon dioxide microbubbles. *Radiology*, **179**, 377–82.

Kudo, M., Tomita, S., Tochio, H., *et al.* (1992*a*). Sonography with intraarterial infusion of carbon dioxide microbubbles (sonographic angiography).: value in differential diagnosis of hepatic tumors. *A.J.R.*, **158**, 65–74.

Kudo, M., Tomita, S., Tochio, H., *et al.* (1992*b*). Small hepatocellular carcinoma: diagnosis with US angiography with intraarterial CO_2 microbubbles. *Radiology*, **182**, 155–160.

Kuhlman, J.E., Fishman, E.K., Leichner, P.K., *et al.* (1986). Skeletal metastases from hepatoma: frequency, distribution, and radiographic features. *Radiology*, **160**, 175–8.

Kuroda, C., Iwasaki, M., Tanaka, T., *et al.* (1983). Gallbladder infarction following hepatic transcatheter arterial embolization: angiographic study. *Radiology*, **149**, 85–9.

Kurdziel, J.C., Stines, J., Parache, R.M., Chaulieu, C. (1984). Adenolipoma of the liver. A unique case with ultrasound and CT patterns. *Europ. J. Radiol.*, **4**, 45–6.

Lack, E.E., Neave, C. and Vawter, G.F. (1982). Hepatoblastoma. A clinical and pathological study of 54 cases. *Am. J. Surg. Pathol.*, **6**, 693–705.

Lam, K.C., Ho, J.C.I. and Yeung, R.T.T. (1982). Spontaneous regression of hepatocellular carcinoma. A case study. *Cancer*, **50**, 332–6.

Lammer, J. and Neumayer, K. (1986). Biliary drainage endoprostheses: experience with 201 placements. *Radiology*, **159**, 625–9.

Lange, J.F., Leese, T., Castaing, D. and Bismuth, H. (1976). Repeat hepatectomy for recurrent malignant tumors of the liver. *Surg. Gynecol. Ostet.*, **169**, 119–26.

Lange, J.F., Leese, T., Castaing, D., and Bismuth, H. (1989). Repeat hepatectomy for recurrent malignant tumours of the liver. *Surg. Gynecol. Obstet.*, **169**, 119–126

Lansing, A.M., David, W.M., and Brizel, H.E. (1968). Radiation hepatitis. *Arch. Surg.*, **96**, 878–882.

Lederman, S.M., Martin, E.C., Laffey, K.T. and Lefkowitch, J.H. (1987). Hepatic neurofibromatosis, malignant schwannoma, and angiosarcoma in von Recklinghausen's disease. *Gastroenterology*, **92**, 234–9.

Lee, M.J., Saini, S., Hamm, B., *et al.* (1991). Focal nodular hyperplasia of the liver: MR findings in 35 proved cases. *A.J.R.*, **156**, 317–20.

Leevy, C.M., Popper, H. and Sherlock, S. (1976). *Diseases of the liver and biliary tract. Standarization of nomenclature, diagnostic criteria, and diagnostic methodology*. DHEW Publications, NIH., Bethesda.

Leevy, C.M., Sherlock, S., Tygstrup, N. and Zetterman, R. (1994). *Diseases of the liver and biliary tract. Standarization of nomenclature, diagnostic criteria and prognosis*. Ravin Press, New York.

Letourneau, J.G., Steely, J.W., Crass, J.R., *et al.* (1988). CT findings following partial hepatectomy. *Radiology*, **166**, 139–41.

Leyman, P., Baert, A.L., Marchal, G. and Fevery, J. (1989). Ultrasound and CT of multifocal liver abscesses caused by *Yersubua enterocolitica*. *J. Comput. Assist. Tomogr.*, **13**, 913–5.

Lieberman, F.L., Hidemura, R., Peters, R.L. and Reynolds, T.B. (1966). Pathogenesis and treatment of hydrothorax complicating cirrhosis with ascites. *Ann. Intern. Med.*, **64**, 341–51.

Lin, T.Y., Chen, K.M., Chen, Y.R., *et al.* (1975). Icteric type hepatoma. *Med. Chir. Digest.*, **4**, 267–70.

Lisa, J., Solomon, C., Gordon, E. (1942). Secondary carcinoma in cirrhosis of liver. *Am. J. Pathol.*, **18**, 137–40.

Liver Cancer Study Group of Japan (1987). *The general rules for the clinical and pathological study of primary liver cancer*, 2nd edn., Kanehara, Tokyo.

Liver Cancer Study Group of Japan (1989). The general rules for the clinical and pathological study of primary liver cancer. *Japan. J. Surg.*, **19**, 98–129.

Liver Cancer Study Group of Japan (1990). Primary liver cancer in Japan. Clinico-pathological features and results of surgical treatment. *Ann. Surg.* 211, 277–87.

Liver Cancer Study Group of Japan (1992). *The general rules for the clinical and pathological study of primary liver cancer*, 3rd edn., Kanehara, Tokyo.

Liver Cancer Study Group of Japan (1995). Survey and follow-up of primary liver cancer in Japan—Report 11. *Acta Hepatol. Japan*, **36**, 208–18 (in Japanese).

Livraghi, T., Festi, D., Monti, F., *et al.* (1986). US-guided percutaneous alcohol injection of small hepatic and abdominal tumors. *Radiology*, **161**, 309–12.

Livraghi, T., Sangalli, G. and Vettori C. (1989). Adenomatous hyperplastic nodules in the cirrhotic liver: a therapeutic approach. *Radiology*, **170**, 155–7.

Livraghi, T., Grigioni, W., Mazziotti, A., *et al.* (1990). Percutaneous alcohol injection of portal thrombosis in hepatocellular carcinoma: a new possible treatment. Tumori, **76**, 394–7.

Livraghi, T., Bolondi, L., Lazzaroni, S., *et al.* (1992). Percutaneous ethanol injection in the treatment of hepatocellular carcinoma in cirrhosis. A study on 207 patients. *Cancer*, **69**, 925–9.

Locker, G,Y., Doroshow, J.H., Zwelling, L.A. and Chabner, B.A. (1979). The clinical features of hepatic angiosarcoma. *Medicine*, **58**, 48–64.

Long, J.A., Jr, Krudy, A., Dunnick, N.R., *et al.* (1980). False aneurysm formation following arteriographic intimal dissection. *Radiology*, **135**, 323–326.

Looney, W.B. (1960). An investigation of the late clinical findings following Thorotrast (thorium dixoide) administration. *Am. J. Roentgenol. Radium Ther. Nucl. Med.*, **83**, 163–85.

Lubbers, P.R., Ros, P.R., Goodman, Z.D. and Ishak, K.G. (1987). Accumulation of technetium-99m sulfur colloid by hepatocellular adenoma: a scintigraphic-pathologic correlation. *A.J.R.*, **148**, 1105–8.

Lunderquist, A. and Vang, J. (1974). Transhepatic catheterization and obliteration of the coronary vein in patients with portal hypertension and esophageal varices. *New Engl. J. Med.* **291**, 646–9.

Lundstedt, C., Holmin, T., and Thorvinger, B. (1992). Peritoneal ovarian metastases simulating liver parenchymal metastases. *Gastrointest. Radiol.*, **17**, 250–2.

MacCarty, R.L., LaRusso, N.F., May, G.R., *et al.* (1985). Cholangiocarcinoma complicating primary sclerosing cholangitis: cholangiographic appearances. *Radiology*, **156**, 43–6.

MacDonald, R.A. (1957). Primary carcinoma of the liver: a clinicopathological study of one hundred and eight cases. *Arch. Int. Med.*, **99**, 266–9.

Magari S. (1990). Hepatic lymphatic system: structure and function. *J. Gastroenterol. Hepatol.*, **5**, 82–93.

Maguire, R. and Doppman, J.L. (1977). Angiographic abnormalities in partial Budd–Chiari syndrome. *Radiology*, **122**, 629–35.

Makuuchi, M., Hasegawa, H., Yamazaki, S., *et al.* (1983). The inferior right hepatic vein: ultrasonic demonstration. *Radiology*, **148**, 213–7.

Makuuchi, M., Hasegawa, H., Yamazaki, S., *et al.* (1984). Primary Budd–Chiari syndrome: ultrasonic demonstration. *Radiology*, **152**, 775–9.

Makuuchi, M., Hasegawa, H. and Yamazaki, S. (1985*a*). Ultrasonically guided subsegmentectomy. *Surg. Gynecol. Obstet.* **161**, 346–50.

Makuuchi, M., Sugihara, M., Mori, T., *et al.* (1985*b*). Bile duct necrosis: complication of transcatheter hepatic arterial embolization. *Radiology*, **156**, 331–4.

Makuuchi, M., Hasegawa, H., Yamazaki, S., *et al.* (1987*a*). The use of operative ultrasound as an aid to liver resection in patients with hepatocellular carcinoma. *World J. Surg.*, **11**, 615–621.

Makuuchi, M. Hasegawa, H., Yamazaki, S., and Takayasu, K. (1987*b*). Four new hepatectomy procedures for resection of the right hepatic vein and preservation of the inferior right hepatic vein. *Surg. Gynecol. Obstet.* 164, 68–72.

Makuuchi, M., Le Thai, B., Takayasu, K., *et al.* (1990). Preoperative portal embolization to increase safety of major hepatetomy for hilar bile duct carcinoma: a preliminary report. *Surgery*, **107**, 521–7.

Makuuchi, M., Takayama, T., Kosuge, T., *et al.* (1991). The value of ultrasonography for hepatic surgery. *Hepatol-Gastroenterology*, **38**, 64–70.

Mallory, F.B. (1932). Cirrhosis of the liver. *New Engl. J. Med.* 206, 1231–9.

Marchal, G., Tshibwabwa-Tumba, E., Verbelem, E. *et al.* (1986). 'Skip areas' in hepatic steatosis: a sonographic-angiographic study. *Gastrointest. Radiol.*, **11**, 151–7.

Mathieu, D., Grenier, P., Larde, D., *et al.* (1984). Portal vein involvement in hepatocellular carcinoma: dynamic CT features. *Radiology*, **152**, 127–32.

Mathieu, D., Vasile, N., Dibie, C., *et al.* (1985). Portal cavernoma: dynamic CT features and transient differences in hepatic attenuation. *Radiology*, **154**, 743–8.

Mathieu, D., Guinet, C., Bouklia-Hassane, A., *et al.* (1988). Hepatic vein involvement in hepatocellular carcinoma. *Gastrointest. Radiol.*, **13**, 55–60.

Matsuda, Y. and Yabuuchi, I. (1986). Hepatic tumors: US contrast enhancement with CO_2 microbubbles. *Radiology*, **161**, 701–5.

Matsui, O., Kadoya, M., Suzuki, M., *et al.* (1983). Dynamic sequential computed tomography during arterial portography in the detection of hepatic neoplasms. *Radiology*, **146**, 721–7.

Matsui, O., Takashima, T., Kadoya, M., *et al.* (1984). Segmental staining on hepatic arteriography as a sign of intrahepatic portal vein obstruction. *Radiology*, **152**, 601–6.

Matsui, O., Takashima, T., Kadoya, M., *et al.* (1987*a*). Staining in the liver surrounding gallbladder fossa on hepatic arteriography caused by increased cystic vanous drainage. *Gastrointest. Radiol.*, **12**, 307–12.

Matsui, O., Takashima, T., Kadoya, M., *et al.* (1987*b*). Liver metastases from colorectal cancers: detection with CT during arterial portography. *Radiology*, **165**, 65–9.

Matsui, O., Takashima, T., Kadoya, M. (1988). CT anatomy of the paracaval portion of the caudate lobe of the liver. *J. Japan Radiol. Soc.*, **48**, 841–6 (in Japanese).

Matsui, O., Kadoya, M., Kameyama, T., *et al.* (1989). Adenomatous hyperplastic nodules in the cirrhotic liver: differentiation from hepatocellular carcinoma with MR imaging. *Radiology*, **173**, 123–6.

Matsui, O., Kadoya, M., Kameyama, J., *et al.* (1990). Benign and malignant nodules in cirrhotic livers; distinction based on blood supply. *Radiology*, **178**, 493–7.

Matsui, O., Kadoya, M., Kameyama, T., *et al.* (1991). Benign and malignant nodules in cirrhotic livers: distinction based on blood supply. *Radiology*, **178**, 493–7.

Matsui, O., Kadoya, M., Yoshikawa, J., *et al.* (1993). Small hepatocellular carcinoma: treatment with subsegmental transcatheter arterial embolization. *Radiology*, **188**, 79–83.

Matsui, O., Takahashi, S., Kadoya, M., *et al.* (1994). Pseudolesion in segment IV of the liver at CT during arterial portography: correlation with aberrant gastric venous drainage. *Radiology*, **193**, 31–5.

Matsuzaki, Y., Osuga, T., Saito, Y., *et al.* (1994). A new, effective, and safe therapeutic option using proton irradiation for hepatocellular carcinoma. *Gastroenterology*, **106**, 1032–41.

Mattison, G.R., Glazer, G.M., Quint LE., *et al.* (1987). MR imaging of hepatic focal nodular hyperplasia: characterization and distinction from primary malignant tumors. *A.J.R.*, **148**, 711–5.

Mayes, G.B., Chuang, V.P and Fisher, R.G. (1981). CT of pseudomyxoma peritonei. *A.J.R.*, **136**, 807–8.

McLoughlin, M.J. (1971). Angiography in cavernous hemangioma of the liver. *A.J.R.*, **113**, 50–5.

Melato, M., Laurino, L., Mucli, E., *et al.* (1989). Relationship between cirrhosis, liver cancer, and hepatic metastases. *Cancer*, **64**, 455–9.

Melnick, P.J. (1955). Polycystic liver. *AMA Arch. Pathol.*, **59**, 162–72.

Merine, D., Takayasu, K., Wakao, F. (1990). Detection of hepatocellular carcinoma: comparison of CT during arterial portography with CT after intraarterial injection of iodized oil. *Radiology*, **175**, 707–10.

Michels, N.A. (1951). The hepatic, cystic and retroduodenal arteries and their relations to the biliary ducts. *Ann. Surg.*, **133**, 503.

Michels, N.A. (1955). *Blood supply and anatomy of the upper abdominal organs.* Lippincott, Philadelphia.

Miki, H., Mogami, H., Tanada, S., and Hamamoto, K. (1991). Comparison of MR angiography and conventional angiography in cerebral aneurysms. *Radiology*, 181 (P) 324.

Mikkonen, R., Kontkanen, T., and Kivisaari, L. (1995). Acute and late adverse reactions to low-osmolas contrast media. *Acta Radiologica*, **36**, 72–76.

Miller, J.H. and Greenspan, B.S. (1985). Integrated imaging of hepatic tumors in childhood: I. Malignant lesions (primary and metastatic). *Radiology*, **145**, 83–90.

Miller, W.J., Dodd, G.D. III, Federle, M.P., and Baron, R.L. (1993). Epithelioid hemangioendothelioma of the liver: imaging findings with pathologic correlation. *A.J.R.* 160, 422–3.

Mills, S.R., Doppman, J.L., and Nienhuis, A.W. (1977). Computed tomography in the diagnosis of disorders of excessive iron storage of the liver. *J. Comput. Assist. Tomogr*, **1**, 101–4.

Mitchell, D.G., Rubin, R., Siegelman, E.S., *et al.* (1991). Hepatocellular carcinoma within siderotic regenerative nodules: appearance as a nodule within a nodule on MRI images. *Radiology*, **178**, 101–3.

Miura, K. and Shirasawa, H. (1988). Primary carcinoid tumor of the liver. *Am. J. Clin. Pathol*, **89**, 561–4.

Moore, G.E. and Bridenbauch, R.B. (1950). Portal venography. *Surgery*, **28**, 827–31.

Moreno, A.H., Burchell, A.R., Reddy, R.V., *et al.* (1975). Spontaneous reversal of portal blood flow. The case for and against its occurrence in patients with cirrhosis of the liver. *Ann. Surg.*, **181**, 346–58.

Mori, H., Hayashi, K., Uetani, M., *et al.* (1987). High-attenuation recent thrombus of the portal vein: CT demonstration and clinical significance. *Radiology*, **163**, 353–6.

Morimoto, K., Shimoi, M., Shirakawa, T., *et al.* (1992). Biliary obstruction: evaluation with three-dimensional MR cholangiography. *Radiology*, **183**, 578–80.

Moriyama, N. (1980). Angiographic computed tomography. *Japan. J. Cancer Clin.*, **26**, 1037–40 (in Japanese).

Moriyasu, F., Ban, N., and Igarashi, A. (1983). A new method of transcutaneous measurement of portal blood flow by an ultrasonic 'Duplex' system composed of a pulsed Doppler flowmeter and a linear-type real time B mode electroscanner. *Acta Hepatol. Japan*, **24**, 537–44.

Moriyasu, F., Ban, N., Nishida, O., *et al.* (1986). Portal hemodynamics in patients with hepatocellular carcinoma. *Radiology*, **161**, 707–11.

Morrow, C.S., Kantor, M., and Armen, R.N. (1958). Hepatic hydrothorax. *Ann. Intern. Med.*, **49**, 193–203.

Moss, A.A., Dean, P.B., Axel, L., *et al.* (1982). Dynamic CT of hepatic masses with intravenous and intraarterial contrast material. *A.J.R.* 138, 847–52.

Muhler, A., Clement, O., Vexler, V., *et al.* (1992). Hepatobiliary enhancement with Gd-EOB-DTPA: comparison of spin-echo and STIR imaging for detection of experimental liver metastases. *Radiology*, **184**, 207–13.

Mukai, H., Nakajima, M., Yasuda, K., *et al.* (1992). Evaluation of endoscopic ultrasonography in the preoperative staging of carcinoma of the ampulla of Vater and common bile duct. *Gastrointest. Endosc.*, **38**, 676–83.

Murakami, T., Nakamura, H., Hori, S., *et al.* (1992). CT and MRI of siderotic regenerating nodules in hepatic cirrhosis. *J. Comput. Assist. Tomogr.*, **16**, 578–82.

Murakami, T., Nakamura, H., Hori, S., *et al.* (1993). Detection of viable tumor cells in hepatocellular carcinoma following transcatheter arterial chemoembolization with iodized oil. *Acta Radiol.*, **34**, 398 403.

Murakami, T., Igarashi, H., Oi, H., *et al.* (1994). Time-of-flight MR angiography of portal system and collaterals in portal hypertension using a 2–DFT fast spoiled gradient recalled steady-state precession technique. *Acta Radiol.*, **35**, 581–5.

Muramatsu, Y., Takayasu, K., Moriyama, N., *et al.* (1986). Peripheral low-density area of hepatic tumors: CT-pathologic correlation. *Radiology*, **160**, 49–52.

Muramatsu, Y., Nawano, S., Takayasu, K., *et al.* (1991). Early hepatocellular carcinoma: MR imaging. *Radiology*, **181**, 209–13.

Mutou, H. (1980). Simultaneous radiographic visualization of all hepatic veins by a single lumen balloon catheter. *Nippon Acta Radiol.*, **40**, 1017–37 (in Japanese).

Nagasue, N., Inokuchi, K., Kobayashi, M., *et al.* (1976). Hepatic dearterialiation for nonresectable primary and secondary tumors of the liver. *Cancer*, **38**, 2593–603.

Nagasue, N., Yukays, H., Ogawa, Y., *et al.* (1986). Second hepatic resection for recurrent hepatocellular carcinoma. *Br. J. Surg.*, **73**, 434–8.

Nagasue, N., Galizia, G., Kohno, H., *et al.* (1989). Adverse effects of preoperative hepatic artery chemoembolization for resectable hepatocellular carcinoma: a retrospective comparison of 138 liver resections. *Surgery*, **106**, 81–6.

Nakamura, H., Uchida, H., Kuroda, C., *et al.* (1980). Accessory left gastric artery arising from the left hepatic artery: angiographic study. *Am. J. Radiol.*, **134**, 529–32.

Nakamura, H., Choi, S., Tanaka, T., *et al.* (1984). CT of hepatoma: dilatation of the intrahepatic bile ducts and intraductal tumor growth. *Eur. J. Radiol.*, **4**, 276–8.

Nakamura, H., Hashimoto, T., Oi, H., and Sawada, S. (1988). Iodized oil in the portal vein after arterial embolization. *Radiology*, **167**, 415–17.

Nakamura, H., Hashimoto, T., Oi, H., *et al.* (1989). Transcatheter oily chemoembolization of hepatocellular carcinoma. *Radiology*, **170**, 783–6.

Nakamura, H., Hashimoto, T., Oi, H., *et al.* (1990). Treatment of hepatocellular carcinoma by segmental hepatic arterial injection of adriamycin-in-oil emulsion with overflow to segmental portal veins. *Acta Radiol.*, **31**, 347–9.

Nakamura, S., and Tuzuki, T. (1981). Surgical anatomy of the hepatic veins and the inferior vena cava. *Surg. Gynecol. Obstet.* **152**, 43–50.

Nakamura, T., Nakamura, S., Aikawa, T., *et al.* (1968). Obstruction of the inferior vena cava in the hepatic portion and the hepatic veins. Report of 18 cases and review of the Japanese literature. *Angiology*, **19**, 479–98.

Nakanuma, Y., Kurumaya, H., and Ohta, G. (1984). Multiple cysts in the hepatic hilum and their pathogenesis: a suggestion of periductal gland origin. *Virchows Arch. (A)*, **404**, 341–50.

Nakao, N., Miura, M., Takahashi, H., *et al.* (1986). Heptocellular carcinoma: combined hepatic, arterial, and portal venous embolization. *Radiology*, **161**, 303–7.

Nakao, N., Kotake, M., Miura, K., *et al.* (1988). Rupture of hepatocellular carcinoma following transcatheter arterial embolization. *Pediat. Med.*, **6**, 147–9.

Nakashima, T. (1976). Vascular changes and hemodynamics in hepatocellular carcinoma. In *Hepatocellular carcinoma* (ed. K. Okuda and R.L. Peters), pp.169–203. Wiley, New York.

Nakashima, T., and Kojiro, M. (1987). *Hepatocellular carcinoma. An atlas of its pathology*. Springer, Tokyo.

Nakashima, T., Kojiro, M., Sakamoto, K., *et al.* (1974). Studies of primary liver carcinoma. I. Proposal of new gross anatomical classification of primary liver cell carcinoma. *Acta Hepatol. Japan*, **15**, 279–91 (in Japanese with English abstract).

Nakashima, T., Okuda, K., Kojiro, M., *et al.* (1975). Primary liver cancer coexistent with schistosomiasis japonica. *Cancer*, **36**, 1483–9.

Nakashima, T., Okuda, K., Kojiro, M., *et al.* (1983). Pathology of hepatocellular carcinoma in Japan, 232 consecutive cases autopsied in ten years. *Cancer*, **51**, 863–877.

Nakayama, T., Hiyama, Y., Ohnishi,, K., *et al.* (1983). Arterioportal shunts on dynamic computed tomography. *A.J.R.*, **140**, 953–957.

Nakayama, T., Ikeda, A., and Okuda, K. (1978). Percutaneous transhepatic drainage of the biliary tract. Technique and results in 104 cases. *Gastroenterology*, **74**, 554–9.

Nelson, R.C., Thompson, G.H., Chezmar, J.L., *et al.* (1992). CT during arterial portography: diagnostic pitfalls. *Radio Graphics*, **12**, 705–18.

Netter, F.H. (1967). *The CIBA collection of medical illustrations. Vol. 3. Digestive system. Part III, Liver, biliary tract and pancreas.* CIBA Publications, Summit.

Nevin, J.E., Moran, T.J., Kay, S., and King, R. (1976). Carcinoma of the gallbladder: staging, treatment and prognosis. *Cancer*, **37**, 141–8.

Niederau, C., Fisher, R., Sonnenberg, A., *et al.* (1985). Survival and causes of death in cirrhotic and in noncirrhotic patients with primary hemochromatosis. *New Engl. J. Med.*, **313**, 1256–83.

Nimura, Y. (1988). *Surgical treatment. In: Hepatobiliary and pancreatic cancer.* Suemasu, K., Moriyama, N., (ed.) *Medical view*, Tokyo (Japanese).

Noguchi, M., Upton, M.P., Hirohashi, S., *et al.* (1987). A case of epithelioid hemangioendothelioma of the liver. *Jpn. J. Clin. Oncol.*, **17**, 275–84.

Nomura, Y., Matsuda, Y., Yabuuchi, I., *et al.* (1993). Hepatocellular carcinoma in adenomatous hyperplasia: detection with contrast-enhanced US with carbon dioxide microbubbles. *Radiology*, **187**, 353–6.

Nornha, R. and Gonzalez-Crussi, F. (1984). Hepatic angiosarcoma in childhood. *Am. J. Surg. Pathol.*, **8**, 863–71.

Numata, K., Takayasu, K., Muramatsu, Y., *et al.* (1989). Clinicopathological study of cholangiocellular carcinoma. *Japan. J. Gastroenterol. Surg.*, **22**, 2375–82 (in Japanese).

Nusbaum, M. and Baum, S. (1963). Radiographic demonstration of unknown sites of gastrointestinal bleeding. *Surg. Forum*, **14**, 374–5.

Obata, H., Hayashi, N., Motoike, Y., *et al.* (1980). A prospective study on the development of hepatocellular carcinoma from liver cirrhosis with persistent hepatitis B virus infection. *Int. J. Cancer*, **25**, 741–7.

Ohishi, H., Uchida, H., Yoshimura, H., *et al.* (1985). Hepatocellular carcinoma detected by iodized oil: use of anticancer agents. *Radiology*, **154**, 25–9.

Ohkubo, H., Okuda, K., Takayasu, K., *et al.* (1978). Cruveilhier–Baumgarten syndrome presenting with precordial murmur and thrill. Report of a case diagnosed by percutaneous transhepatic portography. *Digest. Dis.*, **23**, 65–8.

Ohnishi, K., Nakayama, T., Nomura, F., *et al.* (1984*a*) Reduction of portal vein pressure with the enlargement of portal-systemic shunt: observation made in one patient. *J. Clin. Gastroenterol.*, **6**, 447–51.

Ohnishi, K., Okuda, K., Ohtsuki, T., *et al.* (1984*b*) Formation of hilar collaterals or cavernous transformation after portal vein obstruction by hepatocellular carcinoma. Observations in ten patients. *Gastroenterology*, **87**, 1150–3.

Ohnishi, K., Tsuchiya, S., Nakayama, T., *et al.* (1984*c*) Arterial chemoembolization of hepatocellular carcinoma with mitomycin C microcapsules. *Radiology*, **152**, 51–5.

Ohnishi, K., Nakayama, T., Koen, H., *et al.* (1985*a*) Interrelationship between types of spontaneous portal systemic shunt and portal vein pressure in patients with liver disease. *Am. J. Gastroenterol.*, **80**, 561–4.

Ohnishi, K., Saito, M., Saito, M., *et al.* (1985*b*) Hepatic encephalopathy associated with extensive portal hepatic venous shunts. *Am. J. Gastroenterol*, **80**, 60–3.

Ohnishi, K., Tanabe, Y., Ryu, M., *et al.* (1987). Prognosis of hepatocellular carcinoma smaller than 5 cm in relation to treatment: study of 100 patients. *Hepatology*, **7**, 1285–90.

Ohnishi, K., Ohyama, N., Ito, S., *et al.* (1994). Small hepatocellular carcinoma: treatment with US-guided intratumoral injection of acetic acid. *Radiology*, **193**, 747–52.

Ohto, M., Ono, T., Tsuchiya, Y., and Saisho, H. (1978). *Cholangiography and pancreatography*. Igaku-Shoin, Tokyo.

Ohto, M., Karasawa, E., Tsuchiya, Y., *et al.* (1980). Ultrasonically guided percutaneous contrast medium injection and aspiration biopsy using a real-time puncture transducer. *Radiology*, **136**, 171–6.

Ohto, M., Ebara, M., Yoshikawa, M., Okuda, K. (1987). Radiation therapy and percutaneous ethanol injection for the treatment of hepatocellular carcinoma. In *Neoplasms of the liver* (ed. K. Okuda and K.G. Ishak), pp.335–41, Springer, Tokyo.

Ohtomo, K., Itai, Y., Furui, S., *et al.* (1985). MR imaging of portal vein thrombus in hepatocellular carcinoma. *J. Comput. Assist. Tomogr.*, **9**, 328–9.

Ohtomo, K., Itai, Y., Yoshikaea, K., *et al.* (1987). Hepatic tumors: dynamic MR imaging. *Radiology*, **163**, 27–31.

Ohtomo, K., Itai, Y., Ohtomo, Y., *et al.* (1990). Regenerating nodules of liver cirrhosis: MR imaging with pathologic correlation. *A.J.R.* 154, 505–7.

Ohtomo, K., Araki, T., Itai, Y., *et al.* (1992). MR imaging of malignant mesenchymal tumors of the liver. *Gastrointest. Radiol.*, **17**, 58–62.

Ohtomo, K., Baron, R.L., Dodd, G.D., *et al.* (1993). Confluent hepatic fibrosis complicating cirrhosis: pathologic-imaging correlation in 420 transplant patients. *Radiology*, **189**, 273–4 (abstract).

Okada, S., Okazaki, N., Nose, H., *et al.* (1992). Prognostic factors in patients with hepatocellular carcinoma receiving systemic chemotherapy. *Hepatology*, **16**, 112–17.

Okamoto, E., Kyo, A., Yamanaka, N., *et al.* (1984). Prediction of the safe limit of hepatectomy by combined volumetric and functional mesurements in patients with impaired hepatic function. *Surgery*, **95**, 586–91.

Okamura, H., Horikawa, S., Fujiyama, T., *et al.* (1982). An appraisal of transcatheter arterial embolization combined with transcatheter arterial infusion of chemotherapeutic agent for hepatic malignancies. *World J. Surg.*, **6**, 352–7.

Okazaki, M., Higashihara, H., Koganemaru, F., *et al.* (1991). Intraperitoneal hemorrhage from hepatocellular carcinoma: emergency chemoembolization or embolization. *Radiology*, **180**, 647–651.

Okazaki, N. (1976). Systemic chemotherapy of hepatocellular carcinoma. In *Hepatocellular carcinoma* (ed. K. Okuda and R.L. Peters). pp.469–475. Wiley, New York.

Okazaki, N., Yoshino, M., Yoshida, T., *et al.* (1985). Bone metastasis in hepatocellular carcinoma. *Cancer*, **55**, 1991–4.

Okazaki, N., Yoshino, M., Yoshida, T., *et al.* (1988). Indication of chemotherapy and prognosis in hepatocellular carcinoma. *Naika*, **61**, 660–4 (in Japanese).

Okazaki, N., Yoshino, M., Yoshida, T., *et al.* (1989). Evaluation of the prognosis for small hepatocellular carcinoma based on tumor volume doubling time. A preliminary report. *Cancer*, **63**, 2207–10.

Okazaki, N., Okada, S., Nose, H., Aoki, K. (1992). Systemic chemotherapy for hepatocellular carcinoma. In *Primary liver cancer in Japan* (ed. T. Tobe, H. Kameda, M. Okudaira, *et al.*). pp.301–305. Springer, Tokyo.

Okuda, H., Nakanishi, T., Furukawa, M., Obata, H. (1991). Vitamin K-dependent proteins and hepatocellular carcinoma. *J. Gastroenterol. Hepatol.*, **6**, 392–9.

Okuda, H., Yamagata, H., Obata, H., *et al.* (1995). Epidemiological and clinical features of Budd–Chiari syndrome in Japan. *J. Hepatol.*, **22**, 1–9.

Okuda, K. (1976). Clinical aspects of hepatocellular carcinoma—analysis of 134 cases. In *Hepatocellular carcinoma* (ed. K.Okuda and R.L. Peters), pp.387–436. Wiley, New York.

Okuda, K. (1981). Advances in hepatobiliary ultrasonography. *Hepatology*, **1**, 662–72.

Okuda, K. (1982). Membranous obstruction of the inferior vena cava : etiology and relation to hepatocellular carcinoma. *Gastroenterology*, **82**, 376–9.

Okuda, K. (1986). Early recognition of hepatocellular carcinoma. *Hepatology*, **6**, 729–38.

Okuda, K. (1993). Intratumor ethanol injection. *J. Surg. Oncol. Suppl.*, 3, 97–9.

Okuda, K. and Iio, M. (1976). *Radiological aspects of the liver and biliary tract. X-ray and radioisotope diagnosis*. Year Book, Chicago.

Okuda, K. and Liver Cancer Study Group of Japan (1980). Primary liver cancers in Japan. Cancer, **45**, 2663–9.

Okuda, K. and Nakashima, T. (1985). Primary carcinoma of the liver. In *Bockus gastroenterology* (ed. J.E. Berk), pp.3315–76. Saunders, Philadelphia.

Okuda, K., Ryu, M. and Tobe, T. (1987). Surgical management of hepatoma. The Japanese experience. In *Hepatic and biliary cancer* (ed. H.J. Wanebo), pp.219–38. Dekker, New York.

Okuda, K. and Tsuchiya, Y. (1982). Ultrasonography of the biliary tract. In *Progress in liver diseases*, Vol. 7 (ed. H. Popper and F. Schaffner), pp.285–97. Grune & Stratton, New York.

Okuda, K., Shimokawa, Y., and Yakushiji, F. (1970). Liver scintillation scanning in the diagnosis of chronic schistosomiasis. *Digestion*, **3**, 269–78.

Okuda, K., Emura, T., Morokuma, K., *et al.* (1973*a*) Clonorchiasis studied by percutaneous cholangiography and a therapeutic trial of toluene-a, 4–diisothiocyanate. *Gastroenterology*, **65**, 457–61.

Okuda, K., Moriyama, M., Yasumoto, M., *et al.* (1973*b*) Roentgenologic demonstration of spontaneous reversal of portal blood flow incirrhosis and primary carcinoma of the liver. *A.J.R.*, 119, 419–28.

Okuda, K., Tanikawa, K., Emura, T., *et al.* (1974). Nonsurgical percutaneous transhepatic cholangiography—diagnostic significance in medical problems of the liver. *Am. J. Digest Dis.*, **19**, 21–36.

Okuda, K., Jinnouchi, S., Arakawa, M., et al.. (1975*a*). Generalized cal-cification of the liver in advanced schistosomiasis. *Acta Hepta-Gastroenterol.*, **12**, 98–102.

Okuda K, Musha, H., Yoshida, T., *et al.* (1975*b*) Demonstration of growing casts of hepatocellular carcinoma in the portal vein by celiac angiography: the thread and streaks sign. *Radiology*, **117**, 303–9.

Okuda, K., Ichinohe, A., Kono, K., *et al.* (1976*a*) Minimal Thorotrast deposition in parapancreatic lymph nodes. *Radiology*, **119**, 23–6.

Okuda, K., Sumikoshi, T., Kanda, Y., *et al.* (1976*b*) Hepatic lymphatics as opacified by percutaneous intrahepatic injection of contrast medium. *Radiology* **120**, 321–6.

Okuda, K., Jinnouchi, S., Nagasaki, Y., *et al.* (1977*a*). Angiographic demonstration of growth of hepatocellular carcinoma in the hepatic vein and inferior vena cava. *Radiology*, **124**, 33–6.

Okuda, K., Kubo, Y., Okazaki, N., *et al.* (1977*b*). Clinical aspects of intrahepatic bile duct carcinoma including hilar carcinoma. A study of 57 autopsy-proven cases. *Cancer*, **39**, 232–46.

Okuda, K., Musha, H., Nakajima, Y., *et al.* (1977*c*) Clinicopathological features of encapsulated hepatocellular carcinoma. *Cancer*, **40**, 1240–45.

Okuda, K., Musha, H., Yamasaki, T., *et al.* (1977*d*) Angiographic demonstration of intrahepatic arterio-portal anastomoses in hepatocellular carcinoma. *Radiology*, **122**, 53–8.

Okuda, K., Nakashima, T., Obata, H., and Kubo, Y. (1977*e*) Clinicopathological studies of minute hepatocellular carcinoma. Analysis of 20 cases, including 4 with hepatic resection. *Gastroenterology*, **73**, 109–15.

Okuda, K., Obata, H., Jinnouchi, S., *et al.* (1977*f*) Angiographic assessment of gross anatomy of hepatocellular carcinoma: comparison of celiac angiograms and liver pathology in 100 cases. *Radiology*, **123**, 21–9.

Okuda, K., Suzuki, K., Musha, H., and Arimizu, N. (1977*g*) Percutaneous transhepatic catheterization of the portal vein for the study of portal hemodynamics and shunts. *Gastroenterology*, **73**, 279–84.

Okuda, K., Musha, H., Nakajima, Y., *et al.* (1978). Frequency of intrahepatic arteriovenous fistula as a sequela to percutaneous needle puncture of the liver. *Gastroenterology*, **74**, 1204–7.

Okuda, K., Nomura, F., Kawai, M., *et al.* (1979). Age related gross changes of the liver and right diaphragm, with special references to partial eventration. *Br. J. Radiol.*, **52**, 870–5.

Okuda, K., Nakashima, T., Okudaira, M., *et al.* (1981*a*) Anatomical basis of hepatic venographic alterations in idiopathic portal hypertension. *Liver*, **1**, 255–63.

Okuda, K., Nogushi, T., Kubo, Y., *et al.* (1981*b*) A clinical and pathological study of diffuse type hepatocellular carcinoma. *Liver*, **1**, 280–9.

Okuda, K., Omata, M., Itoh, Y., *et al.* (1981*c*) Peliosis hepatis as a late and fatal complication of thorotrast liver disease. Report of five cases. *Liver*, **1**, 110–22.

Okuda, K., Kimura, K., and Takayasu, K. (1982*a*). Percutaneous trans-hepatic portography and sclerotherapy. *Semin. Liver Dis.*, **2**, 57–66.

Okuda, K., Nakashima, T., Okudaira, M., *et al.* (1982*b*) Liver pathology of idiopathic poral hypertension. Comparison with non-cirrhotic portal fibrosis of India. *Liver*, **2**, 176–92.

Okuda, K., Kono, K., Ohnishi, K., *et al.* (1984*a*) Clinical study of eighty-six cases of idiopathic portal hypertension and comparison with cirrhosis with splenomegaly. *Gastroenterology*, **86**, 600–10.

Okuda, K., Peters, R. and Simson, I.W. (1984*b*) Gross anatomical features of hepatocellular carcinoma from three disparate geographic areas. Proposal of new classification. *Cancer*, **54**, 2165–73.

Okuda, K., Ohnishi, K., Kimura, K., *et al.* (1985*a*) Incidence of portal vein thrombosis in liver cirrhosis: an angiographic study in 708 patients. *Gastroenterology*, **89**, 279–86.

Okuda, K., Ohtsuki, T., Obata, H., *et al.* (1985*b*) Natural history of hepatocellular carcinoma and prognosis in relation to treatment. Study of 850 patients. *Cancer*, **56**, 918–28.

Okuda, K. and Matsutani, S. (1987). Portal-systemic collaterals: anatomy and clinical implications. In *Portal hypertension. Clinical and physiological aspects* (ed. K. Okuda and J.-P. Benhamou). pp.51–62. Springer, Tokyo.

Okumura, T., Itai, Y., Tsuji, H., *et al.* (1994). Focused radiation hepatitis after Bragg-peak proton therapy for hepatocellular carcinoma: CT findings. *J. Comput. Assist. Tomogr.*, **18**, 821–3.

Oliver, J.H. III., Baron, R.L., Dodd, G. III., *et al.* (1995). Does advanced cirrhosis with portosystemic shunting affect the value of AT arterial portography in the evaluation of the liver? *A.J.R.*, 164, 333–7.

Omata, M., Peters, R.L., and Tatter, D. (1981). Sclerosing hepatic carcinoma: relationship to hypercalcemia. *Liver*, **1**, 33–49.

Ong, G.B. and Taw, J.L. (1972). Spontaneous rupture of hepatocellular carcinoma. *Br. Med. J.*, **4**, 146–9.

Osborne, B.M., Butler, J.J. and Guarda, L.A. (1985). Primary lymphoma of the liver. *Cancer*, **56**, 2909–10.

Oshiro, K. and Feinberg, D.A. (1991). GRASE (gradient-and spin echo) imaging: a novel fast MRI technique. *Magn. Reson. Med.*, **20**, 344–9.

Pagani, J.J. (1983). Intrahepatic vascular territories shown by computed tomography (CT). *Radiology*, **147**, 173–8.

Paltiel, H.J., Patriquin, H.B., Keller, M.S., *et al.* (1992). Infantile hepatic hemangioma: Doppler US. *Radiology*, **182**, 735–42.

Pardes, J.G., Bryan, P.J. and Gauderer, M.W.L. (1982). Spontaneous regression of infantile hemangioendotheliomatosis of the liver: demonstration by ultrasound. *J. Ultrasound Med.*, **1**, 349–53.

Park, C.H., Suh, J.H., Yoo, H.S., *et al.* (1986). Evaluation of intrahepatic I-131 ethiodol on a patient with hepatocellular carcinoma—therapeutic feasibility. *Clin. Nucl. Med.*, **11**, 514–17.

Parke, W.W., Michels, N.A. and Ghosh, G.H. (1963). Blood supply of the common bile duct. *Surg. Gynecol. Obstet.*, **117**, 47–55.

Parker, R.A. and Seal, R.M.E. (1955). Cavernous transformation of the portal vein. *J. Pathol. Bacteriol*, **70**, 97–103.

Parkin, D.M., Ohshima, H., Srivatanakul, P. and Vatanasapt, V. (1993). Cholangiocarcinoma: epidemiology, mechanisms of carcinogenesis and prevention. *Cancer Epidemiol Biomarkers Prevention*, **2**, 537–44.

Paulson, E.K., McClellan, J.S., Washington, K., *et al.* (1994). Hepatic adenoma: MR characteristics and correlation with pathologic findings. *A.J.R.* **163**, 113–16.

Pechoux, C.L., Akine, Y., Tokita, N., *et al.* (1994). Hepatocellular carcinoma diagnosed radiologically, treated by transcatheter arterial embolization and limited-field radiotherapy. *Br. J. Radiol.*, **67**, 591–5.

Peding, R., Buard, J.-L., Lebeau, G. and Launois, B. (1991). Surgical management of 552 carcinomas of the extrahepatic bile ducts (gallbladder and periampullary tumors excluded). *Ann. Surg.*, **213**, 236–41.

Peters, R.L. (1976). Pathology of hepatocellular carcinoma. In *Hepatocellular carcinoma* (ed. K. Okuda and R.L. Peters), pp.107–168. Wiley, New York.

Peters, W.M., Dixon, M.F., Williams, N.S. (1983). Angiomyelolipoma of the liver. *Histopathology*, **7**, 99–106.

Piekarski, J., Goldberg, H.I., Royal SA., *et al.* (1980). Difference between liver and spleen CT numbers in the normal adult: usefulness in predicting the presence of diffuse liver disease. *Radiology*, **137**, 727–9.

Pien, E.H., Zeman, R.K., Benjamin, S.B., *et al.* (1985). Iatrogenic sclerosing cholangitis following hepatic arterial chemotherapy infusion. *Radiology*, **156**, 329–30.

Pradinas, F.J., Melia, W.M., Wilkinson, M.L. *et al.* (1982). High serum vitamin B_{12} binding capacity as a marker of the fibrolamellar variant of hepatocellular carcinoma. *Br. Med. J. Slic. Res.*, **285**, 840–2.

Prando, A., Wallace, S., Bernardino, M.R., and Lindell, M.M., Jr (1979). Computed tomographic arteriography of the liver. *Radiology*, **130**, 697–701.

Primack, A., Vogel, C.L., Kyalwazi, S.K., *et al.* (1975). A. staging system for hepatocellular carcinoma: prognostic factors in Ugandan patients. *Cancer*, **35**, 1357–64.

Radin, D.R., Colletti, P.M., Ralls, P.W., *et al.* (1987). Agenesis of the right lobe of the liver. *Radiology*, **164**, 639–42.

Radin, D.R., Craig, J.R., Colletti, P.M., *et al.* (1988). Hepatic epithelioid hemangioendothelioma. *Radiology*, **169**, 145–8.

Rankin, R.N. (1979). Gas formation after renal tumor embolization without abscess: a benign occurrence. *Radiology*, **130**, 317–20.

Rao, B.K., Brodell, G.K., Haaga, J.R., *et al.* (1986). Visceral CT findings associated with Thorotrast. *J. Comput. Assist. Tomogr*, **19**, 57–61.

Reitemeier, R.J., Butt, H.R., and Baggenstoss, A.H. (1958). Riedel's lobe of the liver. *Gastroenterology*, **34**, LP 1090–1095.

Remy-Jardin, M., Remy, J., Giraud, F., and Marquette, C.H. (1993). Pulmonary nodules: detection with thick section spiral CT versus conventional CT. *Radiology*, **187**, 513–20.

Reuter, K., Raptopoulos, V., Reale, F., *et al.* (1983). Diagnosis of peritoneal mesothelioma: computed tomography, sonography, and fine-needle aspiration biopsy. *A.J.R.*, **140**, 1189–94.

Reuter, S.R. and Redman, H.C. (1977). *Gastrointestinal angiography*, 2nd edn. Saunders, Philadelphia.

Roberts, J.L., Fishman, E.K., Hartman, D.S., *et al.* (1986). Lipomatous tumors of the liver: evaluation with CT and US. *Radiology*, **158**, 613–17.

Rolfes, D.B. (1987). Fibrolamellar carcinoma of the liver. In *Neoplasms of the liver*, (ed. K.Okuda and K.G. Ishak), pp.137–42. Springer, Tokyo.

Rooks, J.B., Ory, H.W., Ishak, K.G., *et al.* (1979). Epidemiology of hepatocellular adenoma. The role of oral contraceptive use. *J.A.M.A.*, **242**, 644–48.

Ros, P.R., Goodman, Z.D., and Ishak, K.G. (1986). Mesenchymal hamartoma of the liver: radiologic-pathologic correlation. *Radiology*, **158**, 619–24.

Ross, D., Pina, J., Mirza, M., *et al.* (1976). Regression of focal nodular hyperplasia after discontinuation of oral contraceptives. *Ann. Intern. Med.*, **85**, 203–4.

Rossle, M., Richter, G.M., Noldge, G., *et al.* (1992). Transjugular intrahepatic portosystemic stent shunt: a 2-year follow-up. *Dig. Surg.*, **9**, 6–12.

Royal, S.A. and Callen, P.W. (1979). CT evaluation of anomalies of the inferior vena cava and left renal vein. *A.J.R.*, **132**, 759–63.

Ruebner, B.M., Green, R., Miyai, K., *et al.* (1961). The rarity of intrahepatic metastasis in cirrhosis of the liver. *Am. J. Pathol.*, **39**, 739–46.

Rummeny, E., Weissleder, R., Sironi, S., *et al.* (1989). Central scars in primary liver tumors: MR features, specificity, and pathologic correlation. *Radiology*, **171**, 323–6.

Sagoh, T., Itoh, K., Togashi, K., *et al.* (1990). Gallbladder carcinoma: evaluation with MR imaging. *Radiology*, **174**, 131–6.

Saini, S., Stark, D.D., Hahn, P.F., *et al.* (1987). Ferrite particles: a superparamagnetic MR contrast agent for the reticuloendotherial system. *Radiology*, **162**, 211–16.

Saitoh, M., Tsai, H.F., and Futagawa, S. (1989). Colonic varices in portal hypertension. *J. Gastroenterol. Hepatol.*, 4, Suppl. 1, 289–90.

Sakamoto, M., Hirohashi, S., and Shimosato, Y. (1991). Early stage of multistep hepatocarcinogenesis: adenomatous hyperplasia and early hepatocellular carcinoma. *Hum. Pathol.*, **22**, 172–8.

Sakamoto, M., Ino, Y., Fujii, T., et al.. (1993). Phenotype changes in tumor vessels associated with the progression of hepatocellular carcinoma. *Japan. J. Clin. Oncol.*, **23**, 98–104.

Sakurai, M., Seki, K., Okamura, J., *et al.* (1983). Needle tract implantation of hepatocellular carcinoma after percutaneous liver biopsy. *Am. J. Surg. Pathol.*, **7**, 191–5.

Sano, A., Kuroda, Y., Moriyasu, F., *et al.* (1982). Porto-pulmonary venous anastomosis in portal hypertension demonstrated by percutaneous transhepatic cine-portography. *Radiology*, **144**, 479–84.

Sasaki, K. (1980). Adenomatous hyperplasia in liver cirrhosis. An approach from a microangiographical point of view. *Gann Monogr. Cancer Res.*, **25**, 127–40.

Sasaki, Y., Imaoka, S., Fujito, M., *et al.* (1987). Regional therapy in the management of intrahepatic recurrence after surgery for hepatoma. *Ann. Surg.*, 206, 40–7.

Sato, T. (1989). Anatomical study of injection corrosion model of the human liver biliary tract. *Tando*, **3**, 227–33 (in Japanese).

Sato, T., Higashi, Y., and Ono, Y. (1986). Sonography of gallbaldder perforation: a complication of transcatheter arterial embolization. *J. Ultrasound Med.*, **5**, 715–18.

Sato, Y., Frey, E.E., Wicklund, B., *et al.* (1987). Embolization therapy in the management of infantile hemangioma with Kasabach Merritt syndrome. *Pediatr. Radiol.*, **17**, 503–4.

Sauerbrei, E.E. and Lopez, M. (1986). Pseudotumor of the quandrate lobe in hepatic sonography: a sign of generalized fatty infiltration. *A.J.R.* **147**, 923–7.

Scatarige, J.C., Kenny, J.M., Fishman, E.K., *et al.* (1987). CT of giant cavernous hemangioma. *A.J.R.*, **149**, 83–5.

Schmidt, D., Harms, D., and Lang, W. (1985). Primary malignant hepatic tumors in children. *Virch. Arch. (Pathol. Anat.)*, **407**, 387–405.

Schumann-Giampieri, G., Schmitt-Willich, H., Press, W.R., *et al.* (1992). Preclinical evaluation of Gd-EOB-DTPA. as a contrast agent in MR imaging of the hepatobiliary system. *Radiology*, **183**, 59–64.

Scott, W.W., Sanders, R.C., Siegelman, S.S., *et al.* (1980). Irregular fatty infiltration of the liver: diagnostic dilemmas. *A.J.R.*, **135**, 67–71.

Seidman, E., Weber, A.M., Morin, C.L., *et al.* (1984). Spinal cord paraly-sis following sclerotherapy for esophageal varices. *Hepatology*, **4**, 950–4.

Seki, T., Wakabayashi, M., Nakagawa, T. *et al.* (1994). Ultrasonically guided percutaneous microwave coagulation therapy for small hepatocellular carcinoma. *Cancer*, **74**, 817–25.

Semelka, R.C., Brown, E.D., Ascher, S.M., *et al.* (1994). Hepatic hemangiomas: a multi-institutional study of appearance on T2-weighted and serial gadolinium-enhanced gradient-echo MR images. *Radiology*, **192**, 401–6.

Sevic, R.J., Tsuruda, T.S., and Schmalbrock, P. (1991). Three-dimensional time-of-flight MR angiography in the evaluation of cerebral aneurysms. *J. Comput. Assist. Tomogr.*, **14**, 874–81.

Sherlock, S., Feldman, C.A., Moran, B., and Scheuer, P.J. (1966). Partial nodular transformation of the liver with portal hypertension. *Am. J. Med.*, **40**, 195–203.

Sheu, J.C., Sung, J.L., Chen, D.S., *et al.* (1985). Growth rate of asymptomatic hepatocellular carcinoma and its clinical implications. *Gastroenterology*, **89**, 259–66.

Sheu, J.C., Huang, G.T., Chen, D.S., *et al.* (1987). Small hepatocellular carcinoma: intratumor ethanol treatment using new needle and guidance systems. *Radiology*, **163**, 43–8.

Shiina, S., Yasuda, H., Moto, H., *et al.* (1987). Percutaneous ethanol injection in the treatment of liver neoplasms. *A.J.R.*, **149**, 949–52.

Shiina, S., Tagawa, K., Unuma, T., *et al.* (1990). Percutaneous ethanol injection therapy of hepatocellular carcinoma: analysis of 77 patients. *A.J.R.*, **155**, 1221–26.

Shimizu, K., Matsuda, T., Sakurai, T., *et al.* (1986). Visualization of moving fluid: quantitative analysis of blood velocity using MR imaging. *Radiology*, **159**, 195–9.

Shinagawa, T., Ohto, M., Kimura, K., *et al.* (1984). Diagnosis and clinical features of small hepatocellular carcinoma with emphasis on the utility of real-time ultrasonography. A. study in 51 patients. *Gastroenterology*, **86**, 495–502.

Simson, I.W. (1982). Membranous obstruction of the inferior vena cava and hepatocellular carcinoma in Southern African blacks. *Gastroenterology*, **82**, 171–8.

Sironi, S., Livraghi, T., Angeli, E., *et al.* (1993). Small hepatocellular carcinoma: MR follow-up of treatment with percutaneous ethanol injection. *Radiology*, **187**, 119–23.

Song, E., Kew, M.C., Grieve, T., *et al.* (1984). Primary squamous cell carcinoma of the liver occurring in association with hepatolithiasis. *Cancer*, **53**, 542–46.

Soo, C.-S., Wallace, S., Chuang, V.P., *et al.* (1982). Injury to the intima of the hepatic artery. *Radiology*, **143**, 373–8.

Sordillo, P.P., Helson, L., Hadju, S.I., *et al.* (1981). Malignant schwannoma—clinical characteristics, survival, and response to therapy. *Cancer*, **47**, 2503–9.

Soyer, P., Roche, A., Gad, M., *et al.* (1991). Preoperative segmental localization of hepatic metastases: utility of three-dimensional CT during arterial portography. *Radiology*, **180**, 653–8.

Soyer, P., Lacheheb, D., and Levesque, M. (1993). False-positive CT portography: correlation with pathologic findings. *A.J.R.*, **160**, 285–9.

Stanley, P., Geer, G.D., Miller, J.H., *et al.* (1989). Infantile hepatic hemangiomas. Clinical features, radiologic investigations, and treatment of 20 patients. *Cancer*, **64**, 936–49.

Stanley, R.L., Dehner, L.P., and Hesker, A.E. (1973). Primary malignant mesenchymal tumors (mesenchymom*a*). of the liver in children. *Cancer*, **32**, 973–84.

Stark, D.D., Felder, R.C., Wittenberg, J., *et al.* (1985). Magnetic resonance imaging of cavernous hemangioma of the liver: tissue specific characterization. *A.J.R.*, **145**, 213–20.

Stark, D.D., Hahn, P.F., Trey, C., *et al.* (1986). MRI of the Budd–Chiari syndrome. *A.J.R.*, **146**, 1141–8.

Stockberger, S., Wass, J.L., Sherman, S., *et al.* (1994). Intravenous cholangiography with helical CT: comparison with endoscopic retrograde cholangiography. *Radiology*, **192**, 675–80.

Stocker, J.T. and Ishak, K.G. (1987). Hepatoblastoma. In *Neoplasms of the liver* (ed. K. Okuda and K.G. Ishak), pp.127–36. Springer, Tokyo.

Stone, H.H., Long, W.D., Smith, R.B., and Haynes, C.D. (1969). Physiologic considerations in major hepatic resections. *Am. J. Surg*, **117**, 78–84.

Stromeyer, F.W. and Ishak, K.G. (1981). Nodular transformation (nodular 'regenerative' hyperplasia). of the liver. A. clinicopathologic study of 30 cases. *Hum. Pathol.*, **12**, 60–71.

Subramanyam, B.R. and Balthazar, E.J. (1984). Hepatocellular carcinoma with venous invation. *Radiology*, **150**, 793–6.

Sugihara, S. and Kojiro, M. (1987). Pathology of cholangiocarcinoma. In *Neoplasms of the liver* (ed. K. Okuda and K.G. Ishak), pp.141–58. Springer, Tokyo.

Sugiura, M. and Futagawa, S. (1984). Results of six hundred and thirty-six esophageal transections with paraesophagogastric devascularization in the treatment of esophageal varices. *J. Vasc. Surg.*, **1**, 254–60.

Sugiura, N., Takara, K., Ohto, M., *et al.* (1983). Treatment of small hepatocellular carcinoma by percutaneous injection of ethanol into tumor with real-time ultrasound monitoring. *Acta Hepatol. Japan.*, **24**, 920 (in Japanese).

Suit, H.D., Goitein, M., Munzenrider, L., *et al.* (1990). Increased efficacy of radiation therapy by use of proton mean. *Strahlenther. Onkol.* **166**, 40–4.

Sumiyoshi, A. and Niho, Y. (1971). Primary osteogenic sarcoma of the liver. *Acta Pathol. Japan*, **21**, 305–12.

Suzuki, H. (1982). Anatomical study of the vasculature within the Glisson's sheath near the hepatic hilum. *Nihon Geka Hokan*, **51**, 713–31 (in Japanese).

Suzuki, K., Okuda, K., Yoshida, T., *et al.* (1976). False-positive liver scan in a patient with hepatic amyloidosis. *J. Nucl. Med.*, **17**, 31–2.

Suzuki, M., Takashima, T., Funaki, H., *et al.* (1982). Low-density stone of the gallbladder on computed tomography. *Gastrointest. Radiol.*, **7**, 65–7.

Suzuki, M., Okazaki, N., Yoshino, M., and Yoshida, T. (1989). Spontaneous regression of a hepatocellular carcinoma—a case report. *Hepato-Gasteroenterology*, **36**, 160–3.

Taboury, J., Porcel, A., Tubiana, J.M., *et al.* (1983). Cavernous hemangioma of the liver studied by ultrasound. *Radiology*, **149**, 781–5.

Tachimori, Y., Makuuchi, M., Asamura, H., *et al.* (1988). A. case of hepatocellular carcinoma with tumor thrombi in the epiploic vein. *Japan. J. Clin. Oncol.*, **18**, 269–73.

Takashi, M., Igarashi, M., Hino, S., *et al.* (1984). Chronic portal-systemic encephalopathy with normal W V portal vein pressure possibly due to noncirrhotic portal fibrosis. *Dig. Dis. Sci.*, **29**, 669–73.

Takashi, M., Igarashi, M., Hino, S., *et al.* (1985*a*). Portal hemodynamics in chronic portal-systemic encephalopathy. *J. Hepatol.*, **1**, 467–76.

Takashi, M., Igarashi, M., Hino, S., *et al.* (1985*b*). Esophageal varices: correlation of left gastric venography and endoscopy in patients with portal hypertension. *Radiology*, **155**, 327–31.

Takashima, T. and Matsui, O. (1980). Infusion hepatic angiography in the detection of small hepatocellular carcinoma. *Radiology*, **136**, 321–25.

Takayama, T., Makuuchi, M., Hirohashi, S., *et al.* (1990). Malignant transformation of adenomatous hyperplasia to hepatocellular carcinoma. Lancet 336, 1150–3.

Takayama, T., Makuuchi, M., Kosuge, T., *et al.* (1991). A. hepatoblastoma originating in the caudate lobe radically resected with the inferior vena cava. *Surgery*, **109**, 208–13.

Takayasu, K., Shima, Y., Kobayashi, C., *et al.* (1981). Significance of combined percutaneous transhepatic portography and CT. (CT-PTP). in the diagnosis of liver cancer. *Acta Hepatol. Japan*, **11**, 299 (in Japanese).

Takayasu, K., Kobayashi, C., Takashi, M., and Okuda, K. (1982*a*). Paraesophageal varices mimicking a mediastinal tumor. *J. Clin. Gastroenterol.*, **4**, 163–6.

Takayasu, K., Takashi, M., Mush, H., *et al.* (1982*b*). Spontaneous reversal of portal blood flow demonstrated by percutaneous transhepatic catheterization: report of two cases. *Gastroenterology*, **82**, 753–7.

Takayasu, K., Moriyama, N., Suzuki, M., *et al.* (1983). False-positive liver scans due to portal hypertension: correlation with percutaneous portograms in 33 patients. *Radiology*, **147**, 211–14.

Takayasu, K., Moriyama, N., Muramatsu, Y., *et al.* (1984*a*). Splenic infarction, a complication of transcatheter hepatic arterial embolization. *Radiology*, **151**, 371–5.

Takayasu, K., Moriyama, N., Muramatsu, Y., *et al.* (1984*b*). Hepatic arterial embolization for hepatocellular carcinoma: comparison of CT scans and resected specimens. *Radiology*, **150**, 661–5.

Takayasu, K., Moriyama, N., Shima, Y., *et al.* (1984*c*). Sonographic detection of large spontaneous spleno-renal shunts and its clinical significance. *Br. J. Radiol.*, **57**, 565–70.

Takayasu, K., Moriyama, N., Shima, Y., *et al.* (1984*d*). Spontaneous portal-hepatic venous shunt via an intrahepatic portal vein aneurysm. *Gastroenterology*, **86**, 945–8.

Takayasu, K., Moriyama, N., Ishikawa, T., *et al.* (1985*a*). Large spontaneous intrahepatic arterioportal fistula demonstrated by rapid sequential computed tomographic scan: report of two cases. *Gastroenterology*, **88**, 564–70.

Takayasu, K., Moriyama, N., Muramatsu, Y., *et al.* (1985*b*). Gallbladder infarction after hepatic artery embolization. *A.J.R.*, **144**, 135–8.

Takayasu, K., Moriyama, N., Muramatsu, Y., *et al.* (1985*c*). Intrahepatic venous collaterals forming via the inferior right hepatic vein in 3 patients with obstruction of the inferior vena cava. *Radiology*, **154**, 323–8.

Takayasu, K., Moriyama, N., Muramatsu, Y., *et al.* (1985d). Intrahepatic portal vein branches studied by percutaneous transhepatic portography. *Radiology*, **154**, 31–6.

Takayasu, K., Muramatsu, Y., Shima, Y., *et al.* (1986*a*). Clinical and radiologic features of hepatocellular carcinoma originating in the caudate lobe. *Cancer*, **58**, 1557–62.

Takayasu, K., Muramatsu, Y., Shima, Y., *et al.* (1986*b*). Necrosis of hepatocellular carcinoma as a result of subintimal injury incurred by hepatic angiography: report of two cases. *Am. J. Gastroenterol.*, **81**, 979–83.

Takayasu, K., Muramatsu, Y., Shima, Y., *et al.* (1986*c*). Hepatic lobar atrophy following obstruction on the ipsilateral portal vein from hilar cholangiocarcinoma. *Radiology*, **160**, 389–93.

Takayasu, K., Moriyama, N., Shima, Y., *et al.* (1986*d*). Atypical radiographic findings in hepatic cavernous hemangioma: correlation with histologic features. *A.J.R.*, **146**, 1149–53.

Takayasu, K., Shima, Y., Muramatsu, Y., *et al.* (1986*e*). Angiography of small hepatocellular carcinoma: analysis of 105 resected tumors. *A.J.R.*, **147**, 525–9.

Takayasu, K., Muramatsu, Y., Moriyama, N., *et al.* (1987*a*). Clinicoradiological evaluation of recurrence in the residual liver following hepatectomy in 97 patients with hepatocellular carcinoma. *Japan. J. Gastroenterol.*, **84**, 1424–32 (in Japanese).

Takayasu, K., Shima, Y., Muramatsu, Y., *et al.* (1987*b*). Imaging characteristics of large lipoma and angiomyolipoma of the liver. Case reports. *Cancer*, **59**, 916–21.

Takayasu, K., Shima, Y., Muramatsu, Y., *et al.* (1987*c*). Hepatocellular carcinoma: treatment with intraarterial iodized oil with and without chemotherapeutic agents. *Radiology*, **163**, 345–51.

Takayasu, K. and Uesaka, K. (1987*d*). Is fine-needle biopsy of liver hemangioma hazardous? *A.J.R.*, **148**, 231–2.

Takayasu, K. and Okuda, K. (1987*e*). Celiac angiography in the diagnosis of small hepatocellular carcinoma. In *Neoplasms of the liver* (ed. K. Okuda and K.G. Ishak), pp.279–87. Springer, Tokyo.

Takayasu, K., Muramatsu, Y., Moriyama, N., *et al.* (1988*a*). Infarction of the ileum and the adrenal gland following therapeutic embolization for hepatic malignancies. Report of two cases. *J. Intervent. Radiol.*, **3**, 37–40.

Takayasu, K., Muramatsu, Y., Moriyama, N., *et al.* (1988*b*). Plastic-coated guide wire for hepatic arteriography. *Radiology*, **166**, 545–6.

Takayasu, K., Muramatsu, Y., Moriyama, N., *et al.* (1988*c*). Imaging diagnosis of bile duct cystadenocarcinoma. *Cancer*, **61**, 941–6.

Takayasu, K., Muramatsu, Y., Moriyama, N., and Yamada, T. (1988*d*). A. new hemostatic procedure for percutaneous transhepatic portal vein catheterization. *Japan. J. Clin. Oncol.*, **18**, 227–30.

Takayasu, K., Makuuchi, M., Hirohashi, S., *et al.* (1989*a*). Imaging of adenomatous hyperplastic lesions containing and not containing hepatocellular carcinoma in the liver. *Japan. J. Gastroenterol.*, **86**, 40–9 (in Japanese, English abstract).

Takayasu, K., Moriyama, N., Muramatsu, Y., and Tajiri, H. (1989*b*). Transient perihilar attenuation difference in the liver on dynamic CT secondary to portal vein thrombosis: report of two cases. *Gastroenterol. Japonica*, **24**, 205–8.

Takayasu, K., Muramatsu, Y., Moriyama, N., *et al.* (1989*c*). Surgical treatment of adrenal metastasis following hepatectomy for hepatocellular carcinoma. *Japan. J. Clin. Oncol.*, **19**, 62–6.

Takayasu, K., Muramatsu, Y., Moriyama, N., *et al.* (1989*d*). Hepatocellular and cholangiocellular carcinoma, double cancer of the liver: report of two cases resected synchronously and metachronously. *Am. J. Gastroenterol.*, **84**, 544–7.

Takayasu, K., Muramatsu, Y., Moriyama, N., *et al.* (1989*e*). Clinical and radiologic assessments of the results of hepatectomy for small hepatocellular carcinoma and therapeutic arterial embolization for postoperative recurrence. *Cancer*, **64**, 1848–52.

Takayasu, K., Suzuki, M., Uesaka, K., *et al.* (1989*f*). Hepatic artery embolization for inoperable hepatocellular carcinoma: prognosis and risk factors. *Cancer Chemother. Pharmacol.* 23, (Suppl), S123–S125.

Takayasu, K., Tajiri, H., Noguchi, M., *et al.* (1989*g*). Imaging diagnosis of portal tumor thrombus secondary to gastric cancer. *Gastrointest. Radiol.*, **14**, 161–3.

Takayasu, K., Aoki, K., Ichikawa, T., *et al.* (1990*a*). Aberrant right gastric vein directly communicating with left portal vein system. *Acta Radiol*, **31**, 575–7.

Takayasu, K., Aoki, K., Ichikawa, T., *et al.* (1990*b*). New plastic-coated coaxial catheter system for superselective catheterization: technical note. *Cardiovasc. Intervent. Radiol.*, **13**, 384–6.

Takayasu, K., Ikeya, S., Mukai, K., *et al.* (1990*c*). CT of cholangiocarcinoma: late contrast enhancement in six patients. *A.J.R.*, 154, 1203–6.

Takayasu, K., Makuuchi, M., and Moriya, Y. (1990*d*). Portal vein obstruction complicating intra-arterial chemo-infusion for hepatic metastases. *J. Gastroenterol. Hepatol.*, **5**, 708–13.

Takayasu, K., Makuuchi, M., and Takayama, T. (1990*e*). Computed tomography of a rapidly growing hepatic hemangioma. *J. Comput. Assist. Tomogr.*, *1990*, 143–5.

Takayasu, K., Moriyama, N., Muramatsu, Y., *et al.* (1990*f*). The diagnosis of small hepatocellular carcinoma: efficacy of various imaging procedures in 100 patients. *A.J.R.*, **155**, 49–54.

Takayasu, K., Kasugai, H., Ikeya, S., *et al.* (1992*a*). A. clinical and radiologic study of primary liver cancer associated with extrahepatic primary cancer. *Cancer*, **69**, 45–51.

Takayasu, K., Muramatsu, Y., Moriyama, N., *et al.* (1992*b*). Focal nodular hyperplasia of the liver: arterial angio-CT and microangiography. *J. Comput. Assist. Tomogr.*, **16**, 212–15.

Takayasu, K., Muramatsu, Y., Sakamoto, M., *et al.* (1992*c*). Findings in primary hepatic carcinoid tumor: US., CT., MRI., and Angiography. *J. Comput. Assist. Tomogr.*, **16**, 99–102.

Takayasu, K., Wakao, F., Moriyama, N., *et al.* (1992*d*). Postresection recurrence of hepatocellular carcinoma treated by arterial embolization: analysis of prognostic factors. *Hepatology*, **16**, 906–11.

Takayasu, K., Wakao, F., Moriyama, N., *et al.* (1993). Response of early-stage hepatocellular carcinoma and borderline lesions to therapeutic arterial embolization. *A.J.R.*, **160**, 301–6.

Takayasu, K., Itabashi, M., and Moriyama, N. (1994*a*). Ectopic hepatocellular carcinoma arising from the left diaphragm. *Clin. Radiol.*, **49**, 579–81.

Takayasu, K., Muramatsu, Y., Moriyama, N., *et al.* (1994*b*). Radiological study of idiopathic Budd–Chiari syndrome complicated by hepatocellular carcinoma. A. report of four cases. *Am. J. Gastroenterol*, **88**, 249–53.

Takayasu, K., Muramatsu, Y., Furukawa, H., *et al.* (1995*a*). Early hepatocellular carcinoma: appearance at CT during arterial portography and CT arteriography with pathologic correlation. *Radiology*, **194**, 101–5.

Takayasu, K., Furukawa, H., Wakao, F., *et al.* (1995*b*). CT diagnosis of early hepatocellular carcinoma: sensitivity, findings, and CT-pathologic correlation. *A.J.R.*, **164**, 885–90.

Taketa, K., Endo, Y., Sekiya, C., *et al.* (1993). A. collaborative study for the evaluation of lectin-reactive α-fetoproteins in early detection of hepatocellular carcinoma. *Cancer Res.*, **53**, 5419–23.

Tamada, T., Moriyasu, F., Ono, S., *et al.* (1989). Portal blood flow: measurement with MR imaging. *Radiology*, **173**, 639–44.

Tanaka, K., Okazaki, H., Nakamura, S., *et al.* (1991). Hepatocellular carcinoma: treatment with combination therapy of transcatheter arterial embolization and percutaneous ethanol injection. *Radiology*, **179**, 713–17.

Tanaka, S., Kitamura, T., Imaoka, S., *et al.* (1983). Hepatocellular carcinoma: sonographic and histologic correlation. *A.J.R.*, **140**, 701–7.

Tanaka, S., Kitamura, T., Fujita, M., *et al.* (1990). Color Doppler flow imaging of liver tumors. *A.J.R.*, **154**, 509–14.

Tanikawa, K. (1992). Multidisciplinary treatment of hepatocellular carcinoma. In *Primary liver cancer in Japan* (ed. T. Tobe, H. Kameda, M. Okudaira, *et al.*). pp.327–34. Springer, Tokyo.

Tartar, V.M. and Balfe, D.M. (1990). Lymphoma in the wall of the bile ducts: radiologic imaging. *Gastrointest Radiol*, **15**, 53–7.

Tavill, A.S., Wood, E.J., Kreel, L., *et al.* (1975). Budd–Chiari syndrome: correlation between hepatic scintigraphy and the clinical, radiological and pathological findings in nineteen cases of hepatic venous outflow obstruction. *Gastroenterology*, **68**, 509–18.

Taylor,, K.J.W. (1978). *Atlas of gray scale ultrasonography*. Churchill Livingstone, New York.

Teefey, S.A., Baron, R.L., Rohrmann, C.A., Shuman, W.P., and Freeny, P.C. (1988). Sclerosing cholangitis: CT findings. *Radiology*, **169**, 635–39.

Tegmeyer, C.J., Smith, T.H., Shaw, A., *et al.* (1977). Renal infarction: a complication of gelfoam embolization of a hemangioendothelioma of the liver. *A.J.R.*, **128**, 305–7.

Terabayashi, H., Okuda, K., Nomura, F., *et al.* (1986). Transformation of inferior vena caval thrombosis to membranous obstruction in a patient with the lupus anticoagulant. *Gastroenterology*, **81**, 219–24.

Terada, T. and Nakanuma, Y. (1989*a*). Survey of iron-accumulative macroregnerative nodules in cirrhotic livers. *Hepatology*, **10**, 851–4.

Terada, T. and Nakanuma, Y. (1989*b*). Iron-negative foci in siderotic macroregenerative nodules in human cirrhotic liver. A. marker of incipient neoplastic lesions. *Arch. Pathol. Lab. Med.*, **113**, 916–20.

Terblanche, J., Northover, J.M.A., Bornman, P., *et al.* (1979). A prospective evaluation of injection sclerotherapy in the treatment of acute bleeding from esophageal varices. *Surgery*, **85**, 239–45.

Terpstra, O.T., Ten Kate, F.J.W., van Urk, H., *et al.* (1984). Long term survival after resection of a hepatocellular carcinoma with lymph node metastasis and discontinuation of contraceptives. *Am. J. Gastroenterol.*, **79**, 474–8.

Theise, N.D., Schwartz, M., Miller, C., *et al.* (1992). Macroregenerative nodules and hepatocellular carcinoma in forty-four sequential adult liver explants with cirrhosis. *Hepatology*, **16**, 949–55.

Thorsen, M.K., Quiroz, F., Lawson, T.L., *et al.* (1984). Primary biliary carcinoma: CT evaluation. *Radiology*, **152**, 479–83.

Titelbaum, D.S., Hatabu, H., Schiebler, M.L., *et al.* (1988). Fibrolamellar hepatocellular carcinoma: MR appearance. *J. Comput. Assist. Tomogr.*, **12**, 588–91.

Todani, T., Watanabe, Y., Fujii, M., *et al.* (1985). Carcinoma arising from the bile duct in choledochal cyst and anomalous arrangement of the pancreatobiliary ductal union. *Biliary Tract and Pancreas (Tan-to Sui)*, **6**, 525–35 (in Japanese).

Todoroki, T., Iwasaki, Y., Okamura, T., *et al.* (1980). Intraoperative radiation therapy for advanced carcinoma of the biliary system. *Cancer*, **46**, 2179–84.

Tompkins, R.K., Saunders, K., Roslyn, J.J., Longmire, W.P. (1990). Changing patterns in diagnosis and management of bile duct cancer. *Ann. Surg.*, **211**, 614–21.

Torres, W.E., Whitmire, L.F., Gegauda-McClees, K., and Bernardino, M.E. (1986). Computed tomography of hepatic morphologic changes in cirrhosis of the liver. *J. Comput. Assist. Tomogr.*, **10**, 47–50.

Tsuchiya, Y. (1991). Early carcinoma of the gallbladder : macroscopic features and US findings. *Radiology*, **179**, 171–5.

Tsuda, H., Hirohashi, S., Shiosato, Y., *et al.* (1988). Clonal origin of atypical adenomatous hyperplasia of the liver and clonal identity with hepatocellular carcinoma. *Gastroenterology*, **95**, 1664–6.

Tsujii, H., Tsuji, H., Inada, T., *et al.* (1992). Clinical results of fractionated proton therapy. *Int. J. Radiat. Oncol. Biol. Phys.*, **25**, 49–60.

Tsukamoto, Y., Nakata, H., Kimoto, T., *et al.* (1984). CT and angiography of peliosis hepatis. *A.J.R.*, **142**, 539–40.

Uchino, A., Ohno, M., and Kitahara, Y. (1987). Myelopathy due to intercostal artery embolization with Lipiodol: a case report. *Japan. J. Clin. Radiol.*, **32**, 531–3 (in Japanese).

Ueda, H., Kitani, K., Kameda, H., *et al.* (1967). Detection of hepatic shunts by the use of ^{131}I macroaggregated albumin. *Gastroenterology*, **52**, 480–87.

Ungar, E.C., Lee, J.K.T., and Weyman, P.J. (1987). CT and MR imaging of radiation hepatitis. *J. Comput. Assist. Tomogr.*, **11**, 264–8.

Van Beers, B., Roche, A., Mathieu, D., *et al.* (1992). Epithelioid hemangioendothelioma of the liver: MR and CT findings. *J. Comput. Assist. Tomogr.*, **16**, 420–4.

Van Stiegmann, G., Cambre, T., and Sun JH. (1986). A new endoscopic elastic band ligating device. *Gastrointest. Endosc.*, **32**, 230–3.

Vianna, A., Hayes, P.C., Moscoso, G., *et al.* (1987). Normal venous circulation of the gastroesophageal junction. A route of understanding varices. *Gastroenterology*, **93**, 876–89.

Vilana, R., Bruix, J., Bru, C., *et al.* (1992). Tumor size determines the efficacy of percutaneous ethanol injection for the treatment of small hepatocellular carcinoma. *Hepatology*, **16**, 353–7.

Vock, P., Soucek, M., Daepp, M., *et al.* (1990). Spiral volumetric CT with single-breath-hold technique. *Radiology*, **176**, 864–7.

von Hochstetter, A.R., Hattenschwiler, J., and Vogt, M. (1987). Primary osteosarcoma of the liver. *Cancer*, **60**, 2312–17.

Wada, K., Kondo, F., Kubosawa, H., and Kondo, Y. (1986). Combined hepatocellular and mucinous carcinoma. *Acta Pathol. Japan*, **36**, 285–91.

Wada, K., Kondo, F., and Kondo, Y. (1988). Large regenerative nodules and dysplastic nodules in cirrhotic livers: a histopathologic study. *Hepatology*, **8**, 1684–8.

Walkey, M.M., Friedman, A.C., Sohotra P and Radecki, P.D. (1988). CT manifestation of peritoneal carcinomatosis. *A.J.R.*, **150**, 1035–41.

Wallace, S. (1976). Interventional radiology. *Cancer*, **37**, 517–31.

Wallner, B.K., Schumacher, K.A., Weidenmaier, W., and Friedrich, J.M. (1991). Dilated biliary tract: evaluation with MR cholangiography with a T2-weighted CE-FAST sequence. *Radiology*, **181**, 805–8.

Walt, A.J. (1977). Cysts and benign tumors of the liver. *Surg. Clin. North Am.*, **57**, 449–64.

Waluch, V. and Bradley, W.G. (1984). NMR even echo rephasing in slow laminar flow. *J. Comput. Assist. Tomogr.*, **8**, 594–8.

Wang, L.Y., Lin, Z.Y., Chang, W.Y., *et al.* (1991). Duplex pulsed Doppler sonography of portal vein thrombosis in hepatocellular carcinoma. *J. Ultrasound Med.*, **10**, 265–9.

Wanless, I.R. (1990). Micronodular transformation (nodular regenerative hyperplasia). of the liver: a report of 64 cases among 2500 autopsies and a new classification of benign hepatocellular nodules. *Hepatology*, **11**, 983–97.

Wanless, I. and International Working Party (1995). Terminology of nodular hepatocellular lesions. *Hepatology*, **22**, 983–93.

Warren, W.D., Zeppa, R., and Fomon, J.J. (1967). Selective trans-splenic decompression of gastroesophageal varices by distal splenorenal shunt. *Ann. Surg.*, **166**, 437–55.

Weinmann, H.J., Brasch, R.C., Press, W.R., and Wesbey, G.E. (1984). Characteristics of gadolinium-DTPA. complex: a potential NMR contrast agent. *A.J.R.*, **142**, 619–24.

Weill, F.S. (1978). *Ultrasonography of digestive diseases.* Mosby, St. Louis.

Weiss, S.W and Enzinger, F.M. (1982). Epithelioid hemangioendothelioma : a vascular tumor often mistaken for a carcinoma. *Cancer*, **50**, 970–81.

Weltin, G., Taylor, K.J.W., Carter, A.R., and Taylor, C.R. (1985). Duplex Doppler: identification of cavernous transformation of the portal vein. *A.J.R.*, **144**, 999–1001.

Westaby, D., Hayes, P.C., Gimson, A.E.S., *et al.* (1989). Controlled clinical trial of injection sclerotherapy for active variceal bleeding. *Hepatology*, **9**, 274–7.

Whelan, T. Jr, Bauch, J.H., and Chandor, S. (1973). Focal nodular hyperplasia of the liver. *Ann. Surg.*, **177**, 150–8.

Whitley, N.O., Brenner, D.E., Antman, K.N., *et al.* (1982). CT of peritoneal mesothelioma: analysis of eight cases. *A.J.R.*, **138**, 531–5.

WHO (1979). *WHO handbook for reporting results of cancer treatment.* WHO., Geneva.

Wiechel, K.L. (1979) Direct selective catheterization of the portal venous system. *Scand. J. Gastroenterol.* **14**, Suppl 53, 123–30.

Williams, D.M., Cho, K.J., Ensminger, W.D., *et al.* (1985). Hepatic falciform artery: anatomy, angiographic appearance, and clinical significance. *Radiology*, **156**, 339–40.

Winter, T.C., III., Freeny, P.C., Nghiem, H.V., *et al.* (1993). MR imaging with IV superparamagnetic iron oxide: efficacy in the detection of focal hepatic lesions. *A.J.R.*, **161**, 1191–8.

Winter, T.C. III., Takayasu, K., Muramatsu, Y., *et al.* (1994). Early advanced hepatocellular carcinoma: evaluation of CT and MR appearance with pathologic correlation. *Radiology*, **192**, 379–87.

Yamada, R., Sato, M., Kawabata, M., *et al.* (1983*a*). Hepatic artery embolization in 120 patients with unresectable hepatoma. *Radiology*, **148**, 397–401.

Yamada, R., Sato, M., Kawabata, M., *et al.* (1983*b*). Segmental obstruction of the hepatic inferior vena cava treated by transluminal angioplasty. *Radiology*, **149**, 91–6.

Yamagiwa, K. (1911). Zur Kenntniss des primaren parenchymatosen Lebercarcinoma (Hepatoma). *Virch. Arch*, **206**, 437–67.

Yamamoto, S. and Reynolds, T.B. (1964). Portal venography and pressure measurement at peritoneoscopy. *Gastroenterology*, **47**, 602–3.

Yamamoto, S., Kojoh, K., Saito, I., *et al.* (1988). Computer tomography of congenital absence of the left lobe of the liver. *J. Comput. Assist. Tomog.*, **12**, 206–8.

Yamamoto, T., Kawarada, Y., Yano, T., et al.. (1991). Spontaneous rupture of hemangioma of the liver: treatment with transcatheter hepatic arterial embolization. *Am. J. Gastroenterol.*, **86**, 1645–9.

Yamanaka, N., Okamoto, E., Kawamura, E., *et al.* (1993). Dynamics of normal and injured human liver regeneration after hepatectomy as assessed on the basis of computed tomography and liver function. *Hepatology*, **18**, 79–85.

Yamasaki, S., Takayama, T., Hasegawa, H., et al.. (1990). Problems with the General Rules for the Clinical and pathological Study of Primary Liver Cancer and UICC TNM classification. *J. Japan. Surg. Soc.*, **91**, 1337–9 (in Japanese).

Yamasaki, S., Makuuchi, M., and Hasegawa, H. (1991). Results of hepatectomy for hepatocellular carcinoma at the National Cancer Center Hospital. *HPB Surg.*, **3**, 235–49.

Yamashita, K., Takayasu, K., Muramatsu, Y., *et al.* (1988). Imaging diagnosis of portal vein thrombosis following splenectomy in 23 patients with hepatocellular carcinoma. *Japan. J. Clin. Radiol.*, **33**, 1561–4 (in Japanese).

Yates, C.K., and Streight RA. (1986). Focal fatty infiltration of the liver simulating metastatic disease. *Radiology*, **159**, 83–4.

Yoshida, H., Itai, Y., Minami, M., *et al.* (1989*a*). Biliary malignancies occurring in choledochal cysts. *Radiology*, **173**, 389–92.

Yoshida, H., Itai, Y., Ohtomo, K., *et al.* (1989*b*). Small hepatocellular carcinoma and cavernous hemangioma: differentiation with dynamic FLASH MR imaging with Gd-DTPA. *Radiology*, **171**, 339–42.

Yoshida, J., Yamasaki, S., Yamamoto, J., *et al.* (1991). Growing cavernous haemangioma of the liver: 11-fold increase in volume in a decade. *J. Gastroenterol. Hepatol.*, **6**, 414–16.

Yoshida, J., Takayama, T., Yamamoto, J., *et al.* (1992). Computed tomography of sclerosing hepatocellular carcinoma. *Comput. Med. Imaging Graphics*, **16**, 125–30.

Yoshida, T., Okazaki, N., Yoshino, M., *et al.* (1982). Minute hepatocellular carcinoma without appreciable change in size for seven years. *Cancer*, **49**, 1491–5.

Yoshikawa, J., Matsui, O., Takashima, T., *et al.* (1987). Focal fatty change of the liver adjacent to the falciform ligament : CT and sonographic findings in five surgically confirmed cases. *A.J.R.*, **149**, 491–4.

Yoshikawa, J., Matsui, O., Takashima, T., *et al.* (1988). Fatty metamorphosis in hepatocellular carcinoma: radiologic features in 10 cases. *A.J.R.*, **151**, 717–20.

Yoshino, M. (1983). Growth kinetics of hepatocellular carcinoma. *Japan. J. Clin. Oncol.*, **13**, 45–52.

Yumoto, Y., Jinno, K., Tokuyama, K., *et al.* (1985). Hepatocellular carcinoma detected by iodized oil. *Radiology*, **154**, 19–24.

Zafrani, E.S., Pinaudeau, Y., and Dhumeaux, D. (1983). Drug-induced vascular lesions of the liver. *Arch. Intern. Med.*, **143**, 495–502.

Zeman, R., Taylor, K.J.W., Burrell, M.I., and Gold, J. (1980). Ultrasound demonstration of anicteric dilatation of the biliary tree. *Radiology*, **134**, 689–92.

Index